Peterson's Nursing Programs 2017

DISCARD

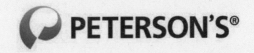

PETERSON'S®

DAYTON MEMORIAL LIBRARY
REGIS UNIVERSITY
3333 REGIS BLVD.,
DENVER, CO 80221

D0406610

Regis University
Library

MAY 2 6 2016

RECEIVED

PETERSON'S®

About Peterson's®

Peterson's®, a Nelnet company, has been your trusted educational publisher for over 50 years. It's a milestone we're quite proud of, as we continue to offer the most accurate, dependable, high-quality education content in the field, providing you with everything you need to succeed. No matter where you are on your academic or professional path, you can rely on Peterson's publications and its online information at **www.petersons.com** for the most up-to-date education exploration data, expert test-prep tools, and the highest quality career success resources—everything you need to achieve your educational goals.

For more information, contact Peterson's, 3 Columbia Circle, Albany, NY 12203-5158; 800-338-3282 Ext. 54229; or visit us online at **www.petersons.com**.

© 2016 Peterson's®, a Nelnet® company. All rights reserved.
Peterson's is a registered service mark of Nelnct, Inc.

Previous editions © 1994, 1996, 1997, 1998, 1999, 2000, 2001, 2002, 2003, 2004, 2005, 2006, 2007, 2008, 2009, 2010, 2011, 2012, 2013, 2014, 2015

Peterson's makes every reasonable effort to obtain accurate, complete, and timely data from reliable sources. Nevertheless, Peterson's and the third-party data suppliers make no representation or warranty, either expressed or implied, as to the accuracy, timeliness, or completeness of the data or the results to be obtained from using the data, including, but not limited to, its quality, performance, merchantability, or fitness for a particular purpose, non-infringement or otherwise.

NOTICE: Certain portions of or information contained in this book have been submitted and paid for by the educational institution identified, and such institutions take full responsibility for the accuracy, timeliness, completeness and functionality of such contents. Such portions or information include (i) each display ad in the "Profiles of Nursing Programs" section from pages 85 through 486 that comprises a full page or half page of information covering a single educational institution, and (ii) each two-page in-depth description in the "Two-Page Descriptions" section from pages 488 through 513.

ALL RIGHTS RESERVED. No part of this work covered by the copyright herein may be reproduced or used in any form or by any means—graphic, electronic, or mechanical, including photocopying, recording, taping, Web distribution, or information storage and retrieval systems—without the prior written permission of the publisher.

For permission to use material from this text or product, complete the Permission Request Form at http://www.petersonspublishing.com/spa/permissions.aspx.

ISSN 1552-7743
ISBN: 978-0-7689-4087-9

Printed in the United States of America

10 9 8 7 6 5 4 3 2 1   18 17 16

Twenty-first Edition

CONTENTS

FOREWORD

The American Association of Colleges of Nursing (AACN) is proud to collaborate on *Peterson's Nursing Programs 2017*.

According to the U.S. Bureau of Labor Statistics' (BLS) Employment Projections 2010–2020 released in February 2012, the registered nursing workforce is the top occupation in terms of job growth through 2020. It is expected that the number of employed nurses will grow from 2.74 million in 2010 to 3.45 million in 2020, an increase of 712,000 or 26 percent. The projections further explain the need for 495,500 replacements in the nursing workforce, bringing the total number of job openings for nurses due to growth and replacements to 1.2 million by 2020. In March 2012, the BLS reported that job growth in the health-care sector was outpacing the growth realized in 2011, accounting for 1 out of every 5 new jobs created in that year. Hospitals, long-term care facilities, and other ambulatory-care settings added 49,000 new jobs in February 2012, up from 43,300 new jobs created in January. As the largest segment of the health-care workforce, RNs likely will be recruited to fill many of these new positions.

As registered nurses find employment beyond hospitals in such areas as home care, community health, and long-term care, newly licensed RNs must have the proper education and training to work in these settings. It is vital that those seeking to enter or advance in a nursing career find the appropriate nursing program. This guide allows readers to find the program that best fits their needs, whether beginning a new career in nursing or attempting to advance one.

According to AACN's most recent annual institutional survey, enrollment in entry-level B.S.N. programs continues to climb. Gains were reported in all parts of the country in 2014, with an overall 4.2 percent increase in enrollments nationwide.

Although the health-care environment is complex and dynamic, there continues to be a significant demand for professional-level nurses. The primary route into professional-level nursing is the four-year baccalaureate degree. The professional nurse with a baccalaureate degree is the only basic nursing graduate prepared to practice in all health-care settings, including critical care, public health, primary care, and mental health. In addition, advanced practice nurses (APNs) deliver essential services as nurse practitioners, certified nurse-midwives, clinical nurse specialists, and nurse anesthetists. APNs typically are prepared in master's degree programs, and the demand for their services is expected to increase substantially.

Higher education in nursing expands the gateway to a variety of career opportunities in the health-care field. In addition to providing primary care to patients, graduates can work as case managers for the growing numbers of managed-care companies or can assume administrative or managerial roles in hospitals, clinics, insurance companies, and other diverse settings.

The Nursing School Adviser section of this guide is instructive and invaluable. Whether you are a high school student looking for a four-year program, an RN returning to school, or a professional in another field contemplating a career change, this section will address your concerns. This information presents various nursing perspectives to benefit students from diverse backgrounds.

Peterson's effort in making this guide well organized and convenient to read cannot be overstated. Peterson's has worked with AACN in producing a publication that is comprehensive and user-friendly. Like the previous editions, this edition is a genuine collaborative work, as AACN provided input from start to finish.

AACN's dedication and achievements in advancing the quality of baccalaureate and graduate nursing education are appreciated by Peterson's. We at AACN are fortunate to work with an organization that prides itself on being the leading publisher of education search and selection.

Furthermore, this publication would not be possible without the cooperation of the institutions included in this guide. We acknowledge the time and effort of those who undertook the task of completing and returning the surveys regarding their programs. We certainly appreciate their contribution.

Peterson's Nursing Programs 2017 is the only comprehensive and concise guide to baccalaureate and graduate nursing education programs in the United States and Canada. We hope its contents will serve as the impetus for those looking for a rewarding and satisfying career in health care. AACN is proud to present this publication to the nursing profession and to those who seek to enter it.

—Juliann Sebastian, Ph.D., RN, FAAN
Chair, AACN

—Deborah E. Trautman, Ph.D., RN, FAAN
President and Chief Executive Officer, AACN

A NOTE FROM THE PETERSON'S EDITORS

For over fifty years, Peterson's has given students and parents the most comprehensive, up-to-date information on undergraduate and graduate institutions in the United States, Canada, and abroad.

Peterson's Nursing Programs 2017 provides prospective nursing students with the most comprehensive information on baccalaureate and graduate nursing education in the United States and Canada. Our goal is to help students find the best nursing program for them.

To this end, Peterson's has joined forces with the American Association of Colleges of Nursing (AACN), the national voice for America's baccalaureate-and higher-degree nursing education programs. AACN's educational, research, governmental advocacy, data collection, publications, and other programs work to establish high-quality standards for bachelor's- and graduate-degree nursing education, assist deans and directors to implement those standards, influence the nursing profession to improve health care, and promote public support of baccalaureate and graduate education, research, and practice in nursing—the nation's largest health-care profession.

For those seeking to enter the nursing profession or to further their nursing careers, *Peterson's Nursing Programs 2017* includes information needed to make important nursing program decisions and to approach the admissions process with knowledge and confidence.

The Nursing School Adviser section contains useful articles to help guide nursing education choices, with information on nursing careers today, selecting a nursing program, financing nursing education, returning to school, and more. It also includes listings that provide valuable contact information for financial aid resources and specialty nursing organizations. And if you are one of the many people interested in accelerated nursing programs, there is an article that offers an in-depth look at this increasingly popular approach to nursing education. It is a must-read for those wishing to enter an accelerated baccalaureate or generic master's degree program.

At the end of **The Nursing School Adviser** is the "How to Use This Guide" article, which explains some of the key factors to consider when choosing a nursing program. In addition, it explains how the book is organized and shows you how to maximize your use of *Peterson's Nursing Programs 2017* to its full potential.

If you already have specifics in mind, such as a particular program or location, turn to the **Quick-Reference Chart.** Here you can search through "Nursing Programs At-a-Glance" for particular degree options offered by schools, listed alphabetically by state.

In the **Profiles of Nursing Programs** section you'll find expanded and updated nursing program descriptions, arranged alphabetically by state. Each profile provides all of the need-to-know information about accredited nursing programs in the United States and Canada. Display ads, which appear near some of the institutions' profiles, have been provided and paid for by those colleges or universities that wished to supplement their profile data with additional information about their institution.

If you are looking for additional information, you can turn to the **Two-Page Descriptions** section. Here you will find in-depth narrative descriptions, with photos, of those nursing programs that chose to pay for and provide additional information.

When you turn to the back of the book, you'll find eight **Indexes** listing institutions offering *baccalaureate, master's degree, concentrations within master's degree, doctoral, post-doctoral, online,* and *continuing education* programs. The last index lists every college and university contained in the guide along with its corresponding page reference.

Peterson's publishes a full line of resources to help guide you and your family through the admission process. Peterson's publications can be found at high school guidance offices, college and university libraries and career centers, your local bookstore or library, and at petersonsbooks.com.

We welcome any comments or suggestions you may have about this publication.

Publishing Department
Peterson's, a Nelnet company
3 Columbia Circle, Suite 205
Albany, NY 12203-5158

Your feedback will help us make your educational dreams possible. The editors at Peterson's wish you great success in your nursing program search.

THE NURSING SCHOOL ADVISER

NURSING FACT SHEET

Misconceptions about nursing have contributed to misinformation about the profession in the media. Here are the real facts:

- **Nursing is the nation's largest health-care profession, with more than 3.1 million registered nurses nationwide.** Of all licensed RNs, 2.6 million or 84.8 percent are employed in nursing.[1]

- **Registered Nurses compose one of the largest segments of the U.S. workforce as a whole and are among the highest paying large occupations.** Nearly 58 percent of RNs worked in general medical and surgical hospitals, where RN salaries averaged $66,700 per year. RNs composed the largest segment of professionals working in the health-care industry.[2]

- **Nurses compose the largest single component of hospital staff, are the primary providers of hospital patient care, and deliver most of the nation's long-term care.**

- **Most health-care services involve some form of care by nurses.** In 1980, 66 percent of all employed RNs worked in hospitals. By 2008, that number had declined slightly to 62.2 percent as more health care moved to sites beyond the hospital, and nurses increased their ranks in a wide range of other settings, including private practices, health maintenance organizations, public health agencies, primary care clinics, home health care, nursing homes, outpatient surgicenters, nursing-school-operated nursing centers, insurance and managed care companies, schools, mental health agencies, hospices, the military, industry, nursing education, and health-care research.[3]

- **Though often working collaboratively, nursing does not "assist" medicine or other fields.** Nursing operates independent of, not auxiliary to, medicine and other disciplines. Nurses' roles range from direct patient care and case management to establishing nursing practice standards, developing quality assurance procedures, and directing complex nursing care systems.

- **With more than four times as many RNs in the United States as physicians, nursing delivers an extended array of health-care services, including primary and preventive care by advanced nurse practitioners in such areas as pediatrics, family health, women's health, and gerontological care.** Nursing's scope also includes services by certified nurse-midwives and nurse anesthetists, as well as care in cardiac, oncology, neonatal, neurological, and obstetric/gynecological nursing and other advanced clinical specialties.

- **The primary pathway to professional nursing, as compared to technical-level practice, is the four-year Bachelor of Science in Nursing (B.S.N.) degree.** Registered nurses are prepared either through a B.S.N. program; a three-year associate degree in nursing; or a three-year hospital training program, receiving a hospital diploma. All take the same state licensing exam. (The number of diploma programs has declined steadily—to less than 10 percent of all basic RN education programs—as nursing education has shifted from hospital-operated instruction into the college and university system.)

- **To meet the more complex demands of today's health-care environment, the National Advisory Council on Nurse Education and Practice has recommended that at least two-thirds of the basic nurse workforce hold baccalaureate or higher degrees in nursing.**[4] Aware of the need, RNs are seeking the B.S.N. degree in increasing numbers. In 1980, almost 55 percent of employed registered nurses held a hospital diploma as their highest educational credential, 22 percent held the bachelor's degree, and 18 percent an associate degree. By 2008, a diploma was the highest educational credential for only 13.9 percent of RNs, while the number with bachelor's degrees as their highest education had climbed to 36.8 percent, with 36.1 percent holding an associate degree as their top academic preparation.[5] In 2010, 22,531 RNs with diplomas or associate degrees graduated from B.S.N. programs.[6]

- **In 2008, 13.2 percent of the nation's registered nurses held either a master's or doctoral degree as their highest educational preparation.**[7] The current demand for master's- and doctorally prepared nurses for advanced practice, clinical specialties, teaching, and research roles far outstrips the supply.

- **According to the U.S. Bureau of Labor Statistics, Registered Nursing is the top occupation in terms of the largest job growth from 2008–2018.**[8] Government analysts project that more than 581,500 new RN jobs will be created through 2018. Other projections indicate that by 2025, the U.S. nursing shortage will grow to more than 260,000 registered nurses.[9] Even as health care continues to shift beyond the hospital to more community-based primary care and other outpatient sites, federal projections say the rising complexity of acute care will see demand for RNs in hospitals climb by 36 percent by 2020.[10]

REFERENCES

1. Health Resources and Services Administration. (September 2010). *The Registered Nurse Population: Findings From the 2008 National Sample Survey of Registered Nurses*. Washington, DC: U.S. Department of Health and Human Services.

2. U.S. Bureau of Labor Statistics, (2010, May). *Occupational Employment and Wages for 2009*. Access online at http://www.bls.gov/oes

3. See Note 1.

4. National Advisory Council on Nurse Education and Practice. (October 1996). *Report to the Secretary of the Department of Health and Human Services on the Basic Registered Nurse Workforce.* Washington, DC: U.S. Department of Health and Human Services, Division of Nursing.

5. See Note 1.

6. American Association of Colleges of Nursing (2011). *2010–2011 Enrollment and graduations in baccalaureate and graduate programs in nursing.* Washington, DC: Author.

7. See Note 1.

8. Lacey, T. A. and B. Wright. (2010). *Occupational Employment Projections to 2018.* Washington, DC: U.S. Department of Labor, Bureau of Labor Statistics.

9. Buerhaus, P. I., D. I. Auerbach, and D. O. Staiger. (2009, July–August). The recent surge in nurse employment: causes and implications. *Health Affairs,* 28(4), w657–w668.

10. See Note 4.

CREATING A MORE HIGHLY QUALIFIED NURSING WORKFORCE

High-quality patient care hinges on having a well-educated nursing workforce. Research has shown that lower mortality rates, fewer medication errors, and positive outcomes are all linked to nurses prepared at the baccalaureate and graduate degree levels. The American Association of Colleges of Nursing (AACN) is committed to working collaboratively to create a more highly qualified nursing workforce since education enhances both clinical competency and care delivery. This fact sheet looks at today's nursing workforce; highlights research connecting education to outcomes; and outlines the capacity of four-year colleges to enhance the level of nursing education in the United States.

Snapshot of Today's Nursing Workforce

According to the National Center for Health Workforce Analysis within the Health Resources and Services Administration (HRSA), approximately 2.8 million registered nurses (RNs) are currently working in nursing (HRSA, 2013). This count reflects an increase from the last *National Sample Survey of Registered Nurses* conducted by HRSA in 2008, which found that 2.6 million RNs were employed in nursing (out of a population of more than 3 million licensed RNs).

HRSA's 2013 report, "The U.S. Nursing Workforce: Trends in Supply and Education," also found that 55 percent of the RN workforce held a baccalaureate or higher degree. In a separate study conducted by the National Council of State Boards of Nursing and The Forum of State Nursing Workforce Centers in 2013, the percentage of nurses in the United States with a baccalaureate or higher degree was 61 percent.

Graduates of entry-level nursing programs (baccalaureate degree, associate degree, and diploma) sit for the NCLEX-RN® licensing examination. The fact that new nurses pass the licensing exam at the same rate does not mean that all entry-level nurses are equally prepared for practice. The NCLEX tests for *minimum technical competency* for safe entry into basic nursing practice. Passing rates *should* be high across all programs preparing new nurses. This exam does not test for differences between graduates of different programs, measure performance over time, or test for all of the knowledge and skills developed through a baccalaureate program.

In October 2010, the Institute of Medicine released its landmark report on *The Future of Nursing*, initiated by the Robert Wood Johnson Foundation, which called for increasing the number of baccalaureate-prepared nurses in the workforce to 80 percent and doubling the population of nurses with doctorates. The expert committee charged with preparing the evidence-based recommendations contained in this report state that to respond "to the demands of an evolving health-care system and meet the changing needs of patients, nurses must achieve higher levels of education."

In March 2005, the American Organization of Nurse Executives (AONE) released a statement calling for all for registered nurses to be educated in baccalaureate programs in an effort to adequately prepare clinicians for their challenging and complex roles. AONE's statement, titled "Practice and Education Partnership for the Future," represents the view of nursing's practice leaders and a desire to create a more highly educated nursing workforce in the interest of improving patient safety and providing enhanced nursing care.

Research Linking Nursing Education to Patient Outcomes

AACN and other authorities believe that education has a strong impact on a nurse's ability to practice, and that patients deserve the best educated nursing workforce possible. A growing body of research reinforces this belief and shows a connection between baccalaureate education and lower mortality rates.

In a study published in the October 2014 issue of *Medical Care,* researcher Olga Yakusheva from the University of Michigan and her colleagues found that a 10 percent increase in the proportion of baccalaureate-prepared nurses on hospital units was associated with lowering the odds of patient mortality by 10.9 percent. Titled "Economic Evaluation of the 80% Baccalaureate Nurse Workforce Recommendation," the study's authors also found that increasing the amount of care provided by BSNs to 80 percent would result in significantly lower readmission rates and shorter lengths of stay. These outcomes translate into cost savings that would more than offset expenses for increasing the number of baccalaureate-prepared nurses in hospital settings.

Posting online in August 2014 by the *International Journal of Nursing Studies*, a team of researchers from several nursing schools in South Korea and the University of Pennsylvania found that a 10 percent increase in baccalaureate-prepared nurses was associated with a 9 percent decrease in patient deaths in South Korean hospitals. The authors concluded that increasing the number of nurses with the BSN would significantly reduce the number of in-hospital deaths.

Published in *The Lancet* in May 2014, authors of the study titled "Nurse Staffing and Education and Hospital Mortality in Nine European Countries: A Retrospective Observational

Study" found that that patients experiencing complications after surgery are more likely to live if treated in hospitals with adequate nurse staffing levels and higher numbers of BSN nurses. Following a review of more than 420,000 patient records in 300 hospitals spanning nine European countries, findings show that a 10 percent increase in the proportion of nurses holding a bachelor's degree in an acute-care setting is associated with a 7 percent decrease in the risk of death in discharged patients following common surgeries.

In an article published in the March 2013 issue of *Health Affairs,* nurse researcher Ann Kutney-Lee and colleagues found that a 10-point increase in the percentage of nurses holding a BSN within a hospital was associated with an average reduction of 2.12 deaths for every 1,000 patients—and for a subset of patients with complications, an average reduction of 7.47 deaths per 1,000 patients.

In the February 2013 issue of the *Journal of Nursing Administration,* Mary Blegen and colleagues published findings from a cross-sectional study of 21 University Health-System Consortium hospitals, which found that hospitals with a higher percentage of RNs with baccalaureate or higher degrees had lower congestive heart failure mortality, decubitus ulcers, failure to rescue, and postoperative deep vein thrombosis or pulmonary embolism and shorter length of stay.

In the October 2012 issue of *Medical Care,* researchers from the University of Pennsylvania found that surgical patients in Magnet hospitals had 14 percent lower odds of inpatient death within 30 days and 12 percent lower odds of failure-to-rescue compared with patients cared for in non-Magnet hospitals. The study authors conclude that these better outcomes were attributed in large part to investments in highly qualified and educated nurses, including a higher proportion of baccalaureate prepared nurses.

In an article published in *Health Services Research* in August 2008 that examined the effect of nursing practice environments on outcomes of hospitalized cancer patients undergoing surgery, Dr. Christopher Friese and colleagues found that nursing education level was significantly associated with patient outcomes. Nurses prepared at the baccalaureate-level were linked with lower mortality and failure-to-rescue rates.

In a study released in the May 2008 issue of the *Journal of Nursing Administration,* Dr. Linda Aiken and her colleagues confirmed the findings from their landmark 2003 study (see below). which show a strong link between RN education level and patient outcomes. The noted nurse researchers found that every 10 percent increase in the proportion of BSN nurses on the hospital staff was associated with a 4 percent decrease in the risk of death.

In the January 2007 *Journal of Advanced Nursing,* a study of 46,993 patients conducted by researchers at the University Toronto found that hospitals with higher proportions of baccalaureate-prepared nurses tended to have lower 30-day mortality rates. The findings indicated that a 10 percent increase in the proportion of baccalaureate-prepared nurses was associated with 9 fewer deaths for every 1,000 discharged patients.

In a study published in the March/April 2005 *Nursing Research*, Dr. Carole Estabrooks and her colleagues at the University of Alberta found that baccalaureate-prepared nurses have a positive impact on mortality rates following an examination of more than 18,000 patient outcomes at 49 Canadian hospitals. This study, "The Impact of Hospital Nursing Characteristics on 30-Day Mortality," confirmed the findings from Dr. Aiken's landmark study from 2003.

In a study published in the September 24, 2003 *Journal of the American Medical Association*, Dr. Linda Aiken and her colleagues at the University of Pennsylvania identified a clear link between higher levels of nursing education and better patient outcomes. This extensive study found that surgical patients have a "substantial survival advantage" if treated in hospitals with higher proportions of nurses educated at the baccalaureate or higher degree level. A 10 percent increase in the proportion of nurses holding BSN degrees decreased the risk of patient death and failure to rescue by 5 percent.

For more information on the link between nursing education and patient outcomes, see http://www.aacn.nche.edu/media-relations/fact-sheets/impact-of-education.

Moving Toward a More Highly Educated Nursing Workforce

AACN stands ready to work with the larger nursing community and representatives from associate degree and diploma programs to expand awareness of degree completion options, facilitate the establishment of articulation agreements, and enhance the educational preparation of the nursing workforce.

In September 2012, the *Joint Statement on Academic Progression for Nursing Students and Graduates* was endorsed by the American Association of Colleges of Nursing, American Association of Community Colleges, Association of Community Colleges Trustees, National League for Nursing, and the National Organization for Associate Degree Nursing. This historic agreement represents the first time leaders from the major national organizations representing community college presidents, boards, and program administrators have joined with representatives from nursing education associations to promote academic progression in nursing. With the common goal of preparing a well-educated, diverse nursing workforce, this statement represents the shared view that nursing students and practicing nurses should be supported in their efforts to pursue higher levels of education. Read the statement at www.aacn.nche.edu/aacn-publications/position/joint-statement-academic-progression.

In March 2012, the Robert Wood Johnson Foundation funded the Academic Progression in Nursing (APIN) Program to advance state and regional strategies to create a more highly educated nursing workforce. A total of $4.3 million in funding was awarded to the Tri-Council for Nursing to steer this initiative. Tri-Council members include the American Association of Colleges of Nursing, National League for Nursing, American Nurses Association, and the American Organization of Nurse Executives. For additional information, visit: www.aone.org/membership/about/press_releases/2012/032312.shtml

The nation's Magnet hospitals, which are recognized for nursing excellence and superior patient outcomes, moved to require all nurse managers and nurse leaders to hold a baccalaureate or graduate degree in nursing by 2013. Settings applying for Magnet designation must also show what plans are in place to achieve the IOM recommendation of having an 80 percent baccalaureate-prepared RN workforce by 2020. Visit www.nursecredentialing.org for more information.

In its October 2010 report, "The Future of Nursing," the Institute of Medicine states, "an increase in the percentage of nurses with a BSN is imperative as the scope of what the public needs from nurses grows, expectations surrounding quality heighten, and the settings where nurses are needed proliferate and become more complex." See http://thefutureofnursing.org

In May 2010, the Tri-Council for Nursing, a coalition of four steering organizations for the nursing profession (AACN, ANA, AONE, and NLN), issued a consensus statement calling for all RNs to advance their education in the interest of enhancing quality and safety across health-care settings. In the statement titled "Education Advancement of Registered Nurses," the Tri-Council organizations present a united view that a more highly educated nursing workforce is critical to meeting the nation's nursing needs and delivering safe, effective patient care. In the policy statement, the Tri-Council finds that "without a more educated nursing workforce, the nation's health will be further at risk." See www.aacn.nche.edu/education-resources/TricouncilEdStatement.pdf.

In December 2009, Dr. Patricia Benner and her team at the Carnegie Foundation for the Advancement of Teaching released a new study titled, "Educating Nurses: A Call for Radical Transformation," which recommended preparing all entry-level registered nurses at the baccalaureate level and requiring all RNs to earn a master's degree within ten years of initial licensure. The authors found that many of today's new nurses are "undereducated" to meet practice demands across settings. Their strong support for high-quality baccalaureate degree programs as the appropriate pathway for RNs entering the profession is consistent with the views of many leading nursing organizations, including AACN. See www.carnegiefoundation.org/elibrary/educating-nurses-highlights.

In the July/August 2009 issue of *Health Affairs,* Dr. Linda Aiken and colleagues call for adapting federal funding mechanisms (i.e. Title VIII and Medicare) to focus on preparing more nurses at the baccalaureate and higher degree levels. This policy emphasis is needed to adequately address the growing need for faculty and nurses to serve in primary care and other advanced practice roles. The researchers reported that new nurses prepared in B.S.N. programs are significantly more likely to complete the graduate-level education needed to fill nursing positions where job growth is expected to be the greatest. See http://content.healthaffairs.org

More than 690 RN-to-Baccalaureate programs are available nationwide, including more than 400 programs that are offered at least partially online. These programs build on the education provided in diploma and associate degree programs and prepare graduates for a broader scope of practice. In addition, 160 RN-to-Master's degree programs are available, which cover the baccalaureate content missing in the other entry-level programs as well as graduate-level course work.

Articulation agreements support education mobility and facilitate the seamless transfer of academic credit between associate degree and baccalaureate nursing programs. In addition to hundreds of individual agreements between community colleges and four-year schools, statewide articulation agreements exist in many areas including Alabama, Arkansas, Connecticut, Florida, Idaho, Iowa, Maryland, Nevada, South Carolina, and Texas to facilitate educational advancement. See www.aacn.nche.edu/media-relations/fact-sheets/articulation-agreements.

References

Aiken, L. (2014, October). Baccalaureate nurses and hospital outcomes: More evidence. *Medical Care,* 52(10), 861–63.

Aiken, L., Sloane, D.M., et al. (2014, May 24). Nurse staffing and education and hospital mortality in nine European countries: a retrospective observational study. *The Lancet,* 383(9931), 1824–30.

Aiken, L.H., Cheung, R.B., and Olds, D.M. (2009, June 12). Education policy initiatives to address the nurse shortage in the United States. *Health Affairs* Web Exclusive. Accessed June 22, 2009 at http://content.healthaffairs.org/cgi/content/abstract/hlthaff.28.4.w646.

Aiken, L.H., Clarke, S.P., Sloane, D.M., Lake, E.T., and Cheney, T. (2008, May). Effects of hospital care environment on patient mortality and nurse outcomes. *Journal of Nursing Administration,* 38(5), 223–29.

Aiken, L.H., Clarke, S.P., Cheung, R.B., Sloane, D.M., and Silber, J.H. (2003, September 24). Educational levels of hospital nurses and surgical patient mortality, *Journal of the American Medical Association,* 290, 1617–23.

American Association of Colleges of Nursing (2013). 2012–2013 Enrollment and graduations in baccalaureate and graduate programs in nursing. Washington, DC: Author.

American Organization of Nurse Executives. (2005). Practice and education partnership for the future. Washington, DC: American Organization of Nurse Executives.

Benner, P., Sutphen, M., Leonard, V., and Day, L. (2009). *Educating Nurses: A Call for Radical Transformation.* Carnegie Foundation for the Advancement of Teaching. San Francisco: Jossey-Bass.

Blegen, M.A., Goode, C.J., Park, S.H., Vaughn, T., and Spetz, J. (2013, February). Baccalaureate education in nursing and patient outcomes. *Journal of Nursing Administration,* 43(2), 89–94.

Budden, J.S., Zhong, E.H., Moulton, P., and Cimiotti, J.P. (2013, July 13). The National Council of State Boards of Nursing and The Forum of State Nursing Workforce Centers 2013 National Workforce Survey of Registered Nurses. *Journal of Nursing Regulation,* 4(2), S1–S72.

Cho, E., Sloane, D.M., Aiken, L., et al. (2014, August). Effects of nurse staffing, work environments, and education on patient mortality: An observational study. *International Journal of Nursing Studies.* In Press. DOI: http://dx.doi.org/10.1016/j.ijnurstu.2014.08.006

Estabrooks, C.A., Midodzi, W.K., Cummings, G.C., Ricker, K.L., and Giovanetti, P. (2005, March/April). The impact of hospital nursing characteristics on 30-day mortality. *Nursing Research*, 54(2), 72–84.

Friese, C.R, Lake, E.T., Aiken, L.H., Silber, J.H., and Sochalski, J. (2008, August). Hospital nurse practice environments and outcomes for surgical oncology patients. *Health Services Research*, 43(4), 1145–63.

Health Resources and Services Administration, National Center for Health Workforce Analysis. (2013, April). The U.S. nursing workforce: Trends in supply and education. Accessible online at http://bhpr.hrsa.gov/healthworkforce/reports/nursingworkforce/index.html.

Institute of Medicine. (2010). *The Future of Nursing: Leading Change, Advancing Health.* Washington, DC: National Academies Press.

Kutney-Lee, A., Sloane, D.M., and Aiken, L. (2003, March). An increase in the number of nurses with baccalaureate degrees is linked to lower rates of post-surgery mortality. *Health Affairs*, 32(3), 579–86.

McHugh, M.D., Kelly, L.A., Smith, H.L., Wu, E.S., Vanak, J.M., and Aiken, L.H. (2012, October). Lower Mortality in Magnet Hospitals. *Medical Care*, Publication forthcoming (published ahead of print).

National Council of State Boards of Nursing (See Budden, et al. reference.).

Tourangeau, A.E., Doran, D.M., et al. (2007, January). Impact of hospital nursing care on 30-day mortality for acute medical patients. *Journal of Advanced Nursing*, 57(1), 32–41.

Tri-Council for Nursing. (2010, May). Educational advancement of registered nurses: A consensus position. Available online at http://www.aacn.nche.edu/Education/pdf/TricouncilEdStatement.pdf.

Van den Heede, K., Lesaffre, E., et al. (2009). The relationship between inpatient cardiac surgery mortality and nurse numbers and educational level: Analysis of administrative data. *International Journal of Nursing Studies,* 46(6), 796–803.

Yakusheva, O., Lindrooth, R., and Weiss, M. (2014, October). Economic evaluation of the 80% baccalaureate nurse workforce recommendation: A patient-level analysis. *Medical Care*, 52(10), 864–69.

COUNSELORS OF CARE IN THE MODERN HEALTH-CARE SYSTEM

Deborah E. Trautman, Ph.D., RN, FAAN
President and Chief Executive Officer
American Association of Colleges of Nursing

A Different Era

The nursing profession is alive and reshaping itself. The role of nurses as those who minister exclusively to a patient's basic-care needs has changed. Much of the effectiveness and productivity of the future health-care industry will derive from the training of and services provided by nurses.

Modern nurses take a proactive role in health care by addressing health issues before they develop into problems. They oversee the continued care of patients who have left the health-care facility. Nurses are expected to make complex decisions in areas ranging from patient screening to diagnosis and education. They explore and document the effects of alternative therapies (e.g., guided imagery) and address public health problems, such as teen pregnancy. They explore and understand new technology and how it relates both to patient care and to their own job performance. They work in a variety of settings and are held accountable for their decisions. In today's health-care environment, health-care administrators must recruit nurses with a broad, well-rounded education.

Health-care providers must change the way they administer care. Instead of focusing on the treatment of illness, they must promote wellness. Nurses will oversee patient treatment and medication and must understand the repercussions of these health-care processes for the patient and his or her family.

Cost is the driving force behind this industry-wide transformation. Insurance companies have, for the most part, instigated changes in the way health-care benefits are paid. The old fee-for-service system is no longer the only option. The trend toward managed care, in which a fixed amount of money is allocated for the care of each patient, is changing the way care is provided. It seems that employers of the future will recruit nurses who understand the overall structure of the health-care industry, who possess highly developed critical-thinking skills, and who bring to their positions a well-rounded understanding of the risks and benefits of every health-care decision.

Counselors of Care

Job prospects for graduates of nursing programs are positive. Although many graduates receive associate degrees as registered nurses (RNs), hospital administrators and other employers want applicants with at least a Bachelor of Science in Nursing degree.

To practice in a fast-changing health system, entry-level RNs must understand community-based primary care and emphasize health promotion and cost-effective coordinated care—all hallmarks of baccalaureate education. In addition to its broad scientific curriculum and focus on leadership and clinical decision-making skills, a Bachelor of Science in Nursing degree education provides specific preparation in community-based care not typically included in associate degree or hospital diploma programs. Moreover, the nurse with a baccalaureate degree is the only basic nursing graduate prepared for all health-care settings—critical care, outpatient care, public health, and mental health—and so has the flexibility to practice in outpatient centers, private homes, and neighborhood clinics where demand is fast expanding as health care moves beyond the hospital to more primary and preventive care throughout the community.

Health-care administrators realize that patients are becoming more sophisticated about the care they receive, requiring an explanation and understanding of their health needs. Nurses will have to be knowledgeable care providers, working with physicians, pharmacists, and public health officials in interdisciplinary settings to satisfy these requirements.

Broader training enables graduates of baccalaureate programs to provide improved and varying types of care, and ensures stability and security in an industry now noted for its instability.

Promising Opportunities

One of the rewards of a baccalaureate education can be a competitive salary. Graduates of four-year degree programs can expect salaries starting around $37,000 per year, a figure that might fluctuate depending on geographic area and, more specifically, by the demand in that area. Obviously, the greater the need for nurses, the higher their salaries.

The baccalaureate degree also serves as a foundation for the pursuit of a master's degree in nursing, which prepares students for the role of advanced practice nurse (APN). Students can earn degrees as clinical nurse specialists in neonatology, oncology, cardiology, and other specialties or as nurse practitioners, nurse-midwives, or nurse anesthetists. Master's-prepared nurses can also enjoy rewarding careers in nursing administration and education.

These programs generally span one to two years. Graduates can expect starting salaries of approximately $50,000 annually in advanced practice nursing settings, and demand for these graduates is expected to be high over the next fifteen years. In some localities, for example, the nurse practitioner may be the sole provider of health care to a family.

Overall Transformation

The nursing field must be transformed to be compatible with the overall changes in the health-care industry. According to 2008 statistics, the average age of nurses was 46, with only 16.6 percent of nurses under the age of 35. It is projected that over the next ten years much of the nursing population will retire. Employment is projected to increase 23 percent by 2020.

The traditional career path of nurses is expected to change. More nurses will enter master's programs directly from baccalaureate programs, and more master's degree graduates will pursue doctoral degrees at a younger age. Since nurses will play a critical role in providing health care, a four-year baccalaureate degree is a crucial first step in preparing nurses to assume increased patient responsibilities within the health-care system.

RNs RETURNING TO SCHOOL: CHOOSING A NURSING PROGRAM

Marilyn Oermann, Ph.D., RN, ANEF, FAAN
Thelma M. Ingles Professor of Nursing and Director of
Evaluation and Educational Research
Duke University School of Nursing

If you are thinking about returning to school to complete your baccalaureate degree or to pursue a graduate degree in nursing, you are not alone. Registered nurses (RNs) are returning to school in record numbers, many seeking advancement or transition to new roles in nursing. Over the last two decades, the number of RNs prepared initially in diploma and associate degree in nursing programs who have graduated from baccalaureate nursing degree programs has more than doubled, according to the AACN. There are expanded opportunities for nurses with baccalaureate degrees in nursing. Although the decision to return to school means considerable investment of time, financial resources, and effort, the benefits can be overwhelmingly positive.

Higher education in nursing opens doors to many opportunities for career growth not otherwise available. By continuing your education, you can do the following:

- Update your knowledge and skills, critical today in light of rapid advances in health care

- Move more easily into a new role within your organization or in other health-care settings

- Pursue a different career path within nursing

Moreover, returning to school brings personal fulfillment and satisfaction gained through learning more about nursing and the changing health-care system and using that knowledge in the delivery and management of patient care.

More Skills and Flexibility Needed

If you are contemplating returning to school, here are some facts to consider. The health-care system continues to undergo dramatic changes. These changes include hospitalized patients who are more acutely ill; an aging population; technological advances that require highly skilled nursing care; a greater role for nurses in primary care, health promotion, and health education; and the need for nurses to care for patients and families in multiple settings, such as schools, workplaces, homes, clinics, and outpatient facilities, as well as hospitals. With the nursing shortage, nurses are in great demand in hospitals. Moreover, as hospitals continue to become centers for acute and critical care, the nurse's role in both patient care and management of other health-care providers in the hospital has become more complex, requiring advanced knowledge and skills.

Because of the complexity of today's health-care environment, AACN and other leading nursing organizations have called for the baccalaureate degree in nursing as the minimum educational requirement for professional nursing practice. In fact, nurse executives in hospitals have indicated their desire for the majority of nurses on staff to be prepared at least at the baccalaureate level to handle the increasingly complex demands of patient care and management of health-care delivery. The baccalaureate nursing degree is essential for nurses to function in different management roles, move across employment settings, have the flexibility to change positions within nursing, and advance in their career. Baccalaureate nursing degree programs prepare the nurse for a broad role within the health-care system and for practice in hospitals, community settings, home health care, neighborhood clinics, and other outpatient settings where opportunities are expanding. Continuing education provides the means for nurses to prepare themselves for a future role in nursing.

The demand for nurses with baccalaureate and more advanced degrees will continue to grow. There is an excess of nurses prepared at the associate degree level, a mounting shortage of baccalaureate-prepared nurses, and only half as many nurses prepared at master's and doctoral levels as needed. Nurses with baccalaureate nursing degrees are needed in all areas of health care, and the demand for nurses with master's and doctoral preparation for advanced practice, management, teaching, and research will continue.

Identifying Strategies

The decision to return to school marks the beginning of a new phase in your career development. It is essential for you to plan this future carefully. Why are you thinking about returning to school, and what do you want to accomplish by doing so? Understanding why you want to go back to school will help you select the best program for you. Knowing what you want to accomplish will help you to focus on your goals and overcome the obstacles that could prevent you from achieving your full potential.

Even if you decide that additional education will help you reach your professional goals, you may also have a list of reasons why you think you cannot return to school—no time, limited financial resources, fear of failure, and concerns about meeting family responsibilities, among others. If you are concerned about the demands of school combined with existing responsibilities, begin by identifying strategies for incorporating classes and study time into your present schedule or consider taking an online course. Remember, you can start your program with one course and reevaluate your time at the end of the term.

Research and anecdotal evidence from adults returning to college indicate that, despite their need to balance school work with a career and often with family responsibilities, these adult learners experience less stress and manage their lives better than they had thought possible. Many of these adult learners report that the satisfaction gained from their education more than compensates for any added stress. Furthermore, studies of nurses who have returned to school suggest that while their education may create stress for them, most nurses cope effectively with the demands of advanced education.

If costs are of concern, it is best to investigate tuition-reimbursement opportunities where you are employed, scholarships from the nursing program and other nursing organizations, and loans. The financial aid officer at the program you are considering is probably the best available resource to answer your financial assistance questions.

If you are unsure of what to expect when returning to school, remember that such feelings are natural for anyone facing a new situation. If you are motivated and committed to pursuing your degree, you will succeed. Most nursing programs offer resources, such as test-taking skills, study skills, and time-management workshops, as well as assistance with academic problems. You can combine school, work, family, and other responsibilities. Even with these greater demands, the benefits of education outweigh the difficulties.

Clarifying Career Goals

Nursing, unlike many other professions, has a variety of educational paths for those who return for advanced education. You should decide if baccalaureate- or graduate-level work is congruent with your career goals. The next step in this process is to reexamine your specific career goals, both immediate and long-term, to determine the level and type of nursing education you will need to meet them. Ask yourself what you want to be doing in the next five to ten years. Discuss your ideas with a counselor in a nursing education program, nurses who are practicing in roles you are considering, and others who are enrolled in a nursing program or who have recently completed a nursing degree.

Baccalaureate degree nursing programs prepare nurses as generalists for practice in all health-care settings. Graduate nursing education occurs at two levels— master's and doctoral. Master's programs vary in length, typically between one and two years. Preparation for roles in advanced practice as nurse practitioners, certified nurse midwives, clinical nurse specialists, certified registered nurse anesthetists, nursing administrators, and nursing educators requires a master's degree in nursing. Many programs meet the needs of RNs by offering options such as accelerated course work, advanced placement, evening and weekend classes, and distance learning courses.

A trend in education for RNs is accelerated programs that combine baccalaureate and master's nursing programs. These combined programs are designed for RNs without degrees whose career goals involve advanced nursing practice and other roles requiring a master's degree. Nurses who complete these combined programs may be awarded both a baccalaureate and a master's degree in nursing or a master's degree only.

At the doctoral level, nurses are prepared for a variety of roles, including research and teaching. Doctoral programs generally consist of three years of full-time study beyond the master's degree, although some programs admit baccalaureate graduates and include the master's-level requirements and degree within the doctoral program.

Matching a Program to Your Needs

Once you have defined your career goals and the level of nursing education they will require, the next step is matching your needs with the offerings and characteristics of specific nursing programs. Some of the criteria you may want to consider in evaluating potential schools of nursing include the types of programs offered, the length of the program and its specific requirements, the availability of full-and part-time study and number of credits required for part-time study, the flexibility of the program, whether distance education courses are available, and the days, times, and sites at which classes and clinical experiences are offered as they relate to your work schedule. Take into consideration the program's accreditation status; faculty qualifications in terms of research, teaching, and practice; and the resources of the school of nursing and of the college/university, such as library holdings, computer services, and statistical consultants. You should also consider the clinical settings used in the curriculum and their relationship to your career goals, as well as the availability of financial aid for nursing students.

Carefully review the admission criteria, including minimum grade point average requirements; scores required on any admission tests, such as the Graduate Record Examinations (GRE) for master's and doctoral programs; and any requirements in terms of work experience. For students returning for a baccalaureate degree, prior nursing knowledge may be validated through testing, transfer of courses, and other mechanisms. Review these options prior to applying to a program.

While the intrinsic quality and characteristics of the program are important, your own personal goals and needs have to be included in your decision. Consider commuting distance, whether courses are offered online, costs in relation to your financial resources, program design, and flexibility of the curriculum in relation to your work, family, and personal responsibilities. While the majority of nursing programs offer part-time study, many programs also schedule classes to accommodate work situations.

Many schools offer nursing courses online, and in some places, the entire baccalaureate and master's programs are available through distance learning. The largest enrollment in nursing distance learning is in baccalaureate programs for RNs. Distance learning allows RNs to further their education no matter where they live. Many nurses prefer online courses because they can learn at times convenient for them, especially considering competing demands associated with their jobs, families, and other commitments.

Ensure Your Success

Once you have made the decision to return to school and have chosen the program that best meets your needs, take an additional step to ensure your success. Identify the support you will need, both academic and personal, to be successful in the nursing program. Academic support is provided by the institution and may include tutoring services, learning resource centers, computer facilities, and other resources to support your learning. You should take advantage of available support services and seek out resources for areas in which you are weak or need review. Academic support services, however, need to be complemented by personal support through family, friends, and peers. With a firm commitment to pursuing advanced education, a clear choice of a nursing program to meet your goals, and support from others, you are certain to find success in returning to school.

BACCALAUREATE PROGRAMS

Linda K. Amos, Ed.D., RN, FAAN
Former Associate Vice President for Health Sciences
Dean Emerita
University of Utah

The health-care industry has continued to change dramatically over the past few years, transforming the roles of nurses and escalating their opportunities. The current shortage of nurses is caused by an increasing number of hospitalized patients who are older and more acutely ill, a growing elderly population with multiple chronic health problems, and expanded opportunities in HMOs, home care, occupational health, surgical centers, and other primary-care settings. Expanding technological advances that prolong life also require more highly skilled personnel.

The increasing scope of nursing opportunities will grow immensely as nurses become the frontline providers of health care. They are assuming important roles in the provision of managed care, and they will be responsible for coordinating and continuing the care outside traditional health-care facilities. Nurses will play a major role in educating the public and addressing the social and economic factors that impact quality of care.

Worldwide Standards

Nursing students of the future will receive a wealth of information. Understanding the technology used to manage that information will be essential to their ability to track and assess care. In this area, nurses will be able to provide care over great distances. In some areas, care is being managed by the nurse via tele-home health over the Internet. Use of the Internet and other computer-oriented systems is now an integral tool used by nurses. Nurses of the future, therefore, will have to become aware of worldwide standards of care. Nevertheless, the primary job of a nurse will be making sure that the right person is providing the right care at the right cost.

This goal will be accomplished as the industry turns away from the hospital as the center of operation. Nurses will work in a broad array of locations, including clinics, outpatient facilities, community centers, schools, and even places of business.

Much of the emphasis in health care will shift to preventive care and the promotion of health. In this system, nurses will take on a broader and more diverse role than they have in the past.

Unlimited Opportunities, Expanded Responsibilities

The four-year baccalaureate programs in today's nursing colleges provide the educational and experiential base not only for entry-level professional practice, but also as the platform on which to build a career through graduate-level study for advanced practice nursing, including careers as nurse practitioners, nurse-midwives, clinical specialists, and nurse administrators and educators. Nurses at this level can be expected to specialize in oncology, pediatrics, neonatology, obstetrics and gynecology, critical care, infection control, psychiatry, women's health, community health, and neuroscience. The potential and responsibilities at this level are great. Increasingly, many families use the nurse practitioner for all health-care needs. In almost all U.S. states, the nurse practitioner can prescribe medications and provide health care for the management of chronic non-acute illnesses and preventive care.

The health-care system demands a lot from nurses. The education of a nurse must transcend the traditional areas of study, such as chemistry and anatomy, to include health promotion, disease prevention, screening, genetic counseling, and immunization. Nurses should understand how health problems may have a social cause, such as poverty and environmental contamination, and they must develop insight into human psychology, behavior, and cultural mores and values.

The transformation of the health-care system offers unlimited opportunities for nurses at the baccalaureate and graduate levels as care in urban and rural settings becomes more accessible. According to the U.S. Bureau of Labor Statistics, employment of RNs will grow more quickly than the average employment for all occupations through 2018, due largely to growing demand in settings such as health maintenance organizations, community health centers, home care, and long-term care. The increased complexity of health problems and increased management of health problems outside of hospitals require highly educated and well-prepared nurses at the baccalaureate and graduate levels. It is an exciting era in nursing that holds exceptional promise for nurses with a baccalaureate nursing degree.

The compensation for new nurses is once again becoming competitive with that of other industries. Entry-level nurses with baccalaureate degrees in nursing can expect a salary range of about $31,000 to $46,000 per year, depending on geographic location and experience. Five years into their careers, the national average for nurses with four-year degrees is more than $50,000 per year, with many earning more than $65,000. The current shortage has prompted some employers to offer sign-on bonuses and other incentives to attract and retain staff.

Applying to College

Meeting your chosen school's general entrance requirements is the first step toward a university or college degree in nursing. Admission requirements may vary, but a high school diploma or equivalent is necessary. Most accredited colleges consider SAT scores along with high school grade point average. A strong preparatory class load in science and mathematics is generally preferred among nursing schools. Students may obtain specific admission information by writing to a school's nursing department.

To apply to a nursing school, contact the admission offices of the colleges or universities you are interested in and request the appropriate application forms. With limited spaces in nursing schools, programs are competitive, and early submission of an application is recommended.

Accreditation

Accreditation of the nursing program is very important, and it should be considered on two levels—the accreditation of the university or college and the accreditation of the nursing program itself. Accreditation is a voluntary process in which the school or the program asks for an external review of its programs, facilities, and faculty. For nursing programs, the review is performed by peers in nursing education to ensure program quality and integrity.

Baccalaureate nursing programs in the United States undergo two types of regular systematic reviews. First, the school must be approved by the state board of nursing. This approval is necessary to ensure that the graduates of the program may sit for the licensing examinations offered through the National Council of State Boards of Nursing, Inc. The second is accreditation administered by a nursing accreditation agency that is recognized by the U.S. Department of Education.

Although accreditation is a voluntary process, access to federal loans and scholarships requires it, and most graduate schools accept only students who have earned degrees from accredited schools. Further, accreditation ensures an ongoing process of quality improvement based on national standards. Canadian nursing school programs are accredited by the Canadian Association of University Schools of Nursing, and the Canadian programs listed in this book must hold this accreditation. There are two recognized accreditation agencies for baccalaureate nursing programs in the United States: the Commission on Collegiate Nursing Education (CCNE) and the National League for Nursing Accrediting Commission (NLNAC).

Focusing Your Education

Academic performance is not the sole basis of acceptance into the upper level of the nursing program. Admission officers also weigh such factors as student activities, employment, and references. Moreover, many require an interview and/or essay in which the nursing candidate offers a goal statement. This part of the admission process can be completed prior to a student's entrance into the college or university or prior to the student's entrance into the school of nursing itself, depending on the program.

In the interview or essay, students may list career preferences and reasons for their choices. This allows admission officers to assess the goals of students and gain insights into their values, integrity, and honesty. One would expect that a goal statement from a student who is just entering college would be more general than that of a student who has had two years of preprofessional nursing studies. The more experienced student would be likely to have a more focused idea of what is to be gained by an education in nursing; there would be more evidence of the student's values and the ways in which she or he relates them to the knowledge gained from preprofessional nursing classes.

Baccalaureate Curriculum

A standard basic or generic baccalaureate program in nursing is a four-year college or university education that incorporates a variety of liberal arts courses with professional education and training. It is designed for high school graduates with no previous nursing experience.

Currently, there are more than 700 baccalaureate programs in the United States. Of the 683 programs that responded to a 2009 survey conducted by the American Association of Colleges of Nursing, total enrollment in all nursing programs leading to a baccalaureate degree was 214,533.

The baccalaureate curriculum is designed to prepare students for work in the growing and changing health-care environment. As nurses take a more active role in all facets of health care, they are expected to develop critical thinking and communication skills in addition to receiving standard nurse training in clinics and hospitals. In a university or college setting, the first two years include classes in the humanities, social sciences, basic sciences, business, psychology, technology, sociology, ethics, and nutrition.

In some programs, nursing classes begin in the sophomore year; others begin in the junior year. Many schools require satisfactory grade point averages before students advance into professional nursing classes. On a 4.0 scale, admission into the last two years of the nursing program may require a minimum GPA of 2.5 to 3.0 in preprofessional nursing classes. The national average is about 2.8, but the cutoff level varies with each program.

In the junior and senior years, the curriculum focuses on the nursing sciences, and emphasis moves from the classroom to health facilities. This is where students are exposed to clinical skills, nursing theory, and the varied roles nurses play in the health-care system. Courses include nurse leadership, health promotion, family planning, mental health, environmental and occupational health, adult and pediatric care, medical and surgical care, psychiatric care, community health, management, and home health care.

This level of education comes in a variety of settings: community hospitals, clinics, social service agencies, schools, and health-maintenance organizations. Training in diverse settings is the best preparation for becoming a vital player in the growing health-care field.

Reentry Programs

Practicing nurses who return to school to earn a baccalaureate degree will have to meet requirements that may include possession of a valid RN license and an associate degree or hospital diploma from an accredited institution. Again, it is best to check with the school's admissions department to determine specifics.

Nurses returning to school will have to consider the rapid rate of change in health care and science. A nurse who passed an undergraduate-level chemistry class ten years ago would probably not receive credit for that class today because of the growth of knowledge in that and all other scientific fields. The need to reeducate applies not only to practicing nurses returning to school, but also to all nurses throughout their careers.

In the same vein, nurses with diplomas from hospital programs who want to work toward a baccalaureate degree must meet the common requirements for more clinical practice, and must develop a deeper understanding of community-based nursing practices such as health prevention and promotion.

Colleges and universities available to the RN in search of a baccalaureate give credit for previous nurse training. These programs are designed to accommodate the needs and career goals of the practicing nurse by providing flexible course schedules and credit for previous experience and education. Some programs lead to a master's-level degree, a process that can take up to three years. Licensed practical nurses (LPNs) can also continue their education through baccalaureate programs.

Nurses considering reentering school may also consider other specialized programs. For example, some programs are aimed at enabling nurses with A.D.N. degrees or LPN/LVN licenses to earn B.S.N.'s. Also, accelerated B.S.N. programs are available for students with degrees in other fields.

Choosing a Program

With more than 700 baccalaureate programs in the United States, the prospective student must do research to determine which programs match his or her needs and career objectives.

If you have no health-care experience, it might be best to gain some insight into the field by volunteering or working part-time in a care facility such as a hospital or an outpatient clinic. Talking to nurse professionals about their work will also help you determine how your attributes may apply to the nursing field.

When considering a nursing education, consider your personal needs. Is it best for you to work in a heavily structured environment or one that offers more flexibility in terms of, say, integrating a part-time work schedule into studies? Do you need to stay close to home? Do you prefer to work in a large health-care system such as a health maintenance organization or a medical center, or do you prefer smaller, community-based operations?

As for nursing programs, ask the following questions: How involved is the faculty in developing students for today's health-

RN-to-Baccalaureate Programs Fact Sheet

More than 692 RN-to-baccalaureate programs are available nationwide, including programs offered in a more intense, accelerated format. Program length varies from one to two years depending upon the school's requirements, program type, and the student's previous academic achievement.

Concerns about the limited availability of RN-to-baccalaureate programs are unfounded. In fact, there are more RN-to-baccalaureate programs available than there are four-year nursing programs or accelerated bachelor's degree programs for non-nursing college graduates. Access to RN-to-baccalaureate programs is further enhanced when programs are offered completely online or on-site at various health-care facilities.

Enrollment in RN-to-baccalaureate programs is increasing in response to calls for a more highly educated nursing workforce. From 2011 to 2012, enrollments increased by 15.5 percent, marking the tenth year of increases in RN-to-baccalaureate programs.

Hundreds of articulation agreements between A.D.N. and diploma programs and four-year institutions exist nationwide (including some statewide agreements), to help students who are seeking baccalaureate-level nursing education. Before enrolling in diploma and A.D.N. programs, students are encouraged to check with school administrators to see what articulation agreements exist with baccalaureate degree–granting schools and to determine which course work will be transferable.

care industry? How strong is the school's affiliation with clinics and hospitals? Is there assurance that a student will gain an up-to-date educational experience for the current job market? Are a variety of care settings available? How much time in clinics is required for graduation? What are the program's resources in terms of computer and science laboratories? Does the school work with hospitals and community-based centers to provide health care? How available is the faculty to oversee a student's curriculum? What kind of student support is available in terms of study groups and audiovisual aids? Moreover, what kind of counseling from faculty members and administrators is available to help students develop well-rounded, effective progress through the program?

Visiting a school and talking to the program's guidance counselors will give you a better understanding of how a particular program or school will fit your needs. You can get a closer look at the faculty, its members' credentials, and the focus of the program. It's also not too early to consider what each program can offer in terms of job placement.

MASTER'S PROGRAMS

Tommie L. Norris, DNS, RN
Professor and Associate Dean/Chair
BSN and MSN Programs
College of Nursing
The University of Tennessee Health Science Center
Memphis, Tennessee

The complexities of the health-care environment accompanied by The Affordable Care Act and the Institute of Medicine's (IOM) report *To Err is Human* have challenged health-care providers, educators, and consumers to redesign healthcare. The IOM report informed health-care providers and consumers that healthcare is fragmented, unsafe, and exists in a crisis situation. The IOM's *Future of Nursing Report* apprised the nation that nurses must practice to the full extent of their scope of practice, training, and education while also pursing higher levels of education. The Affordable Care Act will provide funds to train 600 new nurse practitioners and nurse midwives in just the next year. With improved access to healthcare, consumers will look toward advance practice nurses to manage their health-care needs. As the most trusted profession and largest sector of the health-care workforce, nurses are ready to meet the challenge to be a full partner in redesigning healthcare.

The American Association of Colleges of Nursing's (AACN) *The Essentials of Master's Education in Nursing* describes master's education as a "critical component of the nursing education trajectory to prepare nurses who can address the gaps resulting from growing healthcare needs" and to improve health outcomes. They further define how master's education prepares the nursing graduate to:

- Be the forerunner to improve quality outcomes.
- Exude excellence as a result of lifelong learning.
- Develop and direct interdisciplinary care teams.
- Serve as integrators of patient care across health-care systems.
- Manage innovative nursing practices.
- Incorporate evidenced-based practice.

Consumers of healthcare no longer are content to be passive but are active partners in their healthcare. Consumers can already see the changes in place and those being planned to transform healthcare:

- A Clinical Nurse Leader conducts patient rounds with an interdisciplinary health-care team to brainstorm processes aimed to streamline medication administration, ensuring medications are delivered and administered in a timely, safe, and accurate manner.
- A patient with a pacemaker places the phone's receiver over the implant allowing an advanced practice nurse to evaluate pacemaker function and manage care after oxygen saturation, BMI, and vital signs are transmitted.
- The Certified Nursing Administrator of a home health agency collaborates with the Chief Financial Officer to formulate the agency's budget, then later meets with the Director of the Human Resources Department to review policies related to current hiring practices.
- A Clinical Nurse Specialist consults with other nurses caring for diabetic patients to design cost-effective, patient-centered, high-quality care to reduce recidivism and chronic complications. Clinical Nurse Specialists manage the treatment of specific populations.
- The parents of a child preparing for an appendectomy are visited by a certified registered nurse anesthetist (CRNA) to obtain a preoperative history and answer any questions related to the anesthesia that the CRNA will administer.

Master's Education in Nursing

Master's prepared nurses may assume the role as Advanced Practice Registered Nurses (APRNs), as well as, advanced roles such as Clinical Nurse Leaders (CNLs), nurse administrators, public health nurses, and nurse educators. The demand for master's prepared nurses is expected to remain high. There are more than 536 master's degree programs accredited by the Commission on Collegiate Nursing Education (CCNE) or by the National League for Nursing Accrediting Commission (NLNAC).

The Advanced Practice Registered Nurse (APRN) Consensus Model defines advance practice nurses as being educated at the Master's or Doctoral level and certified to prescribe, treat, and manage all aspects of patient care. AACN recognizes Clinical Nurse Specialists (CNS), Certified Nurse Practitioners (CNP), Certified Registered Nurse Anesthetists (CRNA), and Certified Nurse Midwives (CNM) as APRNs with advanced clinical skills and knowledge. With the Affordable Care Act improving access to healthcare for many Americans who were previously uninsurable or without affordable healthcare, it is clear more APRNs are needed.

APRNs practice in a wide range of practice arenas to provide primary and specialty care.

Nurse Practitioners (NP) manage care for patients across the lifespan with acute and chronic conditions and are key to providing access to care in underserved areas. NPs manage care across the wellness-illness continuum to include health screening and examinations/assessments, diagnosing, treating, health education, and disease prevention/promotion. Family/individual, pediatrics, adult-gerontology, neonatal, psychiatric/mental health, and women's health/gender-related are the six population foci.

Nurse-Midwives provide primary care that includes care of gynecologic and obstetric patients, newborns, and childbirth. Preventative and primary care are managed across diverse settings and could include screening for sexually transmitted diseases and risk factors that increase birth defects or infertility.

Registered Nurse Anesthetists deliver anesthesia across the lifespan in both acute and outpatient settings for general surgery, specialties such as trauma, pain management, and childbirth and outpatient procedures.

Clinical Nurse Specialists (CNS) focus nursing practice by populations, disease, and or practice venue. A CNS is responsible for the management of disease, health promotion/prevention, and assessment of risk behaviors in areas such as adult health, critical care, community health, psychiatric nursing, or neonatal nursing.

Master's-prepared nurses who are not APRNs also have many opportunities. Roles and practice settings are diverse and ever evolving with the dynamic healthcare environment. Such roles may include, but are not limited to, direct care foci such as the Clinical Nurse Leaders and nurse educators. Other roles include nurse administrators, public health nurses, nurse informaticists, and public policy.

In 2003, the American Association of Colleges of Nursing (AACN) in partnership with other national leaders and professionals developed the new Clinical Nurse Leader (CNL) role aimed to improve health-care outcomes by reducing fragmentation of care, decreasing the number of errors, and improving quality outcomes of care. The CNL is a master's-prepared generalist who works across health-care settings as a lateral care integrator. However, it is important to point out that the CNL role is not one of manager or administration—rather, the CNL is responsible for patient care outcomes whether by providing the care directly in complex situations or managing care in a microsystem. Their advanced skills and knowledge allow them to facilitate care in complex and dynamic systems.

Nurse educators advance the knowledge and skills of nurses entering the field, novice nurses, and experienced nurses. With an emphasis on lifelong learning and advancing education, there is a growing demand for nurse educators. Educators may choose to teach theory courses or supervise nursing students in a clinical setting, advance the knowledge of practicing nurses by offering classes on new technologies or evidence-based practice, or they may even serve as consultants to health-care agencies seeking better patient outcomes. The preparation for the nurse educator varies; however, those seeking faculty positions are advised to specialize in a clinical area such as adult health, women's health, pediatrics, psychiatric mental health, or community health. In addition, those seeking faculty roles will need formal course work in curriculum development, pedagogy, and student/program evaluation.

Nurse administrators practice in managerial and leadership roles to ensure high-quality patient care is delivered in a cost-effective manner. Entry-level nurse administrators may manage a microsystem; whereas, experienced nurse administrators may lead an entire organization. Certification programs are available for graduates of accredited nursing administration programs from the American Nurses Credentialing Center and the American Organization of Nurse Executives.

Public health nurses are specialists with an emphasis on the health and well- being of the public. Their diverse roles are applicable to many settings and may include epidemiology, managing a clinic that provides immunizations and health screenings, investigating and managing communicable disease, providing programs to address environmental risks, and working with government and community leaders to improve and or eliminate health risks.

Nurse informaticists apply the nursing process to computer and information science to support patients and health-care providers in clinical decisions. The need to share health-care information across care venues to provide patient-centered care along with the need to ensure privacy provides the perfect environment to promote the role of the nurse informaticist.

Public policy nurses interested in this role use nursing knowledge to educate the public and legislators concerning health-care issues to shape policy. Nurses with advanced education in public policy are poised to serve as consultants to local, state, and national policy-making bodies and associations that influence healthcare.

Overview of the Master's Curriculum

Those looking to earn a master's degree in nursing have many options for entry:

- **Entry-level or Generic degree**—allows individuals who are non-nurses to meet the baccalaureate-level requirements gaining eligibility to sit for the initial RN licensure and earn a master's degree. The new Clinical Nurse Leader role is one popular choice that utilizes this option.

- **RN to Master's Degree**—allows registered nurses (RN) who have an earned an associate degree in nursing to complete the missing baccalaureate content and progress through the master's-level curriculum. The online delivery format is gaining popularity to accommodate the working RN's schedule. The time for completion varies depending whether the part-time or full-time program of study is selected.

- **Baccalaureate to Master's Degree**—thought of as the traditional postbaccalaureate master's degree, this option remains the most popular. Since the undergraduate content has been mastered, students focus solely on graduate-level course work, with most degrees awarded in 18 to 24 months. The Master of Science in Nursing (M.S.N.), Master of Nursing (M.N.), or Master of Science (M.S.) may be offered, all of which prepare students to meet the master's degree competencies.

- **Dual Master's Degree Programs**—provide an extensive concentration in a related field of study that is combined with nursing courses. More than 120 dual master's degrees are available that combine nursing coursework with business (MSN/MBA); public administration (MSN/MPA), and health administration (MSN/MSA).

- **Post Master's Certificate Programs**—allow nurses who have a master's degree in nursing to gain advanced skills and knowledge in an additional area of nursing. Nursing education, administration, informatics, and clinical nurse leader are such options. A current trend is for nurses certified as Family Nurse Practitioners to return to earn certification as an Acute Care Nurse Practitioner to deliver care in such areas as the emergency department or intensive care.

The master's nursing curriculum builds on the skills and competencies gained in the baccalaureate nursing program. Content related to health-care economics/policy, genetics, organizational sciences, information sciences, complexity science, bioethics, and quality improvement science might be included. The master's curriculum includes three components:

1. Foundational core content for all individuals pursing a master's degree regardless of functional focus

2. Essential content aimed at advanced direct patient care

3. The functional area focus (clinical and didactic) experiences required by certification bodies and professional nursing organization as essential for specific roles.

Graduates of any one of the four APRN roles (CNP, CNS, CNM, or CRNA) must complete three separate graduate-level courses in physiology/pathophysiology, health assessment, and pharmacology (known as the direct care core or 3 Ps). Graduates pursing non-APRN roles but who have a direct care focus (CNL and nurse educator) must have content/course work in the 3 Ps, although three separate graduate-level courses are not required. Master's degrees preparing students for a practice profession must provide planned clinical experiences to ensure competence to enter nursing practice.

Admission Requirements

The admissions requirements for master's programs in nursing vary depending on entry point and even by specialty. Schools may elect to use standardized admission exams such as the Graduate Record Examinations (GRE®) or Miller Analogies Test (MAT®). Others may choose to base admission on grade point average, letters of reference, college transcripts, and personal statements/essays. Schools may choose to give more importance to certain requirements—for example a school may weigh grade point average more heavily than the standardized exam score. Carefully select individuals to write letters of reference; faculty and employers may be seen as having more value than those written by personal friends or coworkers. When beginning the application process or just considering which master's programs is right, take the time to research any specific requirements. Some CRNA programs require a year of experience in critical care, and some neonatal nurse practitioner programs require a year in the neonatal ICU or related area for admission eligibility.

RN-to-Master's Degree Programs Fact Sheet

Currently, there are 159 programs available nationwide to transition RNs with diplomas and associate degrees to the master's-degree level (M.S.N., M.S., or Master of Science in Nursing degree). These programs prepare nurses to assume positions requiring graduate preparation, including roles in administration, teaching, research, and as Clinical Nurse Leaders. Master's degree-prepared nurses are in high demand as expert clinicians, nurse executives, clinical educators, health-policy consultants, and research assistants.

RN-to-M.S.N. programs generally take about three years to complete, with specific requirements varying by institution and the student's previous course work. Though the majority of these programs are offered in traditional classroom settings, some RN-to-M.S.N. programs are offered largely online or in a blended classroom/online format.

The baccalaureate-level content missing from diploma and ADN programs is built into the front-end of the RN-to-M.S.N. program. Mastery of this upper-level basic nursing content is necessary for students to move on to graduate study. Upon completion, many programs award both the baccalaureate and master's degree.

The number of RN-to-M.S.N. programs has more than doubled in the past 15 years, from 70 programs in 1994 to 159 programs today. According to AACN's 2012 survey of nursing schools, 29 new RN-to-M.S.N. programs are in the planning stages.

When considering a master's program, consider the program length, delivery format such as face-to-face or online, accreditation status, financial aid availability, and employment rates. If considering transitioning into a doctoral program, determine if an articulation plan is in place. Career fairs, webinars, and college websites provide valuable information related to admission requirements.

Benefits of a Master's Degree in Nursing

The perceived benefits of a master's degree in nursing vary from person to person. However, there is evidence that earning a master's degree boosts your nursing career and earning potential. A master's degree in nursing provides greater knowledge and fulfills the requirement for lifelong learning needed to keep pace with the complex dynamic healthcare system. A master's degree provides entry into leadership and managerial roles while broadening the scope of practice. With the aging of our nation and improved access to healthcare, advanced practice nurses will be pivotal to transform the health-care system. Faculty shortages at nursing schools are limiting the number of nurses when a shortage of nurses exists. A master's degree in nursing is the entry point into a nursing faculty position. The master's degree also provides the foundation for doctoral education whether it is advanced practice or research focused.

For the most part, nurses prepared at the master's-level garner higher wages than those with a bachelor's degree. Salaries differ by geographic regions and specializations. When comparing the salary of the four APN roles, the CRNA has the highest average salary, with an average yearly income of $156,000. Comparably, the average salary of a nurse practitioner is $94,050, with the median salary of a nurse midwife at $92,806. Clinical nurse specialists have an average yearly salary of $94,487. Master's-prepared nurses with a direct care focus but who are not APRNs, such as nursing faculty, are receiving $80,690. Chief nursing officers command $194,477 on average, with nurse informaticist earning $80,500.

THE CLINICAL NURSE LEADER

The Clinical Nurse Leader or CNL® is a rapidly emerging nursing role developed by the American Association of Colleges of Nursing (AACN) in collaboration with leaders from the nursing education and practice arenas. The national movement to advance the CNL is fueled by the critical need to improve the quality of patient care and better prepare nurses to thrive across the health-care system. The CNL role was developed following research and discussion with stakeholder groups as a way to engage highly skilled clinicians as leaders in outcome-based practices.

CNL provide lateral integration at the point of care and combine evidence-based practice with the following:

- Microsystems-level advocacy
- Centralized care coordination
- Outcomes measurement
- Risk assessment
- Quality improvement
- Interprofessional communication

In practice, the CNL oversees the care coordination of a distinct group of patients and actively provides direct patient care in complex situations. CNLs have master's degrees and are advanced generalists, evaluating patient outcomes, assessing risks, and using their authority to change care plans when necessary. CNLs are leaders in the health-care delivery system; the implementation of their roles will vary across settings.

Connecting Nursing Practice and Education

To support the creation of this new nursing role, AACN launched a national initiative involving more than 100 education-practice partnerships across the nation. Partners from schools of nursing and nursing practice sites are working together to transform care delivery by educating new CNLs and integrating them into the health delivery system.

More than seventy schools of nursing are now preparing CNLs for advanced generalist programs offered at the graduate level. Students may choose from traditional post-baccalaureate master's programs, degree completion programs for registered nurses (RNs), and accelerated programs for those seeking to make the transition into nursing. Most CNL programs are directly connected with practice sites interested in employing graduates to enhance care delivery, patient safety, and quality outcomes.

The Veterans Health Administration, the nation's largest employer of RNs, has embraced the CNL role and is planning to introduce it into all Veterans Affairs hospitals nationwide. Support for the clinical role is gaining momentum as many practice sites are reporting on the pioneering outcomes of the CNL staff.

The Key to Positive Patient Outcomes

CNLs provide efficient and cost-effective patient care services, as well as the leadership needed to repair fragmented health-care delivery systems. CNLs are having a measurable impact on the quality of nursing services with practice sites reporting that CNLs are

- quickly making significant progress on raising patient, nurse, and physician satisfaction; improving care outcomes; and realizing sizable cost-savings.

- elevating the level of practice for all nurses on the unit by promoting critical thinking and innovation in nursing care.

- constructively managing change and promoting a team-based approach to care.

- understanding the bigger picture, including outcomes and patient satisfaction, when considering next steps, needed changes, and improvements to the practice setting.

The CNL Mark of Excellence

The CNL Mark of Excellence certification is a unique credential that recognizes graduates of master's and post-master's CNL programs who have demonstrated accepted standards of practice. The CNL Mark of Excellence promotes safe, quality practice through its ongoing requirements for personal and professional growth. In 2007, AACN established a new certification commission—the Commission on Nurse Certification (CNC)—to oversee all aspects of the CNL certification program.

Becoming a CNL

Those interested in becoming a CNL are encouraged to visit the AACN website, www.aacn.nche.edu/CNL, to find out more about this nursing career option. Detailed information is available online, including frequently asked questions, the white paper on the CNL role, and a directory of Web links for related programs.

ACCELERATED BACCALAUREATE AND MASTER'S DEGREES IN NURSING

With the Bureau of Labor Statistics projecting the need for more than one million new and replacement registered nurses by the year 2020, nursing schools around the country are exploring creative ways to increase student capacity and reach out to new student populations. One innovative approach to nursing education that is gaining momentum is the accelerated degree program for non-nursing graduates. Offered at the baccalaureate and master's degree levels, these programs build on previous learning experiences and provide a way for individuals with undergraduate degrees in other disciplines to transition into nursing.

Program Basics

- Accelerated baccalaureate programs offer the quickest route to licensure as a registered nurse (RN) for adults who have already completed a bachelor's or graduate degree in a non-nursing discipline.

- Fast-track baccalaureate programs take between 11 and 18 months to complete, including prerequisites. Fast-track master's degree programs generally take about 3 years to complete.

- Accelerated nursing programs are available in 46 states plus the District of Columbia and Puerto Rico. In 2012, there were 255 accelerated baccalaureate programs and 71 accelerated master's programs available at nursing schools nationwide. In addition, 25 new accelerated baccalaureate programs are in the planning stages, and 7 new accelerated master's programs are also taking shape. See www.aacn.nche.edu/education-resources/nursing-education-programs for a list of accelerated nursing programs.

Fast-Track Nursing Education

- Accelerated baccalaureate programs accomplish programmatic objectives in a short time by building on previous learning experiences. Instruction is intense with courses offered full-time with no breaks between sessions. Students receive the same number of clinical hours as their counterparts in traditional entry-level nursing programs.

- Admission standards for accelerated programs are high, with programs typically requiring a minimum of a 3.0 GPA and a thorough prescreening process. Identifying students who will flourish in this environment is a priority for administrators. Students enrolled in accelerated programs are encouraged NOT to work given the rigor associated with completing degree requirements.

- Accelerated baccalaureate and master's programs in nursing are appropriately geared to individuals who have already proven their ability to succeed at a senior college or university. Having already completed a bachelor's degree, many second-degree students are attracted to the fast-track master's program as the natural next step in their higher education.

Accelerated Program Graduates

- The typical second-degree nursing student is motivated, older, and has higher academic expectations than traditional entry-level nursing students. Accelerated students excel in class and are eager to gain clinical experiences. Faculty members find the accelerated students to be excellent learners who are not afraid to challenge their instructors.

- Graduates of accelerated programs are prized by nurse employers who value the many layers of skill and education they bring to the workplace. Employers report that these graduates are more mature, possess strong clinical skills, and are quick studies on the job.

- Given their experience and level of educational achievement, many graduates of accelerated master's programs are being encouraged to pursue roles as nurse educators to help stem the growing shortage of nurse faculty.

Supporting Accelerated Programs

- Financial aid for students enrolled in accelerated baccalaureate and master's programs in nursing is limited. Many practice settings are partnering with schools and offering tuition repayment to graduates as a mechanism to recruit highly qualified nurses.

- Hospitals, health-care systems, and other practice settings are encouraged to form partnerships with schools offering accelerated programs to remove the student's financial burden in exchange for a steady stream of new nurse recruits. Nurse employers including Tenet Healthcare, Carondelet Health Network, University of Missouri Health Care, North Carolina Baptist Hospital, Duke University Health System, and many others are actively supporting the development and growth of accelerated baccalaureate programs in nursing.

- Legislators on the state and federal levels are encouraged to increase scholarship and grant funding for these programs that produce entry-level nurses faster than any other basic nursing education program. These programs are ideal career transition vehicles for those segments of the labor force impacted by fluctuations in the economy.

Research on Accelerated Nursing Programs

Bentley, R. Comparison of traditional and accelerated baccalaureate nursing graduates. *Nurse Educator*, 31(2), 79–83, May/June 2006.

Brewer, C. S., C. T. Kovner, S. Poornima, S. Fairchild, H. Kim, and M. Djukic. A comparison of second-degree baccalaureate and traditional-baccalaureate new graduate RNs: Implications for the workforce. *Journal of Professional Nursing*, 25 (1), 5–14, January-February 2009.

Kearns, L. E., J. R. Shoaf, and M. B. Summey. Performance and satisfaction of second-degree BSN students in Web-based and traditional course delivery environments. *Journal of Nursing Education*, 43(6), 280–284, June 2004.

Meyer, G. A., K. G. Hoover, and S. Maposa. A profile of accelerated BSN graduates, 2004. *Journal of Nursing Education*, 45(8), 324–327, August 2006.

Oermann, M.H., K. Poole-Dawkins, M. T. Alvarez, B. B. Foster, and R. O'Sullivan. Managers' perspectives of new graduates of accelerated nursing programs: How do they compare with other graduates? *Journal of Continuing Education in Nursing*, 41(9), 394–399, October 2010.

Ouellet, L. L., J. MacIntosh, C. H. Gibson, and S. Jefferson. Evaluation of selected outcomes of an accelerated nursing degree program. *Nursing Education Today*, 28(2), 194–201, February 2008.

Raines, D. A. and A. Spies. One year later: Reflections and work activities of accelerated second-degree Bachelor of Science in Nursing graduates. *Journal of Professional Nursing*, 23(6), 329–334, November/December 2007.

Roberts, K., J. Mason, and P. Wood. A comparison of a traditional and an accelerated basic nursing education program. *Contemporary Nurse*, 11(2/3), 283–287, December 2001.

Rouse, S. M. and L. A. Rooda. Factors for attrition in an accelerated baccalaureate nursing program. *Journal of Nursing Education*, 49(6), 359–362, June 1, 2010.

Seldomridge, L. A. and M. C. DiBartolo. The changing face of accelerated second bachelor's degree students. *Nurse Educator*, 32(6), 240–245, November/December 2007.

Seldomridge, L. A. and M. C. DiBartolo. A profile of accelerated second bachelor's degree nursing students. *Nurse Educator*, 30(2), 65–68, March-April 2005.

White, K., W. Wax, and A. Berrey. Accelerated second degree advanced practice nurses: how do they fare in the job market? *Nursing Outlook*, 48(5), 218–222, September-October 2000.

Ziehm, S. R., I. C. Uibel, D. K. Fontaine, and T. Scherzer. Success indicators for an accelerated masters entry nursing program: Staff RN performance. *Journal of Nursing Education*, 49(7), 395–403, July 2011.

THE DOCTOR OF NURSING PRACTICE (DNP)

On October 25, 2004, the member schools affiliated with the American Association of Colleges of Nursing (AACN) voted to endorse the *Position Statement on the Practice Doctorate in Nursing*. This decision called for moving the current level of preparation necessary for advanced nursing practice from the master's degree to the doctorate-level by the year 2015. This endorsement was preceded by almost four years of research and consensus-building by an AACN task force charged with examining the need for the practice doctorate with a variety of stakeholder groups.

Introducing the Doctor of Nursing Practice (DNP)

- In many institutions, advanced practice registered nurses (APRNs), including Nurse Practitioners, Clinical Nurse Specialists, Certified Nurse Midwives, and Certified Nurse Anesthetists, are prepared in master's-degree programs that often carry a credit load equivalent to doctoral degrees in the other health professions. AACN's position statement calls for educating APRNs and other nurses seeking top leadership/organizational roles in DNP programs.

- DNP curricula build on traditional master's programs by providing education in evidence-based practice, quality improvement, and systems leadership, among other key areas.

- The DNP is designed for nurses seeking a terminal degree in nursing practice and offers an alternative to research-focused doctoral programs. DNP-prepared nurses are well-equipped to fully implement the science developed by nurse researchers prepared in PhD, DNS, and other research-focused nursing doctorates.

Why Move to the DNP?

- The changing demands of this nation's complex health-care environment require the highest level of scientific knowledge and practice expertise to assure high-quality patient outcomes. The Institute of Medicine, Joint Commission, Robert Wood Johnson Foundation, and other authorities have called for reconceptualizing educational programs that prepare today's health professionals.

- Some of the many factors building momentum for change in nursing education at the graduate level include: the rapid expansion of knowledge underlying practice; increased complexity of patient care; national concerns about the quality of care and patient safety; shortages of nursing personnel, which demands a higher level of preparation for leaders who can design and assess care; shortages of doctorally prepared nursing faculty; and increasing educational expectations for the preparation of other members of the health-care team.

- In a 2005 report titled *Advancing the Nation's Health Needs: NIH Research Training Programs*, the National Academy of Sciences called for nursing to develop a non-research clinical doctorate to prepare expert practitioners who can also serve as clinical faculty. AACN's work to advance the DNP is consistent with this call to action.

- Nursing is moving in the direction of other health professions in the transition to the DNP. Medicine (MD), Dentistry (DDS), Pharmacy (PharmD), Psychology (PsyD), Physical Therapy (DPT), and Audiology (AudD) all require or offer practice doctorates.

Sustaining Momentum for the DNP

- After a two-year consensus-building process, AACN member institutions voted to endorse the *Essentials of Doctoral Education for Advanced Nursing Practice* on October 30, 2006. Schools developing a DNP are encouraged to use this document, which defines the curricular elements and competencies that must be present in a practice doctorate in nursing. The *DNP Essentials* are posted online at http://www.aacn.nche.edu/DNP/pdf/Essentials.pdf.

- In July 2006, the AACN Board of Directors endorsed the final report of the *Task Force on the Roadmap to the DNP,* which was developed to assist schools navigating the DNP program approval process. This report includes recommendations for securing institutional approval to transition an MSN into a DNP program; preparing faculty to teach in DNP programs; addressing regulatory, licensure, accreditation, and certification issues; and collecting evaluation data. The Roadmap report and accompanying tool kit are posted at http://www.aacn.nche.edu/DNP.

- Schools nationwide that have initiated the DNP are reporting sizable and competitive student enrollment. Employers are quickly recognizing the unique contribution these expert nurses are making in the practice arena, and the demand for DNP-prepared nurses continues to grow. According to the 2011 salary survey conducted by *ADVANCE for Nurse Practitioners* magazine, DNP-prepared NPs earned $8,576 more than master's-prepared NPs.

- The Commission on Collegiate Nursing Education (CCNE), the leading accrediting agency for baccalaureate-

and graduate-degree nursing programs in the United States, began accrediting DNP programs in fall of 2008. To date, 125 DNP programs have been accredited by CCNE.

Current DNP Program Statistics

- 243 DNP programs are currently enrolling students at schools of nursing nationwide, and an additional 59 new DNP programs are in the planning stages.

- DNP programs are now available in 48 states plus the District of Columbia. States with the most programs (more than 5) include Florida, Illinois, Massachusetts, Minnesota, New York, Ohio, Pennsylvania, and Texas.

- From 2012 to 2013, the number of students enrolled in DNP programs increased from 11,575 to 14,688. During that same period, the number of DNP graduates increased from 1,858 to 2,443.

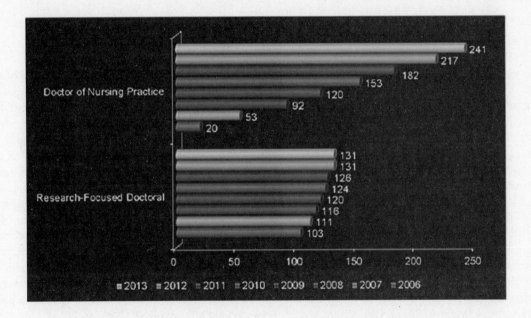

THE PH.D.-PREPARED NURSE: A VITAL LEADER FOR NURSING EDUCATION, HEALTHCARE, AND THE NATION'S HEALTH

Bernadette Mazurek Melnyk, Ph.D., RN, CPNP/PMHNP, FAANP, FNAP, FAAN
Associate Vice President for Health Promotion
University Chief Wellness Officer
Dean and Professor, College of Nursing
Professor of Pediatrics and Psychiatry, College of Medicine
The Ohio State University
Columbus, Ohio

The current state of health and healthcare in America calls for Ph.D.-prepared nurses as never before in our history. Even though the United States spends more than $3.1 trillion every year on healthcare, of which $1.2 trillion is wasteful health-care spending, it ranks low in performance, health, and safety outcomes compared to other industrialized countries (American Hospital Association, 2007; Chernew, Baicker, & Hsu, 2010). Further, gaps in evidence to guide clinical practice, inconsistent implementation of evidence-based practices and recommendations, fragmentation of care, and long lag times between the generation of research evidence and its translation into practice exist (Melnyk et al., 2012; Melnyk & Fineout-Overholt, 2014).

As a result of a health-care system in crisis, the overall health of the American people also is suffering. Behaviors are the number one killer of Americans due to smoking, overeating, lack of physical activity, non-adherence to medications, and suicidal gestures (Melnyk, 2011). Overweight and obesity will soon surpass tobacco as the number one cause of preventable death and disease in the United States (Stewart, Cutler, & Rosen, 2009). With the rapid increase in the prevalence of overweight and obesity, the Centers for Disease Control and Prevention predict that 1 out of 3 Americans will have diabetes by 2050 (Boyle, et al., 2010). One out of 4 children, adolescents, and adults has a mental health disorder, yet less than 25 percent receive treatment (National Institute of Mental Health, 2009). Further, 1 out of 2 Americans has a preventable chronic condition, and 1 out of 4 has multiple chronic conditions, which account for approximately 75 percent of the total U.S. health-care spending (Carter, 2010).

Immediate solutions are needed to improve the current state of healthcare and health in America. Many of these solutions can be generated and led by Ph.D.-prepared nurses who are needed to fill a gap in the education of future generations of nurses for a variety of important roles; to conduct research that generates the best evidence to guide practice, policy, and education; and to assume leadership roles in healthcare and academia. Although many nurses with Ph.D. degrees make the natural transition into an academic career, there are many other career opportunities available for doctorally prepared nurses.

Doctoral Education in Nursing

In the landmark 2010 document, *The Future of Nursing: Leading Change, Advancing Health*, the Institute of Medicine recommended increased education for nurses, specifically a doubling of the number of nurses with doctoral education in order to "add to the cadre of nurse faculty and researchers, with attention to increasing diversity." For decades, doctoral education in nursing focused on the Ph.D., with an emphasis on the generation of evidence through rigorous research to provide a sound knowledge base for nursing practice (Edwardson, 2010). However, in 2004, the American Association of Colleges of Nursing endorsed the Doctor of Nursing Practice (DNP) degree as the single-entry degree for advanced practice nurses (APNs), which led to the rapid expansion of DNP programs across the country. Although both types of doctorally prepared nurses are tremendously needed, there is still much confusion in the role and academic preparation between the Ph.D. and DNP (Melnyk, 2013).

According to the American Association of Colleges of Nursing and the DNP Essentials, the DNP is a practice-focused doctorate that should prepare clinicians for leadership in evidence-based practice (EBP) (AACN, 2006), while the Ph.D. is a research-focused doctorate that prepares nurses to generate new knowledge through rigorous research to ultimately guide practice. Ph.D.-prepared nurses should be the best generators of external evidence (i.e., evidence generated through rigorous research and intended for generalized use in practice), while DNP-prepared nurses should be the best translators of research evidence into practice to improve quality of care and patient outcomes (Melnyk, 2013). Ph.D.-prepared nurses typically seek roles as tenure-track faculty in academic institutions where they engage in teaching, research, and service or are health-care administrators or researchers for hospitals or health-care systems. Conversely, DNP-prepared nurses often seek clinical faculty roles in academia or advanced practice roles in health-care systems, such as direct health-care providers or clinical nurse specialists and directors of evidence-based practice or health-care quality and outcomes management. Another doctoral degree also offered by some colleges of nursing is the Doctor of Nursing Science degree (DNS, DNSc), which is comparable to the Ph.D. degree.

Although the number of both Ph.D. and DNP programs has continued to increase over recent years, DNP programs have expanded at a rapid rate. Currently, there are 243 DNP and 131 Ph.D. programs, with another 59 DNP programs in the planning stages (AACN, 2014a). Enrollment in Ph.D. programs has remained fairly constant while there has been an explosion of nurses enrolled in DNP programs.

Most nurses receive their doctorate in their 40s or 50s in comparison to the other health sciences professions where individuals obtain their Ph.D. at much younger ages (Cleary, Hunt, & Jackson, 2011). As a result, the average age of doctorally prepared nursing faculty in academia in the ranks of full professor, associate professor, and assistant professor is 61.3 years, 57.7 years, and 51.5 years respectively (AACN, 2014b). Therefore, it is critical to encourage nurses to pursue their Ph.D. degrees at younger ages so that they will have decades ahead to have a positive impact on outcomes after completion of their terminal degrees.

There is currently a shortage of doctorally prepared faculty in nursing colleges across the United States (AACN, 2014b). Less than 1 percent of nurses have a doctoral degree, and only 25 percent of full-time nurse faculty have doctoral degrees (Nickitas & Feeg, 2011). In 2013, over 78,000 qualified applicants were turned away from admission to baccalaureate and graduate nursing programs due to the faculty shortage and other factors, such as competition for clinical sites and inadequate numbers of preceptors (AACN, 2014b). This shortage is likely to grow as an aging nursing faculty workforce retires over the next decade.

Ph.D. Admission Criteria and Curricula

Many programs across the United States have two pathways to obtain the doctoral degree: a bachelor's degree to the Ph.D. and a master's degree to the Ph.D. Admission criteria varies, but most programs require RN licensure, academic transcripts, scores from the Graduate Record Examination (GRE®), reference letters, and a personal statement that outlines the applicant's area of research interest and reasons for obtaining the Ph.D. degree. Most programs also require an interview with 2 or 3 members of the doctoral program faculty. Ph.D. programs are typically four years of full-time study.

Ph.D. programs in nursing prepare individuals as experts and leaders in their field, including careers in academia, health-care administration, research, advanced clinical practice, or health policy. Curricula vary, but since the emphasis in a Ph.D. program is on research, these programs typically include courses on theory, research methods, statistics, ethics, leadership, and health policy. Courses in the area of a student's

research interest also are taken as part of the program of study. Students in Ph.D. programs are typically prepared as rigorous independent researchers who are able to tackle the most pressing problems in health and healthcare. Conversely, educational doctorates (Ed.D.) prepare students as expert educators who are equipped to conduct research to advance the field of education. Students in a Ph.D. program are expected to work individually on research projects and complete a dissertation (a written document that describes the research completed as part of the Ph.D. program). Many programs permit either full-time or part-time study. Over twenty Ph.D. programs across the country have institutional T32 pre-doctoral fellowship grants in a certain area of research, which are funded by the National Institutes of Health/National Institute of Nursing Research (e.g., child health, symptom management, aging, health disparities). Students awarded one of these pre-doctoral fellowships receive full tuition and a living stipend. For a full list of funded NIH/NINR T32 grants, visit http://www.ninr.nih.gov/.

Selecting a Ph.D. Program

Selecting a doctoral program comes down to personal choice (Anderson, 2011). However, one very important area for consideration is whether the program has expert faculty who have a track record of research funding and publications in the student's area of interest. Having an expert research mentor to work closely with the student during the Ph.D. program is as vital as the quality of the facilities. The most important question to ask when choosing a program is whether there is a strong "match" between the student's research interest and the faculty's research expertise. Many programs give strong consideration to match when selecting students for admission (Megginson, 2011). In a doctoral program, the contact with professors, the use of research equipment and facilities, and the program's flexibility in allowing the student to choose the course of study are critical questions to pose when investigating programs. Other questions to consider include the following:

- What is the average length of time that students complete their degree?

- How many active researchers with funding are on the faculty?

- How successful are the program's graduates in research funding and publication?

- What opportunities exist for students to work with faculty as research assistants?

- Does the university have adequate support and resources for students, including assistance with statistical analysis of data?

- Does the college have a funded institutional training grant for doctoral study?

Research Conducted by Ph.D.-prepared Nurses

Ph.D.-prepared nurses have the opportunity to engage in a multitude of exciting research projects that extend the science and improve health-care quality and health outcomes. Research opportunities to prevent and solve the major morbidities affecting the nation's health and health-care system, as previously described, abound. Although many people tend to think that nurses primarily focus their research on nurses and nursing care (Anderson, 2011), the truth is that nurses conduct clinical research in real-world practice settings and biomedical research in laboratories in a variety of areas, including cancer, diabetes, palliative care, child health, aging, and wellness.

Since the majority of studies conducted by nurses are descriptive in nature and do not generate the strongest level of evidence to guide clinical practice (Melnyk &d Fineout-Overholt, 2014), there is an urgent need for more nurse researchers to conduct experimental research that develops and tests the effects of interventions designed to improve the quality of healthcare and patient outcomes (Melnyk & Morrison-Beedy, 2012). Comparative effectiveness trials, a type of experimental research that tests the efficacy of one intervention versus another intervention, is especially needed. In addition, more translational research is necessary. Translational research determines how best to take research findings and move them more rapidly into clinical practice settings to ultimately improve patient outcomes. It is also important for nurses to collaborate with scientists from other fields (e.g., medicine, microbiology, pharmacy, public health) when conducting research, as various viewpoints and expertise bring strength to projects.

Finally, nurse researchers must remember that dissemination of research through publications alone is often not sufficient to ensure that the findings are adopted in practice. It is critical that Ph.D.- and DNP-prepared nurses form close collaborations with each other, as well as with other disciplines and policy makers, so that the findings generated from research move quickly to real-world practice settings to ultimately improve health systems and enhance health outcomes in the nation's people.

References

American Association of Colleges of Nursing. (2004). *AACN Position Statement on the Practice Doctorate in Nursing.* Retrieved from www.aacn.nche.edu/dnp/position-statement.

American Association of Colleges of Nursing. (2006). *The Essentials of Doctoral Education for Advanced Nursing Practice.* Retrieved from http://www.aacn.nche.edu/publications/position/DNPEssentials.pdf.

American Association of Colleges of Nursing. *DNP Fact Sheet* (2014a). Retrieved from http://www.aacn.nche.edu/media-relations/fact-sheets/dnp.

American Association of Colleges of Nursing. *Nursing Faculty Shortage* (2014b). Retrieved from http://www.aacn.nche.edu/media-relations/fact-sheets/nursing-faculty-shortage.

American Hospital Association. *TrendWatch Chartbook 2007: Trends Affecting Hospitals and Health Systems.* Retrieved from http://www.aha.org/aha/trendwatch/chartbook/2007/07chapter4.ppt#10.

Anderson, C. A. The Nurse Ph.D.: A Vital Profession Needs Leaders. Association of American Colleges of Nursing. *Peterson's Nursing Programs 2011,* pp. 22–23. Lawrenceville, NJ: Peterson's, 2010.

Boyle, J. P., et al. Projection of the year 2050 burden of diabetes in the US adult population: dynamic modeling of incidence, mortality, and prediabetes prevalence. *Population Health Metrics,* 8(29): 2010. doi: 10.1186/1478-7954-8-29.

Carter, A. Innovation and experimentation in chronic care management will drive enduring healthcare reform. *Home Healthcare Nurse,* 28(8): 508–9, 2010. doi: 10.1097/NHH.0b013e3181ed759d.

Chernew, M. E., K. Baicker, and J. Hsu. The Specter of Financial Armageddon—Health Care and Federal Debt in the United States. *New England Journal of Medicine,* 362(13): 1166–68, 2010.

Cleary, M., G. E. Hunt, and D. Jackson. Demystifying PhDs: A review of doctorate programs designed to fulfil the needs of the next generation of nursing professionals. *Contemporary Nurse: A Journal for the Australian Nursing Profession,* 39(2): 273–80, 2011.

Edwardson, S. R. Doctor of Philosophy and Doctor of Nursing Practice as Complementary Degrees. *Journal of Professional Nursing,* 26(3): 137–40, 2010.

IOM (Institute of Medicine). *The Future of Nursing: Leading Change, Advancing Health.* Washington, DC: The National Academies Press, 2011.

Megginson, L. Exploration of nursing doctoral admissions and performance outcomes. *The Journal of Nursing Education,* 50(9): 502–12, 2011.

Melnyk, B. M. *Evidence-Based Practice in Nursing & Healthcare. A Guide to Best Practice* (2nd edition). Philadelphia: Wolters Kluwer/Lippincott, Williams & Wilkins, 2011.

Melnyk, B. M., et al. US Preventive Services Task Force. USPSTF perspective on evidence-based preventive recommendations for children. *Pediatrics,* 130(2): 399–407, 2012.

Melnyk, B. M., and E. Fineout-Overholt. *Evidence-Based Practice in Nursing & Healthcare: A Guide to Best Practice.* Philadelphia: Wolters Kluwer/Lippincott Williams & Wilkins, 2012.

Melnyk, B. M., and D. Morrison-Beedy. *Designing, Conducting, Analyzing and Funding Intervention Research. A Practical Guide for Success.* New York, NY: Springer Publishing Company, 2012.

Melnyk, B. M. Distinguishing the preparation and roles of the PhD and DNP graduate: National implications for academic curricula and healthcare systems. *Journal of Nursing Education,* 52(8): 442–48, 2013.

National Institute of Mental Health. *The numbers count: mental disorders in America.* Retrieved from http://www.nimh.nih.gov/health/publications/the-numbers-count-mentaldisorders-in-america/index.shtml.

Nickitas, D. M., and V. Feeg. Doubling the number of nurses with a doctorate by 2020: Predicting the right number or getting it right? *Nursing Economics,* 29(3): 109–11, 2011.

Stewart, S. T., D. M. Cutler, and A. B. Rosen. Forecasting the effects of obesity and smoking on U.S. life expectancy. *The New England Journal of Medicine, 361*(23) 2252–60, 2009.

AACN Indicators of Quality in Research-Focused Doctoral Programs in Nursing

Schools of nursing must consider the indicators of quality in evaluating their ability to mount research-focused doctoral programs. High-quality programs require a large number of increasingly scarce resources and a critical mass of faculty members and students. The "AACN Indicators of Quality in Research-Focused Doctoral Programs in Nursing" represent those indicators that should be present in a research-focused program.

There is considerable consensus within the discipline that while there are differences in the purpose and curricula of Ph.D. and Doctor of Nursing/Doctor of Nursing Science programs; most programs emphasize preparation for research. Therefore, AACN recommends continuing with a single set of quality indicators for research-focused doctoral programs in nursing, whether the program leads to a Ph.D. or to a Doctor of Nursing or Doctor of Nursing Science degree.

The following indicators apply to the Doctor of Philosophy (Ph.D.) in nursing, Doctor of Nursing Science (D.N.S. or D.N.Sc.), and Doctor of Nursing (N.D.) degrees.

Faculty

I.   Represent and value a diversity of backgrounds and intellectual perspectives.

II. Meet the requirements of the parent institution for graduate research and doctoral education; a substantial proportion of faculty hold earned doctorates in nursing.

III. Conceptualize and implement productive programs of research and scholarship that are developed over time and build upon previous work, are at the cutting edge of the field of inquiry, are congruent with research priorities within nursing and its constituent communities, include a substantial proportion of extramural funding, and attract and engage students.

IV. Create an environment in which mentoring, socialization of students, and the existence of a community of scholars is evident.

V.   Assist students in understanding the value of programs of research and scholarship that continue over time and build upon previous work.

VI. Identify, generate, and utilize resources within the university and the broader community to support program goals.

VII. Devote a significant proportion of time to dissertation advisement. Generally, each faculty member should serve as the major adviser/chair for no more than 3 to 5 students during the dissertation phase.

Programs of Study

The emphasis of the program of study is consistent with the mission of the parent institution, the discipline of nursing, and the degree awarded. The faculty's areas of expertise and scholarship determine specific foci in the program of study. Requirements and their sequence for progression in the program are clear and available to students in writing. Common elements of the program of study are outlined below.

I.   Core and related course content—the distribution between nursing and supporting content is consistent with the mission and goals of the program, and the student's area of focus and course work are included in the following:

   A. Historical and philosophical foundations to the development of nursing knowledge

   B. Existing and evolving substantive nursing knowledge

   C. Methods and processes of theory/knowledge development

   D. Research methods and scholarship appropriate to inquiry

   E. Development related to roles in academic, research, practice, or policy environments

II. Elements for formal and informal teaching and learning focus on the following:

   A. Analytical and leadership strategies for dealing with social, ethical, cultural, economic, and political issues related to nursing, health care, and research

   B. Progressive and guided student scholarship

research experiences, including exposure to faculty's interdisciplinary research programs

C. Immersion experiences that foster the student's development as a nursing leader, scholarly practitioner, educator, and/or nurse scientist

D. Socialization opportunities for scholarly development in roles that complement students' career goals

III. Outcome indicators for the programs of study include the following:

A. Advancement to candidacy requires faculty's satisfactory evaluation (e.g., comprehensive exam) of the student's basic knowledge of elements I-A through I-E identified above

B. Dissertations represent original contributions to the scholarship of the field

C. Systematic evaluation of graduate outcomes is conducted at regular intervals

D. Within three to five years of completion, graduates have designed and secured funding for a research study, or, within two years of completion, graduates have utilized the research process to address an issue of importance to the discipline of nursing or health care within their employment setting

E. Employers report satisfaction with graduates' leadership and scholarship at regular intervals

F. Graduates' scholarship and leadership are recognized through awards, honors, or external funding within three to five years of completion

Resources

I. Sufficient human, financial, and institutional resources are available to accomplish the goals of the unit for doctoral education and faculty research.

A. The parent institution exhibits the following characteristics:

1) Research is an explicit component of the mission of the parent institution

2) An office of research administration

3) A record of peer-reviewed external funding

4) Postdoctoral programs

5) Internal research funds

6) Mechanisms that value, support, and reward faculty and student scholarship and role preparation

7) A university environment that fosters interdisciplinary research and collaboration

B. The nursing doctoral program exhibits the following characteristics:

1) Research-active faculty as well as other faculty experts to mentor students in other role preparations

2) Provide technical support for the following:

(a) Peer review of proposals and manuscripts in their development phases

(b) Research design expertise

(c) Data management and analysis support

(d) Hardware and software availability

(e) Expertise in grant proposal development and management

3) Procure space sufficient for the following:

(a) Faculty research needs

(b) Doctoral student study, meeting, and socializing

(c) Seminars

(d) Small-group work

C. Schools of exceptional quality also have the following:

1) Centers of research excellence

2) Endowed professorships

3) Mechanisms for financial support to allow full-time study

4) Master teachers capable of preparing graduates for faculty roles

II. State-of-the-art technical and support services are available and accessible to faculty, students, and staff for state-of-the-science information acquisition, communication, and management.

III. Library and database resources are sufficient to support the scholarly endeavors of faculty and students.

Students

I. Students are selected from a pool of highly qualified and motivated applicants who represent diverse populations.

II. Students' research goals and objectives are congruent with faculty research expertise and scholarship and institutional resources.

III. Students are successful in obtaining financial support through competitive intramural and extramural academic and research awards.

IV. Students commit a significant portion of their time to the program and complete the program in a timely fashion.

V. Students establish a pattern of productive scholarship, collaborating with researchers in nursing and other disciplines in scientific endeavors that result in the presentation and publication of scholarly work that continues after graduation.

Evaluation

The evaluation plan includes the following:

I. Is systematic, ongoing, comprehensive, and focuses on the university's and program's specific mission and goals.

II. Includes both process and outcome data related to these indicators of quality in research-focused doctoral programs.

III. Adheres to established ethical and process standards for formal program evaluation, e.g., confidentiality and rigorous quantitative and qualitative analyses.

IV. Involves students and graduates in evaluation activities.

V. Includes data from a variety of internal and external constituencies.

VI. Provides for comparison of program processes and outcomes to the standards of its parent graduate school/ university and selected peer groups within nursing.

VII. Includes ongoing feedback to program faculty, administrators, and external constituents to promote program improvement.

VIII. Provides comprehensive data in order to determine patterns and trends and recommend future directions at regular intervals.

IX. Is supported with adequate human, financial, and institutional resources.

Approved by AACN Membership, November 2001.

WHAT YOU NEED TO KNOW ABOUT ONLINE LEARNING

Sally Kennedy Ph.D., APRN, FNP-C, CNE
Assistant Professor
College of Nursing
Medical University of South Carolina

Today's college students are more diverse than at any time in recent history. Potentially three generations, all with varied life experiences that shaped them, can be found in the classroom. The youngest baby boomers turned 50 in 2014, and their motivation for returning to school ranges from seeking a second career or returning for a graduate degree to finally having the time and money to enter college after having put their own children through school. Realizing the dangers of overgeneralizing, this group may not be particularly tech savvy and may prefer to learn via lecture and taking notes. They are highly motivated and independent thinkers. The GenXers—now between 33 and 50 years of age—may want to be taught only what is necessary to learn a new career, and they consider leisure time as important as school. For them, school is often a means to a career that will support their lifestyles. Millennials, on the other hand, grew up with technology, the Internet, and immediate access to information. They prefer to multi-task. Raised by doting or "helicopter" parents as they are commonly referred to, this generation expects immediate feedback and prefers to work within groups, most likely the result of close family ties.

Because the learning needs of these generations are quite diverse, the classroom experience is much different than in previous generations. The baby boomers may have difficulty with younger students reviewing their Facebook pages, sending e-mails, or chatting during class instead of attending to the instructor or the material. The younger generations may be bored with lectures, want to cut to the chase, and prefer in-class group activities to help them learn the content. The generational differences and many other variables should be considered when deciding whether the classroom experience or an online program is the best choice. Let's explore online education in more depth.

Understanding the Basics

First consider what is meant by **online learning** versus **distance education** as colleges and universities may define them differently. "Distance education" may mean meeting in a classroom with other students to watch a live video feed of a professor lecturing from a remote location. Or, "distance education" may be synonymous with online education. Online education, or e-learning, refers to an online virtual classroom accessed from the Internet that uses a learning management system (LMS), such as Moodle, Blackboard, or Desire2Learn as the platform.

Online education can be delivered synchronously or asynchronously in a fully online or hybrid format—four different variables. **Synchronous delivery** means that students must be online at a specific time to meet with the instructor and classmates. Similar to a classroom-based course, this format removes the flexibility online education typically provides. **Asynchronous course delivery** means "not occurring at the same time." Even if the program is marketed as asynchronous, synchronous meetings could still be required, which will limit flexibility and thus negating a major benefit of online education.

Some programs marketed as online may really be **hybrid**. This means that some of the learning occurs online, but face-to-face meetings are also required. A course delivered **fully online** requires no synchronous meetings, or if they are held, attendance may be optional. Understanding how a school defines "online education" is essential.

The Online Learning Experience

So what is an online class like? Content is typically delivered through reading assignments, posted PowerPoint slides, podcasts (audio recordings), or YouTube videos. Some faculty members will record their lectures on video. However, the actual learning usually takes place in **small group discussions** within the learning management system. Students post their responses to a discussion question posed by the instructor that will help explore the content of the lesson. The assumption is that students will be self-directed and review the materials independently before responding. This approach provides opportunities to learn from both classmates and faculty.

Expectations for the **frequency of participation** in weekly discussions will vary. Some schools prescribe the number of days students must post each week. It is important to understand the expectations of being online and involved in class discussions. Dedicating a few hours, three to five days each week to being online reviewing classmates' posts and then researching and writing a response may be more time on the computer than anticipated.

While **assignments** can vary in online courses, a group project may be required—sometimes in every class. Group projects entail frequent communication, often synchronously, and may entail face-to-face meetings. This removes some of the flexibility of taking classes online. Depending on the group members' comfort with technology, various real-time options are available, such as chat rooms or Skype. Text-based, real-time applications (e.g., GoogleDocs or Wikis) allow students to collaborate on a document and see each other's contribution immediately.

Students who prefer to work independently may find this requirement challenging, especially if **group grades** are given. This means that each student in the group will earn the same grade regardless of how the workload was divided. The flip side of group work is that team-building skills are learned, which will be valuable in the job market. Inquiring about requirements of group work will avoid surprises.

Expectations of **faculty feedback** should be considered. While every student in an online course is required to participate in online discussions, frequent feedback from faculty may not be forthcoming. Faculty may reply to a few posts in each discussion, but not all. Students, on the other hand, will be required to respond to classmates. Students bring a wealth of life experiences to online discussions. Being open to learning from peers may seem foreign, but it can be an enriching experience.

Making the Decision

Before making the decision, students should consider their educational goals as well as personal preferences, such as preferred learning style, learner characteristics, family support, comfort with technology, and a reliable Internet connection.

Understanding **educational goals** and deciding what is important is a first step. If the full college campus experience including attending football games, meeting new people in the student union, and having direct contact with faculty in a classroom setting is desired, online education may not be the best choice. However, if the flexibility of studying "anytime and anywhere" there is an Internet connection is appealing, then earning a degree online can be a viable option. Many adults have other considerations such as family obligations, a full-time job, or the distance to travel to find the right program of study. These variables can make on-campus classroom attendance at the same time each week problematic.

People also have a preferred **learning style,** and it can be visual, auditory, hands-on, or interpersonal. While students can learn from other methods, they typically prefer one over the others. Visual learners prefer pictures and diagrams. Auditory learners prefer to listen to lectures or recordings. Others are hands-on and like to be actively involved doing a task, while others prefer to learn in groups.

Many learning style inventories are available online to determine one's preferred learning style. Googling "learning style inventory" will bring up multiple options. Keep in mind that online education is primarily text-based, so consideration should be given to spending hours reading on the computer. However, more and more faculty members are using technology in their online courses, creating YouTube videos or audio recordings, called podcasts, which can be listened to online or downloaded into an MP3 player. Instructors realize the importance of providing a variety of methods to engage students with various learning style preferences.

Think about the **ideal individual characteristics of online learners.** Students must be motivated to reach their educational goals and be self-directed, organized, and able to meet deadlines. Being committed to completing a degree and having the motivation to do so are key factors in pursuing higher education, regardless of the setting. However, these attributes are essential for taking classes online. Having **support** from family or loved ones is also ideal. Because schoolwork is often done from home, having a dedicated room or space and an atmosphere conducive to studying is essential.

Intimidated by **technology**? Being somewhat familiar with how to use the computer is necessary. How much? When pursuing a college degree, it is important that you are able to focus on your studies and not spend a great deal of time learning technology. Being able to send an e-mail with an attachment and use a word processing program, such as Microsoft Word, is essential. Inquiring about the necessity of using other types of software, such PowerPoint or Excel, is a good idea. Often schools provide support to help students learn program-specific software. Knowing up front what type of software is required and if learning support is available may provide peace of mind.

On the flip side, many students who grew up with technology may have a different set of questions. Knowing whether the learning management system is accessible on an iPad or a smartphone may be a concern. Having an alternate means of accessing the learning management system from work during a lunch break, for example, where the company's firewall may block certain Internet sites may be desired to maximize study time.

A fast and reliable **Internet connection** is a necessity. Dial-up connections (linked to a telephone line) may have download capabilities too slow for today's online courses. With slower connections, the video is often downloaded in pieces resulting in an interrupted feed when listening to a podcast or watching a YouTube Video. Although widespread Internet access exists in most metropolitan areas linked directly via cable, this may not the case in more rural communities.

In addition, many popular gathering places, such as coffee shops and some fast-food restaurant chains provide "hotspots" or free wireless (Wi-Fi) connection. This leads to another consideration for taking classes online, that of having a "Plan B" in place in case problems with the home Internet connection occur.

Finally, consider the cost of online education. Inquire about how tuition is charged—by the course or by the program. Some schools charge an extra fee to take a course online. Ask if financial aide covers this additional fee. Also, having up-to-date hardware including a computer and printer is important. Older computers may not have the processing speed or most current software to access the learning management system or complete assignments effectively and efficiently. Will this be an added cost? Additional technology requirements may be added by the particular program of study, such as a video camera, webcam, headset, or software such as the entire Microsoft Office Suite. Unexpected costs such as these can add up.

In summary, online education offers many advantages. It is flexible, accessible, creates opportunities for great student interaction, helps build team-based skills, provides immediate access to materials, fosters the development of needed technology skills for life, and decreases time and access barriers to achieving educational goals. The disadvantages are best viewed from an individual standpoint. Hopefully, what has been discussed here will assist students in making an informed decision about seeking a higher education online.

THE INTERNATIONAL NURSING STUDENT

For many international students completing baccalaureate, master's, or doctoral nursing programs, their choice of learning institutions is obvious. U.S. and Canadian colleges and universities are thought to offer the finest programs of nursing education available anywhere in the world. U.S. and Canadian nursing programs are renowned for their breadth and flexibility, for the excellence of their basic curriculum structure, and for their commitment to extensive on-site clinical training. Nursing study in the United States and Canada also affords students the opportunity for hands-on learning and practice in the world's most technologically advanced health-care systems. For many international nursing students, and especially for students from countries that are medically underserved, these features make U.S. and Canadian nursing programs unsurpassed.

Applying to Nursing School

The application process for international students often involves the completion of two separate written applications. Many colleges screen international candidates with a brief preliminary application requesting basic biographical and educational information. This document helps the admission officer determine whether the student has the minimum credentials for admission before requiring him or her to begin the lengthy process of completing and submitting final application forms.

Final applications to U.S. and Canadian colleges and universities vary widely in length and complexity, just as specific admission requirements vary from institution to institution. However, international nursing students must typically have a satisfactory scholastic record and demonstrated proficiency in English. To be admitted to any postsecondary institution in the United States or Canada, you must have satisfactorily completed a minimum of twelve years of elementary and secondary education. The customary cycle for this education includes a six-year elementary program, a three-year intermediate program, and a three-year postsecondary program, generally referred to as high school in the United States. In addition, nursing school programs generally require successful completion of several years of high school-level mathematics and science.

The documentation of satisfactory completion of secondary schooling (and university education, in the case of graduate-level applicants) is achieved through submission of school reports, transcripts, and teacher recommendations. Because academic records and systems of evaluation differ widely from one educational system to the next, request that your school include a guide to grading standards. If you have received your secondary education at a school in which English is not the language of instruction, be certain to include official translations of all documents.

International students who have completed some university-level course work in their native country may be eligible to receive credit for equivalent courses at the U.S. or Canadian institution in which they enroll. Under special circumstances, practical nursing experience may also qualify for university credit. Policies regarding the transfer of or qualification for credits based on education or nursing experience outside the United States (or Canada for Canadian schools) vary widely, so be certain to inquire about these policies at the universities or colleges that interest you.

Language skills are a key to scholastic success. "The ability to speak, write, and understand English is an important determinant of success," says Joann Weiss, former Director of the Nursing and Latin American Studies dual-degree programs at the University of New Mexico in Albuquerque. Her advice for potential international applicants is simple: "Develop a true command of written and spoken English." English proficiency for students who have not received formal education in English-speaking schools is usually demonstrated via the Test of English as a Foreign Language (TOEFL®); minimum test scores of 550 to 580 are commonly required. This policy, as well as the level of proficiency required, varies from school to school, so be sure to investigate each college's policies.

In addition, most universities offer some form of English language instruction for international students, often under the rubric ESL (English as a second language). Students who require additional language study to meet admission requirements or students who wish to deepen their skills in written or verbal English should inquire about ESL program availability.

Many colleges and universities also require that all undergraduate applicants take a standardized test—either the SAT® and three SAT Subject Tests™ or the ACT®. Like their U.S. and Canadian counterparts, international applicants to graduate-level nursing programs are required by most institutions to take the standardized Graduate Record Examinations (GRE®).

Applicants should also be aware that financial assistance for international students is usually quite limited. To spare international students economic hardship during their schooling in the United States or Canada, many colleges and universities require them to demonstrate the availability of sufficient financial resources for tuition and minimum living expenses and supplies. As with so many admission requirements, policies regarding financial aid vary considerably; find out early what the policies are at the colleges that interest you.

Attending School in the United States or Canada

Once you are accepted by the college or university of your choice, take full advantage of the academic and personal advising systems offered to international students. Most institutions of higher education in the United States and Canada maintain an international student advisory office staffed with trained counselors. In addition to general academic counseling and planning, an international adviser can assist in a broad range of matters ranging from immigration and visa concerns to employment opportunities and health-care issues.

With few exceptions, all university students also obtain specialized academic counseling from an assigned faculty adviser. Faculty advisers monitor academic performance and progress and try to ensure that students meet the institutional requirements for their degree. Faculty advisers are excellent sources of information regarding course selection, and some advisers offer tutorials or special language or educational support to international students.

Although all university students face academic challenges, international students often find life outside the classroom equally demanding. Suddenly introduced into a new culture where the way of life may be dramatically different from that of their native country, international students often face a variety of social, domestic, medical, religious, or emotional concerns. Questions about social conventions, meal preparation, or other personal concerns can often be addressed by your international or faculty adviser.

Lorraine Rudowski, Assistant Professor and Coordinator of the International Health Program at the College of Health and Human Services at George Mason University in Fairfax, Virginia, emphasizes the benefits of a strong relationship with your advisers: "My job as an adviser is to provide comprehensive support to my students—from academic counseling and opportunities for language development to emotional support and guidance to attending parties or other informal social events to ease the sense of social and personal isolation often experienced by foreign students."

Dr. Rudowski says that international students would do well to find a sponsor or confidant within the university who understands the conventions of the student's native country. "A culturally sensitive sponsor is better equipped to understand the unique needs of each international student and is much more likely to help students obtain the assistance they need, whether we're talking about religious issues, help with study methods or social skills, or simply knowing how to deal with such everyday chores as cooking and cleaning. All of these matters can be sources of deep concern to international students."

Yet for all the academic, social, and personal challenges facing international nursing students, there is good news. Deans of nursing, professors, and advisers typically praise the motivation and determination of their international students, and international nursing students often boast matriculation rates that match or exceed those of their U.S. and Canadian counterparts.

For more information about the rules and regulations governing international students' entrance to U.S. schools, log on to educationUSA, part of the U.S. Department of State's website, at http://educationusa.state.gov.

SPECIALTY NURSING ORGANIZATIONS

Academy of Medical-Surgical Nurses
East Holly Avenue
Box 56
Pitman, NJ 08071-0056
866-877-AMSN (2676) (toll-free)
E-mail: amsn@ajj.com
www.amsn.org

Air & Surface Transport Nurses Association
13918 E. Mississippi Avenue
Suite 215
Aurora, CO 80012
303-344-0457
www.astna.org

American Academy of Ambulatory Care Nursing
East Holly Avenue
Box 56
Pitman, NJ 08071-0056
800-262-6877 (toll-free)
E-mail: aaacn@ajj.com
www.aaacn.org

American Association of Critical-Care Nurses
101 Columbia
Aliso Viejo, CA 92656-4109
949-362-2000
800-899-AACN (2226) (toll-free)
Fax: 949-362-2020
E-mail: info@aacn.org
www.aacn.org

American Association of Diabetes Educators
200 West Madison Street
Suite 800
Chicago, IL 60606
800-338-3633 (toll-free)
Fax: 312-424-2427
E-mail: education@aadenet.org
www.aadenet.org

American Association of Legal Nurse Consultants
330 N. Wabash Avenue
Suite 2000
Chicago, IL 60611
877-402-2562 (toll-free)
Fax: 312-673-6655
E-mail: info@aalnc.org
www.aalnc.org

American Association of Neuroscience Nurses
8735 W. Higgins Road
Suite 300
Chicago, IL 60631
847-375-4733
888-557-2266 (toll-free in the U.S. only)
Fax: 847-375-6430
E-mail: info@aann.org
www.aann.org

American Association of Nurse Anesthetists
222 South Prospect Avenue
Park Ridge, IL 60068-4001
847-692-7050
Fax: 847-692-6968
E-mail: info@aana.com
www.aana.com

The American Association of Nurse Attorneys
3416 Primm Lane
Birmingham, AL 35216
205-824-7615
877-538-2262 (toll-free)
Fax: 205-823-2760
E-mail: taana@primemanagement.net
www.taana.org

American Association of Nurse Practitioners (AANP)
AANP National Administrative Office
PO Box 12846
Austin, TX 78711
512-442-4262
Fax: 512-442-6469
E-mail: admin@aanp.org
www.aanp.org/about-aanp

American Association of Occupational Health Nurses
7794 Grow Drive
Pensacola, FL 32514
850-474-6963
800-241-8014 (toll-free)
Fax: 850-484-8762
E-mail: aaohn@dancyamc.com
www.aaohn.org

American College of Nurse-Midwives
8403 Colesville Road
Suite 1550
Silver Spring, MD 20910
240-485-1800
Fax: 240-485-1818
www.midwife.org

American Holistic Nurses Association
100 SE 9th Street
Suite 3A
Topeka, KS 66612-1213
785-234-1712
800-278-2462 (toll-free)
Fax: 785-234-1713
E-mail: info@ahna.org
www.ahna.org

American Nephrology Nurses' Association
East Holly Avenue
Box 56
Pitman, NJ 08071-0056
856-256-2320
888-600-2662 (toll-free)
Fax: 856-589-7463
E-mail: anna@ajj.com
www.annanurse.org

American Psychiatric Nurses Association
3141 Fairview Park Drive
Suite 625
Falls Church, VA 22042
855-863-APNA (2762; toll-free)
Fax: 855-883-APNA (2762)
www.apna.org

American Public Health Association
800 I Street, NW
Washington, DC 20001-3710
202-777-APHA
Fax: 202-777-2534
E-mail: comments@apha.org
www.apha.org

American Society for Pain Management Nursing
P.O. Box 15473
Lenexa, KS 66285-5473
888-34ASPMN (toll-free)
913-895-4606
Fax: 913-895-4652
E-mail: aspmn@goamp.com
www.aspmn.org

American Society of Ophthalmic Registered Nurses
655 Beach Street
San Francisco, CA 94119-3030
415-561-8513
Fax: 415-561-8531
E-mail: asorn@aao.org
www.asorn.org

American Society of PeriAnesthesia Nurses
90 Frontage Road
Cherry Hill, NJ 08034-1424
877-737-9696 (toll-free)
Fax: 856-616-9601
E-mail: aspan@aspan.org
www.aspan.org

American Society of Plastic Surgical Nurses
500 Cummings Center
Suite 4550
Beverly, MA 01915
877-337-9315 (toll-free)
Fax: 978-524-8890
www.aspsn.org

Association for Death Education and Counseling®
111 Deer Lake Road
Suite 100
Deerfield, IL 60015
847-509-0403
Fax: 847-480-9282
www.adec.org

Association for Professionals in Infection Control and Epidemiology
1275 K Street, NW
Suite 1000
Washington, DC 20005-4006
202-789-1890
800-650-9570 (toll-free)
Fax: 202-789-1899
E-mail: info@apic.org
www.apic.org

Association for Radiologic & Imaging Nursing (ARIN)
2201 Cooperative Way
Suite 600
Herndon, VA 20171
703-884-2229
866-486-2762 (toll-free)
Fax: 703-884-2229
E-mail: info@arinursing.org
www.arinursing.org

Association of Nurses in AIDS Care
3538 Ridgewood Road
Akron, OH 44333-3122
800-260-6780 (toll-free)
330-670-0101
Fax: 330-670-0109
E-mail: anac@anacnet.org
www.anacnet.org

Association of Pediatric Hematology/Oncology Nurses
8735 W. Higgins Road
Suite 300
Chicago, IL 60631
855-202-9760 (toll-free in the U.S. only)
847-375-4724
Fax: 847-375-6478
E-mail: info@aphon.org
www.aphon.org

Association of Perioperative Registered Nurses
2170 South Parker Road
Suite 400
Denver, CO 80231
800-755-2676 (toll-free)
303-755-6300
Fax: 800-847-0045 (toll-free)
E-mail: custsvc@aorn.org
www.aorn.org

Association of Rehabilitation Nurses
8735 W. Higgins Road
Suite 300
Chicago, IL 60631-2738
800-229-7530 (toll-free)
E-mail: info@rehabnurse.org
www.rehabnurse.org

Association of Women's Health, Obstetric and Neonatal Nurses
2000 L Street, NW
Suite 740
Washington, DC 20036
202-261-2400
800-673-8499 (toll-free in the U.S.)
800-245-0231 (toll-free in Canada)
Fax: 202-728-0575
E-mail: customerservice@awhonn.org
www.awhonn.org

Dermatology Nurses' Association
1120 Route 73
Suite 200
Mount Laurel, NJ 08054
800-454-4362 (toll-free)
Fax: 856-439-0525
E-mail: dna@dnanurse.org
www.dnanurse.org

Developmental Disabilities Nurses Association
1501 South Loop 288
Suite 104 – PMB 381
Denton, TX 76205
800-888-6733 (toll-free)
Fax: 844-336-2329
www.ddna.org

Emergency Nurses Association
915 Lee Street
Des Plaines, IL 60016-6569
800-900-9659 (toll-free)
E-mail: www.ena.org/Pages/ContactUs.aspx
www.ena.org

Hospice and Palliative Nurses Association
One Penn Center West
Suite 425
Pittsburgh, PA 15276-0100
412-787-9301
Fax: 412-787-9305
E-mail: hpna@hpna.org
www.hpna.org

Infusion Nurses Society
315 Norwood Park South
Norwood, MA 02062
781-440-9408
Fax: 781-440-9409
E-mail: ins@ins1.org
www.ins1.org

International Nurses Society on Addictions
3416 Primm Lane
Birmingham, Alabama 35216
205-823-6106
E-mail: ntnsa@primemanagement.net
www.intnsa.org

National Association for Home Care & Hospice
228 Seventh Street, SE
Washington, DC 20003
202-547-7424
Fax: 202-547-3540
E-mail: exec@nahc.org
www.nahc.org

National Association of Clinical Nurse Specialists
100 North 20th Street
4th Floor
Philadelphia, PA 19103
215-320-3881
Fax: 215-564-2175
E-mail: info@nacns.org
www.nacns.org

National Association of Directors of Nursing Administration/Long Term Care
11353 Reed Hartman Highway
Suite 210
Cincinnati, OH 45241
800-222-0539 (toll-free)
513-791-3679
Fax: 513-791-3699
www.nadona.org

National Association of Neonatal Nurses
8735 W. Higgins Road
Suite 300
Chicago, IL 60631
847-375-3660
800-451-3795 (toll-free)
Fax: 866-927-5321
E-mail: info@nann.org
www.nann.org

National Association of Nurse Practitioners in Women's Health
505 C Street, NE
Washington, DC 20002
202-543-9693, Ext. 1
E-mail: info@npwh.org
www.npwh.org

National Association of Orthopaedic Nurses
330 N. Wabash Avenue
Suite 2000
Chicago, IL 60611
800-289-NAON (6266) (toll-free)
Fax: 312-673-6941
E-mail: naon@orthonurse.org
www.orthonurse.org

National Association of Pediatric Nurse Practitioners
5 Hanover Square
Suite 1401
New York, NY 10004
917-746-8300
Fax: 212-785-1713
E-mail: info@napnap.org
www.napnap.org

National Association of School Nurses
1100 Wayne Avenue #925
Silver Spring, MD 20910
240-821-1130
E-mail: nasn@nasn.org
www.nasn.org

National Gerontological Nursing Association
3493 Lansdowne Drive
Suite 2
Lexington, KY 40517
800-723-0560 (toll-free)
859-977-7453
Fax: 859-271-0607
E-mail: info@ngna.org
www.ngna.org

National Organization of Nurse Practitioner Faculties
1615 M Street, NW
Suite 270
Washington, DC 20036
202-289-8044
Fax: 202-289-8046
E-mail: nonpf@nonpf.org
www.nonpf.com

Oncology Nursing Society
125 Enterprise Drive
Pittsburgh, PA 15275
866-257-4ONS (4667) (toll-free)
412-859-6100
Fax: 877-369-5497 (toll-free)
E-mail: help@ons.org
www.ons.org

Preventive Cardiovascular Nurses Association
613 Williamson Street
Suite 200
Madison, WI 53703
608-250-2440
E-mail: info@pcna.net
www.pcna.net

Respiratory Nursing Society
Wendy Moore, RN, BSN, N.E.-B.C., President
427 4th Way SE
Dover, MN 44929
E-mail: volkman.tammie@mayo.edu
www.respiratorynursingsociety.org

Society for Vascular Nursing
N83 W13410 Leon Road
Menomonee Falls, WI 53051
Phone: 414-376-0001
Fax: 414-359-1671
E-mail: info@svnnet.org
www.svnnet.org

Society of Gastroenterology Nurses and Associates, Inc.
330 N. Wabash Avenue
Suite 2000
Chicago, IL 60611-7621
800-245-7462 (toll-free)
312-321-5165 (in Illinois)
Fax: 312-673-6694
E-mail: sgna@smithbucklin.com
www.sgna.org

Society of Otorhinolaryngology and Head-Neck Nurses
207 Downing Street
New Smyrna Beach, FL 32168
386-428-1695
Fax: 386-423-7566
E-mail: info@sohnnurse.com
www.sohnnurse.com

Society of Urologic Nurses and Associates
East Holly Avenue
Box 56
Pitman, NJ 08071-0056
888-827-7862 (toll-free)
E-mail: suna@ajj.com
www.suna.org

Wound, Ostomy and Continence Nurses Society™
1120 Rt. 73
Suite 200
Mt. Laurel, NJ 08054
888-224-WOCN (9626) (toll-free)
Fax: 856-439-0525
E-mail: wocn_info@wocn.org
www.wocn.org

PAYING FOR YOUR NURSING EDUCATION

Whether you are considering a baccalaureate degree in nursing or have completed your undergraduate education and are planning to attend graduate school, finding a way to pay for that education is essential.

The cost to attend college is considerable and is increasing each year at a rate faster than most other products and services. In fact, the cost of a nursing education at a public four-year college can be more than $18,000 per year, including tuition, fees, books, room and board, transportation, and miscellaneous expenses. The cost at a private college or university, at either the graduate or undergraduate level, can be more than $40,000 per year.

This is where financial aid comes in. Financial aid is money made available by the government and other sources to help students who otherwise would be unable to attend college. In 2014-15, $238.9 billion in financial aid was distributed to undergraduate and graduate students in the form of grants, Federal Work-Study, federal loans, and federal tax credits and deductions. In addition, students borrowed about $10 billion from private, state, and institutional sources. (College Board, *Trends in Student Aid 2015*). Most college students in this country receive some form of aid, and all prospective students should investigate what may be available. Most of this aid is given to students because neither they nor their families have sufficient personal resources to pay for college. This type of aid is referred to as need-based aid. Recipients of need-based aid include traditional students just out of high school or college and older, nontraditional students who are returning to college or graduate school.

There is also merit-based aid, which is awarded to students who display a particular ability. Merit scholarships are based primarily on academic merit, but may include other special talents. Many colleges and graduate schools offer merit-based aid in addition to need-based aid to their students.

Types and Sources of Financial Aid

There are four types of aid:

1. Scholarships
2. Grants
3. Loans
4. Student employment (including fellowships and assistantships)

Scholarships and grants are outright gifts and do not have to be repaid. Loans are borrowed money that must be repaid with interest, usually after graduation. Student employment provides jobs during the academic year for which students are paid. For graduate students, student employment may include fellowships and assistantships in which students work, receive free or reduced tuition, and may be paid a stipend for living expenses.

Most of the aid available to students is need-based and comes from the federal government through nine financial aid programs. Four of these programs are grant-based and are only available to undergraduate students:

1. Federal Pell Grants
2. Academic Competitive Grants
3. SMART Grants
4. Federal Supplemental Educational Opportunity Grants

Four are loan programs:

1. Federal Perkins Loan
2. Direct Stafford Loans (subsidized and unsubsidized)
3. Federal Direct Graduate PLUS loans
4. Federal Direct PLUS Loans

The final program is a student employment program called the Federal Work-Study Program, which is also awarded to undergraduate and graduate students based on financial need.

The federal government also offers a number of programs especially for nursing students. For example, the U.S. Department of Health and Human Services offers Nursing Student Scholarships, Nursing Student Loans, the Nursing Education Loan Repayment Program, and the Scholarship for Disadvantaged Students (SDS) program. Some of these programs require that the student work in a designated nursing shortage area for a period of time. These programs are administered by the nursing school's financial aid office. For more information, log on to http://bhpr.hrsa.gov/nursing.

The second-largest source of aid is from the colleges and universities themselves. Almost all colleges have aid programs from institutional resources, most of which are grants, scholarships, and fellowships. These can be either need-or merit-based.

A third source of aid is from state governments. Nearly every state provides aid for students attending college in their home state, although most only have programs for undergraduates. Most state aid programs are scholarships and grants, but many states now have low-interest loan and work-study programs. Most state grants and scholarships are not "portable," meaning that they cannot be used outside of your home state of residence.

A fourth source of aid is from private sources such as corporations, hospitals, civic associations, unions, fraternal organizations, foundations, and religious groups that give scholarships, grants, and fellowships to students. Most of these are not based on need, although the amount of the scholarship may vary depending upon financial need. The competition for these scholarships can be formidable, but the rewards are well worth the process. Many companies also offer tuition reimbursement to employees and their dependents. Check with the personnel or human resources department at your or your parents' place of employment for benefit and eligibility information.

Eligibility for Financial Aid

Since most of the financial aid that college students receive is need-based, colleges employ a process called "need analysis" to determine student awards. For most applicants, the student and parents (if the student is a dependent) fill out one form on which family income, assets, and household information are reported. This form is the Free Application for Federal Student Aid (FAFSA). The end result of this need analysis is the student's "Expected Family Contribution," or EFC, representing the amount a family should be able to contribute toward education expenses.

Dependent or Independent

The basic principle of financial aid is that the primary responsibility for paying college expenses resides with the family. In determining your EFC, you will first need to know who makes up your "family." That will tell you whose income is counted when the need analysis is done.

Graduate Students: By definition, all graduate nursing students are considered independent for federal aid purposes. Therefore, only your income and assets (and your spouse's if you are married) count in determining your expected family contribution. (Due to the recent Supreme Court ruling, the use of "marriage" and "spouse" now includes same-sex marriages.)

Undergraduate Students: If you are financially dependent upon your parents, their income and assets, as well as yours, are counted toward the family contribution. If you are financially independent of your parents, only your income (and your spouse's if you are married) counts in the calculation.

According to the U.S. Department of Education, in order to be considered independent for financial aid for 2016–17, you must meet any ONE of the following:

- You were born before January 1, 1992.
- You are or will be enrolled in a master's or doctoral program (beyond a bachelor's degree) during the 2016–17 school year.
- You are married on the day you apply (even if you are separated but not divorced).
- You now have—or will have—children who receive more than half their support from you between July 1, 2016 and June 30, 2017.
- You have dependents (other than your children or spouse) who live with you and who receive more than half of their support from you, now and through June 30, 2017.
- Both your parents are deceased, or you are an orphan, in foster care, or ward of the court (or were a ward of the court until age 18).
- You are engaged in active duty in the U.S. Armed Forces or are a National Guard or Reserves enlistee and are called to active duty for purposes other than training.
- You are a veteran of the U.S. Armed Forces. ("Veteran" includes students who attended a U.S. service academy and who were released under a condition other than dishonorable. Contact your financial aid office for more information.)
- You were verified on or after the start of the award year for which the FAFSA is filed, as either an unaccompanied youth who is homeless or at risk of being homeless and self-supporting.

If you meet any one of these conditions, you are considered independent and only your income and assets (and your spouse's if you are married) count toward your family contribution. Remember, if you are attending school as a graduate student, you are automatically independent for federal aid consideration.

If there are extraordinary circumstances, the financial aid administrator at the college you will be attending has the authority to make a change to your dependency status. You will need to provide extensive documentation of your family situation.

Determining Cost and Need

Now that you know approximately how much you and your family will be expected to contribute toward your college expenses, you can subtract the EFC from the total cost of attending a college or graduate school to determine the amount of need-based financial aid for which you will be eligible. The average cost listed assumes that you will be attending nursing school full-time. If you will be attending part-time, you should adjust costs accordingly. For a more accurate estimate of the cost of attendance at a particular college, check the financial aid information usually available on the college's website or in its publications.

Applying for Financial Aid

After you have subtracted your EFC from the cost of your education and determined your financial need, you will have a better understanding of how much assistance you will need. Even if you do not demonstrate financial need, you are still encouraged to file the FAFSA, as you may be eligible for assistance that is not based on need..

The Free Application for Federal Student Aid or FAFSA (https://fafsa.ed.gov/FAFSA/app/fafsa) is a critical form that anyone seeking college financial aid must complete.

Why You Must File the FAFSA

The FAFSA is required in order for a student to be considered for any type of federal financial aid, including grants and loans.

Federal Financial Aid Programs

Program	Who Benefits?	Maximum/Year
Federal Pell Grants	Undergraduate Students	$5815 / July 1, 2016– June 30, 2017
Federal Supplemental Educational Opportunity Grants (FSEOG)	Undergraduate Students	$4000, depending on financial need
Iraq and Afghanistan Service Grant	Students whose parent or guardian was a member of the U.S. armed forces and died as a result of performing military service in Iraq or Afghanistan after the events of 9/11	$5382.30 / October 1, 2015– October 1, 2016
Federal Perkins Loans	Undergraduate Students	$5500
	Graduate Students	$8000
Federal Direct Loans (subsidized)	Undergraduate Students	$3500 (first-year students) $4500 (second-year students) $5500 (third-year students and above)
	Graduate Students*	$8500
Federal Direct Loans (unsubsidized)	Dependent undergraduate students	$2000
	Independent undergraduate students	$6000 (first- and second-year students) $7000 (third-year students and above)
	Graduate Student Veterinary Students	$20,500 $40,500
Federal Direct PLUS Loans	Graduate and Professional students	Up to cost of attendance (less other financial aid received)
Federal Direct Graduate PLUS Loans	Graduate and Professional students	Up to cost of attendance (less other financial aid received)

Only eligible if period(s) of enrollment began prior to 7/1/2012.

The unsubsidized Federal Direct Loan amounts provided are in addition to the subsidized Federal Direct Loan amounts.

Even if you think your family makes too much for you to qualify for need-based aid, you should still complete the FAFSA. For one thing, you may be surprised to find that you actually qualify for need-based aid—the eligibility for which is determined by a number of factors, in addition to household income.

Also, the FAFSA is required to apply for students loans (for which there is no need-based element such as income limits). If you don't initially think you want to apply for student loans but later change your mind, having a completed FAFSA already on file will help speed up the process.

In addition, most schools will require a student to have a completed FAFSA on file before they can be considered for any school-based aid programs such as scholarships. A completed FAFSA is also required for federal work study jobs.

It's Easier to File Online

While you can opt to print and complete a paper version of the FAFSA, it is much quicker and easier to complete the online version. The system walks you through the process and can alert you to sections you can skip if they don't apply to you.

If you have completed a FAFSA in the past, some of your information will be automatically entered when you start to do the newest one, giving you a head start. You will further save a lot of time by using the IRS data retrieval tool, which will be discussed later in this article.

Filing online means your form will be processed faster, and it also eliminates the worry that your paperwork will be lost or delayed in the mail.

For those who want or need to print and submit a paper version of the FAFSA, you can print a PDF version of the FAFSA online. Students and parents can request up to three copies of the paper FAFSA (in English or Spanish) by calling the Federal Student Aid Information Center toll-free at 800-4-FED-AID.

NEW Federal Student Aid ID

In order for a student to complete the online FAFSA, he or she will need a Federal Student Aid (FSA) ID. You can get this online at https://fsaid.ed.gov/npas/index.htm. Since May 2015, the FSA ID has replaced the PIN system that was previously used. Parents of dependent students also need to obtain their own FSA ID in order to sign their child's FAFSA electronically online.

The FSA ID can be used to access several federal aid-related websites, including FAFSA.gov and StudentLoans.gov. It consists of a username and password and can be used to electronically sign Federal Student Aid documents, access your personal records, and make binding legal obligations. The FSA ID is beneficial in several ways:

- It removes your personal identifiable personally identifiable information (PII), such as your Social Security number, from your log-in credentials.

- It creates a more secure and efficient way to verify your information when you log in to access to your federal student aid information online.

- It gives you the ability to easily update your personal information.

- It allows you to easily retrieve your username and password by requesting a secure code be sent to your e-mail address or by answering challenge questions.

It's relatively simple to create an FSA ID and should only take a few minutes. In addition, you will have an opportunity to link your current Federal Student Aid PIN (if you already have one) to your FSA ID. The final step is to confirm your e-mail address. You will receive a secure code to the e-mail address you provided when you set up your FSA ID. Once you retrieve the code from your e-mail account and enter it—to confirm your e-mail address is valid—you will be able to use this e-mail address instead of your username to log in to any of the federal aid-related websites, making the log-in process EVEN simpler.

When you initially create your FSA ID, your information will need to be verified with the Social Security Administration. This process can take anywhere from one to three days. For that reason, it's a good idea to take care of setting up your FSA ID as early as possible, so it will be all set when you are ready to begin completing your FAFSA.

IMPORTANT NOTE: Since your FSA ID provides access to your personal information and is used to sign online documents, it's imperative that you protect this ID. Don't share it with *anyone* or write it down in an insecure location—you could place yourself at great risk for identify theft.

Information You Will Need

Completing your FAFSA (or updating one you have already started) will be much easier if you have some basic information and documentation handy when you prepare to complete the form. The first section of the FAFSA involves your basic personal information that you should know offhand, such as your name, address, and Social Security number. After that, you will need to provide details about your income, assets, and other financial issues. If you file taxes, much of this information will be taken from your tax return. If you haven't yet completed your taxes for that year, you can enter estimated figures and update the form with the final numbers later.

If you're a student who is married, you will also need to provide information about your spouse and their finances. If you're a dependent student, information about one or both or your parents and their finances will be required.

You will also need to provide information about the school(s) you attend or plan to attend. If you haven't made your final school choices yet, you can list the ones you know at this point and add others later.

Be Mindful of Deadlines

Currently, the FAFSA filing system requires students and parents to complete the federal form as soon as possible after January 1st, usually before they've been able to file the previous year's taxes that are not due until April 15, so students/parents must estimate their income and other data and then update their information later.

The new procedure will begin with those who apply for financial aid for the 2017–18 academic year. You will be able to start the FAFSA in October 2016, using the same data you reported on your 2015 tax returns. The use of older data means families can start the process earlier and won't need to rely on estimates.

For federal aid, the final deadline to submit your FAFSA is June 30 at the end of the school year for which you are applying. So for the 2017–18 school year, the final deadline to submit your FAFSA would be June 30, 2018. However, you would normally want to apply for aid before the start of a semester—and ideally, as far in advance as possible. That's because schools frequently require all of your financial aid to be processed (or at least be in process) before your registration is considered official.

It can sometimes be tricky to keep track of other financial aid deadlines because the deadlines for different types of aid can vary by state and school. Be sure to check with your school—or the schools you are considering attending—to find out their financial aid deadlines so you can get all of your forms submitted in time.

Other Applications

The FAFSA is the required form for applying for federal and most state financial aid programs. Most schools also use the FASFA to determine eligibility for institutional aid; however, some colleges and graduate schools require additional information to determine eligibility for institutional aid. Nearly 300 colleges and scholarship programs employ a form called the CSS/Financial Aid PROFILE® (PROFILE) from the College Board's College Scholarship Service (CSS). While the form is similar to the FAFSA, several additional questions must be answered for colleges that award their own funds. You may file the PROFILE as early as October 1. The PROFILE is filed online at www.collegeboard.org. Select "CSS/PROFILE" under "Pay for College" to get started. You'll need to have all tax forms and other pertinent documents, and you should use a secure browser. The fee for the initial application and one college or program report is $25. Additional reports are $16. Payment may be made via credit or debit card. Fee waivers are granted on an individual basis. For more information, visit https://student.collegeboard.org/css-financial-aid-profile.

Financial Aid Offer

If you qualify for need-based aid, a college will typically offer a combination of different types of assistance— scholarship, grant, loan, and work-study—to meet this need. An offer of aid usually is made after you have been admitted to the college or program. You may accept all or part of the financial aid package. If you will be enrolling part-time (fewer than 12 credits per term), be sure to contact the financial aid office in advance since this may have impact on your overall aid eligibility.

If you are awarded Federal Work-Study Program aid, the amount you are awarded represents your earnings limit for the academic year under the program. In general, schools assume you will earn this money on an hourly basis, so it cannot be used to pay your term bill charges. On most campuses there are many jobs available for students. Not all of these are limited to students in the Federal Work-Study Program. Check with your placement office or financial aid office for more information.

Keep in mind that the student budget used to establish eligibility for financial aid is based on averages. It may not reflect your actual expenses. Student budgets usually reflect most expenses for categories of students (for example, single students living in their parents' home, campus-provided housing, or living in an apartment or house near campus, etc.). But if you have unusual expenses that are not included, you should consult with your school's financial aid office regarding a budget adjustment.

If Your Family or Job Situation Changes

Because a family contribution is based on the previous year's income, many nursing students find they do not qualify for need-based aid (or not enough to pay their full expenses). This is particularly true of older students who were working full-time last year but are no longer doing so or who will not work during the academic year. If this is your situation, you should speak to a counselor in the financial aid office about making an adjustment in your family contribution need analysis. Financial aid administrators may make changes to any of the elements

that go into the need analysis if there are conditions that merit a change. Contact the financial aid office for more information.

Don't Qualify for Need-Based Aid?

If you don't qualify for need-based aid but feel you do not have the resources necessary to pay for college or graduate school, you still have several options available.

First, there is a student loan program for which need is not a consideration. This is the Federal Direct Loan (unsubsidized) program. There is also a non-need-based loan program for parents of dependent students or for graduate or professional students called the Direct PLUS Loan program. If you or your parents are interested in borrowing through one of these programs, you should check with the financial aid office for more information. There are also numerous private or alternative loan sources available. For many students, borrowing to pay for a nursing education can be an excellent investment in one's future. At the same time, be sure that you do not overburden yourself when it comes to paying back the loans. Before you accept a federal student loan, the financial aid office will schedule a counseling session to make certain that you know the terms of the loan and that you understand the ramifications of borrowing. If you can do without, it is often suggested that you postpone student loans until they are absolutely necessary.

For graduate nursing students, Federal Direct PLUS Loans are available to graduate and professional students. Students who are looking into alternative loan programs should be sure to compare any terms and conditions with this federal program. Students can borrow Federal Direct Graduate PLUS loans and alternative loan funds up to the cost of attendance less any other financial aid received.

A second option if you do not qualify for need-based aid is to search for scholarships. Be wary of scholarship search companies that promise to find you scholarships but require you to pay a fee. There are many resources that provide lists of scholarships, including the annually published *Peterson's Scholarships, Grants & Prizes* and *How to Get Money for College,* which are available in libraries, counselors' offices, and bookstores. Non-need scholarships require application forms and are extremely competitive; only a handful of students from thousands of applicants receive awards.

Another option is to work more hours at an existing job or to find a paying position if you do not already have one. The student employment or placement office at your college should be able to help you find a job, either on or off campus. Many colleges have vacancies remaining after they have placed Federal Work-Study Program eligible students in their jobs.

You should always contact the financial aid office at the school you plan to attend for advice concerning sources of college-based and private aid.

Employer-Paid Financial Aid

Robert Atwater is a certified personnel consultant and certified medical staff recruiter and founder of Atwater Consulting in Lilburn, Georgia, a consulting firm for the employment and recruitment of physician assistants, nurse practitioners, certified nurse midwives, nurses, and nursing managers.

Health-care administrators, Atwater says, have coined a phrase to characterize their efforts to meet the growing demand for nurses with better skills and training: "Grow your own."

"Constant training through the course of a nursing career is the only way to keep pace with the technological and medical advances, but it can be a financial burden on the nurse," Atwater says.

That is why many employers now give qualified employees a benefits package that includes a continuing education allowance.

For the employer, this type of benefits package can help to recruit candidates willing to further their careers through edu-cation. Administrators feel it is the best way to build a staff of nurses with up-to-date certifications in all areas.

In a constantly expanding field, nurses should be required to continue and update their education. The nurses get a paid edu-cation, can keep their job, and work flexible hours while they are going to school. Inquiries about these allowances should be made during an interview with the company's human resources department. Additional information can be obtained from the nursing school, local hospitals in the area, or from other health-care professionals. There are many attractive options available because of the nationwide shortage of qualified nurses. Check with a number of potential employers before agreeing to any long-term contract.

SOURCES OF FINANCIAL AID FOR NURSING STUDENTS

The largest proportion of financial aid for college expenses comes from the federal government and is given on the basis of financial need. Beyond this federal need-based aid—which should always be the primary source of financial aid that a prospective student investigates and which is given regardless of one's field of study—a sizable amount of scholarship assistance specifically meant to help students in nursing programs is also available from government agencies, associations, civic or fraternal organizations, and corporations. These sources of aid can be particularly attractive for students who may not be eligible for need-based aid. The following list presents some of the major sources of financial aid specifically for nursing students. Not listed are scholarships that are specific to individual colleges and universities or are limited to residents of a particular place or to individuals who have relatively unusual qualifications. Students seeking financial aid should investigate all appropriate possibilities, including sources not listed here. You can find this information in libraries, bookstores, and guidance offices guides, including two of Peterson's annually updated publications: *Peterson's How to Get Money for College: Go Beyond Federal Aid: Get Money from Your School and State,* for information about undergraduate awards given by the federal government, state governments, and specific colleges, and *Peterson's Scholarships, Grants & Prizes,* for information about awards from private sources.

Air Force Institute of Technology

Award Name: Air Force Active Duty Health Professions Loan Repayment Program
Program Description: Program provides up to $40,000 (2009) to repay qualified educational loans in exchange for active duty service in the U.S. armed forces.
Application Contact:
Air Force Institute of Technology
AFIT/ENEM
2950 P. Street
Bldg. 642
Wright Patterson AFB, OH 45433-7765
800-543-3490, Ext. 3036 (toll-free)
E-mail: enem.adhplrp@afit.edu

Alaska Native Tribal Health Consortium

Award Name: ANTHC Scholarship Program
Program Description: Provides undergraduate and graduate scholarships for Alaska Native/American Indian students pursuing an education in the health-care field. Must be enrolled in a formal education or training program, interested in working in the health-care field, be a permanent Alaska resident, and be enrolled in or descended from a federally recognized tribe.
Application Contact:
Claudia Tiepelman, Associate Trainer
Education, Development & Training Department
Alaska Native Tribal Health Consortium
3900 Ambassador Drive
Suite 101
Anchorage, Alaska 99508
907-729-1301
800-684-8361 (toll-free)
E-mail: learning@anthc.org
http://anthctoday.org/business/int.html

American Association of Colleges of Nursing (AACN)

Award Name: AfterCollege/AACN Scholarship Fund
Program Description: The AfterCollege-AACN Scholarship Fund supports students who are seeking a baccalaureate, master's, or doctoral degree in nursing. Special consideration is given to students in a graduate program with the goal of becoming a nurse educator; students completing an RN-to-B.S.N. or RN-to-M.S.N. program; and those enrolled in an accelerated program.
Application Contact:
American Association of Colleges of Nursing
One Dupont Circle, NW
Suite 530
Washington, DC 20036
202-463-6930
Fax: 202-785-8320
E-mail: scholarships@aftercollege.com
https://www.aftercollege.com/content/article/scholarship-official-rules/

American Association of Critical-Care Nurses

Award Name: AACN Educational Advancement Scholarships
Program Description: Nonrenewable scholarships for AACN members who are RNs currently enrolled in undergraduate or graduate NLNAC-accredited programs. The undergraduate award is for use in the junior or senior year. Minimum 3.0 GPA.
Application Contact:
American Association of Critical-Care Nurses
Scholarships
101 Columbia
Aliso Viejo, CA 92656-4109
800-899-2226 (toll-free)
E-mail: scholarships@aacn.org

American Cancer Society

Award Name: Scholarships in Cancer Nursing

Program Description: Renewable awards for graduate students in nursing pursuing advanced preparation in cancer nursing: research, education, administration, or clinical practice. Must be U.S. citizen.

Application Contact:
American Cancer Society
Extramural Grants Program
250 Williams Street, NW
Atlanta, GA 30303-1002
800-ACS-2345 (toll-free)
Fax: 404-417-5974
E-mail: grants@cancer.org
www.cancer.org

American Holistic Nurses' Association (AHNA)

Award Name: Charlotte McGuire Scholarship Program

Program Description: Open to any licensed nurse or nursing student pursuing holistic education. Experience in holistic health care or alternative health practices is preferred. Must be an AHNA member with a minimum 3.0 GPA.

Application Contact:
Charlotte McGuire Scholarships
American Holistic Nurses' Association
100 SE 9th Street
Suite 3A
Topeka, KS 66612
800-278-2462 Ext. 10 (toll-free)
E-mail: info@ahna.org
www.ahna.org/About-Us/Donate-Sponsor/Charlotte-McGuire-Scholarships

American Indian Graduate Center (AIGC)

Award Name: AIGC Fellowships

Program Description: Graduate fellowships available for American Indian and Alaska Native students from federally recognized U.S. tribes. Applicants must be pursuing a postbaccalaureate graduate or professional degree as a full-time student at an accredited institution in the U.S., demonstrate financial need, and be enrolled in a federally recognized American Indian tribe or Alaska Native group or provide documentation of Indian descent.

Application Contact:
American Indian Graduate Center Fellowships
American Indian Graduate Center
3701 San Mateo, NE
Suite 200
Albuquerque, NM 87110
800-628-1920 (toll-free)
505-881-4584
E-mail: web@aigcs.org
www.aigcs.org/scholarships/graduate-fellowships/

Association of Perioperative Registered Nurses (AORN)

Award Name: AORN Foundation Scholarships

Program Description: Applicant must be an active RN and a member of AORN for twelve consecutive months prior to application. Reapplication for each period is required. For baccalaureate, master's of nursing, or doctoral degree at an accredited institution. Minimum 3.0 GPA required.

Application Contact:
AORN Foundation Scholarship Program
2170 South Parker Road
Suite 400
Denver, CO 80231-5711
800-755-2676 (toll-free)
E-mail: foundation@aorn.org
www.aorn.org/AORNFoundation/Grants

Bethesda Lutheran Communities

Award Name: Nursing Scholastic Achievement Scholarship

Program Description: Award for college nursing students with a minimum 3.0 GPA who are Lutheran and have completed their sophomore year of a four-year nursing program or one year of a two-year program. Must be interested in working with people with developmental disabilities.

Application Contact:
Chris Dovnik, Program Coordinator
Bethesda Lutheran Communities
600 Hoffmann Drive
Watertown, WI 53094
800-383-8743, Ext. 4428 (toll-free)
E-mail: chris.dovnik@mailblc.org
http://bethesdalutherancommunities.org/scholarships

Foundation of the National Student Nurses' Association, Inc.

Award Names: Scholarship Program

Program Description: One-time awards available to nursing students in various educational situations: enrolled in programs leading to an RN license, RNs enrolled in programs leading to a bachelor's or master's degree in nursing, enrolled in a state approved school in a specialty area of nursing, and minority students enrolled in nursing or prenursing programs. High school students are not eligible. Funds for graduate study are available only for a first degree in nursing. Based on financial need, academic ability, and health-related nursing and community activities. Application fee of $10. Send self-addressed stamped envelope with two stamps along with application request.

Application Contact:
Scholarship Chairperson
Foundation of the National Student Nurses' Association, Inc.
45 Main Street
Suite 606
Brooklyn, NY 11201
718-210-0705
E-mail: nsna@nsna.org
www.nsna.org/FoundationScholarships/FNSNASchlarships.aspx

Heart and Stroke Foundation of Canada

Award Name: Nursing Research Fellowships

Program Description: In-training awards for study in an area of cardiovascular or cerebrovascular nursing. Award is directed toward preparing nurses who have completed their doctoral degree and who intend to undertake independent research programs. For master's degree candidates, the programs must include a thesis or project requirement.

Application Contact:
Heart and Stroke Foundation of Canada
1402-222 Queen Street, Suite 1402
Ottawa, Ontario K1P-5V9
Canada
613-691-4047
E-mail: research@hsf.ca
www.hsf.ca/research/en/grants-aid

International Order of the King's Daughters and Sons, Inc.

Award Name: International Order of King's Daughters and Sons Health Careers Scholarships
Program Description: For study in the health fields. B.A./B.S. students are eligible in junior year. Application must be for at least third year of college. RN students must have completed first year of schooling. Send #10 self-addressed stamped envelope for application and information.
Application Contact: Director
Health Careers Scholarship Department
P.O. Box 1040
Chautauqua, NY 14722
716-357-4951
E-mail: healthcareersdirector.kds@gmail.com
www.iokds.org/index.php/scholarship/health-career-scholarships

March of Dimes

Award Name: Graduate Scholarships
Program Description: Scholarships for registered nurses enrolled in graduate programs in maternal-child nursing. Must be a member of the Association of Women's Health, Obstetric and Neonatal Nurses; the American College of Nurse-Midwives; or the National Association of Neonatal Nurses (NANN).
Application Contact: Education Services
March of Dimes
1275 Mamaroneck Avenue
White Plains, NY 10605
914-997-4609
E-mail: mlavan@marchofdimes.com
http://www.marchofdimes.org/professionals/graduate-nursing-scholarships.aspx

National Association of Hispanic Nurses® (NAHN)

Award Name: NAHN Nursing Scholarships
Program Description: One-time award to an outstanding Hispanic nursing student. Must have at least a 3.0 GPA and be a member of NAHN. Based on academic merit, potential contribution to nursing, and financial need.
Application Contact:
National Association of Hispanic Nurses
Awards/Scholarship Committee
10 G Street NE
Suite 605

Washington, DC 20002
501-673-1131
E-mail: info@thehispanicnurses.org
www.thehispanicnurses.org
    National Black Nurses Association, Inc. (NBNA)
Award Names: NBNA Scholarships
Program Description: Scholarships available to nursing students who are members of NBNA and are enrolled in an accredited school of nursing. Must demonstrate involvement in African-American community and present letter of recommendation from local chapter of NBNA.
Application Contact:
National Black Nurses Association, Inc.
Scholarship Committee
8630 Fenton Street, Suite 330
Silver Spring, MD 20910
301-589-3200
E-mail: info@nbna.org
www.nbna.org/

National Student Nurses' Association (NSNA)

Award Name: Educational Advancement Scholarships
Program Description: Scholarships are awarded based on academic achievement and demonstrated commitment to nursing through involvement in student organizations and school and community activities related to health care.
Application Contact:
National Student Nurses' Association Foundation
45 Main Street
Suite 606
Brooklyn, NY 11201
718-210-0705
E-mail: nsna@nsna.org
www.nsna.org

Nurses' Educational Funds, Inc.

Award Name: Nurses' Educational Fund Scholarships
Program Description: Awards for full-time students at master's level, full-time or part-time at doctoral level, or RNs who are U.S. citizens and members of a national professional nursing association. Application fee: $10.
Application Contact:
Nurses' Educational Funds, Inc.
304 Park Avenue South
11th Floor
New York, NY 10010
212-590-2443
E-mail: info@n-e-f.org
www.n-e-f.org

Oncology Nursing Society

Award Name: Scholarships

Program Description: ONF offers nearly a dozen one-time scholarships and awards at all levels of study, with various requirements and purposes, to nursing students who are interested in pursuing oncology nursing. Contact the foundation for details about appropriate awards. Application fee: $5.

Application Contact:

Oncology Nursing Society

Development Coordinator

125 Enterprise Drive

Pittsburgh, PA 15275-1214

866-257-4667 (toll-free)

E-mail: awards@ons.org

www.ons.org/awards

United States Air Force Reserve Officer Training Corps

Award Name: Air Force ROTC Nursing Scholarships

Program Description: One- to four-year programs available to students of nursing and high school seniors. Nursing graduates agree to accept a commission in the Air Force Nurse Corps and serve four years on active duty after successfully completing their licensing examination. Must have at least a 2.5 GPA for one- and four-year scholarships or at least a 2.65 GPA for two- and three-year scholarships. Two exam failures result in a four-year assignment as an Air Force line officer.

Application Contact:

Air Force ROTC

551 East Maxwell Boulevard

Maxwell AFB, AL 36112

866-423-7682 (toll-free)

www.afrotc.com/scholarships

United States Army Reserve Officers' Training Corps

Award Name: Army ROTC Nursing Scholarships

Program Description: Two- to four-year programs available to students of nursing and high school seniors. Nursing graduates agree to accept a commission in the Army Nurse Corps and serve in the military for a period of eight years. This may be fulfilled by serving on active duty for two to four years, followed by service in the Army National Guard or the United States Army Reserve or in the Inactive Ready Reserve for the remainder of the eight-year obligation.

Application Contact:

Army ROTC Cadet Command

Army ROTC Scholarship

Fort Monroe, VA 23651-1052

800-USA-ROTC (toll-free)

www.goarmy.com/rotc/scholarships.html

United States Department of Health and Human Services, Health Resources and Services Administration

Award Names: NURSE Corps Scholarship Program

Program Description: Awards for U.S. citizens enrolled or accepted for enrollment as a full- or part-time student in an accredited school of nursing in a professional registered nurse program (baccalaureate, graduate, associate degree, or diploma)

Application Contact:

Division of Nursing

U.S. Dept. of Health and Human Services

5600 Fishers Lane, Room 8-37

Parklawn Building

Rockville, MD 20857

800-221-9393 (toll-free)

GetHelp@hrsa.gov

www.hrsa.gov/loanscholarships/scholarships/Nursing

HOW TO USE THIS GUIDE

The following includes an overview of the various components of *Peterson's Nursing Programs 2017*, along with background information on the criteria used for including institutions and nursing programs in the guide, and explanatory material to help users interpret details presented within the guide.

Profiles of Nursing Programs

The **Profiles of Nursing Programs** section contains detailed profiles of schools that responded to our online survey and the nursing programs they offer. This section is organized geographically; U.S. schools are listed alphabetically by state or territory, followed by Canadian schools listed alphabetically by province.

The profiles contain basic information about the colleges and universities, along with details specific to the nursing school or department, the nursing student body, and the nursing programs offered.

Schools that are members of a consortium appear with an abbreviated profile. The abbreviated profile lists only the school heading and the specific college or university information, followed by a reference line that refers readers to the consortium profile, which contains detailed program information.

An outline of the profile follows. The items of information found under each section heading are defined and displayed. Any item discussed below that is omitted from an individual profile either does not apply to that particular college or university or is one for which no information was supplied. Each profile begins with a heading with the name of the institution (the college or university), the nursing college or unit, the location of the nursing facilities, the school's Web address, and the institution's founding date, specifically the year in which it was chartered or the year when instruction actually began, whichever date is earlier. In most cases, the location is identical to the main campus of the institution. However, in a few instances, the nursing facilities are not located in the same city or state as the main campus of the college or university.

Basic information about the college follows:

Nursing Program Faculty: The total number of full-time and part-time faculty members, followed by, if provided, the percentage of faculty members holding doctoral degrees.

Baccalaureate Enrollment: The total number of matriculated full-time and part-time baccalaureate program students as of fall 2015 is given. This snapshot of the nursing student body indicates the total number of matriculated students, both full-time and part-time, in the baccalaureate-level nursing program; the school's estimate of the percentage of nursing students in each of the following categories is provided, if applicable: Women, Men, Minority, International, and Part-time.

Graduate Enrollment: The total number of matriculated full-time and part-time students in graduate programs in fall 2015 and the percentages of **Women, Men, Minority, International,** and **Part-time** students are given.

Distance Learning Courses: This section appears if distance learning courses are available.

Nursing Student Activities: This section lists organizations open only to nursing students, including nursing clubs, Sigma Theta Tau (the international honor society for nursing), recruiter clubs, and Student Nurses' Association.

Nursing Student Resources: This section lists special learning resources available for nursing students within the nursing school's (or unit's) facilities.

Library Facilities: Figures are provided for the total number of bound volumes held by the college or university, the number of those volumes in health-related subjects, and the number in nursing and the number of periodical subscriptions held and the number of those in health-related subjects.

BACCALAUREATE PROGRAMS

Degree: Baccalaureate degree or degrees awarded are specified.

Available Programs: If, in addition to a generic baccalaureate program in nursing, a school has other baccalaureate nursing programs (e.g., accelerated programs or programs for RNs, LPNs, or college graduates with non-nursing degrees) they are specified here.

Site Options: Locations other than the nursing program's main campus at which baccalaureate programs may be taken are listed. Off-campus classes generally are held in health-care facilities or other educational facilities that are part of or affiliated with the college or nursing school.

Study Options: Lists full-time and part-time options.

Online Degree Options: This section appears if online baccalaureate degrees are available. It also specifies if the distance learning options are only available online.

Program Entrance Requirements: Lists special requirements typically required to enter a program of nursing leading to a baccalaureate degree, including completion of a specific program of prerequisite courses, sometimes called prenursing courses. These are specific course credits that must be earned by students who wish to enter the generic baccalaureate program. Students entering into other tracks may be required to prove that they have completed analogous courses. Often the minimum GPA requirement for prerequisite courses differs from that expected for general college courses. Other requirements are generally self-explanatory. This paragraph also indicates if transfer students are accepted into the program. Special tracks will require appropriate proof of experience, diplomas, or other credentials. Finally, application deadlines and fees are given.

Advanced Placement: This entry indicates that program credits may be granted on the basis of examinations or evaluations of earned credits at other facilities by the program's faculty and administrators.

Expenses: In this section, figures are provided for tuition, mandatory and other fees, and room and board, as well as an estimate of costs for books and supplies, based on the 2015–16 academic year. If a school did not return a survey, expenses for the 2013–14 or 2014–15 academic year are listed. Unless otherwise indicated, tuition is for one full academic year. If applicable, distinct tuition figures are given for state residents and nonresidents. Part-time tuition is expressed in terms of the per-unit rate (per credit, per semester hour, etc.) specified by the institution. The tuition structure at some institutions is very complex, with different rates for freshmen and sophomores than for juniors and seniors or with part-time tuition prorated on a sliding scale according to the number of credit hours taken. Mandatory fees include such items as activity fees, health insurance, and malpractice insurance.

Financial Aid: This section combines data from our online nursing survey with data received on available financial aid programs. It provides information on college-administered aid for baccalaureate-level students, including the percentage of undergraduate nursing students receiving financial aid, all types of aid offered, and application deadlines. Financial aid programs are organized into these categories: gift aid (need-based), awards based on a student's formally designated inability to pay some or all of the cost of education; gift aid (non-need-based), scholarships given on the basis of a student's special achievements, abilities, or personal characteristics; loans, subsidized low-interest student loans that can be need-based or not; and work-study, a need-based program of part-time work offered to help pay educational expenditures. The application deadline is the deadline by which application forms and need calculations, such as the FAFSA, must be submitted to the institution in order to qualify for need-based and institutional aid.

Contact: This section lists the name, title, mailing address, telephone number, and, if available, fax number and e-mail address of the person to contact for admission information about the baccalaureate program.

GRADUATE PROGRAMS

The first three paragraphs provide information that is common to the college's graduate programs in nursing.

Expenses: In this section, figures are provided for tuition, room and board, and required fees based on the 2015–16 academic year. If a school did not return a survey, expenses for the 2013–14 or 2014–15 academic year are listed. Unless otherwise indicated, tuition is for one full academic year. If applicable, distinct tuition figures are given for state residents and nonresidents. Part-time tuition is expressed in terms of the per-

unit rate (per credit, per semester hour, etc.) specified by the institution.

Financial Aid: This section combines data from our online nursing survey with data received on available financial aid programs. It provides information on college-administered aid including the percentage of graduate nursing students receiving financial aid, all types of aid offered, and application deadlines. The major kinds of aid available are listed, including traineeships, low-interest student loans, fellowships, research assistantships, teaching assistantships, and full and partial tuition waivers. If aid is available to part-time students, this is indicated. The application deadline is the deadline by which application forms must be submitted to the college's financial aid office.

Contact: Lists the name, title, mailing address, telephone number, and, if available, fax number and e-mail address of the person to contact for admission information about graduate programs.

MASTER'S DEGREE PROGRAM

Degree(s): Master's degree or degrees awarded are specified. Joint degrees specify which two degrees are given, e.g., M.S.N./Ed. D., M.S.N./M.B.A., M.S./M.H.A., M.S.N./M.P.H., in programs that combine a master's degree (or doctorate) in nursing with a master's degree in another discipline, such as business administration, hospital administration, or public health.

Available Programs: If a college has special tracks that give credit, accelerated programs, or advanced courses designed for students with previous nursing experience or higher education credentials that enable students to complete programs in less time than regularly required, these are specified here in three categories:

❶ For RNs—programs that admit registered nurses with associate degrees or diplomas in nursing and award a master's degree. These include RN-to-master's programs that combine the baccalaureate and master's degrees into one program for nurses who are graduates of associate or hospital diploma programs and programs that admit registered nurses with non-nursing baccalaureate degrees.

❷ For LPNs—programs that admit licensed practical nurses and award a master's degree.

❸ For College Graduates with Non-Nursing Degrees— programs that admit students with baccalaureate or master's degrees in areas other than nursing and award a master's degree in nursing.

Concentrations Available: Specific areas of study and concentrations offered by the school are listed. Areas of specialization in case management, health-care administration, legal nurse consultant, nurse anesthesia, nurse-midwifery, nursing administration, nursing education, and nursing informatics are noted. Clinical nurse specialist and nurse practitioner programs and areas of specialization within them are noted.

Site Options: Locations other than the nursing program's main campus at which the master's degree programs are offered are listed. Off-campus classes generally are held in health-care facilities or other educational facilities that are part of or affiliated with the nursing school.

Study Options: Lists full-time and part-time options.

Online Degree Options: This section appears if online master's degrees are available. It also specifies if the distance learning options are only available online.

Program Entrance Requirements: Lists generally self-explanatory requirements.

Advanced Placement: Indicates that program credits may be granted on the basis of examinations or evaluations of earned credits at other facilities by the program's faculty and administrators.

Degree Requirements: Indicates the number of master's program credit hours required to earn the master's degree and the need for a thesis or qualifying score on a comprehensive examination.

POST-MASTER'S PROGRAM

Areas of Study: Listed here are the specific areas of clinical nurse specialist programs, nurse practitioner programs, and other specializations offered as postmaster's programs.

DOCTORAL DEGREE PROGRAM

Degree: Doctoral degree awarded is specified.

Areas of Study: Lists specific areas of study and concentration offered by the school.

Program Entrance Requirements: Lists generally self-explanatory requirements.

Degree Requirements: Indicates the number of program credit hours required to earn the doctorate and the need for a dissertation, oral examination, written examination, or residency.

POSTDOCTORAL PROGRAM

Areas of Study: Lists areas of study currently reported. These may change, dependent upon the individuals in the program.

Postdoctoral Program Contact: Lists the name, title, mailing address, telephone number, and, if available, fax number and e-mail address of the person to contact for information about postdoctoral programs.

CONTINUING EDUCATION PROGRAM

Contact: The appearance of this heading indicates that the nursing school has a program of continuing education. If provided, the name, title, mailing address, telephone number, fax number, and e-mail address of the person to contact regarding the program are given.

Display Ads

Display ads, which appear near some of the institutions' profiles, have been provided by those colleges or universities that wished to pay for and supplement the profile data with information about their institutions or nursing programs.

Two-Page Descriptions

The **Two-Page Descriptions** section is an open forum for nursing schools to communicate their particular message to prospective students. The absence of any college or university from this section does not constitute an editorial decision on the part of Peterson's Publishing. Those who have submitted and paid for these inclusions are responsible for the accuracy of the content. Statements regarding a school's objectives and accomplishments represent its own beliefs and are not the opinions of the editors. The **Two-Page Descriptions** are arranged alphabetically by the official institution name.

Indexes

Indexes at the back of the book provide references to profiles by baccalaureate, master's, doctoral, postdoctoral, online, and continuing education programs offered; for master's-level programs, by area of study or concentration; and by institution name.

Abbreviations Used in This Guide

AACN	American Association of Colleges of Nursing
AACSB	AACSB International—The Association to Advance Collegiate Schools of Business
AAHC	Association of Academic Health Centers
AAS	Associate in Applied Science
ABSN	Accelerated Bachelor of Science in Nursing
ACT	American College Testing, Inc.
ACT ASSET	American College Testing Assessment of Skills for Successful Entry and Transfer
AD	Associate Degree
ADN	Associate Degree in Nursing
AHNP	Adult Health Nurse Practitioner
AMEDD	Army Medical Department
ANA	American Nurses Association
ANEE	Advanced Nurse Education Expansion
ANP	Adult Nurse Practitioner
APN	Advanced Practice Nurse
ARNP	Advanced Registered Nurse Practitioner
AS	Associate of Science
ASN	Associate of Science in Nursing
BA	Bachelor of Arts
BAA	Bachelor of Applied Arts
BN	Bachelor of Nursing
BNSc	Bachelor of Nursing Science
BRN	Baccalaureate for the Registered Nurse
BS	Bachelor of Science
BScMH	Bachelor of Science in Mental Health
BScN	Bachelor of Science in Nursing

BSEd	Bachelor of Science in Education
BSN	Bachelor of Science in Nursing
CAI	computer-assisted instruction
CAUSN	Canadian Association of University Schools of Nursing
CCNE	Commission on Collegiate Nursing Education
CCRN	Critical-Care Registered Nurse
CFNP	Certified Family Nurse Practitioner
CGFNS	Commission on Graduates of Foreign Nursing Schools
CINAHL	Cumulative Index to Nursing and Allied Health Literature
CLEP	College-Level Examination Program
CNA	Certified Nurse Assistant, Certified Nursing Assistant, Certified Nurses' Aide
CNAT	Canadian Nurses Association Testing
CNL	Clinical Nurse Leader
CNM	Certified Nurse-Midwife
CNS	Clinical Nurse Specialist
CODEC	coder/decoder
CPNP	Certified Pediatric Nurse Practitioner
CPR	cardiopulmonary resuscitation
CRNA	Certified Registered Nurse Anesthetist
CS	Certified Specialist
CSS	College Scholarship Service
DAP	Doctor of Anesthesia Practice
DNP	Doctor of Nursing Practice
DNS	Doctor of Nursing Science
DNSc	Doctor of Nursing Science
DOE	U.S. Department of Education
DrPH	Doctor of Public Health
DSN	Doctor of Science in Nursing
EdD	Doctor of Education
EFC	expected family contribution
ERIC	Educational Resources Information Center
ESL	English as a second language
ETN	Enterostomal Nurse
FAAN	Fellow in the American Academy of Nursing
FAANP	Fellows of the American Association of Nurse Practitioners
FAF	Financial Aid Form
FAFSA	Free Application for Federal Student Aid
FC	family contribution
FNAP	Fellow of the National Academies of Practice
FNP	Family Nurse Practitioner
FSEOG	Federal Supplemental Educational Opportunity Grants
GED	General Educational Development test
GMAT	Graduate Management Admission Test
GPA	grade point average
GPO	Government Printing Office
GRE	Graduate Record Examinations
Gyn	gynecology
HIV	human immunodeficiency virus
HMO	health maintenance organization
ICU	intensive care unit

ISP	Internet service provider
LD	Licensed Dietician
LPN	Licensed Practical Nurse
LVN	Licensed Vocational Nurse
MA	Master of Arts
MAEd	Master of Arts in Education
MAT	Miller Analogies Test
MBA	Master of Business Administration
MCSc	Master of Clinical Science
MDiv	Master of Divinity
MEd	Master of Education
MEDLINE	Medical Literature Analysis and Retrieval System Online
MELAB	Michigan English Language Assessment Battery
MHA	Master of Hospital Administration Master of Health Administration
MHD	Master of Human Development
MHSA	Master of Health Services Administration
MN	Master of Nursing
MNSc	Master of Nursing Science
MOM	Master of Organizational Management
MPA	Master of Public Affairs
MPH	Master of Public Health
MPS	Master of Public Service
MS	Master of Science
MSBA	Master of Science in Business Administration
M Sc	Master of Science
MSc(A)	Master of Science (Applied)
MScN	Master of Science in Nursing
MTS	Master of Theological Studies
MSEd	Master of Science in Education
MSN	Master of Science in Nursing
MSOB	Master of Science in Organizational Behavior
NCAA	National Collegiate Athletic Association
NCLEX-RN	National Council Licensure Examination for Registered Nurses
ND	Doctor of Nursing
NLN	National League for Nursing
NNP	Neonatal Nurse Practitioner
NP	Nurse Practitioner
NSNA	National Student Nurses' Association
OB	Organizational Behavior
OB/GYN	obstetrics/gynecology
OCLC	Online Computer Library Center
OM	Organizational Management
PEP	Proficiency Examination Program
PhD	Doctor of Philosophy
PHS	Public Health Service
PLUS	Parents' Loan for Undergraduate Students
PMHNP	Psychiatric-Mental Health Nurse Practitioner
PNNP	Perinatal Nurse Practitioner
PNP	Pediatric Nurse Practitioner
RD	Registered Dietician
RN	Registered Nurse
RN, C	Registered Nurse, Certified

RN, CAN	Registered Nurse, Certified in Nursing Administration
RN, CNAA	Registered Nurse, Certified in Nursing Administration, Advanced
RN, CS	Registered Nurse, Certified Specialist
ROTC	Reserve Officers' Training Corps
RPN	Registered Psychiatric Nurse
SAR	Student Aid Report
SAT	SAT and SAT Subject Tests
SNA	Student Nurses' Association
SNAP	Student Nurses Acting for Progress
SNO	Student Nurses Organization
SUNY	State University of New York
TAP	Tuition Assistance Program
TB	tuberculosis
TOEFL	Test of English as a Foreign Language
TSE	Test of Spoken English
TWE	Test of Written English
USIS	United States Information Service
WHNP	Women's Health Nurse Practitioner

Data Collection Procedures

The data contained in the preponderant number of nursing college profiles, as well as in the indexes to them, were collected through *Peterson's Survey of Nursing Programs* during winter 2015–16. Questionnaires were posted online for more than 900 colleges and universities with baccalaureate and graduate programs in nursing. With minor exceptions, data for those colleges or schools of nursing that responded to the questionnaires were submitted by officials at the schools themselves. All usable information received in time for publication has been included. The omission of a particular item from a profile means that it is either not applicable to that institution or was not available or usable. In the handful of instances in which no information regarding an eligible nursing program was submitted and research of reliable secondary sources was unable to elicit the desired information, the name, location, and some general information regarding the nursing program appear in the profile section to indicate the existence of the program. Because of the extensive system of checks performed on the data collected by Peterson's, we believe that the information presented in this guide is accurate. Nonetheless, errors and omissions are possible in a data collection and processing endeavor of this scope. Also, facts and figures, such as tuition and fees, can suddenly change. Therefore, students should check with a specific college or university at the time of application to verify all pertinent information.

Criteria for Inclusion in This Book

Peterson's Nursing Programs 2017 covers accredited institutions in the United States, U.S. territories, and Canada that grant baccalaureate and graduate degrees. The institutions that sponsor the nursing programs must be accredited by accrediting agencies approved by the U.S. Department of Education (USDE) or the Council for Higher Education Accreditation (CHEA) or be candidates for accreditation with an agency recognized by the USDE for its preaccreditation category. Canadian schools may be provincially chartered instead of accredited.

Baccalaureate-level and master's-level nursing programs represented by a profile within the guide are accredited by the National League for Nursing Accrediting Commission (NLNAC) or the Commission on Collegiate Nursing Education (CCNE). Canadian nursing schools are members of the Canadian Association of University Schools of Nursing (CAUSN).

Doctoral, postdoctoral, continuing education, and other nursing programs included in the profiles are offered by nursing schools or departments affiliated with colleges or universities that meet the criteria outlined above.

NOTICE: Certain portions of or information contained in this book have been submitted and paid for by the educational institution identified, and such institutions take full responsibility for the accuracy, timeliness, completeness and functionality of such contents. Such portions or information include (i) each display ad in the "Profiles of Nursing Programs" section from pages 85 through 486 that comprises a full page or half page of information covering a single educational institution, and (ii) each two-page in-depth description in the "Two-Page Descriptions" section from Pages 488 through 513.

QUICK REFERENCE CHART

Nursing Programs At-a-Glance

	Baccalaureate	Masters	Accelerated	Joint Degree	Post-Masters	Doctoral	Postdoctoral	Continuing Education
UNITED STATES								
Alabama								
Auburn University	•	•						
Auburn University at Montgomery	•	•						
Jacksonville State University	•	•						•
Oakwood University	•							
Samford University	•	•	B		•	•		•
Spring Hill College	•	•	M					
Troy University	•	•			•	•		
Tuskegee University	•							
The University of Alabama	•	•			•	•		
The University of Alabama at Birmingham	•	•	M	•	•	•	•	•
The University of Alabama in Huntsville	•	•			•	•		•
University of Mobile	•	•						•
University of North Alabama	•	•	B					•
University of South Alabama	•	•	B,M		•			
Alaska								
University of Alaska Anchorage	•	•						
Arizona								
Arizona State University at the Downtown Phoenix campus	•	•	B	•	•	•		•
Brookline College	•		B					
Chamberlain College of Nursing	•	•	B			•		
Grand Canyon University	•	•		•	•			•
Northern Arizona University	•	•	B		•	•		
The University of Arizona	•	•	M		•	•		•
University of Phoenix–Online Campus	•	•	B	•	•	•		•
University of Phoenix–Phoenix Campus	•	•	B	•	•			•
University of Phoenix–Southern Arizona Campus	•	•	B		•			•
Arkansas								
Arkansas State University	•	•	B		•	•		
Arkansas Tech University	•	•						
Harding University	•	•			•			•
Henderson State University	•							
Southern Arkansas University–Magnolia	•							
University of Arkansas	•	•				•		
University of Arkansas at Little Rock	•							
University of Arkansas at Monticello	•							
University of Arkansas for Medical Sciences	•	•	B			•	•	•
University of Arkansas–Fort Smith	•							
University of Central Arkansas	•	•			•			
California								
American University of Health Sciences	•		B					

B = Baccalaureate; M = Masters

	Baccalaureate	Masters	Accelerated	Joint Degree	Post-Masters	Doctoral	Postdoctoral	Continuing Education
Azusa Pacific University	•	•	B,M		•	•		•
Biola University	•							
Brandman University	•					•	•	•
California Baptist University	•	•	M					
California State University, Bakersfield	•							•
California State University Channel Islands	•							
California State University, Chico	•	•						•
California State University, Dominguez Hills	•	•			•			
California State University, East Bay	•							
California State University, Fresno	•	•	M		•		•	•
California State University, Fullerton	•	•				•		
California State University, Long Beach	•	•			•			
California State University, Los Angeles	•	•	M		•			
California State University, Northridge	•		B					
California State University, Sacramento	•	•						•
California State University, San Bernardino	•	•						
California State University, San Marcos	•		B					
California State University, Stanislaus	•							
Charles R. Drew University of Medicine and Science		•	M					
Concordia University Irvine	•		B					
Dominican University of California	•							
Fresno Pacific University	•							
Holy Names University	•	•		•	•			
Loma Linda University	•	•	B				•	
Mount Saint Mary's University	•	•	B					
National University	•	•						
Pacific College	•							
Pacific Union College	•							•
Point Loma Nazarene University	•	•			•			•
Samuel Merritt University	•	•	B		•	•		
San Diego State University	•	•			•			•
San Francisco State University	•	•	B,M		•			•
San Jose State University	•	•			•			
Sonoma State University	•							
Stanbridge College	•							
United States University	•							
Unitek College	•							•
University of California, Davis		•				•	•	•
University of California, Irvine	•	•				•	•	•
University of California, Los Angeles	•	•		•	•	•	•	•
University of California, San Francisco		•			•	•	•	
University of Phoenix–Bay Area Campus	•	•	B	•				
University of Phoenix–Central Valley Campus	•							
University of Phoenix–Sacramento Valley Campus	•	•	B,M		•			•
University of Phoenix–San Diego Campus	•	•	B					

B = Baccalaureate; M = Masters

	Baccalaureate	Masters	Accelerated	Joint Degree	Post-Masters	Doctoral	Postdoctoral	Continuing Education
University of Phoenix–Southern California Campus	•	•	B	•	•			•
University of San Diego		•	M			•		
University of San Francisco	•	•	M		•	•		
Vanguard University of Southern California	•							
West Coast University	•	•	B,M		•			•
Western University of Health Sciences		•	M		•	•		
Colorado								
Adams State University	•							
American Sentinel University	•	•				•		
Aspen University		•						
Colorado Christian University	•							
Colorado Mesa University	•	•				•		
Colorado State University–Pueblo	•	•	B		•			
Colorado Technical University Online	•							
Denver School of Nursing	•		B					
Metropolitan State University of Denver	•		B					
Platt College	•		B					
Regis University	•	•	B					
University of Colorado Colorado Springs	•	•	B		•	•		•
University of Colorado Denver	•	•	B		•	•	•	•
University of Northern Colorado	•	•			•	•		
Connecticut								
Central Connecticut State University	•							
Fairfield University	•	•	B			•		
Quinnipiac University	•	•	B		•	•		
Sacred Heart University	•	•			•	•		•
St. Vincent's College	•		B					
Southern Connecticut State University	•	•	B		•	•		
University of Connecticut	•	•	B		•	•	•	•
University of Hartford	•	•			•			•
University of Saint Joseph	•	•			•	•		
Western Connecticut State University	•	•			•			
Yale University		•		•	•	•	•	
Delaware								
Delaware State University	•	•						
University of Delaware	•	•	B		•	•		•
Wesley College	•	•	M		•			•
Wilmington University	•	•	B,M	•	•			
District of Columbia								
The Catholic University of America	•	•	B		•	•		
Georgetown University	•	•	M			•		
The George Washington University	•	•	B,M		•	•		
Howard University	•	•			•			

B = Baccalaureate; M = Masters

	Baccalaureate	Masters	Accelerated	Joint Degree	Post-Masters	Doctoral	Postdoctoral	Continuing Education
Trinity Washington University	•							
University of the District of Columbia	•							
Florida								
Adventist University of Health Sciences	•							
Barry University	•	•	B	•	•	•		
Bethune-Cookman University	•							
Broward College	•							
Chipola College	•							
ECPI University	•		B					
Florida Agricultural and Mechanical University	•	•			•	•		•
Florida Atlantic University	•	•	B		•	•		
Florida Gulf Coast University	•	•			•			•
Florida International University	•	•	B,M		•	•		
Florida National University	•							
Florida Southern College	•	•	B	•	•			
Florida SouthWestern State College	•							
Florida State College at Jacksonville	•							
Florida State University	•	•	B		•	•		
Fortis College	•							
Gulf Coast State College	•							
Herzing University	•							
Indian River State College	•							
Jacksonville University	•	•	B	•	•	•		
Kaplan University Online	•	•						
Keiser University (Fort Lauderdale)	•	•						
Keiser University (Fort Myers)	•	•						
Keiser University (Jacksonville)	•	•						
Keiser University (Lakeland)	•	•						
Keiser University (Melbourne)	•	•						
Keiser University (Miami)	•	•						
Keiser University (Orlando)	•	•						
Keiser University (Port St. Lucie)	•	•						
Keiser University (Sarasota)	•	•						
Keiser University (Tallahassee)	•	•						
Keiser University (Tampa)	•	•						
Miami Dade College	•							
Northwest Florida State College	•							
Nova Southeastern University	•	•						
Palm Beach Atlantic University	•	•					•	
Polk State College	•							
St. Petersburg College	•							•
Santa Fe College	•							
State College of Florida Manatee-Sarasota	•							
University of Central Florida	•	•	B,M		•	•		

B = Baccalaureate; M = Masters

	Baccalaureate	Masters	Accelerated	Joint Degree	Post-Masters	Doctoral	Postdoctoral	Continuing Education
University of Florida	•	•	B	•	•	•		
University of Miami	•	•	B		•	•		•
University of North Florida	•	•	B		•			
University of Phoenix–North Florida Campus	•	•	B					
University of Phoenix–South Florida Campus	•	•		•				
University of Phoenix–West Florida Learning Center	•		B					
University of South Florida	•	•	B,M	•	•	•		
The University of Tampa	•	•			•			•
University of West Florida	•	•						
Georgia								
Albany State University	•	•	B,M		•			
Armstrong State University	•	•	B		•			
Augusta University	•	•	M		•	•		
Berry College	•							
Brenau University	•	•				•		
Clayton State University	•	•						
College of Coastal Georgia	•							
Columbus State University	•							
Dalton State College	•							
Darton State College	•							
Emory University	•	•	B	•	•	•		
Georgia College & State University	•	•			•	•		
Georgia Highlands College	•							
Georgia Southern University	•					•		
Georgia Southwestern State University	•	•						
Georgia State University	•	•	B		•	•		
Gordon State College	•							
Herzing University	•							
Kennesaw State University	•	•	B					•
LaGrange College	•							
Mercer University	•	•				•		
Middle Georgia College	•							
Piedmont College	•							
Shorter University	•							
Thomas University	•	•	B,M	•	•			
University of North Georgia	•	•			•			
University of Phoenix–Atlanta Campus								
University of West Georgia	•	•	B		•	•		
Valdosta State University	•	•						•
Guam								
University of Guam								
Hawaii								
Chaminade University of Honolulu	•							
Hawai`i Pacific University	•	•		•	•			

B = Baccalaureate; M = Masters

	Baccalaureate	Masters	Accelerated	Joint Degree	Post-Masters	Doctoral	Postdoctoral	Continuing Education
University of Hawaii at Hilo	•							
University of Hawaii at Manoa	•	•	M	•	•	•		
University of Phoenix–Hawaii Campus	•	•	B					
Idaho								
Boise State University	•	•	B					
Brigham Young University–Idaho	•							
Idaho State University	•	•	B		•	•		
Lewis-Clark State College	•							
Northwest Nazarene University	•	•						
Illinois								
Aurora University	•	•						
Benedictine University	•	•	B,M					
Blessing–Rieman College of Nursing and Health Sciences	•	•	B					
Bradley University	•	•	B			•		
Chamberlain College of Nursing	•							
Chicago State University	•	•						
DePaul University	•	•				•		
Eastern Illinois University	•							
Elmhurst College	•	•		•				
Governors State University	•	•			•			
Illinois State University	•	•	B		•	•		
Illinois Wesleyan University	•							
Lakeview College of Nursing	•		B					
Lewis University	•	•	B,M	•	•	•		•
Loyola University Chicago	•	•	B	•	•	•		
MacMurray College	•							
McKendree University	•	•			•	•		
Methodist College	•		B					
Millikin University	•	•	M			•		
Northern Illinois University	•	•		•	•			
North Park University	•	•		•	•			
Olivet Nazarene University	•	•	B					
Resurrection University	•	•	B					
Rockford University	•							
Rush University		•	M		•	•	•	•
Saint Anthony College of Nursing	•	•			•	•		
Saint Francis Medical Center College of Nursing	•	•	M		•	•		
St. John's College	•							
Saint Xavier University	•	•	B	•	•			
Southern Illinois University Edwardsville	•	•	B		•	•		•
Trinity Christian College	•							
Trinity College of Nursing and Health Sciences	•		B					
University of Illinois at Chicago	•	•				•	•	•
University of St. Francis	•	•	B		•	•		

B = Baccalaureate; M = Masters

	Baccalaureate	Masters	Accelerated	Joint Degree	Post–Masters	Doctoral	Postdoctoral	Continuing Education
Western Illinois University	•							
Indiana								
Anderson University	•	•		•	•			
Ball State University	•	•	B		•	•		
Bethel College	•	•			•			
Goshen College	•	•						
Harrison College	•							
Huntington University	•							
Indiana State University	•	•	B		•	•		•
Indiana University Bloomington	•							
Indiana University East	•							
Indiana University Kokomo	•		B					•
Indiana University Northwest	•		B					
Indiana University–Purdue University Fort Wayne	•	•				•		
Indiana University–Purdue University Indianapolis	•	•	B		•	•	•	•
Indiana University South Bend	•	•	B					
Indiana University Southeast	•							
Indiana Wesleyan University	•	•	B		•			
Marian University	•		B					•
Purdue University	•	•	B		•	•		
Purdue University Calumet	•	•	B		•			
Purdue University North Central	•		B					
Saint Joseph's College	•		B					
Saint Mary's College	•					•		
University of Evansville	•							
University of Indianapolis	•	•	B		•	•		
University of Saint Francis	•	•			•			
University of Southern Indiana	•	•			•	•		•
Valparaiso University	•	•	B			•		•
Vincennes University	•							
Iowa								
Allen College	•	•	B		•	•		•
Briar Cliff University	•	•				•		•
Clarke University	•					•		•
Coe College	•							
Dordt College	•							
Grand View University	•	•						•
Iowa Wesleyan College	•							
Luther College	•							•
Mercy College of Health Sciences	•							
Morningside College	•	•			•			
Mount Mercy University	•	•						
Northwestern College	•							
St. Ambrose University	•	•						•

B = Baccalaureate; M = Masters

	Baccalaureate	Masters	Accelerated	Joint Degree	Post-Masters	Doctoral	Postdoctoral	Continuing Education
University of Dubuque	•							
The University of Iowa	•	•	M	•	•	•	•	•
Upper Iowa University	•							
William Penn University	•							
Kansas								
Baker University	•	•						
Benedictine College	•							
Bethel College	•							
Emporia State University	•							
Fort Hays State University	•	•			•			
Kansas Wesleyan University	•							
MidAmerica Nazarene University	•	•	B					
Newman University	•	•						
Ottawa University–Kansas City	•							
Pittsburg State University	•	•				•		•
Tabor College	•	•	B					
The University of Kansas	•	•		•	•	•	•	•
University of Saint Mary	•	•	B					
Washburn University	•	•				•		•
Wichita State University	•		B			•		
Kentucky								
Bellarmine University	•	•	B	•	•	•		•
Berea College	•							
Eastern Kentucky University	•	•	B					
Frontier Nursing University		•	M		•	•		
Kentucky Christian University	•							•
Kentucky State University	•							
Lindsey Wilson College	•							
Midway University	•		B					•
Morehead State University	•							
Murray State University	•	•			•			•
Northern Kentucky University	•	•	B		•	•		•
Spalding University	•	•	B		•	•		
Sullivan University	•		B					
Thomas More College	•		B					
Union College	•							
University of Kentucky	•	•			•	•		•
University of Louisville	•	•	M			•		•
University of Pikeville	•							
Western Kentucky University	•	•	M		•	•		•
Louisiana								
Dillard University	•							•
Grambling State University	•	•			•			
Louisiana College	•							

B = Baccalaureate; M = Masters

	Baccalaureate	Masters	Accelerated	Joint Degree	Post-Masters	Doctoral	Postdoctoral	Continuing Education
Louisiana State University at Alexandria	•							
Louisiana State University Health Sciences Center	•		B			•		•
Loyola University New Orleans	•	•			•	•		
McNeese State University	•	•			•			•
Nicholls State University	•							•
Northwestern State University of Louisiana	•	•			•	•		•
Our Lady of Holy Cross College	•							
Our Lady of the Lake College	•	•	B					•
Southeastern Louisiana University	•	•	B		•	•		
Southern University and Agricultural and Mechanical College	•	•			•	•		
University of Louisiana at Lafayette	•	•	B		•			•
University of Louisiana at Monroe	•							•
University of Phoenix–New Orleans Learning Center	•		B					
Maine								
Husson University	•	•			•			
Saint Joseph's College of Maine	•	•						•
University of Maine	•	•						
University of Maine at Augusta	•							
University of Maine at Fort Kent	•		B					
University of New England	•		B					•
University of Southern Maine	•	•	B		•	•		•
Maryland								
Bowie State University	•	•	B					
Coppin State University	•	•	B		•			
Frostburg State University	•							
Hood College	•							
Johns Hopkins University		•		•	•	•	•	•
Morgan State University	•							
Notre Dame of Maryland University	•		B					
Salisbury University	•	•	B		•	•	•	
Stevenson University	•	•	B,M					
Towson University	•	•			•			
University of Maryland, Baltimore	•	•		•		•		•
Massachusetts								
American International College	•	•	B,M					
Anna Maria College	•							•
Becker College	•							
Boston College	•	•	M	•	•	•		
Curry College	•	•	B					
Elms College	•	•	B	•		•		
Emmanuel College	•	•						
Endicott College	•	•						•
Fitchburg State University	•	•	B					

B = Baccalaureate; M = Masters

	Baccalaureate	Masters	Accelerated	Joint Degree	Post-Masters	Doctoral	Postdoctoral	Continuing Education
Framingham State University	•	•						•
Labouré College	•							
MCPHS University	•		B					•
MGH Institute of Health Professions	•	•	B		•	•		
Northeastern University	•	•	B	•	•	•		•
Regis College	•	•	B,M		•	•		•
Salem State University	•	•	B	•				•
Simmons College	•	•	B,M			•		
University of Massachusetts Amherst	•	•	B			•		•
University of Massachusetts Boston	•	•	B		•	•	•	•
University of Massachusetts Dartmouth	•	•				•		•
University of Massachusetts Lowell	•	•				•		
University of Massachusetts Medical School		•	M		•	•		
Westfield State University	•							
Worcester State University	•	•			•			•
Michigan								
Andrews University	•					•		
Baker College	•		B					
Calvin College	•							
Davenport University	•							
Davenport University	•							
Eastern Michigan University	•	•			•			
Ferris State University	•	•	M	•				
Finlandia University	•							
Grand Valley State University	•	•	B			•		•
Hope College	•							
Lake Superior State University	•							
Madonna University	•	•		•	•	•		
Michigan State University	•	•	B			•	•	•
Northern Michigan University	•					•		•
Oakland University	•	•	B		•	•		•
Rochester College	•							
Saginaw Valley State University	•	•	M		•	•		•
Siena Heights University	•							
Spring Arbor University	•	•		•				
University of Detroit Mercy	•	•	B,M		•			
University of Michigan	•	•	B,M	•	•	•	•	
University of Michigan–Flint	•	•	B,M		•	•		
Wayne State University	•	•	B		•	•		
Western Michigan University	•	•						•
Minnesota								
Augsburg College	•	•						
Bemidji State University	•							•
Bethel University	•	•						

B = Baccalaureate; M = Masters

	Baccalaureate	Masters	Accelerated	Joint Degree	Post-Masters	Doctoral	Postdoctoral	Continuing Education
Capella University	•	•	M			•		
College of Saint Benedict	•							
The College of St. Scholastica	•		B			•		
Concordia College	•	•	B					
Crown College	•							
Globe University–Woodbury	•							
Gustavus Adolphus College	•							
Herzing University	•							
Metropolitan State University	•	•			•	•		
Minnesota State University Mankato	•	•	B,M		•	•		•
Minnesota State University Moorhead	•	•						
Rasmussen College Bloomington	•							
St. Catherine University	•	•			•	•		
St. Cloud State University	•							
Saint Mary's University of Minnesota	•	•						
St. Olaf College	•							
Southwest Minnesota State University	•							
University of Minnesota, Twin Cities Campus	•					•		•
University of Northwestern–St. Paul	•		B					
Walden University	•	•			•	•		
Winona State University	•	•			•	•		
Mississippi								
Alcorn State University	•	•			•			
Delta State University	•	•			•	•		
Mississippi College	•							
Mississippi University for Women	•	•			•	•		
University of Mississippi Medical Center	•	•	B		•	•		•
University of Southern Mississippi	•	•			•	•		
William Carey University	•	•				•		
Missouri								
Avila University	•							
Central Methodist University	•	•	B					
Chamberlain College of Nursing	•		B					
College of the Ozarks	•							
Cox College	•	•	B					•
Goldfarb School of Nursing at Barnes-Jewish College	•	•	B		•	•		
Graceland University	•	•	B		•	•		
Hannibal-LaGrange University	•							
Lincoln University	•							
Maryville University of Saint Louis	•	•	B		•	•		
Missouri Southern State University	•	•						
Missouri State University	•	•	B,M		•	•		•
Missouri Valley College	•							
Missouri Western State University	•	•						•

B = Baccalaureate; M = Masters

	Baccalaureate	Masters	Accelerated	Joint Degree	Post-Masters	Doctoral	Postdoctoral	Continuing Education
Research College of Nursing	•	•	B		•			
Saint Louis University	•	•	B,M		•	•		•
Saint Luke's College of Health Sciences	•							
Southeast Missouri State University	•	•			•			
Southwest Baptist University	•	•						
Truman State University	•							
University of Central Missouri	•	•						
University of Missouri	•	•	B	•	•	•		•
University of Missouri–Kansas City	•	•	B		•	•		•
University of Missouri–St. Louis	•	•	B		•	•		
Webster University	•	•						
William Jewell College	•		B					
Montana								
Carroll College	•							
Montana State University	•	•	B		•	•		
Montana State University–Northern	•							
Montana Tech of The University of Montana	•							
Salish Kootenai College	•							
Nebraska								
Bryan College of Health Sciences	•	•				•		
Clarkson College	•	•	B		•			•
College of Saint Mary	•	•						
Creighton University	•	•	B		•	•		•
Doane College	•							
Midland University	•							
Nebraska Methodist College	•	•	B		•	•		
Nebraska Wesleyan University	•	•	M	•	•			
Union College	•							
University of Nebraska Medical Center	•	•	B		•	•		•
Nevada								
Great Basin College	•							
Nevada State College at Henderson	•		B					
Roseman University of Health Sciences	•		B					
Touro University	•	•				•		
University of Nevada, Las Vegas	•	•	B		•	•		•
University of Nevada, Reno	•	•	B	•	•	•		
New Hampshire								
Colby-Sawyer College	•							
Franklin Pierce University	•	•						
Granite State College	•							
Keene State College	•							
Plymouth State University	•							
Rivier University	•	•			•			

B = Baccalaureate; M = Masters

	Baccalaureate	Masters	Accelerated	Joint Degree	Post-Masters	Doctoral	Postdoctoral	Continuing Education
Saint Anselm College	•							•
Southern New Hampshire University	•	•	B					
University of New Hampshire	•	•	M		•	•		
New Jersey								
Bloomfield College	•							
Caldwell University	•		B					
The College of New Jersey	•	•			•			•
College of Saint Elizabeth	•	•	B		•			•
Fairleigh Dickinson University, Metropolitan Campus	•	•	B,M		•	•		
Felician University	•	•	B,M	•	•			
Georgian Court University	•							
Kean University	•	•	M	•				
Monmouth University	•	•			•			•
New Jersey City University	•		B					
Ramapo College of New Jersey	•	•			•			•
Rider University	•							
Rowan University	•	•						
Rutgers, The State University of New Jersey, Camden	•	•	B			•	•	
Rutgers, The State University of New Jersey, Newark	•	•	B	•	•	•		•
Saint Peter's University	•	•			•			
Seton Hall University	•	•	B,M	•	•	•		
Stockton University	•	•						
Thomas Edison State University	•	•						
William Paterson University of New Jersey	•	•	B		•	•		
New Mexico								
Brookline College	•							
Eastern New Mexico University	•	•						
New Mexico Highlands University								
New Mexico State University	•	•	B			•		
Northern New Mexico College	•							
University of New Mexico	•	•			•	•		
University of Phoenix–New Mexico Campus	•	•	B					
Western New Mexico University	•							
New York								
Adelphi University	•	•	B		•	•		
Binghamton University, State University of New York	•	•	B		•	•		•
The College at Brockport, State University of New York	•							
College of Mount Saint Vincent	•	•						
The College of New Rochelle	•	•	B		•			
College of Staten Island of the City University of New York	•	•			•			
Columbia University	•	•	B,M	•	•	•	•	•
Concordia College–New York	•		B					
Daemen College	•	•	B,M		•	•		
Dominican College	•	•	B					

B = Baccalaureate; M = Masters

	Baccalaureate	Masters	Accelerated	Joint Degree	Post-Masters	Doctoral	Postdoctoral	Continuing Education
D'Youville College	•	•			•	•	
Elmira College	•							•
Excelsior College	•	•			•		
Farmingdale State College	•						
Hartwick College	•		B				
Helene Fuld College of Nursing	•						
Hunter College of the City University of New York	•	•	B	•	•	•		•
Keuka College	•	•	B,M		•		
Lehman College of the City University of New York	•	•	B		•	•		•
Le Moyne College	•	•	B		•			•
Long Island University–LIU Brooklyn	•	•	B		•		
Long Island University–LIU Post	•	•			•		
Maria College	•						
Medgar Evers College of the City University of New York	•		B				
Mercy College	•	•	B,M		•		
Molloy College	•	•	B	•	•	•		•
Mount Saint Mary College	•	•	B		•		
Nazareth College of Rochester	•						
New York City College of Technology of the City University of New York	•						
New York Institute of Technology	•						
New York University	•	•	B	•	•	•	•	•
Niagara University	•		B				
Nyack College	•						
Pace University	•	•	B		•	•	
Roberts Wesleyan College	•	•			•		
The Sage Colleges	•	•	B,M	•	•	•		•
St. Francis College	•						
St. John Fisher College	•	•	B		•	•	
St. Joseph's College, New York	•	•					
State University of New York at Plattsburgh	•						
State University of New York College of Technology at Alfred	•						
State University of New York College of Technology at Canton	•						
State University of New York College of Technology at Delhi	•						
State University of New York Downstate Medical Center	•	•	B	•	•			•
State University of New York Empire State College	•	•					
State University of New York Polytechnic Institute	•	•	B,M		•			•
State University of New York Upstate Medical University	•	•	M		•			•
Stony Brook University, State University of New York	•	•	B		•	•		•
Touro College	•						
Trocaire College	•						
University at Buffalo, the State University of New York	•	•	B			•	
University of Rochester	•		B				
Utica College	•		B				
Wagner College	•	•			•		
York College of the City University of New York	•						

B = Baccalaureate; M = Masters

	Baccalaureate	Masters	Accelerated	Joint Degree	Post-Masters	Doctoral	Postdoctoral	Continuing Education
North Carolina								
Appalachian State University	•							
Barton College	•	•						
Cabarrus College of Health Sciences	•							
Duke University	•	•	B		•	•	•	
East Carolina University	•	•	B,M		•	•		
Fayetteville State University	•							
Gardner-Webb University	•	•		•	•	•		
Lees-McRae College	•							
Lenoir-Rhyne University	•	•						
Methodist University	•							
North Carolina Agricultural and Technical State University	•		B					
North Carolina Central University	•							
Pfeiffer University	•							
Queens University of Charlotte	•	•	B	•				•
University of Mount Olive	•							
The University of North Carolina at Chapel Hill	•	•	B		•	•		
The University of North Carolina at Charlotte	•	•			•			
The University of North Carolina at Greensboro	•	•		•	•	•		
The University of North Carolina at Pembroke	•							
The University of North Carolina Wilmington	•	•			•			
Western Carolina University	•	•	B		•			
Wingate University	•							
Winston-Salem State University	•	•	B					•
North Dakota								
Dickinson State University	•							
Minot State University	•							
North Dakota State University	•					•		
University of Jamestown	•							
University of Mary	•	•		•		•		
University of North Dakota	•	•	B		•	•		
Ohio								
Ashland University	•		B			•		
Baldwin Wallace University	•		B					
Capital University	•	•	B	•	•			
Case Western Reserve University	•	•	M	•	•	•	•	•
Cedarville University	•	•						
Chamberlain College of Nursing	•	•	B					
The Christ College of Nursing and Health Sciences	•							
Cleveland State University	•	•	B	•	•	•		•
Defiance College	•		B					
Fortis College	•							
Franciscan University of Steubenville	•	•						
Franklin University	•		B					

B = Baccalaureate; M = Masters

	Baccalaureate	Masters	Accelerated	Joint Degree	Post-Masters	Doctoral	Postdoctoral	Continuing Education
Good Samaritan College of Nursing and Health Science	•							
Hiram College	•							
Hondros College	•							
Kent State University	•	•	B,M	•	•	•		•
Kettering College	•							
Lourdes University	•	•						
Malone University	•	•						
Mercy College of Ohio	•							
Miami University	•							
Miami University Hamilton	•							
Mount Carmel College of Nursing	•	•	B		•	•		
Mount St. Joseph University	•	•	B,M					
Mount Vernon Nazarene University	•							
Muskingum University	•							
Notre Dame College	•	•						
Ohio Northern University	•		B					
The Ohio State University	•	•		•	•	•		•
Ohio University	•	•						
Otterbein University	•	•	B		•			•
Shawnee State University	•							•
The University of Akron	•	•	B		•	•		•
University of Cincinnati	•	•	B,M		•	•		•
University of Phoenix–Cleveland Campus	•	•	B					
University of Rio Grande	•							
The University of Toledo	•	•			•	•		•
Urbana University	•	•						•
Ursuline College	•	•	B	•	•	•		
Walsh University	•	•	B,M		•	•		
Wright State University	•	•		•	•	•		•
Xavier University	•	•	M	•	•	•		
Youngstown State University	•	•			•			
Oklahoma								
Bacone College	•		B					
East Central University	•							
Langston University	•							
Northeastern State University	•	•	B					
Northwestern Oklahoma State University	•		B					
Oklahoma Baptist University	•	•						
Oklahoma Christian University	•							
Oklahoma City University	•	•	B,M			•		•
Oklahoma Panhandle State University	•							
Oklahoma Wesleyan University	•		B					
Oral Roberts University	•							
Rogers State University	•							
Southern Nazarene University	•	•	M					

B = Baccalaureate; M = Masters

	Baccalaureate	Masters	Accelerated	Joint Degree	Post-Masters	Doctoral	Postdoctoral	Continuing Education
Southwestern Oklahoma State University	•							
University of Central Oklahoma	•	•						
University of Oklahoma Health Sciences Center	•	•	B		•	•		•
University of Phoenix–Oklahoma City Campus								
University of Phoenix–Tulsa Learning Center								
The University of Tulsa	•							
Oregon								
Concordia University	•							
George Fox University	•							
Linfield College	•		B					•
Oregon Health & Science University	•	•	B,M		•	•	•	•
University of Portland	•	•				•		
Pennsylvania								
Alvernia University	•	•						•
Bloomsburg University of Pennsylvania	•	•	B	•				
California University of Pennsylvania	•							
Carlow University	•	•	B	•	•	•		
Cedar Crest College	•	•						
Chatham University	•	•				•		
Clarion University of Pennsylvania	•	•			•	•		
DeSales University	•	•	B,M	•	•	•		•
Drexel University	•	•	B		•	•		•
Duquesne University	•	•	B		•	•		•
Eastern University	•		B					
East Stroudsburg University of Pennsylvania	•							
Edinboro University of Pennsylvania	•		B					
Gannon University	•	•	M		•	•		
Gwynedd Mercy University	•	•	B		•			
Holy Family University	•	•	B,M		•			•
Immaculata University	•	•	B					
Indiana University of Pennsylvania	•	•				•		
La Roche College	•	•	B					•
La Salle University	•	•		•				
Lock Haven University of Pennsylvania	•		B					
Mansfield University of Pennsylvania	•	•						
Marywood University	•	•		•				•
Messiah College	•	•						
Millersville University of Pennsylvania	•	•			•			
Misericordia University	•	•	B		•			
Moravian College	•	•	B					
Mount Aloysius College	•		B					•
Neumann University	•	•	B		•			
Penn State University Park	•	•		•	•	•	•	•
Pennsylvania College of Health Sciences	•							

B = Baccalaureate; M = Masters

	Baccalaureate	Masters	Accelerated	Joint Degree	Post-Masters	Doctoral	Postdoctoral	Continuing Education
Pennsylvania College of Technology	•							
Robert Morris University	•	•				•		
Saint Francis University	•							
Slippery Rock University of Pennsylvania	•							
Temple University	•	•			•	•		•
Thomas Jefferson University	•	•	B,M		•	•		•
University of Pennsylvania	•	•	B,M	•	•	•	•	
University of Pittsburgh	•	•	B		•	•	•	•
University of Pittsburgh at Bradford	•							
The University of Scranton	•	•	M		•			
Villanova University	•	•	B		•	•		•
Waynesburg University	•	•	B,M	•		•		
West Chester University of Pennsylvania	•	•	B					
Widener University	•	•		•	•	•		
Wilkes University	•	•	B,M		•			•
York College of Pennsylvania	•	•			•	•		
Puerto Rico								
Inter American University of Puerto Rico, Aguadilla Campus	•							
Inter American University of Puerto Rico, Arecibo Campus	•	•						
Inter American University of Puerto Rico, Metropolitan Campus	•		B					
Pontifical Catholic University of Puerto Rico	•							
Universidad Adventista de las Antillas	•							•
Universidad del Turabo	•							
Universidad Metropolitana	•							
University of Puerto Rico in Arecibo	•							
University of Puerto Rico in Humacao	•							
University of Puerto Rico, Mayagüez Campus	•							•
University of Puerto Rico, Medical Sciences Campus	•	•						•
Rhode Island								
New England Institute of Technology	•							
Rhode Island College	•	•						
Salve Regina University	•							•
University of Rhode Island	•	•				•	•	
South Carolina								
Anderson University	•	•	B					
Charleston Southern University	•	•						
Clemson University	•	•	B		•			
Coastal Carolina University	•							
Francis Marion University	•							
Lander University	•		B					
Medical University of South Carolina	•	•	B			•		
Newberry College	•							
University of South Carolina	•	•	B,M		•	•	•	•
University of South Carolina Aiken	•							

B = Baccalaureate; M = Masters

	Baccalaureate	Masters	Accelerated	Joint Degree	Post-Masters	Doctoral	Postdoctoral	Continuing Education
University of South Carolina Beaufort	•							
University of South Carolina Upstate	•	•						
South Dakota								
Augustana University	•		B					
Dakota Wesleyan University	•							
Mount Marty College	•	•	B		•			
National American University	•							
Presentation College	•							
South Dakota State University	•	•	B		•	•		•
University of Sioux Falls	•		B					
The University of South Dakota	•							
Tennessee								
Aquinas College	•	•			•			
Austin Peay State University	•	•			•			
Baptist College of Health Sciences	•							
Belmont University	•	•	B		•	•		
Bethel University	•							
Carson-Newman University	•	•	B		•			
Christian Brothers University	•							
Cumberland University	•		B					
East Tennessee State University	•	•	B		•	•		•
Freed-Hardeman University	•							
King University	•	•	B,M	•				
Lincoln Memorial University	•	•	B		•			
Lipscomb University	•							
Martin Methodist College	•							
Middle Tennessee State University	•	•	M		•			
Milligan College	•							
South College	•							
Southern Adventist University	•	•	M	•	•	•		•
Tennessee State University	•	•			•			
Tennessee Technological University	•	•						
Tennessee Wesleyan College	•							
Union University	•	•	B		•			•
University of Memphis	•	•	B,M		•			
The University of Tennessee	•	•	B	•	•	•		•
The University of Tennessee at Chattanooga	•	•			•	•		
The University of Tennessee at Martin	•							
The University of Tennessee Health Science Center	•	•	B,M			•		•
Vanderbilt University		•		•	•	•	•	
Texas								
Abilene Christian University	•							
Angelo State University	•	•						
Baptist Health System School of Health Professions	•							

B = Baccalaureate; M = Masters

	Baccalaureate	Masters	Accelerated	Joint Degree	Post-Masters	Doctoral	Postdoctoral	Continuing Education
Baylor University	•	•	B				•	
Concordia University Texas	•	•	M					
East Texas Baptist University	•							
Houston Baptist University	•							
Lamar University	•	•		•	•			•
Lubbock Christian University	•							
Midwestern State University	•	•	B		•			•
Patty Hanks Shelton School of Nursing	•	•			•			•
Prairie View A&M University	•	•			•			
Sam Houston State University	•							
Schreiner University	•							
Southwestern Adventist University	•							
Stephen F. Austin State University	•							
Tarleton State University	•	•						•
Texas A&M Health Science Center	•	•	B,M					•
Texas A&M International University	•	•						
Texas A&M University–Commerce	•							
Texas A&M University–Corpus Christi	•	•	B		•			•
Texas A&M University–Texarkana	•	•						
Texas Christian University	•	•	B		•	•		•
Texas State University	•	•						
Texas Tech University Health Sciences Center	•	•	B		•	•		
Texas Tech University Health Sciences Center El Paso	•		B					
Texas Woman's University	•	•		•	•	•		
University of Houston	•	•	B					
University of Mary Hardin-Baylor	•	•			•			
University of St. Thomas	•							
The University of Texas at Arlington	•	•	B	•	•	•		
The University of Texas at Austin	•	•	M		•	•		
The University of Texas at Brownsville	•	•						•
The University of Texas at El Paso	•	•	B		•	•		
The University of Texas at Tyler	•	•	B,M	•	•	•		
The University of Texas Health Science Center at Houston	•	•		•	•	•		•
The University of Texas Health Science Center at San Antonio	•	•	B		•	•		•
The University of Texas Medical Branch	•	•	B		•	•		
The University of Texas Rio Grande Valley	•	•			•			
University of the Incarnate Word	•	•	M		•	•		
Wayland Baptist University	•							
West Texas A&M University	•	•			•			
Utah								
Brigham Young University	•	•						
Dixie State University	•							
Southern Utah University	•							

B = Baccalaureate; M = Masters

	Baccalaureate	Masters	Accelerated	Joint Degree	Post-Masters	Doctoral	Postdoctoral	Continuing Education
University of Phoenix–Utah Campus								
University of Utah	•	•			•	•	•	
Utah Valley University	•							
Weber State University	•	•			•			
Western Governors University	•	•	B,M					
Westminster College	•	•			•			
Vermont								
Castleton State College	•							
Norwich University	•							
Southern Vermont College	•							
University of Vermont	•	•			•	•		
Virgin Islands								
University of the Virgin Islands	•							
Virginia								
Bluefield College	•							
Bon Secours Memorial College of Nursing	•							
Eastern Mennonite University	•	•	B					
ECPI University	•							
George Mason University	•	•	B		•	•		•
Hampton University	•	•	B			•		
James Madison University	•	•				•		
Jefferson College of Health Sciences	•	•						•
Liberty University	•	•						
Longwood University	•							
Lynchburg College	•	•	B					
Marymount University	•	•	B		•	•		
Norfolk State University	•		B					
Old Dominion University	•	•			•	•		
Radford University	•	•			•	•		
Sentara College of Health Sciences	•							
Shenandoah University	•	•	B		•	•		•
Stratford University	•							
University of Virginia	•	•		•	•	•	•	
The University of Virginia's College at Wise	•							
Virginia Commonwealth University	•	•	B		•	•		
Washington								
Bellevue College	•							
Gonzaga University	•	•	M		•	•		
Northwest University	•							
Olympic College	•							
Pacific Lutheran University	•	•	M	•		•		•
Saint Martin's University	•							
Seattle Pacific University	•	•			•			

B = Baccalaureate; M = Masters

	Baccalaureate	Masters	Accelerated	Joint Degree	Post-Masters	Doctoral	Postdoctoral	Continuing Education
Seattle University	•	•	M		•	•		
University of Washington	•	•	B	•	•	•	•	•
Walla Walla University	•							
Western Washington University	•							
WSU College of Nursing	•	•	M		•	•		•
West Virginia								
Alderson Broaddus University	•							
American Public University System	•							
Bluefield State College	•							
Fairmont State University	•		B					•
Marshall University	•	•			•			
Shepherd University	•							•
University of Charleston	•							
West Liberty University	•		B					
West Virginia University	•	•	B,M		•	•		•
West Virginia Wesleyan College	•	•						
Wheeling Jesuit University	•	•	B		•			
Wisconsin								
Alverno College	•	•						•
Bellin College	•	•	B					
Cardinal Stritch University	•	•	B					
Carroll University	•							
Columbia College of Nursing	•	•						
Concordia University Wisconsin	•	•	M		•	•		
Edgewood College	•	•	B	•				
Herzing University Online	•	•						
Maranatha Baptist University	•							
Marian University	•	•			•			
Marquette University	•	•		•	•	•		
Milwaukee School of Engineering	•	•	B					•
Silver Lake College of the Holy Family	•							
University of Phoenix–Milwaukee Campus	•	•				•		
University of Wisconsin–Eau Claire	•	•	B		•	•		•
University of Wisconsin–Green Bay	•	•						
University of Wisconsin–Madison	•					•	•	•
University of Wisconsin–Milwaukee	•	•				•		
University of Wisconsin–Oshkosh	•	•	B		•	•		•
Viterbo University	•					•		
Wisconsin Lutheran College	•							•
Wyoming								
University of Wyoming	•	•	B		•	•		

B = Baccalaureate; M = Masters

	Baccalaureate	Masters	Accelerated	Joint Degree	Post-Masters	Doctoral	Postdoctoral	Continuing Education
CANADA								
Alberta								
Athabasca University	•	•			•			
University of Alberta	•	•	B		•	•		
University of Calgary	•	•	B		•	•		'
University of Lethbridge	•	•	B					
British Columbia								
British Columbia Institute of Technology	•							•
Kwantlen Polytechnic University	•		B					
Thompson Rivers University	•							•
Trinity Western University	•	•						
The University of British Columbia	•	•	B	•		•	•	
University of Northern British Columbia	•	•					•	
University of Victoria	•	•				•		
Vancouver Island University	•							•
Manitoba								
Brandon University	•	•						
University of Manitoba	•	•				•		
New Brunswick								
Université de Moncton	•	•						•
University of New Brunswick Fredericton	•	•	B					•
Newfoundland and Labrador								
Memorial University of Newfoundland	•	•	B		•	•		
Nova Scotia								
St. Francis Xavier University	•		B					•
Ontario								
Brock University	•							
Lakehead University	•		B					
Laurentian University	•	•						•
McMaster University	•	•		•		•		
Nipissing University	•							
Queen's University at Kingston	•	•	B			•		
Ryerson University	•	•						•
Trent University	•		B					
University of Ottawa	•	•	B			•	•	
University of Toronto	•	•	B		•	•	•	•
The University of Western Ontario	•	•	B			•	•	
University of Windsor	•	•			•			•
York University	•							•
Prince Edward Island								
University of Prince Edward Island	•							

B = Baccalaureate; M = Masters

	Baccalaureate	Masters	Accelerated	Joint Degree	Post-Masters	Doctoral	Postdoctoral	Continuing Education
Quebec								
McGill University	•	•	B			•	•	
Université de Montréal	•	•	M		•	•	•	•
Université de Sherbrooke	•	•				•	•	
Université du Québec à Chicoutimi	•	•	B					•
Université du Québec à Rimouski	•	•						•
Université du Québec à Trois-Rivières	•	•						
Université du Québec en Abitibi-Témiscamingue	•							
Université du Québec en Outaouais	•	•					•	•
Université Laval	•	•	B,M		•	•	•	•
Saskatchewan								
University of Saskatchewan	•	•	B		•	•		•

B = Baccalaureate; M = Masters

PROFILES OF NURSING PROGRAMS

ALABAMA

Auburn University

School of Nursing
Auburn University, Alabama

http://www.auburn.edu/academic/nursing/
Founded in 1856
DEGREES • BSN • MSN
Nursing Program Faculty 20 (50% with doctorates).
Baccalaureate Enrollment 279 **Women** 90% **Men** 10%
Graduate Enrollment 120 **Women** 96% **Men** 4% **Part-time** 80%
Nursing Student Activities Nursing Honor Society, Sigma Theta Tau, Student Nurses' Association.
Nursing Student Resources Academic advising; academic or career counseling; assistance for students with disabilities; bookstore; campus computer network; career placement assistance; computer lab; computer-assisted instruction; e-mail services; employment services for current students; interactive nursing skills videos; Internet; library services; nursing audiovisuals; placement services for program completers; remedial services; resume preparation assistance; skills, simulation, or other laboratory; tutoring.

BACCALAUREATE PROGRAMS

Degree BSN
Available Programs Generic Baccalaureate.
Study Options Full-time.
Program Entrance Requirements Minimum overall college GPA of 2.5, transcript of college record, CPR certification, health exam, health insurance, immunizations, interview, minimum GPA in nursing prerequisites of 2.5, professional liability insurance/malpractice insurance, prerequisite course work. Transfer students are accepted. *Application deadline:* 2/1 (fall), 5/1 (spring).
Expenses (2015–16) *Tuition, state resident:* full-time $10,424. *Tuition, nonresident:* full-time $28,040.
Contact Pam Hennessey, Academic Advisor, School of Nursing, Auburn University, 108 Miller Hall, Auburn University, AL 36849. *Telephone:* 334-844-5665. *Fax:* 334-844-4177. *E-mail:* hennepp@auburn.edu.

GRADUATE PROGRAMS

Expenses (2015–16) *Tuition, state resident:* part-time $599 per credit hour. *Tuition, nonresident:* part-time $599 per credit hour.
Contact Dr. Barbara Wilder, Director, MSN Program, School of Nursing, Auburn University, 118 Miller Hall, Auburn University, AL 36849. *Telephone:* 334-844-5665. *E-mail:* wildebf@auburn.edu.

MASTER'S DEGREE PROGRAM

Degree MSN
Available Programs Master's.
Concentrations Available Nursing education. *Clinical nurse specialist programs in:* family health. *Nurse practitioner programs in:* family health.
Study Options Full-time and part-time.
Program Entrance Requirements Minimum overall college GPA of 3.0, transcript of college record, immunizations, 3 letters of recommendation, nursing research course, professional liability insurance/malpractice insurance, statistics course. *Application deadline:* 6/1 (fall), 10/1 (spring), 3/1 (summer).
Degree Requirements 43 total credit hours, thesis or project.

Auburn University at Montgomery

School of Nursing
Montgomery, Alabama

http://www.nursing.aum.edu
Founded in 1967
DEGREES • BSN • MSN
Nursing Program Faculty 21 (52% with doctorates).
Baccalaureate Enrollment 648 **Women** 80% **Men** 20% **Part-time** 20%
Nursing Student Activities Nursing Honor Society, Sigma Theta Tau, Student Nurses' Association.
Nursing Student Resources Academic advising; academic or career counseling; assistance for students with disabilities; bookstore; campus computer network; career placement assistance; computer lab; computer-assisted instruction; e-mail services; housing assistance; interactive nursing skills videos; Internet; learning resource lab; library services; nursing audiovisuals; remedial services; resume preparation assistance; skills, simulation, or other laboratory; tutoring.
Library Facilities 6,608 volumes in health, 4,900 volumes in nursing; 479 periodical subscriptions health-care related.

BACCALAUREATE PROGRAMS

Degree BSN
Available Programs ADN to Baccalaureate; Baccalaureate for Second Degree; Generic Baccalaureate; RN Baccalaureate.
Study Options Full-time.
Program Entrance Requirements Transcript of college record, CPR certification, health exam, health insurance, high school transcript, immunizations, interview, minimum GPA in nursing prerequisites of 2.5, professional liability insurance/malpractice insurance, prerequisite course work. Transfer students are accepted. *Application deadline:* 2/1 (fall), 5/1 (spring).
Financial Aid *Gift aid (need-based):* Federal Pell, FSEOG, state, college/university gift aid from institutional funds. *Loans:* Federal Direct (Subsidized and Unsubsidized Stafford PLUS), Perkins. *Work-study:* Federal Work-Study. *Financial aid application deadline (priority):* 3/1.
Contact Mrs. Kris W. Conner, Advising and Recruiting Manager, School of Nursing, Auburn University at Montgomery, PO Box 244023, Montgomery, AL 36124-4023. *Telephone:* 334-244-3431. *Fax:* 334-244-3243. *E-mail:* kconner4@aum.edu.

GRADUATE PROGRAMS

Financial Aid 10% of graduate students in nursing programs received some form of financial aid in 2014–15.
Contact Dr. Donna Beuk, Administrator, EARN Program, School of Nursing, Auburn University at Montgomery, 325A Moore Hall, Montgomery, AL 36124. *Telephone:* 334-244-3953. *Fax:* 334-244-3243. *E-mail:* dbeuk@aum.edu.

MASTER'S DEGREE PROGRAM

Degree MSN
Available Programs Master's.
Concentrations Available Nursing education. *Clinical nurse specialist programs in:* adult health, gerontology, pediatric. *Nurse practitioner programs in:* primary care.
Study Options Full-time and part-time.
Program Entrance Requirements Clinical experience, minimum overall college GPA of 3.0, written essay, 3 letters of recommendation, resume, statistics course. *Application deadline:* 6/1 (fall), 10/1 (spring), 3/1 (summer).
Advanced Placement Credit given for nursing courses completed elsewhere dependent upon specific evaluations.
Degree Requirements 42 total credit hours, thesis or project, comprehensive exam.

Jacksonville State University
College of Nursing and Health Sciences
Jacksonville, Alabama

http://www.jsu.edu/nursing/
Founded in 1883
DEGREES • BSN • MSN
Nursing Program Faculty 34 (38% with doctorates).
Baccalaureate Enrollment 459 **Women** 82% **Men** 18% **Part-time** 19%
Graduate Enrollment 54 **Women** 96% **Men** 4% **Part-time** 81%
Distance Learning Courses Available.
Nursing Student Activities Sigma Theta Tau, Student Nurses' Association.
Nursing Student Resources Academic advising; academic or career counseling; assistance for students with disabilities; campus computer network; computer lab; computer-assisted instruction; e-mail services; employment services for current students; externships; interactive nursing skills videos; Internet; learning resource lab; library services; nursing audiovisuals; remedial services; resume preparation assistance; skills, simulation, or other laboratory; tutoring.
Library Facilities 23,409 volumes in health, 1,633 volumes in nursing; 7,852 periodical subscriptions health-care related.

BACCALAUREATE PROGRAMS

Degree BSN
Available Programs Generic Baccalaureate; RN Baccalaureate.
Study Options Full-time and part-time.
Online Degree Options Yes.
Program Entrance Requirements Transcript of college record, CPR certification, health exam, health insurance, high school transcript, immunizations, minimum GPA in nursing prerequisites, professional liability insurance/malpractice insurance, prerequisite course work. Transfer students are accepted. *Application deadline:* 6/1 (fall), 10/1 (spring).
Expenses (2015–16) *Tuition, area resident:* full-time $7200; part-time $300 per credit hour. *Tuition, state resident:* full-time $8688; part-time $362 per credit hour. *Tuition, nonresident:* full-time $14,400; part-time $600 per credit hour. *International tuition:* $14,400 full-time. *Room and board:* $6900; room only: $3930 per academic year. *Required fees:* full-time $700; part-time $350 per term.
Financial Aid 70% of baccalaureate students in nursing programs received some form of financial aid in 2014–15.
Contact Ms. Kristi Killingsworth, Director, Student Services for BSN, College of Nursing and Health Sciences, Jacksonville State University, 700 Pelham Road North, Jacksonville, AL 36265-1602. *Telephone:* 256-782-5276. *Fax:* 256-782-5406. *E-mail:* killingsworth@jsu.edu.

GRADUATE PROGRAMS

Expenses (2015–16) *Tuition, state resident:* full-time $8298; part-time $461 per credit hour. *Tuition, nonresident:* full-time $8298; part-time $461 per credit hour. *International tuition:* $8298 full-time. *Room and board:* $6900; room only: $3930 per academic year. *Required fees:* full-time $300; part-time $150 per term.
Financial Aid 60% of graduate students in nursing programs received some form of financial aid in 2014–15.
Contact Dr. Rebecca D. Peinhardt, Director, Graduate Nursing Programs, College of Nursing and Health Sciences, Jacksonville State University, 700 Pelham Road North, Jacksonville, AL 36265-1602. *Telephone:* 256-782-5960. *Fax:* 256-782-5406. *E-mail:* rpeinhardt@jsu.edu.

MASTER'S DEGREE PROGRAM

Degree MSN
Available Programs Master's.
Concentrations Available *Clinical nurse specialist programs in:* community health.
Study Options Full-time and part-time.
Online Degree Options Yes (online only).
Program Entrance Requirements Minimum overall college GPA of 3.0, transcript of college record, written essay, interview, 3 letters of recommendation, nursing research course, physical assessment course, statistics course. *Application deadline:* Applications may be processed on a rolling basis for some programs.
Advanced Placement Credit given for nursing courses completed elsewhere dependent upon specific evaluations.
Degree Requirements 36 total credit hours, thesis or project, comprehensive exam.

CONTINUING EDUCATION PROGRAM

Contact Ms. Kristi Killingsworth, Director, Student Services for BSN, College of Nursing and Health Sciences, Jacksonville State University, 700 Pelham Road North, Jacksonville, AL 36265-1602. *Telephone:* 256-782-5276. *Fax:* 256-782-5406. *E-mail:* killingsworth@jsu.edu.

Oakwood University
Department of Nursing
Huntsville, Alabama

http://www.oakwood.edu/academics/academic-departments/nursing
Founded in 1896
DEGREE • BS
Nursing Program Faculty 10 (33% with doctorates).
Baccalaureate Enrollment 85 **Women** 90% **Men** 10%
Nursing Student Activities Nursing club.
Nursing Student Resources Academic advising; academic or career counseling; assistance for students with disabilities; bookstore; campus computer network; computer lab; computer-assisted instruction; e-mail services; interactive nursing skills videos; Internet; learning resource lab; library services; nursing audiovisuals; remedial services; skills, simulation, or other laboratory; tutoring; unpaid internships.
Library Facilities 5,147 volumes in health, 3,474 volumes in nursing; 47 periodical subscriptions health-care related.

BACCALAUREATE PROGRAMS

Degree BS
Available Programs Generic Baccalaureate; RN Baccalaureate.
Study Options Full-time and part-time.
Program Entrance Requirements Minimum overall college GPA of 3.0, transcript of college record, CPR certification, written essay, health exam, health insurance, high school transcript, immunizations, interview, 3 letters of recommendation, minimum high school GPA of 3.0, minimum GPA in nursing prerequisites of 3.0, prerequisite course work. Transfer students are accepted. *Application deadline:* 1/16 (fall), 1/15 (winter).
Contact *Telephone:* 256-726-7287. *Fax:* 256-726-8338.

Samford University
Ida V. Moffett School of Nursing
Birmingham, Alabama

http://www.samford.edu/nursing/
Founded in 1841
DEGREES • BSN • DNP • MSN
Nursing Program Faculty 54 (55% with doctorates).
Baccalaureate Enrollment 422 **Women** 91% **Men** 9% **Part-time** 8%
Graduate Enrollment 323 **Women** 80% **Men** 20% **Part-time** 11%
Distance Learning Courses Available.
Nursing Student Activities Nursing Honor Society, Sigma Theta Tau, Student Nurses' Association, nursing club.
Nursing Student Resources Academic advising; academic or career counseling; assistance for students with disabilities; bookstore; campus computer network; career placement assistance; computer lab; computer-assisted instruction; e-mail services; employment services for current students; externships; housing assistance; interactive nursing skills videos; Internet; learning resource lab; library services; nursing audiovisuals; paid internships; remedial services; resume preparation assistance; skills, simulation, or other laboratory; tutoring; unpaid internships.
Library Facilities 6,376 volumes in health, 805 volumes in nursing; 2,342 periodical subscriptions health-care related.

BACCALAUREATE PROGRAMS

Degree BSN
Available Programs Accelerated Baccalaureate for Second Degree; Baccalaureate for Second Degree; Generic Baccalaureate.
Site Options Birmingham, AL.
Study Options Full-time and part-time.
Program Entrance Requirements Minimum overall college GPA of 3.0, transcript of college record, CPR certification, written essay, health exam, health insurance, high school biology, high school chemistry, 2 years high school math, 2 years high school science, high school tran-

script, immunizations, minimum high school GPA of 3.0, minimum GPA in nursing prerequisites of 2.0, prerequisite course work. Transfer students are accepted. *Application deadline:* 5/1 (fall). Applications may be processed on a rolling basis for some programs. *Application fee:* $40.
Advanced Placement Credit given for nursing courses completed elsewhere dependent upon specific evaluations.
Expenses (2015–16) *Tuition:* full-time $27,520; part-time $920 per credit. *International tuition:* $27,520 full-time. *Room and board:* $9400; room only: $4860 per academic year. *Required fees:* full-time $850; part-time $650 per term.
Contact Mrs. Trisha W. Stovall, Admissions Counselor, School of Nursing, Ida V. Moffett School of Nursing, Samford University, 800 Lakeshore Drive, Birmingham, AL 35229. *Telephone:* 205-726-2264. *Fax:* 205-726-4269. *E-mail:* pstovall@samford.edu.

GRADUATE PROGRAMS

Financial Aid Institutionally sponsored loans, scholarships, and traineeships available.
Contact Mrs. Allyson Maddox, Director, Graduate Student Services, Ida V. Moffett School of Nursing, Samford University, 800 Lakeshore Drive, Birmingham, AL 35229. *Telephone:* 205-726-2047. *Fax:* 205-726-4235. *E-mail:* amaddox@samford.edu.

MASTER'S DEGREE PROGRAM
Degree MSN
Available Programs Master's; RN to Master's.
Concentrations Available Nurse anesthesia; nursing administration; nursing education. *Nurse practitioner programs in:* family health.
Site Options Birmingham, AL.
Study Options Full-time and part-time.
Online Degree Options Yes.
Program Entrance Requirements Clinical experience, computer literacy, minimum overall college GPA of 3.0, transcript of college record, CPR certification, immunizations, interview, 3 letters of recommendation, nursing research course, physical assessment course, professional liability insurance/malpractice insurance, prerequisite course work, MAT; GRE (for nurse anesthesia). *Application deadline:* 6/1 (fall), 9/1 (spring). Applications may be processed on a rolling basis for some programs. *Application fee:* $65.
Advanced Placement Credit given for nursing courses completed elsewhere dependent upon specific evaluations.
Degree Requirements 38 total credit hours, thesis or project.

POST-MASTER'S PROGRAM
Areas of Study *Nurse practitioner programs in:* family health.

DOCTORAL DEGREE PROGRAM
Degree DNP
Available Programs Doctorate.
Areas of Study Advanced practice nursing, nursing administration.
Site Options Birmingham, AL.
Online Degree Options Yes (online only).
Program Entrance Requirements Clinical experience, minimum overall college GPA of 3.5, interview by faculty committee, interview, 3 letters of recommendation, MSN or equivalent, vita, writing sample. Application deadline: 9/1 (spring), 2/1 (summer). Applications may be processed on a rolling basis for some programs. Application fee: $65.
Degree Requirements 38 total credit hours, oral exam, residency.

CONTINUING EDUCATION PROGRAM

Contact Mrs. Suzanne Scharf, Continuing Education Coordinator, Ida V. Moffett School of Nursing, Samford University, 800 Lakeshore Drive, Birmingham, AL 35229. *Telephone:* 205-726-2045. *Fax:* 205-726-2219. *E-mail:* shscharf@samford.edu.

Spring Hill College
Division of Nursing
Mobile, Alabama

http://www.shc.edu/
Founded in 1830
DEGREES • BSN • MSN
Nursing Program Faculty 8 (84% with doctorates).
Baccalaureate Enrollment 124 **Women** 86% **Men** 14%
Graduate Enrollment 62 **Women** 95% **Men** 5% **Part-time** 40%
Distance Learning Courses Available.

Nursing Student Activities Nursing Honor Society, Sigma Theta Tau, Student Nurses' Association.
Nursing Student Resources Academic advising; academic or career counseling; assistance for students with disabilities; bookstore; campus computer network; career placement assistance; computer lab; computer-assisted instruction; e-mail services; employment services for current students; externships; interactive nursing skills videos; Internet; learning resource lab; library services; nursing audiovisuals; placement services for program completers; resume preparation assistance; skills, simulation, or other laboratory; tutoring; unpaid internships.
Library Facilities 330 volumes in health, 300 volumes in nursing; 58 periodical subscriptions health-care related.

BACCALAUREATE PROGRAMS

Degree BSN
Available Programs Baccalaureate for Second Degree; Generic Baccalaureate.
Study Options Full-time.
Program Entrance Requirements Minimum overall college GPA of 2.75, transcript of college record, CPR certification, written essay, health exam, health insurance, high school transcript, immunizations, 1 letter of recommendation, minimum GPA in nursing prerequisites of 2.75, prerequisite course work. Transfer students are accepted. *Application deadline:* 3/1 (spring).
Advanced Placement Credit by examination available.
Contact *Telephone:* 334-380-4492. *Fax:* 334-380-4495.

GRADUATE PROGRAMS

Contact *Telephone:* 251-380-3067. *Fax:* 251-460-2190.

MASTER'S DEGREE PROGRAM
Degree MSN
Available Programs Accelerated AD/RN to Master's; Master's; RN to Master's.
Concentrations Available Clinical nurse leader.
Study Options Full-time and part-time.
Online Degree Options Yes (online only).
Program Entrance Requirements Clinical experience, minimum overall college GPA of 3.0, transcript of college record, immunizations, professional liability insurance/malpractice insurance, prerequisite course work, resume, statistics course. *Application deadline:* Applications may be processed on a rolling basis for some programs.
Advanced Placement Credit by examination available. Credit given for nursing courses completed elsewhere dependent upon specific evaluations.
Degree Requirements 36 total credit hours, thesis or project.

Troy University
School of Nursing
Troy, Alabama

http://www.troy.edu/
Founded in 1887
DEGREES • BSN • DNP • MSN
Nursing Program Faculty 39 (49% with doctorates).
Baccalaureate Enrollment 800 **Women** 88% **Men** 12% **Part-time** 10%
Graduate Enrollment 200 **Women** 97% **Men** 3% **Part-time** 29%
Distance Learning Courses Available.
Nursing Student Activities Sigma Theta Tau, Student Nurses' Association.
Nursing Student Resources Academic advising; academic or career counseling; assistance for students with disabilities; bookstore; campus computer network; career placement assistance; computer lab; computer-assisted instruction; e-mail services; employment services for current students; externships; housing assistance; interactive nursing skills videos; Internet; learning resource lab; library services; nursing audiovisuals; placement services for program completers; resume preparation assistance; skills, simulation, or other laboratory; tutoring; unpaid internships.
Library Facilities 45,006 volumes in health, 3,843 volumes in nursing; 703 periodical subscriptions health-care related.

BACCALAUREATE PROGRAMS

Degree BSN
Available Programs Generic Baccalaureate; RN Baccalaureate.
Site Options Montgomery, AL; Phenix City, AL; Dothan, AL.
Study Options Full-time.

Program Entrance Requirements Minimum overall college GPA of 2.5, transcript of college record, CPR certification, health exam, health insurance, immunizations, professional liability insurance/malpractice insurance, prerequisite course work. Transfer students are accepted. *Application deadline:* 3/15 (fall), 9/15 (spring). *Application fee:* $20.
Advanced Placement Credit by examination available. Credit given for nursing courses completed elsewhere dependent upon specific evaluations.
Contact *Telephone:* 334-670-3428. *Fax:* 334-670-3744.

GRADUATE PROGRAMS

Contact *Telephone:* 334-834-2320. *Fax:* 334-241-8627.

MASTER'S DEGREE PROGRAM
Degree MSN
Available Programs Master's.
Concentrations Available Nursing administration; nursing education; nursing informatics. *Clinical nurse specialist programs in:* adult health, maternity-newborn. *Nurse practitioner programs in:* family health.
Site Options Montgomery, AL; Phenix City, AL.
Study Options Full-time and part-time.
Online Degree Options Yes.
Program Entrance Requirements Minimum overall college GPA of 3.0, transcript of college record, CPR certification, immunizations, 3 letters of recommendation, physical assessment course, professional liability insurance/malpractice insurance. *Application deadline:* Applications may be processed on a rolling basis for some programs. *Application fee:* $20.
Advanced Placement Credit given for nursing courses completed elsewhere dependent upon specific evaluations.
Degree Requirements 39 total credit hours, thesis or project, comprehensive exam.

POST-MASTER'S PROGRAM
Areas of Study *Nurse practitioner programs in:* family health.

DOCTORAL DEGREE PROGRAM
Degree DNP
Available Programs Doctorate; Post-Baccalaureate Doctorate.
Areas of Study Advanced practice nursing.
Site Options Montgomery, AL; Phenix City, AL.
Online Degree Options Yes (online only).
Program Entrance Requirements Clinical experience, minimum overall college GPA of 3.0, interview by faculty committee, 2 letters of recommendation, MSN or equivalent, vita, writing sample. Application deadline: 2/1 (fall). Application fee: $75.
Degree Requirements 74 total credit hours, oral exam, residency.

Tuskegee University
Program in Nursing
Tuskegee, Alabama

http://www.tuskegee.edu/nah
Founded in 1881
DEGREE • BSN
Nursing Program Faculty 9 (33% with doctorates).
Baccalaureate Enrollment 145 **Women** 99% **Men** 1%
Nursing Student Activities Nursing Honor Society, Student Nurses' Association, nursing club.
Nursing Student Resources Academic advising; academic or career counseling; assistance for students with disabilities; bookstore; campus computer network; career placement assistance; computer lab; computer-assisted instruction; e-mail services; interactive nursing skills videos; Internet; learning resource lab; library services; nursing audiovisuals; placement services for program completers; remedial services; resume preparation assistance; skills, simulation, or other laboratory; tutoring; unpaid internships.
Library Facilities 4,500 volumes in health, 600 volumes in nursing; 250 periodical subscriptions health-care related.

BACCALAUREATE PROGRAMS

Degree BSN
Available Programs ADN to Baccalaureate; Generic Baccalaureate; RN Baccalaureate.
Study Options Full-time and part-time.

Program Entrance Requirements Minimum overall college GPA of 3.0, transcript of college record, CPR certification, written essay, health exam, health insurance, high school biology, high school chemistry, 2 years high school math, 1 year of high school science, high school transcript, immunizations, interview, minimum high school GPA of 3.0, minimum GPA in nursing prerequisites of 3.0, professional liability insurance/malpractice insurance, prerequisite course work. Transfer students are accepted. *Application deadline:* 5/30 (fall), 11/30 (spring), 4/30 (summer). Applications may be processed on a rolling basis for some programs. *Application fee:* $35.
Expenses (2015–16) *Tuition:* full-time $18,560; part-time $2055 per credit hour. *International tuition:* $18,560 full-time. *Room and board:* $11,304; room only: $5480 per academic year. *Required fees:* full-time $1605; part-time $802 per term.
Financial Aid 90% of baccalaureate students in nursing programs received some form of financial aid in 2014–15.
Contact Dr. Doris S. Holeman, Associate Dean and Director, Program in Nursing, Tuskegee University, 209 Basil O'Connor Hall, Tuskegee, AL 36083. *Telephone:* 334-727-8382. *Fax:* 334-727-5461. *E-mail:* dholeman@tuskegee.edu.

The University of Alabama
Capstone College of Nursing
Tuscaloosa, Alabama

http://nursing.ua.edu/
Founded in 1831
DEGREES • BSN • DNP • MSN • MSN/ED D
Nursing Program Faculty 70 (75% with doctorates).
Baccalaureate Enrollment 1,721 **Women** 90% **Men** 10% **Part-time** 6%
Graduate Enrollment 322 **Women** 85% **Men** 15% **Part-time** 60%
Distance Learning Courses Available.
Nursing Student Activities Sigma Theta Tau, Student Nurses' Association.
Nursing Student Resources Academic advising; academic or career counseling; assistance for students with disabilities; bookstore; campus computer network; career placement assistance; computer lab; computer-assisted instruction; e-mail services; interactive nursing skills videos; Internet; learning resource lab; library services; paid internships; placement services for program completers; skills, simulation, or other laboratory; tutoring; unpaid internships.
Library Facilities 21,000 volumes in health, 350 volumes in nursing; 1,500 periodical subscriptions health-care related.

BACCALAUREATE PROGRAMS

Degree BSN
Available Programs Baccalaureate for Second Degree; Generic Baccalaureate; RN Baccalaureate.
Study Options Full-time.
Program Entrance Requirements Minimum overall college GPA of 3.0, transcript of college record, CPR certification, health exam, health insurance, 4 years high school math, 4 years high school science, high school transcript, immunizations, minimum high school GPA of 2.5, minimum GPA in nursing prerequisites of 3.0, professional liability insurance/malpractice insurance, prerequisite course work. Transfer students are accepted. *Application deadline:* 6/1 (fall), 3/1 (summer). *Application fee:* $40.
Expenses (2015–16) *Tuition, state resident:* full-time $10,170; part-time $770 per credit hour. *Tuition, nonresident:* full-time $25,950; part-time $1455 per credit hour. *Room and board:* $12,880; room only: $8800 per academic year. *Required fees:* full-time $800; part-time $400 per term.
Financial Aid 80% of baccalaureate students in nursing programs received some form of financial aid in 2014–15.
Contact Ms. Rebekah Welch, Director of Nursing Student Services, Capstone College of Nursing, The University of Alabama, Box 870358, Tuscaloosa, AL 35487-0358. *Telephone:* 205-348-6639. *Fax:* 205-348-6589. *E-mail:* rebekah.welch@ua.edu.

GRADUATE PROGRAMS

Expenses (2015–16) *Tuition, state resident:* part-time $360 per credit hour. *Tuition, nonresident:* part-time $360 per credit hour. *Required fees:* part-time $400 per term.
Financial Aid 48% of graduate students in nursing programs received some form of financial aid in 2014–15.
Contact Dr. Alice March, Assistant Dean, Graduate Program, Capstone College of Nursing, The University of Alabama, Box 870358,

Tuscaloosa, AL 35487-0358. *Telephone:* 205-348-1020. *Fax:* 205-348-6674. *E-mail:* almarch@ua.edu.

MASTER'S DEGREE PROGRAM
Degrees MSN; MSN/Ed D
Available Programs Master's; RN to Master's.
Concentrations Available Clinical nurse leader; nurse case management; nursing education. *Nurse practitioner programs in:* family health, psychiatric/mental health.
Study Options Full-time and part-time.
Online Degree Options Yes (online only).
Program Entrance Requirements Computer literacy, minimum overall college GPA of 3.0, transcript of college record, CPR certification, written essay, immunizations, 2 letters of recommendation, professional liability insurance/malpractice insurance, resume. *Application deadline:* 6/1 (fall). *Application fee:* $50.
Degree Requirements 38 total credit hours.

POST-MASTER'S PROGRAM
Areas of Study Clinical nurse leader; nurse case management.

DOCTORAL DEGREE PROGRAM
Degree DNP
Available Programs Doctorate.
Areas of Study Individualized study.
Online Degree Options Yes (online only).
Program Entrance Requirements Minimum overall college GPA of 3.0, interview by faculty committee, interview, 3 letters of recommendation, MSN or equivalent, vita, writing sample. Application deadline: 4/1 (fall). Applications may be processed on a rolling basis for some programs. Application fee: $50.
Degree Requirements 40 total credit hours.

The University of Alabama at Birmingham
School of Nursing
Birmingham, Alabama

http://www.uab.edu/nursing
Founded in 1969

DEGREES • BSN • DNP • MSN • MSN/MPH • PHD
Nursing Program Faculty 127 (71% with doctorates).
Baccalaureate Enrollment 547 **Women** 84% **Men** 16% **Part-time** 39.9%
Graduate Enrollment 1,545 **Women** 85% **Men** 15% **Part-time** 66%
Distance Learning Courses Available.
Nursing Student Activities Sigma Theta Tau.
Nursing Student Resources Academic advising; academic or career counseling; assistance for students with disabilities; bookstore; campus computer network; career placement assistance; computer lab; computer-assisted instruction; e-mail services; housing assistance; interactive nursing skills videos; Internet; learning resource lab; library services; nursing audiovisuals; paid internships; placement services for program completers; resume preparation assistance; skills, simulation, or other laboratory; tutoring.
Library Facilities 109,021 volumes in health, 5,746 volumes in nursing; 22,555 periodical subscriptions health-care related.

BACCALAUREATE PROGRAMS
Degree BSN
Available Programs ADN to Baccalaureate; Baccalaureate for Second Degree; Generic Baccalaureate; RN Baccalaureate.
Study Options Full-time.
Program Entrance Requirements Minimum overall college GPA of 2.75, transcript of college record, CPR certification, written essay, health exam, health insurance, high school transcript, immunizations, minimum high school GPA of 2.75, minimum GPA in nursing prerequisites of 2.75, prerequisite course work. Transfer students are accepted. *Application deadline:* 4/8 (fall), 9/11 (spring). *Application fee:* $30.
Expenses (2015–16) *Tuition, state resident:* full-time $12,536. *Tuition, nonresident:* full-time $28,673. *Room and board:* room only: $5900 per academic year. *Required fees:* full-time $2062.
Financial Aid 55% of baccalaureate students in nursing programs received some form of financial aid in 2014–15. *Gift aid (need-based):* Federal Pell, FSEOG, state, private, college/university gift aid from insti-

tutional funds, United Negro College Fund. *Loans:* Federal Direct (Subsidized and Unsubsidized Stafford PLUS), Perkins, state, college/university. *Work-study:* Federal Work-Study. *Financial aid application deadline (priority):* 3/1.
Contact Mr. Peter Tofani, Assistant Dean for Student Affairs, School of Nursing, The University of Alabama at Birmingham, NB 1003, 1720 2nd Avenue South, Birmingham, AL 35294-1210. *Telephone:* 205-975-7529. *Fax:* 205-934-5490. *E-mail:* tofanip@uab.edu.

GRADUATE PROGRAMS
Expenses (2015–16) *Tuition, state resident:* full-time $11,515. *Tuition, nonresident:* full-time $11,515. *Required fees:* full-time $2762.
Financial Aid 58% of graduate students in nursing programs received some form of financial aid in 2014–15. Fellowships, research assistantships, teaching assistantships available.
Contact Ms. Charlene Bender, Program Manager II, School of Nursing, The University of Alabama at Birmingham, NB 1002A, 1720 2nd Avenue South, Birmingham, AL 35294-1210. *Telephone:* 205-975-7529. *Fax:* 205-934-5490. *E-mail:* cbender@uab.edu.

MASTER'S DEGREE PROGRAM
Degrees MSN; MSN/MPH
Available Programs Accelerated AD/RN to Master's; Accelerated Master's for Non-Nursing College Graduates; Master's; Master's for Non-Nursing College Graduates; Master's for Nurses with Non-Nursing Degrees; RN to Master's.
Concentrations Available Clinical nurse leader; nurse anesthesia; nursing administration; nursing education; nursing informatics. *Nurse practitioner programs in:* adult-gerontology acute care, family health, neonatal health, occupational health, oncology, pediatric primary care, psychiatric/mental health, women's health.
Program Entrance Requirements Clinical experience, computer literacy, minimum overall college GPA of 3.0, transcript of college record, CPR certification, written essay, immunizations, 3 letters of recommendation, prerequisite course work, resume, statistics course, GRE, GMAT, or MAT. *Application deadline:* 2/29 (fall), 11/2 (summer). *Application fee:* $65.
Advanced Placement Credit given for nursing courses completed elsewhere dependent upon specific evaluations.
Degree Requirements 45 total credit hours, comprehensive exam.

DOCTORAL DEGREE PROGRAM
Degree DNP
Available Programs Doctorate.
Areas of Study Advanced practice nursing, health-care systems, nursing administration.
Program Entrance Requirements Minimum overall college GPA of 3.0, clinical experience, 3 letters of recommendation, statistics course, vita, writing sample. Application deadline: 1/18 (fall). Application fee: $45.
Degree Requirements 66 total credit hours, dissertation, residency, written exam.

Degree PhD
Available Programs Doctorate; Post-Baccalaureate Doctorate.
Areas of Study Nursing research, nursing science.
Program Entrance Requirements Clinical experience, minimum overall college GPA of 3.0, interview by faculty committee, interview, 3 letters of recommendation, scholarly papers, statistics course, vita, writing sample, GRE General Test. Application deadline: 1/15 (fall), 3/15 (summer). Application fee: $65.
Degree Requirements 74 total credit hours, dissertation, oral exam, written exam, residency.

POSTDOCTORAL PROGRAM
Areas of Study Nursing research, nursing science.
Postdoctoral Program Contact Dr. Karen Heaton, PhD Program Coordinator, Assoc Prof Nursing, School of Nursing, The University of Alabama at Birmingham, 1720 2nd Avenue South, Birmingham, AL 35294-1210. *Telephone:* 205-996-9467. *Fax:* 205-934-5490. *E-mail:* kharnp@uab.edu.

CONTINUING EDUCATION PROGRAM
Contact Dr. Joy Deupree, Assistant Professor and Director of Professional Development, School of Nursing, The University of Alabama at Birmingham, School of Nursing, 1720 2nd Avenue South, Birmingham, AL 35294-1210. *Telephone:* 205-934-6487. *Fax:* 205-996-6585. *E-mail:* deupreej@uab.edu.

The University of Alabama in Huntsville
College of Nursing
Huntsville, Alabama

http://www.uah.edu/nursing/
Founded in 1950
DEGREES • BSN • DNP • MSN
Nursing Program Faculty 58 (43% with doctorates).
Baccalaureate Enrollment 726 **Women** 85% **Men** 15% **Part-time** 11%
Graduate Enrollment 371 **Women** 83% **Men** 17% **Part-time** 75%
Distance Learning Courses Available.
Nursing Student Activities Sigma Theta Tau, Student Nurses' Association.
Nursing Student Resources Academic advising; academic or career counseling; assistance for students with disabilities; bookstore; campus computer network; career placement assistance; computer lab; computer-assisted instruction; daycare for children of students; e-mail services; employment services for current students; housing assistance; interactive nursing skills videos; Internet; learning resource lab; library services; nursing audiovisuals; placement services for program completers; remedial services; resume preparation assistance; skills, simulation, or other laboratory; tutoring.
Library Facilities 13,004 volumes in health, 3,480 volumes in nursing; 3,200 periodical subscriptions health-care related.

BACCALAUREATE PROGRAMS

Degree BSN
Available Programs Baccalaureate for Second Degree; Generic Baccalaureate; RN Baccalaureate.
Study Options Full-time.
Program Entrance Requirements Minimum overall college GPA of 3.0, transcript of college record, CPR certification, health exam, health insurance, immunizations, minimum GPA in nursing prerequisites of 3.0, professional liability insurance/malpractice insurance, prerequisite course work. Transfer students are accepted. *Application deadline:* 3/1 (fall), 6/15 (spring). *Application fee:* $30.
Advanced Placement Credit by examination available.
Expenses (2015–16) *Tuition, state resident:* full-time $9604; part-time $453 per credit hour. *Tuition, nonresident:* full-time $21,870; part-time $1041 per credit hour. *International tuition:* $21,870 full-time. *Room and board:* $8720; room only: $5800 per academic year. *Required fees:* full-time $768; part-time $42 per credit.
Financial Aid 92% of baccalaureate students in nursing programs received some form of financial aid in 2014–15.
Contact Mrs. Laura Mann, Director, Nursing Undergraduate Programs, College of Nursing, The University of Alabama in Huntsville, 207 Nursing Building, Huntsville, AL 35899. *Telephone:* 256-824-6742. *Fax:* 256-824-2850. *E-mail:* laura.mann@uah.edu.

GRADUATE PROGRAMS

Expenses (2015–16) *Tuition, state resident:* full-time $9548; part-time $675 per credit hour. *Tuition, nonresident:* full-time $21,402; part-time $1500 per credit hour. *International tuition:* $21,402 full-time. *Room and board:* $6140; room only: $5160 per academic year. *Required fees:* full-time $768; part-time $42 per credit.
Financial Aid 72% of graduate students in nursing programs received some form of financial aid in 2014–15. 19 teaching assistantships with full tuition reimbursements available (averaging $7,876 per year) were awarded; career-related internships or fieldwork, Federal Work-Study, institutionally sponsored loans, scholarships, traineeships, and unspecified assistantships also available. Aid available to part-time students. *Financial aid application deadline:* 4/1.
Contact Mr. Charles Davis, Director of Nursing Graduate Program Student Affairs, College of Nursing, The University of Alabama in Huntsville, Huntsville, AL 35899. *Telephone:* 256-824-6742. *Fax:* 256-824-6026. *E-mail:* charles.davis@uah.edu.

MASTER'S DEGREE PROGRAM
Degree MSN
Available Programs Master's; RN to Master's.
Concentrations Available Health-care administration. *Clinical nurse specialist programs in:* adult health. *Nurse practitioner programs in:* adult-gerontology acute care, family health.
Study Options Full-time and part-time.
Online Degree Options Yes.

Program Entrance Requirements Minimum overall college GPA of 3.2, transcript of college record, CPR certification, immunizations, 3 letters of recommendation, professional liability insurance/malpractice insurance, statistics course, MAT or GRE. *Application deadline:* 4/1 (fall). *Application fee:* $60.
Advanced Placement Credit given for nursing courses completed elsewhere dependent upon specific evaluations.
Degree Requirements 42 total credit hours, thesis or project, comprehensive exam.

POST-MASTER'S PROGRAM
Areas of Study Nursing education. *Nurse practitioner programs in:* adult-gerontology acute care, family health.

DOCTORAL DEGREE PROGRAM
Degree DNP
Available Programs Doctorate.
Areas of Study Advanced practice nursing, health-care systems, nursing administration.
Online Degree Options Yes (online only).
Program Entrance Requirements Minimum overall college GPA of 3.2, interview by faculty committee, 2 letters of recommendation, MSN or equivalent, vita, writing sample. Application deadline: 4/15 (fall), 11/1 (spring), 4/1 (summer). Application fee: $60.
Degree Requirements 40 total credit hours, dissertation, oral exam, written exam.

CONTINUING EDUCATION PROGRAM

Contact Dr. Marsha Howell Adams, Director of Continuing Education, College of Nursing, The University of Alabama in Huntsville, 301 Sparkman Drive, Huntsville, AL 35899. *Telephone:* 256-824-6345. *Fax:* 256-824-6026. *E-mail:* marsha.adams@uah.edu.

University of Mobile
School of Nursing
Mobile, Alabama

http://www.umobile.edu/
Founded in 1961
DEGREES • BSN • MSN
Nursing Program Faculty 14 (22% with doctorates).
Baccalaureate Enrollment 105 **Women** 93% **Men** 7%
Graduate Enrollment 19 **Women** 90% **Men** 10% **Part-time** 21%
Nursing Student Activities Sigma Theta Tau, Student Nurses' Association.
Nursing Student Resources Academic advising; academic or career counseling; assistance for students with disabilities; bookstore; campus computer network; career placement assistance; computer lab; computer-assisted instruction; e-mail services; employment services for current students; interactive nursing skills videos; Internet; learning resource lab; library services; nursing audiovisuals; remedial services; resume preparation assistance; skills, simulation, or other laboratory; tutoring; unpaid internships.
Library Facilities 10,000 volumes in health, 6,500 volumes in nursing; 4,373 periodical subscriptions health-care related.

BACCALAUREATE PROGRAMS

Degree BSN
Available Programs ADN to Baccalaureate; Generic Baccalaureate; RN Baccalaureate.
Study Options Full-time.
Program Entrance Requirements Minimum overall college GPA of 2.75, transcript of college record, CPR certification, health exam, health insurance, high school transcript, immunizations, minimum GPA in nursing prerequisites of 2.75, prerequisite course work. Transfer students are accepted. *Application deadline:* 3/1 (fall).
Advanced Placement Credit given for nursing courses completed elsewhere dependent upon specific evaluations.
Contact *Telephone:* 251-442-2337. *Fax:* 251-442-2520.

GRADUATE PROGRAMS

Contact *Telephone:* 251-442-2446. *Fax:* 251-442-2520.

MASTER'S DEGREE PROGRAM
Degree MSN
Available Programs Master's.
Concentrations Available Nursing administration; nursing education.

Study Options Full-time and part-time.

Program Entrance Requirements Minimum overall college GPA of 3.0, transcript of college record, CPR certification, immunizations, 3 letters of recommendation, statistics course. *Application deadline:* Applications may be processed on a rolling basis for some programs. *Application fee:* $40.

Advanced Placement Credit given for nursing courses completed elsewhere dependent upon specific evaluations.

Degree Requirements 39 total credit hours, thesis or project, comprehensive exam.

CONTINUING EDUCATION PROGRAM

Contact *Telephone:* 251-442-2446. *Fax:* 251-442-2520.

University of North Alabama
College of Nursing and Allied Health
Florence, Alabama

http://www.una.edu/nursing/
Founded in 1830
DEGREES • BSN • MSN
Nursing Program Faculty 50 (67% with doctorates).
Baccalaureate Enrollment 390 **Women** 87% **Men** 13% **Part-time** 31%
Graduate Enrollment 65 **Women** 90% **Men** 10% **Part-time** 25%
Distance Learning Courses Available.
Nursing Student Activities Nursing Honor Society, Sigma Theta Tau, Student Nurses' Association.
Nursing Student Resources Academic advising; academic or career counseling; assistance for students with disabilities; bookstore; campus computer network; career placement assistance; computer lab; e-mail services; employment services for current students; externships; housing assistance; interactive nursing skills videos; Internet; learning resource lab; library services; nursing audiovisuals; remedial services; resume preparation assistance; skills, simulation, or other laboratory; tutoring; unpaid internships.

BACCALAUREATE PROGRAMS

Degree BSN
Available Programs Accelerated Baccalaureate; Generic Baccalaureate; RN Baccalaureate.
Study Options Full-time and part-time.
Online Degree Options Yes (online only).
Program Entrance Requirements Minimum overall college GPA of 2.5, transcript of college record, CPR certification, health exam, health insurance, high school transcript, immunizations, minimum GPA in nursing prerequisites of 2.5, professional liability insurance/malpractice insurance, prerequisite course work. Transfer students are accepted. *Application fee:* $25.
Expenses (2014–15) *Tuition, state resident:* full-time $5592; part-time $233 per credit hour. *Tuition, nonresident:* full-time $10,000; part-time $466 per credit hour. *Room and board:* $5694; room only: $2780 per academic year.
Financial Aid 75% of baccalaureate students in nursing programs received some form of financial aid in 2013–14.
Contact Dr. Birdie Bailey, Dean, College of Nursing and Allied Health, University of North Alabama, PO Box 5054, Florence, AL 35632-0001. *Telephone:* 256-765-4984. *Fax:* 256-765-4935. *E-mail:* pamcguire@una.edu.

GRADUATE PROGRAMS

Expenses (2014–15) *Tuition, state resident:* full-time $4968; part-time $276 per credit hour. *Tuition, nonresident:* full-time $4968; part-time $276 per credit hour.
Financial Aid 40% of graduate students in nursing programs received some form of financial aid in 2013–14.
Contact Dr. Lynn Aquadro, Chair of Online Department, College of Nursing and Allied Health, University of North Alabama, PO Box 5127, Florence, AL 35632-0001. *Telephone:* 256-765-4931. *Fax:* 256-765-4701. *E-mail:* shthompson@una.edu.

MASTER'S DEGREE PROGRAM

Degree MSN
Available Programs Master's; RN to Master's.
Concentrations Available Nursing administration; nursing education.
Study Options Full-time and part-time.

Online Degree Options Yes (online only).

Program Entrance Requirements Clinical experience, computer literacy, minimum overall college GPA of 3.0, transcript of college record, CPR certification, immunizations, professional liability insurance/malpractice insurance. *Application deadline:* Applications may be processed on a rolling basis for some programs. *Application fee:* $25.

Degree Requirements 42 total credit hours, thesis or project.

CONTINUING EDUCATION PROGRAM

Contact Dr. Craig Robertson, Director, Continuing Education, College of Nursing and Allied Health, University of North Alabama, East Campus, 1640 Tune Avenue, Florence, AL 35630. *Telephone:* 256-765-4787. *Fax:* 256-765-4872. *E-mail:* ctrobertson@una.edu.

University of South Alabama
College of Nursing
Mobile, Alabama

http://www.southalabama.edu/nursing/
Founded in 1963
DEGREES • BSN • MSN
Nursing Program Faculty 57 (30% with doctorates).
Baccalaureate Enrollment 316 **Women** 82% **Men** 18% **Part-time** 11%
Graduate Enrollment 368 **Women** 86% **Men** 14% **Part-time** 22%
Nursing Student Activities Sigma Theta Tau, Student Nurses' Association.
Nursing Student Resources Academic advising; academic or career counseling; assistance for students with disabilities; bookstore; campus computer network; career placement assistance; computer lab; learning resource lab; library services; nursing audiovisuals; resume preparation assistance.
Library Facilities 2,406 volumes in health, 2,300 volumes in nursing; 299 periodical subscriptions health-care related.

BACCALAUREATE PROGRAMS

Degree BSN
Available Programs ADN to Baccalaureate; Accelerated Baccalaureate; Generic Baccalaureate; RN Baccalaureate.
Site Options Fairhope, AL.
Study Options Full-time and part-time.
Program Entrance Requirements Minimum overall college GPA of 2.5, transcript of college record, CPR certification, health exam, health insurance, immunizations, minimum GPA in nursing prerequisites of 2.5, professional liability insurance/malpractice insurance, prerequisite course work. Transfer students are accepted.
Advanced Placement Credit given for nursing courses completed elsewhere dependent upon specific evaluations.
Contact *Telephone:* 251-434-3410. *Fax:* 251-434-3413.

GRADUATE PROGRAMS

Contact *Telephone:* 251-434-3410. *Fax:* 251-434-3413.

MASTER'S DEGREE PROGRAM
Degree MSN
Available Programs Accelerated Master's; Master's; Master's for Nurses with Non-Nursing Degrees.
Concentrations Available Nursing administration; nursing education. *Clinical nurse specialist programs in:* acute care, community health, family health, gerontology, maternity-newborn, pediatric, psychiatric/mental health, women's health. *Nurse practitioner programs in:* acute care, family health, gerontology, neonatal health, pediatric, psychiatric/mental health, women's health.
Study Options Full-time and part-time.
Program Entrance Requirements Computer literacy, minimum overall college GPA of 3.0, transcript of college record, immunizations, nursing research course, physical assessment course, resume.
Advanced Placement Credit given for nursing courses completed elsewhere dependent upon specific evaluations.
Degree Requirements 30 total credit hours, thesis or project.

POST-MASTER'S PROGRAM
Areas of Study Nursing administration; nursing education. *Clinical nurse specialist programs in:* acute care, community health, family health, gerontology, maternity-newborn, pediatric, psychiatric/mental health, women's health. *Nurse practitioner programs in:* acute care,

family health, gerontology, neonatal health, pediatric, psychiatric/mental health, women's health.

ALASKA

University of Alaska Anchorage

School of Nursing
Anchorage, Alaska

http://www.uaa.alaska.edu/schoolofnursing/
Founded in 1954
DEGREES • BS • MS
Nursing Program Faculty 26 (42% with doctorates).
Baccalaureate Enrollment 224 **Women** 80% **Men** 20% **Part-time** 18%
Graduate Enrollment 60 **Women** 94% **Men** 6% **Part-time** 12%
Nursing Student Activities Sigma Theta Tau, Student Nurses' Association.
Nursing Student Resources Academic advising; academic or career counseling; assistance for students with disabilities; bookstore; campus computer network; career placement assistance; computer lab; computer-assisted instruction; daycare for children of students; e-mail services; interactive nursing skills videos; Internet; learning resource lab; library services; nursing audiovisuals; placement services for program completers; remedial services; resume preparation assistance; skills, simulation, or other laboratory; tutoring.
Library Facilities 23,000 volumes in health, 150 volumes in nursing; 780 periodical subscriptions health-care related.

BACCALAUREATE PROGRAMS

Degree BS
Available Programs Generic Baccalaureate; RN Baccalaureate.
Study Options Full-time and part-time.
Program Entrance Requirements Minimum overall college GPA of 2.7, transcript of college record, CPR certification, written essay, immunizations, 3 letters of recommendation, minimum GPA in nursing prerequisites of 2.7, professional liability insurance/malpractice insurance, prerequisite course work. Transfer students are accepted.
Advanced Placement Credit given for nursing courses completed elsewhere dependent upon specific evaluations.
Contact *Telephone:* 907-786-4550. *Fax:* 907-786-4558.

GRADUATE PROGRAMS

Contact *Telephone:* 907-786-4570. *Fax:* 907-786-4559.

MASTER'S DEGREE PROGRAM
Degree MS
Available Programs Master's.
Concentrations Available Health-care administration; nursing education. *Clinical nurse specialist programs in:* community health, psychiatric/mental health. *Nurse practitioner programs in:* family health, psychiatric/mental health.
Study Options Full-time and part-time.
Program Entrance Requirements Clinical experience, minimum overall college GPA of 3.0, transcript of college record, written essay, 3 letters of recommendation, nursing research course, prerequisite course work, statistics course, GRE or MAT.
Advanced Placement Credit given for nursing courses completed elsewhere dependent upon specific evaluations.
Degree Requirements 50 total credit hours, thesis or project.

ARIZONA

Arizona State University at the Downtown Phoenix campus

College of Nursing
Phoenix, Arizona

https://campus.asu.edu/downtown
Founded in 2006
DEGREES • BSN • DNP • MS • MS/MPH
Nursing Program Faculty 119 (44% with doctorates).
Baccalaureate Enrollment 1,085 **Women** 88% **Men** 12% **Part-time** 18%
Graduate Enrollment 363 **Women** 91% **Men** 9% **Part-time** 46%
Distance Learning Courses Available.
Nursing Student Activities Nursing Honor Society, Sigma Theta Tau, Student Nurses' Association, nursing club.
Nursing Student Resources Academic advising; academic or career counseling; assistance for students with disabilities; bookstore; campus computer network; career placement assistance; computer lab; computer-assisted instruction; daycare for children of students; e-mail services; employment services for current students; housing assistance; interactive nursing skills videos; Internet; learning resource lab; library services; nursing audiovisuals; paid internships; placement services for program completers; remedial services; resume preparation assistance; skills, simulation, or other laboratory; tutoring; unpaid internships.
Library Facilities 77,814 volumes in health, 7,501 volumes in nursing; 755 periodical subscriptions health-care related.

BACCALAUREATE PROGRAMS

Degree BSN
Available Programs Accelerated Baccalaureate; Accelerated Baccalaureate for Second Degree; Accelerated RN Baccalaureate; Baccalaureate for Second Degree; Generic Baccalaureate; RN Baccalaureate.
Site Options Phoenix, AZ; Scottsdale, AZ.
Study Options Full-time.
Online Degree Options Yes.
Program Entrance Requirements Minimum overall college GPA of 3.25, transcript of college record, CPR certification, health exam, health insurance, high school biology, high school chemistry, high school foreign language, 4 years high school math, 3 years high school science, high school transcript, immunizations, minimum high school GPA of 3.25, minimum high school rank 25%, minimum GPA in nursing prerequisites of 3.25, professional liability insurance/malpractice insurance, prerequisite course work. Transfer students are accepted. *Application deadline:* 2/1 (fall), 9/1 (spring), 2/1 (summer). *Application fee:* $65.
Financial Aid 70% of baccalaureate students in nursing programs received some form of financial aid in 2013–14.
Contact Nancy Kiernan, Senior Director Student Services, College of Nursing, Arizona State University at the Downtown Phoenix campus, 502 East Monroe Street, Suite C 250, Phoenix, AZ 85004-4431. *Telephone:* 602-496-0712. *Fax:* 602-496-0705. *E-mail:* nancy.kiernan@asu.edu.

GRADUATE PROGRAMS

Financial Aid 75% of graduate students in nursing programs received some form of financial aid in 2013–14.
Contact Dr. Katherine Kenny, Clinical Associate Professor, College of Nursing, Arizona State University at the Downtown Phoenix campus, 550 North 3rd Street, Phoenix, AZ 85004. *Telephone:* 602-496-1719. *E-mail:* katherine.kenny@asu.edu.

MASTER'S DEGREE PROGRAM
Degrees MS; MS/MPH
Available Programs Master's.
Concentrations Available *Clinical nurse specialist programs in:* acute care, adult health, community health, pediatric, psychiatric/mental health. *Nurse practitioner programs in:* acute care, adult health, family health, neonatal health, pediatric, psychiatric/mental health, women's health.
Site Options Phoenix, AZ.
Study Options Full-time and part-time.
Program Entrance Requirements Clinical experience, minimum overall college GPA of 3.0, transcript of college record, immunizations,

interview, 3 letters of recommendation, physical assessment course, prerequisite course work, resume, statistics course, GRE.
Advanced Placement Credit given for nursing courses completed elsewhere dependent upon specific evaluations.
Degree Requirements 40 total credit hours, thesis or project.

POST-MASTER'S PROGRAM
Areas of Study *Clinical nurse specialist programs in:* acute care, adult health, community health, pediatric, psychiatric/mental health. *Nurse practitioner programs in:* acute care, adult health, family health, neonatal health, pediatric, psychiatric/mental health, women's health.

DOCTORAL DEGREE PROGRAM
Degree DNP
Available Programs Doctorate.
Areas of Study Advanced practice nursing.
Site Options Phoenix, AZ.

CONTINUING EDUCATION PROGRAM
Contact Amy Fitzgerald, RN, Assistant Director, College of Nursing, Arizona State University at the Downtown Phoenix campus, 550 North 3rd Street, Phoenix, AZ 85004. *Telephone:* 602-496-2175. *E-mail:* Amy.Fitzgerald@asu.edu.

Brookline College
Baccalaureate Nursing Program
Phoenix, Arizona

http://brooklinecollege.edu/
Founded in 1979
DEGREE • BSN

BACCALAUREATE PROGRAMS
Degree BSN
Available Programs Accelerated Baccalaureate for Second Degree; Generic Baccalaureate.
Contact *Telephone:* 602-242-6265. *Fax:* 602-973-2572.

Chamberlain College of Nursing
Chamberlain College of Nursing
Phoenix, Arizona

DEGREES • BSN • DNP • MSN
Nursing Program Faculty 83
Baccalaureate Enrollment 198 **Women** 85% **Men** 15% **Part-time** 28%
Distance Learning Courses Available.
Nursing Student Activities Sigma Theta Tau.
Nursing Student Resources Academic advising; academic or career counseling; assistance for students with disabilities; bookstore; computer lab; e-mail services; library services; skills, simulation, or other laboratory; tutoring.

BACCALAUREATE PROGRAMS
Degree BSN
Available Programs Accelerated Baccalaureate; Accelerated Baccalaureate for Second Degree; RN Baccalaureate.
Study Options Full-time and part-time.
Online Degree Options Yes.
Program Entrance Requirements Minimum overall college GPA of 2.75, interview, minimum high school GPA of 2.75. Transfer students are accepted. *Application deadline:* Applications may be processed on a rolling basis for some programs.
Advanced Placement Credit given for nursing courses completed elsewhere dependent upon specific evaluations.
Expenses (2015–16) *Tuition:* full-time $17,560; part-time $665 per credit hour. *International tuition:* $17,560 full-time. *Required fees:* full-time $600; part-time $300 per term.
Contact Admissions, Chamberlain College of Nursing, 2149 West Dunlap Avenue, Phoenix, AZ 85021. *Telephone:* 888-556-8226.

GRADUATE PROGRAMS
Expenses (2015–16) *Tuition:* part-time $650 per credit hour. *Required fees:* part-time $300 per term.

Contact Admissions, Chamberlain College of Nursing, 2149 West Dunlap Avenue, Phoenix, AZ 85021. *Telephone:* 888-556-8226.

MASTER'S DEGREE PROGRAM
Degree MSN
Available Programs Master's.
Study Options Full-time and part-time.
Online Degree Options Yes (online only).
Program Entrance Requirements Minimum overall college GPA of 3.0, transcript of college record, interview. *Application deadline:* Applications may be processed on a rolling basis for some programs. *Application fee:* $60.

DOCTORAL DEGREE PROGRAM
Degree DNP
Available Programs Doctorate.
Areas of Study Advanced practice nursing.
Online Degree Options Yes (online only).
Program Entrance Requirements Application deadline: Applications may be processed on a rolling basis for some programs. Application fee: $60.

Grand Canyon University
College of Nursing and Health Sciences
Phoenix, Arizona

http://www.gcu.edu/
Founded in 1949
DEGREES • BSN • MS • MSN/MBA
Nursing Program Faculty 122 (3% with doctorates).
Baccalaureate Enrollment 1,067 **Women** 90% **Men** 10% **Part-time** 58%
Graduate Enrollment 297 **Women** 93% **Men** 7% **Part-time** 89%
Distance Learning Courses Available.
Nursing Student Activities Sigma Theta Tau, Student Nurses' Association.
Nursing Student Resources Academic advising; academic or career counseling; assistance for students with disabilities; bookstore; campus computer network; career placement assistance; computer lab; computer-assisted instruction; e-mail services; employment services for current students; housing assistance; Internet; learning resource lab; library services; nursing audiovisuals; other; paid internships; remedial services; resume preparation assistance; skills, simulation, or other laboratory; tutoring; unpaid internships.
Library Facilities 9,663 volumes in health; 177 periodical subscriptions health-care related.

BACCALAUREATE PROGRAMS
Degree BSN
Available Programs ADN to Baccalaureate; RN Baccalaureate.
Site Options Phoenix, AZ; Tucson, AZ; Albuquerque, NM.
Study Options Full-time.
Online Degree Options Yes.
Program Entrance Requirements Minimum overall college GPA of 3.0, transcript of college record, CPR certification, health exam, health insurance, high school transcript, immunizations, minimum GPA in nursing prerequisites of 3.0, prerequisite course work. Transfer students are accepted. *Application deadline:* 5/15 (fall), 9/15 (spring), 1/15 (summer).
Advanced Placement Credit by examination available. Credit given for nursing courses completed elsewhere dependent upon specific evaluations.
Contact *Telephone:* 602-639-6429.

GRADUATE PROGRAMS
Contact *Telephone:* 602-639-7982.

MASTER'S DEGREE PROGRAM
Degrees MS; MSN/MBA
Available Programs Master's.
Concentrations Available Nursing administration; nursing education. *Clinical nurse specialist programs in:* adult health. *Nurse practitioner programs in:* acute care, family health.
Site Options Phoenix, AZ; Tucson, AZ.
Study Options Full-time and part-time.
Online Degree Options Yes.

Program Entrance Requirements Clinical experience, computer literacy, minimum overall college GPA of 3.0, transcript of college record, CPR certification, written essay, immunizations, interview, nursing research course, physical assessment course, professional liability insurance/malpractice insurance, prerequisite course work, resume, statistics course. *Application deadline:* Applications may be processed on a rolling basis for some programs.
Advanced Placement Credit given for nursing courses completed elsewhere dependent upon specific evaluations.
Degree Requirements 52 total credit hours, thesis or project.

POST-MASTER'S PROGRAM

Areas of Study Nursing education. *Clinical nurse specialist programs in:* adult health. *Nurse practitioner programs in:* acute care, family health.

CONTINUING EDUCATION PROGRAM

Contact *Telephone:* 602-639-7982. *Fax:* 602-639-7982.

Northern Arizona University
School of Nursing
Flagstaff, Arizona

http://www.nau.edu/chhs/nursing/
Founded in 1899
DEGREES • BSN • DNP • MS
Nursing Program Faculty 100 (40% with doctorates).
Baccalaureate Enrollment 1,600 **Women** 80% **Men** 20% **Part-time** 50%
Graduate Enrollment 150 **Women** 95% **Men** 5% **Part-time** 80%
Distance Learning Courses Available.
Nursing Student Activities Sigma Theta Tau, Student Nurses' Association.
Nursing Student Resources Academic advising; academic or career counseling; assistance for students with disabilities; bookstore; campus computer network; computer lab; computer-assisted instruction; e-mail services; interactive nursing skills videos; Internet; learning resource lab; library services; nursing audiovisuals; remedial services; skills, simulation, or other laboratory; tutoring.

BACCALAUREATE PROGRAMS

Degree BSN
Available Programs ADN to Baccalaureate; Accelerated Baccalaureate for Second Degree; Generic Baccalaureate; RN Baccalaureate.
Site Options Yuma, AZ; Fort Defiance, AZ; Tucson, AZ.
Study Options Full-time.
Online Degree Options Yes.
Program Entrance Requirements Transcript of college record, CPR certification, health exam, health insurance, high school transcript, immunizations, 2 letters of recommendation, minimum GPA in nursing prerequisites of 2.75, professional liability insurance/malpractice insurance, prerequisite course work. Transfer students are accepted. *Application deadline:* 3/1 (fall), 10/1 (spring).
Advanced Placement Credit given for nursing courses completed elsewhere dependent upon specific evaluations.
Expenses (2015–16) *Tuition, state resident:* full-time $7500; part-time $400 per credit hour. *Tuition, nonresident:* full-time $18,500; part-time $809 per credit hour. *International tuition:* $18,500 full-time. *Room and board:* room only: $5000 per academic year. *Required fees:* full-time $2196; part-time $120 per credit.
Contact Mr. Gregg Schneider, Senior Academic Advisor, School of Nursing, Northern Arizona University, Box 15035, Flagstaff, AZ 86011. *Telephone:* 928-523-6717. *Fax:* 928-523-7171. *E-mail:* gregg.schneider@nau.edu.

GRADUATE PROGRAMS

Expenses (2015–16) *Tuition, state resident:* full-time $9000; part-time $431 per credit hour. *Tuition, nonresident:* full-time $20,500; part-time $1130 per credit hour. *International tuition:* $20,500 full-time. *Room and board:* room only: $5000 per academic year. *Required fees:* full-time $2500; part-time $40 per credit.
Financial Aid Career-related internships or fieldwork, Federal Work-Study, scholarships, traineeships, tuition waivers, and unspecified assistantships available.
Contact Dr. Dorothy Dunn, Graduate Program Coordinator, School of Nursing, Northern Arizona University, Box 15035, Flagstaff, AZ 86011.

Telephone: 928-523-6455. *Fax:* 928-523-7171. *E-mail:* dorothy.dunn@nau.edu.

MASTER'S DEGREE PROGRAM

Degree MS
Available Programs Master's.
Concentrations Available *Nurse practitioner programs in:* family health.
Study Options Full-time and part-time.
Online Degree Options Yes (online only).
Program Entrance Requirements Clinical experience, computer literacy, minimum overall college GPA of 3.0, transcript of college record, CPR certification, written essay, immunizations, 3 letters of recommendation, nursing research course, physical assessment course, professional liability insurance/malpractice insurance, prerequisite course work, resume, statistics course, GRE General Test or minimum GPA of 3.0. *Application deadline:* 10/15 (fall), 1/15 (spring). *Application fee:* $50.
Advanced Placement Credit given for nursing courses completed elsewhere dependent upon specific evaluations.
Degree Requirements 40 total credit hours, thesis or project.

POST-MASTER'S PROGRAM

Areas of Study *Nurse practitioner programs in:* family health.

DOCTORAL DEGREE PROGRAM

Degree DNP
Available Programs Doctorate.
Areas of Study Clinical practice, health policy.
Online Degree Options Yes (online only).
Program Entrance Requirements Clinical experience, minimum overall college GPA of 3.0, interview by faculty committee, 3 letters of recommendation, MSN or equivalent, statistics course, vita. Application deadline: 3/15 (fall). Application fee: $50.
Degree Requirements 31 total credit hours.

The University of Arizona
College of Nursing
Tucson, Arizona

http://www.nursing.arizona.edu/
Founded in 1885
DEGREES • BSN • MSN • PHD
Nursing Program Faculty 96 (51% with doctorates).
Baccalaureate Enrollment 214 **Women** 91% **Men** 9%
Graduate Enrollment 857 **Women** 85% **Men** 15% **Part-time** 42%
Distance Learning Courses Available.
Nursing Student Activities Nursing Honor Society, Sigma Theta Tau, Student Nurses' Association, nursing club.
Nursing Student Resources Academic advising; academic or career counseling; assistance for students with disabilities; bookstore; campus computer network; career placement assistance; computer lab; computer-assisted instruction; e-mail services; employment services for current students; externships; housing assistance; interactive nursing skills videos; Internet; learning resource lab; library services; nursing audiovisuals; other; placement services for program completers; remedial services; resume preparation assistance; skills, simulation, or other laboratory; tutoring; unpaid internships.
Library Facilities 145,500 volumes in health, 5,400 volumes in nursing; 11,185 periodical subscriptions health-care related.

BACCALAUREATE PROGRAMS

Degree BSN
Available Programs Generic Baccalaureate.
Study Options Full-time.
Program Entrance Requirements Minimum overall college GPA of 3.0, transcript of college record, CPR certification, written essay, health insurance, high school transcript, immunizations, interview, minimum GPA in nursing prerequisites of 3.0, prerequisite course work. Transfer students are accepted. *Application deadline:* 2/1 (fall), 9/1 (spring).
Advanced Placement Credit by examination available. Credit given for nursing courses completed elsewhere dependent upon specific evaluations.
Expenses (2015–16) *Tuition, state resident:* full-time $12,890; part-time $885 per credit hour. *Tuition, nonresident:* full-time $32,044; part-time $1389 per credit hour. *International tuition:* $32,044 full-time. *Room and board:* $9840; room only: $6460 per academic year.

Financial Aid *Gift aid (need-based):* Federal Pell, FSEOG, state, private, college/university gift aid from institutional funds, Federal Nursing. *Loans:* Federal Nursing Student Loans, Federal Direct (Subsidized and Unsubsidized Stafford PLUS), Perkins, college/university. *Work-study:* Federal Work-Study, part-time campus jobs. *Financial aid application deadline:* Continuous.

Contact Dr. Thomas M. Dickson, Assistant Dean for Student Affairs, College of Nursing, The University of Arizona, 1305 North Martin, PO Box 210203, Tucson, AZ 85721-0203. *Telephone:* 520-626-3808. *Fax:* 520-626-6424. *E-mail:* thomas.dickson@arizona.edu.

GRADUATE PROGRAMS

Expenses (2015–16) *Tuition, state resident:* full-time $16,120; part-time $1088 per credit hour. *Tuition, nonresident:* full-time $31,992; part-time $1803 per credit hour. *International tuition:* $31,992 full-time. *Room and board:* $9840; room only: $6460 per academic year.

Financial Aid 11 research assistantships (averaging $18,220 per year), 3 teaching assistantships (averaging $18,327 per year) were awarded; career-related internships or fieldwork, institutionally sponsored loans, scholarships, traineeships, tuition waivers (full), and unspecified assistantships also available.

Contact Dr. Thomas Matthew Dickson, Assistant Dean for Student Affairs, College of Nursing, The University of Arizona, 1305 North Martin, PO Box 210203, Tucson, AZ 85721-0203. *Telephone:* 520-626-3808. *Fax:* 520-626-6424. *E-mail:* advanced@nursing.arizona.edu.

MASTER'S DEGREE PROGRAM

Degree MSN

Available Programs Accelerated AD/RN to Master's; Accelerated Master's; Accelerated Master's for Non-Nursing College Graduates; Accelerated RN to Master's; Master's; RN to Master's.

Concentrations Available Clinical nurse leader.

Site Options Phoenix, AZ.

Study Options Full-time.

Online Degree Options Yes.

Program Entrance Requirements Minimum overall college GPA of 3.0, transcript of college record, CPR certification, written essay, immunizations, interview, prerequisite course work, statistics course. *Application deadline:* 12/15 (fall). *Application fee:* $75.

Advanced Placement Credit given for nursing courses completed elsewhere dependent upon specific evaluations.

Degree Requirements 56 total credit hours, thesis or project, comprehensive exam.

POST-MASTER'S PROGRAM

Areas of Study *Nurse practitioner programs in:* adult-gerontology acute care, family health, gerontology, pediatric, psychiatric/mental health.

DOCTORAL DEGREE PROGRAM

Degree PhD

Available Programs Doctorate; Post-Baccalaureate Doctorate.

Areas of Study Addiction/substance abuse, advanced practice nursing, aging, bio-behavioral research, biology of health and illness, clinical practice, clinical research, community health, critical care, faculty preparation, family health, gerontology, health policy, health promotion/disease prevention, health-care systems, human health and illness, illness and transition, individualized study, information systems, neuro-behavior, nursing research, nursing science, oncology, palliative care, urban health, women's health.

Online Degree Options Yes (online only).

Program Entrance Requirements Minimum overall college GPA of 3.0, interview by faculty committee, interview, 3 letters of recommendation, statistics course, vita. Application deadline: 12/15 (fall). Application fee: $75.

Degree Requirements 64 total credit hours, dissertation, oral exam, written exam, residency.

POSTDOCTORAL PROGRAM

Postdoctoral Program Contact Mr. Thomas Matthew Dickson, Director of Student Affairs, College of Nursing, The University of Arizona, 1305 North Martin, PO Box 210203, Tucson, AZ 85721-0203. *Telephone:* 520-626-3808. *E-mail:* tdickson@email.arizona.edu.

CONTINUING EDUCATION PROGRAM

Contact Dr. Mary Koithan, Associate Dean for Professional and Community Development, College of Nursing, The University of Arizona, 1305 North Martin, PO Box 210203, Tucson, AZ 85721-0203.

Telephone: 520-626-3808. *Fax:* 520-626-6424. *E-mail:* mkoithan@ arizona.edu.

University of Phoenix–Online Campus
Online Campus
Phoenix, Arizona

http://www.uopxonline.com/
Founded in 1989

DEGREES • BSN • MSN • MSN/MBA • MSN/MHA • PHD

Nursing Program Faculty 444 (29% with doctorates).

Baccalaureate Enrollment 5,644 **Women** 92.2% **Men** 7.8%

Graduate Enrollment 5,878 **Women** 92.5% **Men** 7.5%

Distance Learning Courses Available.

Nursing Student Activities Sigma Theta Tau.

Nursing Student Resources Academic advising; academic or career counseling; assistance for students with disabilities; bookstore; campus computer network; computer lab; computer-assisted instruction; e-mail services; interactive nursing skills videos; Internet; learning resource lab; library services; nursing audiovisuals; remedial services; skills, simulation, or other laboratory; tutoring.

Library Facilities 1,300 periodical subscriptions health-care related.

BACCALAUREATE PROGRAMS

Degree BSN

Available Programs Accelerated Baccalaureate.

Study Options Full-time.

Online Degree Options Yes.

Program Entrance Requirements Transcript of college record, CPR certification, immunizations, 1 letter of recommendation, RN licensure. Transfer students are accepted. *Application deadline:* Applications may be processed on a rolling basis for some programs.

Advanced Placement Credit by examination available. Credit given for nursing courses completed elsewhere dependent upon specific evaluations.

Contact *Telephone:* 602-387-7000.

GRADUATE PROGRAMS

Contact *Telephone:* 602-387-7000.

MASTER'S DEGREE PROGRAM

Degrees MSN; MSN/MBA; MSN/MHA

Available Programs Master's; Master's for Nurses with Non-Nursing Degrees.

Concentrations Available Health-care administration; nursing administration; nursing education. *Nurse practitioner programs in:* family health.

Study Options Full-time.

Online Degree Options Yes.

Program Entrance Requirements Clinical experience, computer literacy, minimum overall college GPA of 3.0, transcript of college record, CPR certification. *Application deadline:* Applications may be processed on a rolling basis for some programs.

Advanced Placement Credit given for nursing courses completed elsewhere dependent upon specific evaluations.

Degree Requirements 39 total credit hours, thesis or project.

POST-MASTER'S PROGRAM

Areas of Study *Nurse practitioner programs in:* family health.

DOCTORAL DEGREE PROGRAM

Degree PhD

Available Programs Doctorate.

Areas of Study Nursing administration, nursing education.

Online Degree Options Yes (online only).

Program Entrance Requirements Minimum overall college GPA of 3.0, MSN or equivalent. Application deadline: Applications may be processed on a rolling basis for some programs. Application fee: $45.

Degree Requirements 62 total credit hours, dissertation, residency.

CONTINUING EDUCATION PROGRAM

Contact *Telephone:* 602-387-7000.

University of Phoenix–Phoenix Campus
College of Health Sciences and Nursing
Tempe, Arizona

http://www.phoenix.edu/
Founded in 1976

DEGREES • BSN • MSN • MSN/MBA • MSN/MHA
Nursing Program Faculty 38 (32% with doctorates).
Baccalaureate Enrollment 239 **Women** 89.5% **Men** 10.5%
Graduate Enrollment 148 **Women** 91.9% **Men** 8.1%
Nursing Student Activities Sigma Theta Tau.
Nursing Student Resources Academic advising; academic or career counseling; assistance for students with disabilities; bookstore; campus computer network; computer lab; computer-assisted instruction; interactive nursing skills videos; Internet; learning resource lab; library services; nursing audiovisuals; skills, simulation, or other laboratory; tutoring.
Library Facilities 1,300 periodical subscriptions health-care related.

BACCALAUREATE PROGRAMS

Degree BSN
Available Programs Accelerated Baccalaureate; LPN to Baccalaureate.
Site Options Scottsdale, AZ; Mesa, AZ; Chandler, AZ.
Study Options Full-time.
Online Degree Options Yes.
Program Entrance Requirements Transcript of college record, CPR certification, immunizations, 1 letter of recommendation, RN licensure. Transfer students are accepted. *Application deadline:* Applications may be processed on a rolling basis for some programs.
Advanced Placement Credit by examination available. Credit given for nursing courses completed elsewhere dependent upon specific evaluations.
Contact *Telephone:* 480-804-7600.

GRADUATE PROGRAMS

Contact *Telephone:* 480-804-7600.

MASTER'S DEGREE PROGRAM
Degrees MSN; MSN/MBA; MSN/MHA
Available Programs Master's.
Concentrations Available Health-care administration; nursing administration; nursing education. *Nurse practitioner programs in:* family health.
Site Options Scottsdale, AZ; Mesa, AZ; Chandler, AZ.
Study Options Full-time.
Online Degree Options Yes.
Program Entrance Requirements Clinical experience, computer literacy, minimum overall college GPA of 2.5, transcript of college record. *Application deadline:* Applications may be processed on a rolling basis for some programs. *Application fee:* $45.
Advanced Placement Credit given for nursing courses completed elsewhere dependent upon specific evaluations.
Degree Requirements 39 total credit hours, thesis or project.

POST-MASTER'S PROGRAM
Areas of Study *Nurse practitioner programs in:* family health.

CONTINUING EDUCATION PROGRAM
Contact *Telephone:* 480-557-2279. *Fax:* 480-557-2338.

University of Phoenix–Southern Arizona Campus
College of Social Sciences
Tucson, Arizona

http://www.phoenix.edu/campus-locations/az/southern-arizona-campus/southern-arizona-campus.html
Founded in 1979

DEGREES • BSN • MSN
Nursing Program Faculty 19 (32% with doctorates).
Baccalaureate Enrollment 67 **Women** 85.1% **Men** 14.9%

Graduate Enrollment 97 **Women** 80.4% **Men** 19.6%
Nursing Student Activities Sigma Theta Tau.
Nursing Student Resources Academic advising; academic or career counseling; assistance for students with disabilities; bookstore; campus computer network; computer lab; computer-assisted instruction; e-mail services; interactive nursing skills videos; Internet; learning resource lab; library services; nursing audiovisuals; remedial services; skills, simulation, or other laboratory; tutoring.
Library Facilities 1,300 periodical subscriptions health-care related.

BACCALAUREATE PROGRAMS

Degree BSN
Available Programs Accelerated Baccalaureate; LPN to Baccalaureate.
Site Options Sierra Vista, AZ; Yuma, AZ; Nogales, AZ.
Study Options Full-time.
Online Degree Options Yes.
Program Entrance Requirements Transcript of college record, CPR certification, immunizations, 1 letter of recommendation, RN licensure. Transfer students are accepted. *Application deadline:* Applications may be processed on a rolling basis for some programs.
Advanced Placement Credit by examination available. Credit given for nursing courses completed elsewhere dependent upon specific evaluations.
Contact *Telephone:* 520-881-6512.

GRADUATE PROGRAMS

Contact *Telephone:* 520-881-6512.

MASTER'S DEGREE PROGRAM
Degree MSN
Available Programs Master's.
Concentrations Available Health-care administration; nursing administration; nursing education. *Nurse practitioner programs in:* family health.
Site Options Sierra Vista, AZ; Yuma, AZ; Nogales, AZ.
Study Options Full-time.
Online Degree Options Yes.
Program Entrance Requirements Clinical experience, computer literacy, minimum overall college GPA of 2.5, transcript of college record. *Application deadline:* Applications may be processed on a rolling basis for some programs. *Application fee:* $45.
Advanced Placement Credit given for nursing courses completed elsewhere dependent upon specific evaluations.
Degree Requirements 39 total credit hours, thesis or project.

POST-MASTER'S PROGRAM
Areas of Study *Nurse practitioner programs in:* family health.

CONTINUING EDUCATION PROGRAM

Contact *Telephone:* 520-881-6512.

ARKANSAS

Arkansas State University
Department of Nursing
Jonesboro, State University, Arkansas

http://www.astate.edu/
Founded in 1909

DEGREES • BSN • DNP • MSN
Nursing Program Faculty 91 (17% with doctorates).
Baccalaureate Enrollment 357 **Women** 81% **Men** 19% **Part-time** 35%
Graduate Enrollment 202 **Women** 55% **Men** 45% **Part-time** 50%
Distance Learning Courses Available.
Nursing Student Activities Sigma Theta Tau, Student Nurses' Association.
Nursing Student Resources Academic advising; academic or career counseling; assistance for students with disabilities; bookstore; campus computer network; computer lab; computer-assisted instruction; daycare for children of students; e-mail services; housing assistance; Internet; learning resource lab; library services; nursing audiovisuals; resume preparation assistance; skills, simulation, or other laboratory; tutoring.

BACCALAUREATE PROGRAMS

Degree BSN

Available Programs Accelerated Baccalaureate for Second Degree; Generic Baccalaureate; LPN to Baccalaureate; RN Baccalaureate.

Site Options West Memphis, AR; Mountain Home, AR; Beebe, AR.

Study Options Full-time.

Online Degree Options Yes.

Program Entrance Requirements Minimum overall college GPA of 2.8, transcript of college record, CPR certification, written essay, immunizations, 3 letters of recommendation, professional liability insurance/malpractice insurance, prerequisite course work. Transfer students are accepted. *Application deadline:* 6/15 (fall).

Advanced Placement Credit by examination available. Credit given for nursing courses completed elsewhere dependent upon specific evaluations.

Expenses (2015–16) *Tuition, area resident:* part-time $200 per credit hour. *Tuition, state resident:* part-time $200 per credit. *Tuition, nonresident:* part-time $400 per credit hour. *Room and board:* $8140 per academic year.

Contact Jenafer Wray, Nursing Advisor, Department of Nursing, Arkansas State University, PO Box 910, State University, AR 72467. *Telephone:* 870-972-3074. *Fax:* 870-972-2954. *E-mail:* jwray@astate.edu.

GRADUATE PROGRAMS

Expenses (2015–16) *Tuition, state resident:* part-time $254 per credit. *Tuition, nonresident:* part-time $508 per credit. *Required fees:* part-time $279 per credit.

Contact Dr. Jill Detty Oswaks, MSN Program Director, Department of Nursing, Arkansas State University, PO Box 910, MSN Program, State University, AR 72467. *Telephone:* 870-972-3701. *Fax:* 870-972-2954. *E-mail:* jdettyoswaks@astate.edu.

MASTER'S DEGREE PROGRAM

Degree MSN

Available Programs Master's.

Concentrations Available Nurse anesthesia; nursing administration; nursing education. *Clinical nurse specialist programs in:* adult health. *Nurse practitioner programs in:* primary care.

Study Options Part-time.

Program Entrance Requirements Clinical experience, minimum overall college GPA of 3.0, transcript of college record, CPR certification, written essay, immunizations, physical assessment course, professional liability insurance/malpractice insurance, statistics course. *Application deadline:* 2/1 (fall). *Application fee:* $30.

Degree Requirements 45 total credit hours, thesis or project, comprehensive exam.

POST-MASTER'S PROGRAM

Areas of Study Nursing education. *Nurse practitioner programs in:* primary care.

DOCTORAL DEGREE PROGRAM

Degree DNP

Available Programs Doctorate.

Online Degree Options Yes (online only).

Program Entrance Requirements Clinical experience, minimum overall college GPA of 3.0, interview, MSN or equivalent, statistics course, vita. Application deadline: 10/1 (spring).

Degree Requirements 41 total credit hours.

Arkansas Tech University
Program in Nursing
Russellville, Arkansas

https://www.atu.edu/nursing/
Founded in 1909

DEGREES • BSN • MSN

Nursing Program Faculty 24 (38% with doctorates).

Baccalaureate Enrollment 262 **Women** 84% **Men** 16% **Part-time** 3%

Graduate Enrollment 26 **Women** 92% **Men** 8%

Distance Learning Courses Available.

Nursing Student Activities Nursing Honor Society, Sigma Theta Tau, Student Nurses' Association.

Nursing Student Resources Academic advising; academic or career counseling; assistance for students with disabilities; bookstore; campus computer network; career placement assistance; computer lab; computer-assisted instruction; e-mail services; employment services for current students; housing assistance; interactive nursing skills videos; Internet; learning resource lab; library services; nursing audiovisuals; other; paid internships; placement services for program completers; remedial services; resume preparation assistance; skills, simulation, or other laboratory; tutoring.

Library Facilities 16,900 volumes in health, 2,100 volumes in nursing; 130 periodical subscriptions health-care related.

BACCALAUREATE PROGRAMS

Degree BSN

Available Programs ADN to Baccalaureate; Baccalaureate for Second Degree; Generic Baccalaureate; LPN to Baccalaureate; RN Baccalaureate.

Site Options Russellville, AR.

Study Options Full-time and part-time.

Online Degree Options Yes.

Program Entrance Requirements Transcript of college record, CPR certification, health exam, immunizations, minimum GPA in nursing prerequisites of 3.0, professional liability insurance/malpractice insurance, prerequisite course work. Transfer students are accepted. *Application deadline:* 3/1 (fall), 10/1 (spring).

Advanced Placement Credit by examination available. Credit given for nursing courses completed elsewhere dependent upon specific evaluations.

Expenses (2015–16) *Tuition, state resident:* full-time $5160; part-time $215 per credit hour. *Tuition, nonresident:* full-time $6456; part-time $430 per credit hour. *Room and board:* $3433; room only: $2169 per academic year. *Required fees:* full-time $1032.

Financial Aid *Gift aid (need-based):* Federal Pell, FSEOG, state, private. *Loans:* Federal Direct (Subsidized and Unsubsidized Stafford PLUS). *Work-study:* Federal Work-Study, part-time campus jobs. *Financial aid application deadline (priority):* 3/15.

Contact Dr. Rebecca F. Burris, Professor and Department Chair, Program in Nursing, Arkansas Tech University, 402 West O Street, Russellville, AR 72801. *Telephone:* 479-968-0383. *Fax:* 479-968-0219. *E-mail:* rburris@atu.edu.

GRADUATE PROGRAMS

Expenses (2015–16) *Tuition, state resident:* full-time $7740; part-time $430 per credit hour. *Tuition, nonresident:* full-time $15,480; part-time $860 per credit hour. *Required fees:* full-time $774.

Contact Dr. Mary Gunter, Dean of Graduate College, Program in Nursing, Arkansas Tech University, Tomlinson Graduate College, Russellville, AR 72801. *Telephone:* 479-968-0398. *E-mail:* mgunter@atu.edu.

MASTER'S DEGREE PROGRAM

Degree MSN

Available Programs Master's; Master's for Nurses with Non-Nursing Degrees; RN to Master's.

Concentrations Available Nursing administration.

Site Options Russellville, AR.

Study Options Full-time and part-time.

Program Entrance Requirements Clinical experience, computer literacy, minimum overall college GPA of 3.0, transcript of college record, immunizations, statistics course. *Application deadline:* 5/1 (fall). Applications may be processed on a rolling basis for some programs. *Application fee:* $25.

Advanced Placement Credit given for nursing courses completed elsewhere dependent upon specific evaluations.

Degree Requirements 39 total credit hours, thesis or project.

Harding University
College of Nursing
Searcy, Arkansas

http://www.harding.edu/nursing
Founded in 1924

DEGREES • BSN • MSN

Nursing Program Faculty 17 (35% with doctorates).

Baccalaureate Enrollment 92 **Women** 90% **Men** 10% **Part-time** 1%

Graduate Enrollment 17 **Women** 82% **Men** 18% **Part-time** 41%

Nursing Student Activities Nursing Honor Society, Sigma Theta Tau, Student Nurses' Association.

Nursing Student Resources Academic advising; academic or career counseling; assistance for students with disabilities; bookstore; campus computer network; career placement assistance; computer lab; computer-assisted instruction; e-mail services; employment services for current students; externships; housing assistance; interactive nursing skills videos; Internet; learning resource lab; library services; nursing audiovisuals; placement services for program completers; remedial services; resume preparation assistance; skills, simulation, or other laboratory; tutoring.

Library Facilities 5,000 volumes in health, 1,729 volumes in nursing; 120 periodical subscriptions health-care related.

BACCALAUREATE PROGRAMS

Degree BSN

Available Programs Generic Baccalaureate.

Site Options Searcy, AR.

Study Options Full-time and part-time.

Program Entrance Requirements Minimum overall college GPA of 2.0, transcript of college record, CPR certification, health exam, high school transcript, immunizations, 2 letters of recommendation, minimum GPA in nursing prerequisites of 2.5, prerequisite course work. Transfer students are accepted. *Application deadline:* 3/1 (fall), 10/1 (spring).

Advanced Placement Credit by examination available. Credit given for nursing courses completed elsewhere dependent upon specific evaluations.

Expenses (2015–16) *Tuition:* full-time $17,610; part-time $8805 per credit hour. *International tuition:* $17,610 full-time. *Room and board:* $6628; room only: $3398 per academic year.

Financial Aid 95% of baccalaureate students in nursing programs received some form of financial aid in 2014–15. *Gift aid (need-based):* Federal Pell, FSEOG, state, private, college/university gift aid from institutional funds. *Loans:* Federal Nursing Student Loans, Federal Direct (Subsidized and Unsubsidized Stafford PLUS), Perkins, state, college/university. *Work-study:* Federal Work-Study, part-time campus jobs. *Financial aid application deadline (priority):* 4/15.

Contact Ms. Jeanne L. Castleberry, Director of Admissions, College of Nursing, Harding University, 915 East Market Avenue, Box 12265, Searcy, AR 72149-2265. *Telephone:* 501-279-4682. *Fax:* 501-279-4669. *E-mail:* nursing@harding.edu.

GRADUATE PROGRAMS

Expenses (2015–16) *Tuition:* full-time $10,240; part-time $7478 per credit hour. *International tuition:* $10,240 full-time. *Required fees:* full-time $2240.

Financial Aid 92% of graduate students in nursing programs received some form of financial aid in 2014–15.

Contact Dr. Greg Brooks, Associate Dean, College of Nursing, Harding University, Box 12265, Searcy, AR 72149-2265. *Telephone:* 501-279-4859. *Fax:* 501-279-4669. *E-mail:* gradnursing@harding.edu.

MASTER'S DEGREE PROGRAM

Degree MSN

Available Programs Master's.

Concentrations Available *Nurse practitioner programs in:* family health.

Site Options Searcy, AR.

Study Options Full-time and part-time.

Online Degree Options Yes (online only).

Program Entrance Requirements Clinical experience, minimum overall college GPA of 3.0, transcript of college record, CPR certification, written essay, immunizations, interview, 3 letters of recommendation, nursing research course, physical assessment course, professional liability insurance/malpractice insurance, prerequisite course work, resume, statistics course. *Application deadline:* 3/1 (fall). *Application fee:* $50.

Degree Requirements 45 total credit hours, thesis or project.

POST-MASTER'S PROGRAM

Areas of Study *Nurse practitioner programs in:* family health.

CONTINUING EDUCATION PROGRAM

Contact Dr. Susan Kehl, Dean and Associate Professor, College of Nursing, Harding University, 915 East Market Avenue, Box 12265, Searcy, AR 72149-5615. *Telephone:* 501-279-4476. *Fax:* 501-279-4669. *E-mail:* nursing@harding.edu.

Henderson State University
Department of Nursing
Arkadelphia, Arkansas

http://www.hsu.edu/nursing/
Founded in 1890

DEGREE • BSN

Nursing Program Faculty 7 (3% with doctorates).

Baccalaureate Enrollment 43 **Women** 79% **Men** 21%

Nursing Student Activities Sigma Theta Tau, Student Nurses' Association, nursing club.

Nursing Student Resources Academic advising; academic or career counseling; assistance for students with disabilities; bookstore; campus computer network; career placement assistance; computer lab; computer-assisted instruction; e-mail services; employment services for current students; housing assistance; interactive nursing skills videos; Internet; learning resource lab; library services; nursing audiovisuals; remedial services; resume preparation assistance; skills, simulation, or other laboratory; tutoring.

Library Facilities 1,000 volumes in health, 200 volumes in nursing; 15 periodical subscriptions health-care related.

BACCALAUREATE PROGRAMS

Degree BSN

Available Programs ADN to Baccalaureate; Generic Baccalaureate; LPN to Baccalaureate.

Study Options Full-time.

Program Entrance Requirements Minimum overall college GPA of 2.5, transcript of college record, CPR certification, written essay, immunizations, minimum GPA in nursing prerequisites of 2.50, prerequisite course work. Transfer students are accepted. *Application deadline:* 2/15 (fall). *Application fee:* $57.

Advanced Placement Credit given for nursing courses completed elsewhere dependent upon specific evaluations.

Expenses (2014–15) *Tuition, state resident:* full-time $5970. *Room and board:* $7022; room only: $4000 per academic year. *Required fees:* full-time $2592.

Financial Aid 80% of baccalaureate students in nursing programs received some form of financial aid in 2013–14. *Gift aid (need-based):* Federal Pell, FSEOG, state, private. *Loans:* Federal Direct (Subsidized and Unsubsidized Stafford PLUS), Perkins. *Work-study:* Federal Work-Study, part-time campus jobs. *Financial aid application deadline (priority):* 6/1.

Contact Dr. Barbara J. Landrum, Professor and Department Chair, Department of Nursing, Henderson State University, Box 7803, 1100 Henderson Street, Arkadelphia, AR 71999-0001. *Telephone:* 870-230-5508. *Fax:* 870-230-5390. *E-mail:* landrub@hsu.edu.

Southern Arkansas University–Magnolia
Department of Nursing
Magnolia, Arkansas

http://web.saumag.edu/nursing/
Founded in 1909

DEGREE • BSN

Nursing Program Faculty 13 (23% with doctorates).

Baccalaureate Enrollment 51 **Women** 90% **Men** 10% **Part-time** 58%

Distance Learning Courses Available.

Nursing Student Activities Student Nurses' Association.

Nursing Student Resources Academic advising; academic or career counseling; assistance for students with disabilities; bookstore; campus computer network; career placement assistance; computer lab; computer-assisted instruction; e-mail services; employment services for current students; housing assistance; interactive nursing skills videos; Internet; learning resource lab; library services; nursing audiovisuals; remedial services; resume preparation assistance; skills, simulation, or other laboratory; tutoring.

Library Facilities 800 volumes in health, 200 volumes in nursing; 2,000 periodical subscriptions health-care related.

BACCALAUREATE PROGRAMS

Degree BSN

Available Programs ADN to Baccalaureate; Generic Baccalaureate; RN Baccalaureate.
Study Options Full-time.
Online Degree Options Yes.
Program Entrance Requirements Minimum overall college GPA of 2.5, transcript of college record, CPR certification, high school chemistry, immunizations, minimum GPA in nursing prerequisites of 2.5, prerequisite course work. Transfer students are accepted. *Application deadline:* 2/28 (fall). Applications may be processed on a rolling basis for some programs.
Advanced Placement Credit given for nursing courses completed elsewhere dependent upon specific evaluations.
Contact *Telephone:* 870-235-4331. *Fax:* 870-235-5058.

University of Arkansas
Eleanor Mann School of Nursing
Fayetteville, Arkansas

http://nurs.uark.edu/
Founded in 1871

DEGREES • BSN • DNP • MSN
Nursing Program Faculty 30 (50% with doctorates).
Baccalaureate Enrollment 400 **Women** 92% **Men** 8%
Graduate Enrollment 70 **Women** 93% **Men** 7% **Part-time** 51%
Distance Learning Courses Available.
Nursing Student Activities Nursing Honor Society, Sigma Theta Tau, Student Nurses' Association.
Nursing Student Resources Academic advising; academic or career counseling; assistance for students with disabilities; bookstore; campus computer network; career placement assistance; computer lab; computer-assisted instruction; e-mail services; employment services for current students; housing assistance; interactive nursing skills videos; Internet; learning resource lab; library services; nursing audiovisuals; other; placement services for program completers; remedial services; resume preparation assistance; skills, simulation, or other laboratory; tutoring.
Library Facilities 60,000 volumes in health, 20,000 volumes in nursing; 130,000 periodical subscriptions health-care related.

BACCALAUREATE PROGRAMS

Degree BSN
Available Programs ADN to Baccalaureate; Generic Baccalaureate; LPN to Baccalaureate; LPN to RN Baccalaureate; RN Baccalaureate.
Study Options Full-time.
Online Degree Options Yes.
Program Entrance Requirements Minimum overall college GPA of 3.0, transcript of college record, CPR certification, health insurance, immunizations, minimum GPA in nursing prerequisites of 3.00, professional liability insurance/malpractice insurance, prerequisite course work. Transfer students are accepted. *Application deadline:* 12/1 (fall), 5/1 (spring). *Application fee:* $45.
Financial Aid *Gift aid (need-based):* Federal Pell, FSEOG, state, private, college/university gift aid from institutional funds. *Loans:* Federal Nursing Student Loans, Federal Direct (Subsidized and Unsubsidized Stafford PLUS), Perkins, state, college/university, alternative loans. *Work-study:* Federal Work-Study. *Financial aid application deadline (priority):* 3/15.
Contact Dr. Pegge Bell, Director, Eleanor Mann School of Nursing, University of Arkansas, 606 North Razorback Road, Fayetteville, AR 72701. *Telephone:* 479-575-3907. *Fax:* 479-575-3218. *E-mail:* plbell@uark.edu.

GRADUATE PROGRAMS

Contact Dr. Pegge Bell, Director, Eleanor Mann School of Nursing, University of Arkansas, 606 North Razorback Road, Fayetteville, AR 72701. *Telephone:* 479-575-3907. *Fax:* 479-575-3218. *E-mail:* plbell@uark.edu.

MASTER'S DEGREE PROGRAM
Degree MSN
Available Programs Master's.
Concentrations Available Nursing education. *Clinical nurse specialist programs in:* acute care, medical-surgical.
Study Options Full-time and part-time.
Online Degree Options Yes (online only).
Program Entrance Requirements Computer literacy, minimum overall college GPA of 3.0, transcript of college record, CPR certification, immu-

nizations, nursing research course, physical assessment course, statistics course. *Application deadline:* 7/15 (fall), 10/1 (spring). *Application fee:* $45.
Degree Requirements 42 total credit hours, thesis or project, comprehensive exam.

DOCTORAL DEGREE PROGRAM
Degree DNP
Available Programs Doctorate; Post-Baccalaureate Doctorate.
Areas of Study Advanced practice nursing, gerontology, health promotion/disease prevention.
Online Degree Options Yes (online only).
Program Entrance Requirements Clinical experience, minimum overall college GPA of 3.0, statistics course. Application deadline: 2/1 (fall), 10/1 (spring). Application fee: $45.

University of Arkansas at Little Rock
BSN Programs
Little Rock, Arkansas

http://ualr.edu/
Founded in 1927

DEGREE • BSN

BACCALAUREATE PROGRAMS

Degree BSN
Available Programs RN Baccalaureate.
Contact *Telephone:* 501-569-8081.

University of Arkansas at Monticello
School of Nursing
Monticello, Arkansas

http://www.uamont.edu/Nursing/
Founded in 1909

DEGREE • BSN
Nursing Program Faculty 10 (27% with doctorates).
Baccalaureate Enrollment 52 **Women** 83% **Men** 17%
Nursing Student Activities Sigma Theta Tau, Student Nurses' Association.
Nursing Student Resources Academic advising; academic or career counseling; assistance for students with disabilities; bookstore; campus computer network; computer lab; computer-assisted instruction; e-mail services; interactive nursing skills videos; Internet; learning resource lab; library services; nursing audiovisuals; remedial services; resume preparation assistance; skills, simulation, or other laboratory; tutoring.
Library Facilities 3,888 volumes in health, 539 volumes in nursing; 5,015 periodical subscriptions health-care related.

BACCALAUREATE PROGRAMS

Degree BSN
Available Programs ADN to Baccalaureate; Generic Baccalaureate; LPN to Baccalaureate; RN Baccalaureate.
Study Options Full-time.
Program Entrance Requirements Minimum overall college GPA of 2.5, transcript of college record, CPR certification, immunizations, minimum GPA in nursing prerequisites of 2.5, prerequisite course work. Transfer students are accepted. *Application deadline:* 3/1 (spring).
Advanced Placement Credit given for nursing courses completed elsewhere dependent upon specific evaluations.
Expenses (2015–16) *Tuition, state resident:* full-time $4500; part-time $150 per credit. *Tuition, nonresident:* full-time $5850; part-time $195 per credit. *International tuition:* $5850 full-time.
Contact Dr. Laura K. Evans, Dean, School of Nursing, University of Arkansas at Monticello, 124 University Place, PO Box 3606, Monticello, AR 71656. *Telephone:* 870-460-1069. *Fax:* 870-460-1969. *E-mail:* evansl@uamont.edu.

University of Arkansas for Medical Sciences
College of Nursing
Little Rock, Arkansas

http://www.nursing.uams.edu/
Founded in 1879
DEGREES • BSN • DNP • MN SC • PHD
Nursing Program Faculty 85 (38% with doctorates).
Baccalaureate Enrollment 384 **Women** 83.07% **Men** 16.93%
Graduate Enrollment 262 **Women** 85.5% **Men** 14.5%
Distance Learning Courses Available.
Nursing Student Activities Nursing Honor Society, Sigma Theta Tau, Student Nurses' Association.
Nursing Student Resources Academic advising; academic or career counseling; assistance for students with disabilities; bookstore; campus computer network; computer lab; computer-assisted instruction; e-mail services; externships; interactive nursing skills videos; Internet; learning resource lab; library services; nursing audiovisuals; remedial services; skills, simulation, or other laboratory; tutoring.
Library Facilities 183,975 volumes in health; 1,567 periodical subscriptions health-care related.

BACCALAUREATE PROGRAMS

Degree BSN
Available Programs ADN to Baccalaureate; Accelerated RN Baccalaureate; Baccalaureate for Second Degree; Generic Baccalaureate; LPN to Baccalaureate; RN Baccalaureate.
Site Options Texarkana, AR; Helena, AR; Jonesboro, AR; Fayetteville, AR; El Dorado, AR; Hope, AR.
Study Options Full-time.
Online Degree Options Yes.
Program Entrance Requirements Minimum overall college GPA of 2.5, transcript of college record, CPR certification, health insurance, immunizations, interview, minimum high school GPA of 2.5, minimum GPA in nursing prerequisites of 2.5, prerequisite course work. Transfer students are accepted. *Application deadline:* 3/1 (summer). *Application fee:* $60.
Advanced Placement Credit by examination available. Credit given for nursing courses completed elsewhere dependent upon specific evaluations.
Financial Aid 90% of baccalaureate students in nursing programs received some form of financial aid in 2013–14.
Contact Dr. Donna Middaugh, Associate Dean for Academic Programs, College of Nursing, University of Arkansas for Medical Sciences, 4301 West Markham, #529, Little Rock, AR 72205-7199. *Telephone:* 501-686-5374. *Fax:* 501-686-8350. *E-mail:* middaughdonnaj@uams.edu.

GRADUATE PROGRAMS

Expenses (2014–15) *Tuition, state resident:* part-time $366 per credit hour. *Tuition, nonresident:* part-time $632 per credit hour.
Financial Aid 90% of graduate students in nursing programs received some form of financial aid in 2013–14. Career-related internships or fieldwork and traineeships available. Aid available to part-time students.
Contact Dr. Donna Middaugh, Associate Dean for Academic Programs, College of Nursing, University of Arkansas for Medical Sciences, 4301 West Markham, #529, Little Rock, AR 72205-7199. *Telephone:* 501-686-8349. *Fax:* 501-686-8350. *E-mail:* middaughdonnaj@uams.edu.

MASTER'S DEGREE PROGRAM

Degree MN Sc
Available Programs Master's; Master's for Nurses with Non-Nursing Degrees; RN to Master's.
Concentrations Available Nursing administration; nursing education. *Clinical nurse specialist programs in:* acute care, adult health, pediatric. *Nurse practitioner programs in:* acute care, family health, pediatric, psychiatric/mental health.
Site Options Texarkana, AR; Helena, AR; Jonesboro, AR; Fayetteville, AR; El Dorado, AR.
Study Options Full-time and part-time.
Program Entrance Requirements Clinical experience, minimum overall college GPA of 2.85, transcript of college record, CPR certification, immunizations, physical assessment course, professional liability insurance/malpractice insurance, statistics course. *Application deadline:* 4/1 (fall), 9/1 (spring). *Application fee:* $60.

Advanced Placement Credit given for nursing courses completed elsewhere dependent upon specific evaluations.
Degree Requirements 39 total credit hours, thesis or project, comprehensive exam.

DOCTORAL DEGREE PROGRAM
Degree DNP
Available Programs Doctorate.
Areas of Study Clinical practice.
Program Entrance Requirements Minimum overall college GPA of 3.4, clinical experience, interview, interview by faculty committee, 3 letters of recommendation, MSN or equivalent, statistics course. Application deadline: 3/1 (spring). Application fee: $60.
Degree Requirements 29 total credit hours, oral exam, written exam.

Degree PhD
Available Programs Doctorate; Post-Baccalaureate Doctorate.
Areas of Study Advanced practice nursing, clinical practice, gerontology, health-care systems, nursing administration, nursing education, nursing research, nursing science, oncology.
Program Entrance Requirements Minimum overall college GPA of 3.65, interview by faculty committee, interview, 4 letters of recommendation, MSN or equivalent, scholarly papers, statistics course, writing sample, GRE. Application deadline: 3/1 (spring). Application fee: $60.
Degree Requirements 60 total credit hours, dissertation, oral exam, written exam.

POSTDOCTORAL PROGRAM
Areas of Study Aging, cancer care, gerontology, nursing research, nursing science.
Postdoctoral Program Contact Dr. Jean McSweeney, Postdoctoral Contact, College of Nursing, University of Arkansas for Medical Sciences, 4301 West Markham, #529, Little Rock, AR 72205-7199. *Telephone:* 501-686-5374. *Fax:* 501-686-8350. *E-mail:* mcsweeneyjeanc@uams.edu.

CONTINUING EDUCATION PROGRAM

Contact Dr. Jean McSweeney, Interim Dean, College of Nursing, University of Arkansas for Medical Sciences, 4301 West Markham, #529, Little Rock, AR 72205-7199. *Telephone:* 501-686-5374. *Fax:* 501-686-8350. *E-mail:* McSweeneyJeanC@uams.edu.

University of Arkansas–Fort Smith
Carol McKelvey Moore School of Nursing
Fort Smith, Arkansas

http://uafs.edu/
Founded in 1928
DEGREE • BSN
Nursing Program Faculty 18
Baccalaureate Enrollment 20 **Women** 60% **Men** 40%
Distance Learning Courses Available.
Nursing Student Activities Student Nurses' Association.
Nursing Student Resources Academic advising; academic or career counseling; assistance for students with disabilities; bookstore; campus computer network; career placement assistance; computer lab; computer-assisted instruction; e-mail services; housing assistance; interactive nursing skills videos; Internet; learning resource lab; library services; nursing audiovisuals; remedial services; resume preparation assistance; skills, simulation, or other laboratory; tutoring.
Library Facilities 2,231 volumes in health, 1,183 volumes in nursing; 5,350 periodical subscriptions health-care related.

BACCALAUREATE PROGRAMS

Degree BSN
Available Programs ADN to Baccalaureate; Generic Baccalaureate.
Study Options Full-time.
Online Degree Options Yes (online only).
Program Entrance Requirements Minimum overall college GPA of 2.5, transcript of college record, CPR certification, health exam, health insurance, immunizations, interview, minimum GPA in nursing prerequisites of 2.5, prerequisite course work. Transfer students are accepted.

Advanced Placement Credit given for nursing courses completed elsewhere dependent upon specific evaluations.
Contact *Telephone:* 479-788-7840. *Fax:* 479-788-7869.

University of Central Arkansas

Department of Nursing
Conway, Arkansas

http://www.uca.edu/nursing/
Founded in 1907
DEGREES • BSN • MSN
Nursing Program Faculty 32 (28% with doctorates).
Baccalaureate Enrollment 245 **Women** 84.9% **Men** 15.1% **Part-time** 23.67%
Graduate Enrollment 136 **Women** 95.59% **Men** 4.41% **Part-time** 95.59%
Distance Learning Courses Available.
Nursing Student Activities Sigma Theta Tau, Student Nurses' Association.
Nursing Student Resources Academic advising; academic or career counseling; assistance for students with disabilities; bookstore; campus computer network; career placement assistance; computer lab; computer-assisted instruction; e-mail services; employment services for current students; externships; housing assistance; interactive nursing skills videos; Internet; learning resource lab; library services; nursing audiovisuals; paid internships; placement services for program completers; remedial services; resume preparation assistance; skills, simulation, or other laboratory; tutoring; unpaid internships.

BACCALAUREATE PROGRAMS

Degree BSN
Available Programs ADN to Baccalaureate; Generic Baccalaureate; LPN to Baccalaureate; LPN to RN Baccalaureate; RN Baccalaureate.
Study Options Full-time and part-time.
Program Entrance Requirements Minimum overall college GPA of 2.5, transcript of college record, health exam, health insurance, immunizations, minimum GPA in nursing prerequisites, prerequisite course work. Transfer students are accepted. *Application deadline:* 3/1 (fall). *Application fee:* $50.
Advanced Placement Credit given for nursing courses completed elsewhere dependent upon specific evaluations.
Contact *Telephone:* 501-450-5526. *Fax:* 501-450-5560.

GRADUATE PROGRAMS

Contact *Telephone:* 501-450-5532. *Fax:* 501-450-5560.

MASTER'S DEGREE PROGRAM
Degree MSN
Available Programs Master's; RN to Master's.
Concentrations Available Nursing education. *Clinical nurse specialist programs in:* medical-surgical. *Nurse practitioner programs in:* adult health, family health.
Site Options Russelville, AR; Pine Bluff, AR; Fort Smith, AR.
Study Options Full-time and part-time.
Online Degree Options Yes (online only).
Program Entrance Requirements Clinical experience, minimum overall college GPA of 2.7, transcript of college record, CPR certification, immunizations, professional liability insurance/malpractice insurance, prerequisite course work, resume, statistics course, GRE General Test. *Application deadline:* 4/1 (fall), 8/1 (spring). *Application fee:* $50.
Degree Requirements 39 total credit hours, comprehensive exam.

POST-MASTER'S PROGRAM
Areas of Study Nursing education. *Clinical nurse specialist programs in:* medical-surgical. *Nurse practitioner programs in:* adult health, family health.

CALIFORNIA

American University of Health Sciences
School of Nursing
Signal Hill, California

http://www.auhs.edu/
DEGREE • BSN
Nursing Program Faculty 17 (37% with doctorates).
Baccalaureate Enrollment 195 **Women** 72% **Men** 28%
Nursing Student Activities Nursing Honor Society, Student Nurses' Association, nursing club.
Nursing Student Resources Academic advising; academic or career counseling; assistance for students with disabilities; campus computer network; career placement assistance; computer lab; computer-assisted instruction; e-mail services; interactive nursing skills videos; Internet; learning resource lab; library services; nursing audiovisuals; other; placement services for program completers; remedial services; resume preparation assistance; skills, simulation, or other laboratory; tutoring; unpaid internships.
Library Facilities 1,881 volumes in health, 783 volumes in nursing; 71 periodical subscriptions health-care related.

BACCALAUREATE PROGRAMS

Degree BSN
Available Programs ADN to Baccalaureate; Accelerated RN Baccalaureate.
Study Options Full-time.
Program Entrance Requirements Minimum overall college GPA of 2.5, transcript of college record, CPR certification, written essay, health exam, high school foreign language, 3 years high school math, high school transcript, immunizations, interview, 2 letters of recommendation, minimum high school GPA of 2.5, minimum GPA in nursing prerequisites of 2.50, professional liability insurance/malpractice insurance, prerequisite course work. Transfer students are accepted. *Application deadline:* Applications may be processed on a rolling basis for some programs. *Application fee:* $80.
Advanced Placement Credit by examination available. Credit given for nursing courses completed elsewhere dependent upon specific evaluations.
Contact School of Nursing, School of Nursing, American University of Health Sciences, 1600 East Hill Street, Building #1, Signal Hill, CA 90755. *Telephone:* 562-988-2278. *E-mail:* bsninfo@auhs.edu.

Azusa Pacific University
School of Nursing
Azusa, California

http://www.apu.edu/nursing/
Founded in 1899
DEGREES • BSN • MSN • PHD
Nursing Program Faculty 77 (22% with doctorates).
Baccalaureate Enrollment 236 **Women** 90% **Men** 10% **Part-time** 2%
Graduate Enrollment 110 **Women** 89% **Men** 11%
Nursing Student Activities Sigma Theta Tau, Student Nurses' Association, nursing club.
Nursing Student Resources Academic advising; academic or career counseling; bookstore; campus computer network; career placement assistance; computer lab; computer-assisted instruction; e-mail services; employment services for current students; housing assistance; interactive nursing skills videos; Internet; learning resource lab; library services; nursing audiovisuals; remedial services; resume preparation assistance; skills, simulation, or other laboratory; tutoring.
Library Facilities 14,206 volumes in health, 4,712 volumes in nursing; 432 periodical subscriptions health-care related.

BACCALAUREATE PROGRAMS

Degree BSN
Available Programs ADN to Baccalaureate; Accelerated Baccalaureate; Accelerated RN Baccalaureate; Generic Baccalaureate.
Study Options Full-time and part-time.

Program Entrance Requirements Minimum overall college GPA of 3.0, transcript of college record, CPR certification, written essay, health exam, high school biology, high school chemistry, 2 years high school math, high school transcript, immunizations, 3 letters of recommendation, minimum high school GPA of 3.0, minimum GPA in nursing prerequisites of 3.0. Transfer students are accepted.
Advanced Placement Credit by examination available. Credit given for nursing courses completed elsewhere dependent upon specific evaluations.
Contact *Telephone:* 626-815-6000 Ext. 5501. *Fax:* 626-815-5414.

GRADUATE PROGRAMS

Contact *Telephone:* 626-815-5386. *Fax:* 626-815-5414.

MASTER'S DEGREE PROGRAM
Degree MSN
Available Programs Accelerated Master's for Non-Nursing College Graduates; Accelerated Master's for Nurses with Non-Nursing Degrees; Master's.
Concentrations Available Nursing administration; nursing education. *Clinical nurse specialist programs in:* adult health, medical-surgical, parent-child, pediatric, school health. *Nurse practitioner programs in:* adult health, family health, pediatric, primary care.
Study Options Full-time and part-time.
Program Entrance Requirements Clinical experience, computer literacy, minimum overall college GPA of 3.0, transcript of college record, CPR certification, written essay, immunizations, 3 letters of recommendation, nursing research course, physical assessment course, professional liability insurance/malpractice insurance, prerequisite course work, resume, statistics course.
Advanced Placement Credit by examination available. Credit given for nursing courses completed elsewhere dependent upon specific evaluations.
Degree Requirements 42 total credit hours, thesis or project, comprehensive exam.

POST-MASTER'S PROGRAM
Areas of Study Nursing administration; nursing education. *Clinical nurse specialist programs in:* adult health, medical-surgical, parent-child, pediatric, school health. *Nurse practitioner programs in:* adult health, family health, pediatric, primary care.

DOCTORAL DEGREE PROGRAM
Degree PhD
Available Programs Doctorate.
Areas of Study Community health, family health, nursing education.
Program Entrance Requirements Clinical experience, minimum overall college GPA of 3.5, interview by faculty committee, interview, 3 letters of recommendation, MSN or equivalent, scholarly papers, statistics course, vita, writing sample.
Degree Requirements 64 total credit hours, dissertation, oral exam, written exam.

CONTINUING EDUCATION PROGRAM

Contact *Telephone:* 626-815-5385. *Fax:* 626-815-5414.

Biola University
Department of Nursing
La Mirada, California

http://www.biola.edu/
Founded in 1908
DEGREE • BSN
Nursing Program Faculty 24 (13% with doctorates).
Baccalaureate Enrollment 119 **Women** 91.6% **Men** 8.4%
Nursing Student Activities Student Nurses' Association.
Nursing Student Resources Academic advising; academic or career counseling; assistance for students with disabilities; bookstore; campus computer network; career placement assistance; computer lab; computer-assisted instruction; e-mail services; employment services for current students; housing assistance; Internet; learning resource lab; library services; nursing audiovisuals; placement services for program completers; remedial services; resume preparation assistance; skills, simulation, or other laboratory; tutoring.
Library Facilities 20,000 volumes in health, 10,000 volumes in nursing; 750 periodical subscriptions health-care related.

BACCALAUREATE PROGRAMS
Degree BSN
Available Programs ADN to Baccalaureate; Generic Baccalaureate; LPN to Baccalaureate; RN Baccalaureate.
Study Options Full-time.
Program Entrance Requirements Minimum overall college GPA of 3.0, transcript of college record, written essay, high school chemistry, 2 years high school math, high school transcript, interview, 2 letters of recommendation, minimum high school GPA of 3.5, minimum GPA in nursing prerequisites of 2.5, prerequisite course work. *Application deadline:* 1/15 (fall). *Application fee:* $85.
Advanced Placement Credit given for nursing courses completed elsewhere dependent upon specific evaluations.
Expenses (2015–16) *Tuition:* full-time $34,498; part-time $1438 per credit. *International tuition:* $34,498 full-time. *Room and board:* $10,224; room only: $7906 per academic year. *Required fees:* full-time $400; part-time $200 per term.
Financial Aid 98% of baccalaureate students in nursing programs received some form of financial aid in 2014–15.
Contact Ms. Shannon Gramatky, Nursing Department Advisor, Department of Nursing, Biola University, 13800 Biola Avenue, La Mirada, CA 90639. *Telephone:* 562-903-4850. *Fax:* 562-903-4803. *E-mail:* shannon.gramatky@biola.edu.

Brandman University
School of Nursing and Health Professions
Irvine, California

https://www.brandman.edu/nursing-health-professions
Founded in 2009
DEGREES • BSN • DNP
Nursing Program Faculty 32 (78% with doctorates).
Baccalaureate Enrollment 41 **Women** 90.24% **Men** 9.76% **Part-time** 85.4%
Graduate Enrollment 245 **Women** 82.04% **Men** 17.96% **Part-time** 44.5%
Distance Learning Courses Available.
Nursing Student Activities Nursing Honor Society, Student Nurses' Association.
Nursing Student Resources Academic advising; academic or career counseling; assistance for students with disabilities; bookstore; campus computer network; computer lab; computer-assisted instruction; e-mail services; employment services for current students; interactive nursing skills videos; Internet; learning resource lab; library services; nursing audiovisuals; other; remedial services; resume preparation assistance; skills, simulation, or other laboratory; tutoring; unpaid internships.
Library Facilities 1,609 volumes in health, 269 volumes in nursing; 875 periodical subscriptions health-care related.

BACCALAUREATE PROGRAMS
Degree BSN
Available Programs RN Baccalaureate.
Study Options Full-time and part-time.
Online Degree Options Yes (online only).
Program Entrance Requirements Minimum overall college GPA of 2.0, transcript of college record, CPR certification, immunizations, 3 letters of recommendation, minimum GPA in nursing prerequisites of 2.0, professional liability insurance/malpractice insurance, prerequisite course work, RN licensure. *Application deadline:* 8/15 (fall), 12/1 (winter). Applications may be processed on a rolling basis for some programs.
Expenses (2015–16) *Tuition:* full-time $18,000; part-time $500 per credit hour. *International tuition:* $18,000 full-time. *Required fees:* full-time $580; part-time $60 per term.
Contact Deann Avila, Enrollment Coach, School of Nursing and Health Professions, Brandman University, 16355 Laguna Canyon Road, Irvine, CA 92618. *Telephone:* 866-685-8793. *E-mail:* nursingcoaches@brandman.edu.

GRADUATE PROGRAMS
Expenses (2015–16) *Tuition:* full-time $79,570; part-time $1090 per credit hour. *International tuition:* $79,570 full-time. *Required fees:* full-time $2380; part-time $60 per term.
Contact Deann Avila, Enrollment Coach, School of Nursing and Health Professions, Brandman University, 16355 Laguna Canyon Road, Irvine, CA 92618. *Telephone:* 866-685-8793. *E-mail:* nursingcoaches@brandman.edu.

MASTER'S DEGREE PROGRAM

Program Entrance Requirements *Application deadline:* 8/1 (fall), 12/1 (winter).

DOCTORAL DEGREE PROGRAM

Degree DNP
Available Programs Doctorate; Post-Baccalaureate Doctorate.
Areas of Study Advanced practice nursing, family health, gerontology.
Online Degree Options Yes (online only).
Program Entrance Requirements interview by faculty committee, interview, 3 letters of recommendation, statistics course, writing sample. Application deadline: 8/15 (fall), 12/1 (winter). Applications may be processed on a rolling basis for some programs.
Degree Requirements 73 total credit hours.

POSTDOCTORAL PROGRAM

Areas of Study Adolescent health, chronic illness, family health, gerontology, neuro-behavior.
Postdoctoral Program Contact Deann Avila, Enrollment Coach, School of Nursing and Health Professions, Brandman University, 16355 Laguna Canyon Road, Irvine, CA 92618. *Telephone:* 866-685-8793. *E-mail:* nursingcoaches@brandman.edu.

CONTINUING EDUCATION PROGRAM

Contact Nursing Representative, School of Nursing and Health Professions, Brandman University, 16355 Laguna Canyon Road, Irvine, CA 92618. *Telephone:* 949-341-9940. *E-mail:* nursing@brandman.edu.

California Baptist University

School of Nursing
Riverside, California

http://www.calbaptist.edu/nursing
Founded in 1950
DEGREES • BSN • MSN
Nursing Program Faculty 26 (4% with doctorates).
Baccalaureate Enrollment 180 **Women** 87.78% **Men** 12.22%
Graduate Enrollment 16 **Women** 87.5% **Men** 12.5%
Nursing Student Activities Student Nurses' Association.
Nursing Student Resources Academic advising; academic or career counseling; bookstore; campus computer network; career placement assistance; computer lab; e-mail services; employment services for current students; interactive nursing skills videos; Internet; learning resource lab; library services; nursing audiovisuals; resume preparation assistance; skills, simulation, or other laboratory; tutoring.
Library Facilities 335 volumes in health, 236 volumes in nursing; 286 periodical subscriptions health-care related.

BACCALAUREATE PROGRAMS

Degree BSN
Available Programs ADN to Baccalaureate; Generic Baccalaureate; RN Baccalaureate.
Site Options Corona, CA; San Bernardino, CA; Fullerton, CA.
Study Options Full-time.
Program Entrance Requirements Minimum overall college GPA of 2.7, transcript of college record, CPR certification, written essay, health exam, health insurance, immunizations, 2 letters of recommendation, minimum GPA in nursing prerequisites of 2.7, professional liability insurance/malpractice insurance, prerequisite course work. Transfer students are accepted. *Application deadline:* 3/11 (fall), 8/31 (spring). *Application fee:* $50.
Contact *Telephone:* 951-343-4336.

GRADUATE PROGRAMS

Contact *Telephone:* 951-343-4336. *Fax:* 951-343-4703.

MASTER'S DEGREE PROGRAM

Degree MSN
Available Programs Accelerated Master's for Non-Nursing College Graduates; Master's.
Concentrations Available Clinical nurse leader; nursing education. *Clinical nurse specialist programs in:* adult health.
Study Options Part-time.
Program Entrance Requirements Computer literacy, minimum overall college GPA of 3.25, transcript of college record, CPR certification, written essay, immunizations, interview, 3 letters of recommendation, professional liability insurance/malpractice insurance, prerequisite course work, resume, statistics course. *Application deadline:* Applications may be processed on a rolling basis for some programs. *Application fee:* $45.
Degree Requirements 42 total credit hours, thesis or project, comprehensive exam.

California State University, Bakersfield

Program in Nursing
Bakersfield, California

http://www.csub.edu/nursing
Founded in 1970
DEGREE • BSN
Nursing Program Faculty 24 (15% with doctorates).
Baccalaureate Enrollment 208 **Women** 86% **Men** 14% **Part-time** 6%
Distance Learning Courses Available.
Nursing Student Activities Nursing Honor Society, Sigma Theta Tau, Student Nurses' Association, nursing club.
Nursing Student Resources Academic advising; academic or career counseling; assistance for students with disabilities; bookstore; campus computer network; career placement assistance; computer lab; computer-assisted instruction; daycare for children of students; e-mail services; employment services for current students; externships; housing assistance; interactive nursing skills videos; Internet; learning resource lab; library services; nursing audiovisuals; paid internships; placement services for program completers; remedial services; resume preparation assistance; skills, simulation, or other laboratory; tutoring; unpaid internships.
Library Facilities 20,000 volumes in health, 1,850 volumes in nursing; 255 periodical subscriptions health-care related.

BACCALAUREATE PROGRAMS

Degree BSN
Available Programs ADN to Baccalaureate; Generic Baccalaureate.
Site Options Visalia, CA; Lancaster, CA.
Study Options Full-time.
Program Entrance Requirements Minimum overall college GPA of 2.0, transcript of college record, CPR certification, health exam, health insurance, high school transcript, immunizations, interview, minimum GPA in nursing prerequisites of 2.8, professional liability insurance/malpractice insurance, prerequisite course work. Transfer students are accepted. *Application deadline:* 4/30 (fall), 12/31 (spring). *Application fee:* $25.
Advanced Placement Credit by examination available. Credit given for nursing courses completed elsewhere dependent upon specific evaluations.
Contact *Telephone:* 661-654-2508. *Fax:* 661-654-6347.

CONTINUING EDUCATION PROGRAM

Contact *Telephone:* 661-654-2446. *Fax:* 661-664-2447.

California State University Channel Islands

Nursing Program
Camarillo, California

http://www.csuci.edu/
Founded in 2002
DEGREE • BSN
Nursing Program Faculty 13 (20% with doctorates).
Baccalaureate Enrollment 120
Nursing Student Activities Student Nurses' Association.
Nursing Student Resources Academic advising; academic or career counseling; assistance for students with disabilities; bookstore; campus computer network; career placement assistance; computer lab; e-mail services; housing assistance; interactive nursing skills videos; Internet; learning resource lab; library services; nursing audiovisuals; remedial services; skills, simulation, or other laboratory; tutoring.

BACCALAUREATE PROGRAMS

Degree BSN
Available Programs Generic Baccalaureate; RN Baccalaureate.
Contact *Telephone:* 805-437-3307.

California State University, Chico

School of Nursing
Chico, California

http://www.csuchico.edu/nurs/
Founded in 1887

DEGREES • BSN • MSN

Nursing Program Faculty 39 (28% with doctorates).
Baccalaureate Enrollment 198 **Women** 78% **Men** 22%
Graduate Enrollment 12 **Women** 92% **Men** 8% **Part-time** 100%
Distance Learning Courses Available.
Nursing Student Activities Nursing Honor Society, Sigma Theta Tau, Student Nurses' Association, nursing club.
Nursing Student Resources Academic advising; academic or career counseling; assistance for students with disabilities; bookstore; campus computer network; career placement assistance; computer lab; computer-assisted instruction; daycare for children of students; e-mail services; employment services for current students; externships; housing assistance; interactive nursing skills videos; Internet; learning resource lab; library services; nursing audiovisuals; placement services for program completers; remedial services; resume preparation assistance; skills, simulation, or other laboratory; tutoring; unpaid internships.
Library Facilities 15,600 volumes in health, 2,330 volumes in nursing; 246 periodical subscriptions health-care related.

BACCALAUREATE PROGRAMS

Degree BSN
Available Programs ADN to Baccalaureate; Baccalaureate for Second Degree; Generic Baccalaureate; RN Baccalaureate.
Site Options Paradise, CA; Oroville, CA; Redding, CA.
Study Options Full-time.
Program Entrance Requirements Minimum overall college GPA of 3.0, transcript of college record, CPR certification, health insurance, immunizations, minimum GPA in nursing prerequisites of 3.0, prerequisite course work. Transfer students are accepted. *Application deadline:* 4/1 (fall), 11/1 (spring). *Application fee:* $50.
Advanced Placement Credit by examination available. Credit given for nursing courses completed elsewhere dependent upon specific evaluations.
Expenses (2015–16) *Tuition, state resident:* full-time $7026; part-time $2364 per semester. *Tuition, nonresident:* full-time $15,954; part-time $4596 per semester. *International tuition:* $15,954 full-time. *Room and board:* $11,000; room only: $1984 per academic year. *Required fees:* full-time $1554; part-time $777 per term.
Financial Aid 66% of baccalaureate students in nursing programs received some form of financial aid in 2014–15.
Contact Dr. Margaret J. Rowberg, Director, School of Nursing, California State University, Chico, Holt Hall 369, Chico, CA 95929-0200. *Telephone:* 530-898-5891. *Fax:* 530-898-6709. *E-mail:* mrowberg@csuchico.edu.

GRADUATE PROGRAMS

Expenses (2015–16) *Tuition, state resident:* full-time $8292; part-time $2730 per semester. *Tuition, nonresident:* full-time $11,640; part-time $6078 per semester. *International tuition:* $11,640 full-time. *Room and board:* $11,200; room only: $9200 per academic year. *Required fees:* full-time $1554; part-time $777 per term.
Financial Aid 30% of graduate students in nursing programs received some form of financial aid in 2014–15. Career-related internships or fieldwork and scholarships available. *Financial aid application deadline:* 3/1.
Contact Irene Morgan, Graduate Coordinator, School of Nursing, California State University, Chico, Holt Hall 369, Chico, CA 95929-0200. *Telephone:* 530-898-5891. *Fax:* 530-898-6709. *E-mail:* imorgan@csuchico.edu.

MASTER'S DEGREE PROGRAM

Degree MSN
Available Programs Master's.
Concentrations Available Nursing administration; nursing education.
Study Options Part-time.

Program Entrance Requirements Clinical experience, minimum overall college GPA of 3.0, transcript of college record, CPR certification, written essay, immunizations, prerequisite course work, statistics course, GRE. *Application deadline:* 5/1 (fall), 5/1 (spring). *Application fee:* $50.
Advanced Placement Credit given for nursing courses completed elsewhere dependent upon specific evaluations.
Degree Requirements 30 total credit hours, thesis or project.

CONTINUING EDUCATION PROGRAM

Contact Dr. Margaret J. Rowberg, Director, School of Nursing, School of Nursing, California State University, Chico, Holt Hall 369, Chico, CA 95929-0200. *Telephone:* 530-898-5891. *Fax:* 530-898-6709. *E-mail:* mrowberg@csuchico.edu.

California State University, Dominguez Hills

Program in Nursing
Carson, California

http://www4.csudh.edu/son/
Founded in 1960

DEGREES • BSN • MSN

Nursing Program Faculty 50 (64% with doctorates).
Baccalaureate Enrollment 485 **Women** 86% **Men** 14% **Part-time** 85%
Graduate Enrollment 275 **Women** 91% **Men** 9% **Part-time** 96%
Distance Learning Courses Available.
Nursing Student Activities Sigma Theta Tau, nursing club.
Nursing Student Resources Academic advising; academic or career counseling; assistance for students with disabilities; bookstore; campus computer network; career placement assistance; computer lab; computer-assisted instruction; e-mail services; interactive nursing skills videos; Internet; learning resource lab; library services; nursing audiovisuals; remedial services; skills, simulation, or other laboratory; tutoring.
Library Facilities 11,085 volumes in health, 1,242 volumes in nursing; 3,361 periodical subscriptions health-care related.

BACCALAUREATE PROGRAMS

Degree BSN
Available Programs Baccalaureate for Second Degree; RN Baccalaureate.
Site Options Ventura, CA.
Study Options Full-time and part-time.
Program Entrance Requirements Minimum overall college GPA of 2.0, transcript of college record, minimum GPA in nursing prerequisites of 2.0, prerequisite course work, RN licensure. Transfer students are accepted. *Application fee:* $55.
Advanced Placement Credit by examination available. Credit given for nursing courses completed elsewhere dependent upon specific evaluations.
Expenses (2015–16) *Tuition, area resident:* part-time $1587 per semester. *Required fees:* part-time $558 per term.
Financial Aid *Gift aid (need-based):* Federal Pell, FSEOG, state, private, college/university gift aid from institutional funds. *Loans:* Federal Direct (Subsidized and Unsubsidized Stafford PLUS), Perkins, college/university. *Work-study:* Federal Work-Study. *Financial aid application deadline:* 5/15(priority: 3/2).
Contact Dr. Nop Ratanasiripong, BSN Coordinator, Program in Nursing, California State University, Dominguez Hills, 1000 East Victoria Street, WH 335, Carson, CA 90747. *Telephone:* 310-243-3225. *Fax:* 310-516-3542. *E-mail:* nratanasiripong@csudh.edu.

GRADUATE PROGRAMS

Expenses (2015–16) *Tuition, area resident:* part-time $1953 per semester. *Required fees:* part-time $558 per term.
Contact Dr. Terri Ares, MSN Coordinator, Program in Nursing, California State University, Dominguez Hills, 1000 East Victoria Street, WH A320, Carson, CA 90747. *Telephone:* 310-243-2644. *Fax:* 310-516-3542. *E-mail:* tares@csudh.edu.

MASTER'S DEGREE PROGRAM

Degree MSN
Available Programs Master's; Master's for Nurses with Non-Nursing Degrees.

Concentrations Available Nursing administration; nursing education. *Clinical nurse specialist programs in:* adult-gerontology acute care, parent-child. *Nurse practitioner programs in:* family health.

Study Options Full-time and part-time.

Online Degree Options Yes (online only).

Program Entrance Requirements Minimum overall college GPA of 3.0, transcript of college record, written essay, nursing research course, physical assessment course, prerequisite course work, resume, statistics course. *Application deadline:* 4/1 (fall), 11/1 (spring). *Application fee:* $55.

Advanced Placement Credit given for nursing courses completed elsewhere dependent upon specific evaluations.

Degree Requirements 40 total credit hours, comprehensive exam.

POST-MASTER'S PROGRAM

Areas of Study Nursing administration; nursing education. *Clinical nurse specialist programs in:* adult-gerontology acute care, parent-child. *Nurse practitioner programs in:* family health.

California State University, East Bay

Department of Nursing and Health Sciences
Hayward, California

http://www20.csueastbay.edu/csci/departments/nursing/
Founded in 1957

DEGREE • BS

Nursing Program Faculty 68 (15% with doctorates).

Baccalaureate Enrollment 496 **Women** 80% **Men** 20% **Part-time** 15%

Distance Learning Courses Available.

Nursing Student Activities Sigma Theta Tau, Student Nurses' Association.

Nursing Student Resources Academic advising; academic or career counseling; assistance for students with disabilities; bookstore; campus computer network; career placement assistance; computer lab; computer-assisted instruction; e-mail services; employment services for current students; externships; interactive nursing skills videos; Internet; learning resource lab; library services; nursing audiovisuals; other; paid internships; placement services for program completers; remedial services; resume preparation assistance; skills, simulation, or other laboratory; tutoring; unpaid internships.

BACCALAUREATE PROGRAMS

Degree BS

Available Programs ADN to Baccalaureate; Generic Baccalaureate.

Site Options Concord, CA.

Study Options Full-time and part-time.

Program Entrance Requirements Minimum overall college GPA, transcript of college record, CPR certification, health exam, health insurance, immunizations, minimum GPA in nursing prerequisites of 3.0, prerequisite course work, RN licensure. Transfer students are accepted. *Application deadline:* 11/30 (fall).

Advanced Placement Credit by examination available. Credit given for nursing courses completed elsewhere dependent upon specific evaluations.

Expenses (2015–16) *Tuition, state resident:* full-time $5500; part-time $1000 per quarter. *Tuition, nonresident:* full-time $10,000. *International tuition:* $10,000 full-time. *Required fees:* full-time $500.

Financial Aid *Gift aid (need-based):* Federal Pell, FSEOG, state, private, college/university gift aid from institutional funds. *Loans:* Federal Direct (Subsidized and Unsubsidized Stafford PLUS), Perkins, college/university. *Work-study:* Federal Work-Study. *Financial aid application deadline (priority):* 3/2.

Contact Nursing Admissions Advisor, Department of Nursing and Health Sciences, California State University, East Bay, Nursing Department, 25800 Carlos Bee Boulevard, Hayward, CA 94542. *Telephone:* 510-885-3481. *Fax:* 510-885-2156. *E-mail:* nursing@csueastbay.edu.

California State University, Fresno

Department of Nursing
Fresno, California

http://www.csufresno.edu/chhs/depts_programs/nursing/
Founded in 1911

DEGREES • BSN • DNP • MSN

Nursing Program Faculty 55 (30% with doctorates).

Baccalaureate Enrollment 450 **Women** 80% **Men** 20% **Part-time** 5%

Graduate Enrollment 270 **Women** 86% **Men** 14% **Part-time** 36%

Distance Learning Courses Available.

Nursing Student Activities Sigma Theta Tau, Student Nurses' Association.

Nursing Student Resources Academic advising; academic or career counseling; assistance for students with disabilities; bookstore; campus computer network; career placement assistance; computer lab; computer-assisted instruction; daycare for children of students; e-mail services; externships; housing assistance; interactive nursing skills videos; Internet; learning resource lab; library services; nursing audiovisuals; paid internships; placement services for program completers; remedial services; skills, simulation, or other laboratory; tutoring.

Library Facilities 28,197 volumes in health, 1,287 volumes in nursing; 1,700 periodical subscriptions health-care related.

BACCALAUREATE PROGRAMS

Degree BSN

Available Programs ADN to Baccalaureate; Generic Baccalaureate.

Study Options Full-time.

Program Entrance Requirements Minimum overall college GPA of 3.0, transcript of college record, CPR certification, health exam, immunizations, minimum GPA in nursing prerequisites of 3.0, professional liability insurance/malpractice insurance, prerequisite course work. Transfer students are accepted. *Application deadline:* 3/31 (fall), 8/31 (spring).

Advanced Placement Credit by examination available. Credit given for nursing courses completed elsewhere dependent upon specific evaluations.

Contact *Telephone:* 559-278-2041. *Fax:* 559-278-6360.

GRADUATE PROGRAMS

Contact *Telephone:* 559-278-6697. *Fax:* 559-278-6360.

MASTER'S DEGREE PROGRAM

Degree MSN

Available Programs Accelerated Master's; Master's.

Concentrations Available Nursing education. *Clinical nurse specialist programs in:* adult health, gerontology, pediatric. *Nurse practitioner programs in:* family health, pediatric.

Study Options Full-time.

Program Entrance Requirements Clinical experience, computer literacy, minimum overall college GPA of 3.0, transcript of college record, CPR certification, written essay, 3 letters of recommendation, nursing research course, physical assessment course, professional liability insurance/malpractice insurance, prerequisite course work, resume, statistics course, GRE General Test. *Application deadline:* 4/1 (fall).

Advanced Placement Credit given for nursing courses completed elsewhere dependent upon specific evaluations.

Degree Requirements 40 total credit hours, thesis or project.

POST-MASTER'S PROGRAM

Areas of Study *Nurse practitioner programs in:* family health, pediatric.

DOCTORAL DEGREE PROGRAM

Degree DNP

Available Programs Doctorate.

Online Degree Options Yes (online only).

Program Entrance Requirements Clinical experience, minimum overall college GPA of 3.0, interview by faculty committee, 3 letters of recommendation, MSN or equivalent, vita, writing sample. Application deadline: 1/31 (fall).

Degree Requirements 37 total credit hours, oral exam.

CONTINUING EDUCATION PROGRAM

Contact *Telephone:* 559-278-2691. *Fax:* 559-278-0333.

California State University, Fullerton

Department of Nursing
Fullerton, California

http://www.fullerton.edu/
Founded in 1957
DEGREES • BSN • DNP • MSN
Nursing Program Faculty 71 (28% with doctorates).
Baccalaureate Enrollment 464 **Women** 83.2% **Men** 16.8% **Part-time** 69%
Graduate Enrollment 372 **Women** 84.9% **Men** 15.1% **Part-time** 46.5%
Distance Learning Courses Available.
Nursing Student Activities Nursing Honor Society, Sigma Theta Tau, Student Nurses' Association.
Nursing Student Resources Academic advising; academic or career counseling; assistance for students with disabilities; bookstore; campus computer network; computer lab; computer-assisted instruction; daycare for children of students; e-mail services; housing assistance; Internet; learning resource lab; library services; resume preparation assistance; skills, simulation, or other laboratory; tutoring.
Library Facilities 17,340 volumes in health, 837 volumes in nursing; 8,145 periodical subscriptions health-care related.

BACCALAUREATE PROGRAMS

Degree BSN
Available Programs ADN to Baccalaureate; Baccalaureate for Second Degree; Generic Baccalaureate; LPN to Baccalaureate; RN Baccalaureate.
Site Options Los Angeles, CA; Riverside, CA; Mission Viejo, CA.
Study Options Full-time.
Program Entrance Requirements Minimum overall college GPA, transcript of college record, minimum GPA in nursing prerequisites, prerequisite course work. *Application deadline:* 2/15 (fall).
Advanced Placement Credit given for nursing courses completed elsewhere dependent upon specific evaluations.
Contact *Telephone:* 657-278-3217. *Fax:* 657-278-2096.

GRADUATE PROGRAMS

Contact *Telephone:* 714-278-3217. *Fax:* 714-278-2096.

MASTER'S DEGREE PROGRAM
Degree MSN
Available Programs Master's; Master's for Non-Nursing College Graduates.
Concentrations Available Nurse anesthesia; nurse-midwifery; nursing administration; nursing education. *Clinical nurse specialist programs in:* school health. *Nurse practitioner programs in:* women's health.
Study Options Full-time and part-time.
Online Degree Options Yes.
Program Entrance Requirements Clinical experience, minimum overall college GPA of 3.0, transcript of college record, CPR certification, written essay, immunizations, interview, 3 letters of recommendation, nursing research course, professional liability insurance/malpractice insurance, prerequisite course work, statistics course. *Application deadline:* 11/30 (fall). Applications may be processed on a rolling basis for some programs. *Application fee:* $55.
Advanced Placement Credit given for nursing courses completed elsewhere dependent upon specific evaluations.
Degree Requirements 71 total credit hours, thesis or project, comprehensive exam.

DOCTORAL DEGREE PROGRAM
Degree DNP
Available Programs Doctorate; Doctorate for Nurses with Non-Nursing Degrees; Post-Baccalaureate Doctorate.
Areas of Study Advanced practice nursing, clinical practice, community health, critical care, family health, nursing administration, nursing education, nursing research, nursing science, women's health.
Program Entrance Requirements Clinical experience, minimum overall college GPA of 3.5, interview, 3 letters of recommendation, MSN or equivalent, statistics course, writing sample. Application deadline: 12/15 (fall). Application fee: $55.
Degree Requirements 36 total credit hours, dissertation, written exam.

California State University, Long Beach

School of Nursing
Long Beach, California

http://www.csulb.edu/colleges/chhs/departments/nursing/
Founded in 1949
DEGREES • BSN • MSN
Nursing Program Faculty 76 (40% with doctorates).
Baccalaureate Enrollment 458 **Women** 77% **Men** 23% **Part-time** 33%
Graduate Enrollment 429 **Women** 86% **Men** 14%
Nursing Student Activities Nursing Honor Society, Sigma Theta Tau, Student Nurses' Association.
Nursing Student Resources Academic advising; academic or career counseling; assistance for students with disabilities; bookstore; campus computer network; e-mail services; interactive nursing skills videos; Internet; learning resource lab; library services; nursing audiovisuals; remedial services; resume preparation assistance; skills, simulation, or other laboratory; tutoring; unpaid internships.

BACCALAUREATE PROGRAMS

Degree BSN
Available Programs ADN to Baccalaureate; Generic Baccalaureate.
Site Options Huntington Beach, CA.
Study Options Full-time.
Program Entrance Requirements Transcript of college record, CPR certification, health exam, health insurance, immunizations, interview, minimum GPA in nursing prerequisites of 3.0, professional liability insurance/malpractice insurance, prerequisite course work. Transfer students are accepted. *Application deadline:* 1/31 (fall), 8/31 (spring). *Application fee:* $55.
Advanced Placement Credit given for nursing courses completed elsewhere dependent upon specific evaluations.
Expenses (2015–16) *Tuition, state resident:* full-time $6452.
Contact Dr. Beth R. Keely, Assistant Director, Undergraduate Nursing Programs, School of Nursing, California State University, Long Beach, 1250 Bellflower Boulevard, Long Beach, CA 90840. *Telephone:* 562-985-4478. *Fax:* 562-985-2382. *E-mail:* bkeely@csulb.edu.

GRADUATE PROGRAMS

Expenses (2015–16) *Tuition, state resident:* full-time $9672.
Financial Aid Federal Work-Study, institutionally sponsored loans, and scholarships available.
Contact Alison Kliachko-Trafas, Administrative Assistant, School of Nursing, California State University, Long Beach, 1250 Bellflower Boulevard, Long Beach, CA 90840. *Telephone:* 562-985-4473. *Fax:* 562-985-2382. *E-mail:* akliachk@csulb.edu.

MASTER'S DEGREE PROGRAM
Degree MSN
Available Programs Master's.
Concentrations Available Health-care administration; nursing administration; nursing education. *Nurse practitioner programs in:* adult health, family health, gerontology, pediatric, psychiatric/mental health, women's health.
Site Options Long Beach, CA; Huntington Beach, CA.
Study Options Full-time and part-time.
Program Entrance Requirements Clinical experience, minimum overall college GPA of 2.75, transcript of college record, written essay, 3 letters of recommendation, physical assessment course, prerequisite course work, resume, statistics course. *Application deadline:* 3/15 (fall). *Application fee:* $55.
Advanced Placement Credit given for nursing courses completed elsewhere dependent upon specific evaluations.
Degree Requirements 37 total credit hours, thesis or project, comprehensive exam.

POST-MASTER'S PROGRAM
Areas of Study Nursing administration. *Nurse practitioner programs in:* adult health, family health, gerontology, pediatric, psychiatric/mental health, women's health.

California State University, Los Angeles

School of Nursing
Los Angeles, California

http://web.calstatela.edu/academic/hhs/nursing/
Founded in 1947

DEGREES • BSN • MSN
Nursing Program Faculty 31 (39% with doctorates).
Baccalaureate Enrollment 300
Graduate Enrollment 100
Nursing Student Resources Academic advising.

BACCALAUREATE PROGRAMS

Degree BSN
Available Programs Generic Baccalaureate; LPN to RN Baccalaureate; RN Baccalaureate.
Study Options Full-time.
Program Entrance Requirements Minimum overall college GPA of 2.75, CPR certification, health exam, health insurance, high school biology, immunizations, minimum GPA in nursing prerequisites of 2.75, professional liability insurance/malpractice insurance, prerequisite course work. Transfer students are accepted. *Application deadline:* 12/1 (fall).
Advanced Placement Credit given for nursing courses completed elsewhere dependent upon specific evaluations.
Contact *Telephone:* 323-343-4700. *Fax:* 323-343-6454.

GRADUATE PROGRAMS

Contact *Telephone:* 323-343-4700. *Fax:* 323-343-6454.

MASTER'S DEGREE PROGRAM
Degree MSN
Available Programs Accelerated Master's for Nurses with Non-Nursing Degrees; Accelerated RN to Master's; Master's; Master's for Non-Nursing College Graduates.
Concentrations Available Nursing administration; nursing education. *Clinical nurse specialist programs in:* psychiatric/mental health. *Nurse practitioner programs in:* acute care, adult health, family health, pediatric, primary care, psychiatric/mental health.
Study Options Full-time and part-time.
Program Entrance Requirements Clinical experience, minimum overall college GPA of 3.0, transcript of college record, written essay, immunizations, letters of recommendation, nursing research course, physical assessment course, professional liability insurance/malpractice insurance, resume, statistics course. *Application deadline:* 11/15 (fall), 5/15 (spring).
Advanced Placement Credit given for nursing courses completed elsewhere dependent upon specific evaluations.
Degree Requirements 45 total credit hours, comprehensive exam.

POST-MASTER'S PROGRAM
Areas of Study *Nurse practitioner programs in:* acute care, adult health, family health, pediatric, primary care.

California State University, Northridge

Nursing Program
Northridge, California

http://www.csun.edu/~nursing/
Founded in 1958

DEGREE • BSN
Nursing Program Faculty 18 (3.6% with doctorates).
Baccalaureate Enrollment 140 **Women** 92% **Men** 8% **Part-time** 66%
Nursing Student Activities Sigma Theta Tau, Student Nurses' Association.
Nursing Student Resources Academic advising; academic or career counseling; assistance for students with disabilities; bookstore; campus computer network; career placement assistance; computer lab; computer-assisted instruction; daycare for children of students; e-mail services; housing assistance; interactive nursing skills videos; Internet; learning resource lab; library services; nursing audiovisuals; remedial services; resume preparation assistance; skills, simulation, or other laboratory; tutoring.
Library Facilities 61,848 volumes in health, 1,401 volumes in nursing; 303 periodical subscriptions health-care related.

BACCALAUREATE PROGRAMS

Degree BSN
Available Programs ADN to Baccalaureate; Accelerated Baccalaureate.
Site Options Panorama City, CA; Ventura , CA; Antelope Valley, CA.
Study Options Full-time and part-time.
Program Entrance Requirements Minimum overall college GPA of 3.0, transcript of college record, CPR certification, written essay, health exam, health insurance, immunizations, interview, 3 letters of recommendation, minimum GPA in nursing prerequisites of 3.0, professional liability insurance/malpractice insurance, prerequisite course work, RN licensure. Transfer students are accepted. *Application deadline:* 11/30 (fall), 11/30 (summer). *Application fee:* $55.
Advanced Placement Credit by examination available. Credit given for nursing courses completed elsewhere dependent upon specific evaluations.
Contact *Telephone:* 818-677-3101. *Fax:* 818-677-2045.

California State University, Sacramento

Division of Nursing
Sacramento, California

http://www.hhs.csus.edu/nrs
Founded in 1947

DEGREES • BSN • MS
Nursing Program Faculty 75 (45% with doctorates).
Baccalaureate Enrollment 380 **Women** 89% **Men** 11%
Graduate Enrollment 140 **Women** 95% **Men** 5% **Part-time** 100%
Distance Learning Courses Available.
Nursing Student Activities Sigma Theta Tau, Student Nurses' Association.
Nursing Student Resources Academic advising; academic or career counseling; assistance for students with disabilities; bookstore; campus computer network; computer lab; computer-assisted instruction; daycare for children of students; e-mail services; externships; housing assistance; interactive nursing skills videos; Internet; learning resource lab; library services; nursing audiovisuals; paid internships; remedial services; resume preparation assistance; skills, simulation, or other laboratory; tutoring.
Library Facilities 33,000 volumes in health; 327 periodical subscriptions health-care related.

BACCALAUREATE PROGRAMS

Degree BSN
Available Programs ADN to Baccalaureate; Baccalaureate for Second Degree; Generic Baccalaureate.
Study Options Full-time.
Program Entrance Requirements Transcript of college record, CPR certification, health exam, health insurance, high school biology, high school math, immunizations, minimum GPA in nursing prerequisites of 3.3, professional liability insurance/malpractice insurance, prerequisite course work. Transfer students are accepted. *Application deadline:* 3/1 (fall), 10/1 (spring).
Advanced Placement Credit by examination available. Credit given for nursing courses completed elsewhere dependent upon specific evaluations.
Expenses (2015–16) *Tuition, state resident:* full-time $3436. *Tuition, nonresident:* part-time $372 per unit. *Required fees:* full-time $300.
Contact Sara J. Niekamp, Administrative Support Coordinator, Division of Nursing, California State University, Sacramento, 6000 J Street, Sacramento, CA 95819-6096. *Telephone:* 916-278-6714. *Fax:* 916-278-6311. *E-mail:* Sara.niekamp@csus.edu.

GRADUATE PROGRAMS

Expenses (2015–16) *Tuition, state resident:* full-time $4069.
Financial Aid Research assistantships, teaching assistantships, career-related internships or fieldwork and Federal Work-Study available.
Contact Dr. Kitty Kelly, RN, Graduate Coordinator, Division of Nursing, California State University, Sacramento, 6000 J Street, Sacramento, CA 95819-6096. *Fax:* 916-278-6311. *E-mail:* kkelly@csus.edu.

MASTER'S DEGREE PROGRAM

Degree MS
Available Programs Master's; Master's for Nurses with Non-Nursing Degrees.
Concentrations Available Clinical nurse leader; nursing administration; nursing education.
Study Options Part-time.
Program Entrance Requirements Clinical experience, computer literacy, minimum overall college GPA of 3.0, transcript of college record, CPR certification, immunizations, nursing research course, professional liability insurance/malpractice insurance, prerequisite course work, statistics course, GRE. *Application deadline:* 11/30 (fall).
Advanced Placement Credit given for nursing courses completed elsewhere dependent upon specific evaluations.
Degree Requirements 33 total credit hours, comprehensive exam.

CONTINUING EDUCATION PROGRAM

Contact Dr. Dian Baker, RN, School Nursing Program Coordinator, Division of Nursing, California State University, Sacramento, 6000 J Street, Sacramento, CA 95819-6096. *Fax:* 916-278-6311. *E-mail:* dibaker@csus.edu.

California State University, San Bernardino

Department of Nursing
San Bernardino, California

https://www.csusb.edu/
Founded in 1965

DEGREES • BSN • MSN

Nursing Program Faculty 42 (19% with doctorates).
Baccalaureate Enrollment 457 **Women** 81% **Men** 19%
Graduate Enrollment 19 **Women** 89% **Men** 11%
Distance Learning Courses Available.
Nursing Student Activities Sigma Theta Tau, Student Nurses' Association.
Nursing Student Resources Academic advising; academic or career counseling; assistance for students with disabilities; bookstore; campus computer network; computer lab; computer-assisted instruction; daycare for children of students; e-mail services; Internet; learning resource lab; library services; nursing audiovisuals; remedial services; skills, simulation, or other laboratory.
Library Facilities 1,500 volumes in health, 1,000 volumes in nursing; 5,000 periodical subscriptions health-care related.

BACCALAUREATE PROGRAMS

Degree BSN
Available Programs Generic Baccalaureate; LPN to Baccalaureate; RN Baccalaureate.
Site Options Palm Desert, CA.
Study Options Full-time.
Program Entrance Requirements Minimum overall college GPA of 2.5, transcript of college record, 3 letters of recommendation, minimum GPA in nursing prerequisites of 2.5, prerequisite course work. Transfer students are accepted. *Application deadline:* 3/1 (fall), 10/1 (winter).
Advanced Placement Credit given for nursing courses completed elsewhere dependent upon specific evaluations.
Contact *Telephone:* 909-537-5381.

GRADUATE PROGRAMS

Contact *Telephone:* 909-537-7241.

MASTER'S DEGREE PROGRAM

Degree MSN
Available Programs Master's.
Concentrations Available Nursing administration; nursing education. *Clinical nurse specialist programs in:* community health.
Study Options Full-time and part-time.
Program Entrance Requirements Clinical experience, minimum overall college GPA of 3.0, transcript of college record, letters of recommendation, prerequisite course work, resume, statistics course. *Application deadline:* 6/10 (fall).
Advanced Placement Credit given for nursing courses completed elsewhere dependent upon specific evaluations.

Degree Requirements 65 total credit hours, thesis or project, comprehensive exam.

California State University, San Marcos

School of Nursing
San Marcos, California

http://www.csusm.edu/
Founded in 1990
DEGREE • BSN
Nursing Student Activities Student Nurses' Association.

BACCALAUREATE PROGRAMS

Degree BSN
Available Programs Accelerated Baccalaureate; Generic Baccalaureate.
Contact *Telephone:* 706-750-7550. *Fax:* 706-750-3646.

California State University, Stanislaus

Department of Nursing
Turlock, California

http://www.csustan.edu/academics/CHHS/Nursing.html
Founded in 1957
DEGREE • BSN
Nursing Program Faculty 17 (24% with doctorates).
Baccalaureate Enrollment 164 **Women** 88% **Men** 12% **Part-time** 30%
Nursing Student Activities Sigma Theta Tau, Student Nurses' Association.
Nursing Student Resources Academic advising; academic or career counseling; assistance for students with disabilities; bookstore; campus computer network; career placement assistance; computer lab; computer-assisted instruction; daycare for children of students; e-mail services; employment services for current students; externships; interactive nursing skills videos; Internet; learning resource lab; library services; nursing audiovisuals; resume preparation assistance; skills, simulation, or other laboratory; tutoring.
Library Facilities 12,642 volumes in health, 1,338 volumes in nursing; 93 periodical subscriptions health-care related.

BACCALAUREATE PROGRAMS

Degree BSN
Available Programs ADN to Baccalaureate; Generic Baccalaureate; LPN to Baccalaureate.
Study Options Full-time.
Program Entrance Requirements Minimum overall college GPA of 3.0, transcript of college record, CPR certification, health exam, immunizations, minimum GPA in nursing prerequisites of 3.0, professional liability insurance/malpractice insurance, prerequisite course work. Transfer students are accepted.
Advanced Placement Credit given for nursing courses completed elsewhere dependent upon specific evaluations.
Contact *Telephone:* 209-667-3141. *Fax:* 209-667-3690.

Charles R. Drew University of Medicine and Science

School of Nursing
Los Angeles, California

Founded in 1966
DEGREE • MSN

GRADUATE PROGRAMS

Contact *Telephone:* 323-568-3301.

MASTER'S DEGREE PROGRAM

Degree MSN

Available Programs Accelerated Master's for Nurses with Non-Nursing Degrees; Master's.
Program Entrance Requirements Minimum overall college GPA of 3.0, written essay, 3 letters of recommendation, resume. *Application fee:* $100.

Concordia University Irvine
Bachelor of Science in Nursing Program
Irvine, California

http://www.cui.edu/academicprograms/nursing
Founded in 1972
DEGREE • BSN
Nursing Program Faculty 27 (7% with doctorates).
Baccalaureate Enrollment 170 **Women** 83% **Men** 17% **Part-time** 52%
Distance Learning Courses Available.
Nursing Student Activities Nursing Honor Society, Student Nurses' Association.
Nursing Student Resources Academic advising; academic or career counseling; assistance for students with disabilities; bookstore; campus computer network; computer lab; computer-assisted instruction; e-mail services; Internet; learning resource lab; library services; nursing audiovisuals; remedial services; resume preparation assistance; skills, simulation, or other laboratory; tutoring.
Library Facilities 234 volumes in health, 91 volumes in nursing; 5,380 periodical subscriptions health-care related.

BACCALAUREATE PROGRAMS

Degree BSN
Available Programs ADN to Baccalaureate; Accelerated Baccalaureate for Second Degree.
Site Options Irvine, CA.
Study Options Full-time.
Program Entrance Requirements Minimum overall college GPA of 3.0, transcript of college record, CPR certification, written essay, health exam, health insurance, immunizations, interview, 2 letters of recommendation, minimum GPA in nursing prerequisites of 3.0, professional liability insurance/malpractice insurance, prerequisite course work. *Application deadline:* 6/1 (fall), 1/15 (summer). *Application fee:* $50.
Expenses (2014–15) *Tuition:* full-time $42,000; part-time $700 per unit. *International tuition:* $42,000 full-time. *Required fees:* full-time $5000.
Financial Aid 91% of baccalaureate students in nursing programs received some form of financial aid in 2013–14. *Gift aid (need-based):* Federal Pell, FSEOG, state, private, college/university gift aid from institutional funds. *Loans:* Federal Direct (Subsidized and Unsubsidized Stafford PLUS), private loans. *Work-study:* Federal Work-Study, part-time campus jobs. *Financial aid application deadline:* 3/2.
Contact Ms. Henny Halim, Assistant Director of Admissions, Nursing ABSN, Bachelor of Science in Nursing Program, Concordia University Irvine, 1530 Concordia West, Irvine, CA 92612. *Telephone:* 949-214-3022. *Fax:* 949-214-3022. *E-mail:* henny.halim@cui.edu.

Dominican University of California
Program in Nursing
San Rafael, California

http://www.dominican.edu/
Founded in 1890
DEGREE • BSN
Nursing Program Faculty 50 (22% with doctorates).
Baccalaureate Enrollment 372 **Women** 86.29% **Men** 13.71% **Part-time** 15.05%
Nursing Student Activities Sigma Theta Tau, Student Nurses' Association, nursing club.
Nursing Student Resources Academic advising; academic or career counseling; assistance for students with disabilities; bookstore; campus computer network; career placement assistance; computer lab; computer-assisted instruction; e-mail services; employment services for current students; housing assistance; interactive nursing skills videos; Internet; learning resource lab; library services; nursing audiovisuals; remedial services; resume preparation assistance; skills, simulation, or other laboratory; tutoring; unpaid internships.

Library Facilities 825 volumes in health, 402 volumes in nursing; 180 periodical subscriptions health-care related.

BACCALAUREATE PROGRAMS

Degree BSN
Available Programs Baccalaureate for Second Degree; Generic Baccalaureate; RN Baccalaureate.
Study Options Full-time and part-time.
Program Entrance Requirements Minimum overall college GPA of 3.25, transcript of college record, written essay, health exam, health insurance, high school biology, high school chemistry, 2 years high school math, high school transcript, immunizations, 1 letter of recommendation, minimum high school GPA of 3.0, minimum GPA in nursing prerequisites of 3.25, prerequisite course work. Transfer students are accepted. *Application deadline:* 2/1 (fall), 9/1 (spring). Applications may be processed on a rolling basis for some programs. *Application fee:* $40.
Advanced Placement Credit given for nursing courses completed elsewhere dependent upon specific evaluations.
Expenses (2015–16) *Tuition:* full-time $42,100; part-time $1760 per unit. *International tuition:* $42,100 full-time. *Room and board:* $13,380; room only: $7880 per academic year. *Required fees:* full-time $450.
Contact Assistant Vice President of Undergraduate Admissions, Program in Nursing, Dominican University of California, 50 Acacia Avenue, San Rafael, CA 94901-2298. *Telephone:* 415-485-3204. *Fax:* 415-485-3214. *E-mail:* enroll@dominican.edu.

Fresno Pacific University
RN to BSN Program
Fresno, California

Founded in 1944
DEGREE • BSN

BACCALAUREATE PROGRAMS

Degree BSN
Available Programs RN Baccalaureate.
Contact *Telephone:* 559-453-2000.

Holy Names University
Department of Nursing
Oakland, California

http://www.hnu.edu/
Founded in 1868
DEGREES • BSN • MSN • MSN/MBA
Nursing Program Faculty 41 (10% with doctorates).
Baccalaureate Enrollment 110 **Women** 83% **Men** 17% **Part-time** 41%
Graduate Enrollment 111 **Women** 85% **Men** 15% **Part-time** 93%
Distance Learning Courses Available.
Nursing Student Activities Nursing Honor Society, Sigma Theta Tau, nursing club.
Nursing Student Resources Academic advising; academic or career counseling; assistance for students with disabilities; bookstore; campus computer network; career placement assistance; computer lab; computer-assisted instruction; e-mail services; employment services for current students; externships; housing assistance; interactive nursing skills videos; Internet; learning resource lab; library services; nursing audiovisuals; placement services for program completers; remedial services; resume preparation assistance; skills, simulation, or other laboratory; tutoring.
Library Facilities 500 volumes in health, 200 volumes in nursing; 200 periodical subscriptions health-care related.

BACCALAUREATE PROGRAMS

Degree BSN
Available Programs LPN to RN Baccalaureate; RN Baccalaureate.
Study Options Full-time and part-time.
Program Entrance Requirements Minimum overall college GPA of 2.7, transcript of college record, written essay, 1 letter of recommendation, prerequisite course work, RN licensure. Transfer students are accepted. *Application deadline:* Applications may be processed on a rolling basis for some programs. *Application fee:* $50.
Advanced Placement Credit given for nursing courses completed elsewhere dependent upon specific evaluations.

Expenses (2014–15) *Tuition:* full-time $34,058; part-time $17,029 per semester. *Room and board:* $11,412; room only: $6048 per academic year. *Required fees:* full-time $430; part-time $215 per term.

Financial Aid 79% of baccalaureate students in nursing programs received some form of financial aid in 2013–14.

Contact Admission Counselor, Department of Nursing, Holy Names University, 3500 Mountain Boulevard, Oakland, CA 94619-1699. *Telephone:* 510-436-1351. *Fax:* 510-436-1376. *E-mail:* admissions@hnu.edu.

GRADUATE PROGRAMS

Expenses (2014–15) *Tuition:* part-time $928 per unit.

Financial Aid 56% of graduate students in nursing programs received some form of financial aid in 2013–14. Career-related internships or fieldwork, Federal Work-Study, scholarships, and unspecified assistantships available. Aid available to part-time students. *Financial aid application deadline:* 3/2.

Contact Ms. Lisa Marie Gibson, Admission Counselor, Department of Nursing, Holy Names University, 3500 Mountain Boulevard, Oakland, CA 94619-1699. *Telephone:* 510-436-1317. *Fax:* 510-436-1376. *E-mail:* lgibson@hnu.edu.

MASTER'S DEGREE PROGRAM

Degrees MSN; MSN/MBA

Available Programs Master's; Master's for Nurses with Non-Nursing Degrees; RN to Master's.

Concentrations Available Nursing administration; nursing education; nursing informatics. *Nurse practitioner programs in:* family health.

Site Options Stanford, CA; Arroyo Grande.

Study Options Full-time and part-time.

Program Entrance Requirements Minimum overall college GPA of 2.8, transcript of college record, written essay, 2 letters of recommendation, resume. *Application deadline:* Applications may be processed on a rolling basis for some programs. *Application fee:* $65.

Degree Requirements 45 total credit hours, thesis or project.

POST-MASTER'S PROGRAM

Areas of Study Nursing administration; nursing education. *Nurse practitioner programs in:* family health.

Loma Linda University
School of Nursing
Loma Linda, California

http://www.llu.edu/nursing
Founded in 1905

DEGREES • BS • DNP • MS

Nursing Program Faculty 60 (55% with doctorates).
Baccalaureate Enrollment 509 **Women** 80% **Men** 20% **Part-time** 16%
Graduate Enrollment 191 **Women** 98% **Men** 2% **Part-time** 73%
Nursing Student Activities Nursing Honor Society, Sigma Theta Tau, Student Nurses' Association, nursing club.
Nursing Student Resources Academic advising; academic or career counseling; assistance for students with disabilities; bookstore; campus computer network; computer lab; computer-assisted instruction; e-mail services; employment services for current students; externships; housing assistance; interactive nursing skills videos; Internet; learning resource lab; library services; nursing audiovisuals; paid internships; remedial services; resume preparation assistance; skills, simulation, or other laboratory; tutoring.
Library Facilities 73,702 volumes in health, 4,965 volumes in nursing; 6,516 periodical subscriptions health-care related.

BACCALAUREATE PROGRAMS

Degree BS

Available Programs ADN to Baccalaureate; Accelerated Baccalaureate for Second Degree; Accelerated RN Baccalaureate; Baccalaureate for Second Degree; Generic Baccalaureate; LPN to Baccalaureate; RN Baccalaureate.

Study Options Full-time and part-time.

Program Entrance Requirements Minimum overall college GPA of 3.0, transcript of college record, CPR certification, written essay, health exam, high school transcript, immunizations, interview, 3 letters of recommendation, minimum GPA in nursing prerequisites of 3.0, prerequisite course work. Transfer students are accepted. *Application deadline:* 3/31

(fall), 8/15 (winter), 11/1 (spring). Applications may be processed on a rolling basis for some programs. *Application fee:* $120.

Advanced Placement Credit by examination available. Credit given for nursing courses completed elsewhere dependent upon specific evaluations.

Expenses (2015–16) *Tuition:* full-time $29,520; part-time $615 per quarter hour. *International tuition:* $29,520 full-time. *Required fees:* full-time $4089; part-time $1363 per term.

Financial Aid 95% of baccalaureate students in nursing programs received some form of financial aid in 2014–15.

Contact Mrs. Heather Krause, Director of Admissions, Marketing, and Recruitment, School of Nursing, Loma Linda University, 11262 Campus Street, Loma Linda, CA 92350. *Telephone:* 909-558-4923. *Fax:* 909-558-0175. *E-mail:* hkrause@llu.edu.

GRADUATE PROGRAMS

Expenses (2015–16) *Tuition:* part-time $785 per quarter hour. *Required fees:* part-time $763 per term.

Financial Aid 26% of graduate students in nursing programs received some form of financial aid in 2014–15.

Contact Mr. K.C. Larsen, Assistant Director of Admissions, Marketing, and Recruitment, School of Nursing, Loma Linda University, 11262 Campus Street, Loma Linda, CA 92350. *Telephone:* 909-558-4923. *E-mail:* graduatenursing@llu.edu.

MASTER'S DEGREE PROGRAM

Degree MS

Available Programs Master's.

Concentrations Available Nurse anesthesia; nursing administration; nursing education. *Clinical nurse specialist programs in:* adult health, maternity-newborn, parent-child, pediatric, perinatal.

Study Options Full-time and part-time.

Program Entrance Requirements Clinical experience, minimum overall college GPA of 3.0, transcript of college record, immunizations, interview, 3 letters of recommendation, nursing research course, prerequisite course work, resume, statistics course. *Application deadline:* 4/1 (fall), 8/15 (winter). *Application fee:* $60.

Advanced Placement Credit given for nursing courses completed elsewhere dependent upon specific evaluations.

Degree Requirements Comprehensive exam.

DOCTORAL DEGREE PROGRAM

Degree DNP

Available Programs Doctorate.

Areas of Study Addiction/substance abuse, advanced practice nursing, aging, clinical nurse leader, clinical practice, clinical research, community health, critical care, ethics, faculty preparation, family health, gerontology, health policy, health promotion/disease prevention, health-care systems, human health and illness, individualized study, maternity-newborn, neuro-behavior, nurse case management, nursing administration, nursing education, nursing policy, nursing research, nursing science, oncology, palliative care, women's health.

Program Entrance Requirements Minimum overall college GPA of 3.2, interview by faculty committee, interview, 3 letters of recommendation, statistics course, vita, writing sample. Application deadline: 4/1 (fall), 8/15 (winter). Applications may be processed on a rolling basis for some programs. Application fee: $60.

Degree Requirements Dissertation, written exam.

Mount Saint Mary's University
Department of Nursing
Los Angeles, California

https://www.msmu.edu/undergraduate-bachelor-programs/nursing/
Founded in 1925

DEGREES • BSN • BSC PN • MSN

Nursing Program Faculty 112 (10% with doctorates).
Baccalaureate Enrollment 326 **Women** 87% **Men** 13%
Graduate Enrollment 51 **Women** 91% **Men** 9%
Distance Learning Courses Available.
Nursing Student Activities Nursing Honor Society, Student Nurses' Association, nursing club.
Nursing Student Resources Academic advising; academic or career counseling; assistance for students with disabilities; bookstore; campus computer network; career placement assistance; computer lab; computer-

assisted instruction; daycare for children of students; e-mail services; employment services for current students; housing assistance; interactive nursing skills videos; Internet; learning resource lab; library services; nursing audiovisuals; remedial services; resume preparation assistance; skills, simulation, or other laboratory; tutoring.
Library Facilities 4,000 volumes in health, 1,000 volumes in nursing; 150 periodical subscriptions health-care related.

BACCALAUREATE PROGRAMS

Degrees BSN; BSc PN
Available Programs ADN to Baccalaureate; Accelerated Baccalaureate; Generic Baccalaureate.
Study Options Full-time.
Program Entrance Requirements Minimum overall college GPA of 2.7, transcript of college record, CPR certification, written essay, health exam, high school chemistry, high school transcript, immunizations, 1 letter of recommendation, minimum GPA in nursing prerequisites of 2.5, professional liability insurance/malpractice insurance, prerequisite course work. Transfer students are accepted. *Application deadline:* 2/1 (fall). *Application fee:* $20.
Advanced Placement Credit by examination available. Credit given for nursing courses completed elsewhere dependent upon specific evaluations.
Contact *Telephone:* 310-954-4279. *Fax:* 310-954-4229.

GRADUATE PROGRAMS

Contact *Telephone:* 213-477-2980. *Fax:* 213-477-2639.

MASTER'S DEGREE PROGRAM

Degree MSN
Available Programs Master's; RN to Master's.
Concentrations Available Nursing administration; nursing education. *Clinical nurse specialist programs in:* adult health, community health.
Study Options Full-time and part-time.
Program Entrance Requirements Minimum overall college GPA of 3.0, transcript of college record, CPR certification, written essay, immunizations, interview, professional liability insurance/malpractice insurance, statistics course. *Application deadline:* Applications may be processed on a rolling basis for some programs. *Application fee:* $50.
Advanced Placement Credit given for nursing courses completed elsewhere dependent upon specific evaluations.
Degree Requirements 39 total credit hours, thesis or project.

National University
Department of Nursing
La Jolla, California

http://www.nu.edu
Founded in 1971
DEGREES • BSN • MSN
Nursing Program Faculty 167 (10% with doctorates).
Baccalaureate Enrollment 734 **Women** 80% **Men** 20%
Graduate Enrollment 21 **Women** 43% **Men** 57%
Distance Learning Courses Available.
Nursing Student Activities Nursing Honor Society, Student Nurses' Association.
Nursing Student Resources Academic advising; academic or career counseling; assistance for students with disabilities; bookstore; campus computer network; computer lab; Internet; library services; nursing audiovisuals; other; remedial services; resume preparation assistance; skills, simulation, or other laboratory; tutoring.
Library Facilities 5,000 volumes in health, 2,500 volumes in nursing; 1,400 periodical subscriptions health-care related.

BACCALAUREATE PROGRAMS

Degree BSN
Available Programs Baccalaureate for Second Degree; Generic Baccalaureate; LPN to Baccalaureate; RN Baccalaureate.
Site Options Fresno, CA; Los Angeles, CA.
Study Options Full-time.
Program Entrance Requirements Minimum overall college GPA of 2.75, transcript of college record, CPR certification, written essay, health exam, health insurance, immunizations, minimum GPA in nursing prerequisites of 2.75, professional liability insurance/malpractice insurance, prerequisite course work. Transfer students are accepted. *Application deadline:* 4/17 (fall), 7/18 (winter), 10/16 (spring), 1/16 (summer). Appli-

cations may be processed on a rolling basis for some programs. *Application fee:* $60.
Advanced Placement Credit given for nursing courses completed elsewhere dependent upon specific evaluations.
Contact *Telephone:* 800-628-8648 Ext. 3906. *Fax:* 858-521-3995.

GRADUATE PROGRAMS

Contact *Telephone:* 858-521-3906. *Fax:* 858-521-3995.

MASTER'S DEGREE PROGRAM

Degree MSN
Available Programs RN to Master's.
Concentrations Available Nurse anesthesia; nursing administration; nursing informatics. *Clinical nurse specialist programs in:* forensic nursing.
Site Options Fresno, CA.
Study Options Full-time.
Program Entrance Requirements Clinical experience, computer literacy, minimum overall college GPA of 3.0, transcript of college record, CPR certification, written essay, immunizations, interview, 3 letters of recommendation, nursing research course, physical assessment course, professional liability insurance/malpractice insurance, prerequisite course work, statistics course. *Application deadline:* Applications may be processed on a rolling basis for some programs. *Application fee:* $60.
Advanced Placement Credit given for nursing courses completed elsewhere dependent upon specific evaluations.
Degree Requirements 59 total credit hours, thesis or project.

DOCTORAL DEGREE PROGRAM

Program Entrance Requirements Application deadline: Applications may be processed on a rolling basis for some programs. Application fee: $60.

Pacific College
Bachelor of Science in Nursing
Costa Mesa, California

http://www.pacific-college.edu/
DEGREE • BSN

BACCALAUREATE PROGRAMS

Degree BSN
Available Programs RN Baccalaureate.
Program Entrance Requirements *Application deadline:* Applications may be processed on a rolling basis for some programs.
Contact Donna Beuk, Program Director, Bachelor of Science in Nursing, Pacific College, 3160 Red Hill Avenue, Costa Mesa, CA 92626. *Telephone:* 714-662-4402. *E-mail:* dbeuk@pacific-college.edu.

Pacific Union College
Department of Nursing
Angwin, California

http://www.puc.edu
Founded in 1882
DEGREE • BSN
Nursing Program Faculty 16 (14% with doctorates).
Baccalaureate Enrollment 56 **Women** 77% **Men** 23% **Part-time** 59%
Nursing Student Activities Student Nurses' Association.
Nursing Student Resources Academic advising; academic or career counseling; assistance for students with disabilities; bookstore; campus computer network; career placement assistance; computer lab; daycare for children of students; e-mail services; employment services for current students; externships; housing assistance; Internet; learning resource lab; library services; nursing audiovisuals; skills, simulation, or other laboratory; tutoring.
Library Facilities 125 volumes in health, 75 volumes in nursing; 109 periodical subscriptions health-care related.

BACCALAUREATE PROGRAMS

Degree BSN
Available Programs ADN to Baccalaureate.
Site Options Napa, CA.

Study Options Full-time and part-time.

Program Entrance Requirements Transcript of college record, CPR certification, health exam, health insurance, immunizations, interview, 2 letters of recommendation, minimum GPA in nursing prerequisites of 2.0, professional liability insurance/malpractice insurance, prerequisite course work, RN licensure. Transfer students are accepted.

Advanced Placement Credit given for nursing courses completed elsewhere dependent upon specific evaluations.

Contact *Telephone:* 707-965-7618. *Fax:* 707-965-6499.

CONTINUING EDUCATION PROGRAM

Contact *Telephone:* 707-965-7262. *Fax:* 707-965-6499.

Point Loma Nazarene University

School of Nursing
San Diego, California

http://www.pointloma.edu/

DEGREES • BSN • MSN

Nursing Program Faculty 28 (40% with doctorates).
Baccalaureate Enrollment 170 **Women** 90% **Men** 10% **Part-time** 2%
Graduate Enrollment 43 **Women** 92% **Men** 8% **Part-time** 5%
Nursing Student Activities Sigma Theta Tau, Student Nurses' Association.
Nursing Student Resources Academic advising; academic or career counseling; bookstore; campus computer network; computer lab; computer-assisted instruction; daycare for children of students; e-mail services; employment services for current students; externships; housing assistance; interactive nursing skills videos; Internet; learning resource lab; library services; nursing audiovisuals; paid internships; resume preparation assistance; skills, simulation, or other laboratory; tutoring; unpaid internships.

BACCALAUREATE PROGRAMS

Degree BSN
Available Programs ADN to Baccalaureate; Generic Baccalaureate; LPN to RN Baccalaureate; RN Baccalaureate.
Site Options San Diego, CA.
Study Options Full-time.
Program Entrance Requirements Minimum overall college GPA of 2.7, transcript of college record, CPR certification, written essay, health exam, health insurance, 2 years high school math, immunizations, 1 letter of recommendation, minimum GPA in nursing prerequisites of 2.7, prerequisite course work. Transfer students are accepted. *Application deadline:* 2/1 (fall), 2/1 (winter).
Advanced Placement Credit by examination available. Credit given for nursing courses completed elsewhere dependent upon specific evaluations.
Contact *Telephone:* 619-849-7055. *Fax:* 619-849-2672.

GRADUATE PROGRAMS

Contact *Telephone:* 619-849-2863. *Fax:* 619-849-2672.

MASTER'S DEGREE PROGRAM
Degree MSN
Available Programs Master's; RN to Master's.
Concentrations Available Nursing education. *Clinical nurse specialist programs in:* family health, gerontology, medical-surgical, psychiatric/mental health.
Site Options San Diego, CA.
Study Options Full-time and part-time.
Program Entrance Requirements Clinical experience, computer literacy, minimum overall college GPA of 3.0, transcript of college record, CPR certification, written essay, immunizations, interview, 3 letters of recommendation, professional liability insurance/malpractice insurance, resume. *Application deadline:* 8/1 (fall), 12/1 (winter), 8/1 (summer). *Application fee:* $40.
Degree Requirements 43 total credit hours, thesis or project.

POST-MASTER'S PROGRAM
Areas of Study Nursing education. *Clinical nurse specialist programs in:* family health, gerontology, medical-surgical, psychiatric/mental health.

CONTINUING EDUCATION PROGRAM

Contact *Telephone:* 619-849-7055. *Fax:* 619-849-2672.

Samuel Merritt University

School of Nursing
Oakland, California

http://www.samuelmerritt.edu/nursing
Founded in 1909

DEGREES • BSN • DNP • MSN

Nursing Program Faculty 201 (27% with doctorates).
Baccalaureate Enrollment 459 **Women** 82% **Men** 18% **Part-time** 2%
Graduate Enrollment 484 **Women** 79% **Men** 21% **Part-time** 11%
Distance Learning Courses Available.
Nursing Student Activities Sigma Theta Tau, Student Nurses' Association.
Nursing Student Resources Academic advising; academic or career counseling; assistance for students with disabilities; bookstore; campus computer network; computer lab; computer-assisted instruction; e-mail services; housing assistance; interactive nursing skills videos; Internet; learning resource lab; library services; nursing audiovisuals; remedial services; resume preparation assistance; skills, simulation, or other laboratory; tutoring; unpaid internships.

BACCALAUREATE PROGRAMS

Degree BSN
Available Programs Accelerated Baccalaureate; Generic Baccalaureate.
Site Options Sacramento, CA; San Mateo, CA.
Study Options Full-time and part-time.
Program Entrance Requirements Transcript of college record, CPR certification, written essay, health exam, health insurance, immunizations, 2 letters of recommendation, minimum GPA in nursing prerequisites of 3.0, prerequisite course work. Transfer students are accepted. *Application deadline:* 3/1 (fall), 7/1 (spring), 9/1 (summer). *Application fee:* $50.
Advanced Placement Credit by examination available. Credit given for nursing courses completed elsewhere dependent upon specific evaluations.
Expenses (2015–16) *Tuition:* full-time $44,166; part-time $1861 per unit. *International tuition:* $44,166 full-time. *Required fees:* full-time $1327.
Financial Aid 77% of baccalaureate students in nursing programs received some form of financial aid in 2014–15. *Gift aid (need-based):* Federal Pell, FSEOG, state, private, college/university gift aid from institutional funds, Federal Nursing. *Loans:* Federal Nursing Student Loans, Federal Direct (Subsidized and Unsubsidized Stafford PLUS), Perkins. *Work-study:* Federal Work-Study, part-time campus jobs. *Financial aid application deadline (priority):* 3/2.
Contact Mr. Timothy Cranford, Dean of Admission, School of Nursing, Samuel Merritt University, 3100 Telegraph Avenue, Office of Admissions, Oakland, CA 94609. *Telephone:* 510-869-1508. *Fax:* 510-869-6525. *E-mail:* admission@samuelmerritt.edu.

GRADUATE PROGRAMS

Expenses (2015–16) *Tuition:* part-time $1251 per unit.
Financial Aid 82% of graduate students in nursing programs received some form of financial aid in 2014–15. Career-related internships or fieldwork, Federal Work-Study, scholarships, and traineeships available. Aid available to part-time students. *Financial aid application deadline:* 3/2.
Contact Mr. Timothy Cranford, Dean of Admission, School of Nursing, Samuel Merritt University, 3100 Telegraph Avenue, Office of Admissions, Oakland, CA 94609. *Telephone:* 510-869-1508. *Fax:* 510-869-6525. *E-mail:* admission@samuelmerritt.edu.

MASTER'S DEGREE PROGRAM
Degree MSN
Available Programs Master's; Master's for Non-Nursing College Graduates; Master's for Nurses with Non-Nursing Degrees.
Concentrations Available Nurse anesthesia; nurse case management. *Nurse practitioner programs in:* family health.
Site Options Sacramento, CA.
Study Options Full-time and part-time.
Program Entrance Requirements Clinical experience, computer literacy, minimum overall college GPA of 3.0, transcript of college record, CPR certification, written essay, immunizations, interview, 2 letters of

recommendation, prerequisite course work, resume, statistics course. *Application deadline:* 11/1 (fall), 7/1 (spring), 1/1 (summer). *Application fee:* $50.

Advanced Placement Credit by examination available. Credit given for nursing courses completed elsewhere dependent upon specific evaluations.

Degree Requirements Comprehensive exam.

POST-MASTER'S PROGRAM

Areas of Study Nurse anesthesia; nurse case management. *Nurse practitioner programs in:* family health.

DOCTORAL DEGREE PROGRAM

Degree DNP

Available Programs Doctorate; Post-Baccalaureate Doctorate.

Areas of Study Advanced practice nursing, aging, bio-behavioral research, biology of health and illness, clinical practice, clinical research, ethics, family health, health policy, health promotion/disease prevention, health-care systems, human health and illness, illness and transition, information systems, nursing research, women's health.

Program Entrance Requirements Clinical experience, minimum overall college GPA of 3.0, interview by faculty committee, interview, 3 letters of recommendation, MSN or equivalent, scholarly papers, statistics course, vita, writing sample. Application deadline: 8/1 (spring). Applications may be processed on a rolling basis for some programs. Application fee: $50.

Degree Requirements 36 total credit hours, residency.

San Diego State University

School of Nursing
San Diego, California

http://www.nursing.sdsu.edu/
Founded in 1897

DEGREES • BSN • MSN

Nursing Program Faculty 65 (30% with doctorates).

Baccalaureate Enrollment 419 **Women** 85% **Men** 15% **Part-time** 2%

Graduate Enrollment 96 **Women** 95% **Men** 5% **Part-time** 77%

Distance Learning Courses Available.

Nursing Student Activities Sigma Theta Tau, Student Nurses' Association.

Nursing Student Resources Academic advising; academic or career counseling; assistance for students with disabilities; bookstore; campus computer network; career placement assistance; computer lab; daycare for children of students; e-mail services; housing assistance; Internet; learning resource lab; library services; nursing audiovisuals; paid internships; placement services for program completers; remedial services; resume preparation assistance; skills, simulation, or other laboratory; unpaid internships.

Library Facilities 36,000 volumes in health, 14,000 volumes in nursing; 335 periodical subscriptions health-care related.

BACCALAUREATE PROGRAMS

Degree BSN

Available Programs ADN to Baccalaureate; Generic Baccalaureate; RN Baccalaureate.

Study Options Full-time and part-time.

Program Entrance Requirements Minimum overall college GPA of 2.8, transcript of college record, high school transcript, minimum GPA in nursing prerequisites of 2.8, prerequisite course work. Transfer students are accepted. *Application deadline:* 11/30 (fall). Applications may be processed on a rolling basis for some programs.

Advanced Placement Credit by examination available. Credit given for nursing courses completed elsewhere dependent upon specific evaluations.

Contact *Telephone:* 619-594-2540. *Fax:* 619-594-2765.

GRADUATE PROGRAMS

Contact *Telephone:* 619-594-2766. *Fax:* 619-594-2765.

MASTER'S DEGREE PROGRAM

Degree MSN

Available Programs Master's.

Concentrations Available Nurse-midwifery; nursing administration; nursing education. *Clinical nurse specialist programs in:* adult health, community health, critical care, gerontology, maternity-newborn, school

health, women's health. *Nurse practitioner programs in:* acute care, adult health, gerontology, women's health.

Study Options Full-time and part-time.

Program Entrance Requirements Clinical experience, minimum overall college GPA of 3.0, transcript of college record, written essay, 3 letters of recommendation, nursing research course, physical assessment course, professional liability insurance/malpractice insurance, resume, statistics course, GRE General Test. *Application deadline:* 2/1 (fall), 2/1 (spring). Applications may be processed on a rolling basis for some programs.

Advanced Placement Credit by examination available. Credit given for nursing courses completed elsewhere dependent upon specific evaluations.

Degree Requirements 39 total credit hours, thesis or project, comprehensive exam.

POST-MASTER'S PROGRAM

Areas of Study Nurse-midwifery.

CONTINUING EDUCATION PROGRAM

Contact *Telephone:* 619-594-2766. *Fax:* 619-594-2765.

San Francisco State University

School of Nursing
San Francisco, California

http://www.nursing.sfsu.edu/
Founded in 1899

DEGREES • BSN • MSN

Nursing Program Faculty 40 (50% with doctorates).

Baccalaureate Enrollment 250 **Women** 88% **Men** 12% **Part-time** 5%

Graduate Enrollment 180 **Women** 80% **Men** 20% **Part-time** 20%

Nursing Student Activities Sigma Theta Tau, Student Nurses' Association.

Nursing Student Resources Academic advising; academic or career counseling; assistance for students with disabilities; bookstore; campus computer network; career placement assistance; computer lab; computer-assisted instruction; daycare for children of students; e-mail services; employment services for current students; externships; housing assistance; interactive nursing skills videos; Internet; learning resource lab; library services; nursing audiovisuals; other; placement services for program completers; remedial services; resume preparation assistance; skills, simulation, or other laboratory; tutoring.

Library Facilities 11,000 volumes in health, 1,500 volumes in nursing; 200 periodical subscriptions health-care related.

BACCALAUREATE PROGRAMS

Degree BSN

Available Programs ADN to Baccalaureate; Accelerated LPN to Baccalaureate; Generic Baccalaureate; RN Baccalaureate.

Study Options Full-time.

Program Entrance Requirements Minimum overall college GPA of 2.5, transcript of college record, CPR certification, health exam, health insurance, immunizations, minimum GPA in nursing prerequisites of 2.5, professional liability insurance/malpractice insurance, prerequisite course work. Transfer students are accepted.

Advanced Placement Credit by examination available. Credit given for nursing courses completed elsewhere dependent upon specific evaluations.

Contact *Telephone:* 415-338-2315 Ext. 1. *Fax:* 415-338-0555.

GRADUATE PROGRAMS

Contact *Telephone:* 415-338-1802. *Fax:* 415-338-0555.

MASTER'S DEGREE PROGRAM

Degree MSN

Available Programs Accelerated Master's for Non-Nursing College Graduates; Accelerated Master's for Nurses with Non-Nursing Degrees; Master's; Master's for Non-Nursing College Graduates; Master's for Nurses with Non-Nursing Degrees.

Concentrations Available Nurse case management; nursing administration. *Clinical nurse specialist programs in:* adult health, perinatal, public health. *Nurse practitioner programs in:* family health.

Study Options Full-time and part-time.

Program Entrance Requirements Minimum overall college GPA of 3.0, transcript of college record, CPR certification, written essay, immu-

nizations, 3 letters of recommendation, nursing research course, professional liability insurance/malpractice insurance, resume, statistics course.
Advanced Placement Credit by examination available. Credit given for nursing courses completed elsewhere dependent upon specific evaluations.
Degree Requirements 36 total credit hours, thesis or project.

POST-MASTER'S PROGRAM
Areas of Study Nursing administration. *Nurse practitioner programs in:* family health.

CONTINUING EDUCATION PROGRAM

Contact *Telephone:* 415-405-3660. *Fax:* 415-338-0555.

San Jose State University
The Valley Foundation School of Nursing
San Jose, California

http://www.sjsu.edu/nursing
Founded in 1857
DEGREES • BS • MS
Nursing Program Faculty 57 (43% with doctorates).
Baccalaureate Enrollment 433 **Women** 80% **Men** 20% **Part-time** 3%
Graduate Enrollment 43 **Women** 86% **Men** 14% **Part-time** 100%
Nursing Student Activities Nursing Honor Society, Sigma Theta Tau, Student Nurses' Association, nursing club.
Nursing Student Resources Academic advising; academic or career counseling; assistance for students with disabilities; bookstore; campus computer network; computer lab; computer-assisted instruction; daycare for children of students; e-mail services; employment services for current students; housing assistance; interactive nursing skills videos; Internet; learning resource lab; library services; nursing audiovisuals; remedial services; resume preparation assistance; skills, simulation, or other laboratory; tutoring.
Library Facilities 27,400 volumes in health, 2,100 volumes in nursing; 92 periodical subscriptions health-care related.

BACCALAUREATE PROGRAMS

Degree BS
Available Programs Generic Baccalaureate; RPN to Baccalaureate.
Study Options Full-time.
Program Entrance Requirements Transcript of college record, health exam, health insurance, high school biology, high school chemistry, high school foreign language, 3 years high school math, 3 years high school science, immunizations, minimum high school GPA of 3.0, minimum GPA in nursing prerequisites of 3.0, professional liability insurance/malpractice insurance, prerequisite course work. Transfer students are accepted. *Application deadline:* 2/15 (fall), 9/15 (spring). *Application fee:* $150.
Expenses (2015–16) *Tuition, state resident:* full-time $3689. *Tuition, nonresident:* full-time $6479. *Room and board:* $13,454; room only: $13,074 per academic year. *Required fees:* full-time $3174.
Contact Dr. Suzanne Malloy, Professor, The Valley Foundation School of Nursing, San Jose State University, One Washington Square, San Jose, CA 95192-0057. *Telephone:* 408-924-3142. *Fax:* 408-924-3135. *E-mail:* suzanne.malloy@sjsu.edu.

GRADUATE PROGRAMS

Expenses (2015–16) *Tuition, state resident:* part-time $2906 per semester. *Tuition, nonresident:* part-time $5138 per semester.
Contact Dr. Daryl Canham, Graduate Coordinator, The Valley Foundation School of Nursing, San Jose State University, One Washington Square, San Jose, CA 95192-0057. *Telephone:* 408-924-1323. *Fax:* 408-924-3135. *E-mail:* daryl.canham@sjsu.edu.

MASTER'S DEGREE PROGRAM
Degree MS
Available Programs Master's.
Concentrations Available Health-care administration; nursing administration; nursing education.
Study Options Full-time and part-time.
Program Entrance Requirements Minimum overall college GPA of 3.0, transcript of college record, CPR certification, written essay, immunizations, 3 letters of recommendation, nursing research course, physical assessment course, professional liability insurance/malpractice insurance,

prerequisite course work, resume, statistics course. *Application deadline:* 5/1 (fall), 11/1 (spring). *Application fee:* $150.
Degree Requirements 36 total credit hours, thesis or project.

POST-MASTER'S PROGRAM
Areas of Study Nursing education.

Sonoma State University
Department of Nursing
Rohnert Park, California

http://www.sonoma.edu/nursing
Founded in 1960
DEGREE • BSN

BACCALAUREATE PROGRAMS

Degree BSN
Available Programs Generic Baccalaureate.
Study Options Full-time.
Program Entrance Requirements Written essay, health exam, high school biology, high school chemistry, high school foreign language, 3 years high school math, 2 years high school science, high school transcript, immunizations, minimum high school GPA of 3.5. Transfer students are accepted. *Application deadline:* 2/28 (fall).
Contact *Telephone:* 707-664-2465. *Fax:* 707-664-2653.

Stanbridge College
Nursing Program
Irvine, California

https://www.stanbridge.edu/
DEGREE • BSN

BACCALAUREATE PROGRAMS

Degree BSN
Available Programs RN Baccalaureate.
Contact Bobbi-Ann Murphy, Assistant Director, Nursing Program, Stanbridge College, 2041 Business Center Drive, Suite 107, Irvine, CA 92612. *Telephone:* 949-794-9090. *E-mail:* bmurphy@stanbridge.edu.

United States University
School of Nursing
Chula Vista, California

http://www.usuniversity.edu/
DEGREE • BSN

BACCALAUREATE PROGRAMS

Degree BSN
Available Programs RN Baccalaureate.
Contact Renee McLeod, Dean, School of Nursing, United States University, 830 Bay Boulevard, Chula Vista, CA 91911. *Telephone:* 619-477-6310 Ext. 2036. *E-mail:* rmcleod@usuniversity.edu.

Unitek College
School of Nursing and Allied Health
Fremont, California

http://www.unitekcollege.edu
DEGREE • BSN
Nursing Program Faculty 38 (90% with doctorates).
Baccalaureate Enrollment 36
Distance Learning Courses Available.
Nursing Student Resources Academic advising; academic or career counseling; assistance for students with disabilities; campus computer network; career placement assistance; computer lab; computer-assisted instruction; e-mail services; employment services for current students; interactive nursing skills videos; Internet; learning resource lab; library

services; nursing audiovisuals; placement services for program completers; remedial services; resume preparation assistance; skills, simulation, or other laboratory; tutoring.

BACCALAUREATE PROGRAMS

Degree BSN
Available Programs ADN to Baccalaureate.
Study Options Full-time and part-time.
Online Degree Options Yes (online only).
Program Entrance Requirements Minimum overall college GPA of 2.5, transcript of college record, 2 letters of recommendation, minimum GPA in nursing prerequisites of 2.5, prerequisite course work, RN licensure. Transfer students are accepted. *Application deadline:* Applications may be processed on a rolling basis for some programs. *Application fee:* $150.
Advanced Placement Credit given for nursing courses completed elsewhere dependent upon specific evaluations.
Expenses (2015–16) *Tuition:* full-time $20,000. *International tuition:* $20,000 full-time. *Required fees:* full-time $150.
Contact Jason Ho, Director of Academic Operations, School of Nursing and Allied Health, Unitek College, 4670 Auto Mall Parkway, Fremont, CA 94538. *Telephone:* 510-249-1060. *E-mail:* jasonho@unitekcollege.edu.

CONTINUING EDUCATION PROGRAM

Contact Jason Ho, School of Nursing and Allied Health, Unitek College, 4670 Auto Mall Parkway, Fremont, CA 94538. *Telephone:* 510-249-1060. *Fax:* 510-249-1060. *E-mail:* jasonho@unitekcollege.edu.

University of California, Davis
The Betty Irene Moore School of Nursing
Davis, California

http://www.ucdmc.ucdavis.edu/nursing/
Founded in 1905
DEGREES • MS • PHD
Nursing Program Faculty 29 (100% with doctorates).
Graduate Enrollment 94 **Women** 83% **Men** 17%
Distance Learning Courses Available.
Nursing Student Activities Sigma Theta Tau.
Nursing Student Resources Academic advising; academic or career counseling; assistance for students with disabilities; bookstore; campus computer network; career placement assistance; computer lab; computer-assisted instruction; e-mail services; employment services for current students; Internet; learning resource lab; library services; remedial services; resume preparation assistance; skills, simulation, or other laboratory; tutoring.
Library Facilities 371,673 volumes in health, 1,700 volumes in nursing; 8,662 periodical subscriptions health-care related.

GRADUATE PROGRAMS

Expenses (2015–16) *Tuition, state resident:* full-time $21,249. *Tuition, nonresident:* full-time $33,494. *International tuition:* $33,494 full-time. *Required fees:* full-time $1945.
Financial Aid 100% of graduate students in nursing programs received some form of financial aid in 2014–15.
Contact Anna Libonati, Student Affairs Officer, The Betty Irene Moore School of Nursing, University of California, Davis, 4610 X Street, Suite 4202, Sacramento, CA 95817. *Telephone:* 916-734-2145. *Fax:* 916-734-3257. *E-mail:* HS-BettyIreneMooreSON@ucdavis.edu.

MASTER'S DEGREE PROGRAM
Degree MS
Available Programs Master's.
Study Options Full-time.
Program Entrance Requirements Minimum overall college GPA of 3.0, transcript of college record, CPR certification, written essay, immunizations, interview, 3 letters of recommendation, prerequisite course work. *Application deadline:* 1/15 (fall). *Application fee:* $90.
Degree Requirements 60 total credit hours, thesis or project.

DOCTORAL DEGREE PROGRAM
Degree PhD
Available Programs Doctorate; Doctorate for Nurses with Non-Nursing Degrees; Post-Baccalaureate Doctorate.

Areas of Study Nursing research, nursing science.
Program Entrance Requirements Minimum overall college GPA of 3.0, interview, 3 letters of recommendation, vita, writing sample. Application deadline: 1/15 (fall). Application fee: $90.
Degree Requirements 144 total credit hours, dissertation.

POSTDOCTORAL PROGRAM
Areas of Study Individualized study, nursing research, nursing science.
Postdoctoral Program Contact Lisa Reevesman, Academic Personnel Coordinator, The Betty Irene Moore School of Nursing, University of California, Davis, 4610 X Street, Suite 4202, Sacramento, CA 95817. *Telephone:* 916-734-4737. *Fax:* 916-734-3257. *E-mail:* lareevesman@ucdavis.edu.

CONTINUING EDUCATION PROGRAM

Contact Ms. Jacqueline Kelly Tobar, Manager, The Betty Irene Moore School of Nursing, University of California, Davis, 4900 Broadway, Suite 1630, Sacramento, CA 95820. *Telephone:* 916-734-9790. *E-mail:* jktobar@ucdavis.edu.

University of California, Irvine
Program in Nursing Science
Irvine, California

http://www.nursing.uci.edu/
Founded in 1965
DEGREES • BS • MS • PHD
Nursing Program Faculty 36 (25% with doctorates).
Baccalaureate Enrollment 161 **Women** 84% **Men** 16%
Graduate Enrollment 40 **Women** 88% **Men** 12%
Nursing Student Activities Student Nurses' Association, nursing club.
Nursing Student Resources Academic advising; academic or career counseling; assistance for students with disabilities; bookstore; campus computer network; computer lab; computer-assisted instruction; daycare for children of students; e-mail services; employment services for current students; housing assistance; interactive nursing skills videos; Internet; learning resource lab; library services; nursing audiovisuals; skills, simulation, or other laboratory; tutoring.
Library Facilities 342,244 volumes in health, 3,296 volumes in nursing; 12,346 periodical subscriptions health-care related.

BACCALAUREATE PROGRAMS

Degree BS
Available Programs Baccalaureate for Second Degree; Generic Baccalaureate.
Study Options Full-time.
Program Entrance Requirements Written essay, high school biology, high school chemistry, 2 years high school science. Transfer students are accepted. *Application deadline:* 11/30 (fall). *Application fee:* $70.
Financial Aid *Gift aid (need-based):* Federal Pell, FSEOG, state, private, college/university gift aid from institutional funds. *Loans:* Federal Direct (Subsidized and Unsubsidized Stafford PLUS), Perkins, college/university, private loans. *Work-study:* Federal Work-Study, part-time campus jobs. *Financial aid application deadline:* 6/20(priority: 3/3).
Contact Baccalaureate Program, Program in Nursing Science, University of California, Irvine, 106 Berk Hall, Building 802, Irvine, CA 92697-3959. *Telephone:* 949-824-1514. *Fax:* 949-824-0470. *E-mail:* nssao@uci.edu.

GRADUATE PROGRAMS

Contact Master's Program, Program in Nursing Science, University of California, Irvine, 106 Berk Hall, Irvine, CA 92697-3959. *Telephone:* 949-824-1514. *Fax:* 949-824-0470. *E-mail:* gsnao@uci.edu.

MASTER'S DEGREE PROGRAM
Degree MS
Available Programs Master's.
Concentrations Available *Nurse practitioner programs in:* adult health, family health, gerontology.
Study Options Full-time.
Program Entrance Requirements Clinical experience, transcript of college record, written essay, interview, 3 letters of recommendation, nursing research course, physical assessment course, resume, statistics course. *Application deadline:* 2/1 (fall). *Application fee:* $90.
Degree Requirements 72 total credit hours, comprehensive exam.

POST-MASTER'S PROGRAM

Areas of Study *Nurse practitioner programs in:* adult health, family health, gerontology.

DOCTORAL DEGREE PROGRAM

Degree PhD
Available Programs Doctorate.
Areas of Study Addiction/substance abuse, advanced practice nursing, aging, bio-behavioral research, biology of health and illness, clinical practice, clinical research, community health, critical care, ethics, faculty preparation, family health, forensic nursing, gerontology, health policy, health promotion/disease prevention, health-care systems, human health and illness, illness and transition, individualized study, information systems, maternity-newborn, neuro-behavior, nurse case management, nursing administration, nursing education, nursing policy, nursing research, nursing science, oncology, palliative care, women's health.
Program Entrance Requirements interview by faculty committee, 3 letters of recommendation, statistics course, vita, writing sample. Application deadline: 3/1 (fall). Application fee: $90.
Degree Requirements 44 total credit hours, dissertation, oral exam.

CONTINUING EDUCATION PROGRAM

Contact Continuing Education, Program in Nursing Science, University of California, Irvine, 106 Berk Hall, Irvine, CA 92697-3959. *Telephone:* 949-824-1514. *Fax:* 949-824-0470. *E-mail:* gnsao@uci.edu.

University of California, Los Angeles
School of Nursing
Los Angeles, California

http://www.nursing.ucla.edu
Founded in 1919

DEGREES • BS • MSN • MSN/MBA • PHD

Nursing Program Faculty 87 (54% with doctorates).
Baccalaureate Enrollment 186 **Women** 91% **Men** 9%
Graduate Enrollment 382 **Women** 86% **Men** 14%
Nursing Student Activities Nursing Honor Society, Sigma Theta Tau, Student Nurses' Association, nursing club.
Nursing Student Resources Academic advising; academic or career counseling; assistance for students with disabilities; bookstore; campus computer network; computer lab; daycare for children of students; e-mail services; housing assistance; Internet; library services; nursing audiovisuals; skills, simulation, or other laboratory.
Library Facilities 760,000 volumes in health, 8,000 volumes in nursing; 600,000 periodical subscriptions health-care related.

BACCALAUREATE PROGRAMS

Degree BS
Available Programs Generic Baccalaureate.
Study Options Full-time.
Program Entrance Requirements Transcript of college record, written essay, high school transcript, 2 letters of recommendation, minimum high school GPA, prerequisite course work. Transfer students are accepted. *Application deadline:* 11/30 (fall). *Application fee:* $70.
Expenses (2015–16) *Tuition, state resident:* full-time $15,183. *Tuition, nonresident:* full-time $39,891. *International tuition:* $39,891 full-time. *Room and board:* $14,090; room only: $12,328 per academic year.
Financial Aid 80% of baccalaureate students in nursing programs received some form of financial aid in 2014–15. *Gift aid (need-based):* Federal Pell, FSEOG, state, private, college/university gift aid from institutional funds, United Negro College Fund, Federal Nursing. *Loans:* Federal Nursing Student Loans, Federal Direct (Subsidized and Unsubsidized Stafford PLUS), Perkins, state, college/university. *Work-study:* Federal Work-Study, part-time campus jobs. *Financial aid application deadline (priority):* 3/2.
Contact Ms. Rhonda Flenoy-Younger, Director of Recruitment, Outreach, and Admissions, School of Nursing, University of California, Los Angeles, Box 951702, Los Angeles, CA 90095-1702. *Telephone:* 310-825-9193. *Fax:* 310-206-7433. *E-mail:* rflenoy@sonnet.ucla.edu.

GRADUATE PROGRAMS

Expenses (2015–16) *Tuition, state resident:* full-time $25,858. *Tuition, nonresident:* full-time $38,103. *International tuition:* $38,103 full-time.

Financial Aid 244 fellowships, 14 research assistantships, 44 teaching assistantships were awarded; Federal Work-Study, scholarships, tuition waivers (full and partial), and unspecified assistantships also available.
Contact Ms. Rhonda Flenoy-Younger, Director of Recruitment, Outreach, and Admissions, School of Nursing, University of California, Los Angeles, Box 951702, Los Angeles, CA 90095-1702. *Telephone:* 310-825-9193. *Fax:* 310-267-0330. *E-mail:* rflenoy@sonnet.ucla.edu.

MASTER'S DEGREE PROGRAM

Degrees MSN; MSN/MBA
Available Programs Master's; Master's for Non-Nursing College Graduates.
Concentrations Available Clinical nurse leader; nursing administration. *Clinical nurse specialist programs in:* acute care, pediatric. *Nurse practitioner programs in:* adult-gerontology acute care, family health, gerontology, occupational health, pediatric.
Study Options Full-time.
Program Entrance Requirements Minimum overall college GPA of 3.0, transcript of college record, written essay, 3 letters of recommendation, nursing research course, physical assessment course, prerequisite course work, resume, statistics course. *Application deadline:* 12/1 (fall). *Application fee:* $90.
Degree Requirements 72 total credit hours, comprehensive exam.

POST-MASTER'S PROGRAM

Areas of Study Nursing administration. *Clinical nurse specialist programs in:* acute care, pediatric. *Nurse practitioner programs in:* adult-gerontology acute care, family health, gerontology, occupational health, pediatric.

DOCTORAL DEGREE PROGRAM

Degree PhD
Available Programs Doctorate; Post-Baccalaureate Doctorate.
Areas of Study Addiction/substance abuse, advanced practice nursing, aging, bio-behavioral research, biology of health and illness, clinical practice, community health, critical care, family health, gerontology, health policy, health promotion/disease prevention, health-care systems, human health and illness, illness and transition, neuro-behavior, nursing administration, nursing research, nursing science, oncology, women's health.
Program Entrance Requirements Minimum overall college GPA of 3.5, interview, 3 letters of recommendation, scholarly papers, statistics course, vita, writing sample. Application deadline: 12/1 (fall). Application fee: $90.
Degree Requirements 127 total credit hours, dissertation, oral exam, written exam, residency.

POSTDOCTORAL PROGRAM

Areas of Study Addiction/substance abuse, adolescent health, aging, cancer care, gerontology, health promotion/disease prevention, nursing research, vulnerable population, women's health.
Postdoctoral Program Contact Dr. Lynn Doering, Associate Dean for Academic Affairs, School of Nursing, University of California, Los Angeles, Box 951702, Los Angeles, CA 90095-1702. *Telephone:* 310-825-4890. *Fax:* 310-206-7433. *E-mail:* ldoering@sonnet.ucla.edu.

CONTINUING EDUCATION PROGRAM

Contact Ms. Salpy Akaragian, Education Specialist, School of Nursing, University of California, Los Angeles, Box 951701, Los Angeles, CA 90095-1701. *Telephone:* 310-206-9581. *E-mail:* nssa@mednet.ucla.edu.

University of California, San Francisco
School of Nursing
San Francisco, California

http://www.nurseweb.ucsf.edu/
Founded in 1864

DEGREES • MS • PHD

Nursing Program Faculty 151 (72% with doctorates).
Graduate Enrollment 721 **Women** 87% **Men** 13% **Part-time** 1%
Distance Learning Courses Available.
Nursing Student Activities Nursing Honor Society, Sigma Theta Tau, Student Nurses' Association, nursing club.
Nursing Student Resources Academic advising; academic or career counseling; assistance for students with disabilities; bookstore; campus

computer network; career placement assistance; computer lab; computer-assisted instruction; daycare for children of students; e-mail services; employment services for current students; housing assistance; interactive nursing skills videos; Internet; learning resource lab; library services; nursing audiovisuals; other; paid internships; placement services for program completers; remedial services; resume preparation assistance; skills, simulation, or other laboratory; tutoring; unpaid internships.

Library Facilities 856,169 volumes in health, 131,046 volumes in nursing; 3,270 periodical subscriptions health-care related.

GRADUATE PROGRAMS

Contact *Telephone:* 415-476-1435. *Fax:* 415-476-9707.

MASTER'S DEGREE PROGRAM

Degree MS

Available Programs Master's; Master's for Non-Nursing College Graduates; Master's for Nurses with Non-Nursing Degrees.

Concentrations Available Nurse-midwifery; nursing administration. *Clinical nurse specialist programs in:* cardiovascular, community health, critical care, gerontology, occupational health, oncology, pediatric, perinatal, psychiatric/mental health. *Nurse practitioner programs in:* acute care, adult health, family health, gerontology, neonatal health, occupational health, pediatric, psychiatric/mental health.

Study Options Full-time.

Program Entrance Requirements Clinical experience, computer literacy, minimum overall college GPA of 3.0, transcript of college record, written essay, immunizations, 4 letters of recommendation, statistics course, GRE General Test. *Application deadline:* 2/1 (fall). *Application fee:* $60.

Advanced Placement Credit given for nursing courses completed elsewhere dependent upon specific evaluations.

Degree Requirements 44 total credit hours, comprehensive exam.

POST-MASTER'S PROGRAM

Areas of Study *Clinical nurse specialist programs in:* cardiovascular, community health, critical care, gerontology, occupational health, oncology, pediatric, perinatal, psychiatric/mental health. *Nurse practitioner programs in:* acute care, adult health, family health, gerontology, neonatal health, occupational health, pediatric, psychiatric/mental health.

DOCTORAL DEGREE PROGRAM

Degree PhD

Available Programs Doctorate; Post-Baccalaureate Doctorate.

Areas of Study Addiction/substance abuse, aging, bio-behavioral research, biology of health and illness, community health, critical care, ethics, family health, gerontology, health policy, health promotion/disease prevention, health-care systems, human health and illness, illness and transition, individualized study, information systems, maternity-newborn, nursing administration, nursing policy, nursing research, nursing science, oncology, urban health, women's health.

Program Entrance Requirements Minimum overall college GPA of 3.0, 4 letters of recommendation, statistics course, writing sample, GRE General Test. Application deadline: 12/15 (fall). Application fee: $60.

Degree Requirements Dissertation, oral exam, written exam, residency.

POSTDOCTORAL PROGRAM

Areas of Study Individualized study.

Postdoctoral Program Contact *Telephone:* 415-476-1435. *Fax:* 415-476-9707.

University of Phoenix–Bay Area Campus

College of Nursing
San Jose, California

DEGREES • BSN • MSN • MSN/MBA • MSN/MHA

Nursing Program Faculty 12 (58% with doctorates).
Baccalaureate Enrollment 39 **Women** 92.3% **Men** 7.7%
Graduate Enrollment 22 **Women** 86.4% **Men** 13.6%
Nursing Student Activities Sigma Theta Tau.

Nursing Student Resources Academic advising; academic or career counseling; assistance for students with disabilities; bookstore; campus computer network; computer lab; computer-assisted instruction; e-mail services; interactive nursing skills videos; Internet; learning resource lab; library services; nursing audiovisuals; remedial services; skills, simulation, or other laboratory; tutoring.

Library Facilities 1,300 periodical subscriptions health-care related.

BACCALAUREATE PROGRAMS

Degree BSN

Available Programs Accelerated Baccalaureate.

Site Options Oakland, CA; San Francisco, CA; Novato, CA.

Study Options Full-time.

Program Entrance Requirements Transcript of college record, CPR certification, immunizations, 1 letter of recommendation, RN licensure. Transfer students are accepted. *Application deadline:* Applications may be processed on a rolling basis for some programs.

Advanced Placement Credit by examination available. Credit given for nursing courses completed elsewhere dependent upon specific evaluations.

Contact *Telephone:* 877-416-4100.

GRADUATE PROGRAMS

Contact *Telephone:* 877-416-4100.

MASTER'S DEGREE PROGRAM

Degrees MSN; MSN/MBA; MSN/MHA

Available Programs Master's.

Concentrations Available Health-care administration; nursing administration; nursing education.

Site Options Oakland, CA; San Francisco, CA; Novato, CA.

Study Options Full-time.

Program Entrance Requirements Clinical experience, computer literacy, minimum overall college GPA of 2.5, transcript of college record. *Application deadline:* Applications may be processed on a rolling basis for some programs. *Application fee:* $45.

Advanced Placement Credit given for nursing courses completed elsewhere dependent upon specific evaluations.

Degree Requirements 39 total credit hours, thesis or project.

University of Phoenix–Central Valley Campus

College of Health and Human Services
Fresno, California

Founded in 2004

DEGREE • BSN

Nursing Program Faculty 8 (13% with doctorates).
Baccalaureate Enrollment 53 **Women** 94.3% **Men** 5.7%
Nursing Student Activities Sigma Theta Tau.

Nursing Student Resources Academic advising; academic or career counseling; bookstore; campus computer network; computer lab; computer-assisted instruction; e-mail services; interactive nursing skills videos; Internet; learning resource lab; library services; nursing audiovisuals; remedial services; skills, simulation, or other laboratory; tutoring.

Library Facilities 1,300 periodical subscriptions health-care related.

BACCALAUREATE PROGRAMS

Degree BSN

Available Programs RN Baccalaureate.

Site Options Fresno, CA; Visalia, CA; Bakersfield, CA.

Study Options Full-time.

Program Entrance Requirements Transcript of college record, CPR certification, immunizations, 1 letter of recommendation, RN licensure. Transfer students are accepted.

Advanced Placement Credit by examination available. Credit given for nursing courses completed elsewhere dependent upon specific evaluations.

Contact *Telephone:* 661-663-0300. *Fax:* 661-633-2711.

University of Phoenix–Sacramento Valley Campus
College of Nursing
Sacramento, California

Founded in 1993

DEGREES • BSN • MSN • MSN/MHA
Nursing Program Faculty 29 (28% with doctorates).
Baccalaureate Enrollment 250 **Women** 88.8% **Men** 11.2%
Graduate Enrollment 53 **Women** 90.6% **Men** 9.4%
Nursing Student Activities Sigma Theta Tau.
Nursing Student Resources Academic advising; academic or career counseling; assistance for students with disabilities; bookstore; campus computer network; computer lab; computer-assisted instruction; e-mail services; interactive nursing skills videos; Internet; learning resource lab; library services; nursing audiovisuals; skills, simulation, or other laboratory; tutoring.
Library Facilities 1,300 periodical subscriptions health-care related.

BACCALAUREATE PROGRAMS

Degree BSN
Available Programs Accelerated Baccalaureate; LPN to Baccalaureate.
Site Options Lathrop, CA; Modesto, CA; Fairfield, CA.
Study Options Full-time.
Online Degree Options Yes.
Program Entrance Requirements Transcript of college record, CPR certification, immunizations, 1 letter of recommendation, RN licensure. Transfer students are accepted. *Application deadline:* Applications may be processed on a rolling basis for some programs.
Advanced Placement Credit by examination available. Credit given for nursing courses completed elsewhere dependent upon specific evaluations.
Contact *Telephone:* 800-266-2107.

GRADUATE PROGRAMS

Contact *Telephone:* 800-266-2107.

MASTER'S DEGREE PROGRAM
Degrees MSN; MSN/MHA
Available Programs Accelerated Master's.
Concentrations Available Health-care administration; nursing administration; nursing education. *Nurse practitioner programs in:* family health.
Site Options Lathrop, CA; Modesto, CA; Fairfield, CA.
Study Options Full-time and part-time.
Program Entrance Requirements Clinical experience, computer literacy, minimum overall college GPA of 2.5, transcript of college record. *Application deadline:* Applications may be processed on a rolling basis for some programs. *Application fee:* $45.
Advanced Placement Credit given for nursing courses completed elsewhere dependent upon specific evaluations.
Degree Requirements 39 total credit hours, thesis or project.

POST-MASTER'S PROGRAM
Areas of Study *Nurse practitioner programs in:* family health.

CONTINUING EDUCATION PROGRAM

Contact *Telephone:* 800-266-2107.

University of Phoenix–San Diego Campus
College of Nursing
San Diego, California

Founded in 1988

DEGREES • BSN • MSN • MSN/ED D
Nursing Program Faculty 30 (37% with doctorates).
Baccalaureate Enrollment 103 **Women** 81.6% **Men** 18.4%
Graduate Enrollment 46 **Women** 89.1% **Men** 10.9%
Nursing Student Activities Sigma Theta Tau.
Nursing Student Resources Academic advising; academic or career counseling; assistance for students with disabilities; bookstore; campus computer network; computer lab; computer-assisted instruction; e-mail services; interactive nursing skills videos; Internet; learning resource lab; library services; nursing audiovisuals; skills, simulation, or other laboratory; tutoring.
Library Facilities 1,300 periodical subscriptions health-care related.

BACCALAUREATE PROGRAMS

Degree BSN
Available Programs Accelerated Baccalaureate.
Site Options Chula Vista, CA; Imperial, CA; Palm Desert, CA.
Study Options Full-time.
Program Entrance Requirements Transcript of college record, CPR certification, immunizations, 1 letter of recommendation, RN licensure. Transfer students are accepted. *Application deadline:* Applications may be processed on a rolling basis for some programs.
Advanced Placement Credit by examination available. Credit given for nursing courses completed elsewhere dependent upon specific evaluations.
Contact *Telephone:* 888-867-4636.

GRADUATE PROGRAMS

Contact *Telephone:* 888-867-4636.

MASTER'S DEGREE PROGRAM
Degrees MSN; MSN/Ed D
Available Programs Master's.
Concentrations Available Health-care administration; nursing administration; nursing education.
Site Options Chula Vista, CA; Imperial, CA; Palm Desert, CA.
Study Options Full-time.
Program Entrance Requirements Clinical experience, computer literacy, minimum overall college GPA of 2.5, transcript of college record. *Application deadline:* Applications may be processed on a rolling basis for some programs. *Application fee:* $45.
Advanced Placement Credit given for nursing courses completed elsewhere dependent upon specific evaluations.
Degree Requirements 39 total credit hours, thesis or project.

University of Phoenix–Southern California Campus
College of Health Sciences and Nursing
Costa Mesa, California

Founded in 1980

DEGREES • BSN • MSN • MSN/MBA • MSN/MHA
Nursing Program Faculty 109 (23% with doctorates).
Baccalaureate Enrollment 563 **Women** 89.2% **Men** 10.8%
Graduate Enrollment 379 **Women** 90.2% **Men** 9.8%
Nursing Student Activities Sigma Theta Tau.
Nursing Student Resources Academic advising; academic or career counseling; assistance for students with disabilities; bookstore; campus computer network; computer lab; computer-assisted instruction; e-mail services; interactive nursing skills videos; Internet; learning resource lab; library services; nursing audiovisuals; remedial services; skills, simulation, or other laboratory; tutoring.
Library Facilities 1,300 periodical subscriptions health-care related.

BACCALAUREATE PROGRAMS

Degree BSN
Available Programs Accelerated Baccalaureate.
Site Options Diamond Bar, CA; La Marada, CA; Lancaster, CA.
Study Options Full-time.
Program Entrance Requirements Transcript of college record, CPR certification, immunizations, 1 letter of recommendation, RN licensure. Transfer students are accepted. *Application deadline:* Applications may be processed on a rolling basis for some programs.
Advanced Placement Credit by examination available. Credit given for nursing courses completed elsewhere dependent upon specific evaluations.
Contact *Telephone:* 800-697-8223.

GRADUATE PROGRAMS

Contact *Telephone:* 800-697-8223.

MASTER'S DEGREE PROGRAM
Degrees MSN; MSN/MBA; MSN/MHA

Available Programs Master's.
Concentrations Available Health-care administration; nursing administration; nursing education. *Nurse practitioner programs in:* family health.
Site Options Diamond Bar, CA; La Marada, CA; Lancaster, CA.
Study Options Full-time.
Program Entrance Requirements Clinical experience, computer literacy, minimum overall college GPA of 2.5, transcript of college record, 1 letter of recommendation. *Application deadline:* Applications may be processed on a rolling basis for some programs. *Application fee:* $45.
Advanced Placement Credit given for nursing courses completed elsewhere dependent upon specific evaluations.
Degree Requirements 39 total credit hours, thesis or project.

POST-MASTER'S PROGRAM

Areas of Study *Nurse practitioner programs in:* family health.

CONTINUING EDUCATION PROGRAM

Contact *Telephone:* 714-338-1720.

University of San Diego
Hahn School of Nursing and Health Science
San Diego, California

http://www.sandiego.edu/nursing
Founded in 1949
DEGREES • DNP • MSN • PHD
Nursing Program Faculty 66 (90% with doctorates).
Baccalaureate Enrollment 335
Graduate Enrollment 335 **Women** 84% **Men** 16% **Part-time** 25%
Nursing Student Activities Nursing Honor Society, Sigma Theta Tau, Student Nurses' Association.
Nursing Student Resources Academic advising; academic or career counseling; assistance for students with disabilities; bookstore; campus computer network; career placement assistance; computer lab; computer-assisted instruction; daycare for children of students; e-mail services; employment services for current students; externships; interactive nursing skills videos; Internet; learning resource lab; library services; nursing audiovisuals; resume preparation assistance; skills, simulation, or other laboratory; tutoring.
Library Facilities 47,500 volumes in health, 24,600 volumes in nursing; 2,200 periodical subscriptions health-care related.

GRADUATE PROGRAMS

Expenses (2015–16) *Tuition:* full-time $33,360; part-time $1390 per unit. *International tuition:* $33,360 full-time. *Room and board:* $12,000 per academic year. *Required fees:* full-time $352; part-time $176 per term.
Financial Aid 90% of graduate students in nursing programs received some form of financial aid in 2014–15. Scholarships and traineeships available. Aid available to part-time students. *Financial aid application deadline:* 4/1.
Contact Ms. Cathleen Mumper, Director of Admission and Student Services, Hahn School of Nursing and Health Science, University of San Diego, 5998 Alcala Park, San Diego, CA 92110-2492. *Telephone:* 619-260-4163. *Fax:* 619-260-6814. *E-mail:* cmm@sandiego.edu.

MASTER'S DEGREE PROGRAM

Degree MSN
Available Programs Accelerated Master's for Non-Nursing College Graduates; Master's.
Concentrations Available Clinical nurse leader; nursing administration; nursing education; nursing informatics. *Clinical nurse specialist programs in:* acute care, adult health, adult-gerontology acute care, critical care, gerontology, medical-surgical, palliative care. *Nurse practitioner programs in:* adult health, adult-psychiatric mental health, family health, gerontology, pediatric primary care, primary care, psychiatric/mental health.
Study Options Full-time and part-time.
Program Entrance Requirements Clinical experience, computer literacy, minimum overall college GPA of 3.0, transcript of college record, CPR certification, written essay, immunizations, interview, 3 letters of recommendation, prerequisite course work, resume, statistics course, GRE General Test (for entry-level nursing). *Application deadline:* 3/1 (fall), 11/1 (spring) 11/1 (direct-entry program MSN for non-RNs). *Application fee:* $45.

Advanced Placement Credit by examination available. Credit given for nursing courses completed elsewhere dependent upon specific evaluations.
Degree Requirements 33-71 total credit hours.

DOCTORAL DEGREE PROGRAM

Degree DNP
Available Programs Doctorate, Post-Baccalaureate Doctorate.
Areas of Study Adult-gerontology acute care, advanced practice nursing, family health, pediatric, psychiatric/mental health.
Program Entrance Requirements Minimum overall college GPA of 3.5, APRN clinical experience, interview, 3 letters of recommendation, writing sample. For BSN to DNP: Minimum overall college GPA of 3.0, RN clinical experience, interview, 3 letters of recommendation, writing sample. Application deadline: 3/1 (fall).

Degree PhD
Available Programs Doctorate; Post-Baccalaureate Doctorate.
Areas of Study Addiction/substance abuse, advanced practice nursing, aging, bio-behavioral research, clinical practice, community health, critical care, ethics, faculty preparation, family health, gerontology, health policy, health promotion/disease prevention, health-care systems, human health and illness, illness and transition, individualized study, information systems, maternity-newborn, nurse case management, nurse executive, nursing administration, nursing education, nursing policy, nursing research, nursing science, oncology, palliative care, urban health, women's health.
Program Entrance Requirements Clinical experience, minimum overall college GPA of 3.5, interview by faculty committee, interview, 3 letters of recommendation, MSN or equivalent, statistics course, vita, writing sample. Application deadline: 2/1 (fall). Application fee: $45.
Degree Requirements 48 total credit hours, dissertation, residency.

University of San Francisco
School of Nursing and Health Professions
San Francisco, California

http://www.usfca.edu/nursing/
Founded in 1855
DEGREES • BSN • DNP • MSN
Nursing Program Faculty 112 (75% with doctorates).
Baccalaureate Enrollment 756 **Women** 86% **Men** 14% **Part-time** 1%
Graduate Enrollment 378 **Women** 84% **Men** 16% **Part-time** 5%
Distance Learning Courses Available.
Nursing Student Activities Nursing Honor Society, Sigma Theta Tau, Student Nurses' Association, nursing club.
Nursing Student Resources Academic advising; academic or career counseling; assistance for students with disabilities; bookstore; campus computer network; career placement assistance; computer lab; computer-assisted instruction; e-mail services; employment services for current students; housing assistance; interactive nursing skills videos; Internet; learning resource lab; library services; nursing audiovisuals; remedial services; resume preparation assistance; skills, simulation, or other laboratory; tutoring; unpaid internships.
Library Facilities 200 periodical subscriptions health-care related.

BACCALAUREATE PROGRAMS

Degree BSN
Available Programs Generic Baccalaureate.
Study Options Full-time.
Online Degree Options Yes.
Program Entrance Requirements Minimum overall college GPA of 3.0, transcript of college record, written essay, health insurance, high school biology, high school chemistry, 3 years high school math, 2 years high school science, high school transcript, immunizations, 2 letters of recommendation, minimum high school GPA of 3.9, prerequisite course work. Transfer students are accepted. *Application deadline:* 1/15 (fall), 12/15 (winter). *Application fee:* $55.
Advanced Placement Credit given for nursing courses completed elsewhere dependent upon specific evaluations.
Contact *Telephone:* 800-422-6563. *Fax:* 415-422-6877.

GRADUATE PROGRAMS

Contact *Telephone:* 415-422-6681. *Fax:* 415-422-6877.

MASTER'S DEGREE PROGRAM

Degree MSN

Available Programs Accelerated AD/RN to Master's; Accelerated Master's for Non-Nursing College Graduates; Master's for Nurses with Non-Nursing Degrees; RN to Master's.

Concentrations Available Clinical nurse leader.

Site Options San Jose, CA; San Ramon, CA; Santa Rosa, CA.

Study Options Full-time.

Online Degree Options Yes.

Program Entrance Requirements Clinical experience, minimum overall college GPA of 3.5, transcript of college record, written essay, 2 letters of recommendation, prerequisite course work, resume, statistics course. *Application deadline:* 6/15 (fall), 10/15 (spring), 2/15 (summer). *Application fee:* \$55.

Advanced Placement Credit given for nursing courses completed elsewhere dependent upon specific evaluations.

Degree Requirements 40 total credit hours, thesis or project, comprehensive exam.

POST-MASTER'S PROGRAM

Areas of Study Clinical nurse leader.

DOCTORAL DEGREE PROGRAM

Degree DNP

Available Programs Doctorate; Post-Baccalaureate Doctorate.

Areas of Study Advanced practice nursing, family health, health-care systems.

Program Entrance Requirements Clinical experience, minimum overall college GPA of 3.0, 3 letters of recommendation, vita, writing sample. Application deadline: 6/15 (fall), 10/15 (spring). Application fee: \$55.

Degree Requirements Dissertation, oral exam, residency.

Vanguard University of Southern California

Nursing Program
Costa Mesa, California

Founded in 1920

DEGREE • BSN

Baccalaureate Enrollment 75

BACCALAUREATE PROGRAMS

Degree BSN

Available Programs RN Baccalaureate.

Contact *Telephone:* 714-668-6130 Ext. 3902. *Fax:* 714-668-6194.

West Coast University

Nursing Programs
North Hollywood, California

http://westcoastuniversity.edu/

Founded in 1909

DEGREES • BSN • MSN

Nursing Program Faculty 347 (7% with doctorates).

Baccalaureate Enrollment 2,890 **Women** 80% **Men** 20%

Graduate Enrollment 93 **Women** 80% **Men** 20%

Distance Learning Courses Available.

Nursing Student Activities Sigma Theta Tau, Student Nurses' Association.

Nursing Student Resources Academic or career counseling; assistance for students with disabilities; bookstore; campus computer network; career placement assistance; computer lab; computer-assisted instruction; e-mail services; interactive nursing skills videos; Internet; learning resource lab; library services; nursing audiovisuals; placement services for program completers; remedial services; resume preparation assistance; skills, simulation, or other laboratory; tutoring.

Library Facilities 4,696 volumes in health, 2,586 volumes in nursing; 15,867 periodical subscriptions health-care related.

BACCALAUREATE PROGRAMS

Degree BSN

Available Programs ADN to Baccalaureate; Accelerated Baccalaureate; Accelerated LPN to Baccalaureate; Accelerated RN Baccalaureate.

Site Options Ontario, CA; Dallas, TX; Anaheim, CA; Miami, FL.

Study Options Full-time.

Online Degree Options Yes.

Program Entrance Requirements Transcript of college record, CPR certification, health exam, health insurance, high school chemistry, immunizations, minimum GPA in nursing prerequisites of 2.25, prerequisite course work, RN licensure. Transfer students are accepted. *Application deadline:* Applications may be processed on a rolling basis for some programs. *Application fee:* \$75.

Advanced Placement Credit by examination available. Credit given for nursing courses completed elsewhere dependent upon specific evaluations.

Expenses (2015–16) *Tuition:* full-time \$132,400. *Required fees:* full-time \$6997.

Contact Dr. Robyn Nelson, College of Nursing, Nursing Programs, West Coast University, 151 Innovation Drive, Irvine, CA 92617. *Telephone:* 866-508-2684. *E-mail:* rnelson@westcoastuniversity.edu.

GRADUATE PROGRAMS

Expenses (2015–16) *Tuition:* full-time \$8700. *Required fees:* full-time \$920.

Contact Dr. Robyn Nelson, Dean, College of Nursing, Nursing Programs, West Coast University, 12215 Victory Boulevard, North Hollywood, CA 91606. *Telephone:* 866-508-2684. *E-mail:* rnelson@westcoastuniversity.edu.

MASTER'S DEGREE PROGRAM

Degree MSN

Available Programs Accelerated Master's; Accelerated Master's for Nurses with Non-Nursing Degrees; Accelerated RN to Master's.

Concentrations Available Nursing education. *Nurse practitioner programs in:* family health.

Study Options Full-time.

Online Degree Options Yes.

Program Entrance Requirements Clinical experience, minimum overall college GPA of 3.0, transcript of college record, interview, statistics course. *Application deadline:* Applications may be processed on a rolling basis for some programs. *Application fee:* \$75.

Advanced Placement Credit by examination available. Credit given for nursing courses completed elsewhere dependent upon specific evaluations.

Degree Requirements 36 total credit hours, thesis or project.

POST-MASTER'S PROGRAM

Areas of Study Nursing education. *Nurse practitioner programs in:* family health.

CONTINUING EDUCATION PROGRAM

Contact Dr. Robyn Nelson, Dean, College of Nursing, Nursing Programs, West Coast University, 151 Innovation Drive, Irvine, CA 92617. *Telephone:* 949-783-4814.

E-mail: rnelson@westcoastuniversity.edu.

Western University of Health Sciences

College of Graduate Nursing
Pomona, California

http://www.westernu.edu/nursing-visitor

Founded in 1975

DEGREES • DNP • MSN

Nursing Program Faculty 25 (76% with doctorates).

Graduate Enrollment 285 **Women** 85% **Men** 15% **Part-time** 5%

Distance Learning Courses Available.

Nursing Student Activities Nursing Honor Society, Sigma Theta Tau, Student Nurses' Association, nursing club.

Nursing Student Resources Academic advising; academic or career counseling; assistance for students with disabilities; bookstore; campus computer network; career placement assistance; computer lab; computer-assisted instruction; e-mail services; interactive nursing skills videos; Internet; learning resource lab; library services; nursing audiovisuals; other; remedial services; resume preparation assistance; skills, simulation, or other laboratory; tutoring.

Library Facilities 17,171 volumes in health, 322 volumes in nursing; 5,000 periodical subscriptions health-care related.

GRADUATE PROGRAMS

Expenses (2015–16) *Tuition:* part-time $831 per credit. *International tuition:* $831 full-time. *Required fees:* full-time $1876.
Financial Aid 69% of graduate students in nursing programs received some form of financial aid in 2014–15. Institutionally sponsored loans, scholarships, and veterans' educational benefits available. *Financial aid application deadline:* 3/2.
Contact Ms. Mitzi McKay, Assistant Dean of Student Affairs, College of Graduate Nursing, Western University of Health Sciences, 309 East Second Street, Pomona, CA 91766-1854. *Telephone:* 909-469-5255. *Fax:* 909-469-5521. *E-mail:* mmckay@westernu.edu.

MASTER'S DEGREE PROGRAM

Degree MSN
Available Programs Accelerated AD/RN to Master's; Accelerated Master's; Accelerated Master's for Non-Nursing College Graduates; Accelerated RN to Master's; Master's; RN to Master's.
Concentrations Available Clinical nurse leader; nursing administration. *Nurse practitioner programs in:* family health.
Study Options Full-time and part-time.
Online Degree Options Yes (online only).
Program Entrance Requirements Clinical experience, computer literacy, minimum overall college GPA of 3.0, transcript of college record, CPR certification, written essay, immunizations, interview, 3 letters of recommendation, prerequisite course work, resume, statistics course. *Application deadline:* 3/1 (fall). Applications may be processed on a rolling basis for some programs. *Application fee:* $60.
Advanced Placement Credit given for nursing courses completed elsewhere dependent upon specific evaluations.
Degree Requirements 50 total credit hours, thesis or project.

POST-MASTER'S PROGRAM

Areas of Study *Nurse practitioner programs in:* family health.

DOCTORAL DEGREE PROGRAM

Degree DNP
Available Programs Doctorate.
Online Degree Options Yes (online only).
Program Entrance Requirements Minimum overall college GPA of 3.0, 3 letters of recommendation, MSN or equivalent, scholarly papers, statistics course, vita, writing sample. Application deadline: 3/1 (fall). Applications may be processed on a rolling basis for some programs. Application fee: $60.
Degree Requirements 30 total credit hours.

COLORADO

Adams State University

Nursing Program
Alamosa, Colorado

http://www.adams.edu/
Founded in 1921
DEGREE • BSN
Nursing Program Faculty 10 (10% with doctorates).
Baccalaureate Enrollment 83 **Women** 87% **Men** 13% **Part-time** 39%
Distance Learning Courses Available.
Nursing Student Activities Sigma Theta Tau, Student Nurses' Association.
Nursing Student Resources Academic advising; academic or career counseling; assistance for students with disabilities; bookstore; campus computer network; computer lab; computer-assisted instruction; e-mail services; employment services for current students; housing assistance; interactive nursing skills videos; Internet; learning resource lab; library services; nursing audiovisuals; remedial services; resume preparation assistance; skills, simulation, or other laboratory; tutoring; unpaid internships.
Library Facilities 565 volumes in health, 565 volumes in nursing; 200 periodical subscriptions health-care related.

BACCALAUREATE PROGRAMS

Degree BSN
Available Programs Generic Baccalaureate; RN Baccalaureate.
Study Options Full-time.
Online Degree Options Yes (online only).
Program Entrance Requirements Minimum overall college GPA of 3.0, transcript of college record, written essay, immunizations, 2 letters of recommendation, minimum high school GPA of 2.0, minimum GPA in nursing prerequisites of 3.0, prerequisite course work. Transfer students are accepted. *Application deadline:* 7/15 (fall), 7/15 (spring), 7/15 (summer).
Advanced Placement Credit by examination available. Credit given for nursing courses completed elsewhere dependent upon specific evaluations.
Contact Dr. Shawn Elliott, Director of Nursing, Nursing Program, Adams State University, 208 Edgemont Boulevard, Alamosa, CO 81102. *Telephone:* 719-587-8134. *Fax:* 719-587-7522. *E-mail:* selliott@adams.edu.

American Sentinel University

RN to Bachelor of Science Nursing
Aurora, Colorado

http://www.americansentinel.edu
Founded in 1988
DEGREES • BSN • DNP • MSN
Nursing Program Faculty 45 (40% with doctorates).
Baccalaureate Enrollment 1,551 **Women** 92.5% **Men** 7.5% **Part-time** 100%
Graduate Enrollment 1,310 **Women** 91.1% **Men** 8.9% **Part-time** 100%
Distance Learning Courses Available.
Nursing Student Activities Nursing Honor Society, Sigma Theta Tau.
Nursing Student Resources Academic advising; assistance for students with disabilities; library services; resume preparation assistance.

BACCALAUREATE PROGRAMS

Degree BSN
Available Programs ADN to Baccalaureate; International Nurse to Baccalaureate; RN Baccalaureate.
Online Degree Options Yes (online only).
Program Entrance Requirements Transcript of college record, RN licensure. Transfer students are accepted. *Application deadline:* Applications may be processed on a rolling basis for some programs.
Advanced Placement Credit given for nursing courses completed elsewhere dependent upon specific evaluations.
Expenses (2014–15) *Tuition:* full-time $6750; part-time $375 per credit hour. *International tuition:* $6750 full-time. *Required fees:* full-time $240.
Financial Aid 26% of baccalaureate students in nursing programs received some form of financial aid in 2013–14.
Contact Dr. Judy Burckhardt, Dean, Nursing Programs, RN to Bachelor of Science Nursing, American Sentinel University, 2260 South Xanadu Way, Suite 310, Aurora, CO 80014. *Telephone:* 303-557-9948. *Fax:* 866-505-2450. *E-mail:* judy.burckhardt@americansentinel.edu.

GRADUATE PROGRAMS

Expenses (2014–15) *Tuition:* full-time $8820; part-time $490 per credit hour. *International tuition:* $8820 full-time. *Required fees:* full-time $240.
Financial Aid 33% of graduate students in nursing programs received some form of financial aid in 2013–14.
Contact Dr. Judy Burckhardt, Dean, Nursing Programs, RN to Bachelor of Science Nursing, American Sentinel University, 2260 South Xanadu Way, Suite 310, Aurora, CO 80014. *Telephone:* 303-557-9948. *Fax:* 866-505-2450. *E-mail:* judy.burckhardt@americansentinel.edu.

MASTER'S DEGREE PROGRAM

Degree MSN
Available Programs Master's; RN to Master's.
Concentrations Available Nurse case management; nursing administration; nursing education; nursing informatics.
Study Options Part-time.
Online Degree Options Yes (online only).

Program Entrance Requirements Computer literacy, minimum overall college GPA of 2.0, transcript of college record. *Application deadline:* Applications may be processed on a rolling basis for some programs.
Advanced Placement Credit given for nursing courses completed elsewhere dependent upon specific evaluations.
Degree Requirements 36 total credit hours.

DOCTORAL DEGREE PROGRAM
Degree DNP
Available Programs Doctorate.
Areas of Study Nursing administration, nursing education.
Program Entrance Requirements Clinical experience, minimum overall college GPA of 2.5, MSN or equivalent, vita. Application deadline: Applications may be processed on a rolling basis for some programs.
Degree Requirements 42 total credit hours, dissertation, residency.

Aspen University
Graduate School of Health Professions and Studies
Denver, Colorado

http://www.aspen.edu
Founded in 1987
DEGREE • MSN
Nursing Program Faculty 4 (100% with doctorates).
Graduate Enrollment 206
Distance Learning Courses Available.
Nursing Student Resources Academic advising; computer-assisted instruction.

GRADUATE PROGRAMS
Contact *Telephone:* 800-373-7814.

MASTER'S DEGREE PROGRAM
Degree MSN
Available Programs Master's; RN to Master's.
Concentrations Available Nursing administration; nursing education.
Study Options Full-time and part-time.
Online Degree Options Yes (online only).
Program Entrance Requirements Clinical experience, minimum overall college GPA of 3.0, transcript of college record, written essay, resume. *Application deadline:* Applications may be processed on a rolling basis for some programs.
Advanced Placement Credit given for nursing courses completed elsewhere dependent upon specific evaluations.
Degree Requirements 36 total credit hours, thesis or project, comprehensive exam.

Colorado Christian University
Nursing Programs
Lakewood, Colorado

Founded in 1914
DEGREE • BSN

BACCALAUREATE PROGRAMS
Degree BSN
Available Programs Generic Baccalaureate; RN Baccalaureate.
Online Degree Options Yes.
Contact *Telephone:* 303-963-3311.

Colorado Mesa University
Department of Nursing and Radiologic Sciences
Grand Junction, Colorado

http://www.coloradomesa.edu/healthsciences/index.html
Founded in 1925
DEGREES • BSN • DNP • MSN
Nursing Program Faculty 55 (15% with doctorates).

Baccalaureate Enrollment 190 **Women** 88% **Men** 12% **Part-time** 8%
Graduate Enrollment 45 **Women** 90% **Men** 10% **Part-time** 50%
Distance Learning Courses Available.
Nursing Student Activities Nursing Honor Society, Sigma Theta Tau, Student Nurses' Association.
Nursing Student Resources Academic advising; academic or career counseling; assistance for students with disabilities; bookstore; campus computer network; career placement assistance; computer lab; computer-assisted instruction; daycare for children of students; e-mail services; employment services for current students; housing assistance; interactive nursing skills videos; Internet; learning resource lab; library services; nursing audiovisuals; placement services for program completers; resume preparation assistance; skills, simulation, or other laboratory; tutoring; unpaid internships.
Library Facilities 7,500 volumes in health, 6,576 volumes in nursing; 100 periodical subscriptions health-care related.

BACCALAUREATE PROGRAMS
Degree BSN
Available Programs ADN to Baccalaureate; Generic Baccalaureate; LPN to RN Baccalaureate; RN Baccalaureate.
Study Options Full-time and part-time.
Online Degree Options Yes.
Program Entrance Requirements Minimum overall college GPA of 2.5, transcript of college record, CPR certification, health exam, health insurance, immunizations, interview, minimum GPA in nursing prerequisites of 2.5, professional liability insurance/malpractice insurance, prerequisite course work. Transfer students are accepted. *Application deadline:* 3/1 (fall), 10/1 (spring). *Application fee:* $30.
Advanced Placement Credit by examination available.
Financial Aid 90% of baccalaureate students in nursing programs received some form of financial aid in 2013–14.
Contact Dr. Diana Bailey, Program Director, Department of Nursing and Radiologic Sciences, Colorado Mesa University, 1100 North Avenue, Grand Junction, CO 81501. *Telephone:* 970-248-1772. *Fax:* 970-248-1133. *E-mail:* dlbailey@coloradomesa.edu.

GRADUATE PROGRAMS
Financial Aid 70% of graduate students in nursing programs received some form of financial aid in 2013–14.
Contact Dr. Debra K. Bailey, Director of Health Sciences/DNP Program Director, Department of Nursing and Radiologic Sciences, Colorado Mesa University, 1100 North Avenue, Grand Junction, CO 81501. *Telephone:* 970-248-1772. *Fax:* 970-248-1133. *E-mail:* dbailey@coloradomesa.edu.

MASTER'S DEGREE PROGRAM
Degree MSN
Available Programs Master's.
Concentrations Available Nursing education. *Clinical nurse specialist programs in:* family health.
Study Options Full-time and part-time.
Online Degree Options Yes (online only).
Program Entrance Requirements Minimum overall college GPA of 3.0, transcript of college record, CPR certification, written essay, immunizations, letters of recommendation, professional liability insurance/malpractice insurance. *Application deadline:* 10/15 (fall), 2/15 (spring). Applications may be processed on a rolling basis for some programs. *Application fee:* $50.
Advanced Placement Credit given for nursing courses completed elsewhere dependent upon specific evaluations.
Degree Requirements 34 total credit hours, thesis or project, comprehensive exam.

DOCTORAL DEGREE PROGRAM
Degree DNP
Available Programs Doctorate.
Areas of Study Family health.
Online Degree Options Yes (online only).
Program Entrance Requirements Minimum overall college GPA of 3.0, letters of recommendation, writing sample. Application deadline: 10/15 (fall), 2/15 (spring). Applications may be processed on a rolling basis for some programs. Application fee: $50.
Degree Requirements 72 total credit hours, oral exam, written exam.

Colorado State University–Pueblo
Department of Nursing
Pueblo, Colorado

http://www.colostate-pueblo.edu/Pages/default.aspx
Founded in 1933
DEGREES • BSN • MS
Nursing Program Faculty 30 (17% with doctorates).
Baccalaureate Enrollment 200 **Women** 90% **Men** 10% **Part-time** 2%
Graduate Enrollment 90 **Women** 73% **Men** 27% **Part-time** 92%
Nursing Student Activities Sigma Theta Tau, Student Nurses' Association.
Nursing Student Resources Academic advising; academic or career counseling; assistance for students with disabilities; bookstore; campus computer network; career placement assistance; computer lab; computer-assisted instruction; daycare for children of students; e-mail services; employment services for current students; housing assistance; Internet; learning resource lab; library services; nursing audiovisuals; remedial services; resume preparation assistance; skills, simulation, or other laboratory; tutoring.
Library Facilities 2,891 volumes in health, 1,168 volumes in nursing; 3,745 periodical subscriptions health-care related.

BACCALAUREATE PROGRAMS

Degree BSN
Available Programs ADN to Baccalaureate; Accelerated Baccalaureate for Second Degree; Accelerated RN Baccalaureate; Baccalaureate for Second Degree; Generic Baccalaureate; LPN to Baccalaureate; LPN to RN Baccalaureate; RN Baccalaureate.
Study Options Full-time.
Program Entrance Requirements Minimum overall college GPA of 3.0, transcript of college record, CPR certification, health exam, health insurance, immunizations, minimum GPA in nursing prerequisites of 3.0, professional liability insurance/malpractice insurance, prerequisite course work. Transfer students are accepted. *Application deadline:* 5/25 (fall), 10/1 (summer). *Application fee:* $25.
Advanced Placement Credit by examination available. Credit given for nursing courses completed elsewhere dependent upon specific evaluations.
Financial Aid 80% of baccalaureate students in nursing programs received some form of financial aid in 2013–14. *Gift aid (need-based):* Federal Pell, FSEOG, state, private, college/university gift aid from institutional funds, Federal Nursing, TEACH Grants. *Loans:* Federal Nursing Student Loans, Federal Direct (Subsidized and Unsubsidized Stafford PLUS), Perkins. *Work-study:* Federal Work-Study, part-time campus jobs. *Financial aid application deadline (priority):* 3/1.
Contact Dr. Donna Wofford, Associate Dean of Nursing, Department of Nursing, Colorado State University–Pueblo, 2200 Bonforte Boulevard, Pueblo, CO 81001. *Telephone:* 719-549-2871. *Fax:* 719-549-2113. *E-mail:* donna.wofford@csupueblo.edu.

GRADUATE PROGRAMS

Financial Aid 50% of graduate students in nursing programs received some form of financial aid in 2013–14.
Contact Dr. Joe Franta, Nursing Graduate Coordinator, Department of Nursing, Colorado State University–Pueblo, 2200 Bonforte Boulevard, Pueblo, CO 81001. *Telephone:* 719-549-2459. *Fax:* 719-549-2949. *E-mail:* joe.franta@csupueblo.edu.

MASTER'S DEGREE PROGRAM
Degree MS
Available Programs Master's.
Concentrations Available Nursing education. *Nurse practitioner programs in:* acute care, family health, psychiatric/mental health.
Study Options Full-time and part-time.
Program Entrance Requirements Clinical experience, computer literacy, minimum overall college GPA of 3.0, transcript of college record, CPR certification, written essay, immunizations, 3 letters of recommendation, nursing research course, professional liability insurance/malpractice insurance, prerequisite course work, resume, statistics course. *Application deadline:* 4/15 (fall). *Application fee:* $35.
Advanced Placement Credit given for nursing courses completed elsewhere dependent upon specific evaluations.
Degree Requirements Thesis or project, comprehensive exam.

POST-MASTER'S PROGRAM
Areas of Study Nursing education. *Nurse practitioner programs in:* acute care, family health, psychiatric/mental health.

Colorado Technical University Online
Nursing Program
Colorado Springs, Colorado

http://www.coloradotech.edu/
DEGREE • BSN

BACCALAUREATE PROGRAMS

Degree BSN
Available Programs RN Baccalaureate.
Online Degree Options Yes.
Program Entrance Requirements *Application deadline:* Applications may be processed on a rolling basis for some programs.
Contact Admissions, Nursing Program, Colorado Technical University Online, 4435 North Chestnut Street, Suite E, Colorado Springs, CO 80907. *Telephone:* 800-416-8904. *E-mail:* enroll@ctuonline.edu.

Denver School of Nursing
Denver School of Nursing
Denver, Colorado

DEGREE • BSN
Nursing Program Faculty 78 (5% with doctorates).
Baccalaureate Enrollment 270 **Women** 80% **Men** 20%
Distance Learning Courses Available.
Nursing Student Activities Student Nurses' Association.
Nursing Student Resources Academic advising; academic or career counseling; assistance for students with disabilities; bookstore; campus computer network; career placement assistance; computer lab; computer-assisted instruction; e-mail services; employment services for current students; externships; interactive nursing skills videos; Internet; learning resource lab; library services; nursing audiovisuals; placement services for program completers; remedial services; resume preparation assistance; skills, simulation, or other laboratory; tutoring; unpaid internships.
Library Facilities 1,000 volumes in health, 1,000 volumes in nursing; 26,000 periodical subscriptions health-care related.

BACCALAUREATE PROGRAMS

Degree BSN
Available Programs ADN to Baccalaureate; Accelerated Baccalaureate; Accelerated Baccalaureate for Second Degree; Generic Baccalaureate; LPN to RN Baccalaureate; RN Baccalaureate.
Site Options Denver, CO.
Study Options Full-time.
Program Entrance Requirements Transcript of college record, CPR certification, written essay, health exam, health insurance, immunizations, interview, 3 letters of recommendation, minimum high school GPA of 2.0, minimum GPA in nursing prerequisites of 2.0, prerequisite course work. Transfer students are accepted. *Application deadline:* 4/1 (fall), 7/1 (winter), 10/1 (spring), 1/1 (summer). Applications may be processed on a rolling basis for some programs. *Application fee:* $50.
Advanced Placement Credit given for nursing courses completed elsewhere dependent upon specific evaluations.
Contact *Telephone:* 303-292-0015 Ext. 3611. *Fax:* 720-974-0290.

Metropolitan State University of Denver
Department of Health Professions
Denver, Colorado

https://www.msudenver.edu/nursing/
Founded in 1963
DEGREE • BSN
Nursing Program Faculty 19 (10% with doctorates).

Baccalaureate Enrollment 124 **Women** 89% **Men** 11% **Part-time** 63%
Distance Learning Courses Available.
Nursing Student Activities Nursing club.
Nursing Student Resources Academic advising; academic or career counseling; assistance for students with disabilities; bookstore; campus computer network; computer lab; computer-assisted instruction; daycare for children of students; e-mail services; interactive nursing skills videos; Internet; library services; nursing audiovisuals; remedial services; resume preparation assistance; skills, simulation, or other laboratory.
Library Facilities 21,503 volumes in health; 204 periodical subscriptions health-care related.

BACCALAUREATE PROGRAMS

Degree BSN

Available Programs ADN to Baccalaureate; Accelerated Baccalaureate for Second Degree.
Study Options Full-time and part-time.
Program Entrance Requirements Transcript of college record, CPR certification, written essay, immunizations, minimum GPA in nursing prerequisites of 2.5, professional liability insurance/malpractice insurance, prerequisite course work, RN licensure. Transfer students are accepted. *Application deadline:* 4/15 (spring). *Application fee:* $25.
Advanced Placement Credit given for nursing courses completed elsewhere dependent upon specific evaluations.
Contact *Telephone:* 303-556-4391. *Fax:* 303-556-5165.

Platt College
School of Nursing
Aurora, Colorado

http://www.plattcolorado.edu/
Founded in 1986
DEGREE • BSN
Nursing Program Faculty 8 (37% with doctorates).
Baccalaureate Enrollment 218 **Women** 87% **Men** 13%
Distance Learning Courses Available.
Nursing Student Activities Student Nurses' Association.
Nursing Student Resources Academic advising; academic or career counseling; assistance for students with disabilities; bookstore; campus computer network; career placement assistance; computer lab; computer-assisted instruction; e-mail services; employment services for current students; housing assistance; Internet; learning resource lab; library services; nursing audiovisuals; placement services for program completers; resume preparation assistance; skills, simulation, or other laboratory; tutoring; unpaid internships.

BACCALAUREATE PROGRAMS

Degree BSN

Available Programs Accelerated Baccalaureate.
Study Options Full-time.
Program Entrance Requirements Transcript of college record, CPR certification, written essay, health exam, health insurance, high school transcript, immunizations, interview, professional liability insurance/malpractice insurance. Transfer students are accepted. *Application deadline:* 9/12 (fall), 1/4 (winter), 3/28 (spring), 6/20 (summer). Applications may be processed on a rolling basis for some programs. *Application fee:* $75.
Advanced Placement Credit by examination available. Credit given for nursing courses completed elsewhere dependent upon specific evaluations.
Expenses (2015–16) *Tuition:* full-time $68,265. *Required fees:* full-time $8880.
Contact Ms. Rachael Hornbostel, Admissions Coordinator, School of Nursing, Platt College, 3100 South Parker Road, Suite 200, Aurora, CO 80014. *Telephone:* 303-369-5151. *E-mail:* rachael.hornbostel@ plattcolorado.edu.

Regis University
School of Nursing
Denver, Colorado

http://www.regis.edu/
Founded in 1877
DEGREES • BSN • MS
Nursing Program Faculty 18 (55% with doctorates).
Distance Learning Courses Available.
Nursing Student Activities Nursing Honor Society, Sigma Theta Tau, Student Nurses' Association.
Nursing Student Resources Academic advising; academic or career counseling; assistance for students with disabilities; bookstore; campus computer network; computer lab; computer-assisted instruction; e-mail services; interactive nursing skills videos; Internet; learning resource lab; library services; nursing audiovisuals; resume preparation assistance; skills, simulation, or other laboratory; tutoring; unpaid internships.

BACCALAUREATE PROGRAMS

Degree BSN

Available Programs Accelerated Baccalaureate; Generic Baccalaureate; RN Baccalaureate.
Site Options Cheyenne, WY.
Study Options Full-time.
Program Entrance Requirements Minimum overall college GPA of 2.5, transcript of college record, written essay, 2 letters of recommendation, prerequisite course work. Transfer students are accepted.
Advanced Placement Credit by examination available.
Contact *Telephone:* 303-964-5178. *Fax:* 303-964-5400.

GRADUATE PROGRAMS

Contact *Telephone:* 303-458-3534. *Fax:* 303-964-5400.

MASTER'S DEGREE PROGRAM
Degree MS
Available Programs Master's; RN to Master's.
Concentrations Available Health-care administration; nursing administration; nursing education. *Nurse practitioner programs in:* family health, neonatal health.
Study Options Full-time and part-time.
Online Degree Options Yes.
Program Entrance Requirements Minimum overall college GPA of 2.75, transcript of college record, written essay, 3 letters of recommendation, prerequisite course work, statistics course.
Advanced Placement Credit by examination available.
Degree Requirements 42 total credit hours, thesis or project.

University of Colorado Colorado Springs
Helen and Arthur E. Johnson Beth-El College of Nursing & Health Sciences
Colorado Springs, Colorado

http://www.uccs.edu/~bethel/
Founded in 1965
DEGREES • BSN • DNP • MSN
Nursing Program Faculty 62 (24% with doctorates).
Baccalaureate Enrollment 430 **Women** 88% **Men** 12% **Part-time** 52%
Graduate Enrollment 183 **Women** 94% **Men** 6% **Part-time** 89%
Distance Learning Courses Available.
Nursing Student Activities Nursing Honor Society, Sigma Theta Tau, Student Nurses' Association, nursing club.
Nursing Student Resources Academic advising; academic or career counseling; assistance for students with disabilities; bookstore; campus computer network; career placement assistance; computer lab; computer-assisted instruction; daycare for children of students; e-mail services; employment services for current students; externships; housing assistance; interactive nursing skills videos; Internet; learning resource lab; library services; nursing audiovisuals; remedial services; resume preparation assistance; skills, simulation, or other laboratory; tutoring; unpaid internships.
Library Facilities 15,858 volumes in health, 1,724 volumes in nursing; 331 periodical subscriptions health-care related.

BACCALAUREATE PROGRAMS

Degree BSN

Available Programs Accelerated Baccalaureate for Second Degree; Generic Baccalaureate; RN Baccalaureate.

Study Options Full-time.

Online Degree Options Yes.

Program Entrance Requirements Minimum overall college GPA of 3.0, transcript of college record, CPR certification, health insurance, high school biology, high school chemistry, high school foreign language, 3 years high school math, 1 year of high school science, high school transcript, immunizations, minimum high school GPA of 3.3, minimum GPA in nursing prerequisites of 3.0. Transfer students are accepted. *Application deadline:* 3/1 (fall), 3/1 (spring). Applications may be processed on a rolling basis for some programs. *Application fee:* $50.

Advanced Placement Credit given for nursing courses completed elsewhere dependent upon specific evaluations.

Expenses (2015–16) *Tuition, state resident:* full-time $11,070; part-time $369 per credit hour. *Tuition, nonresident:* full-time $22,410; part-time $747 per credit hour. *Room and board:* $9690; room only: $8300 per academic year. *Required fees:* full-time $1588.

Contact Linda Goodwin, Advisor, Baccalaureate Nursing and Health Sciences, Helen and Arthur E. Johnson Beth-El College of Nursing & Health Sciences, University of Colorado Colorado Springs, 1420 Austin Bluffs Parkway, Colorado Springs, CO 80918. *Telephone:* 719-255-3867. *Fax:* 719-255-3645. *E-mail:* lgoodwin@uccs.edu.

GRADUATE PROGRAMS

Expenses (2015–16) *Tuition, state resident:* full-time $11,734; part-time $652 per credit hour. *Tuition, nonresident:* full-time $20,068; part-time $1115 per credit hour. *Room and board:* $9500; room only: $8300 per academic year. *Required fees:* full-time $600; part-time $33 per credit.

Contact Diane Busch, Program Assistant, Nursing Department, Helen and Arthur E. Johnson Beth-El College of Nursing & Health Sciences, University of Colorado Colorado Springs, 1420 Austin Bluffs Parkway, Colorado Springs, CO 80918. *Telephone:* 719-255-4424. *Fax:* 719-255-4496. *E-mail:* dbusch@uccs.edu.

MASTER'S DEGREE PROGRAM

Degree MSN

Available Programs Master's.

Concentrations Available *Nurse practitioner programs in:* adult health, family health, primary care.

Study Options Full-time and part-time.

Online Degree Options Yes (online only).

Program Entrance Requirements Computer literacy, minimum overall college GPA of 3.3, transcript of college record, CPR certification, written essay, immunizations, 3 letters of recommendation, nursing research course, physical assessment course, prerequisite course work, resume, statistics course. *Application deadline:* 3/15 (fall), 8/15 (spring). *Application fee:* $60.

Advanced Placement Credit given for nursing courses completed elsewhere dependent upon specific evaluations.

Degree Requirements 46 total credit hours, thesis or project, comprehensive exam.

POST-MASTER'S PROGRAM

Areas of Study Nursing education. *Nurse practitioner programs in:* adult health, family health, primary care.

DOCTORAL DEGREE PROGRAM

Degree DNP

Available Programs Doctorate; Post-Baccalaureate Doctorate.

Areas of Study Individualized study.

Online Degree Options Yes (online only).

Program Entrance Requirements Clinical experience, minimum overall college GPA of 3.3, 3 letters of recommendation, MSN or equivalent, statistics course, vita, writing sample. Application deadline: 2/3 (summer). Application fee: $60.

Degree Requirements 35 total credit hours, residency.

CONTINUING EDUCATION PROGRAM

Contact Derek Wilson, Director, Extended Studies, Helen and Arthur E. Johnson Beth-El College of Nursing & Health Sciences, University of Colorado Colorado Springs, 1420 Austin Bluffs Parkway, Colorado Springs, CO 80918. *Telephone:* 719-255-4651. *Fax:* 719-255-4284. *E-mail:* dwilson6@uccs.edu.

University of Colorado Denver
College of Nursing
Aurora, Colorado

http://www.nursing.ucdenver.edu/
Founded in 1912
DEGREES • BS • DNP • MS • PHD
Nursing Program Faculty 87 (57% with doctorates).
Baccalaureate Enrollment 487 **Women** 86.25% **Men** 13.75% **Part-time** 13.9%
Graduate Enrollment 466 **Women** 92.92% **Men** 7.08% **Part-time** 30.9%
Distance Learning Courses Available.
Nursing Student Activities Nursing Honor Society, Sigma Theta Tau, Student Nurses' Association, nursing club.
Nursing Student Resources Academic advising; academic or career counseling; assistance for students with disabilities; bookstore; campus computer network; computer lab; computer-assisted instruction; e-mail services; housing assistance; interactive nursing skills videos; Internet; learning resource lab; library services; nursing audiovisuals; resume preparation assistance; skills, simulation, or other laboratory; tutoring.
Library Facilities 107,073 volumes in health, 4,552 volumes in nursing; 8,948 periodical subscriptions health-care related.

BACCALAUREATE PROGRAMS

Degree BS

Available Programs Accelerated Baccalaureate; Generic Baccalaureate; RN Baccalaureate.

Study Options Full-time and part-time.

Online Degree Options Yes.

Program Entrance Requirements Minimum overall college GPA of 3.0, transcript of college record, CPR certification, written essay, health exam, health insurance, immunizations, interview, minimum GPA in nursing prerequisites of 2.0, professional liability insurance/malpractice insurance, prerequisite course work. Transfer students are accepted. *Application deadline:* 6/15 (spring), 10/15 (summer). *Application fee:* $65.

Contact *Telephone:* 303-724-1812. *Fax:* 303-724-1710.

GRADUATE PROGRAMS

Contact *Telephone:* 303-724-1812. *Fax:* 303-724-1710.

MASTER'S DEGREE PROGRAM

Degree MS

Available Programs Master's.

Concentrations Available Nurse-midwifery; nursing administration; nursing informatics. *Clinical nurse specialist programs in:* adult health. *Nurse practitioner programs in:* adult health, family health, pediatric, psychiatric/mental health, women's health.

Study Options Full-time and part-time.

Online Degree Options Yes.

Program Entrance Requirements Computer literacy, minimum overall college GPA of 3.0, transcript of college record, written essay, immunizations, 4 letters of recommendation, nursing research course, prerequisite course work, resume, statistics course, GRE if cumulative undergraduate GPA is less than 3.0. *Application deadline:* 7/1 (fall), 2/1 (spring). *Application fee:* $50.

Degree Requirements 30 total credit hours, thesis or project, comprehensive exam.

POST-MASTER'S PROGRAM

Areas of Study Nurse-midwifery; nursing administration; nursing informatics. *Clinical nurse specialist programs in:* adult health. *Nurse practitioner programs in:* adult health, family health, pediatric, psychiatric/mental health, women's health.

DOCTORAL DEGREE PROGRAM

Degree DNP

Available Programs Doctorate.

Areas of Study Advanced practice nursing, clinical nurse specialist--general, nurse anesthesia, nurse-midwifery.

Online Degree Options Yes (online only).

Program Entrance Requirements Minimum overall college GPA of 3.0, essay, interview, letters of recommendation, MSN or equivalent, vita. Application deadline: 2/1 (fall), 7/1 (spring). Application fee: $65.

Degree Requirements 41 total credit hours, Capstone project.

Degree PhD
Available Programs Doctorate.
Areas of Study Bio-behavioral research, health-care systems.
Program Entrance Requirements Minimum overall college GPA of 3.0, interview by faculty committee, interview, 4 letters of recommendation, MSN or equivalent, statistics course, vita, writing sample, GRE. Application deadline: 3/1 (fall). Application fee: $50.
Degree Requirements 72 total credit hours, dissertation, oral exam, written exam.

POSTDOCTORAL PROGRAM

Postdoctoral Program Contact *Telephone:* 303-724-1812. *Fax:* 303-724-1710.

CONTINUING EDUCATION PROGRAM

Contact *Telephone:* 303-724-1372.

University of Northern Colorado
School of Nursing
Greeley, Colorado

http://www.unco.edu/nhs/nursing/
Founded in 1890
DEGREES • BS • MS • PHD
Nursing Program Faculty 55 (36% with doctorates).
Baccalaureate Enrollment 340
Graduate Enrollment 180
Distance Learning Courses Available.
Nursing Student Activities Sigma Theta Tau, Student Nurses' Association.
Nursing Student Resources Academic advising; academic or career counseling; assistance for students with disabilities; bookstore; campus computer network; career placement assistance; computer lab; computer-assisted instruction; e-mail services; employment services for current students; housing assistance; interactive nursing skills videos; Internet; learning resource lab; library services; nursing audiovisuals; paid internships; placement services for program completers; resume preparation assistance; skills, simulation, or other laboratory; tutoring.

BACCALAUREATE PROGRAMS

Degree BS
Available Programs Baccalaureate for Second Degree; Generic Baccalaureate; RN Baccalaureate.
Site Options Greeley, CO.
Study Options Full-time.
Program Entrance Requirements Minimum overall college GPA of 3.0, transcript of college record, CPR certification, health exam, immunizations, minimum GPA in nursing prerequisites of 3.0, professional liability insurance/malpractice insurance, prerequisite course work. Transfer students are accepted.
Contact Dr. Melissa Henry, Assistant Director of Undergraduate Programs, School of Nursing, University of Northern Colorado, Gunter Hall, Box 125, Greeley, CO 80639. *Telephone:* 970-351-2293. *Fax:* 970-351-1707. *E-mail:* melissa.henry@unco.edu.

GRADUATE PROGRAMS

Financial Aid 7 research assistantships (averaging $6,274 per year), 5 teaching assistantships (averaging $6,362 per year) were awarded; fellowships, unspecified assistantships also available.
Contact Dr. Karen Hessler, Assistant Director of Graduate Programs, School of Nursing, University of Northern Colorado, Gunter Hall, Box 125, Greeley, CO 80639. *Telephone:* 970-351-2293. *Fax:* 970-351-1707. *E-mail:* karen.hessler@unco.edu.

MASTER'S DEGREE PROGRAM

Degree MS
Available Programs Master's.
Concentrations Available *Nurse practitioner programs in:* adult-gerontology acute care, family health.
Site Options Greeley, CO.
Study Options Full-time and part-time.
Online Degree Options Yes (online only).
Program Entrance Requirements Clinical experience, minimum overall college GPA of 3.0, transcript of college record, CPR certification, immunizations, 2 letters of recommendation, GRE General Test.

Advanced Placement Credit given for nursing courses completed elsewhere dependent upon specific evaluations.
Degree Requirements Thesis or project, comprehensive exam.

POST-MASTER'S PROGRAM

Areas of Study Nursing education. *Nurse practitioner programs in:* adult-gerontology acute care, family health.

DOCTORAL DEGREE PROGRAM

Degree PhD
Available Programs Doctorate.
Areas of Study Advanced practice nursing, nursing education.
Site Options Greeley, CO.
Online Degree Options Yes (online only).
Program Entrance Requirements Minimum overall college GPA of 3.0, 2 letters of recommendation, MSN or equivalent, vita, writing sample, GRE General Test.
Degree Requirements Dissertation, written exam.

CONNECTICUT

Central Connecticut State University
Department of Nursing
New Britain, Connecticut

Founded in 1849
DEGREE • BSN
Nursing Program Faculty 4 (100% with doctorates).
Nursing Student Activities Sigma Theta Tau, nursing club.
Nursing Student Resources Academic advising; academic or career counseling; assistance for students with disabilities; bookstore; campus computer network; career placement assistance; computer lab; computer-assisted instruction; e-mail services; employment services for current students; externships; Internet; learning resource lab; library services; nursing audiovisuals; resume preparation assistance; skills, simulation, or other laboratory; tutoring.

BACCALAUREATE PROGRAMS

Degree BSN
Available Programs Generic Baccalaureate; RN Baccalaureate.
Site Options New Britain, CT.
Study Options Full-time and part-time.
Program Entrance Requirements Minimum overall college GPA of 2.7, CPR certification, health exam, high school transcript, immunizations, minimum GPA in nursing prerequisites of 2.7, prerequisite course work. Transfer students are accepted.
Advanced Placement Credit given for nursing courses completed elsewhere dependent upon specific evaluations.
Contact *Telephone:* 860-832-2147. *Fax:* 860-832-2188.

Fairfield University
School of Nursing
Fairfield, Connecticut

http://www.fairfield.edu/son
Founded in 1942
DEGREES • BSN • DNP • MSN
Nursing Program Faculty 98 (81% with doctorates).
Baccalaureate Enrollment 425 **Women** 93% **Men** 7% **Part-time** 8%
Graduate Enrollment 218 **Women** 88% **Men** 12% **Part-time** 80%
Distance Learning Courses Available.
Nursing Student Activities Sigma Theta Tau, Student Nurses' Association, nursing club.
Nursing Student Resources Academic advising; academic or career counseling; assistance for students with disabilities; bookstore; campus computer network; career placement assistance; computer lab; computer-assisted instruction; daycare for children of students; e-mail services; housing assistance; interactive nursing skills videos; Internet; learning resource lab; library services; nursing audiovisuals; placement services

for program completers; remedial services; resume preparation assistance; skills, simulation, or other laboratory; tutoring; unpaid internships.
Library Facilities 8,963 volumes in health, 4,433 volumes in nursing; 7,429 periodical subscriptions health-care related.

BACCALAUREATE PROGRAMS

Degree BSN

Available Programs Accelerated Baccalaureate for Second Degree; Generic Baccalaureate; RN Baccalaureate.

Study Options Full-time and part-time.

Program Entrance Requirements Written essay, health exam, high school chemistry, high school foreign language, 3 years high school math, 3 years high school science, high school transcript, immunizations, letters of recommendation, minimum high school GPA of 3.0. *Application deadline:* 1/15 (fall). *Application fee:* $60.

Advanced Placement Credit by examination available. Credit given for nursing courses completed elsewhere dependent upon specific evaluations.

Expenses (2015–16) *Tuition:* full-time $44,250; part-time $725 per credit hour. *Room and board:* $13,520 per academic year. *Required fees:* full-time $625.

Financial Aid 84% of baccalaureate students in nursing programs received some form of financial aid in 2014–15. *Gift aid (need-based):* Federal Pell, FSEOG, state, private, college/university gift aid from institutional funds, Federal Nursing. *Loans:* Federal Nursing Student Loans, Federal Direct (Subsidized and Unsubsidized Stafford PLUS), Perkins, alternative loans. *Work-study:* Federal Work-Study. *Financial aid application deadline:* 2/15.

Contact Audrey Beauvais, Associate Dean for Undergraduate Studies, School of Nursing, Fairfield University, 1073 North Benson Road, School of Nuring, Fairfield, CT 06824. *Telephone:* 203-254-4000 Ext. 2719. *E-mail:* abeauvais@fairfield.edu.

GRADUATE PROGRAMS

Expenses (2015–16) *Tuition:* part-time $850 per credit hour. *Room and board:* room only: $11,340 per academic year.

Financial Aid 37% of graduate students in nursing programs received some form of financial aid in 2014–15. Unspecified assistantships available.

Contact Joyce Shea, Associate Dean for School Of Nursing, School of Nursing, Fairfield University, 1073 North Benson Road, School of Nuring, Fairfield, CT 06824. *Telephone:* 203-254-4000 Ext. 2575. *Fax:* 203-254-4126. *E-mail:* jshea@fairfield.edu.

MASTER'S DEGREE PROGRAM

Degree MSN

Available Programs Master's.

Concentrations Available Clinical nurse leader. *Nurse practitioner programs in:* family health, psychiatric/mental health.

Site Options Norwalk, CT; Danbury, CT.

Study Options Full-time and part-time.

Program Entrance Requirements Computer literacy, minimum overall college GPA of 3.0, transcript of college record, CPR certification, written essay, immunizations, interview, 2 letters of recommendation, professional liability insurance/malpractice insurance, resume. *Application deadline:* Applications may be processed on a rolling basis for some programs. *Application fee:* $60.

Advanced Placement Credit given for nursing courses completed elsewhere dependent upon specific evaluations.

Degree Requirements 53 total credit hours.

DOCTORAL DEGREE PROGRAM

Degree DNP

Available Programs Doctorate; Post-Baccalaureate Doctorate.

Areas of Study Advanced practice nursing, family health.

Site Options Bridgeport, CT.

Program Entrance Requirements Minimum overall college GPA of 3.0, interview, 2 letters of recommendation, vita, writing sample, GRE (nurse anesthesia applicants only). Application deadline: Applications may be processed on a rolling basis for some programs. Application fee: $60.

Degree Requirements 75 total credit hours.

Quinnipiac University
School of Nursing
Hamden, Connecticut

http://www.quinnipiac.edu/nursing
Founded in 1929
DEGREES • BSN • DNP • MSN
Nursing Program Faculty 77 (90% with doctorates).
Baccalaureate Enrollment 600 **Women** 97% **Men** 3%
Graduate Enrollment 182 **Women** 98% **Men** 2% **Part-time** 60%
Distance Learning Courses Available.
Nursing Student Activities Sigma Theta Tau, Student Nurses' Association.
Nursing Student Resources Academic advising; academic or career counseling; bookstore; campus computer network; career placement assistance; computer lab; computer-assisted instruction; e-mail services; employment services for current students; externships; housing assistance; interactive nursing skills videos; Internet; learning resource lab; library services; nursing audiovisuals; paid internships; placement services for program completers; resume preparation assistance; skills, simulation, or other laboratory; tutoring; unpaid internships.
Library Facilities 1,700 volumes in nursing.

BACCALAUREATE PROGRAMS

Degree BSN

Available Programs Accelerated Baccalaureate for Second Degree; Generic Baccalaureate; RN Baccalaureate.

Site Options North Haven, CT.

Study Options Full-time.

Program Entrance Requirements Minimum overall college GPA of 3.0, transcript of college record, written essay, health exam, high school biology, high school chemistry, 4 years high school math, 4 years high school science, high school transcript, immunizations, 1 letter of recommendation, minimum high school GPA of 3.0, minimum high school rank 35%, minimum GPA in nursing prerequisites of 3.0. Transfer students are accepted. *Application deadline:* 11/15 (fall), 12/1 (spring). Applications may be processed on a rolling basis for some programs. *Application fee:* $65.

Advanced Placement Credit given for nursing courses completed elsewhere dependent upon specific evaluations.

Expenses (2015–16) *Tuition:* full-time $40,820; part-time $965 per credit. *International tuition:* $40,820 full-time. *Room and board:* $14,820 per academic year. *Required fees:* full-time $1550; part-time $38 per credit.

Financial Aid 86% of baccalaureate students in nursing programs received some form of financial aid in 2014–15. *Gift aid (need-based):* Federal Pell, FSEOG, state, private, college/university gift aid from institutional funds. *Loans:* Federal Direct (Subsidized and Unsubsidized Stafford PLUS), Perkins. *Work-study:* Federal Work-Study. *Financial aid application deadline (priority):* 3/1.

Contact Ms. Carla Knowlton, Director of Undergraduate Admissions, School of Nursing, Quinnipiac University, 275 Mount Carmel Avenue, Hamden, CT 06518. *Telephone:* 203-582-8600. *Fax:* 203-582-8906. *E-mail:* admissions@quinnipiac.edu.

GRADUATE PROGRAMS

Expenses (2015–16) *Tuition:* full-time $30,082; part-time $955 per credit. *International tuition:* $30,082 full-time. *Required fees:* full-time $720; part-time $38 per credit.

Financial Aid 65% of graduate students in nursing programs received some form of financial aid in 2014–15.

Contact Ms. Kristin Parent, Senior Associate Director of Graduate Admissions, School of Nursing, Quinnipiac University, 275 Mount Carmel Avenue, Hamden, CT 06518. *Telephone:* 203-582-8672. *Fax:* 203-582-3443. *E-mail:* graduate@quinnipiac.edu.

MASTER'S DEGREE PROGRAM

Degree MSN

Available Programs Master's.

Concentrations Available *Nurse practitioner programs in:* adult health, family health.

Site Options North Haven, CT.

Study Options Full-time and part-time.

Program Entrance Requirements Clinical experience, minimum overall college GPA of 3.0, transcript of college record, written essay, 2 letters of recommendation. *Application deadline:* 6/1 (fall). Applications

may be processed on a rolling basis for some programs. *Application fee:* $45.
Degree Requirements 43 total credit hours.

POST-MASTER'S PROGRAM
Areas of Study Nurse anesthesia. *Nurse practitioner programs in:* adult health, family health.

DOCTORAL DEGREE PROGRAM
Degree DNP
Available Programs Doctorate; Post-Baccalaureate Doctorate.
Areas of Study Advanced practice nursing.
Site Options North Haven, CT.
Program Entrance Requirements Minimum overall college GPA of 3.0, interview, 2 letters of recommendation, vita, writing sample. Application deadline: 6/1 (fall). Applications may be processed on a rolling basis for some programs. Application fee: $45.
Degree Requirements 75 total credit hours, residency.

See display below and full description on page 506.

Sacred Heart University
College of Nursing
Fairfield, Connecticut

http://www.sacredheart.edu/nursing.cfm
Founded in 1963

DEGREES • BSN • DNP • MSN
Nursing Program Faculty 101 (21% with doctorates).
Baccalaureate Enrollment 709 **Women** 94% **Men** 6% **Part-time** 36%
Graduate Enrollment 796 **Women** 92% **Men** 8% **Part-time** 90%
Distance Learning Courses Available.
Nursing Student Activities Nursing Honor Society, Sigma Theta Tau, Student Nurses' Association.
Nursing Student Resources Academic advising; academic or career counseling; assistance for students with disabilities; bookstore; campus computer network; career placement assistance; computer lab; computer-assisted instruction; e-mail services; employment services for current stu-

dents; housing assistance; interactive nursing skills videos; Internet; learning resource lab; library services; nursing audiovisuals; placement services for program completers; resume preparation assistance; skills, simulation, or other laboratory; tutoring.

BACCALAUREATE PROGRAMS
Degree BSN
Available Programs Generic Baccalaureate; RN Baccalaureate.
Site Options New Haven, CT; Norwalk, CT.
Study Options Full-time and part-time.
Online Degree Options Yes.
Program Entrance Requirements Minimum overall college GPA of 2.8, written essay, 3 years high school math, 3 years high school science, high school transcript, 1 letter of recommendation, minimum GPA in nursing prerequisites of 2.33. Transfer students are accepted. *Application deadline:* Applications may be processed on a rolling basis for some programs. *Application fee:* $50.
Advanced Placement Credit given for nursing courses completed elsewhere dependent upon specific evaluations.
Expenses (2015–16) *Tuition:* full-time $36,920; part-time $600 per credit. *Required fees:* full-time $250.
Financial Aid 64% of baccalaureate students in nursing programs received some form of financial aid in 2014–15.
Contact Mr. Kevin O'Sullivan, Executive Director of Admissions, College of Nursing, Sacred Heart University, 5151 Park Avenue, Fairfield, CT 06825-1000. *Telephone:* 203-365-7560. *E-mail:* osullivank6@sacredheart.edu.

GRADUATE PROGRAMS
Expenses (2015–16) *Tuition:* part-time $765 per credit.
Financial Aid 52% of graduate students in nursing programs received some form of financial aid in 2014–15.
Contact Mr. Bill Sweeney, Director of Graduate Admissions, College of Nursing, Sacred Heart University, 5151 Park Avenue, Fairfield, CT 06825-1000. *Telephone:* 203-365-4827. *E-mail:* sweeneyw@sacredheart.edu.

MASTER'S DEGREE PROGRAM
Degree MSN
Available Programs Master's; RN to Master's.

QUINNIPIAC UNIVERSITY
Hamden, Connecticut

Experience an education that sets your passion ablaze.

Our unique blend of classroom and practical experience helps give your fire a focus, preparing you for a promising future in the real world. Quinnipiac University's attentive faculty create a personalized and empowering experience, giving you access to opportunities made possible by our professional connections and our long record of success.

Fuel your ambition at www.quinnipiac.edu

Concentrations Available Clinical nurse leader; nursing administration; nursing education. *Nurse practitioner programs in:* family health.
Site Options Norwalk, CT.
Study Options Full-time and part-time.
Online Degree Options Yes.
Program Entrance Requirements Clinical experience, minimum overall college GPA of 3.0, transcript of college record, written essay, immunizations, 2 letters of recommendation, resume. *Application deadline:* 2/15 (fall). Applications may be processed on a rolling basis for some programs. *Application fee:* $75.
Advanced Placement Credit given for nursing courses completed elsewhere dependent upon specific evaluations.
Degree Requirements 42 total credit hours, thesis or project.

POST-MASTER'S PROGRAM

Areas of Study *Nurse practitioner programs in:* family health.

DOCTORAL DEGREE PROGRAM

Degree DNP
Available Programs Doctorate.
Areas of Study Clinical practice, nursing administration.
Program Entrance Requirements Minimum overall college GPA of 3.2, interview by faculty committee, interview, 2 letters of recommendation, MSN or equivalent, scholarly papers. Application deadline: 4/1 (fall). Application fee: $75.
Degree Requirements 39 total credit hours, dissertation.

CONTINUING EDUCATION PROGRAM

Contact Mr. Jon DeBenedictis, Recruiter/Admissions Coordinator, College of Nursing, Sacred Heart University, 5151 Park Avenue, Fairfield, CT 06825-1000. *Telephone:* 203-365-7678. *E-mail:* debenedictisj2700@sacredheart.edu.

St. Vincent's College

Nursing Program
Bridgeport, Connecticut

Founded in 1991
DEGREE • BSN

BACCALAUREATE PROGRAMS

Degree BSN
Available Programs Accelerated Baccalaureate.
Online Degree Options Yes (online only).
Contact *Telephone:* 203-576-5478.

Southern Connecticut State University

Department of Nursing
New Haven, Connecticut

http://www.southernct.edu/nursing/
Founded in 1893
DEGREES • BSN • EDD • MSN
Nursing Program Faculty 45 (65% with doctorates).
Baccalaureate Enrollment 220 **Women** 85% **Men** 15% **Part-time** 5%
Graduate Enrollment 40 **Women** 97% **Men** 3% **Part-time** 97%
Distance Learning Courses Available.
Nursing Student Activities Nursing Honor Society, Sigma Theta Tau, Student Nurses' Association.
Nursing Student Resources Academic advising; academic or career counseling; assistance for students with disabilities; bookstore; campus computer network; career placement assistance; computer lab; daycare for children of students; e-mail services; employment services for current students; housing assistance; Internet; learning resource lab; library services; nursing audiovisuals; resume preparation assistance; skills, simulation, or other laboratory; tutoring.
Library Facilities 35,540 volumes in health, 2,279 volumes in nursing; 318 periodical subscriptions health-care related.

BACCALAUREATE PROGRAMS

Degree BSN
Available Programs ADN to Baccalaureate; Accelerated Baccalaureate; Generic Baccalaureate; RN Baccalaureate.
Study Options Full-time and part-time.
Program Entrance Requirements Minimum overall college GPA of 3.0, transcript of college record, CPR certification, health exam, high school transcript, immunizations, minimum GPA in nursing prerequisites, prerequisite course work. Transfer students are accepted. *Application deadline:* 11/1 (fall), 2/1 (spring). Applications may be processed on a rolling basis for some programs.
Advanced Placement Credit given for nursing courses completed elsewhere dependent upon specific evaluations.
Expenses (2015–16) *Tuition, area resident:* full-time $4800; part-time $2400 per semester. *Tuition, state resident:* full-time $6000; part-time $3000 per semester. *Tuition, nonresident:* full-time $10,935; part-time $5000 per semester. *International tuition:* $10,935 full-time. *Room and board:* $4692 per academic year. *Required fees:* part-time $210 per credit; part-time $339 per term.
Financial Aid 90% of baccalaureate students in nursing programs received some form of financial aid in 2014–15. *Gift aid (need-based):* Federal Pell, FSEOG, state, private, college/university gift aid from institutional funds. *Loans:* Federal Direct (Subsidized and Unsubsidized Stafford PLUS), Perkins. *Work-study:* Federal Work-Study, part-time campus jobs. *Financial aid application deadline:* 3/9(priority: 3/5).
Contact Dr. Christine Denhup, Coordinator, BSN Program in Nursing, Department of Nursing, Southern Connecticut State University, 501 Crescent Street, New Haven, CT 06515-1355. *Telephone:* 203-392-6479. *Fax:* 203-392-6493. *E-mail:* Denhupc1@southernct.edu.

GRADUATE PROGRAMS

Expenses (2015–16) *Tuition, area resident:* full-time $10,704; part-time $5352 per semester. *Tuition, state resident:* full-time $22,916; part-time $8620 per semester. *Tuition, nonresident:* full-time $22,916; part-time $8620 per semester. *International tuition:* $22,916 full-time. *Required fees:* part-time $420 per credit; part-time $1811 per term.
Financial Aid 50% of graduate students in nursing programs received some form of financial aid in 2014–15. *Application deadline:* 4/15.
Contact Dr. Cynthia O'Sullivan, Coordinator, Graduate Programs in Nursing, Department of Nursing, Southern Connecticut State University, 501 Crescent Street, New Haven, CT 06515. *Telephone:* 203-392-6486. *Fax:* 203-392-6493. *E-mail:* osullivanc2@southernct.edu.

MASTER'S DEGREE PROGRAM

Degree MSN
Available Programs Master's; RN to Master's.
Concentrations Available Clinical nurse leader; nursing education. *Nurse practitioner programs in:* family health.
Study Options Full-time and part-time.
Program Entrance Requirements Clinical experience, minimum overall college GPA of 3.0, transcript of college record, CPR certification, written essay, immunizations, interview, 2 letters of recommendation, nursing research course, physical assessment course, professional liability insurance/malpractice insurance, prerequisite course work, resume, statistics course, GRE, MAT. *Application deadline:* 10/1 (fall), 3/1 (spring). Applications may be processed on a rolling basis for some programs.
Advanced Placement Credit given for nursing courses completed elsewhere dependent upon specific evaluations.
Degree Requirements 42 total credit hours, thesis or project.

POST-MASTER'S PROGRAM

Areas of Study Nursing education. *Nurse practitioner programs in:* family health.

DOCTORAL DEGREE PROGRAM

Degree EdD
Available Programs Doctorate.
Areas of Study Nursing education.
Online Degree Options Yes (online only).
Program Entrance Requirements Minimum overall college GPA of 3.0, interview, 2 letters of recommendation, MSN or equivalent, vita, writing sample. Application deadline: 3/1 (spring). Applications may be processed on a rolling basis for some programs.
Degree Requirements 51 total credit hours, dissertation, written exam, residency.

University of Connecticut
School of Nursing
Storrs, Connecticut

http://www.nursing.uconn.edu/
Founded in 1881
DEGREES • BS • DNP • MS • PHD
Nursing Program Faculty 110 (69% with doctorates).
Baccalaureate Enrollment 611 **Women** 86% **Men** 14%
Graduate Enrollment 189 **Women** 90% **Men** 10% **Part-time** 60%
Distance Learning Courses Available.
Nursing Student Activities Nursing Honor Society, Sigma Theta Tau, Student Nurses' Association, nursing club.
Nursing Student Resources Academic advising; academic or career counseling; assistance for students with disabilities; bookstore; campus computer network; career placement assistance; computer lab; e-mail services; housing assistance; interactive nursing skills videos; Internet; learning resource lab; library services; nursing audiovisuals; remedial services; resume preparation assistance; skills, simulation, or other laboratory; tutoring; unpaid internships.
Library Facilities 46,250 volumes in health, 1,170 volumes in nursing; 9,041 periodical subscriptions health-care related.

BACCALAUREATE PROGRAMS

Degree BS
Available Programs Accelerated Baccalaureate for Second Degree; Generic Baccalaureate.
Site Options Waterbury, CT; Groton, CT; Stamford, CT.
Study Options Full-time.
Program Entrance Requirements Minimum overall college GPA of 3.3, transcript of college record, written essay, health exam, health insurance, high school chemistry, high school foreign language, 3 years high school math, 2 years high school science, high school transcript, immunizations, 3 letters of recommendation, minimum high school GPA of 3.0, minimum GPA in nursing prerequisites of 3.0, prerequisite course work. Transfer students are accepted. *Application deadline:* 1/15 (fall). *Application fee:* $70.
Advanced Placement Credit by examination available.
Expenses (2015–16) *Tuition, state resident:* full-time $10,524; part-time $967 per credit. *Tuition, nonresident:* full-time $32,066; part-time $1337 per credit. *Room and board:* $12,436; room only: $6660 per academic year. *Required fees:* full-time $2842; part-time $826 per term.
Financial Aid *Gift aid (need-based):* Federal Pell, FSEOG, state, private, college/university gift aid from institutional funds. *Loans:* Federal Nursing Student Loans, Federal Direct (Subsidized and Unsubsidized Stafford PLUS), Perkins. *Work-study:* Federal Work-Study, part-time campus jobs. *Financial aid application deadline (priority):* 3/1.
Contact Ms. Dorine Nagy, Admissions Coordinator, School of Nursing, University of Connecticut, 231 Glenbrook Road, Unit 4026, Storrs, CT 06269-4026. *Telephone:* 860-486-1937. *Fax:* 860-486-0906.
E-mail: Dorine.Nagy@uconn.edu.

GRADUATE PROGRAMS

Expenses (2015–16) *Tuition, state resident:* full-time $13,026; part-time $724 per credit. *Tuition, nonresident:* full-time $33,812; part-time $1879 per credit. *Room and board:* $12,436; room only: $6660 per academic year. *Required fees:* full-time $2270; part-time $782 per term.
Financial Aid 24% of graduate students in nursing programs received some form of financial aid in 2014–15. 9 research assistantships with full tuition reimbursements available, 12 teaching assistantships with full tuition reimbursements available were awarded; fellowships, Federal Work-Study, scholarships, and unspecified assistantships also available. *Financial aid application deadline:* 2/1.
Contact Ms. Dorine Nagy, Graduate Program Contact, School of Nursing, University of Connecticut, 231 Glenbrook Road, Unit 4026, Storrs, CT 06269-4026. *Telephone:* 860-486-1937. *Fax:* 860-486-0906.
E-mail: Dorine.Nagy@uconn.edu.

MASTER'S DEGREE PROGRAM
Degree MS
Available Programs Master's; RN to Master's.
Concentrations Available Clinical nurse leader. *Nurse practitioner programs in:* adult-gerontology acute care, family health, neonatal health, primary care.
Study Options Full-time and part-time.
Online Degree Options Yes.

Program Entrance Requirements Clinical experience, computer literacy, minimum overall college GPA of 3.0, transcript of college record, interview, 3 letters of recommendation, nursing research course, physical assessment course, resume, statistics course. *Application deadline:* 2/1 (fall). *Application fee:* $75.
Advanced Placement Credit given for nursing courses completed elsewhere dependent upon specific evaluations.
Degree Requirements 37 total credit hours, comprehensive exam.

POST-MASTER'S PROGRAM
Areas of Study *Nurse practitioner programs in:* adult-gerontology acute care, neonatal health, primary care.

DOCTORAL DEGREE PROGRAM
Degree DNP
Available Programs Doctorate, Post-Baccalaureate Doctorate.
Areas of Study Advanced practice nursing, critical care, family health, gerontology, health promotion/disease prevention, human health and illness, maternity-newborn, nursing policy, palliative care.
Program Entrance Requirements Minimum overall college GPA of 3.0, clinical experience, interview, interview by faculty committee, 3 letters of recommendation, statistics course, vita, writing sample. Application deadline: 2/1 (fall). Applications may be processed on a rolling basis for some programs. Application fee: $75.
Degree Requirements 38 total credit hours, dissertation, oral exam, residency, written exam.

Degree PhD
Available Programs Doctorate; Post-Baccalaureate Doctorate.
Areas of Study Nursing research, nursing science.
Program Entrance Requirements Minimum overall college GPA of 3.25, interview by faculty committee, interview, 3 letters of recommendation, statistics course, vita, writing sample. Application deadline: 2/1 (fall). Application fee: $75.
Degree Requirements 52 total credit hours, dissertation, oral exam, written exam, residency.

POSTDOCTORAL PROGRAM
Areas of Study Neonatal health, neuro-behavior, nursing interventions, nursing research, nursing science, vulnerable population.
Postdoctoral Program Contact Dr. Jacqueline McGrath, Associate Dean for Research and Scholarship, School of Nursing, University of Connecticut, 231 Glenbrook Road, U-4026, Storrs, CT 06269-4026. *Telephone:* 860-486-0537. *Fax:* 860-486-9085.
E-mail: Jacqueline.Mcgrath@uconn.edu.

CONTINUING EDUCATION PROGRAM

Contact Ms. Joyce McSweeney, School of Nursing, University of Connecticut, 231 Glenbrook Road, U-4026, Storrs, CT 06269-4026. *Telephone:* 860-486-0508. *Fax:* 860-486-0001.
E-mail: Joyce.Mcsweeney@uconn.edu.

University of Hartford
College of Education, Nursing, and Health Professions
West Hartford, Connecticut

http://www.hartford.edu/enhp
Founded in 1877
DEGREES • BSN • MSN
Nursing Program Faculty 5 (80% with doctorates).
Baccalaureate Enrollment 73 **Women** 88% **Men** 12% **Part-time** 100%
Graduate Enrollment 159 **Women** 94% **Men** 6% **Part-time** 100%
Distance Learning Courses Available.
Nursing Student Activities Nursing Honor Society, Sigma Theta Tau.
Nursing Student Resources Academic advising; academic or career counseling; assistance for students with disabilities; bookstore; campus computer network; computer lab; e-mail services; interactive nursing skills videos; Internet; library services; nursing audiovisuals; resume preparation assistance; skills, simulation, or other laboratory; tutoring.

BACCALAUREATE PROGRAMS

Degree BSN
Available Programs ADN to Baccalaureate; RN Baccalaureate.
Study Options Part-time.

Program Entrance Requirements Transcript of college record, professional liability insurance/malpractice insurance, prerequisite course work, RN licensure. Transfer students are accepted. *Application deadline:* Applications may be processed on a rolling basis for some programs. *Application fee:* $35.

Advanced Placement Credit by examination available. Credit given for nursing courses completed elsewhere dependent upon specific evaluations.

Expenses (2014–15) *Tuition:* part-time $500 per credit.

Financial Aid 20% of baccalaureate students in nursing programs received some form of financial aid in 2013–14. *Gift aid (need-based):* Federal Pell, FSEOG, state, private, college/university gift aid from institutional funds. *Loans:* Federal Direct (Subsidized and Unsubsidized Stafford PLUS), Perkins. *Work-study:* Federal Work-Study, part-time campus jobs. *Financial aid application deadline (priority):* 2/1.

Contact Kim Groot, Nursing Faculty, College of Education, Nursing, and Health Professions, University of Hartford, 200 Bloomfield Avenue, West Hartford, CT 06117-1599. *Telephone:* 860-768-5408. *Fax:* 860-768-5043. *E-mail:* groot@hartford.edu.

GRADUATE PROGRAMS

Expenses (2014–15) *Tuition:* part-time $525 per credit.

Financial Aid 20% of graduate students in nursing programs received some form of financial aid in 2013–14. 4 research assistantships (averaging $4,500 per year) were awarded; teaching assistantships, institutionally sponsored loans and unspecified assistantships also available. *Financial aid application deadline:* 6/1.

Contact Susan Eichar, Associate Professor of Nursing, College of Education, Nursing, and Health Professions, University of Hartford, 200 Bloomfield Avenue, West Hartford, CT 06117-1599. *Telephone:* 860-768-4214. *Fax:* 860-768-5346. *E-mail:* seichar@hartford.edu.

MASTER'S DEGREE PROGRAM

Degree MSN

Available Programs Master's; Master's for Nurses with Non-Nursing Degrees.

Concentrations Available Nursing administration; nursing education.

Study Options Part-time.

Program Entrance Requirements Clinical experience, minimum overall college GPA of 3.0, transcript of college record, written essay, immunizations, 2 letters of recommendation, nursing research course, physical assessment course, professional liability insurance/malpractice insurance, resume. *Application deadline:* 4/15 (fall), 11/15 (spring). *Application fee:* $50.

Advanced Placement Credit given for nursing courses completed elsewhere dependent upon specific evaluations.

Degree Requirements 34 total credit hours, thesis or project.

POST-MASTER'S PROGRAM

Areas of Study Nursing education.

DOCTORAL DEGREE PROGRAM

Program Entrance Requirements MAT.

CONTINUING EDUCATION PROGRAM

Contact Dr. Susan Eichar, Associate Professor, Department of Health Sciences and Nursing, College of Education, Nursing, and Health Professions, University of Hartford, 200 Bloomfield Avenue, West Hartford, CT 06117-1599. *Telephone:* 860-768-4214. *Fax:* 860-768-5346. *E-mail:* seichar@hartford.edu.

University of Saint Joseph

Department of Nursing
West Hartford, Connecticut

http://www.usj.edu/
Founded in 1932

DEGREES • BS • DNP • MS

Nursing Program Faculty 18 (72% with doctorates).

Baccalaureate Enrollment 333 **Women** 98% **Part-time** 11%

Graduate Enrollment 137 **Women** 93% **Men** 7% **Part-time** 93%

Distance Learning Courses Available.

Nursing Student Activities Sigma Theta Tau, Student Nurses' Association, nursing club.

Nursing Student Resources Academic advising; academic or career counseling; assistance for students with disabilities; bookstore; campus computer network; career placement assistance; computer lab; computer-assisted instruction; daycare for children of students; e-mail services; employment services for current students; externships; housing assistance; interactive nursing skills videos; Internet; learning resource lab; library services; nursing audiovisuals; paid internships; placement services for program completers; remedial services; resume preparation assistance; skills, simulation, or other laboratory; tutoring; unpaid internships.

Library Facilities 7,058 volumes in health, 1,949 volumes in nursing; 1,495 periodical subscriptions health-care related.

BACCALAUREATE PROGRAMS

Degree BS

Available Programs Baccalaureate for Second Degree; Generic Baccalaureate; RN Baccalaureate.

Site Options Middletown, CT.

Study Options Full-time.

Program Entrance Requirements Minimum overall college GPA of 2.8, transcript of college record, CPR certification, written essay, health exam, health insurance, high school biology, high school chemistry, high school transcript, immunizations, minimum high school GPA of 3.0, minimum GPA in nursing prerequisites of 3.0, prerequisite course work. Transfer students are accepted. *Application deadline:* 4/1 (fall), 12/1 (spring). Applications may be processed on a rolling basis for some programs. *Application fee:* $50.

Advanced Placement Credit given for nursing courses completed elsewhere dependent upon specific evaluations.

Contact *Telephone:* 860-231-5304.

GRADUATE PROGRAMS

Program Entrance Requirements Clinical experience, transcript of college record, CPR certification, written essay, immunizations, interview, 2 letters of recommendation, professional liability insurance/malpractice insurance, resume. *Application deadline:* 3/1 (fall), 10/1 (spring). for some programs. *Application fee:* $50.

Contact *Telephone:* 860-231-5304. *Fax:* 860-231-8396.

MASTER'S DEGREE PROGRAM

Degree MS

Available Programs Master's; Master's for Nurses with Non-Nursing Degrees.

Concentrations Available Nursing education. *Nurse practitioner programs in:* family health, psychiatric/mental health.

Study Options Full-time and part-time.

Program Entrance Requirements Clinical experience, transcript of college record, CPR certification, written essay, immunizations, interview, 2 letters of recommendation, professional liability insurance/malpractice insurance, resume. *Application deadline:* 3/1 (fall), 10/1 (spring). *Application fee:* $50.

Advanced Placement Credit given for nursing courses completed elsewhere dependent upon specific evaluations.

Degree Requirements 44 total credit hours, comprehensive exam.

POST-MASTER'S PROGRAM

Areas of Study *Nurse practitioner programs in:* psychiatric/mental health.

DOCTORAL DEGREE PROGRAM

Degree DNP

Available Programs Doctorate.

Areas of Study Nursing administration.

Program Entrance Requirements Minimum overall college GPA of 3.2, interview, 3 letters of recommendation, vita, writing sample, MSN or equivalent.

Application deadline: Applications may be processed on a rolling basis for some programs. *Application fee:* $50.

Western Connecticut State University

Department of Nursing
Danbury, Connecticut

http://www.wcsu.edu/
Founded in 1903
DEGREES • BS • MS
Nursing Program Faculty 18 (50% with doctorates).
Baccalaureate Enrollment 160 **Women** 95% **Men** 5%
Graduate Enrollment 35 **Women** 100% **Part-time** 100%
Distance Learning Courses Available.
Nursing Student Activities Sigma Theta Tau, Student Nurses' Association.
Nursing Student Resources Academic advising; academic or career counseling; assistance for students with disabilities; bookstore; campus computer network; career placement assistance; computer lab; computer-assisted instruction; daycare for children of students; e-mail services; employment services for current students; externships; housing assistance; interactive nursing skills videos; Internet; learning resource lab; library services; nursing audiovisuals; paid internships; remedial services; resume preparation assistance; skills, simulation, or other laboratory; tutoring.

BACCALAUREATE PROGRAMS

Degree BS
Available Programs Generic Baccalaureate; RN Baccalaureate.
Site Options Waterbury, CT.
Study Options Full-time.
Program Entrance Requirements Minimum overall college GPA of 2.5, transcript of college record, CPR certification, health exam, health insurance, high school biology, high school chemistry, high school foreign language, 3 years high school math, 2 years high school science, high school transcript, immunizations, minimum GPA in nursing prerequisites of 2.5, prerequisite course work. Transfer students are accepted. *Application deadline:* Applications may be processed on a rolling basis for some programs. *Application fee:* $60.
Advanced Placement Credit by examination available. Credit given for nursing courses completed elsewhere dependent upon specific evaluations.
Contact *Telephone:* 203-837-8556. *Fax:* 203-837-8550.

GRADUATE PROGRAMS

Contact *Telephone:* 203-837-8556. *Fax:* 203-837-8550.

MASTER'S DEGREE PROGRAM
Degree MS
Available Programs Master's.
Concentrations Available *Clinical nurse specialist programs in:* adult health. *Nurse practitioner programs in:* adult health.
Study Options Part-time.
Program Entrance Requirements Clinical experience, computer literacy, minimum overall college GPA of 3.0, transcript of college record, CPR certification, immunizations, interview, 2 letters of recommendation, nursing research course, physical assessment course, professional liability insurance/malpractice insurance, prerequisite course work, resume, statistics course. *Application deadline:* Applications may be processed on a rolling basis for some programs. *Application fee:* $60.
Advanced Placement Credit by examination available. Credit given for nursing courses completed elsewhere dependent upon specific evaluations.
Degree Requirements 36 total credit hours, thesis or project.

POST-MASTER'S PROGRAM
Areas of Study *Clinical nurse specialist programs in:* adult health. *Nurse practitioner programs in:* adult health.

Yale University

School of Nursing
West Haven, Connecticut

http://www.nursing.yale.edu/
Founded in 1701
DEGREES • DNP • MSN • MSN/MDIV • MSN/MPH • PHD
Nursing Program Faculty 66 (50% with doctorates).
Graduate Enrollment 327 **Women** 87% **Men** 13% **Part-time** 19%
Distance Learning Courses Available.
Nursing Student Activities Nursing Honor Society, Sigma Theta Tau.
Nursing Student Resources Academic advising; academic or career counseling; assistance for students with disabilities; bookstore; campus computer network; career placement assistance; computer lab; computer-assisted instruction; daycare for children of students; e-mail services; employment services for current students; housing assistance; interactive nursing skills videos; Internet; learning resource lab; library services; nursing audiovisuals; placement services for program completers; remedial services; resume preparation assistance; skills, simulation, or other laboratory; tutoring; unpaid internships.
Library Facilities 416,262 volumes in health; 22,212 periodical subscriptions health-care related.

GRADUATE PROGRAMS

Expenses (2015–16) *Tuition:* full-time $18,414; part-time $12,241 per semester. *Required fees:* full-time $2951.
Financial Aid 239 fellowships (averaging $5,905 per year), 13 research assistantships (averaging $28,450 per year) were awarded; Federal Work-Study, scholarships, and traineeships also available.
Contact Ms. Melissa Pucci, Director of Admissions, School of Nursing, Yale University, PO Box 27399, West Haven, CT 06516. *Telephone:* 203-737-1793. *Fax:* 203-737-5409. *E-mail:* melissa.pucci@yale.edu.

MASTER'S DEGREE PROGRAM
Degrees MSN; MSN/MDIV; MSN/MPH
Available Programs Master's; Master's for Non-Nursing College Graduates; Master's for Nurses with Non-Nursing Degrees.
Concentrations Available Nurse-midwifery. *Nurse practitioner programs in:* acute care, adult health, adult-gerontology acute care, family health, pediatric primary care, psychiatric/mental health, women's health.
Study Options Full-time.
Program Entrance Requirements Minimum overall college GPA of 3.0, transcript of college record, CPR certification, written essay, immunizations, interview, 3 letters of recommendation, resume, GRE General Test. *Application deadline:* 11/1 (fall). *Application fee:* $100.
Advanced Placement Credit by examination available. Credit given for nursing courses completed elsewhere dependent upon specific evaluations.
Degree Requirements 48 total credit hours.

POST-MASTER'S PROGRAM
Areas of Study *Nurse practitioner programs in:* adult-gerontology acute care, family health, pediatric primary care, psychiatric/mental health.

DOCTORAL DEGREE PROGRAM
Degree DNP
Available Programs Doctorate.
Areas of Study Health policy, health-care systems, nursing administration, nursing policy.
Program Entrance Requirements Clinical experience, minimum overall college GPA of 3.0, interview by faculty committee, interview, 3 letters of recommendation, MSN or equivalent, vita, GRE General Test. Application deadline: 3/1 (fall). Application fee: $100.
Degree Requirements 40 total credit hours.

Degree PhD
Available Programs Doctorate.
Areas of Study Aging, critical care, family health, gerontology, health policy, health promotion/disease prevention, health-care systems, human health and illness, maternity-newborn, neuro-behavior, nursing policy, nursing research, oncology.
Program Entrance Requirements Minimum overall college GPA of 3.0, clinical experience, interview, interview by faculty committee, 3 letters of recommendation, MSN or equivalent, statistics course, vita, writing sample. Application deadline: 1/2 (fall). Application fee: $100.
Degree Requirements 60 total credit hours, dissertation, oral exam, written exam.

POSTDOCTORAL PROGRAM

Areas of Study Adolescent health, cancer care, chronic illness, health promotion/disease prevention, nursing interventions, nursing research, nursing science, self-care, vulnerable population, women's health.

Postdoctoral Program Contact Ms. Sarah Zaino, Assistant Director, Research Activities, School of Nursing, Yale University, PO Box 27399, West Haven, CT 06516. *Telephone:* 203-737-2420. *Fax:* 203-737-4480. *E-mail:* sarah.zaino@yale.edu.

DELAWARE

Delaware State University
Department of Nursing
Dover, Delaware

http://www.desu.edu/department-nursing
Founded in 1891

DEGREES • BSN • MS
Nursing Program Faculty 11
Baccalaureate Enrollment 72 **Women** 93% **Men** 7%
Nursing Student Activities Sigma Theta Tau, Student Nurses' Association.
Nursing Student Resources Academic advising; assistance for students with disabilities; bookstore; campus computer network; computer lab; daycare for children of students; e-mail services; interactive nursing skills videos; library services; nursing audiovisuals; skills, simulation, or other laboratory.

BACCALAUREATE PROGRAMS

Degree BSN
Available Programs Generic Baccalaureate; LPN to Baccalaureate; RN Baccalaureate.
Study Options Full-time and part-time.
Program Entrance Requirements CPR certification, health exam, high school biology, high school chemistry, high school transcript, immunizations, minimum high school GPA of 2.0, professional liability insurance/malpractice insurance, prerequisite course work. Transfer students are accepted. *Application deadline:* 2/25 (winter).
Contact *Telephone:* 302-857-6700.

GRADUATE PROGRAMS

Contact *Telephone:* 302-857-6700.

MASTER'S DEGREE PROGRAM

Degree MS
Available Programs Master's.
Concentrations Available Nursing education. *Clinical nurse specialist programs in:* public health.
Study Options Full-time.
Program Entrance Requirements Clinical experience, minimum overall college GPA of 3.0, transcript of college record, CPR certification, written essay, immunizations, 3 letters of recommendation, professional liability insurance/malpractice insurance, resume. *Application deadline:* 2/1 (winter). *Application fee:* $35.
Advanced Placement Credit given for nursing courses completed elsewhere dependent upon specific evaluations.
Degree Requirements 39 total credit hours, thesis or project.

University of Delaware
School of Nursing
Newark, Delaware

http://www.udel.edu/nursing/
Founded in 1743

DEGREES • BSN • MSN • PHD
Nursing Program Faculty 38 (65% with doctorates).
Baccalaureate Enrollment 753 **Women** 92% **Men** 8% **Part-time** 10%
Graduate Enrollment 138 **Women** 94% **Men** 6% **Part-time** 88%
Distance Learning Courses Available.

Nursing Student Activities Sigma Theta Tau, Student Nurses' Association.
Nursing Student Resources Academic advising; academic or career counseling; assistance for students with disabilities; bookstore; campus computer network; career placement assistance; computer lab; computer-assisted instruction; e-mail services; employment services for current students; externships; housing assistance; interactive nursing skills videos; Internet; learning resource lab; library services; nursing audiovisuals; paid internships; remedial services; resume preparation assistance; skills, simulation, or other laboratory; tutoring; unpaid internships.
Library Facilities 2.7 million volumes in health, 40,000 volumes in nursing; 407 periodical subscriptions health-care related.

BACCALAUREATE PROGRAMS

Degree BSN
Available Programs Accelerated Baccalaureate for Second Degree; Generic Baccalaureate; RN Baccalaureate.
Study Options Full-time.
Online Degree Options Yes.
Program Entrance Requirements Written essay, high school biology, high school chemistry, high school foreign language, 3 years high school math, 4 years high school science, high school transcript, 1 letter of recommendation, minimum high school GPA of 3.0. Transfer students are accepted. *Application deadline:* 1/15 (fall). *Application fee:* $75.
Advanced Placement Credit given for nursing courses completed elsewhere dependent upon specific evaluations.
Expenses (2014–15) *Tuition, state resident:* full-time $23,900; part-time $454 per credit hour. *Tuition, nonresident:* full-time $42,250; part-time $1219 per credit hour. *Room and board:* $11,558; room only: $7514 per academic year. *Required fees:* full-time $1000; part-time $160 per term.
Financial Aid 75% of baccalaureate students in nursing programs received some form of financial aid in 2013–14. *Gift aid (need-based):* Federal Pell, FSEOG, state, private, college/university gift aid from institutional funds. *Loans:* Federal Nursing Student Loans, Federal Direct (Subsidized and Unsubsidized Stafford PLUS), Perkins. *Work-study:* Federal Work-Study, part-time campus jobs. *Financial aid application deadline:* 3/15(priority: 2/1).
Contact Ms. Anne DeCaire, Nursing Recruiter, School of Nursing, University of Delaware, 385 McDowell Hall, Newark, DE 19716. *Telephone:* 302-831-0442. *Fax:* 302-831-2382. *E-mail:* aderb@udel.edu.

GRADUATE PROGRAMS

Expenses (2014–15) *Tuition, state resident:* part-time $731 per credit hour. *Tuition, nonresident:* part-time $731 per credit hour. *Required fees:* part-time $30 per term.
Financial Aid 100% of graduate students in nursing programs received some form of financial aid in 2013–14. Research assistantships with tuition reimbursements available (averaging $15,000 per year); scholarships, traineeships, tuition waivers (full), and unspecified assistantships also available. Aid available to part-time students. *Financial aid application deadline:* 7/1.
Contact Ms. Joanne Marra, Office Coordinator, School of Nursing, University of Delaware, 349 McDowell Hall, Newark, DE 19716. *Telephone:* 302-831-8386. *Fax:* 302-831-2382. *E-mail:* ud-gradnursing@udel.edu.

MASTER'S DEGREE PROGRAM

Degree MSN
Available Programs Master's; RN to Master's.
Concentrations Available Health-care administration. *Clinical nurse specialist programs in:* adult-gerontology acute care, pediatric. *Nurse practitioner programs in:* adult health, family health.
Study Options Full-time and part-time.
Online Degree Options Yes.
Program Entrance Requirements Clinical experience, minimum overall college GPA of 3.0, transcript of college record, CPR certification, written essay, immunizations, interview, 3 letters of recommendation, resume. *Application deadline:* 3/1 (fall), 10/1 (spring). *Application fee:* $75.
Advanced Placement Credit given for nursing courses completed elsewhere dependent upon specific evaluations.
Degree Requirements 46 total credit hours.

POST-MASTER'S PROGRAM

Areas of Study Health-care administration. *Clinical nurse specialist programs in:* adult-gerontology acute care, pediatric. *Nurse practitioner programs in:* adult health, family health.

DOCTORAL DEGREE PROGRAM

Degree PhD
Available Programs Doctorate.
Areas of Study Advanced practice nursing, aging, bio-behavioral research, community health, faculty preparation, family health, gerontology, health policy, health promotion/disease prevention, human health and illness, illness and transition, individualized study, neuro-behavior, nursing education, nursing research, nursing science, oncology, women's health.
Program Entrance Requirements Clinical experience, minimum overall college GPA of 3.5, interview by faculty committee, 3 letters of recommendation, MSN or equivalent, statistics course, vita, writing sample. Application deadline: 2/1 (fall). Application fee: $75.
Degree Requirements 50 total credit hours, dissertation, oral exam, written exam, residency.

CONTINUING EDUCATION PROGRAM

Contact Dr. Soma Chakrabanti, Division of Professional and Continuing Studies, School of Nursing, University of Delaware, Clayton Hall, Newark, DE 19716. *Telephone:* 302-831-6442. *Fax:* 302-831-1077. *E-mail:* continuing-ed@udel.edu.

Wesley College
Nursing Program
Dover, Delaware

http://www.wesley.edu/
Founded in 1873

DEGREES • BSN • MSN
Nursing Program Faculty 32 (22% with doctorates).
Baccalaureate Enrollment 131 **Women** 92% **Men** 8%
Graduate Enrollment 26 **Women** 96% **Men** 4% **Part-time** 10%
Distance Learning Courses Available.
Nursing Student Activities Sigma Theta Tau, Student Nurses' Association.
Nursing Student Resources Academic advising; academic or career counseling; assistance for students with disabilities; bookstore; campus computer network; career placement assistance; computer lab; computer-assisted instruction; e-mail services; employment services for current students; externships; housing assistance; interactive nursing skills videos; Internet; learning resource lab; library services; nursing audiovisuals; placement services for program completers; remedial services; resume preparation assistance; skills, simulation, or other laboratory; tutoring; unpaid internships.
Library Facilities 15,000 volumes in health, 1,500 volumes in nursing; 40 periodical subscriptions health-care related.

BACCALAUREATE PROGRAMS

Degree BSN
Available Programs Generic Baccalaureate; International Nurse to Baccalaureate; LPN to Baccalaureate.
Study Options Full-time and part-time.
Program Entrance Requirements Minimum overall college GPA of 2.5, transcript of college record, CPR certification, health exam, health insurance, high school biology, high school chemistry, 2 years high school math, 3 years high school science, high school transcript, immunizations, minimum high school GPA of 2.5, minimum GPA in nursing prerequisites of 2.5, professional liability insurance/malpractice insurance. Transfer students are accepted. *Application deadline:* Applications may be processed on a rolling basis for some programs. *Application fee:* $25.
Advanced Placement Credit by examination available. Credit given for nursing courses completed elsewhere dependent upon specific evaluations.
Expenses (2015–16) *Tuition:* full-time $25,020; part-time $950 per credit hour. *Room and board:* $11,000 per academic year. *Required fees:* full-time $1200.
Financial Aid 100% of baccalaureate students in nursing programs received some form of financial aid in 2014–15.
Contact Dr. Karen Panunto, Program Director, Nursing Program, Wesley College, 120 North State Street, Dover, DE 19901. *Telephone:* 302-736-2511. *E-mail:* karen.panunto@wesley.edu.

GRADUATE PROGRAMS

Expenses (2015–16) *Tuition:* part-time $595 per credit hour.
Financial Aid 50% of graduate students in nursing programs received some form of financial aid in 2014–15. Traineeships available.

Contact Dr. Nancy Rubino, MSN Program Director, Nursing Program, Wesley College, 120 North State Street, Dover, DE 19901. *Telephone:* 302-736-2550. *E-mail:* nancy.rubino@wesley.edu.

MASTER'S DEGREE PROGRAM

Degree MSN
Available Programs Accelerated AD/RN to Master's; Master's; RN to Master's.
Concentrations Available *Clinical nurse specialist programs in:* gerontology.
Study Options Full-time and part-time.
Program Entrance Requirements Clinical experience, computer literacy, minimum overall college GPA of 3.0, transcript of college record, interview, 2 letters of recommendation, professional liability insurance/malpractice insurance, resume, statistics course, GRE or MAT. *Application deadline:* Applications may be processed on a rolling basis for some programs. *Application fee:* $25.
Advanced Placement Credit by examination available. Credit given for nursing courses completed elsewhere dependent upon specific evaluations.
Degree Requirements 39 total credit hours, thesis or project.

POST-MASTER'S PROGRAM
Areas of Study Nursing education.

CONTINUING EDUCATION PROGRAM

Contact Dr. Robert Contino, Professor of Nursing and Chair, Nursing Program, Wesley College, 120 North State Street, Dover, DE 19901. *Telephone:* 302-736-2482. *E-mail:* robert.contino@wesley.edu.

Wilmington University
College of Health Professions
New Castle, Delaware

http://www.wilmu.edu/health/index.aspx
Founded in 1967

DEGREES • BSN • MSN • MSN/MBA • MSN/MS
Nursing Program Faculty 13 (50% with doctorates).
Baccalaureate Enrollment 620 **Women** 95% **Men** 5% **Part-time** 88%
Graduate Enrollment 253 **Women** 97% **Men** 3% **Part-time** 50%
Distance Learning Courses Available.
Nursing Student Activities Sigma Theta Tau.
Nursing Student Resources Academic advising; academic or career counseling; assistance for students with disabilities; bookstore; campus computer network; career placement assistance; computer lab; computer-assisted instruction; e-mail services; employment services for current students; housing assistance; interactive nursing skills videos; learning resource lab; library services; nursing audiovisuals; remedial services; resume preparation assistance; skills, simulation, or other laboratory; tutoring.
Library Facilities 6,000 volumes in health, 3,500 volumes in nursing; 60 periodical subscriptions health-care related.

BACCALAUREATE PROGRAMS

Degree BSN
Available Programs Accelerated RN Baccalaureate; International Nurse to Baccalaureate; RN Baccalaureate.
Site Options Georgetown, DE; New Castle, DE; Dover, DE.
Online Degree Options Yes.
Program Entrance Requirements Transfer students are accepted. *Application deadline:* 8/31 (fall), 1/1 (spring), 5/1 (summer). Applications may be processed on a rolling basis for some programs. *Application fee:* $35.
Contact *Telephone:* 302-356-6915. *Fax:* 302-322-7081.

GRADUATE PROGRAMS

Contact *Telephone:* 302-295-1121.

MASTER'S DEGREE PROGRAM
Degrees MSN; MSN/MBA; MSN/MS
Available Programs Accelerated AD/RN to Master's; Accelerated Master's for Nurses with Non-Nursing Degrees; Master's.
Concentrations Available Legal nurse consultant; nursing administration; nursing education. *Nurse practitioner programs in:* adult health, family health, gerontology.
Site Options Georgetown, DE; New Castle, DE.

Study Options Full-time and part-time.
Online Degree Options Yes.
Program Entrance Requirements Minimum overall college GPA of 3.0, transcript of college record, prerequisite course work. *Application deadline:* Applications may be processed on a rolling basis for some programs. *Application fee:* $35.
Advanced Placement Credit given for nursing courses completed elsewhere dependent upon specific evaluations.
Degree Requirements 36 total credit hours, thesis or project.

POST-MASTER'S PROGRAM

Areas of Study Legal nurse consultant; nursing administration; nursing education. *Nurse practitioner programs in:* adult health, family health, gerontology.

DISTRICT OF COLUMBIA

The Catholic University of America
School of Nursing
Washington, District of Columbia

http://www.cua.edu/
Founded in 1887
DEGREES • BSN • DNP • MSN • PHD
Nursing Program Faculty 67 (27% with doctorates).
Baccalaureate Enrollment 149 **Women** 95% **Men** 5% **Part-time** 7%
Graduate Enrollment 247 **Women** 93% **Men** 7% **Part-time** 86%
Distance Learning Courses Available.
Nursing Student Activities Nursing Honor Society, Sigma Theta Tau, Student Nurses' Association, nursing club.
Nursing Student Resources Academic advising; academic or career counseling; assistance for students with disabilities; bookstore; campus computer network; career placement assistance; computer lab; computer-assisted instruction; e-mail services; employment services for current students; externships; housing assistance; interactive nursing skills videos; Internet; learning resource lab; library services; nursing audiovisuals; remedial services; resume preparation assistance; skills, simulation, or other laboratory; tutoring.
Library Facilities 20,500 volumes in health.

BACCALAUREATE PROGRAMS

Degree BSN
Available Programs Accelerated Baccalaureate for Second Degree; Generic Baccalaureate.
Study Options Full-time and part-time.
Program Entrance Requirements Transcript of college record, written essay, health exam, health insurance, high school biology, high school chemistry, 3 years high school math, 3 years high school science, high school transcript, immunizations, 1 letter of recommendation, minimum GPA in nursing prerequisites of 2.75, prerequisite course work. *Application deadline:* 11/1 (fall). Applications may be processed on a rolling basis for some programs. *Application fee:* $55.
Expenses (2015–16) *Tuition:* full-time $40,400; part-time $1600 per credit hour. *Room and board:* $10,000; room only: $7500 per academic year. *Required fees:* full-time $360; part-time $180 per term.
Financial Aid 94% of baccalaureate students in nursing programs received some form of financial aid in 2014–15. *Gift aid (need-based):* Federal Pell, FSEOG, state, private, college/university gift aid from institutional funds. *Loans:* Federal Nursing Student Loans, Federal Direct (Subsidized and Unsubsidized Stafford PLUS), Perkins, private loans. *Work-study:* Federal Work-Study. *Financial aid application deadline:* 4/10(priority: 2/15).
Contact Ms. Megan Podboy, School of Nursing Counselor and Liaison, School of Nursing, The Catholic University of America, 255 Nursing—Biology/Gowan Hall, 620 Michigan Avenue NE, Washington, DC 20064. *Telephone:* 202-319-6462. *Fax:* 202-319-6485.
E-mail: podboy@cua.edu.

GRADUATE PROGRAMS

Expenses (2015–16) *Tuition:* full-time $41,400; part-time $1650 per credit hour. *Required fees:* full-time $100; part-time $50 per term.

Financial Aid 64% of graduate students in nursing programs received some form of financial aid in 2014–15. Fellowships, research assistantships, teaching assistantships, Federal Work-Study, scholarships, tuition waivers (full and partial), and unspecified assistantships available. *Financial aid application deadline:* 2/1.
Contact Jacqueline Tintle, Administrative Assistant, School of Nursing, The Catholic University of America, 118 Gowan Hall, Washington, DC 20064. *Telephone:* 202-319-5403. *Fax:* 202-319-6946.
E-mail: tintlej@cua.edu.

MASTER'S DEGREE PROGRAM

Degree MSN
Available Programs Master's.
Concentrations Available *Nurse practitioner programs in:* acute care, adult health, adult-gerontology acute care, family health, gerontology, pediatric, pediatric primary care, primary care.
Site Options Washington, DC.
Study Options Full-time and part-time.
Online Degree Options Yes (online only).
Program Entrance Requirements Clinical experience, minimum overall college GPA of 3.0, transcript of college record, written essay, immunizations, interview, 3 letters of recommendation, statistics course, GRE General Test. *Application deadline:* 8/1 (fall), 12/1 (spring). Applications may be processed on a rolling basis for some programs. *Application fee:* $55.
Advanced Placement Credit given for nursing courses completed elsewhere dependent upon specific evaluations.
Degree Requirements 48 total credit hours, comprehensive exam.

POST-MASTER'S PROGRAM

Areas of Study *Nurse practitioner programs in:* acute care, adult health, adult-gerontology acute care, family health, gerontology, pediatric, pediatric primary care, primary care.

DOCTORAL DEGREE PROGRAM

Degree DNP
Available Programs Doctorate, Post-Baccalaureate Doctorate.
Areas of Study Advanced practice nursing, aging, clinical practice, clinical research, community health, critical care, ethics, family health, gerontology, health promotion/disease prevention, health-care systems, illness and transition, maternity-newborn, nursing research, oncology, palliative care, women's health.
Online Degree Options Yes (online only).
Program Entrance Requirements Minimum overall college GPA of 3.2, interview, 3 letters of recommendation, MSN or equivalent, vita, writing sample. Application deadline: 8/1 (fall). Applications may be processed on a rolling basis for some programs. Application fee: $55.
Degree Requirements Capstone project, oral exam, residency, written exam.

Degree PhD
Available Programs Doctorate; Post-Baccalaureate Doctorate.
Areas of Study Advanced practice nursing, aging, clinical practice, clinical research, community health, critical care, ethics, family health, gerontology, health promotion/disease prevention, health-care systems, human health and illness, illness and transition, maternity-newborn, nursing science, oncology, palliative care, women's health.
Online Degree Options Yes.
Program Entrance Requirements Clinical experience, minimum overall college GPA of 3.2, interview, 3 letters of recommendation, MSN or equivalent, vita, writing sample, GRE General Test. Application deadline: 8/1 (fall). Applications may be processed on a rolling basis for some programs. Application fee: $55.
Degree Requirements 80 total credit hours, dissertation, oral exam, written exam.

Georgetown University
School of Nursing and Health Studies
Washington, District of Columbia

http://nhs.georgetown.edu/
Founded in 1789
DEGREES • BSN • DNP • MS
Nursing Program Faculty 222 (54% with doctorates).
Baccalaureate Enrollment 184 **Women** 94.1% **Men** 5.9%
Graduate Enrollment 935 **Women** 93.7% **Men** 6.3% **Part-time** 80%

Distance Learning Courses Available.

Nursing Student Activities Nursing Honor Society, Sigma Theta Tau, Student Nurses' Association.

Nursing Student Resources Academic advising; academic or career counseling; assistance for students with disabilities; bookstore; campus computer network; career placement assistance; computer lab; computer-assisted instruction; e-mail services; employment services for current students; externships; housing assistance; interactive nursing skills videos; Internet; learning resource lab; library services; nursing audiovisuals; placement services for program completers; resume preparation assistance; skills, simulation, or other laboratory; tutoring; unpaid internships.

BACCALAUREATE PROGRAMS

Degree BSN

Available Programs Generic Baccalaureate.

Study Options Full-time.

Program Entrance Requirements CPR certification, written essay, health exam, health insurance, 3 years high school math, 4 years high school science, high school transcript, immunizations, interview, 2 letters of recommendation. Transfer students are accepted. *Application deadline:* 1/10 (fall). *Application fee:* $65.

Financial Aid *Gift aid (need-based):* Federal Pell, FSEOG, state, private, college/university gift aid from institutional funds. *Loans:* Federal Nursing Student Loans, Federal Direct (Subsidized and Unsubsidized Stafford PLUS), Perkins, alternative loans. *Work-study:* Federal Work-Study. *Financial aid application deadline:* 2/1.

Contact Office of Undergraduate Admissions, School of Nursing and Health Studies, Georgetown University, 37th and O Street NW, Washington, DC 20057. *Telephone:* 202-687-3600.

GRADUATE PROGRAMS

Financial Aid Scholarships and traineeships available.

Contact Office of Graduate Admissions, School of Nursing and Health Studies, Georgetown University, 37th and O Street NW, Washington, DC 20057. *Telephone:* 202-687-5568.

MASTER'S DEGREE PROGRAM

Degree MS

Available Programs Accelerated Master's for Non-Nursing College Graduates; Master's; Master's for Non-Nursing College Graduates.

Concentrations Available Clinical nurse leader; health-care administration; nurse anesthesia; nurse-midwifery. *Nurse practitioner programs in:* acute care, family health, women's health.

Study Options Full-time and part-time.

Online Degree Options Yes (online only).

Program Entrance Requirements Clinical experience, minimum overall college GPA of 3.0, transcript of college record, CPR certification, written essay, immunizations, interview, 3 letters of recommendation, resume, statistics course, GRE General Test or MAT.

Advanced Placement Credit given for nursing courses completed elsewhere dependent upon specific evaluations.

DOCTORAL DEGREE PROGRAM

Degree DNP

Available Programs Doctorate.

Program Entrance Requirements Clinical experience, minimum overall college GPA of 3.3, interview by faculty committee, 3 letters of recommendation, MSN or equivalent, vita. Application deadline: 4/15 (fall). Applications may be processed on a rolling basis for some programs.

Degree Requirements 38 total credit hours.

The George Washington University

School of Nursing
Washington, District of Columbia

http://www.gwu.edu/
Founded in 1821

DEGREES • BSN • DNP • MSN

Nursing Program Faculty 58
Baccalaureate Enrollment 198 Women 93% Men 7%
Graduate Enrollment 556 Women 95% Men 5% Part-time 50%
Distance Learning Courses Available.

Nursing Student Activities Sigma Theta Tau, Student Nurses' Association.

Nursing Student Resources Academic advising; academic or career counseling; assistance for students with disabilities; bookstore; campus computer network; career placement assistance; computer lab; computer-assisted instruction; e-mail services; interactive nursing skills videos; Internet; learning resource lab; library services; nursing audiovisuals; remedial services; resume preparation assistance; skills, simulation, or other laboratory; tutoring.

Library Facilities 100,000 volumes in health, 5,000 volumes in nursing; 3,031 periodical subscriptions health-care related.

BACCALAUREATE PROGRAMS

Degree BSN

Available Programs ADN to Baccalaureate; Accelerated Baccalaureate for Second Degree; International Nurse to Baccalaureate.

Site Options Ashburn , VA.

Online Degree Options Yes.

Contact Deirdre Hughes, Associate Director of Admissions, School of Nursing, The George Washington University, 45085 University Drive, Suite 201, Ashburn, VA 20147. *Telephone:* 571-553-0138.

E-mail: sonadmit@gwu.edu.

GRADUATE PROGRAMS

Contact Deirdre Hughes, Associate Director of Admissions, School of Nursing, The George Washington University, 45085 University Drive, Suite 201, Ashburn, VA 20147. *Telephone:* 571-553-0138.

E-mail: sonadmit@gwu.edu.

MASTER'S DEGREE PROGRAM

Degree MSN

Available Programs Accelerated AD/RN to Master's; Master's.

Concentrations Available Health-care administration; nurse-midwifery; nursing administration. *Nurse practitioner programs in:* adult health, family health, gerontology, primary care.

Study Options Full-time and part-time.

Online Degree Options Yes (online only).

Program Entrance Requirements Minimum overall college GPA of 3.33, transcript of college record, CPR certification, written essay, immunizations, 2 letters of recommendation, resume.

POST-MASTER'S PROGRAM

Areas of Study Health-care administration; nursing administration; nursing education. *Nurse practitioner programs in:* adult health, family health, gerontology, primary care.

DOCTORAL DEGREE PROGRAM

Degree DNP

Available Programs Doctorate; Post-Baccalaureate Doctorate.

Areas of Study Advanced practice nursing, family health, gerontology, nursing administration, palliative care.

Program Entrance Requirements Minimum overall college GPA of 3.33, 2 letters of recommendation, MSN or equivalent, vita, writing sample.

Howard University

Division of Nursing
Washington, District of Columbia

http://huhealthcare.com/education/schools-and-academics/nursing-allied-health/division-of-nursing
Founded in 1867

DEGREES • BSN • MSN

Nursing Program Faculty 25 (56% with doctorates).
Baccalaureate Enrollment 178 Women 89% Men 11% Part-time 11%
Graduate Enrollment 31 Women 90% Men 10% Part-time 77%
Distance Learning Courses Available.

Nursing Student Activities Nursing Honor Society, Sigma Theta Tau, Student Nurses' Association, nursing club.

Nursing Student Resources Academic advising; academic or career counseling; assistance for students with disabilities; bookstore; campus computer network; career placement assistance; computer lab; computer-assisted instruction; e-mail services; externships; housing assistance; interactive nursing skills videos; Internet; learning resource lab; library services; nursing audiovisuals; paid internships; placement services for

program completers; remedial services; resume preparation assistance; skills, simulation, or other laboratory; tutoring.
Library Facilities 219,448 volumes in health, 4,500 volumes in nursing; 5,247 periodical subscriptions health-care related.

BACCALAUREATE PROGRAMS

Degree BSN
Available Programs Generic Baccalaureate; LPN to Baccalaureate; RN Baccalaureate.
Study Options Full-time.
Online Degree Options Yes.
Program Entrance Requirements Minimum overall college GPA of 2.8, transcript of college record, written essay, health exam, high school biology, high school chemistry, high school foreign language, 3 years high school math, 2 years high school science, high school transcript, immunizations, interview, 2 letters of recommendation, minimum high school GPA of 2.5, minimum high school rank 50%, minimum GPA in nursing prerequisites of 2.8, prerequisite course work. Transfer students are accepted. *Application deadline:* 2/15 (fall), 11/1 (spring), 4/1 (summer). Applications may be processed on a rolling basis for some programs. *Application fee:* $45.
Expenses (2015–16) *Tuition:* full-time $22,740; part-time $980 per credit hour. *International tuition:* $22,740 full-time. *Room and board:* $13,779; room only: $6000 per academic year. *Required fees:* full-time $2193; part-time $617 per term.
Financial Aid 90% of baccalaureate students in nursing programs received some form of financial aid in 2014–15. *Gift aid (need-based):* Federal Pell, FSEOG, state, private, college/university gift aid from institutional funds, Federal Nursing. *Loans:* Federal Nursing Student Loans, Federal Direct (Subsidized and Unsubsidized Stafford PLUS), Perkins, state, college/university. *Work-study:* Federal Work-Study, part-time campus jobs. *Financial aid application deadline:* 5/1(priority: 2/1).
Contact Miss Melissa L. Weir, Interim Chairperson, Undergraduate Program, Division of Nursing, Howard University, 516 Bryant Street NW, Annex 1, Washington, DC 20059. *Telephone:* 202-806-7854. *Fax:* 202-806-5085. *E-mail:* melissa.weir@howard.edu.

GRADUATE PROGRAMS

Expenses (2015–16) *Tuition:* full-time $30,545; part-time $1700 per credit hour. *International tuition:* $30,545 full-time. *Room and board:* $18,213; room only: $8812 per academic year. *Required fees:* full-time $1343; part-time $1343 per term.
Financial Aid Teaching assistantships (averaging $16,000 per year); career-related internships or fieldwork, institutionally sponsored loans, and scholarships also available.
Contact Dr. Tammi L. Damas, Interim Chairperson, Graduate Program, Division of Nursing, Howard University, 516 Bryant Street NW, Annex 1, Washington, DC 20059. *Telephone:* 202-806-5021. *Fax:* 202-806-5085. *E-mail:* Tammi.damas@howard.edu.

MASTER'S DEGREE PROGRAM
Degree MSN
Available Programs Master's.
Concentrations Available Nursing education. *Nurse practitioner programs in:* family health.
Study Options Full-time and part-time.
Program Entrance Requirements Clinical experience, computer literacy, minimum overall college GPA of 3.0, transcript of college record, written essay, interview, 3 letters of recommendation, resume, statistics course. *Application deadline:* 7/1 (fall), 11/15 (spring). Applications may be processed on a rolling basis for some programs. *Application fee:* $45.
Advanced Placement Credit given for nursing courses completed elsewhere dependent upon specific evaluations.
Degree Requirements 47 total credit hours.

POST-MASTER'S PROGRAM
Areas of Study Nursing education. *Nurse practitioner programs in:* family health.

Trinity Washington University
Nursing Program
Washington, District of Columbia

Founded in 1897
DEGREE • BSN
Nursing Program Faculty 9 (4% with doctorates).

Baccalaureate Enrollment 80
Nursing Student Activities Sigma Theta Tau, Student Nurses' Association.
Nursing Student Resources Academic advising; academic or career counseling; assistance for students with disabilities; bookstore; campus computer network; career placement assistance; computer lab; computer-assisted instruction; e-mail services; employment services for current students; housing assistance; Internet; learning resource lab; library services; nursing audiovisuals; paid internships; remedial services; resume preparation assistance; skills, simulation, or other laboratory; tutoring; unpaid internships.
Library Facilities 1,200 volumes in health, 200 volumes in nursing; 40 periodical subscriptions health-care related.

BACCALAUREATE PROGRAMS

Degree BSN
Available Programs Generic Baccalaureate; RN Baccalaureate.
Study Options Full-time and part-time.
Program Entrance Requirements Transcript of college record, CPR certification, written essay, health exam, health insurance, high school transcript, immunizations, interview, 1 letter of recommendation, minimum GPA in nursing prerequisites of 2.0, professional liability insurance/malpractice insurance, prerequisite course work, RN licensure. Transfer students are accepted. *Application deadline:* Applications may be processed on a rolling basis for some programs.
Advanced Placement Credit by examination available. Credit given for nursing courses completed elsewhere dependent upon specific evaluations.
Contact *Telephone:* 202-884-9245. *Fax:* 202-884-9308.

University of the District of Columbia
Nursing Education Program
Washington, District of Columbia

Founded in 1976
DEGREE • BSN
Nursing Program Faculty 6 (3% with doctorates).
Baccalaureate Enrollment 40 **Women** 97% **Men** 3% **Part-time** 50%
Nursing Student Activities Student Nurses' Association.
Nursing Student Resources Academic advising; academic or career counseling; assistance for students with disabilities; bookstore; campus computer network; career placement assistance; computer lab; computer-assisted instruction; daycare for children of students; e-mail services; employment services for current students; Internet; learning resource lab; library services; nursing audiovisuals; remedial services; resume preparation assistance; skills, simulation, or other laboratory; tutoring.
Library Facilities 500 volumes in health, 250 volumes in nursing; 75 periodical subscriptions health-care related.

BACCALAUREATE PROGRAMS

Degree BSN
Available Programs RN Baccalaureate.
Site Options Washington, DC.
Study Options Full-time and part-time.
Program Entrance Requirements Minimum overall college GPA of 2.7, transcript of college record, CPR certification, written essay, health exam, health insurance, immunizations, 2 letters of recommendation, minimum GPA in nursing prerequisites of 2.7, professional liability insurance/malpractice insurance, prerequisite course work, RN licensure. Transfer students are accepted. *Application deadline:* 6/15 (fall), 11/15 (spring), 4/15 (summer).
Advanced Placement Credit by examination available. Credit given for nursing courses completed elsewhere dependent upon specific evaluations.
Contact *Telephone:* 202-274-5916. *Fax:* 202-274-5952.

FLORIDA

Adventist University of Health Sciences

Department of Nursing
Orlando, Florida

Founded in 1913
DEGREE • BSN
Nursing Program Faculty 21 (23% with doctorates).
Baccalaureate Enrollment 562
Distance Learning Courses Available.
Nursing Student Activities Nursing Honor Society, Student Nurses' Association.
Nursing Student Resources Academic advising; academic or career counseling; bookstore; campus computer network; computer lab; computer-assisted instruction; e-mail services; interactive nursing skills videos; Internet; learning resource lab; library services; nursing audiovisuals; skills, simulation, or other laboratory; tutoring.

BACCALAUREATE PROGRAMS

Degree BSN
Available Programs Generic Baccalaureate; RN Baccalaureate.
Study Options Full-time and part-time.
Online Degree Options Yes (online only).
Program Entrance Requirements Minimum overall college GPA of 3.0, transcript of college record, CPR certification, written essay, health exam, high school transcript, immunizations, 2 letters of recommendation, minimum high school GPA of 3.0, prerequisite course work, RN licensure. Transfer students are accepted. *Application deadline:* 4/15 (fall).
Advanced Placement Credit by examination available. Credit given for nursing courses completed elsewhere dependent upon specific evaluations.
Contact *Telephone:* 407-303-5762. *Fax:* 407-303-1872.

Barry University

Division of Nursing
Miami Shores, Florida

http://www.barry.edu/nursing
Founded in 1940
DEGREES • BSN • MSN • MSN/MBA • PHD
Nursing Program Faculty 30 (50% with doctorates).
Baccalaureate Enrollment 431 **Women** 87% **Men** 13% **Part-time** 20%
Graduate Enrollment 161 **Women** 93% **Men** 7% **Part-time** 99%
Nursing Student Activities Sigma Theta Tau, Student Nurses' Association.
Nursing Student Resources Academic advising; academic or career counseling; assistance for students with disabilities; bookstore; campus computer network; career placement assistance; computer lab; computer-assisted instruction; e-mail services; employment services for current students; housing assistance; interactive nursing skills videos; Internet; learning resource lab; library services; nursing audiovisuals; paid internships; remedial services; resume preparation assistance; skills, simulation, or other laboratory; tutoring.
Library Facilities 15,000 volumes in health, 8,500 volumes in nursing; 400 periodical subscriptions health-care related.

BACCALAUREATE PROGRAMS

Degree BSN
Available Programs ADN to Baccalaureate; Accelerated Baccalaureate; Accelerated Baccalaureate for Second Degree; Baccalaureate for Second Degree; Generic Baccalaureate; LPN to Baccalaureate; LPN to RN Baccalaureate; RN Baccalaureate.
Site Options Kendall, FL.
Study Options Full-time and part-time.
Program Entrance Requirements Minimum overall college GPA of 3.0, transcript of college record, CPR certification, health exam, health insurance, high school biology, high school chemistry, high school math, high school science, high school transcript, immunizations, 2 letters of recommendation, minimum high school GPA of 3.0, minimum GPA in nursing prerequisites of 3.0, professional liability insurance/malpractice insurance. Transfer students are accepted. *Application deadline:* Applications may be processed on a rolling basis for some programs. *Application fee:* $30.
Advanced Placement Credit given for nursing courses completed elsewhere dependent upon specific evaluations.
Contact *Telephone:* 305-899-3813. *Fax:* 305-899-3831.

GRADUATE PROGRAMS

Contact *Telephone:* 305-899-3814. *Fax:* 305-899-3831.

MASTER'S DEGREE PROGRAM
Degrees MSN; MSN/MBA
Available Programs Master's.
Concentrations Available Nursing administration; nursing education. *Nurse practitioner programs in:* acute care, family health.
Site Options Kendall, FL.
Study Options Part-time.
Program Entrance Requirements Clinical experience, computer literacy, minimum overall college GPA of 3.0, transcript of college record, written essay, 2 letters of recommendation, nursing research course, professional liability insurance/malpractice insurance, statistics course, GRE General Test or MAT. *Application deadline:* Applications may be processed on a rolling basis for some programs.
Advanced Placement Credit given for nursing courses completed elsewhere dependent upon specific evaluations.
Degree Requirements 45 total credit hours.

POST-MASTER'S PROGRAM
Areas of Study Nursing administration; nursing education. *Nurse practitioner programs in:* acute care, family health.

DOCTORAL DEGREE PROGRAM
Degree PhD
Available Programs Doctorate.
Areas of Study Nursing research, nursing science.
Site Options Orlando, FL; Kendall, FL; Palm Beach, FL.
Program Entrance Requirements Clinical experience, minimum overall college GPA of 3.0, interview, 2 letters of recommendation, MSN or equivalent, statistics course, writing sample, GRE General Test or MAT. Application deadline: Applications may be processed on a rolling basis for some programs.
Degree Requirements 45 total credit hours, dissertation, written exam, residency.

Bethune-Cookman University

School of Nursing
Daytona Beach, Florida

http://www.cookman.edu/academics/schools/sn/index.html
Founded in 1904
DEGREE • BSN
Nursing Program Faculty 11 (2% with doctorates).
Baccalaureate Enrollment 137 **Women** 93% **Men** 7%
Nursing Student Activities Nursing Honor Society, Student Nurses' Association.
Nursing Student Resources Academic advising; bookstore; campus computer network; computer lab; computer-assisted instruction; e-mail services; interactive nursing skills videos; Internet; learning resource lab; library services; nursing audiovisuals; resume preparation assistance; skills, simulation, or other laboratory; tutoring; unpaid internships.

BACCALAUREATE PROGRAMS

Degree BSN
Available Programs Generic Baccalaureate; RN Baccalaureate.
Study Options Full-time.
Program Entrance Requirements Minimum overall college GPA of 2.8, transcript of college record, CPR certification, written essay, health exam, high school transcript, immunizations, interview, 2 letters of recommendation, minimum GPA in nursing prerequisites of 2.8, prerequisite course work. Transfer students are accepted.
Advanced Placement Credit by examination available. Credit given for nursing courses completed elsewhere dependent upon specific evaluations.
Contact *Telephone:* 386-481-2000.

Broward College
Nursing Program
Fort Lauderdale, Florida

Founded in 1960
DEGREE • BSN

BACCALAUREATE PROGRAMS

Degree BSN
Available Programs RN Baccalaureate.
Program Entrance Requirements Minimum overall college GPA of 2.5, RN licensure.
Contact *Telephone:* 954-201-4880.

Chipola College
School of Health Sciences
Marianna, Florida

http://www.chipola.edu/
Founded in 1947
DEGREE • BSN

BACCALAUREATE PROGRAMS

Degree BSN
Available Programs RN Baccalaureate.
Program Entrance Requirements Minimum overall college GPA of 2.5, prerequisite course work. *Application deadline:* 8/20 (fall).
Contact Dr. Karen Lipford, Dean, School of Health Sciences, School of Health Sciences, Chipola College, 3094 Indian Circle, Marianna, FL 32446. *Telephone:* 850-718-2278. *E-mail:* lipfordk@chipola.edu.

ECPI University
ECPI University
Lake Mary, Florida

DEGREE • BSN
Nursing Program Faculty 17 (18% with doctorates).
Baccalaureate Enrollment 86 **Women** 80% **Men** 20%
Distance Learning Courses Available.
Nursing Student Activities Student Nurses' Association.
Nursing Student Resources Academic advising; academic or career counseling; assistance for students with disabilities; campus computer network; career placement assistance; computer-assisted instruction; e-mail services; interactive nursing skills videos; Internet; learning resource lab; library services; nursing audiovisuals; other; remedial services; resume preparation assistance; skills, simulation, or other laboratory; tutoring.
Library Facilities 990 volumes in health, 880 volumes in nursing; 905 periodical subscriptions health-care related.

BACCALAUREATE PROGRAMS

Degree BSN
Available Programs Accelerated Baccalaureate for Second Degree.
Study Options Full-time.
Program Entrance Requirements Minimum overall college GPA of 2.5, transcript of college record, CPR certification, written essay, health exam, health insurance, immunizations, interview, 2 letters of recommendation, prerequisite course work. *Application deadline:* 12/1 (winter), 6/1 (summer). Applications may be processed on a rolling basis for some programs. *Application fee:* $50.
Advanced Placement Credit given for nursing courses completed elsewhere dependent upon specific evaluations.
Financial Aid 38% of baccalaureate students in nursing programs received some form of financial aid in 2013–14.
Contact Melissa Nash, Admissions Coordinator, ECPI University, 660 Century Point, Suite 1050, Lake Mary, FL 32746. *Telephone:* 800-294-4434. *E-mail:* nursing.info@remingtoncollege.edu.

Florida Agricultural and Mechanical University
School of Nursing
Tallahassee, Florida

http://www.famu.edu/index.cfm?a=nursing
Founded in 1887
DEGREES • BSN • MSN • PHD
Nursing Program Faculty 28 (18% with doctorates).
Baccalaureate Enrollment 161 **Women** 90% **Men** 10%
Graduate Enrollment 17 **Women** 83% **Men** 17% **Part-time** 12%
Nursing Student Activities Sigma Theta Tau, Student Nurses' Association.
Nursing Student Resources Academic advising; academic or career counseling; bookstore; campus computer network; career placement assistance; computer lab; computer-assisted instruction; daycare for children of students; e-mail services; employment services for current students; externships; interactive nursing skills videos; Internet; library services; nursing audiovisuals; placement services for program completers; remedial services; resume preparation assistance; skills, simulation, or other laboratory; tutoring.
Library Facilities 5,000 volumes in health, 4,091 volumes in nursing; 385 periodical subscriptions health-care related.

BACCALAUREATE PROGRAMS

Degree BSN
Available Programs Generic Baccalaureate.
Study Options Part-time.
Program Entrance Requirements CPR certification, health exam, immunizations, 3 letters of recommendation, minimum high school GPA of 2.5, prerequisite course work. Transfer students are accepted.
Contact *Telephone:* 850-599-3458. *Fax:* 850-599-3508.

GRADUATE PROGRAMS

Contact *Telephone:* 850-599-3017. *Fax:* 850-599-3508.

MASTER'S DEGREE PROGRAM
Degree MSN
Available Programs Master's.
Concentrations Available *Nurse practitioner programs in:* adult health, gerontology, women's health.
Study Options Full-time and part-time.
Program Entrance Requirements Clinical experience, minimum overall college GPA of 3.0, CPR certification, immunizations, interview, nursing research course, physical assessment course, professional liability insurance/malpractice insurance, statistics course.
Degree Requirements 42 total credit hours, thesis or project.

POST-MASTER'S PROGRAM
Areas of Study *Nurse practitioner programs in:* adult health, gerontology, women's health.

DOCTORAL DEGREE PROGRAM
Degree PhD
Program Entrance Requirements Minimum overall college GPA of 3.5, 3 letters of recommendation, MSN or equivalent.
Degree Requirements 90 total credit hours, dissertation, oral exam, written exam.

CONTINUING EDUCATION PROGRAM

Contact *Telephone:* 850-599-3017. *Fax:* 850-599-3508.

Florida Atlantic University
Christine E. Lynn College of Nursing
Boca Raton, Florida

http://nursing.fau.edu/
Founded in 1961
DEGREES • BSN • DNP • MSN
Nursing Program Faculty 61 (70% with doctorates).
Baccalaureate Enrollment 531 **Women** 90% **Men** 10% **Part-time** 54%
Graduate Enrollment 395 **Women** 92% **Men** 8% **Part-time** 58%
Distance Learning Courses Available.

Nursing Student Activities Sigma Theta Tau, Student Nurses' Association, nursing club.

Nursing Student Resources Academic advising; academic or career counseling; assistance for students with disabilities; bookstore; campus computer network; computer lab; computer-assisted instruction; e-mail services; housing assistance; interactive nursing skills videos; Internet; learning resource lab; library services; nursing audiovisuals; remedial services; skills, simulation, or other laboratory; tutoring.

Library Facilities 28,670 volumes in health, 5,749 volumes in nursing; 903 periodical subscriptions health-care related.

BACCALAUREATE PROGRAMS

Degree BSN

Available Programs Accelerated Baccalaureate for Second Degree; Generic Baccalaureate; RN Baccalaureate.

Site Options Davie, FL; Fort Pierce, FL.

Study Options Full-time.

Online Degree Options Yes (online only).

Program Entrance Requirements Minimum overall college GPA of 3.0, transcript of college record, CPR certification, health exam, health insurance, high school transcript, immunizations, interview, minimum GPA in nursing prerequisites of 2.0, prerequisite course work. Transfer students are accepted. *Application deadline:* 1/15 (winter). *Application fee:* $30.

Contact *Telephone:* 561-297-2535. *Fax:* 561-297-3652.

GRADUATE PROGRAMS

Contact *Telephone:* 561-297-3389. *Fax:* 561-297-3652.

MASTER'S DEGREE PROGRAM

Degree MSN

Available Programs Master's.

Concentrations Available Clinical nurse leader; nursing administration; nursing education. *Nurse practitioner programs in:* adult health, family health, gerontology, primary care.

Site Options Davie, FL; Fort Pierce, FL.

Study Options Full-time and part-time.

Online Degree Options Yes.

Program Entrance Requirements Minimum overall college GPA of 3.0, transcript of college record, CPR certification, written essay, immunizations, interview, 2 letters of recommendation, nursing research course, physical assessment course, professional liability insurance/malpractice insurance, prerequisite course work, resume, statistics course, GRE General Test or MAT. *Application deadline:* 6/1 (fall), 10/1 (spring), 2/1 (summer). *Application fee:* $30.

Advanced Placement Credit given for nursing courses completed elsewhere dependent upon specific evaluations.

Degree Requirements 39 total credit hours.

POST-MASTER'S PROGRAM

Areas of Study Clinical nurse leader; nursing administration; nursing education. *Nurse practitioner programs in:* adult health, family health, gerontology, primary care.

DOCTORAL DEGREE PROGRAM

Degree DNP

Available Programs Doctorate; Post-Baccalaureate Doctorate.

Areas of Study Advanced practice nursing, aging, family health, gerontology, health-care systems, nursing administration.

Program Entrance Requirements Minimum overall college GPA of 3.5, interview by faculty committee, interview, 3 letters of recommendation, scholarly papers, statistics course, vita, writing sample, GRE General Test or MAT. Application deadline: 11/1 (fall), 3/1 (spring). Application fee: $30.

Degree Requirements 83 total credit hours, written exam, residency.

Florida Gulf Coast University

School of Nursing
Fort Myers, Florida

http://www.fgcu.edu/chp/nursing/
Founded in 1991

DEGREES • BSN • MSN
Nursing Program Faculty 17 (57% with doctorates).
Baccalaureate Enrollment 141 **Women** 89% **Men** 11% **Part-time** 15%
Graduate Enrollment 75 **Women** 88% **Men** 12% **Part-time** 10%

Nursing Student Activities Sigma Theta Tau, Student Nurses' Association.

Nursing Student Resources Academic advising; academic or career counseling; assistance for students with disabilities; bookstore; campus computer network; career placement assistance; computer lab; computer-assisted instruction; e-mail services; employment services for current students; Internet; learning resource lab; library services; nursing audiovisuals; skills, simulation, or other laboratory; tutoring.

Library Facilities 13,943 volumes in health, 6,742 volumes in nursing; 471 periodical subscriptions health-care related.

BACCALAUREATE PROGRAMS

Degree BSN

Available Programs Generic Baccalaureate.

Study Options Full-time.

Program Entrance Requirements Minimum overall college GPA of 3.0, transcript of college record, CPR certification, health insurance, high school foreign language, immunizations, professional liability insurance/malpractice insurance, prerequisite course work. Transfer students are accepted. *Application deadline:* 2/1 (fall), 5/15 (spring).

Advanced Placement Credit given for nursing courses completed elsewhere dependent upon specific evaluations.

Contact *Telephone:* 239-590-7454. *Fax:* 239-590-7474.

GRADUATE PROGRAMS

Contact *Telephone:* 239-590-7505. *Fax:* 239-590-7474.

MASTER'S DEGREE PROGRAM

Degree MSN

Available Programs Master's.

Concentrations Available Nurse anesthesia. *Nurse practitioner programs in:* acute care, adult health, family health.

Study Options Full-time and part-time.

Program Entrance Requirements Clinical experience, minimum overall college GPA of 3.0, transcript of college record, interview, physical assessment course, resume, statistics course.

Advanced Placement Credit given for nursing courses completed elsewhere dependent upon specific evaluations.

POST-MASTER'S PROGRAM

Areas of Study *Nurse practitioner programs in:* acute care, family health.

CONTINUING EDUCATION PROGRAM

Contact *Telephone:* 239-590-7513. *Fax:* 239-590-7474.

Florida International University

Nursing Program
Miami, Florida

http://www.fiu.edu/
Founded in 1965

DEGREES • BSN • DNP • MSN • PHD
Nursing Program Faculty 100 (57% with doctorates).
Baccalaureate Enrollment 701 **Women** 76% **Men** 24% **Part-time** 49%
Graduate Enrollment 408 **Women** 69% **Men** 31% **Part-time** 20%
Distance Learning Courses Available.
Nursing Student Activities Sigma Theta Tau, Student Nurses' Association.
Nursing Student Resources Academic advising; academic or career counseling; assistance for students with disabilities; bookstore; campus computer network; career placement assistance; computer lab; computer-assisted instruction; daycare for children of students; e-mail services; externships; housing assistance; interactive nursing skills videos; Internet; learning resource lab; library services; nursing audiovisuals; paid internships; remedial services; resume preparation assistance; skills, simulation, or other laboratory; tutoring.
Library Facilities 26,884 volumes in health, 2,142 volumes in nursing; 2,451 periodical subscriptions health-care related.

BACCALAUREATE PROGRAMS

Degree BSN

Available Programs Accelerated Baccalaureate; Accelerated Baccalaureate for Second Degree; Generic Baccalaureate; RN Baccalaureate.

Site Options North Miami, FL.

Study Options Full-time.

Online Degree Options Yes.

Program Entrance Requirements Minimum overall college GPA of 3.25, transcript of college record, CPR certification, written essay, health exam, health insurance, high school foreign language, high school transcript, immunizations, minimum GPA in nursing prerequisites of 3.25, prerequisite course work. Transfer students are accepted. *Application deadline:* 3/15 (fall). *Application fee:* $30.

Advanced Placement Credit given for nursing courses completed elsewhere dependent upon specific evaluations.

Expenses (2014–15) *Tuition, state resident:* full-time $6110. *Tuition, nonresident:* full-time $18,000. *International tuition:* $18,000 full-time. *Required fees:* full-time $615.

Financial Aid 82% of baccalaureate students in nursing programs received some form of financial aid in 2013–14.

Contact Dr. Maria Olenick, Chair, Undergraduate Nursing, Nursing Program, Florida International University, 11200 SW 8th Street, Modesto A. Maidique Campus, AHC3-329, Miami, FL 33199. *Telephone:* 305-348-7757. *Fax:* 305-348-7764. *E-mail:* molenick@fiu.edu.

GRADUATE PROGRAMS

Expenses (2014–15) *Tuition, state resident:* full-time $13,783. *Tuition, nonresident:* full-time $24,873. *International tuition:* $24,873 full-time. *Required fees:* full-time $577.

Financial Aid 89% of graduate students in nursing programs received some form of financial aid in 2013–14. Institutionally sponsored loans and scholarships available. *Financial aid application deadline:* 3/1.

Contact Dr. Yhovana Gordon, Chair, Graduate Nursing, Nursing Program, Florida International University, 11200 SW 8th Street, Modesto A. Maidique Campus, AHC3, Room 224, Miami, FL 33199. *Telephone:* 305-348-7733. *Fax:* 305-348-7764. *E-mail:* gordony@fiu.edu.

MASTER'S DEGREE PROGRAM

Degree MSN

Available Programs Accelerated AD/RN to Master's; Master's.

Concentrations Available Nurse anesthesia; nursing administration. *Nurse practitioner programs in:* adult health, family health, pediatric primary care, psychiatric/mental health.

Study Options Full-time.

Program Entrance Requirements Computer literacy, minimum overall college GPA of 3.0, transcript of college record, CPR certification, written essay, immunizations, interview, 3 letters of recommendation, professional liability insurance/malpractice insurance, resume, statistics course. *Application deadline:* 3/1 (fall). *Application fee:* $95.

Advanced Placement Credit given for nursing courses completed elsewhere dependent upon specific evaluations.

Degree Requirements 44 total credit hours, thesis or project.

POST-MASTER'S PROGRAM

Areas of Study Nursing administration; nursing education. *Nurse practitioner programs in:* adult health, family health, pediatric primary care, psychiatric/mental health.

DOCTORAL DEGREE PROGRAM

Degree DNP

Available Programs Doctorate.

Areas of Study Clinical practice, faculty preparation, family health, gerontology, health policy, health-care systems, individualized study, nursing education, nursing policy, nursing research, nursing science.

Program Entrance Requirements Minimum overall college GPA of 3.25, clinical experience, interview by faculty committee, 3 letters of recommendation, MSN or equivalent, statistics course, writing sample. Application deadline: 6/1 (fall), 10/1 (spring). Applications may be processed on a rolling basis for some programs. Application fee: $30.

Degree Requirements 36 total credit hours, oral exam, written exam.

Degree PhD

Available Programs Doctorate.

Areas of Study Faculty preparation, health policy, health-care systems, individualized study, nursing administration, nursing education, nursing policy, nursing research, nursing science.

Program Entrance Requirements Minimum overall college GPA of 3.3, interview by faculty committee, 3 letters of recommendation, MSN or equivalent, statistics course, vita, writing sample, GRE. Application deadline: 6/1 (fall), 10/1 (spring), 3/1 (summer). Applications may be processed on a rolling basis for some programs. Application fee: $30.

Degree Requirements 60 total credit hours, dissertation, oral exam, written exam.

Florida National University
Nursing Division
Hialeah, Florida

http://www.fnu.edu/
Founded in 1982
DEGREE • BSN

BACCALAUREATE PROGRAMS

Degree BSN

Available Programs Generic Baccalaureate; RN Baccalaureate.

Program Entrance Requirements *Application deadline:* Applications may be processed on a rolling basis for some programs.

Contact Hialeah Campus, Nursing Division, Florida National University, 4425 West Jose Regueiro (20th) Avenue, Hialeah, FL 33012. *Telephone:* 305-821-3333. *Fax:* 305-362-0595.

Florida Southern College
School of Nursing & Health Sciences
Lakeland, Florida

http://www.flsouthern.edu/KCMS/Nursing-Health-Sciences.aspx
Founded in 1885
DEGREES • BSN • MSN • MSN/MBA

Nursing Program Faculty 12 (75% with doctorates).

Baccalaureate Enrollment 149

Graduate Enrollment 89

Nursing Student Activities Nursing Honor Society, Sigma Theta Tau, Student Nurses' Association.

Nursing Student Resources Academic advising; academic or career counseling; assistance for students with disabilities; bookstore; campus computer network; career placement assistance; computer lab; computer-assisted instruction; e-mail services; externships; interactive nursing skills videos; Internet; learning resource lab; library services; nursing audiovisuals; paid internships; placement services for program completers; remedial services; resume preparation assistance; skills, simulation, or other laboratory; tutoring.

Library Facilities 4,000 volumes in health, 3,500 volumes in nursing; 40 periodical subscriptions health-care related.

BACCALAUREATE PROGRAMS

Degree BSN

Available Programs Accelerated Baccalaureate; Accelerated Baccalaureate for Second Degree; Baccalaureate for Second Degree; Generic Baccalaureate; RN Baccalaureate.

Study Options Full-time.

Program Entrance Requirements Minimum overall college GPA of 3.2, transcript of college record, CPR certification, written essay, health exam, health insurance, immunizations, minimum high school GPA of 3.2, minimum GPA in nursing prerequisites of 3.0, prerequisite course work. Transfer students are accepted. *Application deadline:* 5/1 (fall). Applications may be processed on a rolling basis for some programs.

Advanced Placement Credit by examination available. Credit given for nursing courses completed elsewhere dependent upon specific evaluations.

Contact *Telephone:* 863-680-3951. *Fax:* 863-680-3860.

GRADUATE PROGRAMS

Contact *Telephone:* 863-680-3951. *Fax:* 863-680-3860.

MASTER'S DEGREE PROGRAM

Degrees MSN; MSN/MBA

Available Programs Master's; Master's for Nurses with Non-Nursing Degrees.

Concentrations Available Nursing administration; nursing education. *Clinical nurse specialist programs in:* adult health, gerontology. *Nurse practitioner programs in:* adult health, primary care.

Study Options Full-time and part-time.

Program Entrance Requirements Clinical experience, computer literacy, minimum overall college GPA of 3.0, transcript of college record, CPR certification, written essay, immunizations, 3 letters of recommendation, nursing research course, physical assessment course, professional liability insurance/malpractice insurance, prerequisite course work, resume, statistics course. *Application deadline:* 6/1 (fall), 11/1 (spring). *Application fee:* $30.

Advanced Placement Credit given for nursing courses completed elsewhere dependent upon specific evaluations.

Degree Requirements 42 total credit hours, thesis or project.

POST-MASTER'S PROGRAM

Areas of Study Nursing administration; nursing education. *Clinical nurse specialist programs in:* adult health, gerontology. *Nurse practitioner programs in:* adult health, primary care.

Florida SouthWestern State College

Bachelor of Science in Nursing Program
Fort Myers, Florida

Founded in 1962

DEGREE • BSN

BACCALAUREATE PROGRAMS

Degree BSN

Available Programs RN Baccalaureate.

Program Entrance Requirements Minimum overall college GPA of 2.0, transcript of college record, prerequisite course work, RN licensure. *Application deadline:* 8/1 (fall), 12/1 (spring), 4/1 (summer).

Contact *Telephone:* 800-749-2322.

Florida State College at Jacksonville

Nursing Department
Jacksonville, Florida

http://www.fscj.edu/
Founded in 1963

DEGREE • BSN

Nursing Program Faculty 4 (100% with doctorates).

Baccalaureate Enrollment 81 **Women** 98% **Men** 2%

Distance Learning Courses Available.

Nursing Student Activities Student Nurses' Association.

Nursing Student Resources Academic advising; academic or career counseling; assistance for students with disabilities; bookstore; campus computer network; career placement assistance; computer lab; computer-assisted instruction; daycare for children of students; e-mail services; employment services for current students; interactive nursing skills videos; Internet; learning resource lab; library services; nursing audiovisuals; resume preparation assistance; skills, simulation, or other laboratory; tutoring.

Library Facilities 50,000 volumes in health, 5,000 volumes in nursing; 148 periodical subscriptions health-care related.

BACCALAUREATE PROGRAMS

Degree BSN

Available Programs RN Baccalaureate.

Study Options Part-time.

Program Entrance Requirements Minimum overall college GPA of 2.0, transcript of college record, CPR certification, written essay, health exam, high school transcript, immunizations, 1 letter of recommendation, minimum GPA in nursing prerequisites of 2.0, professional liability insurance/malpractice insurance, prerequisite course work, RN licensure. Transfer students are accepted. *Application deadline:* 6/1 (fall), 10/1 (winter), 2/1 (spring). *Application fee:* $25.

Advanced Placement Credit given for nursing courses completed elsewhere dependent upon specific evaluations.

Contact *Telephone:* 904-713-6015. *Fax:* 904-713-4850.

Florida State University

College of Nursing
Tallahassee, Florida

http://www.nursing.fsu.edu/
Founded in 1851

DEGREES • BSN • DNP • MSN

Nursing Program Faculty 40 (78% with doctorates).

Baccalaureate Enrollment 194 **Women** 97% **Men** 3%

Graduate Enrollment 90 **Women** 89% **Men** 11% **Part-time** 24%

Distance Learning Courses Available.

Nursing Student Activities Sigma Theta Tau, Student Nurses' Association.

Nursing Student Resources Academic advising; academic or career counseling; assistance for students with disabilities; bookstore; campus computer network; computer lab; computer-assisted instruction; e-mail services; interactive nursing skills videos; Internet; library services; nursing audiovisuals; skills, simulation, or other laboratory; unpaid internships.

BACCALAUREATE PROGRAMS

Degree BSN

Available Programs Accelerated Baccalaureate; Generic Baccalaureate.

Study Options Full-time.

Program Entrance Requirements Minimum overall college GPA of 3.4, CPR certification, health exam, health insurance, immunizations, minimum GPA in nursing prerequisites of 3.0, prerequisite course work. Transfer students are accepted. *Application deadline:* 2/1 (fall). *Application fee:* $35.

Advanced Placement Credit given for nursing courses completed elsewhere dependent upon specific evaluations.

Expenses (2015–16) *Tuition, state resident:* part-time $216 per credit. *Tuition, nonresident:* part-time $721 per credit. *Room and board:* $10,208; room only: $6160 per academic year.

Financial Aid *Gift aid (need-based):* Federal Pell, FSEOG, state, private, college/university gift aid from institutional funds, Academic Competitiveness Grants, National SMART Grants. *Loans:* Federal Direct (Subsidized and Unsubsidized Stafford PLUS), Perkins, college/university. *Work-study:* Federal Work-Study, part-time campus jobs. *Financial aid application deadline:* Continuous.

Contact Mr. Carlos Urrutia, Director of Student Services, College of Nursing, Florida State University, 98 Varsity Way, 103 SCN, Tallahassee, FL 32306-4310. *Telephone:* 850-644-5638. *Fax:* 850-645-7249. *E-mail:* currutia@admin.fsu.edu.

GRADUATE PROGRAMS

Expenses (2015–16) *Tuition, state resident:* part-time $479 per credit. *Tuition, nonresident:* part-time $1111 per credit.

Financial Aid Fellowships (averaging $6,300 per year), research assistantships (averaging $3,000 per year), 3 teaching assistantships (averaging $3,000 per year) were awarded; career-related internships or fieldwork, Federal Work-Study, institutionally sponsored loans, scholarships, traineeships, and tuition waivers (partial) also available.

Contact Mr. Carlos Urrutia, Director of Student Services, College of Nursing, Florida State University, 98 Varsity Way, 103 SCN, Tallahassee, FL 32306-4310. *Telephone:* 850-644-5638. *Fax:* 850-645-7249. *E-mail:* currutia@admin.fsu.edu.

MASTER'S DEGREE PROGRAM
Degree MSN

Available Programs Master's.

Concentrations Available Nursing education.

Study Options Part-time.

Online Degree Options Yes (online only).

Program Entrance Requirements Minimum overall college GPA of 3.0, transcript of college record, CPR certification, immunizations, 2 letters of recommendation, GRE General Test, MAT. *Application deadline:* 5/1 (fall). *Application fee:* $35.

Advanced Placement Credit given for nursing courses completed elsewhere dependent upon specific evaluations.

Degree Requirements 38 total credit hours.

POST-MASTER'S PROGRAM
Areas of Study Nursing education.

DOCTORAL DEGREE PROGRAM
Degree DNP

Available Programs Doctorate; Post-Baccalaureate Doctorate.
Areas of Study Advanced practice nursing.
Site Options Sarasota, FL; Panama City, FL.
Program Entrance Requirements Minimum overall college GPA of 3.0, interview by faculty committee, interview, 3 letters of recommendation, GRE General Test, MAT. Application deadline: 4/15 (fall). Application fee: $35.
Degree Requirements 90 total credit hours, residency.

Fortis College
Nursing Department
Cutler Bay, Florida

https://www.fortis.edu/
DEGREE • BSN

BACCALAUREATE PROGRAMS

Degree BSN
Available Programs RN Baccalaureate.
Contact Admissions, Nursing Department, Fortis College, 19600 South Dixie Highway Suite B, Cutler Bay, FL 33157. *Telephone:* 786-345-5300.

Gulf Coast State College
Nursing Program
Panama City, Florida

http://www.gulfcoast.edu/
Founded in 1957
DEGREE • BSN

BACCALAUREATE PROGRAMS

Degree BSN
Available Programs RN Baccalaureate.
Program Entrance Requirements Minimum overall college GPA of 2.5, prerequisite course work, RN licensure.
Contact Health Sciences Division, Nursing Program, Gulf Coast State College, 5230 West Highway 98, Panama City, FL 32401. *Telephone:* 850-769-1551 Ext. 3827.

Herzing University
Nursing Program
Winter Park, Florida

https://www.herzing.edu/career-programs/undergraduate-degrees/healthcare/nursing
Founded in 1989
DEGREE • BSN

BACCALAUREATE PROGRAMS

Degree BSN
Available Programs RN Baccalaureate.
Contact Nursing Program, Nursing Program, Herzing University, 1865 SR 436, Winter Park, FL 32792. *Telephone:* 407-478-0500.

Indian River State College
Bachelor of Science in Nursing Program
Fort Pierce, Florida

Founded in 1960
DEGREE • BSN

BACCALAUREATE PROGRAMS

Degree BSN
Available Programs RN Baccalaureate.
Contact *Telephone:* 772-462-7415.

Jacksonville University
School of Nursing
Jacksonville, Florida

http://www.jacksonvilleu.com/?loc=logo
Founded in 1934
DEGREES • BSN • DNP • MSN • MSN/MBA
Nursing Program Faculty 85 (65% with doctorates).
Baccalaureate Enrollment 1,113 **Women** 88% **Men** 12% **Part-time** 26%
Graduate Enrollment 568 **Women** 91% **Men** 9% **Part-time** 32%
Distance Learning Courses Available.
Nursing Student Activities Sigma Theta Tau, Student Nurses' Association.
Nursing Student Resources Academic advising; academic or career counseling; assistance for students with disabilities; bookstore; campus computer network; career placement assistance; computer lab; computer-assisted instruction; e-mail services; employment services for current students; externships; interactive nursing skills videos; Internet; learning resource lab; library services; nursing audiovisuals; placement services for program completers; remedial services; resume preparation assistance; skills, simulation, or other laboratory; tutoring.
Library Facilities 6,608 volumes in health, 1,573 volumes in nursing; 2,958 periodical subscriptions health-care related.

BACCALAUREATE PROGRAMS

Degree BSN
Available Programs ADN to Baccalaureate; Accelerated Baccalaureate; Accelerated Baccalaureate for Second Degree; Baccalaureate for Second Degree; Generic Baccalaureate.
Site Options Jacksonville, FL.
Study Options Full-time.
Online Degree Options Yes.
Program Entrance Requirements Minimum overall college GPA of 2.5, transcript of college record, CPR certification, written essay, health exam, health insurance, high school biology, high school chemistry, high school transcript, immunizations, interview, 3 letters of recommendation, minimum high school GPA of 3.5, minimum GPA in nursing prerequisites of 2.0, prerequisite course work. Transfer students are accepted. *Application deadline:* 4/1 (fall), 9/15 (spring), 1/15 (summer). *Application fee:* $30.
Advanced Placement Credit given for nursing courses completed elsewhere dependent upon specific evaluations.
Expenses (2015–16) *Tuition:* full-time $32,620; part-time $1085 per credit hour. *International tuition:* $32,620 full-time. *Room and board:* $13,323; room only: $7800 per academic year.
Financial Aid 90% of baccalaureate students in nursing programs received some form of financial aid in 2014–15.
Contact Mrs. Stephanie Bloom, Director of Enrollment and Program Development, School of Nursing, Jacksonville University, 2800 University Boulevard North, Jacksonville, FL 32211. *Telephone:* 904-256-7286. *Fax:* 904-256-7287. *E-mail:* slbloom@ju.edu.

GRADUATE PROGRAMS

Expenses (2015–16) *Tuition:* full-time $13,080; part-time $545 per credit hour. *International tuition:* $13,080 full-time. *Room and board:* $13,323; room only: $7800 per academic year.
Contact Ms. Stephanie Bloom, Director of Admissions and Enrollment CHS, School of Nursing, Jacksonville University, 2800 University Boulevard North, Jacksonville, FL 32211. *Telephone:* 904-256-7286. *Fax:* 904-256-7287. *E-mail:* slbloom@ju.edu.

MASTER'S DEGREE PROGRAM
Degrees MSN; MSN/MBA
Available Programs Master's; RN to Master's.
Concentrations Available Nursing administration; nursing education; nursing informatics. *Nurse practitioner programs in:* family health, psychiatric/mental health.
Site Options Jacksonville, FL.
Study Options Full-time and part-time.
Online Degree Options Yes.
Program Entrance Requirements Clinical experience, minimum overall college GPA of 3.0, transcript of college record, CPR certification, written essay, immunizations, interview, 3 letters of recommendation, physical assessment course, professional liability insurance/malpractice insurance, resume, statistics course. *Application*

deadline: 3/15 (fall), 11/15 (spring), 4/15 (summer). Applications may be processed on a rolling basis for some programs. *Application fee:* $50.

Advanced Placement Credit given for nursing courses completed elsewhere dependent upon specific evaluations.

Degree Requirements 30 total credit hours.

POST-MASTER'S PROGRAM

Areas of Study Nursing informatics. *Nurse practitioner programs in:* adult-gerontology acute care, family health, psychiatric/mental health.

DOCTORAL DEGREE PROGRAM

Degree DNP

Available Programs Doctorate; Post-Baccalaureate Doctorate.

Areas of Study Advanced practice nursing, nursing administration.

Site Options Jacksonville, FL.

Program Entrance Requirements Clinical experience, minimum overall college GPA of 3.3, interview by faculty committee, 3 letters of recommendation, MSN or equivalent, statistics course, vita, writing sample. Application deadline: 7/15 (fall), 11/15 (spring), 4/15 (summer). Applications may be processed on a rolling basis for some programs. Application fee: $50.

Degree Requirements 39 total credit hours, residency.

Kaplan University Online

The School of Nursing Online
Fort Lauderdale, Florida

DEGREES • BSN • MSN

BACCALAUREATE PROGRAMS

Degree BSN

Available Programs Generic Baccalaureate.

Contact *Telephone:* 866-527-5268.

GRADUATE PROGRAMS

Contact *Telephone:* 866-527-5268.

MASTER'S DEGREE PROGRAM

Degree MSN

Available Programs Master's; RN to Master's.

Concentrations Available Health-care administration; nursing education; nursing informatics. *Nurse practitioner programs in:* adult health, family health.

Keiser University

Nursing Programs
Fort Lauderdale, Florida

Founded in 1977

DEGREES • BSN • MSN

BACCALAUREATE PROGRAMS

Degree BSN

Available Programs RN Baccalaureate.

Contact *Telephone:* 954-776-4456. *Fax:* 954-771-4894.

GRADUATE PROGRAMS

Contact *Telephone:* 954-776-4456. *Fax:* 954-771-4894.

MASTER'S DEGREE PROGRAM

Degree MSN

Available Programs Master's.

Program Entrance Requirements Minimum overall college GPA of 2.7.

Degree Requirements 33 total credit hours.

Keiser University

Nursing Programs
Fort Myers, Florida

DEGREES • BSN • MSN

BACCALAUREATE PROGRAMS

Degree BSN

Available Programs RN Baccalaureate.

Contact *Telephone:* 239-277-1336. *Fax:* 239-277-1259.

GRADUATE PROGRAMS

Contact *Telephone:* 239-277-1336. *Fax:* 239-277-1259.

MASTER'S DEGREE PROGRAM

Degree MSN

Available Programs Master's.

Program Entrance Requirements Minimum overall college GPA of 2.7.

Degree Requirements 33 total credit hours.

Keiser University

Nursing Programs
Jacksonville, Florida

DEGREES • BSN • MSN

BACCALAUREATE PROGRAMS

Degree BSN

Available Programs RN Baccalaureate.

Contact *Telephone:* 904-296-3440. *Fax:* 904-296-3407.

GRADUATE PROGRAMS

Contact *Telephone:* 904-296-3440. *Fax:* 904-296-3407.

MASTER'S DEGREE PROGRAM

Degree MSN

Available Programs Master's.

Program Entrance Requirements Minimum overall college GPA of 2.7.

Degree Requirements 33 total credit hours.

Keiser University

Nursing Programs
Lakeland, Florida

DEGREES • BSN • MSN

BACCALAUREATE PROGRAMS

Degree BSN

Available Programs RN Baccalaureate.

Contact *Telephone:* 863-682-6020. *Fax:* 863-688-6196.

GRADUATE PROGRAMS

Contact *Telephone:* 863-682-6020. *Fax:* 863-688-6196.

MASTER'S DEGREE PROGRAM

Degree MSN

Available Programs Master's.

Program Entrance Requirements Minimum overall college GPA of 2.7.

Degree Requirements 33 total credit hours.

Keiser University
Nursing Programs
Melbourne, Florida

Founded in 1989
DEGREES • BSN • MSN

BACCALAUREATE PROGRAMS

Degree BSN
Available Programs RN Baccalaureate.
Contact *Telephone:* 321-409-4800. *Fax:* 321-725-3766.

GRADUATE PROGRAMS

Contact *Telephone:* 321-409-4800. *Fax:* 321-725-3766.

MASTER'S DEGREE PROGRAM

Degree MSN
Available Programs Master's.
Program Entrance Requirements Minimum overall college GPA of 2.7.
Degree Requirements 33 total credit hours.

Keiser University
Nursing Programs
Miami, Florida

DEGREES • BSN • MSN

BACCALAUREATE PROGRAMS

Degree BSN
Available Programs RN Baccalaureate.
Contact *Telephone:* 305-596-2226. *Fax:* 305-596-7077.

GRADUATE PROGRAMS

Contact *Telephone:* 305-596-2226. *Fax:* 305-596-7077.

MASTER'S DEGREE PROGRAM

Degree MSN
Available Programs Master's.
Program Entrance Requirements Minimum overall college GPA of 2.7.
Degree Requirements 33 total credit hours.

Keiser University
Nursing Programs
Orlando, Florida

DEGREES • BSN • MSN

BACCALAUREATE PROGRAMS

Degree BSN
Available Programs RN Baccalaureate.
Contact *Telephone:* 407-273-5800. *Fax:* 407-381-1233.

GRADUATE PROGRAMS

Contact *Telephone:* 407-273-5800. *Fax:* 407-381-1233.

MASTER'S DEGREE PROGRAM

Degree MSN
Available Programs Master's.
Program Entrance Requirements Minimum overall college GPA of 2.7.
Degree Requirements 33 total credit hours.

Keiser University
Nursing Programs
Port St. Lucie, Florida

Founded in 1999
DEGREES • BSN • MSN

BACCALAUREATE PROGRAMS

Degree BSN
Available Programs RN Baccalaureate.
Contact *Telephone:* 772-398-9990. *Fax:* 772-335-9619.

GRADUATE PROGRAMS

Contact *Telephone:* 772-398-9990. *Fax:* 772-335-9619.

MASTER'S DEGREE PROGRAM

Degree MSN
Available Programs Master's.
Program Entrance Requirements Minimum overall college GPA of 2.7.
Degree Requirements 33 total credit hours.

Keiser University
Nursing Programs
Sarasota, Florida

Founded in 1995
DEGREES • BSN • MSN

BACCALAUREATE PROGRAMS

Degree BSN
Available Programs RN Baccalaureate.
Contact *Telephone:* 941-907-3900. *Fax:* 941-907-2016.

GRADUATE PROGRAMS

Contact *Telephone:* 941-907-3900. *Fax:* 941-907-2016.

MASTER'S DEGREE PROGRAM

Degree MSN
Available Programs Master's.
Program Entrance Requirements Minimum overall college GPA of 2.7.
Degree Requirements 33 total credit hours.

Keiser University
Nursing Programs
Tallahassee, Florida

Founded in 1992
DEGREES • BSN • MSN

BACCALAUREATE PROGRAMS

Degree BSN
Available Programs RN Baccalaureate.
Contact *Telephone:* 850-906-9494. *Fax:* 850-906-9497.

GRADUATE PROGRAMS

Contact *Telephone:* 850-906-9494. *Fax:* 850-906-9497.

MASTER'S DEGREE PROGRAM

Degree MSN
Available Programs Master's.
Program Entrance Requirements Minimum overall college GPA of 2.7.
Degree Requirements 33 total credit hours.

Keiser University
Nursing Programs
Tampa, Florida

DEGREES • BSN • MSN

BACCALAUREATE PROGRAMS

Degree BSN
Available Programs RN Baccalaureate.
Contact *Telephone:* 813-885-4900. *Fax:* 813-885-4911.

GRADUATE PROGRAMS

Contact *Telephone:* 813-885-4900. *Fax:* 813-885-4911.

MASTER'S DEGREE PROGRAM
Degree MSN
Available Programs Master's.
Program Entrance Requirements Minimum overall college GPA of 2.7.
Degree Requirements 33 total credit hours.

Miami Dade College
School of Nursing
Miami, Florida

http://mdc.edu
Founded in 1960
DEGREE • BSN
Nursing Program Faculty 14 (73% with doctorates).
Baccalaureate Enrollment 578 **Women** 88% **Men** 12% **Part-time** 92%
Distance Learning Courses Available.
Nursing Student Activities Nursing Honor Society, Student Nurses' Association.
Nursing Student Resources Academic advising; academic or career counseling; assistance for students with disabilities; bookstore; campus computer network; computer lab; computer-assisted instruction; e-mail services; interactive nursing skills videos; Internet; learning resource lab; library services; nursing audiovisuals; remedial services; resume preparation assistance; skills, simulation, or other laboratory; tutoring.
Library Facilities 14,000 volumes in health, 3,580 volumes in nursing; 14,090 periodical subscriptions health-care related.

BACCALAUREATE PROGRAMS

Degree BSN
Available Programs RN Baccalaureate.
Site Options Miami, FL.
Program Entrance Requirements CPR certification, health exam, immunizations, minimum GPA in nursing prerequisites of 2.5, prerequisite course work, RN licensure. Transfer students are accepted. *Application deadline:* 5/1 (fall), 9/1 (spring). *Application fee:* $200.
Contact *Telephone:* 305-237-4039.

Northwest Florida State College
RN to BSN Degree Program
Niceville, Florida

http://www.fsw.edu/academics/programs/bsnursing
Founded in 1963
DEGREE • BSN
Nursing Program Faculty 6 (50% with doctorates).
Baccalaureate Enrollment 98 **Women** 89% **Men** 11% **Part-time** 94%
Distance Learning Courses Available.
Nursing Student Activities Student Nurses' Association, nursing club.
Nursing Student Resources Academic advising; academic or career counseling; assistance for students with disabilities; bookstore; campus computer network; career placement assistance; computer lab; computer-assisted instruction; daycare for children of students; e-mail services; employment services for current students; interactive nursing skills videos; Internet; learning resource lab; library services; nursing audiovisuals; placement services for program completers; remedial services; resume preparation assistance; skills, simulation, or other laboratory; tutoring; unpaid internships.
Library Facilities 3,951 volumes in health, 645 volumes in nursing; 2,143 periodical subscriptions health-care related.

BACCALAUREATE PROGRAMS

Degree BSN
Available Programs ADN to Baccalaureate.
Study Options Full-time and part-time.
Program Entrance Requirements Transcript of college record, CPR certification, health exam, immunizations, minimum GPA in nursing prerequisites of 2.75, RN licensure. Transfer students are accepted. *Application deadline:* 7/1 (fall), 11/1 (spring), 3/15 (summer). Applications may be processed on a rolling basis for some programs.
Advanced Placement Credit given for nursing courses completed elsewhere dependent upon specific evaluations.
Expenses (2015–16) *Tuition, state resident:* part-time $123 per credit hour. *Tuition, nonresident:* part-time $451 per credit hour.
Contact Dr. Marty L. Walker, Director of Nursing, RN to BSN Degree Program, Northwest Florida State College, 100 College Boulevard, Niceville, FL 32578. *Telephone:* 850-729-6400. *Fax:* 850-729-6484. *E-mail:* walkerm@nwfsc.edu.

Nova Southeastern University
College of Health Care Sciences
Fort Lauderdale, Florida

http://www.nova.edu/nursing
Founded in 1964
DEGREES • BSN • MSN
Distance Learning Courses Available.
Nursing Student Activities Sigma Theta Tau, Student Nurses' Association.
Nursing Student Resources Academic advising; academic or career counseling; assistance for students with disabilities; bookstore; campus computer network; career placement assistance; computer lab; computer-assisted instruction; e-mail services; employment services for current students; housing assistance; interactive nursing skills videos; Internet; learning resource lab; library services; placement services for program completers; resume preparation assistance; skills, simulation, or other laboratory; tutoring.

BACCALAUREATE PROGRAMS

Degree BSN
Available Programs Generic Baccalaureate; RN Baccalaureate.
Site Options Fort Myers, FL; Kendall, FL.
Study Options Full-time.
Online Degree Options Yes.
Program Entrance Requirements Minimum overall college GPA of 3.0, transcript of college record, health insurance, immunizations, interview, minimum GPA in nursing prerequisites of 2.75, prerequisite course work. *Application deadline:* 4/1 (fall), 10/1 (winter). *Application fee:* $50.
Contact *Telephone:* 800-338-4723. *Fax:* 954-262-8000 Ext. 7184.

GRADUATE PROGRAMS

Contact *Telephone:* 954-262-1101. *Fax:* 877-640-0218.

MASTER'S DEGREE PROGRAM
Degree MSN
Available Programs Master's; RN to Master's.
Concentrations Available Nursing administration; nursing education; nursing informatics.
Study Options Full-time and part-time.
Online Degree Options Yes (online only).
Program Entrance Requirements Minimum overall college GPA of 3.0, transcript of college record, written essay, immunizations, 2 letters of recommendation, statistics course, GRE General Test, MCAT. *Application deadline:* 8/1 (fall), 12/1 (winter). *Application fee:* $50.
Degree Requirements 36 total credit hours, thesis or project.

DOCTORAL DEGREE PROGRAM
Program Entrance Requirements GRE General Test.

Palm Beach Atlantic University

School of Nursing
West Palm Beach, Florida

http://www.pba.edu/school-of-nursing
Founded in 1968
DEGREES • BSN • DNP • MSN
Nursing Program Faculty 28 (7% with doctorates).
Baccalaureate Enrollment 109 **Women** 92% **Men** 8%
Graduate Enrollment 60 **Women** 90% **Men** 10%
Distance Learning Courses Available.
Nursing Student Activities Nursing Honor Society, Sigma Theta Tau, Student Nurses' Association.
Nursing Student Resources Academic advising; academic or career counseling; bookstore; campus computer network; career placement assistance; computer lab; computer-assisted instruction; e-mail services; employment services for current students; Internet; learning resource lab; library services; nursing audiovisuals; placement services for program completers; remedial services; resume preparation assistance; skills, simulation, or other laboratory; tutoring.
Library Facilities 6,151 volumes in health, 560 volumes in nursing; 8,402 periodical subscriptions health-care related.

BACCALAUREATE PROGRAMS

Degree BSN
Available Programs ADN to Baccalaureate; Baccalaureate for Second Degree.
Study Options Full-time.
Online Degree Options Yes.
Program Entrance Requirements Transcript of college record, written essay, health insurance, 3 letters of recommendation, minimum high school GPA of 3.0, minimum GPA in nursing prerequisites of 3.0, prerequisite course work. Transfer students are accepted. *Application deadline:* 10/1 (spring), 3/1 (summer). *Application fee:* $50.
Expenses (2015–16) *Tuition:* full-time $26,750; part-time $900 per credit hour. *Room and board:* $8000; room only: $4000 per academic year. *Required fees:* full-time $1300.
Financial Aid *Gift aid (need-based):* Federal Pell, FSEOG, state, private, college/university gift aid from institutional funds. *Loans:* Federal Direct (Subsidized and Unsubsidized Stafford PLUS), Perkins. *Work-study:* Federal Work-Study, part-time campus jobs. *Financial aid application deadline:* 8/1(priority: 5/1).
Contact BSN Program, School of Nursing, Palm Beach Atlantic University, 901 South Flagler Drive, PO Box 24708, West Palm Beach, FL 33416-4708. *Telephone:* 561-803-2825. *Fax:* 561-803-2828. *E-mail:* admit@pba.edu.

GRADUATE PROGRAMS

Contact Graduate Admissions, Coordinator for Evening and Graduate Admissions, School of Nursing, Palm Beach Atlantic University, 901 South Flagler Drive, West Palm Beach, FL 33416. *Telephone:* 561-803-2122. *E-mail:* grad@pba.edu.

MASTER'S DEGREE PROGRAM

Degree MSN
Available Programs Master's; RN to Master's.
Concentrations Available Health-care administration.
Study Options Full-time and part-time.
Program Entrance Requirements Clinical experience, computer literacy, minimum overall college GPA of 3.8, transcript of college record, written essay, immunizations, 3 letters of recommendation, resume. *Application deadline:* 8/21 (fall), 12/24 (spring). Applications may be processed on a rolling basis for some programs. *Application fee:* $45.
Advanced Placement Credit by examination available. Credit given for nursing courses completed elsewhere dependent upon specific evaluations.
Degree Requirements 39 total credit hours, thesis or project.

DOCTORAL DEGREE PROGRAM

Degree DNP
Available Programs Doctorate; Post-Baccalaureate Doctorate.
Areas of Study Advanced practice nursing.
Program Entrance Requirements Clinical experience, minimum overall college GPA of 3.8, interview by faculty committee, 3 letters of recommendation, vita, writing sample. Application deadline: 8/21 (fall), 12/24 (spring). Applications may be processed on a rolling basis for some programs. Application fee: $45.
Degree Requirements 74 total credit hours.

Polk State College

RN to BSN Program
Winter Haven, Florida

Founded in 1964
DEGREE • BSN

BACCALAUREATE PROGRAMS

Degree BSN
Available Programs RN Baccalaureate.
Contact *Telephone:* 863-297-1039.

St. Petersburg College

Department of Nursing
St. Petersburg, Florida

http://www.spcollege.edu/
Founded in 1927
DEGREE • BSN
Nursing Program Faculty 27 (56% with doctorates).
Baccalaureate Enrollment 688 **Women** 85% **Men** 15%
Distance Learning Courses Available.
Nursing Student Activities Sigma Theta Tau, Student Nurses' Association.
Nursing Student Resources Academic advising; academic or career counseling; assistance for students with disabilities; bookstore; campus computer network; computer lab; computer-assisted instruction; e-mail services; employment services for current students; interactive nursing skills videos; Internet; learning resource lab; library services; nursing audiovisuals; placement services for program completers; remedial services; resume preparation assistance; skills, simulation, or other laboratory; tutoring; unpaid internships.
Library Facilities 1,390 volumes in health, 484 volumes in nursing; 77 periodical subscriptions health-care related.

BACCALAUREATE PROGRAMS

Degree BSN
Available Programs ADN to Baccalaureate; RN Baccalaureate.
Site Options Pinellas Park, FL.
Online Degree Options Yes.
Program Entrance Requirements Minimum overall college GPA of 2.0, transcript of college record, high school transcript, prerequisite course work, RN licensure. Transfer students are accepted. *Application deadline:* 7/13 (fall), 11/9 (spring). *Application fee:* $40.
Contact *Telephone:* 727-341-3640. *Fax:* 727-341-3646.

CONTINUING EDUCATION PROGRAM

Contact *Telephone:* 727-341-3374. *Fax:* 727-341-4197.

Santa Fe College

Bachelor of Science in Nursing
Gainesville, Florida

http://www.sfcollege.edu/healthsciences/nursing/
Founded in 1966
DEGREE • BSN

BACCALAUREATE PROGRAMS

Degree BSN
Available Programs RN Baccalaureate.
Contact Nursing Program, Bachelor of Science in Nursing, Santa Fe College, 3000 NW 83rd Street, Gainesville, FL 32606. *Telephone:* 352-395-5000.

State College of Florida Manatee-Sarasota
Nursing Degree Program
Bradenton, Florida

http://scf.edu/Academics/Nursing/NursingA_S_/default.asp
Founded in 1957
DEGREE • BSN
Nursing Program Faculty 12 (92% with doctorates).
Baccalaureate Enrollment 313 **Women** 87% **Men** 13% **Part-time** 70%
Distance Learning Courses Available.
Nursing Student Activities Nursing Honor Society, Student Nurses' Association.
Nursing Student Resources Academic advising; academic or career counseling; assistance for students with disabilities; bookstore; campus computer network; career placement assistance; computer lab; computer-assisted instruction; e-mail services; interactive nursing skills videos; Internet; learning resource lab; library services; nursing audiovisuals; remedial services; resume preparation assistance; skills, simulation, or other laboratory; tutoring.
Library Facilities 1,500 volumes in health, 750 volumes in nursing; 110 periodical subscriptions health-care related.

BACCALAUREATE PROGRAMS

Degree BSN
Available Programs ADN to Baccalaureate; RN Baccalaureate.
Site Options Sarasota, FL.
Study Options Full-time and part-time.
Online Degree Options Yes.
Program Entrance Requirements Minimum overall college GPA of 2.0, prerequisite course work, RN licensure. Transfer students are accepted. *Application deadline:* 6/1 (fall), 10/1 (spring), 3/1 (summer).
Advanced Placement Credit given for nursing courses completed elsewhere dependent upon specific evaluations.
Expenses (2015–16) *Tuition, state resident:* part-time $112 per credit hour. *Tuition, nonresident:* part-time $442 per credit hour.
Financial Aid 90% of baccalaureate students in nursing programs received some form of financial aid in 2014–15. *Gift aid (need-based):* Federal Pell, FSEOG, state, private, college/university gift aid from institutional funds. *Loans:* college/university. *Work-study:* Federal Work-Study. *Financial aid application deadline:* 8/15.
Contact Admissions, Nursing Degree Program, State College of Florida Manatee-Sarasota, 5840 26th Street West, Bradenton, FL 34206. *Telephone:* 941-752-5050. *Fax:* 941-727-6380. *E-mail:* admissions@scf.edu.

University of Central Florida
College of Nursing
Orlando, Florida

http://www.nursing.ucf.edu/
Founded in 1963
DEGREES • BSN • DNP • MSN • PHD
Nursing Program Faculty 117 (39% with doctorates).
Baccalaureate Enrollment 1,484 **Women** 85% **Men** 15% **Part-time** 70%
Graduate Enrollment 337 **Women** 90% **Men** 10% **Part-time** 86%
Distance Learning Courses Available.
Nursing Student Activities Nursing Honor Society, Sigma Theta Tau, Student Nurses' Association.
Nursing Student Resources Academic advising; academic or career counseling; assistance for students with disabilities; bookstore; campus computer network; career placement assistance; computer lab; computer-assisted instruction; daycare for children of students; e-mail services; employment services for current students; externships; housing assistance; interactive nursing skills videos; Internet; learning resource lab; library services; nursing audiovisuals; paid internships; remedial services; resume preparation assistance; skills, simulation, or other laboratory; tutoring.
Library Facilities 81,762 volumes in health, 3,757 volumes in nursing; 8,673 periodical subscriptions health-care related.

BACCALAUREATE PROGRAMS

Degree BSN

Available Programs ADN to Baccalaureate; Accelerated Baccalaureate for Second Degree; Generic Baccalaureate; RN Baccalaureate.
Site Options Cocoa Beach, FL; Daytona Beach, FL; Leesburg, FL.
Study Options Full-time and part-time.
Program Entrance Requirements Minimum overall college GPA of 3.0, transcript of college record, CPR certification, health exam, health insurance, high school foreign language, high school math, high school transcript, immunizations, minimum high school GPA of 3.0, minimum GPA in nursing prerequisites of 3.0, prerequisite course work. Transfer students are accepted. *Application deadline:* 2/15 (fall), 8/16 (spring). *Application fee:* $30.
Advanced Placement Credit given for nursing courses completed elsewhere dependent upon specific evaluations.
Expenses (2015–16) *Tuition, state resident:* full-time $3700; part-time $105 per credit hour. *Tuition, nonresident:* full-time $22,470; part-time $616 per credit hour. *International tuition:* $22,470 full-time. *Room and board:* $9700; room only: $6000 per academic year. *Required fees:* full-time $3150.
Financial Aid *Gift aid (need-based):* Federal Pell, FSEOG, state, private, college/university gift aid from institutional funds. *Loans:* Federal Direct (Subsidized and Unsubsidized Stafford PLUS), Perkins. *Work-study:* Federal Work-Study, part-time campus jobs. *Financial aid application deadline:* 6/30(priority: 3/1).
Contact Dr. Kelly Allred, Undergraduate Program Coordinator, College of Nursing, University of Central Florida, 12201 Research Parkway, Suite 300, Orlando, FL 32826. *Telephone:* 407-823-2744. *Fax:* 407-823-5675. *E-mail:* ucfnurse@mail.ucf.edu.

GRADUATE PROGRAMS

Expenses (2015–16) *Tuition, state resident:* part-time $288 per credit hour. *Tuition, nonresident:* part-time $1073 per credit hour. *Required fees:* part-time $80 per credit.
Contact Dr. Susan Chase, Associate Dean for Graduate Affairs, College of Nursing, University of Central Florida, PO Box 162210, Orlando, FL 32816-2210. *Telephone:* 407-823-3079. *Fax:* 407-823-5675. *E-mail:* susan.chase@ucf.edu.

MASTER'S DEGREE PROGRAM
Degree MSN
Available Programs Accelerated RN to Master's; Master's; Master's for Nurses with Non-Nursing Degrees.
Concentrations Available Nursing administration; nursing education. *Clinical nurse specialist programs in:* acute care. *Nurse practitioner programs in:* adult health, family health.
Study Options Full-time and part-time.
Online Degree Options Yes.
Program Entrance Requirements Clinical experience, minimum overall college GPA of 3.5, transcript of college record, written essay, resume, statistics course. *Application deadline:* 2/15 (fall), 9/15 (spring). *Application fee:* $30.
Advanced Placement Credit given for nursing courses completed elsewhere dependent upon specific evaluations.
Degree Requirements 46 total credit hours.

POST-MASTER'S PROGRAM
Areas of Study *Clinical nurse specialist programs in:* acute care. *Nurse practitioner programs in:* adult health, family health.

DOCTORAL DEGREE PROGRAM
Degree DNP
Available Programs Doctorate.
Areas of Study Advanced practice nursing, family health, nursing administration.
Online Degree Options Yes.
Program Entrance Requirements Minimum overall college GPA of 3.5, 3 letters of recommendation, statistics course, vita.
Degree Requirements 43-86 total credit hours, project.

Degree PhD
Available Programs Doctorate.
Areas of Study Individualized study, nursing research.
Program Entrance Requirements Minimum overall college GPA of 3.5, interview by faculty committee, interview, 3 letters of recommendation, MSN or equivalent, statistics course, vita, writing sample. Application deadline: 2/15 (fall), 9/15 (spring), 1/15 (summer). Application fee: $30.
Degree Requirements 60 total credit hours, dissertation, oral exam.

University of Florida
College of Nursing
Gainesville, Florida

http://www.nursing.ufl.edu/
Founded in 1853
DEGREES • BSN • MSN • MSN/PHD • PHD
Nursing Program Faculty 62 (50% with doctorates).
Baccalaureate Enrollment 374 **Women** 94% **Men** 6%
Graduate Enrollment 364 **Women** 97% **Men** 3% **Part-time** 56%
Distance Learning Courses Available.
Nursing Student Activities Nursing Honor Society, Sigma Theta Tau, Student Nurses' Association.
Nursing Student Resources Academic advising; academic or career counseling; assistance for students with disabilities; bookstore; campus computer network; career placement assistance; computer lab; computer-assisted instruction; daycare for children of students; e-mail services; employment services for current students; housing assistance; interactive nursing skills videos; Internet; learning resource lab; library services; nursing audiovisuals; placement services for program completers; remedial services; resume preparation assistance; skills, simulation, or other laboratory; tutoring.
Library Facilities 260,000 volumes in health, 3,000 volumes in nursing; 200 periodical subscriptions health-care related.

BACCALAUREATE PROGRAMS

Degree BSN
Available Programs Accelerated Baccalaureate for Second Degree; Generic Baccalaureate.
Study Options Full-time.
Program Entrance Requirements Minimum overall college GPA of 2.8, transcript of college record, CPR certification, written essay, health exam, health insurance, high school biology, high school chemistry, high school foreign language, high school transcript, immunizations, 2 letters of recommendation, minimum GPA in nursing prerequisites of 2.8, pre-requisite course work. Transfer students are accepted. *Application deadline:* 3/15 (fall), 1/15 (summer). *Application fee:* $30.
Advanced Placement Credit by examination available. Credit given for nursing courses completed elsewhere dependent upon specific evaluations.
Contact *Telephone:* 352-273-6383. *Fax:* 352-273-6440.

GRADUATE PROGRAMS

Contact *Telephone:* 352-273-6331. *Fax:* 352-273-6440.

MASTER'S DEGREE PROGRAM
Degrees MSN; MSN/PhD
Available Programs Master's.
Concentrations Available Clinical nurse leader; nurse-midwifery. *Clinical nurse specialist programs in:* psychiatric/mental health, public health. *Nurse practitioner programs in:* acute care, adult health, family health, neonatal health, pediatric, psychiatric/mental health.
Site Options Jacksonville, FL.
Study Options Full-time and part-time.
Online Degree Options Yes.
Program Entrance Requirements Minimum overall college GPA of 3.0, transcript of college record, CPR certification, written essay, immunizations, 2 letters of recommendation, resume, GRE General Test. *Application deadline:* 3/15 (fall). Applications may be processed on a rolling basis for some programs. *Application fee:* $30.
Advanced Placement Credit given for nursing courses completed elsewhere dependent upon specific evaluations.
Degree Requirements 46 total credit hours, comprehensive exam.

POST-MASTER'S PROGRAM
Areas of Study Clinical nurse leader; nurse-midwifery. *Clinical nurse specialist programs in:* psychiatric/mental health, public health. *Nurse practitioner programs in:* acute care, adult health, family health, neonatal health, pediatric, psychiatric/mental health.

DOCTORAL DEGREE PROGRAM
Degree PhD
Available Programs Doctorate; Post-Baccalaureate Doctorate.
Areas of Study Aging, bio-behavioral research, health policy, nursing policy, nursing science, oncology, women's health.
Site Options Jacksonville, FL.
Online Degree Options Yes.

Program Entrance Requirements Minimum overall college GPA of 3.5, 3 letters of recommendation, MSN or equivalent, vita, writing sample, GRE General Test. Application deadline: 3/15 (fall). Applications may be processed on a rolling basis for some programs. Application fee: $30.
Degree Requirements 62 total credit hours, dissertation.

University of Miami
School of Nursing and Health Studies
Coral Gables, Florida

http://www.miami.edu/sonhs
Founded in 1925
DEGREES • BSN • DNP • MSN
Nursing Program Faculty 75 (61% with doctorates).
Baccalaureate Enrollment 280 **Women** 88.21% **Men** 11.79% **Part-time** 2.5%
Graduate Enrollment 253 **Women** 82.61% **Men** 17.39% **Part-time** 67.19%
Distance Learning Courses Available.
Nursing Student Activities Nursing Honor Society, Sigma Theta Tau, Student Nurses' Association.
Nursing Student Resources Academic advising; academic or career counseling; assistance for students with disabilities; bookstore; campus computer network; career placement assistance; computer lab; computer-assisted instruction; e-mail services; employment services for current students; externships; housing assistance; interactive nursing skills videos; Internet; learning resource lab; library services; nursing audiovisuals; placement services for program completers; remedial services; resume preparation assistance; skills, simulation, or other laboratory; tutoring; unpaid internships.
Library Facilities 89,500 volumes in health, 1,700 volumes in nursing.

BACCALAUREATE PROGRAMS

Degree BSN
Available Programs Accelerated Baccalaureate for Second Degree; Baccalaureate for Second Degree; Generic Baccalaureate; RN Baccalaureate.
Study Options Full-time.
Program Entrance Requirements Minimum overall college GPA of 3.5, transcript of college record, written essay, high school transcript, 1 letter of recommendation. Transfer students are accepted. *Application deadline:* 11/1 (fall), 11/1 (spring). Applications may be processed on a rolling basis for some programs. *Application fee:* $70.
Expenses (2015–16) *Tuition:* full-time $44,400; part-time $1850 per credit. *International tuition:* $44,400 full-time. *Room and board:* $12,908; room only: $7556 per academic year. *Required fees:* full-time $1324; part-time $396 per term.
Financial Aid 69% of baccalaureate students in nursing programs received some form of financial aid in 2014–15.
Contact Mr. Sean Kilpatrick, Assistant Dean for Student Services, School of Nursing and Health Studies, University of Miami, PO Box 248153-3850, Coral Gables, FL 33124-3850. *Telephone:* 305-284-4199. *Fax:* 305-284-4827. *E-mail:* smkilpatrick@miami.edu.

GRADUATE PROGRAMS

Expenses (2015–16) *Tuition:* full-time $40,700; part-time $1850 per credit. *International tuition:* $40,700 full-time. *Required fees:* full-time $1718; part-time $910 per term.
Financial Aid 85% of graduate students in nursing programs received some form of financial aid in 2014–15. 1 fellowship (averaging $36,000 per year), 6 research assistantships with tuition reimbursements available (averaging $36,000 per year), 4 teaching assistantships with tuition reimbursements available (averaging $36,000 per year) were awarded; Federal Work-Study, institutionally sponsored loans, scholarships, and unspecified assistantships also available. Aid available to part-time students. *Financial aid application deadline:* 3/1.
Contact Mr. Sean Kilpatrick, Assistant Dean for Student Services, School of Nursing and Health Studies, University of Miami, PO Box 248153, M. Christine Schwartz Center, Coral Gables, FL 33124-3850. *Telephone:* 305-284-4199. *Fax:* 305-284-5686. *E-mail:* smkilpatrick@miami.edu.

MASTER'S DEGREE PROGRAM
Degree MSN
Available Programs Master's.

Concentrations Available Nursing informatics. *Nurse practitioner programs in:* adult-gerontology acute care, family health, primary care.
Study Options Full-time and part-time.
Program Entrance Requirements Clinical experience, minimum overall college GPA of 3.0, transcript of college record, CPR certification, written essay, immunizations, interview, 3 letters of recommendation, resume, statistics course, GRE General Test. *Application deadline:* 4/1 (fall), 9/1 (spring). Applications may be processed on a rolling basis for some programs. *Application fee:* $65.
Degree Requirements 37 total credit hours, comprehensive exam.

POST-MASTER'S PROGRAM

Areas of Study *Nurse practitioner programs in:* adult-gerontology acute care, family health, primary care, psychiatric/mental health.

DOCTORAL DEGREE PROGRAM

Degree DNP
Available Programs Doctorate; Post-Baccalaureate Doctorate.
Areas of Study Advanced practice nursing, nurse executive.
Program Entrance Requirements Clinical experience, minimum overall college GPA of 3.0, interview by faculty committee, interview, 2 letters of recommendation, MSN or equivalent, statistics course, vita, writing sample, GRE General Test. Application deadline: 4/1 (fall), 9/1 (spring). Applications may be processed on a rolling basis for some programs. Application fee: $65.
Degree Requirements 41 total credit hours, written exam.

CONTINUING EDUCATION PROGRAM

Contact Mr. Sean Kilpatrick, Assistant Dean, School of Nursing and Health Studies, University of Miami, PO Box 248153, M. Christine Schwartz Center, Room 152, Coral Gables, FL 33124-3850. *Telephone:* 305-284-4199. *Fax:* 305-284-4827. *E-mail:* smkilpatrick@miami.edu.

University of North Florida
School of Nursing
Jacksonville, Florida

http://www.unf.edu/brooks/nursing/
Founded in 1965
DEGREES • BSN • MSN
Nursing Program Faculty 19 (50% with doctorates).
Baccalaureate Enrollment 279 **Women** 85% **Men** 15% **Part-time** 27%
Graduate Enrollment 35 **Women** 86% **Men** 14% **Part-time** 70%
Nursing Student Activities Sigma Theta Tau, Student Nurses' Association.
Nursing Student Resources Academic advising; academic or career counseling; assistance for students with disabilities; bookstore; campus computer network; career placement assistance; computer lab; computer-assisted instruction; e-mail services; interactive nursing skills videos; Internet; learning resource lab; library services; nursing audiovisuals; resume preparation assistance; skills, simulation, or other laboratory.
Library Facilities 30,466 volumes in health, 3,000 volumes in nursing; 200 periodical subscriptions health-care related.

BACCALAUREATE PROGRAMS

Degree BSN
Available Programs Accelerated Baccalaureate for Second Degree; Generic Baccalaureate; RN Baccalaureate.
Study Options Full-time.
Program Entrance Requirements Minimum overall college GPA of 2.7, CPR certification, written essay, health exam, immunizations, interview, minimum high school GPA, minimum GPA in nursing prerequisites of 3.0, professional liability insurance/malpractice insurance, prerequisite course work. Transfer students are accepted.
Advanced Placement Credit given for nursing courses completed elsewhere dependent upon specific evaluations.
Contact *Telephone:* 904-620-2418.

GRADUATE PROGRAMS

Contact *Telephone:* 904-620-2684. *Fax:* 904-620-2848.

MASTER'S DEGREE PROGRAM

Degree MSN

Available Programs Master's; RN to Master's.
Concentrations Available *Clinical nurse specialist programs in:* adult health, cardiovascular, community health, critical care, gerontology, maternity-newborn, medical-surgical, pediatric, psychiatric/mental health, women's health. *Nurse practitioner programs in:* family health, primary care.
Study Options Full-time and part-time.
Program Entrance Requirements Clinical experience, computer literacy, minimum overall college GPA of 3.0, transcript of college record, CPR certification, written essay, immunizations, 2 letters of recommendation, nursing research course, physical assessment course, professional liability insurance/malpractice insurance, resume, statistics course.
Advanced Placement Credit given for nursing courses completed elsewhere dependent upon specific evaluations.
Degree Requirements 43 total credit hours, thesis or project.

POST-MASTER'S PROGRAM

Areas of Study *Nurse practitioner programs in:* family health, primary care.

University of Phoenix–North Florida Campus
College of Nursing
Jacksonville, Florida

Founded in 1976
DEGREES • BSN • MSN • MSN/ED D • MSN/MHA
Nursing Program Faculty 7 (29% with doctorates).
Baccalaureate Enrollment 13 **Women** 92.3% **Men** 7.7%
Graduate Enrollment 10 **Women** 100%
Nursing Student Activities Sigma Theta Tau.
Nursing Student Resources Academic advising; academic or career counseling; assistance for students with disabilities; bookstore; campus computer network; computer lab; computer-assisted instruction; e-mail services; interactive nursing skills videos; Internet; learning resource lab; library services; nursing audiovisuals; remedial services; skills, simulation, or other laboratory; tutoring.
Library Facilities 1,300 periodical subscriptions health-care related.

BACCALAUREATE PROGRAMS

Degree BSN
Available Programs Accelerated Baccalaureate.
Site Options Orange Park, FL.
Study Options Full-time.
Program Entrance Requirements Transcript of college record, CPR certification, immunizations, 1 letter of recommendation, RN licensure. Transfer students are accepted. *Application deadline:* Applications may be processed on a rolling basis for some programs.
Advanced Placement Credit by examination available. Credit given for nursing courses completed elsewhere dependent upon specific evaluations.
Contact *Telephone:* 904-636-6645.

GRADUATE PROGRAMS

Contact *Telephone:* 904-636-6645.

MASTER'S DEGREE PROGRAM

Degrees MSN; MSN/Ed D; MSN/MHA
Available Programs Master's.
Concentrations Available Health-care administration; nursing administration; nursing education.
Site Options Orange Park, FL.
Study Options Full-time.
Program Entrance Requirements Clinical experience, computer literacy, minimum overall college GPA of 2.5, transcript of college record. *Application deadline:* Applications may be processed on a rolling basis for some programs. *Application fee:* $45.
Advanced Placement Credit given for nursing courses completed elsewhere dependent upon specific evaluations.
Degree Requirements 39 total credit hours, thesis or project.

University of Phoenix–South Florida Campus
College of Nursing
Miramar, Florida

DEGREES • BSN • MSN • MSN/MBA • MSN/MHA
Nursing Program Faculty 24 (21% with doctorates).
Baccalaureate Enrollment 135 **Women** 96.3% **Men** 3.7%
Graduate Enrollment 102 **Women** 91.2% **Men** 8.8%
Nursing Student Activities Sigma Theta Tau.
Nursing Student Resources Academic advising; academic or career counseling; assistance for students with disabilities; bookstore; campus computer network; computer lab; computer-assisted instruction; e-mail services; interactive nursing skills videos; Internet; learning resource lab; library services; nursing audiovisuals; skills, simulation, or other laboratory; tutoring.
Library Facilities 1,300 periodical subscriptions health-care related.

BACCALAUREATE PROGRAMS

Degree BSN
Available Programs RN Baccalaureate.
Site Options Palm Beach Gardens, FL; Ft. Lauderdale, FL; Miramar, FL.
Study Options Full-time.
Online Degree Options Yes.
Program Entrance Requirements Transcript of college record, CPR certification, immunizations, 1 letter of recommendation, RN licensure. Transfer students are accepted. *Application deadline:* Applications may be processed on a rolling basis for some programs.
Advanced Placement Credit by examination available. Credit given for nursing courses completed elsewhere dependent upon specific evaluations.
Contact *Telephone:* 954-382-5303.

GRADUATE PROGRAMS

Contact *Telephone:* 954-382-5303.

MASTER'S DEGREE PROGRAM
Degrees MSN; MSN/MBA; MSN/MHA
Available Programs Master's.
Concentrations Available Health-care administration; nursing administration; nursing education.
Site Options Palm Beach Gardens, FL; Ft. Lauderdale, FL; Miramar, FL.
Study Options Full-time.
Online Degree Options Yes.
Program Entrance Requirements Clinical experience, computer literacy, minimum overall college GPA of 2.5, transcript of college record. *Application deadline:* Applications may be processed on a rolling basis for some programs. *Application fee:* $45.
Advanced Placement Credit given for nursing courses completed elsewhere dependent upon specific evaluations.
Degree Requirements 39 total credit hours, thesis or project.

University of Phoenix–West Florida Learning Center
College of Nursing
Temple Terrace, Florida

DEGREE • BSN
Nursing Program Faculty 5 (60% with doctorates).
Baccalaureate Enrollment 8 **Women** 87.5% **Men** 12.5%
Nursing Student Activities Sigma Theta Tau.
Nursing Student Resources Academic advising; academic or career counseling; assistance for students with disabilities; bookstore; campus computer network; computer lab; computer-assisted instruction; e-mail services; interactive nursing skills videos; Internet; learning resource lab; library services; nursing audiovisuals; remedial services; skills, simulation, or other laboratory; tutoring.
Library Facilities 1,300 periodical subscriptions health-care related.

BACCALAUREATE PROGRAMS

Degree BSN
Available Programs Accelerated Baccalaureate.
Site Options Tampa, FL; Clearwater, FL; Sarasota, FL.

Study Options Full-time.
Online Degree Options Yes.
Program Entrance Requirements Transcript of college record, CPR certification, immunizations, 1 letter of recommendation, RN licensure. Transfer students are accepted. *Application deadline:* Applications may be processed on a rolling basis for some programs.
Advanced Placement Credit by examination available. Credit given for nursing courses completed elsewhere dependent upon specific evaluations.
Contact *Telephone:* 813-626-7911.

University of South Florida
College of Nursing
Tampa, Florida

http://www.hsc.usf.edu/nursing
Founded in 1956

DEGREES • BS • DNP • MS • MS/MPH • PHD
Nursing Program Faculty 81 (70% with doctorates).
Baccalaureate Enrollment 1,051 **Women** 85.26% **Men** 14.74% **Part-time** 69.93%
Graduate Enrollment 789 **Women** 86.95% **Men** 13.05% **Part-time** 84.28%
Distance Learning Courses Available.
Nursing Student Activities Sigma Theta Tau, Student Nurses' Association.
Nursing Student Resources Academic advising; academic or career counseling; assistance for students with disabilities; bookstore; campus computer network; career placement assistance; computer lab; computer-assisted instruction; daycare for children of students; e-mail services; employment services for current students; housing assistance; interactive nursing skills videos; Internet; learning resource lab; library services; nursing audiovisuals; remedial services; resume preparation assistance; skills, simulation, or other laboratory; tutoring.
Library Facilities 2 million volumes in health, 4,000 volumes in nursing.

BACCALAUREATE PROGRAMS

Degree BS
Available Programs ADN to Baccalaureate; Accelerated Baccalaureate for Second Degree; Generic Baccalaureate.
Study Options Full-time.
Online Degree Options Yes.
Program Entrance Requirements Minimum overall college GPA of 3.2, transcript of college record, written essay, interview, prerequisite course work. Transfer students are accepted. *Application deadline:* 3/2 (fall), 6/1 (summer). *Application fee:* $30.
Expenses (2015–16) *Tuition, state resident:* full-time $4728; part-time $630 per semester. *Tuition, nonresident:* full-time $20,320; part-time $2709 per semester. *International tuition:* $20,320 full-time. *Room and board:* $9400; room only: $7200 per academic year. *Required fees:* full-time $3475; part-time $59 per credit; part-time $355 per term.
Financial Aid 62% of baccalaureate students in nursing programs received some form of financial aid in 2014–15.
Contact Ms. Ashley Sanford, Undergraduate Admissions Advisor, College of Nursing, University of South Florida, 12901 Bruce B. Downs Boulevard, MDC Box 22, Tampa, FL 33612. *Telephone:* 813-974-8717. *Fax:* 813-974-3118. *E-mail:* nurstudent@health.usf.edu.

GRADUATE PROGRAMS

Expenses (2015–16) *Tuition, state resident:* full-time $9384; part-time $2087 per semester. *Tuition, nonresident:* full-time $20,856; part-time $4634 per semester. *International tuition:* $20,856 full-time. *Room and board:* $10,550; room only: $8050 per academic year. *Required fees:* full-time $2950; part-time $84 per credit; part-time $501 per term.
Financial Aid 34% of graduate students in nursing programs received some form of financial aid in 2014–15. 7 research assistantships with tuition reimbursements available (averaging $18,935 per year), 29 teaching assistantships with tuition reimbursements available (averaging $30,814 per year) were awarded; tuition waivers (partial) and unspecified assistantships also available. *Financial aid application deadline:* 2/1.
Contact Ms. Stormie Charles, Graduate Admissions Advisor, College of Nursing, University of South Florida, 12901 Bruce B. Downs Boulevard, MDC Box 22, Tampa, FL 33612. *Telephone:* 813-974-9436. *Fax:* 813-974-3118. *E-mail:* nurstudent@health.usf.edu.

MASTER'S DEGREE PROGRAM

Degrees MS; MS/MPH

Available Programs Accelerated RN to Master's; Master's; Master's for Nurses with Non-Nursing Degrees; RN to Master's.

Concentrations Available Nurse anesthesia; nursing education. *Nurse practitioner programs in:* adult-gerontology acute care, adult-gerontology primary care, family health, occupational health, pediatric primary care.

Study Options Full-time and part-time.

Program Entrance Requirements Computer literacy, minimum overall college GPA of 3.0, transcript of college record, CPR certification, written essay, immunizations, 3 letters of recommendation, resume, GRE General Test. *Application deadline:* 2/15 (fall), 10/1 (spring). *Application fee:* $30.

Advanced Placement Credit given for nursing courses completed elsewhere dependent upon specific evaluations.

Degree Requirements 45–72 total credit hours, comprehensive exam.

POST-MASTER'S PROGRAM

Areas of Study Nursing education.

DOCTORAL DEGREE PROGRAM

Degree DNP

Available Programs Doctorate, Post-Baccalaureate Doctorate.

Areas of Study Advanced practice nursing, family health, gerontology, pediatric, women's health.

Program Entrance Requirements Minimum overall college GPA of 3.0, interview, interview by faculty committee, letters of recommendation, MSN or equivalent, statistics course, vita, writing sample. Application deadline: 2/1 (fall). Deadline varies for each admission cycle.

Degree Requirements 30-91 total credit hours, final project, residency.

Degree PhD

Available Programs Doctorate; Doctorate for Nurses with Non-Nursing Degrees; Post-Baccalaureate Doctorate.

Areas of Study Bio-behavioral research, biology of health and illness, clinical research, illness and transition, nursing research, nursing science.

Program Entrance Requirements Minimum overall college GPA of 3.0, interview by faculty committee, interview, 3 letters of recommendation, statistics course, vita, writing sample, GRE General Test (recommended). Application deadline: 12/15 (fall). Application fee: $30.

Degree Requirements 60 total credit hours, dissertation, written exam.

The University of Tampa
Department of Nursing
Tampa, Florida

http://www.ut.edu/nursing
Founded in 1931

DEGREES • BSN • MSN

Nursing Program Faculty 32 (22% with doctorates).

Baccalaureate Enrollment 104 **Women** 89% **Men** 11%

Graduate Enrollment 146 **Women** 86% **Men** 14% **Part-time** 89%

Nursing Student Activities Sigma Theta Tau, Student Nurses' Association.

Nursing Student Resources Academic advising; academic or career counseling; assistance for students with disabilities; bookstore; campus computer network; career placement assistance; computer lab; computer-assisted instruction; e-mail services; employment services for current students; externships; housing assistance; interactive nursing skills videos; Internet; learning resource lab; library services; nursing audiovisuals; paid internships; placement services for program completers; remedial services; resume preparation assistance; skills, simulation, or other laboratory; tutoring; unpaid internships.

Library Facilities 252,152 volumes in health, 3,025 volumes in nursing; 10,870 periodical subscriptions health-care related.

BACCALAUREATE PROGRAMS

Degree BSN

Available Programs Generic Baccalaureate.

Study Options Full-time.

Program Entrance Requirements Minimum overall college GPA of 3.25, transcript of college record, CPR certification, written essay, health exam, health insurance, high school transcript, immunizations, 1 letter of recommendation, minimum GPA in nursing prerequisites of 3.25, professional liability insurance/malpractice insurance, prerequisite course work. Transfer students are accepted. *Application deadline:* 10/15 (spring). *Application fee:* $40.

Expenses (2014–15) *Tuition:* full-time $24,528. *International tuition:* $25,772 full-time. *Room and board:* $9624; room only: $6000 per academic year. *Required fees:* full-time $1802.

Financial Aid 85% of baccalaureate students in nursing programs received some form of financial aid in 2013–14. *Gift aid (need-based):* Federal Pell, FSEOG, state, private, college/university gift aid from institutional funds. *Loans:* Federal Direct (Subsidized and Unsubsidized Stafford PLUS), Perkins, college/university. *Work-study:* Federal Work-Study, part-time campus jobs. *Financial aid application deadline:* Continuous.

Contact Admissions Office, Department of Nursing, The University of Tampa, 401 West Kennedy Boulevard, Box F, Tampa, FL 33606. *Telephone:* 813-253-6211. *Fax:* 813-258-7398. *E-mail:* admissions@ut.edu.

GRADUATE PROGRAMS

Expenses (2014–15) *Tuition:* part-time $558 per credit hour. *Required fees:* part-time $265 per term.

Financial Aid 80% of graduate students in nursing programs received some form of financial aid in 2013–14.

Contact Graduate Studies Office, Department of Nursing, The University of Tampa, 401 West Kennedy Boulevard, Tampa, FL 33606. *Telephone:* 813-258-7409. *Fax:* 813-259-5403. *E-mail:* utgrad@ut.edu.

MASTER'S DEGREE PROGRAM

Degree MSN

Available Programs Master's.

Concentrations Available *Nurse practitioner programs in:* adult health, family health.

Study Options Full-time and part-time.

Program Entrance Requirements Computer literacy, minimum overall college GPA of 3.0, transcript of college record, CPR certification, written essay, immunizations, 2 letters of recommendation, nursing research course, physical assessment course, professional liability insurance/malpractice insurance, prerequisite course work, resume, statistics course. *Application deadline:* Applications may be processed on a rolling basis for some programs. *Application fee:* $40.

Advanced Placement Credit given for nursing courses completed elsewhere dependent upon specific evaluations.

Degree Requirements 47 total credit hours, comprehensive exam.

POST-MASTER'S PROGRAM

Areas of Study *Nurse practitioner programs in:* adult health, family health.

CONTINUING EDUCATION PROGRAM

Contact Dr. Susan Garbutt, Clinical Simulation Coordinator, Department of Nursing, The University of Tampa, 401 West Kennedy Boulevard, Box 10-F, Tampa, FL 33606-1490. *Telephone:* 813-257-3295. *Fax:* 813-258-7214. *E-mail:* sgarbutt@ut.edu.

University of West Florida
Department of Nursing
Pensacola, Florida

http://www.uwf.edu/nursing
Founded in 1963

DEGREES • BSN • MSN

Nursing Program Faculty 13 (64% with doctorates).

Baccalaureate Enrollment 133 **Women** 73% **Men** 27% **Part-time** 60%

Graduate Enrollment 30 **Women** 87% **Men** 13% **Part-time** 60%

Distance Learning Courses Available.

Nursing Student Activities Sigma Theta Tau, Student Nurses' Association.

Nursing Student Resources Academic advising; academic or career counseling; assistance for students with disabilities; bookstore; campus computer network; computer lab; computer-assisted instruction; daycare for children of students; e-mail services; employment services for current students; housing assistance; interactive nursing skills videos; Internet; learning resource lab; library services; nursing audiovisuals; remedial services; resume preparation assistance; skills, simulation, or other laboratory; tutoring; unpaid internships.

Library Facilities 3,500 volumes in health, 1,300 volumes in nursing; 54 periodical subscriptions health-care related.

BACCALAUREATE PROGRAMS

Degree BSN
Available Programs ADN to Baccalaureate; Generic Baccalaureate; RN Baccalaureate.
Study Options Full-time.
Program Entrance Requirements Minimum overall college GPA of 3.0, transcript of college record, CPR certification, health exam, health insurance, immunizations, prerequisite course work. Transfer students are accepted. *Application deadline:* 3/1 (fall).
Contact *Telephone:* 850-473-7757. *Fax:* 850-473-7769.

GRADUATE PROGRAMS

Contact *Telephone:* 850-473-7760. *Fax:* 850-473-7769.

MASTER'S DEGREE PROGRAM

Degree MSN
Available Programs Master's.
Concentrations Available Nursing administration; nursing education.
Study Options Full-time and part-time.
Online Degree Options Yes (online only).
Program Entrance Requirements Clinical experience, computer literacy, minimum overall college GPA of 3.0, transcript of college record, CPR certification, immunizations, 3 letters of recommendation, professional liability insurance/malpractice insurance, resume. *Application deadline:* 6/1 (fall), 10/1 (spring), 3/1 (summer). Applications may be processed on a rolling basis for some programs.
Advanced Placement Credit given for nursing courses completed elsewhere dependent upon specific evaluations.
Degree Requirements 39 total credit hours, thesis or project.

GEORGIA

Albany State University

College of Sciences and Health Professions
Albany, Georgia

http://www.asurams.edu/
Founded in 1903
DEGREES • BSN • MSN
Nursing Program Faculty 16 (40% with doctorates).
Baccalaureate Enrollment 94 **Women** 94% **Men** 6% **Part-time** 33%
Graduate Enrollment 48 **Women** 92% **Men** 8% **Part-time** 46%
Distance Learning Courses Available.
Nursing Student Activities Nursing Honor Society, Student Nurses' Association, nursing club.
Nursing Student Resources Academic advising; academic or career counseling; assistance for students with disabilities; bookstore; campus computer network; career placement assistance; computer lab; computer-assisted instruction; e-mail services; employment services for current students; interactive nursing skills videos; Internet; learning resource lab; library services; nursing audiovisuals; paid internships; placement services for program completers; remedial services; resume preparation assistance; skills, simulation, or other laboratory; tutoring; unpaid internships.
Library Facilities 15,075 volumes in health, 7,032 volumes in nursing; 75 periodical subscriptions health-care related.

BACCALAUREATE PROGRAMS

Degree BSN
Available Programs ADN to Baccalaureate; Accelerated Baccalaureate for Second Degree; Generic Baccalaureate.
Study Options Full-time and part-time.
Online Degree Options Yes.
Program Entrance Requirements Minimum overall college GPA of 2.0, transcript of college record, CPR certification, health exam, health insurance, high school biology, high school foreign language, 4 years high school math, 3 years high school science, high school transcript, immunizations, minimum high school GPA of 2.0, minimum GPA in nursing prerequisites of 2.75, professional liability insurance/malpractice insurance, prerequisite course work. Transfer students are accepted. *Application deadline:* 7/1 (fall), 11/1 (spring), 4/1 (summer). Applications may be processed on a rolling basis for some programs.

Advanced Placement Credit given for nursing courses completed elsewhere dependent upon specific evaluations.
Expenses (2015–16) *Tuition, state resident:* full-time $5488; part-time $162 per credit hour. *Tuition, nonresident:* full-time $7872; part-time $589 per credit hour. *International tuition:* $7872 full-time. *Room and board:* $3849; room only: $2425 per academic year. *Required fees:* full-time $920; part-time $455 per term.
Financial Aid *Gift aid (need-based):* Federal Pell, FSEOG, state, private, college/university gift aid from institutional funds, United Negro College Fund, Federal Nursing. *Loans:* Federal Direct (Subsidized and Unsubsidized Stafford PLUS), Perkins, state. *Work-study:* Federal Work-Study, part-time campus jobs. *Financial aid application deadline:* 6/30(priority: 4/15).
Contact Dr. Cathy H. Williams, Chair, Department of Nursing, College of Sciences and Health Professions, Albany State University, 504 College Drive, Albany, GA 31705. *Telephone:* 229-430-4728. *Fax:* 229-430-3937. *E-mail:* cathy.williams@asurams.edu.

GRADUATE PROGRAMS

Expenses (2015–16) *Tuition, state resident:* full-time $6130. *Tuition, nonresident:* full-time $19,708. *International tuition:* $19,708 full-time. *Room and board:* $6959; room only: $2425 per academic year. *Required fees:* full-time $920.
Financial Aid Scholarships and traineeships available.
Contact Dr. Cathy H. Williams, Chair, Department of Nursing, College of Sciences and Health Professions, Albany State University, 504 College Drive, Albany, GA 31705. *Telephone:* 229-430-4728. *Fax:* 229-430-3937. *E-mail:* cathy.williams@asurams.edu.

MASTER'S DEGREE PROGRAM

Degree MSN
Available Programs Accelerated RN to Master's; Master's.
Concentrations Available Nursing education. *Nurse practitioner programs in:* family health.
Study Options Full-time and part-time.
Online Degree Options Yes (online only).
Program Entrance Requirements Clinical experience, computer literacy, minimum overall college GPA of 3.0, transcript of college record, CPR certification, immunizations, interview, 2 letters of recommendation, nursing research course, physical assessment course, professional liability insurance/malpractice insurance, prerequisite course work, resume, statistics course, GRE or MAT. *Application deadline:* 7/1 (fall), 11/1 (spring), 4/1 (summer). Applications may be processed on a rolling basis for some programs.
Advanced Placement Credit given for nursing courses completed elsewhere dependent upon specific evaluations.
Degree Requirements 36 total credit hours, thesis or project, comprehensive exam.

POST-MASTER'S PROGRAM

Areas of Study Nursing education. *Nurse practitioner programs in:* family health.

Armstrong State University

Program in Nursing
Savannah, Georgia

http://www.armstrong.edu/Health_professions/nursing/nursing_welcome
Founded in 1935
DEGREES • BSN • MSN
Nursing Program Faculty 53 (21% with doctorates).
Baccalaureate Enrollment 350 **Women** 85% **Men** 15% **Part-time** 10%
Graduate Enrollment 45 **Women** 90% **Men** 10% **Part-time** 75%
Distance Learning Courses Available.
Nursing Student Activities Nursing Honor Society, Sigma Theta Tau, Student Nurses' Association.
Nursing Student Resources Academic advising; academic or career counseling; assistance for students with disabilities; bookstore; campus computer network; career placement assistance; computer lab; computer-assisted instruction; e-mail services; employment services for current students; externships; housing assistance; interactive nursing skills videos; Internet; learning resource lab; library services; nursing audiovisuals; remedial services; resume preparation assistance; skills, simulation, or other laboratory; tutoring.

Library Facilities 8,500 volumes in nursing; 200 periodical subscriptions health-care related.

BACCALAUREATE PROGRAMS

Degree BSN

Available Programs ADN to Baccalaureate; Accelerated Baccalaureate; Accelerated Baccalaureate for Second Degree; Generic Baccalaureate; LPN to Baccalaureate; RN Baccalaureate.

Study Options Full-time and part-time.

Program Entrance Requirements Minimum overall college GPA of 3.0, transcript of college record, CPR certification, health exam, health insurance, immunizations, minimum GPA in nursing prerequisites of 3.0, professional liability insurance/malpractice insurance, prerequisite course work. Transfer students are accepted. *Application deadline:* 2/28 (fall), 10/15 (spring). *Application fee:* $35.

Advanced Placement Credit by examination available. Credit given for nursing courses completed elsewhere dependent upon specific evaluations.

Financial Aid 90% of baccalaureate students in nursing programs received some form of financial aid in 2013–14. *Gift aid (need-based):* Federal Pell, FSEOG, state, private, college/university gift aid from institutional funds, Federal Nursing. *Loans:* Federal Direct (Subsidized and Unsubsidized Stafford PLUS), state, college/university, alternative loans. *Work-study:* Federal Work-Study, part-time campus jobs. *Financial aid application deadline (priority):* 3/15.

Contact Ms. Kristy Gose, Administrative Assistant, Program in Nursing, Armstrong State University, 11935 Abercorn Street, Savannah, GA 31419-1997. *Telephone:* 912-344-2575. *Fax:* 912-344-3481. *E-mail:* kristy.gose@armstrong.edu.

GRADUATE PROGRAMS

Financial Aid 85% of graduate students in nursing programs received some form of financial aid in 2013–14. Research assistantships with full tuition reimbursements available (averaging $5,000 per year); Federal Work-Study, scholarships, and unspecified assistantships also available. Aid available to part-time students. *Financial aid application deadline:* 3/1.

Contact Dr. Anita Nivens, Graduate Program Coordinator, Program in Nursing, Armstrong State University, 11935 Abercorn Street, Savannah, GA 31419-1997. *Telephone:* 912-344-2724. *Fax:* 912-344-3481. *E-mail:* anita.nivens@armstrong.edu.

MASTER'S DEGREE PROGRAM

Degree MSN

Available Programs Master's.

Concentrations Available *Nurse practitioner programs in:* acute care, adult health, family health.

Study Options Full-time and part-time.

Program Entrance Requirements Clinical experience, computer literacy, minimum overall college GPA of 3.0, transcript of college record, CPR certification, written essay, immunizations, interview, 3 letters of recommendation, nursing research course, physical assessment course, professional liability insurance/malpractice insurance, prerequisite course work, statistics course, GRE General Test or MAT. *Application deadline:* 5/15 (fall), 11/15 (spring). Applications may be processed on a rolling basis for some programs.

Advanced Placement Credit by examination available. Credit given for nursing courses completed elsewhere dependent upon specific evaluations.

Degree Requirements 47 total credit hours, thesis or project.

POST-MASTER'S PROGRAM

Areas of Study *Nurse practitioner programs in:* acute care, adult health, family health.

Augusta University

School of Nursing
Augusta, Georgia

http://www.gru.edu/nursing/
Founded in 1828

DEGREES • BSN • DNP • MSN • PHD
Nursing Program Faculty 55 (47% with doctorates).
Baccalaureate Enrollment 362 **Women** 86% **Men** 14% **Part-time** 1%
Graduate Enrollment 434 **Women** 85% **Men** 15% **Part-time** 23%
Distance Learning Courses Available.

Nursing Student Activities Nursing Honor Society, Sigma Theta Tau, Student Nurses' Association, nursing club.

Nursing Student Resources Academic advising; academic or career counseling; assistance for students with disabilities; bookstore; campus computer network; career placement assistance; computer lab; computer-assisted instruction; daycare for children of students; e-mail services; employment services for current students; externships; housing assistance; interactive nursing skills videos; Internet; learning resource lab; library services; nursing audiovisuals; paid internships; remedial services; skills, simulation, or other laboratory; tutoring.

Library Facilities 178,650 volumes in health, 14,650 volumes in nursing; 1,307 periodical subscriptions health-care related.

BACCALAUREATE PROGRAMS

Degree BSN

Available Programs Generic Baccalaureate.

Site Options Athens, GA.

Study Options Full-time.

Program Entrance Requirements Minimum overall college GPA of 2.8, transcript of college record, CPR certification, written essay, health insurance, immunizations, 2 letters of recommendation, prerequisite course work. Transfer students are accepted. *Application deadline:* 2/15 (fall). *Application fee:* $50.

Expenses (2014–15) *Tuition, state resident:* full-time $8036; part-time $268 per credit. *Tuition, nonresident:* full-time $26,702; part-time $890 per credit. *International tuition:* $26,702 full-time. *Room and board:* room only: $4300 per academic year. *Required fees:* full-time $2433.

Financial Aid 90% of baccalaureate students in nursing programs received some form of financial aid in 2013–14. *Gift aid (need-based):* Federal Pell, FSEOG, state, private, college/university gift aid from institutional funds, Federal Nursing. *Loans:* Federal Nursing Student Loans, Federal Direct (Subsidized and Unsubsidized Stafford PLUS), Perkins, state, college/university. *Work-study:* Federal Work-Study. *Financial aid application deadline:* 3/1.

Contact Office of Academic Admissions, School of Nursing, Augusta University, 1120 15th Street, Benet House, Augusta, GA 30912. *Telephone:* 706-737-1524. *Fax:* 706-667-4355. *E-mail:* admissions@georgiahealth.edu.

GRADUATE PROGRAMS

Expenses (2014–15) *Tuition, state resident:* full-time $17,418; part-time $484 per credit. *Tuition, nonresident:* full-time $43,551; part-time $1210 per credit. *International tuition:* $43,551 full-time. *Room and board:* room only: $4950 per academic year. *Required fees:* full-time $2728.

Financial Aid 85% of graduate students in nursing programs received some form of financial aid in 2013–14.

Contact Director, Academic Admissions, School of Nursing, Augusta University, 1120 15th Street, Benet House, Augusta, GA 30912. *Telephone:* 706-737-1524. *Fax:* 706-667-4355. *E-mail:* admissions@georgiahealth.edu.

MASTER'S DEGREE PROGRAM

Degree MSN

Available Programs Accelerated Master's for Non-Nursing College Graduates; Master's.

Concentrations Available Clinical nurse leader; nurse anesthesia. *Nurse practitioner programs in:* family health, pediatric.

Site Options Athens, GA; Columbus, GA.

Study Options Full-time and part-time.

Online Degree Options Yes.

Program Entrance Requirements Clinical experience, computer literacy, minimum overall college GPA of 3.0, transcript of college record, CPR certification, written essay, immunizations, interview, 3 letters of recommendation, professional liability insurance/malpractice insurance, prerequisite course work, resume, statistics course. *Application deadline:* 2/1 (fall), 4/2 (spring). *Application fee:* $50.

Degree Requirements 60 total credit hours, thesis or project.

POST-MASTER'S PROGRAM

Areas of Study *Nurse practitioner programs in:* adult-gerontology acute care, family health, pediatric, psychiatric/mental health.

DOCTORAL DEGREE PROGRAM

Degree DNP

Available Programs Doctorate, Post-Baccalaureate Doctorate.

Areas of Study Advanced practice nursing.

Online Degree Options Yes.

Program Entrance Requirements Minimum overall college GPA of 3.3, clinical experience, interview, interview by faculty committee, 3

letters of recommendation, statistics course, vita, writing sample. Application deadline: 2/1 (fall). Application fee: $50.
Degree Requirements Capstone project.

Degree PhD
Available Programs Doctorate; Post-Baccalaureate Doctorate.
Areas of Study Bio-behavioral research, nursing research.
Site Options Athens, GA; Columbus, GA.
Program Entrance Requirements Clinical experience, minimum overall college GPA of 3.2, interview by faculty committee, interview, 3 letters of recommendation, MSN or equivalent, scholarly papers, statistics course, vita, writing sample. Application deadline: 2/1 (fall). Application fee: $50.
Degree Requirements 75 total credit hours, dissertation, oral exam, written exam.

Berry College
Division of Nursing
Mount Berry, Georgia

http://www.berry.edu
Founded in 1902
DEGREE • BSN
Nursing Program Faculty 10 (30% with doctorates).
Baccalaureate Enrollment 58
Nursing Student Activities Student Nurses' Association, nursing club.
Nursing Student Resources Academic advising; academic or career counseling; assistance for students with disabilities; bookstore; campus computer network; career placement assistance; computer lab; computer-assisted instruction; e-mail services; employment services for current students; housing assistance; interactive nursing skills videos; Internet; learning resource lab; library services; nursing audiovisuals; remedial services; resume preparation assistance; skills, simulation, or other laboratory; tutoring; unpaid internships.

BACCALAUREATE PROGRAMS

Degree BSN
Available Programs Generic Baccalaureate.
Study Options Full-time.
Program Entrance Requirements CPR certification, health exam, health insurance, immunizations, interview, minimum GPA in nursing prerequisites of 2.8, professional liability insurance/malpractice insurance, prerequisite course work. *Application deadline:* 2/1 (winter).
Expenses (2015–16) *Tuition:* full-time $64,000. *Room and board:* $16,000 per academic year. *Required fees:* full-time $3000.
Contact Starr Boylan, Admission Counselor, Division of Nursing, Berry College, 2277 Martha Berry Highway, Mount Berry, GA 30149. *Telephone:* 706-232-5374. *E-mail:* Sboylan@berry.edu.

Brenau University
College of Health and Science
Gainesville, Georgia

http://www.brenau.edu/
Founded in 1878
DEGREES • BSN • DNP • MSN
Nursing Program Faculty 15 (65% with doctorates).
Baccalaureate Enrollment 300 **Women** 95% **Men** 5% **Part-time** 50%
Graduate Enrollment 70 **Women** 95% **Men** 5% **Part-time** 100%
Distance Learning Courses Available.
Nursing Student Activities Sigma Theta Tau, Student Nurses' Association.
Nursing Student Resources Academic advising; academic or career counseling; assistance for students with disabilities; bookstore; campus computer network; career placement assistance; computer lab; computer-assisted instruction; e-mail services; housing assistance; interactive nursing skills videos; Internet; learning resource lab; library services; nursing audiovisuals; remedial services; skills, simulation, or other laboratory; tutoring.
Library Facilities 6,000 volumes in health, 5,000 volumes in nursing; 500 periodical subscriptions health-care related.

BACCALAUREATE PROGRAMS

Degree BSN
Available Programs ADN to Baccalaureate; Generic Baccalaureate; RN Baccalaureate.
Study Options Full-time and part-time.
Online Degree Options Yes.
Program Entrance Requirements Minimum overall college GPA of 2.75, transcript of college record, health exam, high school biology, high school chemistry, high school foreign language, 2 years high school math, 1 year of high school science, high school transcript, immunizations, minimum high school GPA of 2.75, minimum GPA in nursing prerequisites of 2.5, prerequisite course work. Transfer students are accepted. *Application deadline:* 7/15 (spring), 11/15 (summer). *Application fee:* $35.
Advanced Placement Credit by examination available. Credit given for nursing courses completed elsewhere dependent upon specific evaluations.
Financial Aid 75% of baccalaureate students in nursing programs received some form of financial aid in 2013–14. *Gift aid (need-based):* Federal Pell, FSEOG, private, college/university gift aid from institutional funds. *Loans:* Federal Nursing Student Loans, Federal Direct (Subsidized and Unsubsidized Stafford PLUS), Perkins, state. *Work-study:* Federal Work-Study. *Financial aid application deadline (priority):* 4/1.
Contact Mr. Nathan Goss, Assistant Vice President for Recruitment, College of Health and Science, Brenau University, 500 Washington Street SE, Gainesville, GA 30501. *Telephone:* 770-534-6162. *Fax:* 770-538-4306. *E-mail:* ngoss@brenau.edu.

GRADUATE PROGRAMS

Financial Aid 90% of graduate students in nursing programs received some form of financial aid in 2013–14. Scholarships and traineeships available. Aid available to part-time students. *Financial aid application deadline:* 7/15.
Contact Dr. Troy Heidesch, Chair, Graduate Programs, College of Health and Science, Brenau University, 500 Washington Street SE, Gainesville, GA 30501. *Telephone:* 770-446-2900.
E-mail: theidesch@brenau.edu.

MASTER'S DEGREE PROGRAM
Degree MSN
Available Programs Master's; RN to Master's.
Concentrations Available Nursing administration; nursing education. *Nurse practitioner programs in:* family health.
Site Options Atlanta, GA.
Study Options Part-time.
Program Entrance Requirements Clinical experience, minimum overall college GPA of 3.0, transcript of college record, CPR certification, immunizations, 2 letters of recommendation, nursing research course, physical assessment course, prerequisite course work, statistics course, GRE General Test or MAT (for some programs). *Application deadline:* Applications may be processed on a rolling basis for some programs.
Degree Requirements Thesis or project.

DOCTORAL DEGREE PROGRAM
Degree DNP
Available Programs Doctorate.
Areas of Study Clinical practice, nursing administration.
Site Options Atlanta, GA.
Program Entrance Requirements Clinical experience, minimum overall college GPA of 3.0, letters of recommendation, MSN or equivalent, statistics course, vita, writing sample. Application deadline: Applications may be processed on a rolling basis for some programs.

Clayton State University
Department of Nursing
Morrow, Georgia

http://www.clayton.edu/health/Nursing
Founded in 1969
DEGREES • BSN • MSN
Nursing Program Faculty 42 (35% with doctorates).
Baccalaureate Enrollment 258 **Women** 85.7% **Men** 14.3% **Part-time** 38%
Graduate Enrollment 25 **Women** 96% **Men** 4% **Part-time** 64%
Distance Learning Courses Available.

Nursing Student Activities Nursing Honor Society, Sigma Theta Tau, Student Nurses' Association.

Nursing Student Resources Academic advising; academic or career counseling; assistance for students with disabilities; bookstore; campus computer network; career placement assistance; computer lab; computer-assisted instruction; e-mail services; employment services for current students; externships; housing assistance; interactive nursing skills videos; Internet; learning resource lab; library services; nursing audiovisuals; paid internships; placement services for program completers; remedial services; resume preparation assistance; skills, simulation, or other laboratory; tutoring.

Library Facilities 3,450 volumes in health, 1,800 volumes in nursing; 151 periodical subscriptions health-care related.

BACCALAUREATE PROGRAMS

Degree BSN

Available Programs Generic Baccalaureate; RN Baccalaureate.
Study Options Full-time.
Online Degree Options Yes.
Program Entrance Requirements Minimum overall college GPA of 2.5, transcript of college record, CPR certification, health exam, health insurance, immunizations, interview, minimum GPA in nursing prerequisites of 2.5, professional liability insurance/malpractice insurance, prerequisite course work. Transfer students are accepted. *Application deadline:* 2/15 (fall), 9/15 (spring). *Application fee:* $25.
Contact *Telephone:* 678-466-4959. *Fax:* 678-466-4999.

GRADUATE PROGRAMS

Contact *Telephone:* 678-466-4953. *Fax:* 678-466-4999.

MASTER'S DEGREE PROGRAM

Degree MSN
Available Programs Master's; RN to Master's.
Concentrations Available Nursing administration; nursing education.
Study Options Full-time and part-time.
Online Degree Options Yes (online only).
Program Entrance Requirements Computer literacy, minimum overall college GPA of 3.0, transcript of college record, CPR certification, written essay, immunizations, interview, 3 letters of recommendation, professional liability insurance/malpractice insurance. *Application deadline:* 7/1 (fall), 11/1 (spring), 3/1 (summer). Applications may be processed on a rolling basis for some programs. *Application fee:* $25.
Advanced Placement Credit given for nursing courses completed elsewhere dependent upon specific evaluations.
Degree Requirements 36 total credit hours, thesis or project.

College of Coastal Georgia
Department of Nursing and Health Sciences
Brunswick, Georgia

http://www.ccga.edu/
Founded in 1961
DEGREE • BSN
Nursing Program Faculty 14 (29% with doctorates).
Baccalaureate Enrollment 91 **Women** 89% **Men** 11% **Part-time** 5%
Distance Learning Courses Available.
Nursing Student Activities Student Nurses' Association.
Nursing Student Resources Academic advising; academic or career counseling; assistance for students with disabilities; bookstore; campus computer network; career placement assistance; computer lab; computer-assisted instruction; e-mail services; employment services for current students; externships; housing assistance; interactive nursing skills videos; Internet; learning resource lab; library services; nursing audiovisuals; placement services for program completers; remedial services; resume preparation assistance; skills, simulation, or other laboratory; tutoring; unpaid internships.
Library Facilities 1,436 volumes in health, 277 volumes in nursing; 94 periodical subscriptions health-care related.

BACCALAUREATE PROGRAMS

Degree BSN
Available Programs Generic Baccalaureate; RN Baccalaureate.
Study Options Full-time.
Online Degree Options Yes.

Program Entrance Requirements Minimum overall college GPA of 2.8, transcript of college record, CPR certification, health exam, health insurance, immunizations, minimum GPA in nursing prerequisites of 2.8, professional liability insurance/malpractice insurance, prerequisite course work. Transfer students are accepted. *Application deadline:* 2/15 (fall).
Expenses (2015–16) *Tuition, state resident:* full-time $3063. *Tuition, nonresident:* full-time $11,322. *Room and board:* $4253; room only: $2528 per academic year. *Required fees:* full-time $1945.
Financial Aid *Gift aid (need-based):* Federal Pell, FSEOG, state, private, college/university gift aid from institutional funds. *Work-study:* Federal Work-Study. *Financial aid application deadline (priority):* 7/1.
Contact Dr. Patricia Kraft, Southeast Georgia Health System Distinguished Dean of Nursing and Health Sciences, Department of Nursing and Health Sciences, College of Coastal Georgia, One College Drive, Brunswick, GA 31520. *Telephone:* 912-279-5860. *Fax:* 912-279-5912. *E-mail:* pkraft@ccga.edu.

Columbus State University
Nursing Program
Columbus, Georgia

http://nursing.columbusstate.edu/
Founded in 1958
DEGREE • BSN
Nursing Program Faculty 31 (12% with doctorates).
Baccalaureate Enrollment 187 **Women** 91% **Men** 9% **Part-time** 3%
Distance Learning Courses Available.
Nursing Student Activities Sigma Theta Tau, Student Nurses' Association.
Nursing Student Resources Academic advising; academic or career counseling; assistance for students with disabilities; bookstore; campus computer network; career placement assistance; computer lab; computer-assisted instruction; e-mail services; housing assistance; interactive nursing skills videos; Internet; learning resource lab; library services; nursing audiovisuals; remedial services; resume preparation assistance; skills, simulation, or other laboratory; tutoring.
Library Facilities 284 volumes in health, 260 volumes in nursing; 81 periodical subscriptions health-care related.

BACCALAUREATE PROGRAMS

Degree BSN
Available Programs Generic Baccalaureate; RN Baccalaureate.
Study Options Full-time.
Online Degree Options Yes.
Program Entrance Requirements Minimum overall college GPA of 2.75, transcript of college record, CPR certification, health exam, health insurance, immunizations, 3 letters of recommendation, minimum GPA in nursing prerequisites of 2.75, professional liability insurance/malpractice insurance, prerequisite course work. *Application deadline:* 2/28 (fall).
Advanced Placement Credit given for nursing courses completed elsewhere dependent upon specific evaluations.
Contact *Telephone:* 706-568-5050. *Fax:* 706-569-3101.

Dalton State College
Department of Nursing
Dalton, Georgia

https://www.daltonstate.edu/
Founded in 1963
DEGREE • BSN

BACCALAUREATE PROGRAMS

Degree BSN
Available Programs RN Baccalaureate.
Program Entrance Requirements Minimum overall college GPA of 2.75, RN licensure. *Application deadline:* 4/1 (fall), 11/1 (spring).
Contact Office of the Registrar, Department of Nursing, Dalton State College, 650 College Drive, Dalton, GA 30720. *Telephone:* 706-272-4436. *E-mail:* registrar@daltonstate.edu.

Darton State College

Division of Nursing
Albany, Georgia

http://www.darton.edu/programs/nursing/bachelors/
Founded in 1965

DEGREE • BSN

Nursing Program Faculty 55 (10% with doctorates).
Baccalaureate Enrollment 150
Distance Learning Courses Available.
Nursing Student Activities Nursing Honor Society, Student Nurses' Association, nursing club.
Nursing Student Resources Academic advising; academic or career counseling; assistance for students with disabilities; bookstore; campus computer network; computer lab; computer-assisted instruction; e-mail services; interactive nursing skills videos; Internet; learning resource lab; library services; nursing audiovisuals; remedial services; skills, simulation, or other laboratory; tutoring.

BACCALAUREATE PROGRAMS

Degree BSN

Available Programs RN Baccalaureate.
Study Options Full-time and part-time.
Online Degree Options Yes (online only).
Program Entrance Requirements CPR certification, immunizations, letters of recommendation, minimum GPA in nursing prerequisites of 2.7, professional liability insurance/malpractice insurance, prerequisite course work, RN licensure. Transfer students are accepted.
Contact Nursing Division, Division of Nursing, Darton State College, 2400 Gillionville Road, Albany, GA 31707. *Telephone:* 229-317-6504. *E-mail:* sherry.koster@darton.edu.

Emory University

Nell Hodgson Woodruff School of Nursing
Atlanta, Georgia

http://www.nursing.emory.edu/
Founded in 1836

DEGREES • BSN • MSN • MSN/MPH • PHD

Nursing Program Faculty 102 (86% with doctorates).
Baccalaureate Enrollment 328 **Women** 94% **Men** 6%
Graduate Enrollment 197 **Women** 91% **Men** 9% **Part-time** 10%
Nursing Student Activities Sigma Theta Tau, Student Nurses' Association.
Nursing Student Resources Academic advising; academic or career counseling; assistance for students with disabilities; bookstore; campus computer network; career placement assistance; computer lab; computer-assisted instruction; daycare for children of students; e-mail services; employment services for current students; externships; housing assistance; interactive nursing skills videos; Internet; learning resource lab; library services; nursing audiovisuals; other; resume preparation assistance; skills, simulation, or other laboratory; tutoring; unpaid internships.
Library Facilities 250,000 volumes in health; 1,800 periodical subscriptions health-care related.

BACCALAUREATE PROGRAMS

Degree BSN

Available Programs Accelerated Baccalaureate; Accelerated Baccalaureate for Second Degree; Baccalaureate for Second Degree; Generic Baccalaureate.
Study Options Full-time.
Program Entrance Requirements Minimum overall college GPA of 3.0, transcript of college record, minimum GPA in nursing prerequisites of 3.0, prerequisite course work. Transfer students are accepted. *Application deadline:* 1/15 (fall), 12/15 (summer). *Application fee:* $50.
Advanced Placement Credit given for nursing courses completed elsewhere dependent upon specific evaluations.

Expenses (2015–16) *Tuition:* full-time $21,000; part-time $1750 per credit hour. *International tuition:* $21,000 full-time. *Required fees:* full-time $600.
Financial Aid 94% of baccalaureate students in nursing programs received some form of financial aid in 2014–15. *Gift aid (need-based):* Federal Pell, FSEOG, private, college/university gift aid from institutional funds. *Loans:* Federal Nursing Student Loans, Federal Direct (Subsidized and Unsubsidized Stafford PLUS), Perkins, state, college/university, alternative loans. *Work-study:* Federal Work-Study, part-time campus jobs. *Financial aid application deadline:* 3/1(priority: 2/15).
Contact Mrs. Katie Kennedy, Office of Enrollment and Student Affairs, Nell Hodgson Woodruff School of Nursing, Emory University, 1520 Clifton Road NE, Atlanta, GA 30322. *Telephone:* 404-727-7980. *Fax:* 404-727-8509. *E-mail:* admit@nursing.emory.edu.

GRADUATE PROGRAMS

Expenses (2015–16) *Tuition:* full-time $21,000; part-time $1750 per credit hour. *International tuition:* $21,000 full-time. *Required fees:* full-time $600.
Financial Aid 94% of graduate students in nursing programs received some form of financial aid in 2014–15. 14 fellowships (averaging $28,000 per year) were awarded; career-related internships or fieldwork, Federal Work-Study, institutionally sponsored loans, and scholarships also available. Aid available to part-time students. *Financial aid application deadline:* 3/1.
Contact Mrs. Katie Kennedy, Office of Enrollment and Student Affairs, Nell Hodgson Woodruff School of Nursing, Emory University, 1520 Clifton Road NE, Atlanta, GA 30322. *Telephone:* 404-727-7980. *Fax:* 404-727-8509. *E-mail:* admit@nursing.emory.edu.

MASTER'S DEGREE PROGRAM

Degrees MSN; MSN/MPH
Available Programs Master's.
Concentrations Available Health-care administration; nurse-midwifery. *Nurse practitioner programs in:* adult health, adult-gerontology acute care, family health, neonatal health, pediatric, pediatric primary care, primary care, women's health.
Study Options Full-time and part-time.
Program Entrance Requirements Clinical experience, minimum overall college GPA of 3.0, transcript of college record, written essay, interview, 3 letters of recommendation, physical assessment course, prerequisite course work, resume, statistics course, GRE General Test or MAT. *Application deadline:* 1/15 (fall), 1/15 (summer). Applications may be processed on a rolling basis for some programs. *Application fee:* $50.
Advanced Placement Credit given for nursing courses completed elsewhere dependent upon specific evaluations.
Degree Requirements 64 total credit hours.

POST-MASTER'S PROGRAM

Areas of Study Health-care administration; nurse-midwifery. *Nurse practitioner programs in:* adult health, adult-gerontology acute care, family health, neonatal health, pediatric, pediatric primary care, primary care, women's health.

DOCTORAL DEGREE PROGRAM

Degree PhD
Available Programs Doctorate; Post-Baccalaureate Doctorate.
Areas of Study Aging, biology of health and illness, ethics, faculty preparation, gerontology, health policy, human health and illness, illness and transition, individualized study, neuro-behavior, nursing policy, nursing research, nursing science, women's health.
Program Entrance Requirements Minimum overall college GPA of 3.0, interview by faculty committee, 3 letters of recommendation, MSN or equivalent, statistics course, vita, writing sample. Application deadline: 1/3 (fall). Applications may be processed on a rolling basis for some programs.
Degree Requirements 50 total credit hours, dissertation, oral exam, written exam, residency.

POSTDOCTORAL PROGRAM

Postdoctoral Program Contact Ms. Teresa Fosque, Senior Business Manager, Nell Hodgson Woodruff School of Nursing, Emory University, 1520 Clifton Road NE, Atlanta, GA 30322. *E-mail:* tfosque@emory.edu.

Georgia College & State University

College of Health Sciences
Milledgeville, Georgia

http://www.gcsu.edu/nursing
Founded in 1889

DEGREES • BSN • DNP • MSN

Nursing Program Faculty 22 (69% with doctorates).
Baccalaureate Enrollment 210 **Women** 86% **Men** 14%
Graduate Enrollment 118 **Women** 92% **Men** 8% **Part-time** 34%
Distance Learning Courses Available.
Nursing Student Activities Nursing Honor Society, Sigma Theta Tau, Student Nurses' Association.
Nursing Student Resources Academic advising; academic or career counseling; assistance for students with disabilities; bookstore; campus computer network; career placement assistance; computer lab; computer-assisted instruction; e-mail services; employment services for current students; housing assistance; interactive nursing skills videos; Internet; learning resource lab; library services; nursing audiovisuals; remedial services; resume preparation assistance; skills, simulation, or other laboratory; tutoring; unpaid internships.
Library Facilities 3,095 volumes in health, 1,465 volumes in nursing; 315 periodical subscriptions health-care related.

BACCALAUREATE PROGRAMS

Degree BSN
Available Programs Generic Baccalaureate; RN Baccalaureate.
Study Options Full-time.
Online Degree Options Yes.
Program Entrance Requirements Minimum overall college GPA of 2.75, transcript of college record, CPR certification, health exam, health insurance, high school foreign language, 4 years high school math, 4 years high school science, high school transcript, immunizations, minimum high school GPA of 2.5, minimum GPA in nursing prerequisites of 2.75, professional liability insurance/malpractice insurance, prerequisite course work. Transfer students are accepted. *Application deadline:* 2/1 (fall), 8/1 (spring). *Application fee:* $10.
Expenses (2015–16) *Tuition, state resident:* full-time $7180. *Tuition, nonresident:* full-time $25,528. *Room and board:* $6284 per academic year. *Required fees:* full-time $1990.
Financial Aid 94% of baccalaureate students in nursing programs received some form of financial aid in 2014–15.
Contact Ms. Michelle Beck, Pre-Nursing Advisor, College of Health Sciences, Georgia College & State University, Campus Box 115, Milledgeville, GA 31061. *Telephone:* 478-445-2634. *E-mail:* michelle.beck@gcsu.edu.

GRADUATE PROGRAMS

Expenses (2015–16) *Tuition, state resident:* part-time $373 per credit hour. *Tuition, nonresident:* part-time $373 per credit hour. *Required fees:* part-time $100 per credit.
Financial Aid 30 research assistantships were awarded; career-related internships or fieldwork and unspecified assistantships also available.
Contact Dr. Sallie Coke, Interim Assistant Director, Graduate Programs, College of Health Sciences, Georgia College & State University, Macon Graduate Center, 433 Cherry Street, Macon, GA 31204. *Telephone:* 478-752-1074. *E-mail:* sallie.coke@gcsu.edu.

MASTER'S DEGREE PROGRAM

Degree MSN
Available Programs Master's.
Concentrations Available Nursing education. *Nurse practitioner programs in:* family health, psychiatric/mental health.
Site Options Macon, GA.
Study Options Full-time and part-time.
Online Degree Options Yes (online only).
Program Entrance Requirements Clinical experience, computer literacy, minimum overall college GPA of 2.75, transcript of college record, CPR certification, written essay, immunizations, interview, 2 letters of recommendation, physical assessment course, professional liability insurance/malpractice insurance, resume, statistics course, GRE, GMAT or MAT. *Application deadline:* 1/12 (summer). *Application fee:* $35.
Advanced Placement Credit given for nursing courses completed elsewhere dependent upon specific evaluations.

Degree Requirements 40 total credit hours, thesis or project, comprehensive exam.

POST-MASTER'S PROGRAM

Areas of Study *Nurse practitioner programs in:* family health.

DOCTORAL DEGREE PROGRAM

Degree DNP
Available Programs Doctorate.
Site Options Macon, GA.
Online Degree Options Yes (online only).
Program Entrance Requirements Clinical experience, minimum overall college GPA of 3.2, interview by faculty committee, interview, 2 letters of recommendation, MSN or equivalent, statistics course, vita, writing sample. Application deadline: 1/12 (spring). Application fee: $10.
Degree Requirements 37 total credit hours.

Georgia Highlands College

RN-BSN Online Completion Program
Rome, Georgia

https://www.highlands.edu/site/bsn
Founded in 1970

DEGREE • BSN

Nursing Program Faculty 4 (50% with doctorates).
Baccalaureate Enrollment 57 **Women** 80% **Men** 20% **Part-time** 20%
Nursing Student Activities Student Nurses' Association.
Nursing Student Resources Academic advising; academic or career counseling; assistance for students with disabilities; bookstore; campus computer network; computer lab; e-mail services; Internet; library services; remedial services; skills, simulation, or other laboratory; tutoring.
Library Facilities 806 volumes in health, 700 volumes in nursing; 4,100 periodical subscriptions health-care related.

BACCALAUREATE PROGRAMS

Degree BSN
Available Programs RN Baccalaureate.
Financial Aid *Gift aid (need-based):* Federal Pell, FSEOG, state, private, college/university gift aid from institutional funds, United Negro College Fund. *Loans:* Federal Nursing Student Loans. *Work-study:* Federal Work-Study. *Financial aid application deadline (priority):* 3/15.
Contact Dr. Janet Alexander, Dean of Health Sciences, RN-BSN Online Completion Program, Georgia Highlands College, 415 East Third Avenue, Heritage Hall, Rome, GA 30161. *Telephone:* 706-295-6326. *Fax:* 706-204-2341. *E-mail:* jalexand@highlands.edu.

Georgia Southern University

School of Nursing
Statesboro, Georgia

http://chhs.georgiasouthern.edu/nursing/
Founded in 1906

DEGREES • BSN • DNP

Nursing Program Faculty 36 (18% with doctorates).
Baccalaureate Enrollment 267 **Women** 86% **Men** 14% **Part-time** .1%
Graduate Enrollment 64 **Women** 95% **Men** 5%
Distance Learning Courses Available.
Nursing Student Activities Sigma Theta Tau, Student Nurses' Association.
Nursing Student Resources Academic advising; academic or career counseling; assistance for students with disabilities; bookstore; campus computer network; career placement assistance; computer lab; computer-assisted instruction; daycare for children of students; e-mail services; employment services for current students; housing assistance; interactive nursing skills videos; Internet; learning resource lab; library services; nursing audiovisuals; placement services for program completers; resume preparation assistance; skills, simulation, or other laboratory; tutoring.
Library Facilities 25,000 volumes in health, 12,000 volumes in nursing; 20,000 periodical subscriptions health-care related.

BACCALAUREATE PROGRAMS

Degree BSN

Available Programs ADN to Baccalaureate; Generic Baccalaureate; LPN to RN Baccalaureate.
Study Options Full-time.
Online Degree Options Yes.
Program Entrance Requirements Minimum overall college GPA of 3.0, transcript of college record, CPR certification, written essay, health exam, health insurance, high school biology, high school chemistry, high school foreign language, 2 years high school math, 4 years high school science, high school transcript, immunizations, minimum GPA in nursing prerequisites of 3.0, professional liability insurance/malpractice insurance, prerequisite course work. Transfer students are accepted. *Application deadline:* 2/4 (fall), 8/5 (spring).
Advanced Placement Credit given for nursing courses completed elsewhere dependent upon specific evaluations.
Expenses (2015–16) *Tuition, state resident:* full-time $2613; part-time $174 per credit hour. *Tuition, nonresident:* full-time $9222; part-time $614 per credit hour. *International tuition:* $9222 full-time. *Room and board:* $9289; room only: $3285 per academic year. *Required fees:* part-time $145 per credit.
Contact Dr. Melissa Garno, BSN Program Director, School of Nursing, Georgia Southern University, PO Box 8158, Statesboro, GA 30460-8158. *Telephone:* 912-478-5454. *Fax:* 912-478-1159.
E-mail: mel@georgiasouthern.edu.

GRADUATE PROGRAMS

Expenses (2015–16) *Tuition, state resident:* full-time $3318; part-time $227 per credit hour. *Tuition, nonresident:* full-time $13,259; part-time $1105 per credit hour. *Room and board:* $9994; room only: $3285 per academic year. *Required fees:* part-time $145 per credit.
Financial Aid Research assistantships (averaging $7,200 per year), teaching assistantships (averaging $7,200 per year) were awarded; career-related internships or fieldwork, Federal Work-Study, scholarships, traineeships, tuition waivers (partial), and unspecified assistantships also available.
Contact Dr. Deborah Allen, Director, Graduate Program, School of Nursing, Georgia Southern University, PO Box 8158, Statesboro, GA 30460-8158. *Telephone:* 912-478-0017. *Fax:* 912-478-1679.
E-mail: debbieallen@georgiasouthern.edu.

MASTER'S DEGREE PROGRAM
Program Entrance Requirements GRE General Test or MAT.

DOCTORAL DEGREE PROGRAM
Degree DNP
Available Programs Doctorate; Post-Baccalaureate Doctorate.
Areas of Study Addiction/substance abuse, advanced practice nursing, clinical practice, family health, neuro-behavior, nursing education.
Online Degree Options Yes (online only).
Program Entrance Requirements Minimum overall college GPA of 3.0, interview by faculty committee, 3 letters of recommendation, vita, writing sample, GRE, MAT. Application deadline: 3/15 (fall).
Degree Requirements 74 total credit hours, oral exam, written exam.

Georgia Southwestern State University
School of Nursing
Americus, Georgia

http://www.gsw.edu/
Founded in 1906

DEGREES • BSN • MSN
Nursing Program Faculty 14 (46% with doctorates).
Baccalaureate Enrollment 134 **Women** 90% **Men** 10% **Part-time** 3%
Graduate Enrollment 48 **Women** 83% **Men** 17% **Part-time** 50%
Distance Learning Courses Available.
Nursing Student Activities Sigma Theta Tau, Student Nurses' Association.
Nursing Student Resources Academic advising; academic or career counseling; assistance for students with disabilities; bookstore; campus computer network; career placement assistance; computer lab; computer-assisted instruction; e-mail services; employment services for current students; interactive nursing skills videos; Internet; learning resource lab; library services; nursing audiovisuals; placement services for program completers; remedial services; resume preparation assistance; skills, simulation, or other laboratory; tutoring.

Library Facilities 627 volumes in health, 528 volumes in nursing; 141 periodical subscriptions health-care related.

BACCALAUREATE PROGRAMS

Degree BSN
Available Programs Baccalaureate for Second Degree; Generic Baccalaureate; LPN to RN Baccalaureate; RN Baccalaureate.
Study Options Full-time and part-time.
Online Degree Options Yes.
Program Entrance Requirements Minimum overall college GPA of 3.0, transcript of college record, CPR certification, written essay, health exam, health insurance, high school foreign language, 4 years high school math, 4 years high school science, high school transcript, immunizations, 2 letters of recommendation, minimum high school GPA of 2.8, minimum GPA in nursing prerequisites of 3.0, professional liability insurance/malpractice insurance, prerequisite course work, RN licensure. Transfer students are accepted. *Application deadline:* 2/15 (fall), 1/15 (summer).
Expenses (2015–16) *Tuition, state resident:* full-time $4860; part-time $162 per credit hour. *Tuition, nonresident:* full-time $17,678; part-time $589 per credit hour. *Room and board:* $8640; room only: $4980 per academic year. *Required fees:* full-time $1376.
Financial Aid *Gift aid (need-based):* Federal Pell, FSEOG, state, private, college/university gift aid from institutional funds. *Loans:* Federal Direct (Subsidized and Unsubsidized Stafford PLUS), Perkins, state. *Work-study:* Federal Work-Study. *Financial aid application deadline:* 6/15(priority: 4/15).
Contact Dr. Sandra Daniel, Dean and Professor, School of Nursing, Georgia Southwestern State University, 800 Georgia Southwestern State University Drive, Americus, GA 31709. *Telephone:* 229-931-2280. *Fax:* 229-931-2288. *E-mail:* sandra.daniel@gsw.edu.

GRADUATE PROGRAMS

Expenses (2015–16) *Tuition, state resident:* full-time $6930; part-time $385 per credit hour. *Tuition, nonresident:* full-time $6930; part-time $385 per credit hour. *Required fees:* full-time $1376; part-time $307 per term.
Contact Dr. Sandra Daniel, Dean, School of Nursing, Georgia Southwestern State University, 800 Georgia Southwestern State University Drive, Americus, GA 31709. *Telephone:* 912-931-2275. *Fax:* 912-931-2288. *E-mail:* Sandra.Daniel@gsw.edu.

MASTER'S DEGREE PROGRAM
Degree MSN
Available Programs Master's.
Concentrations Available Nursing administration; nursing education; nursing informatics. *Nurse practitioner programs in:* family health.
Study Options Full-time and part-time.
Online Degree Options Yes (online only).
Program Entrance Requirements Clinical experience, computer literacy, minimum overall college GPA of 3.0, transcript of college record, CPR certification, written essay, immunizations, interview, 3 letters of recommendation, nursing research course, physical assessment course, professional liability insurance/malpractice insurance, prerequisite course work, resume, statistics course. *Application deadline:* 4/15 (fall), 11/15 (spring). *Application fee:* $25.
Degree Requirements 36 total credit hours, thesis or project, comprehensive exam.

Georgia State University
Byrdine F. Lewis School of Nursing
Atlanta, Georgia

http://snhp.gsu.edu/
Founded in 1913

DEGREES • BS • MS • PHD
Nursing Program Faculty 60 (40% with doctorates).
Baccalaureate Enrollment 297 **Women** 86% **Men** 14% **Part-time** 5%
Graduate Enrollment 300 **Women** 90% **Men** 10% **Part-time** 90%
Distance Learning Courses Available.
Nursing Student Activities Sigma Theta Tau, Student Nurses' Association.
Nursing Student Resources Academic advising; academic or career counseling; assistance for students with disabilities; bookstore; campus computer network; career placement assistance; computer lab; computer-assisted instruction; e-mail services; interactive nursing skills videos;

Internet; learning resource lab; library services; nursing audiovisuals; remedial services; resume preparation assistance; skills, simulation, or other laboratory; tutoring.
Library Facilities 52,835 volumes in health, 20,856 volumes in nursing; 725 periodical subscriptions health-care related.

BACCALAUREATE PROGRAMS

Degree BS
Available Programs ADN to Baccalaureate; Accelerated RN Baccalaureate; Generic Baccalaureate.
Study Options Full-time and part-time.
Program Entrance Requirements Minimum overall college GPA of 3.5, transcript of college record, CPR certification, written essay, health exam, health insurance, immunizations, 2 letters of recommendation, minimum GPA in nursing prerequisites of 3.0, professional liability insurance/malpractice insurance, prerequisite course work. Transfer students are accepted. *Application deadline:* 3/1 (fall), 10/1 (spring).
Advanced Placement Credit given for nursing courses completed elsewhere dependent upon specific evaluations.
Expenses (2015–16) *Tuition, state resident:* part-time $285 per credit hour. *Tuition, nonresident:* part-time $892 per credit hour. *Room and board:* room only: $4952 per academic year.
Financial Aid 72% of baccalaureate students in nursing programs received some form of financial aid in 2014–15.
Contact Mr. Hugh Grant, Admissions Counselor, Byrdine F. Lewis School of Nursing, Georgia State University, School of Nursing and Health Professions, Office of Academic Assistance, Atlanta, GA 30303-3083. *Telephone:* 404-413-1000. *Fax:* 404-413-1001.
E-mail: hgrant@gsu.edu.

GRADUATE PROGRAMS

Expenses (2015–16) *Tuition, state resident:* part-time $388 per credit hour. *Tuition, nonresident:* part-time $1249 per credit hour. *Room and board:* $14,160 per academic year.
Financial Aid 64% of graduate students in nursing programs received some form of financial aid in 2014–15. Research assistantships with full and partial tuition reimbursements available (averaging $1,666 per year), teaching assistantships with full and partial tuition reimbursements available (averaging $1,920 per year) were awarded; scholarships, tuition waivers (full and partial), and unspecified assistantships also available. Aid available to part-time students. *Financial aid application deadline:* 8/1.
Contact Ms. Denisa Reed, Admissions Counselor III, Byrdine F. Lewis School of Nursing, Georgia State University, School of Nursing and Health Professions, PO Box 3995, Atlanta, GA 30302-3995. *Telephone:* 404-413-1000. *Fax:* 404-413-1001. *E-mail:* dmreed@gsu.edu.

MASTER'S DEGREE PROGRAM
Degree MS
Available Programs Master's; RN to Master's.
Concentrations Available Nursing administration; nursing informatics. *Clinical nurse specialist programs in:* adult health, adult-psychiatric mental health, pediatric, perinatal, psychiatric/mental health, women's health. *Nurse practitioner programs in:* adult health, adult-psychiatric mental health, family health, pediatric, psychiatric/mental health, women's health.
Site Options Alpharetta, GA.
Study Options Full-time and part-time.
Program Entrance Requirements Clinical experience, computer literacy, minimum overall college GPA of 3.0, transcript of college record, CPR certification, written essay, interview, 2 letters of recommendation, professional liability insurance/malpractice insurance. *Application deadline:* 3/1 (fall), 10/15 (spring), 3/1 (summer). *Application fee:* $50.
Advanced Placement Credit given for nursing courses completed elsewhere dependent upon specific evaluations.
Degree Requirements 48 total credit hours.

POST-MASTER'S PROGRAM
Areas of Study *Clinical nurse specialist programs in:* adult health, adult-psychiatric mental health, pediatric, perinatal, psychiatric/mental health, women's health. *Nurse practitioner programs in:* adult health, adult-psychiatric mental health, family health, pediatric, psychiatric/mental health, women's health.

DOCTORAL DEGREE PROGRAM
Degree PhD
Available Programs Doctorate; Post-Baccalaureate Doctorate.
Areas of Study Bio-behavioral research, health promotion/disease prevention, individualized study, nursing research, nursing science.

Site Options Alpharetta, GA.
Program Entrance Requirements Minimum overall college GPA of 3.0, interview by faculty committee, interview, 3 letters of recommendation, MSN or equivalent, statistics course, vita, GRE. Application deadline: 3/1 (fall). Application fee: $50.
Degree Requirements 60 total credit hours, dissertation, written exam, residency.

Gordon State College
Division of Nursing and Health Sciences
Barnesville, Georgia

https://www.gordonstate.edu/nhs/
Founded in 1852
DEGREE • BSN
Nursing Program Faculty 2 (50% with doctorates).
Baccalaureate Enrollment 26
Nursing Student Activities Student Nurses' Association.
Nursing Student Resources Academic advising; academic or career counseling; assistance for students with disabilities; bookstore; campus computer network; computer lab; computer-assisted instruction; e-mail services; employment services for current students; externships; interactive nursing skills videos; Internet; learning resource lab; library services; nursing audiovisuals; remedial services; skills, simulation, or other laboratory; tutoring.
Library Facilities 15 volumes in nursing.

BACCALAUREATE PROGRAMS
Degree BSN
Available Programs RN Baccalaureate.
Program Entrance Requirements Transcript of college record.
Contact *Telephone:* 678-359-5085. *Fax:* 678-359-5064.

Herzing University
Nursing Program
Atlanta, Georgia

https://www.herzing.edu/
Founded in 1949
DEGREE • BSN

BACCALAUREATE PROGRAMS
Degree BSN
Available Programs RN Baccalaureate.
Online Degree Options Yes.
Program Entrance Requirements RN licensure. *Application deadline:* Applications may be processed on a rolling basis for some programs.
Contact Atlanta Campus, Nursing Program, Herzing University, Lenox Square, 3393 Peachtree Drive NE, Atlanta, GA 30326. *Telephone:* 404-586-4265.

Kennesaw State University
School of Nursing
Kennesaw, Georgia

http://www.kennesaw.edu/
Founded in 1963
DEGREES • BSN • MSN
Distance Learning Courses Available.
Nursing Student Activities Sigma Theta Tau, Student Nurses' Association.
Nursing Student Resources Academic advising; academic or career counseling; assistance for students with disabilities; bookstore; campus computer network; career placement assistance; computer lab; computer-assisted instruction; e-mail services; employment services for current students; externships; housing assistance; interactive nursing skills videos; Internet; learning resource lab; library services; nursing audiovisuals; paid internships; placement services for program completers; remedial services; resume preparation assistance; skills, simulation, or other laboratory; tutoring.

Library Facilities 20,000 volumes in health, 10,000 volumes in nursing; 503 periodical subscriptions health-care related.

BACCALAUREATE PROGRAMS

Degree BSN
Available Programs ADN to Baccalaureate; Accelerated Baccalaureate; Accelerated Baccalaureate for Second Degree; Baccalaureate for Second Degree; Generic Baccalaureate; RN Baccalaureate.
Site Options Rome, GA; Jasper, GA.
Study Options Full-time and part-time.
Program Entrance Requirements Minimum overall college GPA of 2.7, transcript of college record, CPR certification, health exam, health insurance, 2 years high school math, 2 years high school science, high school transcript, immunizations, interview, 1 letter of recommendation, minimum high school GPA of 2.5, minimum GPA in nursing prerequisites of 2.7, professional liability insurance/malpractice insurance, prerequisite course work. Transfer students are accepted.
Advanced Placement Credit by examination available. Credit given for nursing courses completed elsewhere dependent upon specific evaluations.
Contact *Telephone:* 770-499-3211. *Fax:* 770-423-6627.

GRADUATE PROGRAMS

Contact *Telephone:* 770-423-6061. *Fax:* 770-423-6627.

MASTER'S DEGREE PROGRAM

Degree MSN
Available Programs Master's.
Concentrations Available *Clinical nurse specialist programs in:* adult health. *Nurse practitioner programs in:* adult health, family health, primary care.
Study Options Full-time.
Program Entrance Requirements Clinical experience, minimum overall college GPA of 3.0, transcript of college record, CPR certification, written essay, immunizations, 2 letters of recommendation, nursing research course, physical assessment course, professional liability insurance/malpractice insurance, prerequisite course work, resume.
Advanced Placement Credit given for nursing courses completed elsewhere dependent upon specific evaluations.
Degree Requirements 40 total credit hours, thesis or project.

CONTINUING EDUCATION PROGRAM

Contact *Telephone:* 770-423-6064. *Fax:* 770-423-6627.

LaGrange College
Department of Nursing
LaGrange, Georgia

http://www.lagrange.edu/
Founded in 1831
DEGREE • BSN
Nursing Program Faculty 7 (20% with doctorates).
Baccalaureate Enrollment 96 **Women** 85% **Men** 15%
Nursing Student Activities Nursing Honor Society, Student Nurses' Association.
Nursing Student Resources Academic advising; academic or career counseling; assistance for students with disabilities; bookstore; campus computer network; career placement assistance; computer lab; computer-assisted instruction; e-mail services; employment services for current students; externships; interactive nursing skills videos; Internet; learning resource lab; library services; nursing audiovisuals; paid internships; placement services for program completers; remedial services; resume preparation assistance; skills, simulation, or other laboratory; tutoring; unpaid internships.
Library Facilities 19,000 volumes in health, 10,000 volumes in nursing; 100 periodical subscriptions health-care related.

BACCALAUREATE PROGRAMS

Degree BSN
Available Programs Generic Baccalaureate; RN Baccalaureate.
Study Options Full-time.
Program Entrance Requirements Minimum overall college GPA of 2.5, transcript of college record, CPR certification, written essay, health exam, health insurance, immunizations, interview, 2 letters of recommendation, minimum GPA in nursing prerequisites of 2.5, professional lia-

bility insurance/malpractice insurance, prerequisite course work. Transfer students are accepted. *Application deadline:* 4/15 (fall). *Application fee:* $50.
Advanced Placement Credit given for nursing courses completed elsewhere dependent upon specific evaluations.
Expenses (2015–16) *Tuition:* full-time $38,000. *Room and board:* $10,800; room only: $6310 per academic year. *Required fees:* full-time $1700.
Financial Aid 90% of baccalaureate students in nursing programs received some form of financial aid in 2014–15.
Contact Dr. Celia G. Hay, Chair, Department of Nursing, LaGrange College, 601 Broad Street, LaGrange, GA 30240-2999. *Telephone:* 706-880-8220. *Fax:* 706-880-8029. *E-mail:* chay@lagrange.edu.

Mercer University
Georgia Baptist College of Nursing of Mercer University
Atlanta, Georgia

http://nursing.mercer.edu
Founded in 1968
DEGREES • BSN • DNP • MSN • PHD
Nursing Program Faculty 32 (65% with doctorates).
Baccalaureate Enrollment 297 **Women** 86% **Men** 14% **Part-time** 10%
Graduate Enrollment 110 **Women** 92% **Men** 8% **Part-time** 40%
Distance Learning Courses Available.
Nursing Student Activities Sigma Theta Tau, Student Nurses' Association, nursing club.
Nursing Student Resources Academic advising; academic or career counseling; assistance for students with disabilities; bookstore; campus computer network; career placement assistance; computer lab; computer-assisted instruction; e-mail services; employment services for current students; housing assistance; interactive nursing skills videos; Internet; learning resource lab; library services; nursing audiovisuals; placement services for program completers; remedial services; resume preparation assistance; skills, simulation, or other laboratory; tutoring.
Library Facilities 11,200 volumes in health, 3,300 volumes in nursing; 845 periodical subscriptions health-care related.

BACCALAUREATE PROGRAMS

Degree BSN
Available Programs Generic Baccalaureate; RN Baccalaureate.
Study Options Full-time.
Program Entrance Requirements Minimum overall college GPA, transcript of college record, CPR certification, written essay, health exam, health insurance, immunizations, letters of recommendation, minimum high school GPA of 3.0, minimum GPA in nursing prerequisites of 3.0, prerequisite course work. Transfer students are accepted. *Application deadline:* 4/1 (fall). Applications may be processed on a rolling basis for some programs. *Application fee:* $50.
Expenses (2015–16) *Tuition:* full-time $22,380; part-time $932 per credit hour. *International tuition:* $22,380 full-time. *Room and board:* room only: $8750 per academic year. *Required fees:* full-time $1350.
Financial Aid 63% of baccalaureate students in nursing programs received some form of financial aid in 2014–15. *Gift aid (need-based):* Federal Pell, FSEOG, state, private, college/university gift aid from institutional funds. *Loans:* Federal Direct (Subsidized and Unsubsidized Stafford PLUS), Perkins. *Work-study:* Federal Work-Study. *Financial aid application deadline:* 5/1.
Contact Ms. Janda Anderson, Director of Admissions, Georgia Baptist College of Nursing of Mercer University, Mercer University, 3001 Mercer University Drive, Atlanta, GA 30341-4115. *Telephone:* 678-547-6700. *Fax:* 678-547-6794. *E-mail:* Anderson_J@Mercer.edu.

GRADUATE PROGRAMS

Expenses (2015–16) *Tuition:* full-time $29,784; part-time $1103 per credit hour. *International tuition:* $29,784 full-time. *Room and board:* room only: $10,500 per academic year. *Required fees:* full-time $1460; part-time $750 per term.
Financial Aid 57% of graduate students in nursing programs received some form of financial aid in 2014–15.
Contact Ms. Janda Anderson, Director of Nursing Admissions, Georgia Baptist College of Nursing of Mercer University, Mercer University, 3001 Mercer University Drive, Atlanta, GA 30341. *Telephone:* 678-547-6700. *Fax:* 678-547-6794. *E-mail:* Anderson_J@Mercer.edu.

MASTER'S DEGREE PROGRAM

Degree MSN

Available Programs Master's.

Concentrations Available *Nurse practitioner programs in:* family health.

Study Options Full-time and part-time.

Program Entrance Requirements Clinical experience, computer literacy, minimum overall college GPA of 3.0, transcript of college record, CPR certification, written essay, immunizations, interview, 3 letters of recommendation, nursing research course, physical assessment course, prerequisite course work, statistics course. *Application deadline:* 5/1 (fall), 11/1 (spring), 3/1 (summer). Applications may be processed on a rolling basis for some programs. *Application fee:* $50.

Advanced Placement Credit given for nursing courses completed elsewhere dependent upon specific evaluations.

Degree Requirements 49 total credit hours, thesis or project.

DOCTORAL DEGREE PROGRAM

Degree DNP

Available Programs Doctorate.

Areas of Study Nurse executive.

Online Degree Options Yes (online only).

Program Entrance Requirements Minimum overall college GPA of 3.0, clinical experience, interview by faculty committee, 3 letters of recommendation, MSN or equivalent, statistics course, vita, writing sample. Application deadline: 4/1 (fall). Applications may be processed on a rolling basis for some programs. Application fee: $50.

Degree Requirements 41 total credit hours, residency, scholarly project.

Degree PhD

Available Programs Doctorate.

Areas of Study Ethics, nursing education, nursing research, nursing science.

Online Degree Options Yes (online only).

Program Entrance Requirements Minimum overall college GPA of 3.2, interview by faculty committee, 3 letters of recommendation, MSN or equivalent, statistics course, vita, writing sample. Application deadline: 3/1 (fall). Applications may be processed on a rolling basis for some programs. Application fee: $50.

Degree Requirements 58 total credit hours, dissertation, written exam, residency.

Middle Georgia College

School of Nursing and Health Sciences
Cochran, Georgia

http://www.mga.edu/health-sciences/nursing/default.aspx
Founded in 1884

DEGREE • BSN

Nursing Program Faculty 30 (7% with doctorates).

Baccalaureate Enrollment 104 **Women** 88% **Men** 12%

Nursing Student Activities Student Nurses' Association.

Nursing Student Resources Academic advising; academic or career counseling; assistance for students with disabilities; bookstore; campus computer network; career placement assistance; computer lab; computer-assisted instruction; e-mail services; interactive nursing skills videos; Internet; learning resource lab; library services; nursing audiovisuals; remedial services; resume preparation assistance; skills, simulation, or other laboratory; tutoring.

Library Facilities 4,000 volumes in health, 920 volumes in nursing; 90 periodical subscriptions health-care related.

BACCALAUREATE PROGRAMS

Degree BSN

Available Programs ADN to Baccalaureate; Generic Baccalaureate.

Study Options Full-time and part-time.

Program Entrance Requirements Minimum overall college GPA of 2.0, transcript of college record, CPR certification, health exam, health insurance, immunizations, minimum GPA in nursing prerequisites of 2.5, professional liability insurance/malpractice insurance, prerequisite course work. Transfer students are accepted. *Application deadline:* 2/15 (fall).

Contact *Telephone:* 478-471-2761. *Fax:* 478-471-2983.

Piedmont College

School of Nursing
Demorest, Georgia

http://www.piedmont.edu/pc/index.php/nursing-home
Founded in 1897

DEGREE • BSN

Nursing Program Faculty 8 (25% with doctorates).

Baccalaureate Enrollment 60 **Women** 99% **Men** 1% **Part-time** 20%

Distance Learning Courses Available.

Nursing Student Activities Nursing Honor Society, Student Nurses' Association.

Nursing Student Resources Academic advising; academic or career counseling; assistance for students with disabilities; bookstore; campus computer network; career placement assistance; computer lab; computer-assisted instruction; e-mail services; externships; housing assistance; interactive nursing skills videos; Internet; learning resource lab; library services; nursing audiovisuals; other; paid internships; resume preparation assistance; skills, simulation, or other laboratory; tutoring.

Library Facilities 3,000 volumes in health, 500 volumes in nursing; 75 periodical subscriptions health-care related.

BACCALAUREATE PROGRAMS

Degree BSN

Available Programs Generic Baccalaureate; LPN to Baccalaureate; RN Baccalaureate.

Study Options Full-time.

Program Entrance Requirements Transcript of college record, CPR certification, health exam, health insurance, high school foreign language, 2 years high school math, 3 years high school science, high school transcript, immunizations, minimum GPA in nursing prerequisites of 3.0, professional liability insurance/malpractice insurance, prerequisite course work. Transfer students are accepted. *Application deadline:* 10/15 (fall).

Advanced Placement Credit given for nursing courses completed elsewhere dependent upon specific evaluations.

Contact *Telephone:* 706-776-0116. *Fax:* 706-778-0701.

Shorter University

School of Nursing
Rome, Georgia

http://su.shorter.edu/nursing/
Founded in 1873

DEGREE • BSN

Nursing Program Faculty 10 (10% with doctorates).

Baccalaureate Enrollment 62 **Women** 75% **Men** 25%

Nursing Student Activities Student Nurses' Association, nursing club.

Nursing Student Resources Academic advising; academic or career counseling; assistance for students with disabilities; bookstore; campus computer network; computer lab; e-mail services; housing assistance; interactive nursing skills videos; Internet; learning resource lab; library services; nursing audiovisuals; resume preparation assistance; skills, simulation, or other laboratory; tutoring.

BACCALAUREATE PROGRAMS

Degree BSN

Available Programs Generic Baccalaureate.

Site Options Rome, GA.

Study Options Full-time.

Program Entrance Requirements Minimum overall college GPA of 3.0, transcript of college record, CPR certification, written essay, health exam, health insurance, immunizations, interview, letters of recommendation, minimum GPA in nursing prerequisites of 3.0, professional liability insurance/malpractice insurance, prerequisite course work. Transfer students are accepted. *Application deadline:* 3/1 (fall). *Application fee:* $25.

Contact *Telephone:* 706-233-7464. *Fax:* 706-291-4283.

Thomas University

Division of Nursing
Thomasville, Georgia

http://www.thomasu.edu/nursing.htm
Founded in 1950
DEGREES • BSN • MSN • MSN/MBA
Nursing Program Faculty 8 (75% with doctorates).
Baccalaureate Enrollment 120 **Women** 85% **Men** 15%
Graduate Enrollment 45 **Women** 90% **Men** 10% **Part-time** 50%
Distance Learning Courses Available.
Nursing Student Activities Nursing Honor Society, Sigma Theta Tau.
Nursing Student Resources Academic advising; academic or career counseling; assistance for students with disabilities; bookstore; campus computer network; career placement assistance; computer lab; computer-assisted instruction; e-mail services; housing assistance; interactive nursing skills videos; Internet; learning resource lab; library services; nursing audiovisuals; remedial services; resume preparation assistance; tutoring.
Library Facilities 1,200 volumes in health, 400 volumes in nursing; 150 periodical subscriptions health-care related.

BACCALAUREATE PROGRAMS

Degree BSN

Available Programs ADN to Baccalaureate; Accelerated RN Baccalaureate; International Nurse to Baccalaureate; RN Baccalaureate.
Site Options Tallahassee, FL; Moultrie, GA.
Study Options Full-time and part-time.
Program Entrance Requirements Minimum overall college GPA of 2.5, transcript of college record, CPR certification, health exam, health insurance, immunizations, minimum GPA in nursing prerequisites of 2.5, professional liability insurance/malpractice insurance, prerequisite course work, RN licensure. Transfer students are accepted. *Application deadline:* 8/1 (fall), 12/1 (spring), 4/15 (summer). Applications may be processed on a rolling basis for some programs. *Application fee:* $35.
Advanced Placement Credit by examination available. Credit given for nursing courses completed elsewhere dependent upon specific evaluations.
Financial Aid 90% of baccalaureate students in nursing programs received some form of financial aid in 2013–14.
Contact Rita Gagliano, Director of Admissions, Division of Nursing, Thomas University, 1501 Millpond Road, Thomasville, GA 31792. *Fax:* 229-226-1653. *E-mail:* rgagliano@thomasu.edu.

GRADUATE PROGRAMS

Financial Aid 50% of graduate students in nursing programs received some form of financial aid in 2013–14.
Contact Rita Gagliano, Director of Admissions, Division of Nursing, Thomas University, 1501 Millpond Road, Thomasville, GA 31792. *Fax:* 229-226-1653. *E-mail:* rgagliano@thomasu.edu.

MASTER'S DEGREE PROGRAM

Degrees MSN; MSN/MBA
Available Programs Accelerated Master's; Master's; RN to Master's.
Concentrations Available Health-care administration; nursing administration; nursing education.
Study Options Full-time and part-time.
Program Entrance Requirements Computer literacy, minimum overall college GPA of 3.0, transcript of college record, CPR certification, written essay, immunizations, 3 letters of recommendation, professional liability insurance/malpractice insurance, resume, statistics course. *Application deadline:* 8/1 (fall), 12/1 (spring), 4/15 (summer). Applications may be processed on a rolling basis for some programs. *Application fee:* $50.
Advanced Placement Credit given for nursing courses completed elsewhere dependent upon specific evaluations.
Degree Requirements 36 total credit hours, thesis or project.

POST-MASTER'S PROGRAM

Areas of Study Health-care administration; nursing administration; nursing education.

University of North Georgia

Department of Nursing
Dahlonega, Georgia

http://ung.edu/nursing/index.php
Founded in 1873
DEGREES • BSN • MS
Nursing Program Faculty 42 (17% with doctorates).
Baccalaureate Enrollment 360 **Women** 91% **Men** 9% **Part-time** 40%
Graduate Enrollment 50 **Women** 90% **Men** 10% **Part-time** 5%
Distance Learning Courses Available.
Nursing Student Activities Nursing Honor Society, Sigma Theta Tau, Student Nurses' Association.
Nursing Student Resources Academic advising; academic or career counseling; assistance for students with disabilities; bookstore; campus computer network; career placement assistance; computer lab; computer-assisted instruction; e-mail services; externships; interactive nursing skills videos; Internet; learning resource lab; library services; nursing audiovisuals; remedial services; resume preparation assistance; skills, simulation, or other laboratory; tutoring.
Library Facilities 6,875 volumes in health, 619 volumes in nursing; 2,377 periodical subscriptions health-care related.

BACCALAUREATE PROGRAMS

Degree BSN

Available Programs ADN to Baccalaureate; Generic Baccalaureate; RN Baccalaureate.
Study Options Full-time and part-time.
Online Degree Options Yes (online only).
Program Entrance Requirements Minimum overall college GPA of 2.75, transcript of college record, CPR certification, health exam, health insurance, high school biology, high school chemistry, high school foreign language, 3 years high school math, 2 years high school science, high school transcript, immunizations, 2 letters of recommendation, professional liability insurance/malpractice insurance, prerequisite course work, RN licensure. Transfer students are accepted. *Application deadline:* 12/15 (fall). *Application fee:* $25.
Expenses (2015–16) *Tuition, area resident:* full-time $8560. *Tuition, state resident:* full-time $5350. *Tuition, nonresident:* full-time $18,900. *International tuition:* $18,900 full-time. *Room and board:* room only: $5350 per academic year. *Required fees:* full-time $1826.
Financial Aid 88% of baccalaureate students in nursing programs received some form of financial aid in 2014–15.
Contact Mrs. Patti Simmons, Coordinator, BSN Program, Department of Nursing, University of North Georgia, 82 College Circle, Dahlonega, GA 30597. *Telephone:* 706-864-1937. *Fax:* 706-864-1845. *E-mail:* patti.simmons@ung.edu.

GRADUATE PROGRAMS

Contact Dr. Deborah A Dumphy, Coordinator, MS Program, Department of Nursing, University of North Georgia, 82 College Circle, Dahlonega, GA 30597. *Telephone:* 706-864-1939. *Fax:* 706-864-1845. *E-mail:* deborah.dumphy@ung.edu.

MASTER'S DEGREE PROGRAM

Degree MS
Available Programs Master's.
Concentrations Available Nursing education. *Nurse practitioner programs in:* family health.
Study Options Full-time and part-time.
Program Entrance Requirements Clinical experience, computer literacy, minimum overall college GPA of 3.0, transcript of college record, CPR certification, written essay, immunizations, 3 letters of recommendation, nursing research course, physical assessment course, professional liability insurance/malpractice insurance, prerequisite course work. *Application deadline:* 2/28 (spring). *Application fee:* $40.
Degree Requirements 46 total credit hours, thesis or project, comprehensive exam.

POST-MASTER'S PROGRAM

Areas of Study Nursing education. *Nurse practitioner programs in:* family health.

University of Phoenix–Atlanta Campus

College of Health and Human Services
Sandy Springs, Georgia

Nursing Student Activities Sigma Theta Tau.
Nursing Student Resources Academic advising; academic or career counseling; assistance for students with disabilities; bookstore; campus computer network; computer lab; computer-assisted instruction; e-mail services; interactive nursing skills videos; Internet; learning resource lab; library services; nursing audiovisuals; remedial services; skills, simulation, or other laboratory; tutoring.
Library Facilities 1,300 periodical subscriptions health-care related.

University of West Georgia

School of Nursing
Carrollton, Georgia

http://nursing.westga.edu/
Founded in 1933

DEGREES • BSN • EDD • MSN
Nursing Program Faculty 45 (33% with doctorates).
Baccalaureate Enrollment 357 **Women** 88% **Men** 12% **Part-time** 66%
Graduate Enrollment 118 **Women** 86% **Men** 14% **Part-time** 38%
Distance Learning Courses Available.
Nursing Student Activities Sigma Theta Tau, Student Nurses' Association.
Nursing Student Resources Academic advising; academic or career counseling; assistance for students with disabilities; bookstore; campus computer network; career placement assistance; computer lab; computer-assisted instruction; e-mail services; employment services for current students; externships; housing assistance; interactive nursing skills videos; Internet; learning resource lab; library services; nursing audiovisuals; remedial services; resume preparation assistance; skills, simulation, or other laboratory; tutoring.
Library Facilities 8,842 volumes in health, 460 volumes in nursing; 28 periodical subscriptions health-care related.

BACCALAUREATE PROGRAMS

Degree BSN
Available Programs Accelerated RN Baccalaureate; Generic Baccalaureate.
Site Options Newnan, GA.
Study Options Full-time and part-time.
Program Entrance Requirements Minimum overall college GPA of 3.0, transcript of college record, CPR certification, health exam, health insurance, immunizations, minimum GPA in nursing prerequisites of 3.00, professional liability insurance/malpractice insurance, prerequisite course work. Transfer students are accepted. *Application deadline:* 2/1 (summer). *Application fee:* $40.
Expenses (2015–16) *Tuition, state resident:* full-time $8866; part-time $174 per credit hour. *Tuition, nonresident:* full-time $23,846; part-time $615 per credit hour. *Room and board:* $5049; room only: $3100 per academic year. *Required fees:* full-time $732; part-time $244 per term.
Financial Aid 67% of baccalaureate students in nursing programs received some form of financial aid in 2014–15.
Contact Dr. Cynthia D. Epps, Associate Dean and Undergraduate Program Coordinator, School of Nursing, University of West Georgia, 1601 Maple Street, Carrollton, GA 30118. *Telephone:* 678-839-6552. *Fax:* 678-839-2462. *E-mail:* cepps@westga.edu.

GRADUATE PROGRAMS

Expenses (2015–16) *Tuition, area resident:* full-time $8116; part-time $222 per credit hour.
Financial Aid 42% of graduate students in nursing programs received some form of financial aid in 2014–15.
Contact Dr. Laurie Jowers Ware, Associate Dean and Director of Graduate Program, School of Nursing, University of West Georgia, 1601 Maple Street, Carrollton, GA 30118. *Telephone:* 678-839-6552. *Fax:* 678-839-2462. *E-mail:* lware@westga.edu.

MASTER'S DEGREE PROGRAM
Degree MSN
Available Programs Master's.

Concentrations Available Clinical nurse leader; nursing administration; nursing education.
Study Options Full-time and part-time.
Online Degree Options Yes (online only).
Program Entrance Requirements Clinical experience, computer literacy, minimum overall college GPA of 3.0, transcript of college record, CPR certification, immunizations, 2 letters of recommendation, nursing research course, professional liability insurance/malpractice insurance, prerequisite course work, resume, statistics course. *Application deadline:* 2/1 (fall). *Application fee:* $40.
Degree Requirements 36 total credit hours, thesis or project.

POST-MASTER'S PROGRAM
Areas of Study Clinical nurse leader; nursing administration; nursing education.

DOCTORAL DEGREE PROGRAM
Degree EdD
Available Programs Doctorate.
Areas of Study Nursing education.
Online Degree Options Yes (online only).
Program Entrance Requirements Minimum overall college GPA of 3.0, 3 letters of recommendation, MSN or equivalent, statistics course, vita, writing sample. Application deadline: 2/1 (fall). Application fee: $40.
Degree Requirements 60 total credit hours, dissertation, oral exam, written exam.

Valdosta State University

College of Nursing
Valdosta, Georgia

http://www.valdosta.edu/nursing/
Founded in 1906

DEGREES • BSN • MSN
Nursing Program Faculty 23 (52% with doctorates).
Baccalaureate Enrollment 183 **Women** 87% **Men** 13% **Part-time** 7%
Graduate Enrollment 25 **Women** 99% **Men** 1% **Part-time** 49%
Nursing Student Activities Sigma Theta Tau, Student Nurses' Association.
Nursing Student Resources Academic advising; academic or career counseling; assistance for students with disabilities; bookstore; campus computer network; career placement assistance; computer lab; computer-assisted instruction; e-mail services; employment services for current students; externships; housing assistance; Internet; learning resource lab; library services; nursing audiovisuals; placement services for program completers; resume preparation assistance; skills, simulation, or other laboratory; tutoring; unpaid internships.
Library Facilities 21,688 volumes in health; 75 periodical subscriptions health-care related.

BACCALAUREATE PROGRAMS

Degree BSN
Available Programs Generic Baccalaureate; RN Baccalaureate.
Study Options Full-time.
Program Entrance Requirements Minimum overall college GPA of 2.8, transcript of college record, CPR certification, health exam, health insurance, immunizations, minimum GPA in nursing prerequisites of 2.8, professional liability insurance/malpractice insurance, prerequisite course work. Transfer students are accepted.
Advanced Placement Credit given for nursing courses completed elsewhere dependent upon specific evaluations.
Contact *Telephone:* 229-333-5959. *Fax:* 229-333-7300.

GRADUATE PROGRAMS

Contact *Telephone:* 229-333-5959. *Fax:* 229-333-7300.

MASTER'S DEGREE PROGRAM
Degree MSN
Available Programs Master's; RN to Master's.
Concentrations Available Nurse case management; nursing administration; nursing education. *Clinical nurse specialist programs in:* adult health, family health, psychiatric/mental health.
Study Options Full-time and part-time.
Program Entrance Requirements Minimum overall college GPA of 2.8, transcript of college record, CPR certification, immunizations, 3

letters of recommendation, physical assessment course, professional liability insurance/malpractice insurance, statistics course, GRE General Test.

Advanced Placement Credit given for nursing courses completed elsewhere dependent upon specific evaluations.

Degree Requirements 36 total credit hours, thesis or project, comprehensive exam.

CONTINUING EDUCATION PROGRAM

Contact *Telephone:* 229-333-5960.

GUAM

University of Guam
School of Nursing and Health Sciences
Mangilao, Guam

http://www.uog.edu/
Founded in 1952
DEGREE • BSN
Nursing Program Faculty 10 (30% with doctorates).
Baccalaureate Enrollment 175 **Women** 97% **Men** 3%
Nursing Student Activities Student Nurses' Association.
Nursing Student Resources Academic advising; academic or career counseling; assistance for students with disabilities; bookstore; campus computer network; career placement assistance; computer lab; daycare for children of students; e-mail services; employment services for current students; interactive nursing skills videos; Internet; learning resource lab; library services; nursing audiovisuals; remedial services; skills, simulation, or other laboratory; tutoring.
Library Facilities 5,246 volumes in health, 982 volumes in nursing; 53 periodical subscriptions health-care related.

BACCALAUREATE PROGRAMS

Degree BSN
Available Programs ADN to Baccalaureate; Generic Baccalaureate; RN Baccalaureate.
Study Options Full-time and part-time.
Program Entrance Requirements Transcript of college record, CPR certification, written essay, health exam, high school biology, high school chemistry, 1 year of high school math, 1 year of high school science, high school transcript, immunizations, interview, minimum high school GPA of 2.5, minimum GPA in nursing prerequisites of 2.7, prerequisite course work. Transfer students are accepted.
Advanced Placement Credit by examination available. Credit given for nursing courses completed elsewhere dependent upon specific evaluations.
Contact *Telephone:* 671-735-2210. *Fax:* 671-734-4245.

HAWAII

Chaminade University of Honolulu
Nursing Program
Honolulu, Hawaii

http://www.chaminade.edu/nursing
Founded in 1955
DEGREE • BSN
Nursing Program Faculty 10 (36% with doctorates).
Baccalaureate Enrollment 280 **Women** 74% **Men** 26%
Nursing Student Activities Nursing Honor Society, Sigma Theta Tau, Student Nurses' Association, nursing club.
Nursing Student Resources Academic advising; academic or career counseling; assistance for students with disabilities; bookstore; campus computer network; computer lab; computer-assisted instruction; e-mail services; employment services for current students; interactive nursing skills videos; Internet; learning resource lab; library services; nursing audiovisuals; paid internships; remedial services; resume preparation assistance; skills, simulation, or other laboratory; tutoring; unpaid internships.

BACCALAUREATE PROGRAMS

Degree BSN
Available Programs Generic Baccalaureate.
Study Options Full-time.
Program Entrance Requirements Minimum overall college GPA of 2.75, transcript of college record, written essay, high school chemistry, 4 years high school math, high school transcript, 2 letters of recommendation, minimum high school GPA of 2.75. Transfer students are accepted. *Application deadline:* 2/1 (fall). *Application fee:* $25.
Expenses (2015–16) *Tuition:* full-time $26,600.
Financial Aid *Gift aid (need-based):* Federal Pell, FSEOG, private, college/university gift aid from institutional funds, Academic Competitiveness Grants, National SMART Grants, TEACH Grants, LEAP grants, AAP. *Loans:* Federal Direct (Subsidized and Unsubsidized Stafford PLUS), alternative loans. *Work-study:* Federal Work-Study. *Financial aid application deadline:* Continuous.
Contact Dr. Gwenevere Anderson, Dean, School of Nursing, Nursing Program, Chaminade University of Honolulu, 3140 Waialae Avenue, Henry Hall 110, Honolulu, HI 96816. *Telephone:* 808-735-4813. *Fax:* 808-739-8564. *E-mail:* camille.cabalo@chaminade.edu.

Hawaii Pacific University
College of Nursing and Health Sciences
Honolulu, Hawaii

http://www.hpu.edu/
Founded in 1965
DEGREES • BSN • MSN • MSN/MBA
Nursing Program Faculty 50 (51% with doctorates).
Baccalaureate Enrollment 497 **Women** 80% **Men** 20% **Part-time** 67%
Graduate Enrollment 61 **Women** 87% **Men** 13% **Part-time** 57%
Distance Learning Courses Available.
Nursing Student Activities Nursing Honor Society, Sigma Theta Tau, Student Nurses' Association.
Nursing Student Resources Academic advising; academic or career counseling; assistance for students with disabilities; bookstore; campus computer network; career placement assistance; computer lab; computer-assisted instruction; e-mail services; employment services for current students; externships; housing assistance; Internet; learning resource lab; library services; nursing audiovisuals; paid internships; placement services for program completers; remedial services; resume preparation assistance; skills, simulation, or other laboratory; tutoring.
Library Facilities 4,608 volumes in health, 1,335 volumes in nursing; 7,682 periodical subscriptions health-care related.

BACCALAUREATE PROGRAMS

Degree BSN
Available Programs Generic Baccalaureate; International Nurse to Baccalaureate; LPN to Baccalaureate; RN Baccalaureate.
Site Options Kaneohe, HI.
Study Options Full-time.
Program Entrance Requirements Minimum overall college GPA of 2.75, transcript of college record, CPR certification, written essay, health exam, health insurance, immunizations, 2 letters of recommendation, minimum high school GPA, minimum GPA in nursing prerequisites of 2.75, prerequisite course work. Transfer students are accepted. *Application deadline:* 2/28 (fall), 10/15 (spring). *Application fee:* $50.
Advanced Placement Credit given for nursing courses completed elsewhere dependent upon specific evaluations.
Expenses (2015–16) *Tuition:* full-time $28,460; part-time $955 per credit. *Room and board:* $13,610 per academic year. *Required fees:* full-time $280; part-time $25 per term.
Contact Miss Sara Sato, Director of Admissions, College of Nursing and Health Sciences, Hawai'i Pacific University, 1164 Bishop Street, Honolulu, HI 96813. *Telephone:* 808-544-0238. *Fax:* 808-544-1136. *E-mail:* ssato@hpu.edu.

GRADUATE PROGRAMS

Expenses (2015–16) *Tuition:* part-time $1275 per credit hour. *Room and board:* $13,610 per academic year. *Required fees:* part-time $13 per term.

Financial Aid Career-related internships or fieldwork, Federal Work-Study, scholarships, traineeships, and tuition waivers available.

Contact Dr. Diane Knight, Chair, Department of Graduate and Post-Baccalaureate Nursing Programs, College of Nursing and Health Sciences, Hawai`i Pacific University, 45-045 Kamehameha Highway, Kaneohe, HI 96744-5297. *Telephone:* 808-236-3552. *Fax:* 808-236-5847. *E-mail:* dknight@hpu.edu.

MASTER'S DEGREE PROGRAM

Degrees MSN; MSN/MBA
Available Programs Master's; RN to Master's.
Concentrations Available *Nurse practitioner programs in:* acute care, family health.
Site Options Kaneohe, HI.
Study Options Full-time and part-time.
Program Entrance Requirements Minimum overall college GPA of 3.0, transcript of college record, written essay, 2 letters of recommendation, nursing research course, prerequisite course work, statistics course. *Application deadline:* 4/15 (fall), 10/15 (spring). *Application fee:* $50.
Advanced Placement Credit given for nursing courses completed elsewhere dependent upon specific evaluations.
Degree Requirements 50 total credit hours, thesis or project.

POST-MASTER'S PROGRAM

Areas of Study *Nurse practitioner programs in:* acute care, family health.

See display below and full description on page 496.

University of Hawaii at Hilo
Department in Nursing
Hilo, Hawaii

http://www.uhh.hawaii.edu/
Founded in 1970

DEGREE • BSN
Nursing Program Faculty 10 (50% with doctorates).
Baccalaureate Enrollment 78 **Women** 83% **Men** 17% **Part-time** 18%

Distance Learning Courses Available.
Nursing Student Activities Nursing Honor Society, Sigma Theta Tau, Student Nurses' Association.
Nursing Student Resources Academic advising; academic or career counseling; assistance for students with disabilities; bookstore; campus computer network; career placement assistance; computer lab; computer-assisted instruction; e-mail services; employment services for current students; externships; housing assistance; interactive nursing skills videos; Internet; learning resource lab; library services; nursing audiovisuals; paid internships; remedial services; resume preparation assistance; skills, simulation, or other laboratory; tutoring.
Library Facilities 680 volumes in health, 284 volumes in nursing; 15,000 periodical subscriptions health-care related.

BACCALAUREATE PROGRAMS

Degree BSN
Available Programs ADN to Baccalaureate; Generic Baccalaureate; RN Baccalaureate.
Site Options Kona, HI; Lihue, HI; Kahalui, HI.
Study Options Full-time.
Program Entrance Requirements Minimum overall college GPA of 2.7, transcript of college record, CPR certification, written essay, health exam, health insurance, high school biology, high school chemistry, high school foreign language, 1 year of high school math, 3 years high school science, high school transcript, immunizations, 2 letters of recommendation, minimum high school GPA of 3.0, minimum GPA in nursing prerequisites of 2.7, professional liability insurance/malpractice insurance, prerequisite course work. *Application deadline:* 1/15 (fall).
Contact *Telephone:* 808-974-7760. *Fax:* 808-974-7665.

University of Hawaii at Manoa
School of Nursing and Dental Hygiene
Honolulu, Hawaii

http://www.nursing.hawaii.edu/
Founded in 1907

DEGREES • BSN • MS • MSN/MBA • PHD
Nursing Program Faculty 97 (35% with doctorates).
Baccalaureate Enrollment 336 **Women** 77% **Men** 23% **Part-time** 56%

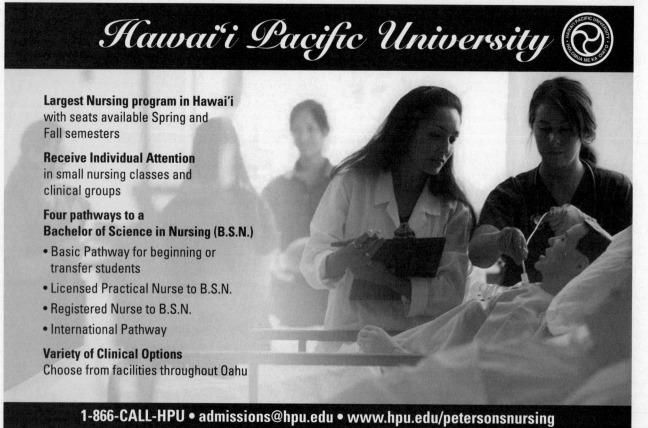

Hawai'i Pacific University

Largest Nursing program in Hawai'i
with seats available Spring and Fall semesters

Receive Individual Attention
in small nursing classes and clinical groups

Four pathways to a Bachelor of Science in Nursing (B.S.N.)
- Basic Pathway for beginning or transfer students
- Licensed Practical Nurse to B.S.N.
- Registered Nurse to B.S.N.
- International Pathway

Variety of Clinical Options
Choose from facilities throughout Oahu

1-866-CALL-HPU • admissions@hpu.edu • www.hpu.edu/petersonsnursing

Graduate Enrollment 170 Women 88% Men 12% Part-time 66%
Distance Learning Courses Available.
Nursing Student Activities Nursing Honor Society, Sigma Theta Tau, Student Nurses' Association, nursing club.
Nursing Student Resources Academic advising; academic or career counseling; assistance for students with disabilities; bookstore; computer lab; computer-assisted instruction; e-mail services; employment services for current students; housing assistance; Internet; learning resource lab; library services; nursing audiovisuals; resume preparation assistance; skills, simulation, or other laboratory.

BACCALAUREATE PROGRAMS

Degree BSN
Available Programs ADN to Baccalaureate; Generic Baccalaureate; RN Baccalaureate.
Study Options Full-time and part-time.
Program Entrance Requirements Minimum overall college GPA of 2.5, transcript of college record, CPR certification, health exam, health insurance, immunizations, minimum GPA in nursing prerequisites of 2.5, prerequisite course work. Transfer students are accepted. *Application deadline:* 3/1 (fall), 10/1 (spring). *Application fee:* $50.
Advanced Placement Credit by examination available. Credit given for nursing courses completed elsewhere dependent upon specific evaluations.
Contact *Telephone:* 808-956-8939. *Fax:* 808-956-5977.

GRADUATE PROGRAMS

Contact *Telephone:* 808-956-3519. *Fax:* 808-956-5977.

MASTER'S DEGREE PROGRAM

Degrees MS; MSN/MBA
Available Programs Accelerated Master's; Master's; Master's for Non-Nursing College Graduates; RN to Master's.
Concentrations Available Nursing administration; nursing education. *Clinical nurse specialist programs in:* psychiatric/mental health. *Nurse practitioner programs in:* adult health, community health, family health, gerontology, pediatric.
Site Options Kahului, HI; Lihue, HI; Kailua Kona, HI.
Study Options Full-time and part-time.
Online Degree Options Yes.
Program Entrance Requirements Minimum overall college GPA of 3.0, transcript of college record, CPR certification, written essay, immunizations, interview, 2 letters of recommendation, resume, statistics course. *Application deadline:* 3/1 (fall). *Application fee:* $60.
Advanced Placement Credit given for nursing courses completed elsewhere dependent upon specific evaluations.
Degree Requirements 52 total credit hours.

POST-MASTER'S PROGRAM

Areas of Study Nursing administration; nursing education. *Clinical nurse specialist programs in:* psychiatric/mental health. *Nurse practitioner programs in:* adult health, community health, family health, gerontology, pediatric.

DOCTORAL DEGREE PROGRAM

Degree PhD
Available Programs Doctorate.
Areas of Study Faculty preparation, nursing education, nursing research, nursing science.
Site Options Kahului, HI; Lihue, HI; Kailua Kona, HI.
Online Degree Options Yes (online only).
Program Entrance Requirements Clinical experience, minimum overall college GPA of 3.0, interview by faculty committee, interview, 3 letters of recommendation, MSN or equivalent, scholarly papers, statistics course, vita, writing sample. Application deadline: 2/1 (fall).
Degree Requirements 46 total credit hours, dissertation, oral exam, residency.

University of Phoenix–Hawaii Campus
College of Nursing
Honolulu, Hawaii

DEGREES • BSN • MSN • MSN/ED D
Nursing Program Faculty 26 (15% with doctorates).
Baccalaureate Enrollment 70 Women 90% Men 10%

Graduate Enrollment 14 Women 71.4% Men 28.6%
Nursing Student Activities Sigma Theta Tau.
Nursing Student Resources Academic advising; academic or career counseling; assistance for students with disabilities; bookstore; campus computer network; computer lab; computer-assisted instruction; e-mail services; interactive nursing skills videos; Internet; learning resource lab; library services; nursing audiovisuals; remedial services; skills, simulation, or other laboratory; tutoring.
Library Facilities 1,300 periodical subscriptions health-care related.

BACCALAUREATE PROGRAMS

Degree BSN
Available Programs Accelerated Baccalaureate; LPN to Baccalaureate.
Site Options Kaneohe, HI; Mililani, HI; Kapolei, HI.
Study Options Full-time.
Program Entrance Requirements Transcript of college record, CPR certification, immunizations, 1 letter of recommendation, RN licensure. Transfer students are accepted. *Application deadline:* Applications may be processed on a rolling basis for some programs.
Advanced Placement Credit by examination available. Credit given for nursing courses completed elsewhere dependent upon specific evaluations.
Contact *Telephone:* 808-536-2686.

GRADUATE PROGRAMS

Contact *Telephone:* 808-536-2686.

MASTER'S DEGREE PROGRAM

Degrees MSN; MSN/Ed D
Available Programs Master's.
Concentrations Available Health-care administration; nursing administration; nursing education. *Nurse practitioner programs in:* family health.
Site Options Kaneohe, HI; Mililani, HI; Kapolei, HI.
Study Options Full-time.
Program Entrance Requirements Clinical experience, computer literacy, minimum overall college GPA of 2.5, transcript of college record. *Application deadline:* Applications may be processed on a rolling basis for some programs. *Application fee:* $45.
Advanced Placement Credit given for nursing courses completed elsewhere dependent upon specific evaluations.
Degree Requirements 39 total credit hours, thesis or project.

IDAHO

Boise State University
Department of Nursing
Boise, Idaho

http://hs.boisestate.edu/nursing/
Founded in 1932
DEGREES • BS • MSN • MSN/MS
Nursing Program Faculty 55 (25% with doctorates).
Baccalaureate Enrollment 540 Women 75% Men 25%
Graduate Enrollment 12
Distance Learning Courses Available.
Nursing Student Activities Nursing Honor Society, Sigma Theta Tau, Student Nurses' Association.
Nursing Student Resources Academic advising; academic or career counseling; assistance for students with disabilities; bookstore; campus computer network; career placement assistance; computer lab; computer-assisted instruction; daycare for children of students; e-mail services; employment services for current students; housing assistance; interactive nursing skills videos; Internet; learning resource lab; library services; nursing audiovisuals; placement services for program completers; remedial services; resume preparation assistance; skills, simulation, or other laboratory; tutoring.
Library Facilities 27,919 volumes in health, 2,617 volumes in nursing; 158 periodical subscriptions health-care related.

BACCALAUREATE PROGRAMS

Degree BS

Available Programs Accelerated RN Baccalaureate; Generic Baccalaureate; LPN to Baccalaureate; RN Baccalaureate.
Site Options Nampa, ID.
Study Options Full-time.
Online Degree Options Yes.
Program Entrance Requirements Transcript of college record, immunizations, minimum GPA in nursing prerequisites of 3.0, professional liability insurance/malpractice insurance, prerequisite course work. Transfer students are accepted. *Application deadline:* 3/1 (fall), 10/1 (spring). *Application fee:* $20.
Advanced Placement Credit by examination available. Credit given for nursing courses completed elsewhere dependent upon specific evaluations.
Contact *Telephone:* 208-426-4143. *Fax:* 208-426-1370.

GRADUATE PROGRAMS

Contact *Telephone:* 208-426-4143.

MASTER'S DEGREE PROGRAM

Degrees MSN; MSN/MS
Available Programs Master's.
Concentrations Available Clinical nurse leader; health-care administration; nurse case management; nursing administration; nursing education.
Study Options Part-time.
Program Entrance Requirements Minimum overall college GPA of 3.0, transcript of college record, CPR certification, written essay, letters of recommendation, nursing research course, professional liability insurance/malpractice insurance, prerequisite course work, resume, statistics course. *Application deadline:* 3/31 (spring).
Degree Requirements 39 total credit hours, thesis or project.

Brigham Young University–Idaho
Department of Nursing
Rexburg, Idaho

http://www.byui.edu
Founded in 1888
DEGREE • BSN

BACCALAUREATE PROGRAMS

Degree BSN
Available Programs RN Baccalaureate.
Program Entrance Requirements RN licensure. Transfer students are accepted. *Application deadline:* 6/1 (fall), 10/1 (winter), 2/1 (spring).
Contact *Telephone:* 208-496-4555. *Fax:* 208-496-4553.

Idaho State University
Department of Nursing
Pocatello, Idaho

http://www.isu.edu/nursing
Founded in 1901
DEGREES • BS • DNP • MS • PHD
Nursing Program Faculty 16 (44% with doctorates).
Baccalaureate Enrollment 159 **Women** 74% **Men** 26%
Graduate Enrollment 65 **Women** 88% **Men** 12% **Part-time** 26%
Distance Learning Courses Available.
Nursing Student Activities Sigma Theta Tau, Student Nurses' Association.
Nursing Student Resources Academic advising; academic or career counseling; assistance for students with disabilities; bookstore; campus computer network; career placement assistance; computer lab; computer-assisted instruction; daycare for children of students; e-mail services; employment services for current students; housing assistance; interactive nursing skills videos; Internet; learning resource lab; library services; nursing audiovisuals; resume preparation assistance; skills, simulation, or other laboratory; tutoring.
Library Facilities 35,948 volumes in health, 1,775 volumes in nursing; 5,312 periodical subscriptions health-care related.

BACCALAUREATE PROGRAMS

Degree BS

Available Programs ADN to Baccalaureate; Accelerated Baccalaureate for Second Degree; Generic Baccalaureate.
Site Options Meridian, ID; Idaho Falls, ID.
Study Options Full-time.
Program Entrance Requirements Minimum overall college GPA of 3.0, transcript of college record, CPR certification, health exam, health insurance, high school transcript, immunizations, minimum high school GPA of 2.0, minimum GPA in nursing prerequisites of 3.0, professional liability insurance/malpractice insurance, prerequisite course work. Transfer students are accepted. *Application deadline:* 2/12 (fall). *Application fee:* $50.
Advanced Placement Credit given for nursing courses completed elsewhere dependent upon specific evaluations.
Expenses (2014–15) *Tuition, state resident:* full-time $3283; part-time $328 per credit. *Tuition, nonresident:* full-time $9663; part-time $535 per credit. *International tuition:* $9663 full-time. *Room and board:* $2665; room only: $1275 per academic year. *Required fees:* full-time $861; part-time $35 per credit; part-time $861 per term.
Financial Aid 75% of baccalaureate students in nursing programs received some form of financial aid in 2013–14.
Contact Dr. Elizabeth D. Rocha, Associate Director of Undergraduate Studies, School of Nursing, Department of Nursing, Idaho State University, 921 South 8th Avenue, Stop 8101, Pocatello, ID 83209-8101. *Telephone:* 208-282-2854. *Fax:* 208-236-4476. *E-mail:* rocheli2@isu.edu.

GRADUATE PROGRAMS

Expenses (2014–15) *Tuition, state resident:* full-time $3867; part-time $387 per credit. *Tuition, nonresident:* full-time $10,247; part-time $594 per credit. *Required fees:* full-time $3766.
Financial Aid 40% of graduate students in nursing programs received some form of financial aid in 2013–14. 1 research assistantship with full and partial tuition reimbursement available (averaging $9,401 per year), 4 teaching assistantships with full and partial tuition reimbursements available (averaging $10,841 per year) were awarded; career-related internships or fieldwork, Federal Work-Study, institutionally sponsored loans, scholarships, tuition waivers (full and partial), and unspecified assistantships also available. Aid available to part-time students. *Financial aid application deadline:* 1/1.
Contact Dr. Karen Neill, Associate Director of Graduate Studies, School of Nursing, Department of Nursing, Idaho State University, 921 South 8th Avenue, Stop 8101, Pocatello, ID 83209-8101. *Telephone:* 208-282-2102. *Fax:* 208-282-4476. *E-mail:* nielkare@isu.edu.

MASTER'S DEGREE PROGRAM

Degree MS
Available Programs Master's.
Concentrations Available Nursing education.
Study Options Full-time and part-time.
Online Degree Options Yes (online only).
Program Entrance Requirements Minimum overall college GPA of 3.0, transcript of college record, CPR certification, written essay, immunizations, interview, 3 letters of recommendation, professional liability insurance/malpractice insurance, prerequisite course work, resume, statistics course, GRE General Test. *Application deadline:* Applications may be processed on a rolling basis for some programs. *Application fee:* $55.
Advanced Placement Credit given for nursing courses completed elsewhere dependent upon specific evaluations.
Degree Requirements 40 total credit hours, comprehensive exam.

POST-MASTER'S PROGRAM

Areas of Study Nursing education.

DOCTORAL DEGREE PROGRAM

Degree DNP
Available Programs Doctorate; Post-Baccalaureate Doctorate.
Areas of Study Advanced practice nursing, family health.
Online Degree Options Yes (online only).
Program Entrance Requirements Minimum overall college GPA of 3.0, 3 letters of recommendation, statistics course, vita, writing sample. Application deadline: Applications may be processed on a rolling basis for some programs. Application fee: $55.
Degree Requirements 76 total credit hours, oral exam, written exam.

Degree PhD
Available Programs Doctorate, Post-Baccalaureate Doctorate.
Areas of Study Nursing science.
Online Degree Options Yes (online only).

Program Entrance Requirements Minimum overall college GPA of 3.0, interview by faculty committee, 3 letters of recommendation, statistics course, vita, writing sample. Application deadline: Applications are processed on a rolling basis. Application fee: $55.

Degree Requirements 59 total credit hours, dissertation, written exam.

Lewis-Clark State College
Division of Nursing and Health Sciences
Lewiston, Idaho

http://www.lcsc.edu/nursing/
Founded in 1893

DEGREE • BSN

Nursing Program Faculty 25 (20% with doctorates).
Baccalaureate Enrollment 267 **Women** 83% **Men** 17% **Part-time** 29%
Distance Learning Courses Available.
Nursing Student Activities Student Nurses' Association.
Nursing Student Resources Academic advising; academic or career counseling; assistance for students with disabilities; bookstore; campus computer network; career placement assistance; computer lab; computer-assisted instruction; daycare for children of students; e-mail services; housing assistance; interactive nursing skills videos; Internet; learning resource lab; library services; nursing audiovisuals; remedial services; resume preparation assistance; skills, simulation, or other laboratory; tutoring; unpaid internships.
Library Facilities 1,492 volumes in health, 542 volumes in nursing; 9,289 periodical subscriptions health-care related.

BACCALAUREATE PROGRAMS

Degree BSN
Available Programs ADN to Baccalaureate; Generic Baccalaureate; LPN to Baccalaureate; LPN to RN Baccalaureate.
Site Options Coeur d'Alene, ID.
Study Options Full-time.
Online Degree Options Yes.
Program Entrance Requirements Minimum overall college GPA of 2.5, transcript of college record, CPR certification, health insurance, immunizations, minimum GPA in nursing prerequisites of 2.5, prerequisite course work. Transfer students are accepted. *Application deadline:* 2/28 (fall), 9/30 (spring). *Application fee:* $35.
Advanced Placement Credit given for nursing courses completed elsewhere dependent upon specific evaluations.
Expenses (2015–16) *Tuition, state resident:* full-time $6000; part-time $307 per credit. *Tuition, nonresident:* full-time $17,000. *Room and board:* $6570 per academic year. *Required fees:* full-time $400.
Financial Aid 75% of baccalaureate students in nursing programs received some form of financial aid in 2014–15.
Contact Advising Center, Division of Nursing and Health Sciences, Lewis-Clark State College, 500 8th Avenue, Lewiston, ID 83501. *Telephone:* 208-792-2688. *Fax:* 208-792-2062. *E-mail:* nhs@lcsc.edu.

Northwest Nazarene University
School of Health and Science
Nampa, Idaho

http://www.nnu.edu/
Founded in 1913

DEGREES • BSN • MSN

Nursing Program Faculty 26 (27% with doctorates).
Baccalaureate Enrollment 120 **Women** 88% **Men** 12% **Part-time** 1%
Graduate Enrollment 17 **Women** 100%
Distance Learning Courses Available.
Nursing Student Activities Student Nurses' Association.
Nursing Student Resources Academic advising; academic or career counseling; assistance for students with disabilities; bookstore; campus computer network; career placement assistance; computer lab; computer-assisted instruction; e-mail services; housing assistance; interactive nursing skills videos; Internet; learning resource lab; library services; nursing audiovisuals; remedial services; resume preparation assistance; skills, simulation, or other laboratory; tutoring; unpaid internships.
Library Facilities 1,500 volumes in health, 950 volumes in nursing; 218 periodical subscriptions health-care related.

BACCALAUREATE PROGRAMS

Degree BSN
Available Programs Generic Baccalaureate.
Study Options Full-time.
Program Entrance Requirements Transcript of college record, CPR certification, health exam, health insurance, high school chemistry, immunizations, minimum GPA in nursing prerequisites of 2.75, professional liability insurance/malpractice insurance, prerequisite course work. Transfer students are accepted. *Application deadline:* 4/15 (fall).
Advanced Placement Credit given for nursing courses completed elsewhere dependent upon specific evaluations.
Contact *Telephone:* 208-467-8650. *Fax:* 208-467-8651.

GRADUATE PROGRAMS

Contact *Telephone:* 208-467-8642. *Fax:* 208-467-8651.

MASTER'S DEGREE PROGRAM

Degree MSN
Available Programs Master's; RN to Master's.
Concentrations Available Nursing education.
Study Options Full-time.
Online Degree Options Yes (online only).
Program Entrance Requirements Computer literacy, minimum overall college GPA of 3.0, transcript of college record, nursing research course, prerequisite course work, resume, statistics course. *Application deadline:* 7/31 (fall). Applications may be processed on a rolling basis for some programs. *Application fee:* $50.
Degree Requirements 36 total credit hours, thesis or project.

ILLINOIS

Aurora University
School of Nursing
Aurora, Illinois

http://www.aurora.edu/
Founded in 1893

DEGREES • BSN • MSN

Nursing Program Faculty 23 (33% with doctorates).
Baccalaureate Enrollment 510 **Women** 90% **Men** 10% **Part-time** 4%
Graduate Enrollment 63 **Women** 97% **Men** 3% **Part-time** 98%
Distance Learning Courses Available.
Nursing Student Activities Sigma Theta Tau, Student Nurses' Association.
Nursing Student Resources Academic advising; academic or career counseling; assistance for students with disabilities; bookstore; campus computer network; career placement assistance; computer lab; computer-assisted instruction; e-mail services; externships; interactive nursing skills videos; Internet; learning resource lab; library services; nursing audiovisuals; remedial services; resume preparation assistance; skills, simulation, or other laboratory; tutoring.
Library Facilities 4,865 volumes in health, 3,000 volumes in nursing; 6,900 periodical subscriptions health-care related.

BACCALAUREATE PROGRAMS

Degree BSN
Available Programs Generic Baccalaureate; RN Baccalaureate.
Site Options Williams Bay, WI; Aurora, IL; Winfield, IL.
Study Options Full-time.
Online Degree Options Yes.
Program Entrance Requirements Minimum overall college GPA of 2.75, transcript of college record, CPR certification, written essay, health exam, health insurance, immunizations, interview, minimum high school GPA, minimum GPA in nursing prerequisites of 2.75, prerequisite course work. Transfer students are accepted. *Application deadline:* 1/15 (fall).
Advanced Placement Credit given for nursing courses completed elsewhere dependent upon specific evaluations.
Expenses (2015–16) *Tuition:* full-time $21,860; part-time $630 per contact hour. *International tuition:* $21,860 full-time. *Room and board:* $10,760; room only: $5980 per academic year. *Required fees:* full-time $220.

Financial Aid 89% of baccalaureate students in nursing programs received some form of financial aid in 2014–15.
Contact Dr. Brenda Shostrom, Executive Director, School of Nursing, School of Nursing, Aurora University, 347 South Gladstone Avenue, Aurora, IL 60506-4892. *Telephone:* 630-844-5135. *Fax:* 630-844-7822. *E-mail:* bshostrom@aurora.edu.

GRADUATE PROGRAMS

Expenses (2015–16) *Tuition:* full-time $12,240; part-time $680 per contact hour. *International tuition:* $12,240 full-time.
Financial Aid 54% of graduate students in nursing programs received some form of financial aid in 2014–15.
Contact Dr. Brenda Shostrom, Executive Director, School of Nursing, School of Nursing, Aurora University, 347 South Gladstone Avenue, Aurora, IL 60506-4892. *Telephone:* 630-844-5135. *Fax:* 630-844-7822. *E-mail:* bshostrom@aurora.edu.

MASTER'S DEGREE PROGRAM

Degree MSN
Available Programs Master's.
Concentrations Available Nursing administration; nursing education.
Site Options Aurora, IL.
Program Entrance Requirements Clinical experience, computer literacy, minimum overall college GPA of 3.0, transcript of college record, CPR certification, written essay, immunizations, interview, 3 letters of recommendation, nursing research course, physical assessment course, professional liability insurance/malpractice insurance, resume, statistics course.
Degree Requirements 36 total credit hours, thesis or project.

Benedictine University
Department of Nursing
Lisle, Illinois

http://www.ben.edu/nursing
Founded in 1887
DEGREES • BSN • MSN
Nursing Program Faculty 30 (80% with doctorates).
Baccalaureate Enrollment 157 **Women** 95% **Men** 5%
Graduate Enrollment 322 **Women** 96% **Men** 4%
Distance Learning Courses Available.
Nursing Student Activities Nursing Honor Society, Sigma Theta Tau.
Nursing Student Resources Academic advising; academic or career counseling; assistance for students with disabilities; bookstore; campus computer network; career placement assistance; computer lab; computer-assisted instruction; e-mail services; interactive nursing skills videos; Internet; learning resource lab; library services; nursing audiovisuals; placement services for program completers; remedial services; resume preparation assistance; skills, simulation, or other laboratory; tutoring.
Library Facilities 1,350 volumes in health, 850 volumes in nursing; 291 periodical subscriptions health-care related.

BACCALAUREATE PROGRAMS

Degree BSN
Available Programs Accelerated RN Baccalaureate.
Site Options Springfield, IL; Glen Ellyn, IL; River Grove, IL.
Study Options Full-time.
Program Entrance Requirements Minimum overall college GPA of 2.5, transcript of college record, 1 letter of recommendation, RN licensure. Transfer students are accepted. *Application deadline:* 7/1 (fall), 11/1 (winter), 2/1 (spring), 5/1 (summer). Applications may be processed on a rolling basis for some programs.
Advanced Placement Credit given for nursing courses completed elsewhere dependent upon specific evaluations.
Contact *Telephone:* 630-829-1152. *Fax:* 630-829-1154.

GRADUATE PROGRAMS

Contact *Telephone:* 866-295-3104 Ext. 5411. *Fax:* 866-789-5608.

MASTER'S DEGREE PROGRAM

Degree MSN
Available Programs Accelerated Master's; Master's.
Study Options Full-time and part-time.
Online Degree Options Yes (online only).
Program Entrance Requirements Minimum overall college GPA of 3.0, transcript of college record, written essay, 1 letter of recommen-

dation, resume. *Application deadline:* Applications may be processed on a rolling basis for some programs.
Advanced Placement Credit given for nursing courses completed elsewhere dependent upon specific evaluations.
Degree Requirements 36 total credit hours, thesis or project.

Blessing–Rieman College of Nursing and Health Sciences
Quincy, Illinois

http://www.brcn.edu/
DEGREES • BSN • MSN
Nursing Program Faculty 28 (21% with doctorates).
Baccalaureate Enrollment 229 **Women** 87% **Men** 13% **Part-time** 18%
Graduate Enrollment 17 **Women** 94% **Men** 6% **Part-time** 100%
Distance Learning Courses Available.
Nursing Student Activities Nursing Honor Society, Sigma Theta Tau, Student Nurses' Association.
Nursing Student Resources Academic advising; academic or career counseling; assistance for students with disabilities; bookstore; campus computer network; computer lab; computer-assisted instruction; daycare for children of students; e-mail services; employment services for current students; externships; interactive nursing skills videos; Internet; learning resource lab; library services; nursing audiovisuals; paid internships; resume preparation assistance; skills, simulation, or other laboratory; tutoring.
Library Facilities 3,752 volumes in health, 3,752 volumes in nursing; 125 periodical subscriptions health-care related.

BACCALAUREATE PROGRAMS

Degree BSN
Available Programs ADN to Baccalaureate; Accelerated Baccalaureate for Second Degree; Generic Baccalaureate; RN Baccalaureate.
Study Options Full-time and part-time.
Online Degree Options Yes.
Program Entrance Requirements Minimum overall college GPA of 2.7, transcript of college record, CPR certification, health insurance, 2 years high school math, 2 years high school science, high school transcript, immunizations, minimum high school GPA of 3.0, minimum GPA in nursing prerequisites of 2.7, prerequisite course work. Transfer students are accepted. *Application deadline:* Applications may be processed on a rolling basis for some programs.
Advanced Placement Credit by examination available. Credit given for nursing courses completed elsewhere dependent upon specific evaluations.
Expenses (2015–16) *Tuition:* full-time $21,810; part-time $727 per credit hour. *Required fees:* full-time $680.
Financial Aid 98% of baccalaureate students in nursing programs received some form of financial aid in 2014–15.
Contact Mrs. Debbie Ann Giesing, Admission Counselor, Blessing–Rieman College of Nursing and Health Sciences, Broadway at 11th Street, PO Box 7005, Quincy, IL 62305-7005. *Telephone:* 217-228-5520 Ext. 6949. *Fax:* 217-223-4661. *E-mail:* admissions@brcn.edu.

GRADUATE PROGRAMS

Expenses (2015–16) *Tuition:* part-time $500 per credit hour.
Financial Aid 100% of graduate students in nursing programs received some form of financial aid in 2014–15.
Contact Mrs. Heather Mutter, Admissions Counselor, Blessing–Rieman College of Nursing and Health Sciences, Broadway at 11th Street, PO Box 7005, Quincy, IL 62305-7005. *Telephone:* 217-228-5520 Ext. 6949. *Fax:* 217-223-4661. *E-mail:* admissions@brcn.edu.

MASTER'S DEGREE PROGRAM

Degree MSN
Available Programs Master's; RN to Master's.
Concentrations Available Nursing administration; nursing education.
Study Options Part-time.
Program Entrance Requirements Clinical experience, computer literacy, minimum overall college GPA of 3.0, transcript of college record, CPR certification, written essay, immunizations, letters of recommendation, nursing research course, physical assessment course, professional liability insurance/malpractice insurance, prerequisite course work, resume, statistics course. *Application deadline:* Applications may be processed on a rolling basis for some programs.

Advanced Placement Credit given for nursing courses completed elsewhere dependent upon specific evaluations.
Degree Requirements 44 total credit hours, thesis or project.

Bradley University
Department of Nursing
Peoria, Illinois

http://www.bradley.edu/academic/departments/nursing/
Founded in 1897
DEGREES • BSN • BSC PN • DNP • MSN
Nursing Program Faculty 42 (14% with doctorates).
Baccalaureate Enrollment 359 **Women** 94% **Men** 6% **Part-time** 1.5%
Graduate Enrollment 110 **Women** 87% **Men** 13% **Part-time** 79%
Distance Learning Courses Available.
Nursing Student Activities Sigma Theta Tau, Student Nurses' Association.
Nursing Student Resources Academic advising; academic or career counseling; assistance for students with disabilities; bookstore; campus computer network; career placement assistance; computer lab; computer-assisted instruction; e-mail services; employment services for current students; externships; housing assistance; Internet; learning resource lab; library services; nursing audiovisuals; placement services for program completers; remedial services; resume preparation assistance; skills, simulation, or other laboratory; tutoring; unpaid internships.
Library Facilities 3,845 volumes in health, 3,624 volumes in nursing; 566 periodical subscriptions health-care related.

BACCALAUREATE PROGRAMS

Degrees BSN; BSc PN
Available Programs ADN to Baccalaureate; Accelerated Baccalaureate; Accelerated Baccalaureate for Second Degree; Baccalaureate for Second Degree; Generic Baccalaureate; LPN to Baccalaureate; RN Baccalaureate.
Study Options Full-time.
Program Entrance Requirements Written essay, high school biology, high school chemistry, 3 years high school math, 3 years high school science, high school transcript, 1 letter of recommendation, minimum high school GPA of 3.25. Transfer students are accepted. *Application deadline:* Applications may be processed on a rolling basis for some programs.
Expenses (2015–16) *Tuition:* full-time $31,100; part-time $830 per credit hour. *Room and board:* $9700 per academic year.
Financial Aid 80% of baccalaureate students in nursing programs received some form of financial aid in 2014–15. *Gift aid (need-based):* Federal Pell, FSEOG, state, private, college/university gift aid from institutional funds. *Loans:* Federal Nursing Student Loans, Federal Direct (Subsidized and Unsubsidized Stafford PLUS), Perkins. *Work-study:* Federal Work-Study. *Financial aid application deadline (priority):* 3/1.
Contact Mr. Justin Ball, Director of Admissions, Department of Nursing, Bradley University, 1501 West Bradley Avenue, Peoria, IL 61625. *Telephone:* 309-677-1000. *Fax:* 309-677-2797. *E-mail:* admissions@bradley.edu.

GRADUATE PROGRAMS

Expenses (2015–16) *Tuition:* part-time $830 per credit hour. *Room and board:* $9700 per academic year.
Financial Aid 5 research assistantships (averaging $19,640 per year) were awarded; scholarships, tuition waivers (partial), and unspecified assistantships also available.
Contact Dr. Deborah Erickson, Graduate Coordinator, Department of Nursing, Bradley University, 1501 West Bradley Avenue, Burgess Hall 312, Peoria, IL 61625. *Telephone:* 309-677-4974. *Fax:* 309-677-2527. *E-mail:* erickson@bradley.edu.

MASTER'S DEGREE PROGRAM

Degree MSN
Available Programs Master's; RN to Master's.
Concentrations Available Nursing administration; nursing education. *Nurse practitioner programs in:* family health.
Study Options Full-time and part-time.
Online Degree Options Yes.
Program Entrance Requirements Clinical experience, minimum overall college GPA of 3.0, transcript of college record, CPR certification, written essay, immunizations, 3 letters of recommendation, nursing research course, resume, statistics course, GRE General Test or

MAT. *Application deadline:* Applications may be processed on a rolling basis for some programs. *Application fee:* $40.
Advanced Placement Credit given for nursing courses completed elsewhere dependent upon specific evaluations.
Degree Requirements 67 total credit hours, thesis or project.

DOCTORAL DEGREE PROGRAM

Degree DNP
Available Programs Doctorate; Post-Baccalaureate Doctorate.
Areas of Study Advanced practice nursing, family health.
Online Degree Options Yes (online only).
Program Entrance Requirements Clinical experience, minimum overall college GPA of 3.0, 3 letters of recommendation, vita. Application deadline: Applications may be processed on a rolling basis for some programs. Application fee: $40.
Degree Requirements 45 total credit hours.

Chamberlain College of Nursing
Nursing Program
Addison, Illinois

http://chamberlain.edu/nursing-schools/campuses/Addison-Illinois
DEGREE • BSN

BACCALAUREATE PROGRAMS

Degree BSN
Available Programs Generic Baccalaureate.
Contact Nursing Program, Nursing Program, Chamberlain College of Nursing, 1221 North Swift Road, Addison, IL 60101-6106. *Telephone:* 877-751-5783. *E-mail:* info@chamberlain.edu.

Chicago State University
Department of Nursing
Chicago, Illinois

http://www.csu.edu/
Founded in 1867
DEGREES • BSN • MSN
Nursing Program Faculty 23 (60% with doctorates).
Baccalaureate Enrollment 348 **Women** 93% **Men** 7% **Part-time** 24%
Nursing Student Activities Student Nurses' Association.
Nursing Student Resources Academic advising; academic or career counseling; assistance for students with disabilities; bookstore; campus computer network; career placement assistance; computer lab; computer-assisted instruction; daycare for children of students; e-mail services; employment services for current students; externships; housing assistance; interactive nursing skills videos; Internet; learning resource lab; library services; nursing audiovisuals; paid internships; remedial services; resume preparation assistance; skills, simulation, or other laboratory; tutoring; unpaid internships.

BACCALAUREATE PROGRAMS

Degree BSN
Available Programs Generic Baccalaureate; LPN to Baccalaureate; RN Baccalaureate.
Site Options Chicago, IL.
Study Options Full-time.
Program Entrance Requirements Minimum overall college GPA of 2.75, transcript of college record, written essay, health exam, health insurance, 3 years high school math, 3 years high school science, high school transcript, immunizations, interview, 3 letters of recommendation, minimum GPA in nursing prerequisites of 2.75, professional liability insurance/malpractice insurance, prerequisite course work. Transfer students are accepted. *Application deadline:* 9/30 (fall), 3/15 (spring).
Advanced Placement Credit by examination available.
Expenses (2015–16) *Tuition, state resident:* full-time $3750; part-time $294 per credit hour. *Tuition, nonresident:* full-time $6940; part-time $584 per credit hour. *Required fees:* full-time $1541; part-time $175 per credit; part-time $516 per term.
Contact Dr. Patricia Prendergast, Chairperson, Department of Nursing, Chicago State University, 9501 South Martin Luther King Drive,

Chicago, IL 60628. *Telephone:* 773-995-3992. *Fax:* 773-821-2438. *E-mail:* nursing@csu.edu.

GRADUATE PROGRAMS

Contact Dr. Patricia Prendergast, Chairperson, Department of Nursing, Chicago State University, 9501 South Martin Luther King Drive, Chicago, IL 60628. *Telephone:* 773-995-3992. *Fax:* 773-821-2438. *E-mail:* nursing@csu.edu.

MASTER'S DEGREE PROGRAM
Degree MSN
Available Programs Master's.
Concentrations Available Nursing administration; nursing education. *Clinical nurse specialist programs in:* community health.
Site Options Chicago, IL.
Program Entrance Requirements *Application deadline:* 3/15 (fall).

DePaul University
School of Nursing
Chicago, Illinois

http://csh.depaul.edu/departments/nursing/Pages/default.asp x
Founded in 1898

DEGREES • BS • DNP • MS
Nursing Program Faculty 156 (30% with doctorates).
Baccalaureate Enrollment 14 **Women** 93% **Men** 7% **Part-time** 7%
Graduate Enrollment 407 **Women** 85% **Men** 15% **Part-time** 13%
Distance Learning Courses Available.
Nursing Student Activities Sigma Theta Tau, Student Nurses' Association.
Nursing Student Resources Academic advising; academic or career counseling; assistance for students with disabilities; bookstore; campus computer network; career placement assistance; computer lab; computer-assisted instruction; e-mail services; employment services for current students; externships; housing assistance; interactive nursing skills videos; Internet; learning resource lab; library services; nursing audiovisuals; remedial services; resume preparation assistance; skills, simulation, or other laboratory; tutoring.
Library Facilities 27,000 volumes in health, 5,800 volumes in nursing; 1,800 periodical subscriptions health-care related.

BACCALAUREATE PROGRAMS

Degree BS
Available Programs ADN to Baccalaureate; Baccalaureate for Second Degree.
Study Options Full-time and part-time.
Online Degree Options Yes (online only).
Program Entrance Requirements Transcript of college record, written essay, 2 letters of recommendation, minimum GPA in nursing prerequisites, prerequisite course work, RN licensure. Transfer students are accepted. *Application deadline:* Applications may be processed on a rolling basis for some programs. *Application fee:* $40.
Advanced Placement Credit given for nursing courses completed elsewhere dependent upon specific evaluations.
Expenses (2015–16) *Tuition:* part-time $680 per quarter hour.
Financial Aid 60% of baccalaureate students in nursing programs received some form of financial aid in 2014–15.
Contact Ms. Alyssa Nagy, Assistant Director, Graduate Admissions, School of Nursing, DePaul University, 2400 North Sheffield Avenue, Chicago, IL 60614. *Telephone:* 773-325-7271. *E-mail:* anagy@depaul.edu.

GRADUATE PROGRAMS

Expenses (2015–16) *Tuition:* part-time $680 per quarter hour.
Financial Aid 60% of graduate students in nursing programs received some form of financial aid in 2014–15. 6 fellowships (averaging $1,500 per year) were awarded; traineeships also available.
Contact Alyssa Nagy, Assistant Director, Graduate Admissions, School of Nursing, DePaul University, 2400 North Sheffield Avenue, Chicago, IL 60614. *Telephone:* 773-325-7271. *E-mail:* anagy@depaul.edu.

MASTER'S DEGREE PROGRAM
Degree MS
Available Programs Master's for Non-Nursing College Graduates.
Site Options North Chicago, IL.

Study Options Full-time and part-time.
Program Entrance Requirements Computer literacy, minimum overall college GPA of 3.0, transcript of college record, written essay, 2 letters of recommendation, prerequisite course work, resume, GRE (if bachelor's GPA less than 3.2). *Application deadline:* Applications may be processed on a rolling basis for some programs. *Application fee:* $40.
Advanced Placement Credit given for nursing courses completed elsewhere dependent upon specific evaluations.
Degree Requirements 107 total credit hours, thesis or project.

DOCTORAL DEGREE PROGRAM
Degree DNP
Available Programs Doctorate; Post-Baccalaureate Doctorate.
Areas of Study Advanced practice nursing, family health, gerontology.
Program Entrance Requirements Clinical experience, minimum overall college GPA of 3.5, interview by faculty committee, interview, 2 letters of recommendation, vita, GRE. Application deadline: Applications may be processed on a rolling basis for some programs. Application fee: $40.
Degree Requirements 100 total credit hours, dissertation.

Eastern Illinois University
Nursing Program
Charleston, Illinois

http://www.eiu.edu/nursing
Founded in 1895

DEGREE • BSN
Nursing Program Faculty 5 (100% with doctorates).
Baccalaureate Enrollment 55 **Women** 65% **Men** 35% **Part-time** 80%
Distance Learning Courses Available.
Nursing Student Resources Academic advising; academic or career counseling; assistance for students with disabilities; bookstore; campus computer network; computer lab; computer-assisted instruction; e-mail services; interactive nursing skills videos; Internet; library services; nursing audiovisuals; remedial services; resume preparation assistance; skills, simulation, or other laboratory; tutoring.
Library Facilities 500 volumes in nursing; 50 periodical subscriptions health-care related.

BACCALAUREATE PROGRAMS

Degree BSN
Available Programs ADN to Baccalaureate.
Study Options Full-time and part-time.
Online Degree Options Yes (online only).
Program Entrance Requirements Minimum overall college GPA of 2.5, transcript of college record, CPR certification, written essay, health exam, health insurance, high school transcript, immunizations, 2 letters of recommendation, professional liability insurance/malpractice insurance, prerequisite course work, RN licensure. *Application deadline:* 11/15 (fall), 7/15 (summer). *Application fee:* $30.
Advanced Placement Credit given for nursing courses completed elsewhere dependent upon specific evaluations.
Contact *Telephone:* 217-581-7049. *Fax:* 217-581-7050.

Elmhurst College
Deicke Center for Nursing Education
Elmhurst, Illinois

Founded in 1871

DEGREES • BS • MS • MSN/MBA
Nursing Program Faculty 13 (55% with doctorates).
Baccalaureate Enrollment 195
Graduate Enrollment 34
Nursing Student Activities Sigma Theta Tau, Student Nurses' Association.
Nursing Student Resources Academic advising; academic or career counseling; assistance for students with disabilities; bookstore; campus computer network; career placement assistance; computer lab; daycare for children of students; e-mail services; employment services for current students; housing assistance; Internet; learning resource lab; library services; nursing audiovisuals; remedial services; resume preparation assistance; skills, simulation, or other laboratory; tutoring.

Library Facilities 6,000 volumes in health; 80 periodical subscriptions health-care related.

BACCALAUREATE PROGRAMS

Degree BS
Available Programs Generic Baccalaureate; RN Baccalaureate.
Study Options Full-time.
Program Entrance Requirements Minimum overall college GPA of 2.75, transcript of college record, CPR certification, written essay, health insurance, immunizations, 2 letters of recommendation, minimum GPA in nursing prerequisites of 2.75, prerequisite course work. Transfer students are accepted. *Application deadline:* 6/1 (fall).
Advanced Placement Credit given for nursing courses completed elsewhere dependent upon specific evaluations.
Contact *Telephone:* 630-617-3344. *Fax:* 630-617-3237.

GRADUATE PROGRAMS

Contact *Fax:* 630-617-3514.

MASTER'S DEGREE PROGRAM

Degrees MS; MSN/MBA
Available Programs Master's.
Concentrations Available Clinical nurse leader; nursing education.
Study Options Full-time.
Program Entrance Requirements Clinical experience, computer literacy, transcript of college record, CPR certification, written essay, immunizations, interview, 3 letters of recommendation, nursing research course, physical assessment course, prerequisite course work, resume, statistics course. *Application deadline:* Applications may be processed on a rolling basis for some programs.
Degree Requirements 33 total credit hours.

Governors State University
College of Health and Human Services
University Park, Illinois

http://www.govst.edu/
Founded in 1969
DEGREES • BS • MS
Nursing Program Faculty 7 (85% with doctorates).
Baccalaureate Enrollment 31 **Women** 98% **Men** 2% **Part-time** 100%
Graduate Enrollment 72 **Women** 97% **Men** 3% **Part-time** 4%
Nursing Student Activities Sigma Theta Tau.
Nursing Student Resources Academic advising; assistance for students with disabilities; bookstore; campus computer network; computer lab; daycare for children of students; e-mail services; Internet; learning resource lab; library services; nursing audiovisuals; tutoring.

BACCALAUREATE PROGRAMS

Degree BS
Available Programs RN Baccalaureate.
Study Options Part-time.
Program Entrance Requirements Transcript of college record, CPR certification, health exam, health insurance, immunizations, minimum GPA in nursing prerequisites of 2.0, professional liability insurance/malpractice insurance, prerequisite course work, RN licensure. Transfer students are accepted.
Contact *Telephone:* 708-534-4053. *Fax:* 708-534-2197.

GRADUATE PROGRAMS

Contact *Telephone:* 708-534-4053. *Fax:* 708-534-2197.

MASTER'S DEGREE PROGRAM

Degree MS
Available Programs Master's.
Concentrations Available *Clinical nurse specialist programs in:* adult health.
Study Options Full-time and part-time.
Program Entrance Requirements Clinical experience, computer literacy, minimum overall college GPA of 3.0, transcript of college record, CPR certification, written essay, immunizations, nursing research course, physical assessment course, professional liability insurance/malpractice insurance, prerequisite course work, statistics course.
Degree Requirements 42 total credit hours, comprehensive exam.

POST-MASTER'S PROGRAM
Areas of Study Nursing education.

Illinois State University
Mennonite College of Nursing
Normal, Illinois

http://www.mcn.illinoisstate.edu/
Founded in 1857
DEGREES • BSN • DNP • MSN • PHD
Nursing Program Faculty 96 (18% with doctorates).
Baccalaureate Enrollment 601 **Women** 91.2% **Men** 8.8% **Part-time** 8.2%
Graduate Enrollment 138 **Women** 89.1% **Men** 10.9% **Part-time** 88.4%
Distance Learning Courses Available.
Nursing Student Activities Nursing Honor Society, Sigma Theta Tau, Student Nurses' Association.
Nursing Student Resources Academic advising; academic or career counseling; assistance for students with disabilities; bookstore; campus computer network; career placement assistance; computer lab; computer-assisted instruction; daycare for children of students; e-mail services; employment services for current students; interactive nursing skills videos; Internet; learning resource lab; library services; nursing audiovisuals; remedial services; resume preparation assistance; skills, simulation, or other laboratory; tutoring.
Library Facilities 28,149 volumes in health, 2,863 volumes in nursing; 415 periodical subscriptions health-care related.

BACCALAUREATE PROGRAMS

Degree BSN
Available Programs Accelerated Baccalaureate for Second Degree; Generic Baccalaureate; RN Baccalaureate.
Site Options Normal, IL.
Study Options Full-time and part-time.
Online Degree Options Yes (online only).
Program Entrance Requirements Minimum overall college GPA of 2.5, transcript of college record, CPR certification, written essay, health exam, health insurance, immunizations, minimum GPA in nursing prerequisites of 2.0, prerequisite course work. Transfer students are accepted. *Application deadline:* 1/15 (fall), 3/15 (winter), 6/15 (summer). *Application fee:* $50.
Advanced Placement Credit given for nursing courses completed elsewhere dependent upon specific evaluations.
Expenses (2015–16) *Tuition, state resident:* full-time $10,784; part-time $359 per credit hour. *Tuition, nonresident:* full-time $18,600; part-time $620 per credit hour. *International tuition:* $18,600 full-time. *Room and board:* $6253; room only: $5282 per academic year. *Required fees:* full-time $2384; part-time $79 per credit.
Financial Aid 84% of baccalaureate students in nursing programs received some form of financial aid in 2014–15. *Gift aid (need-based):* Federal Pell, FSEOG, state, private, college/university gift aid from institutional funds, Federal Nursing. *Loans:* Federal Nursing Student Loans, Federal Direct (Subsidized and Unsubsidized Stafford PLUS), Perkins. *Work-study:* Federal Work-Study, part-time campus jobs. *Financial aid application deadline (priority):* 3/1.
Contact Ms. Nancy Diller, Academic Advisor, Mennonite College of Nursing, Illinois State University, Campus Box 5810, Edwards Hall, Room 112G, Normal, IL 61790-5810. *Telephone:* 309-438-7400. *Fax:* 309-438-7711. *E-mail:* njakubc@ilstu.edu.

GRADUATE PROGRAMS

Expenses (2015–16) *Tuition, state resident:* full-time $6732; part-time $374 per credit hour. *Tuition, nonresident:* full-time $13,986; part-time $777 per credit hour. *International tuition:* $13,986 full-time. *Room and board:* $6253; room only: $5282 per academic year. *Required fees:* full-time $1430; part-time $79 per credit.
Financial Aid 85% of graduate students in nursing programs received some form of financial aid in 2014–15.
Contact Ms. Melissa K. Moody, Academic Advisor, Mennonite College of Nursing, Illinois State University, Campus Box 5810, Edwards Hall, Room 112J, Normal, IL 61790-5810. *Telephone:* 309-438-7035. *Fax:* 309-438-7711. *E-mail:* mkmoody@ilstu.edu.

MASTER'S DEGREE PROGRAM

Degree MSN
Available Programs Master's.
Concentrations Available Clinical nurse leader; nursing administration. *Nurse practitioner programs in:* family health.
Site Options Normal, IL.
Study Options Full-time and part-time.
Online Degree Options Yes (online only).
Program Entrance Requirements Minimum overall college GPA of 3.0, transcript of college record, CPR certification, written essay, immunizations, interview, 3 letters of recommendation, nursing research course, physical assessment course, prerequisite course work, resume, statistics course. *Application deadline:* 2/1 (fall), 5/1 (winter). *Application fee:* $50.
Advanced Placement Credit given for nursing courses completed elsewhere dependent upon specific evaluations.
Degree Requirements 44 total credit hours, thesis or project.

POST-MASTER'S PROGRAM

Areas of Study *Nurse practitioner programs in:* family health.

DOCTORAL DEGREE PROGRAM

Degree DNP
Available Programs Doctorate.
Areas of Study Nursing administration.
Online Degree Options Yes (online only).
Program Entrance Requirements Minimum overall college GPA of 3.0, 3 letters of recommendation, MSN or equivalent, vita. Application deadline: 2/1 (spring). Applications may be processed on a rolling basis for some programs. Application fee: $50.
Degree Requirements 34 total credit hours, dissertation.

Degree PhD
Available Programs Doctorate.
Areas of Study Aging.
Site Options Normal, IL.
Online Degree Options Yes (online only).
Program Entrance Requirements Minimum overall college GPA of 3.0, interview by faculty committee, interview, 3 letters of recommendation, MSN or equivalent, statistics course, vita. Application deadline: 4/1 (fall). Applications may be processed on a rolling basis for some programs. Application fee: $50.
Degree Requirements 66 total credit hours, dissertation, oral exam, written exam, residency.

Illinois Wesleyan University

School of Nursing
Bloomington, Illinois

http://www2.iwu.edu/nursing/
Founded in 1850
DEGREE • BSN
Nursing Program Faculty 29 (38% with doctorates).
Baccalaureate Enrollment 17 **Women** 91% **Men** 9%
Nursing Student Activities Nursing Honor Society, Sigma Theta Tau, Student Nurses' Association, nursing club.
Nursing Student Resources Academic advising; academic or career counseling; assistance for students with disabilities; bookstore; campus computer network; career placement assistance; computer lab; computer-assisted instruction; e-mail services; employment services for current students; externships; housing assistance; interactive nursing skills videos; Internet; learning resource lab; library services; nursing audiovisuals; paid internships; placement services for program completers; resume preparation assistance; skills, simulation, or other laboratory; tutoring; unpaid internships.
Library Facilities 9,957 volumes in health, 7,940 volumes in nursing; 115 periodical subscriptions health-care related.

BACCALAUREATE PROGRAMS

Degree BSN
Available Programs Generic Baccalaureate.
Study Options Full-time and part-time.
Program Entrance Requirements Minimum overall college GPA of 3.0, transcript of college record, written essay, health exam, health insurance, high school biology, high school chemistry, 2 years high school math, 2 years high school science, high school transcript, immuni-

zations, interview, minimum high school GPA of 3.0, minimum high school rank 25%, minimum GPA in nursing prerequisites of 3.0. Transfer students are accepted. *Application deadline:* Applications may be processed on a rolling basis for some programs.
Expenses (2014–15) *Tuition:* full-time $40,664; part-time $5083 per unit. *International tuition:* $40,664 full-time. *Room and board:* $9446; room only: $5926 per academic year. *Required fees:* full-time $180.
Financial Aid 96% of baccalaureate students in nursing programs received some form of financial aid in 2013–14.
Contact Dr. Victoria N. Folse, Director and Associate Professor, School of Nursing, Illinois Wesleyan University, PO Box 2900, Bloomington, IL 61702-2900. *Telephone:* 309-556-3051. *Fax:* 309-556-3043. *E-mail:* vfolse@iwu.edu.

Lakeview College of Nursing
Danville, Illinois

http://www.lakeviewcol.edu/
Founded in 1987
DEGREE • BSN
Nursing Program Faculty 24 (4% with doctorates).
Baccalaureate Enrollment 284 **Women** 87% **Men** 13% **Part-time** 8%
Nursing Student Activities Nursing Honor Society, Sigma Theta Tau, Student Nurses' Association.
Nursing Student Resources Academic advising; academic or career counseling; assistance for students with disabilities; bookstore; campus computer network; career placement assistance; computer lab; Internet; library services; nursing audiovisuals; resume preparation assistance; skills, simulation, or other laboratory; tutoring.
Library Facilities 2,000 volumes in health; 41 periodical subscriptions health-care related.

BACCALAUREATE PROGRAMS

Degree BSN
Available Programs Accelerated RN Baccalaureate; Generic Baccalaureate; RN Baccalaureate.
Site Options Charleston, IL.
Study Options Full-time and part-time.
Program Entrance Requirements Minimum overall college GPA of 2.5, transcript of college record, CPR certification, written essay, health exam, immunizations, 2 letters of recommendation, prerequisite course work. Transfer students are accepted. *Application deadline:* 4/1 (fall), 10/1 (spring). *Application fee:* $100.
Advanced Placement Credit given for nursing courses completed elsewhere dependent upon specific evaluations.
Contact *Telephone:* 217-709-0931. *Fax:* 217-709-0953.

Lewis University
Program in Nursing
Romeoville, Illinois

http://www.lewisu.edu/academics/nursing/index.htm
Founded in 1932
DEGREES • BSN • DNP • MSN • MSN/MBA
Nursing Program Faculty 44 (23% with doctorates).
Baccalaureate Enrollment 636 **Women** 90% **Men** 10% **Part-time** 69%
Graduate Enrollment 289 **Women** 95% **Men** 5% **Part-time** 89%
Distance Learning Courses Available.
Nursing Student Activities Sigma Theta Tau, Student Nurses' Association.
Nursing Student Resources Academic advising; academic or career counseling; assistance for students with disabilities; bookstore; campus computer network; career placement assistance; computer lab; computer-assisted instruction; e-mail services; employment services for current students; externships; interactive nursing skills videos; Internet; learning resource lab; library services; nursing audiovisuals; other; placement services for program completers; remedial services; resume preparation assistance; skills, simulation, or other laboratory; tutoring.
Library Facilities 3,100 volumes in health, 2,038 volumes in nursing; 90 periodical subscriptions health-care related.

BACCALAUREATE PROGRAMS

Degree BSN

Available Programs Accelerated Baccalaureate for Second Degree; Accelerated RN Baccalaureate; Generic Baccalaureate.
Site Options Oak Brook, IL; Tinley Park, IL; Hickory Hills, IL; Shorewood, IL.
Study Options Full-time.
Program Entrance Requirements Minimum overall college GPA of 2.75, transcript of college record, CPR certification, health exam, health insurance, high school biology, high school chemistry, 3 years high school math, high school transcript, immunizations, minimum high school GPA of 2.75, minimum GPA in nursing prerequisites of 2.75, prerequisite course work. Transfer students are accepted. *Application deadline:* Applications may be processed on a rolling basis for some programs. *Application fee:* $40.
Advanced Placement Credit given for nursing courses completed elsewhere dependent upon specific evaluations.
Contact *Telephone:* 815-836-5245. *Fax:* 815-838-8306.

GRADUATE PROGRAMS

Contact *Telephone:* 815-836-5878 Ext. 815. *Fax:* 815-836-5806.

MASTER'S DEGREE PROGRAM
Degrees MSN; MSN/MBA
Available Programs Accelerated Master's; Accelerated Master's for Nurses with Non-Nursing Degrees; Accelerated RN to Master's; Master's; RN to Master's.
Concentrations Available Nursing administration; nursing education. *Clinical nurse specialist programs in:* adult health, gerontology. *Nurse practitioner programs in:* adult health, family health, gerontology.
Site Options Oak Brook, IL; Tinley Park, IL; Hickory Hills, IL; Shorewood, IL.
Study Options Full-time and part-time.
Online Degree Options Yes.
Program Entrance Requirements Minimum overall college GPA of 3.0, transcript of college record, CPR certification, written essay, immunizations, 2 letters of recommendation, nursing research course, prerequisite course work, resume, statistics course. *Application deadline:* 4/1 (fall), 11/15 (spring). Applications may be processed on a rolling basis for some programs. *Application fee:* $40.
Advanced Placement Credit given for nursing courses completed elsewhere dependent upon specific evaluations.
Degree Requirements 40 total credit hours, thesis or project.

POST-MASTER'S PROGRAM
Areas of Study Nursing administration; nursing education. *Clinical nurse specialist programs in:* adult health, gerontology. *Nurse practitioner programs in:* adult health, family health, gerontology.

DOCTORAL DEGREE PROGRAM
Degree DNP
Available Programs Doctorate.
Areas of Study Health-care systems.
Online Degree Options Yes (online only).
Program Entrance Requirements Clinical experience, minimum overall college GPA of 3.25, letters of recommendation, MSN or equivalent, statistics course, vita, writing sample. Application deadline: 4/1 (fall), 11/15 (spring). Applications may be processed on a rolling basis for some programs. Application fee: $40.
Degree Requirements 30 total credit hours, residency.

CONTINUING EDUCATION PROGRAM

Contact *Telephone:* 815-836-5720. *Fax:* 815-838-8306.

Loyola University Chicago
Marcella Niehoff School of Nursing
Maywood, Illinois

http://www.luc.edu/nursing/
Founded in 1870
DEGREES • BSN • DNP • MSN • MSN/MBA • PHD
Nursing Program Faculty 68 (69% with doctorates).
Baccalaureate Enrollment 1,139 **Women** 85.9% **Men** 14.1% **Part-time** 9.3%
Graduate Enrollment 406 **Women** 94% **Men** 6% **Part-time** 54%
Distance Learning Courses Available.
Nursing Student Activities Nursing Honor Society, Sigma Theta Tau, Student Nurses' Association.

Nursing Student Resources Academic advising; academic or career counseling; assistance for students with disabilities; bookstore; campus computer network; computer lab; computer-assisted instruction; e-mail services; interactive nursing skills videos; Internet; learning resource lab; library services; nursing audiovisuals; remedial services; resume preparation assistance; skills, simulation, or other laboratory; tutoring.
Library Facilities 36,709 volumes in health, 6,316 volumes in nursing; 2,630 periodical subscriptions health-care related.

BACCALAUREATE PROGRAMS

Degree BSN
Available Programs Accelerated Baccalaureate for Second Degree; Generic Baccalaureate; RN Baccalaureate.
Site Options Maywood, IL.
Study Options Full-time.
Program Entrance Requirements Transcript of college record, written essay, health exam, health insurance, high school biology, high school chemistry, 2 years high school math, high school transcript, immunizations, 2 letters of recommendation, minimum high school GPA of 3.0, minimum high school rank 25%. *Application deadline:* 12/1 (fall). Applications may be processed on a rolling basis for some programs.
Financial Aid *Gift aid (need-based):* Federal Pell, FSEOG, state, private, college/university gift aid from institutional funds. *Loans:* Federal Nursing Student Loans, Federal Direct (Subsidized and Unsubsidized Stafford PLUS), Perkins. *Work-study:* Federal Work-Study. *Financial aid application deadline:* Continuous.
Contact Ms. Janet Campbell, Director, Student Affairs, Lakeshore Campus, Marcella Niehoff School of Nursing, Loyola University Chicago, 1032 West Sheridan Road, BVM Hall, 801, Chicago, IL 60660. *Telephone:* 773-508-2918. *Fax:* 773-508-3241. *E-mail:* jcampbell2@luc.edu.

GRADUATE PROGRAMS

Expenses (2015–16) *Tuition:* part-time $1060 per credit hour.
Financial Aid 1 fellowship, 4 research assistantships, 1 teaching assistantship were awarded; career-related internships or fieldwork, Federal Work-Study, traineeships, unspecified assistantships, and nurse faculty loan program also available.
Contact Ms. Antoaneta Topalova, Enrollment Advisor, Marcella Niehoff School of Nursing, Loyola University Chicago, 2160 South 1st Avenue, 125-4524, Maywood, IL 60153. *Telephone:* 708-216-3751. *Fax:* 708-216-9555. *E-mail:* atopalova@luc.edu.

MASTER'S DEGREE PROGRAM
Degrees MSN; MSN/MBA
Available Programs Master's; RN to Master's.
Concentrations Available Health-care administration; nursing administration; nursing informatics. *Clinical nurse specialist programs in:* acute care, adult health. *Nurse practitioner programs in:* acute care, adult health, family health, primary care, women's health.
Site Options Maywood, IL.
Study Options Full-time and part-time.
Online Degree Options Yes (online only).
Program Entrance Requirements Clinical experience, minimum overall college GPA of 3.0, transcript of college record, CPR certification, written essay, immunizations, 2 letters of recommendation, physical assessment course, professional liability insurance/malpractice insurance, resume, statistics course. *Application deadline:* 6/1 (fall), 11/15 (spring), 3/15 (summer). Applications may be processed on a rolling basis for some programs.
Advanced Placement Credit given for nursing courses completed elsewhere dependent upon specific evaluations.
Degree Requirements 48 total credit hours.

POST-MASTER'S PROGRAM
Areas of Study Health-care administration; nursing administration; nursing informatics. *Clinical nurse specialist programs in:* acute care, adult health. *Nurse practitioner programs in:* acute care, adult health, family health, primary care, women's health.

DOCTORAL DEGREE PROGRAM
Degree DNP
Available Programs Doctorate, Post-Baccalaureate Doctorate.
Areas of Study Information systems, nursing administration.
Program Entrance Requirements Minimum overall college GPA of 3.0, interview, interview by faculty committee, 3 letters of recommendation, MSN or equivalent, statistics course, vita, writing sample. Application deadline: 7/1 (fall). Applications may be processed on a rolling basis for some programs.

Degree Requirements 45 total credit hours, Capstone project.

Degree PhD
Available Programs Doctorate; Post-Baccalaureate Doctorate.
Areas of Study Nursing research, nursing science.
Site Options Maywood, IL.
Program Entrance Requirements Minimum overall college GPA of 3.0, interview by faculty committee, interview, 3 letters of recommendation, MSN or equivalent, statistics course, vita, writing sample, GRE General Test (for PhD). Application deadline: 4/1 (fall). Applications may be processed on a rolling basis for some programs.
Degree Requirements 45 total credit hours, dissertation, oral exam, written exam.

MacMurray College
Department of Nursing
Jacksonville, Illinois

https://www.mac.edu/oncampus_programs/majors/nursing.asp
Founded in 1846
DEGREE • BSN
Nursing Program Faculty 9 (44% with doctorates).
Baccalaureate Enrollment 105 **Women** 90% **Men** 10% **Part-time** 8%
Distance Learning Courses Available.
Nursing Student Activities Sigma Theta Tau, nursing club.
Nursing Student Resources Academic advising; academic or career counseling; bookstore; campus computer network; career placement assistance; computer lab; computer-assisted instruction; e-mail services; Internet; learning resource lab; library services; nursing audiovisuals; placement services for program completers; resume preparation assistance; skills, simulation, or other laboratory; tutoring.
Library Facilities 1,800 volumes in health, 1,300 volumes in nursing; 50 periodical subscriptions health-care related.

BACCALAUREATE PROGRAMS
Degree BSN
Available Programs ADN to Baccalaureate; Generic Baccalaureate; LPN to RN Baccalaureate.
Study Options Full-time and part-time.
Online Degree Options Yes.
Program Entrance Requirements Minimum overall college GPA of 2.75, transcript of college record, CPR certification, health exam, health insurance, high school chemistry, high school transcript, immunizations, minimum high school GPA of 2.75. Transfer students are accepted. *Application deadline:* 3/1 (fall).
Expenses (2015–16) *Tuition:* full-time $24,390; part-time $750 per credit hour. *Room and board:* $8510 per academic year. *Required fees:* full-time $1120.
Financial Aid 98% of baccalaureate students in nursing programs received some form of financial aid in 2014–15. *Gift aid (need-based):* Federal Pell, FSEOG, state, private, college/university gift aid from institutional funds. *Loans:* Federal Direct (Subsidized and Unsubsidized Stafford PLUS), Perkins, college/university. *Work-study:* Federal Work-Study. *Financial aid application deadline (priority):* 2/1.
Contact Director of Admissions, Department of Nursing, MacMurray College, 447 East College Avenue, Jacksonville, IL 62650. *Telephone:* 800-252-7485. *Fax:* 217-291-0702. *E-mail:* admissions@mac.edu.

McKendree University
Department of Nursing
Lebanon, Illinois

http://www.mckendree.edu/nursing
Founded in 1828
DEGREES • BSN • MSN • MSN/MBA
Nursing Program Faculty 15 (40% with doctorates).
Baccalaureate Enrollment 252 **Women** 91% **Men** 9% **Part-time** 86%
Graduate Enrollment 73 **Women** 96% **Men** 4% **Part-time** 96%
Distance Learning Courses Available.
Nursing Student Activities Nursing Honor Society.
Nursing Student Resources Academic advising; academic or career counseling; assistance for students with disabilities; bookstore; campus computer network; career placement assistance; computer lab; computer-assisted instruction; e-mail services; interactive nursing skills videos; Internet; learning resource lab; library services; nursing audiovisuals; resume preparation assistance; tutoring.
Library Facilities 4,450 volumes in health, 2,880 volumes in nursing; 80 periodical subscriptions health-care related.

BACCALAUREATE PROGRAMS
Degree BSN
Available Programs ADN to Baccalaureate.
Site Options Radcliff, KY; Louisville, KY.
Study Options Full-time and part-time.
Online Degree Options Yes.
Program Entrance Requirements Minimum overall college GPA of 2.0, transcript of college record, CPR certification, health exam, high school transcript, immunizations, prerequisite course work, RN licensure. Transfer students are accepted. *Application deadline:* Applications may be processed on a rolling basis for some programs.
Advanced Placement Credit given for nursing courses completed elsewhere dependent upon specific evaluations.
Expenses (2015–16) *Tuition:* part-time $340 per credit.
Financial Aid 42% of baccalaureate students in nursing programs received some form of financial aid in 2014–15. *Gift aid (need-based):* Federal Pell, FSEOG, state, private, college/university gift aid from institutional funds. *Loans:* Federal Direct (Subsidized and Unsubsidized Stafford PLUS), Perkins. *Work-study:* Federal Work-Study, part-time campus jobs. *Financial aid application deadline (priority):* 5/31.
Contact Carol Fairlie, Director of Nursing Admissions, Department of Nursing, McKendree University, 701 College Road, Lebanon, IL 62254. *Telephone:* 800-232-7228 Ext. 6507. *Fax:* 618-537-6410. *E-mail:* cjfairlie@mckendree.edu.

GRADUATE PROGRAMS
Expenses (2015–16) *Tuition:* part-time $430 per credit hour.
Financial Aid 34% of graduate students in nursing programs received some form of financial aid in 2014–15.
Contact Melissa Meeker, Assistant Dean of Student Services for Online and External Programs, Department of Nursing, McKendree University, 701 College Road, Lebanon, IL 62254. *Telephone:* 618-537-6834. *Fax:* 618-537-6410. *E-mail:* mlmeeker@mckendree.edu.

MASTER'S DEGREE PROGRAM
Degrees MSN; MSN/MBA
Available Programs Master's; RN to Master's.
Concentrations Available Nursing administration; nursing education.
Study Options Full-time and part-time.
Online Degree Options Yes.
Program Entrance Requirements Minimum overall college GPA of 3.0, transcript of college record, CPR certification, written essay, immunizations, interview, 3 letters of recommendation, resume. *Application deadline:* Applications may be processed on a rolling basis for some programs.
Advanced Placement Credit given for nursing courses completed elsewhere dependent upon specific evaluations.
Degree Requirements 38 total credit hours, thesis or project.

POST-MASTER'S PROGRAM
Areas of Study Nursing administration; nursing education.

Methodist College
Methodist College
Peoria, Illinois

DEGREE • BSN
Nursing Program Faculty 44 (13% with doctorates).
Baccalaureate Enrollment 522 **Women** 87% **Men** 13% **Part-time** 12%
Distance Learning Courses Available.
Nursing Student Activities Nursing Honor Society, Student Nurses' Association.
Nursing Student Resources Academic advising; academic or career counseling; assistance for students with disabilities; bookstore; campus computer network; career placement assistance; computer lab; computer-assisted instruction; daycare for children of students; e-mail services; employment services for current students; externships; housing assistance; interactive nursing skills videos; Internet; learning resource lab; library services; nursing audiovisuals; remedial services; resume preparation assistance; skills, simulation, or other laboratory; tutoring; unpaid internships.

Library Facilities 2,425 volumes in health, 1,175 volumes in nursing; 880 periodical subscriptions health-care related.

BACCALAUREATE PROGRAMS

Degree BSN
Available Programs Accelerated Baccalaureate for Second Degree; Baccalaureate for Second Degree; Generic Baccalaureate; RN Baccalaureate.
Study Options Full-time and part-time.
Online Degree Options Yes (online only).
Program Entrance Requirements Transcript of college record, CPR certification, health exam, high school transcript, immunizations, minimum high school GPA of 2.5, minimum GPA in nursing prerequisites of 3.0, professional liability insurance/malpractice insurance. Transfer students are accepted. *Application deadline:* 4/15 (fall), 9/15 (spring). *Application fee:* $35.
Advanced Placement Credit by examination available. Credit given for nursing courses completed elsewhere dependent upon specific evaluations.
Contact *Telephone:* 309-672-5513. *Fax:* 309-671-8303.

Millikin University
School of Nursing
Decatur, Illinois

http://www.millikin.edu/academics/cps/nursing/pages/default .aspx
Founded in 1901

DEGREES • BSN • DNP • MSN
Nursing Program Faculty 30 (50% with doctorates).
Baccalaureate Enrollment 223 **Women** 86% **Men** 14% **Part-time** 1%
Graduate Enrollment 61 **Women** 68% **Men** 32% **Part-time** 15%
Distance Learning Courses Available.
Nursing Student Activities Nursing Honor Society, Sigma Theta Tau, Student Nurses' Association, nursing club.
Nursing Student Resources Academic advising; academic or career counseling; assistance for students with disabilities; bookstore; campus computer network; career placement assistance; computer lab; computer-assisted instruction; e-mail services; employment services for current students; housing assistance; interactive nursing skills videos; Internet; learning resource lab; library services; nursing audiovisuals; other; placement services for program completers; remedial services; resume preparation assistance; skills, simulation, or other laboratory; tutoring; unpaid internships.
Library Facilities 10,000 volumes in health, 6,000 volumes in nursing; 64 periodical subscriptions health-care related.

BACCALAUREATE PROGRAMS

Degree BSN
Available Programs Generic Baccalaureate; RN Baccalaureate.
Study Options Full-time and part-time.
Program Entrance Requirements Minimum overall college GPA of 2.5, transcript of college record, CPR certification, written essay, health exam, high school biology, high school chemistry, 2 years high school math, 2 years high school science, high school transcript, immunizations, 2 letters of recommendation, minimum high school GPA of 3.0, minimum high school rank 75%, minimum GPA in nursing prerequisites of 2.5, prerequisite course work. Transfer students are accepted. *Application deadline:* Applications may be processed on a rolling basis for some programs.
Advanced Placement Credit given for nursing courses completed elsewhere dependent upon specific evaluations.
Expenses (2015–16) *Tuition:* full-time $29,838; part-time $499 per credit. *International tuition:* $29,838 full-time. *Room and board:* $9916; room only: $7726 per academic year. *Required fees:* full-time $660; part-time $22 per credit.
Financial Aid 98% of baccalaureate students in nursing programs received some form of financial aid in 2014–15.
Contact Ms. Dawn Johnson, Administrative Assistant, School of Nursing, Millikin University, 1184 West Main Street, Decatur, IL 62522. *Telephone:* 217-424-6348. *Fax:* 217-420-6731.
E-mail: dejohnson@mail.millikin.edu.

GRADUATE PROGRAMS

Expenses (2015–16) *Tuition:* part-time $750 per credit. *Room and board:* $9916; room only: $7726 per academic year.

Financial Aid 80% of graduate students in nursing programs received some form of financial aid in 2014–15.
Contact Ms. Bonnie Niemeyer, Administrative Assistant I, School of Nursing, Millikin University, 1184 West Main Street, LTSC 101, Decatur, IL 62522. *Telephone:* 217-424-5034. *Fax:* 217-420-6731.
E-mail: bniemeyer@mail.millikin.edu.

MASTER'S DEGREE PROGRAM

Degree MSN
Available Programs Accelerated Master's for Non-Nursing College Graduates; Master's.
Concentrations Available Nursing education.
Study Options Full-time and part-time.
Program Entrance Requirements Clinical experience, computer literacy, minimum overall college GPA of 3.0, transcript of college record, CPR certification, written essay, immunizations, 3 letters of recommendation, nursing research course, professional liability insurance/malpractice insurance, prerequisite course work, resume, statistics course. *Application deadline:* Applications may be processed on a rolling basis for some programs.
Advanced Placement Credit given for nursing courses completed elsewhere dependent upon specific evaluations.
Degree Requirements 36 total credit hours, thesis or project.

DOCTORAL DEGREE PROGRAM

Degree DNP
Available Programs Doctorate; Post-Baccalaureate Doctorate.
Areas of Study Advanced practice nursing.
Program Entrance Requirements Clinical experience, minimum overall college GPA of 3.0, interview by faculty committee, interview, 3 letters of recommendation, statistics course, vita, writing sample. *Application deadline:* 7/1 (fall). *Application fee:* $1000.
Degree Requirements 88 total credit hours, residency.

Northern Illinois University
School of Nursing and Health Studies
De Kalb, Illinois

http://www.chhs.niu.edu/nuhs/
Founded in 1895

DEGREES • BS • MS • MSN/MPH
Nursing Program Faculty 43 (44% with doctorates).
Baccalaureate Enrollment 469 **Women** 92% **Men** 8% **Part-time** 23%
Graduate Enrollment 164 **Women** 96% **Men** 4% **Part-time** 96%
Distance Learning Courses Available.
Nursing Student Activities Nursing Honor Society, Sigma Theta Tau, Student Nurses' Association, nursing club.
Nursing Student Resources Academic advising; academic or career counseling; assistance for students with disabilities; bookstore; campus computer network; career placement assistance; computer lab; computer-assisted instruction; daycare for children of students; e-mail services; employment services for current students; externships; housing assistance; interactive nursing skills videos; Internet; learning resource lab; library services; nursing audiovisuals; paid internships; placement services for program completers; remedial services; resume preparation assistance; skills, simulation, or other laboratory; tutoring; unpaid internships.
Library Facilities 39,869 volumes in health, 7,600 volumes in nursing; 676 periodical subscriptions health-care related.

BACCALAUREATE PROGRAMS

Degree BS
Available Programs ADN to Baccalaureate; Generic Baccalaureate; RN Baccalaureate.
Site Options Rockford, IL; Palatine, IL; Aurora, IL.
Study Options Full-time and part-time.
Program Entrance Requirements Transcript of college record, CPR certification, health exam, health insurance, high school transcript, immunizations, minimum high school GPA of 3.25, minimum high school rank 50%, minimum GPA in nursing prerequisites of 2.5, professional liability insurance/malpractice insurance. Transfer students are accepted.
Advanced Placement Credit given for nursing courses completed elsewhere dependent upon specific evaluations.
Contact *Telephone:* 815-753-0665. *Fax:* 815-753-0814.

GRADUATE PROGRAMS

Contact *Telephone:* 815-753-6551. *Fax:* 815-753-0814.

MASTER'S DEGREE PROGRAM

Degrees MS; MSN/MPH
Available Programs Master's.
Concentrations Available Nursing education. *Clinical nurse specialist programs in:* adult health, community health. *Nurse practitioner programs in:* adult health, family health.
Study Options Full-time and part-time.
Program Entrance Requirements Minimum overall college GPA of 3.0, transcript of college record, CPR certification, written essay, immunizations, 2 letters of recommendation, nursing research course, physical assessment course, professional liability insurance/malpractice insurance, statistics course.
Degree Requirements 48 total credit hours.

POST-MASTER'S PROGRAM

Areas of Study Nursing education. *Nurse practitioner programs in:* family health.

North Park University

School of Nursing
Chicago, Illinois

http://www.northpark.edu/nursing/
Founded in 1891

DEGREES • BS • MS • MSN/MA • MSN/MBA • MSN/MM

Nursing Program Faculty 35 (63% with doctorates).
Baccalaureate Enrollment 278 **Women** 88.4% **Men** 11.6% **Part-time** 36%
Graduate Enrollment 189 **Women** 95% **Men** 5% **Part-time** 80%
Nursing Student Activities Sigma Theta Tau, Student Nurses' Association.
Nursing Student Resources Academic advising; academic or career counseling; assistance for students with disabilities; bookstore; campus computer network; career placement assistance; computer lab; computer-assisted instruction; e-mail services; employment services for current students; interactive nursing skills videos; Internet; learning resource lab; library services; nursing audiovisuals; remedial services; skills, simulation, or other laboratory; tutoring.
Library Facilities 3,959 volumes in health, 1,791 volumes in nursing; 239 periodical subscriptions health-care related.

BACCALAUREATE PROGRAMS

Degree BS
Available Programs Generic Baccalaureate; RN Baccalaureate.
Site Options Evanston, IL; Arlington Heights, IL; Grayslake, IL.
Study Options Full-time.
Program Entrance Requirements Minimum overall college GPA of 2.75, transcript of college record, CPR certification, health exam, health insurance, immunizations, 1 letter of recommendation, minimum GPA in nursing prerequisites of 2.75, prerequisite course work. Transfer students are accepted.
Contact *Telephone:* 773-244-5516.

GRADUATE PROGRAMS

Contact *Telephone:* 773-244-5508. *Fax:* 773-279-7082.

MASTER'S DEGREE PROGRAM

Degrees MS; MSN/MA; MSN/MBA; MSN/MM
Available Programs Master's; RN to Master's.
Concentrations Available Nursing administration. *Clinical nurse specialist programs in:* community health. *Nurse practitioner programs in:* adult health, family health.
Site Options Arlington Heights, IL; Grayslake, IL.
Study Options Full-time and part-time.
Program Entrance Requirements Clinical experience, minimum overall college GPA of 3.0, transcript of college record, CPR certification, immunizations, 2 letters of recommendation, nursing research course, physical assessment course, professional liability insurance/malpractice insurance, prerequisite course work, resume, statistics course.
Degree Requirements 37 total credit hours.

POST-MASTER'S PROGRAM

Areas of Study *Nurse practitioner programs in:* adult health, family health.

Olivet Nazarene University

Division of Nursing
Bourbonnais, Illinois

http://www.olivet.edu/
Founded in 1907

DEGREES • BSN • MSN

Nursing Program Faculty 106 (24% with doctorates).
Baccalaureate Enrollment 449 **Women** 89% **Men** 11% **Part-time** 27%
Graduate Enrollment 442 **Women** 93% **Men** 7% **Part-time** 31%
Distance Learning Courses Available.
Nursing Student Activities Sigma Theta Tau, Student Nurses' Association.
Nursing Student Resources Academic advising; academic or career counseling; assistance for students with disabilities; bookstore; campus computer network; career placement assistance; computer lab; computer-assisted instruction; e-mail services; employment services for current students; externships; housing assistance; interactive nursing skills videos; Internet; learning resource lab; library services; nursing audiovisuals; placement services for program completers; remedial services; resume preparation assistance; skills, simulation, or other laboratory; tutoring.
Library Facilities 3,371 volumes in health, 1,475 volumes in nursing; 5,523 periodical subscriptions health-care related.

BACCALAUREATE PROGRAMS

Degree BSN
Available Programs Accelerated Baccalaureate; Generic Baccalaureate; RN Baccalaureate.
Site Options Rolling Meadows, IL; Oak Brook, IL.
Study Options Full-time.
Program Entrance Requirements Minimum overall college GPA of 2.75, transcript of college record, CPR certification, health exam, health insurance, high school biology, high school chemistry, 2 years high school science, high school transcript, immunizations, minimum GPA in nursing prerequisites of 2.75, prerequisite course work. Transfer students are accepted. *Application deadline:* Applications may be processed on a rolling basis for some programs.
Expenses (2015–16) *Tuition:* full-time $31,950; part-time $1332 per credit. *International tuition:* $31,950 full-time. *Room and board:* $7900; room only: $3950 per academic year. *Required fees:* full-time $840; part-time $420 per term.
Financial Aid *Gift aid (need-based):* Federal Pell, FSEOG, state, private, college/university gift aid from institutional funds. *Loans:* Federal Direct (Subsidized and Unsubsidized Stafford PLUS), Perkins, private loans. *Work-study:* Federal Work-Study, part-time campus jobs. *Financial aid application deadline (priority):* 3/1.
Contact Mrs. Susan Wolff, Director of Admissions, Division of Nursing, Olivet Nazarene University, One University Avenue, Bourbonnais, IL 60914-2345. *Telephone:* 815-939-5203. *Fax:* 815-935-4998. *E-mail:* swolff@olivet.edu.

GRADUATE PROGRAMS

Expenses (2015–16) *Tuition:* full-time $10,800; part-time $675 per credit. *International tuition:* $10,800 full-time.
Contact Dr. Deb Bruley, Director of MSN Programs, Division of Nursing, Olivet Nazarene University, One University Avenue, Bourbonnais, IL 60914-2345. *Telephone:* 815-939-5186. *Fax:* 815-935-4991. *E-mail:* dbruley@olivet.edu.

MASTER'S DEGREE PROGRAM

Degree MSN
Available Programs Master's.
Concentrations Available *Nurse practitioner programs in:* family health.
Site Options Rolling Meadows, IL; Oak Brook, IL.
Study Options Full-time.
Online Degree Options Yes.
Program Entrance Requirements Computer literacy, minimum overall college GPA of 2.75, transcript of college record, nursing research course, statistics course. *Application deadline:* Applications may be processed on a rolling basis for some programs. *Application fee:* $50.

Degree Requirements 36 total credit hours.

Quincy University
Blessing–Rieman College of Nursing
Quincy, Illinois

http://www.quincy.edu/

See description of programs under Blessing–Rieman College of Nursing (Quincy, Illinois).

Resurrection University
Resurrection University
Chicago, Illinois

Founded in 1982
DEGREES • BSN • MSN
Nursing Program Faculty 27 (22% with doctorates).
Baccalaureate Enrollment 392 **Women** 80% **Men** 20% **Part-time** 25%
Graduate Enrollment 97 **Women** 80% **Men** 20% **Part-time** 70%
Nursing Student Activities Nursing Honor Society, Student Nurses' Association.
Nursing Student Resources Academic advising; academic or career counseling; assistance for students with disabilities; campus computer network; career placement assistance; computer lab; computer-assisted instruction; e-mail services; employment services for current students; externships; Internet; learning resource lab; library services; nursing audiovisuals; resume preparation assistance; skills, simulation, or other laboratory; tutoring.
Library Facilities 2,400 volumes in health, 1,100 volumes in nursing; 300 periodical subscriptions health-care related.

BACCALAUREATE PROGRAMS

Degree BSN
Available Programs ADN to Baccalaureate; Accelerated Baccalaureate; Accelerated Baccalaureate for Second Degree; Accelerated RN Baccalaureate; Baccalaureate for Second Degree; RN Baccalaureate.
Site Options Chicago, IL.
Study Options Full-time and part-time.
Program Entrance Requirements Minimum overall college GPA of 2.75, transcript of college record, CPR certification, written essay, health exam, health insurance, immunizations, minimum GPA in nursing prerequisites of 2.75, prerequisite course work. Transfer students are accepted. *Application deadline:* 4/1 (fall), 9/1 (spring), 2/1 (summer). Applications may be processed on a rolling basis for some programs. *Application fee:* $50.
Advanced Placement Credit by examination available. Credit given for nursing courses completed elsewhere dependent upon specific evaluations.
Expenses (2014–15) *Tuition:* full-time $11,923; part-time $808 per credit hour. *International tuition:* $11,923 full-time. *Required fees:* full-time $290; part-time $140 per term.
Financial Aid 72% of baccalaureate students in nursing programs received some form of financial aid in 2013–14.
Contact Mr. Ron de los Santos, Director of Enrollment Management, Resurrection University, 1431 North Claremont, Chicago, IL 60622. *Telephone:* 773-252-5389. *E-mail:* admissions@resu.edu.

GRADUATE PROGRAMS

Expenses (2014–15) *Tuition:* full-time $32,680; part-time $817 per credit hour. *International tuition:* $32,680 full-time. *Required fees:* full-time $290; part-time $140 per term.
Financial Aid 72% of graduate students in nursing programs received some form of financial aid in 2013–14.
Contact Mr. Ron de los Santos, Director of Enrollment Management, Resurrection University, 1431 North Claremont, Chicago, IL 60622. *Telephone:* 773-252-5389. *E-mail:* admissions@resu.edu.

MASTER'S DEGREE PROGRAM
Degree MSN
Available Programs Master's; RN to Master's.
Concentrations Available Clinical nurse leader; nursing administration; nursing education. *Nurse practitioner programs in:* adult health, family health.

Study Options Full-time.
Program Entrance Requirements Computer literacy, minimum overall college GPA of 3.0, transcript of college record, CPR certification, written essay, immunizations, resume. *Application deadline:* 7/15 (fall). Applications may be processed on a rolling basis for some programs. *Application fee:* $50.
Advanced Placement Credit given for nursing courses completed elsewhere dependent upon specific evaluations.
Degree Requirements 40 total credit hours, thesis or project.

Rockford University
Department of Nursing
Rockford, Illinois

http://www.rockford.edu/
Founded in 1847
DEGREE • BSN
Nursing Program Faculty 7
Baccalaureate Enrollment 101 **Women** 94% **Men** 6% **Part-time** 7%
Nursing Student Activities Student Nurses' Association.
Nursing Student Resources Academic advising; academic or career counseling; assistance for students with disabilities; bookstore; campus computer network; career placement assistance; computer lab; computer-assisted instruction; e-mail services; employment services for current students; externships; housing assistance; interactive nursing skills videos; Internet; learning resource lab; library services; nursing audiovisuals; paid internships; placement services for program completers; remedial services; resume preparation assistance; skills, simulation, or other laboratory; tutoring.
Library Facilities 655 volumes in health, 600 volumes in nursing; 55 periodical subscriptions health-care related.

BACCALAUREATE PROGRAMS

Degree BSN
Available Programs ADN to Baccalaureate; Generic Baccalaureate; RN Baccalaureate.
Study Options Full-time.
Program Entrance Requirements Minimum overall college GPA of 2.75, transcript of college record, CPR certification, health exam, health insurance, high school biology, high school chemistry, 4 years high school math, 2 years high school science, high school transcript, immunizations, minimum high school GPA of 2.75, minimum high school rank 50%, minimum GPA in nursing prerequisites of 2.75, prerequisite course work. Transfer students are accepted. *Application deadline:* 3/1 (fall), 9/1 (spring).
Advanced Placement Credit given for nursing courses completed elsewhere dependent upon specific evaluations.
Contact *Telephone:* 815-226-4050.

Rush University
College of Nursing
Chicago, Illinois

http://www.rushu.rush.edu/nursing
Founded in 1969
DEGREES • DNP • MSN
Nursing Program Faculty 159 (47% with doctorates).
Graduate Enrollment 1,036 **Women** 89.48% **Men** 10.52% **Part-time** 70.1%
Distance Learning Courses Available.
Nursing Student Activities Nursing Honor Society, Sigma Theta Tau, Student Nurses' Association.
Nursing Student Resources Academic advising; academic or career counseling; assistance for students with disabilities; bookstore; campus computer network; computer lab; computer-assisted instruction; e-mail services; employment services for current students; housing assistance; interactive nursing skills videos; Internet; learning resource lab; library services; nursing audiovisuals; remedial services; resume preparation assistance; skills, simulation, or other laboratory; tutoring; unpaid internships.
Library Facilities 5,228 periodical subscriptions health-care related.

GRADUATE PROGRAMS

Expenses (2015–16) *Tuition:* part-time $999 per credit hour.

Financial Aid 50% of graduate students in nursing programs received some form of financial aid in 2014–15. Research assistantships, teaching assistantships, Federal Work-Study, scholarships, and traineeships available. Aid available to part-time students. *Financial aid application deadline:* 3/1.
Contact Dr. Lisa Rosenberg, Associate Dean for Admissions and Recruitment, College of Nursing, Rush University, 600 South Paulina Street, Armour Academic Center, Room 440, Chicago, IL 60612. *Telephone:* 312-942-7100. *Fax:* 312-942-3043.
E-mail: rush_admissions@rush.edu.

MASTER'S DEGREE PROGRAM
Degree MSN
Available Programs Accelerated Master's; Master's for Non-Nursing College Graduates.
Concentrations Available Clinical nurse leader.
Study Options Full-time and part-time.
Online Degree Options Yes.
Program Entrance Requirements Clinical experience, minimum overall college GPA of 3.0, transcript of college record, CPR certification, written essay, immunizations, interview, 3 letters of recommendation, resume, GRE General Test (waived if cumulative GPA is 3.25 or greater, nursing GPA is 3.0 or greater, or completed graduate program GPA is 3.5 or greater). *Application deadline:* Applications may be processed on a rolling basis for some programs. *Application fee:* $100.
Advanced Placement Credit given for nursing courses completed elsewhere dependent upon specific evaluations.
Degree Requirements 70 total credit hours, thesis or project.

POST-MASTER'S PROGRAM
Areas of Study Clinical nurse leader.

DOCTORAL DEGREE PROGRAM
Degree DNP
Available Programs Doctorate; Post-Baccalaureate Doctorate.
Areas of Study Advanced practice nursing, clinical practice, critical care, family health, gerontology, health-care systems, maternity-newborn, nurse executive, nursing science.
Online Degree Options Yes.
Program Entrance Requirements Clinical experience, minimum overall college GPA of 3.0, interview by faculty committee, interview, 3 letters of recommendation, statistics course, vita, writing sample, GRE General Test (for DNP in nurse anesthesia and PhD; waived for DNP if cumulative GPA is 3.25 or greater, nursing GPA is 3.0 or greater, or a completed graduate program GPA is 3.5 or greater). Application deadline: Applications may be processed on a rolling basis for some programs. Application fee: $100.
Degree Requirements 70 total credit hours.

POSTDOCTORAL PROGRAM
Areas of Study Neonatal health.
Postdoctoral Program Contact Dr. Lisa Rosenberg, Associate Dean of Students, College of Nursing, Rush University, 600 South Paulina Street, Chicago, IL 60612. *Telephone:* 312-942-7100.
E-mail: lisa_rosenberg@rush.edu.

CONTINUING EDUCATION PROGRAM
Contact Mrs. Angela Moss, Director of Faculty Practice, College of Nursing, Rush University, 600 South Paulina Street, Suite 1080, Chicago, IL 60612-3832. *E-mail:* angela_m_moss@rush.edu.

Saint Anthony College of Nursing
Saint Anthony College of Nursing
Rockford, Illinois

http://www.sacn.edu/
Founded in 1915
DEGREES • BSN • DNP • MSN
Nursing Program Faculty 44 (23% with doctorates).
Baccalaureate Enrollment 233 **Women** 88% **Men** 12% **Part-time** 35%
Graduate Enrollment 73 **Women** 95% **Men** 5% **Part-time** 99%
Nursing Student Activities Sigma Theta Tau, Student Nurses' Association.

Nursing Student Resources Academic advising; academic or career counseling; assistance for students with disabilities; campus computer network; computer lab; computer-assisted instruction; e-mail services; interactive nursing skills videos; Internet; learning resource lab; library services; nursing audiovisuals; skills, simulation, or other laboratory; tutoring.
Library Facilities 1,609 volumes in health, 1,441 volumes in nursing; 60 periodical subscriptions health-care related.

BACCALAUREATE PROGRAMS
Degree BSN
Available Programs Baccalaureate for Second Degree; Generic Baccalaureate; RN Baccalaureate.
Site Options Dixon, IL; Freeport, IL.
Study Options Full-time and part-time.
Program Entrance Requirements Minimum overall college GPA of 2.5, transcript of college record, written essay, 3 letters of recommendation, minimum GPA in nursing prerequisites of 2.7. Transfer students are accepted. *Application deadline:* 2/15 (fall), 9/15 (spring). *Application fee:* $50.
Advanced Placement Credit by examination available. Credit given for nursing courses completed elsewhere dependent upon specific evaluations.
Expenses (2014–15) *Tuition:* full-time $22,144; part-time $692 per credit hour. *Required fees:* full-time $746; part-time $202 per term.
Financial Aid 86% of baccalaureate students in nursing programs received some form of financial aid in 2013–14.
Contact April Lipnitzky, Supervisor of Enrollment Management, Saint Anthony College of Nursing, 5658 East State Street, Rockford, IL 61108-2468. *Telephone:* 815-227-2141. *Fax:* 815-227-2730.
E-mail: Admissions@sacn.edu.

GRADUATE PROGRAMS
Expenses (2014–15) *Tuition:* full-time $15,264; part-time $848 per credit hour. *Required fees:* full-time $327; part-time $163 per term.
Financial Aid 70% of graduate students in nursing programs received some form of financial aid in 2013–14.
Contact Angela Taillet, Student Affairs Specialist, Graduate Program, Saint Anthony College of Nursing, 5658 East State Street, Rockford, IL 61108-2468. *Telephone:* 815-395-5476. *Fax:* 815-395-2275.
E-mail: angelataillet@sacn.edu.

MASTER'S DEGREE PROGRAM
Degree MSN
Available Programs Master's; Master's for Nurses with Non-Nursing Degrees; RN to Master's.
Concentrations Available Clinical nurse leader; nursing education. *Clinical nurse specialist programs in:* adult health. *Nurse practitioner programs in:* adult health, family health.
Study Options Full-time and part-time.
Program Entrance Requirements Minimum overall college GPA of 2.8, transcript of college record, written essay, interview, 3 letters of recommendation, nursing research course, prerequisite course work, resume, statistics course. *Application deadline:* Applications may be processed on a rolling basis for some programs. *Application fee:* $50.
Advanced Placement Credit given for nursing courses completed elsewhere dependent upon specific evaluations.
Degree Requirements 48 total credit hours, thesis or project.

POST-MASTER'S PROGRAM
Areas of Study Nursing education. *Clinical nurse specialist programs in:* adult health. *Nurse practitioner programs in:* adult health, family health.

DOCTORAL DEGREE PROGRAM
Degree DNP
Available Programs Doctorate; Doctorate for Nurses with Non-Nursing Degrees; Post-Baccalaureate Doctorate.
Areas of Study Advanced practice nursing, family health, gerontology, health-care systems.
Program Entrance Requirements Minimum overall college GPA of 3.0, interview, 3 letters of recommendation, statistics course, vita. Application deadline: Applications may be processed on a rolling basis for some programs. Application fee: $50.
Degree Requirements 77 total credit hours.

Saint Francis Medical Center College of Nursing
Baccalaureate Nursing Program
Peoria, Illinois

http://www.sfmccon.edu/
Founded in 1986
DEGREES • BSN • DNP • MSN
Nursing Program Faculty 55 (20% with doctorates).
Baccalaureate Enrollment 408 **Women** 90% **Men** 10% **Part-time** 30%
Graduate Enrollment 277 **Women** 89% **Men** 11% **Part-time** 95%
Distance Learning Courses Available.
Nursing Student Activities Sigma Theta Tau, Student Nurses' Association.
Nursing Student Resources Academic advising; academic or career counseling; campus computer network; computer lab; computer-assisted instruction; e-mail services; housing assistance; interactive nursing skills videos; Internet; learning resource lab; library services; nursing audiovisuals; skills, simulation, or other laboratory; tutoring.
Library Facilities 2,461 volumes in health, 2,097 volumes in nursing; 20 periodical subscriptions health-care related.

BACCALAUREATE PROGRAMS

Degree BSN
Available Programs Generic Baccalaureate; RN Baccalaureate.
Study Options Full-time and part-time.
Program Entrance Requirements Transcript of college record, CPR certification, written essay, health exam, high school transcript, immunizations, minimum GPA in nursing prerequisites of 2.5, professional liability insurance/malpractice insurance, prerequisite course work. Transfer students are accepted. *Application deadline:* 9/15 (fall), 2/15 (spring). *Application fee:* $50.
Advanced Placement Credit given for nursing courses completed elsewhere dependent upon specific evaluations.
Expenses (2015–16) *Tuition:* full-time $18,298; part-time $563 per credit hour. *International tuition:* $18,298 full-time. *Room and board:* room only: $3400 per academic year. *Required fees:* full-time $920; part-time $500 per credit.
Financial Aid *Gift aid (need-based):* Federal Pell, state, private, college/university gift aid from institutional funds. *Loans:* Federal Direct (Subsidized and Unsubsidized Stafford PLUS), college/university. *Financial aid application deadline (priority):* 3/1.
Contact Ms. Janice E. Farquharson, Director of Admissions/Registrar, Baccalaureate Nursing Program, Saint Francis Medical Center College of Nursing, 511 NE Greenleaf Street, Peoria, IL 61603. *Telephone:* 309-624-8980. *Fax:* 309-624-8973.
E-mail: janice.farquharson@osfhealthcare.org.

GRADUATE PROGRAMS

Expenses (2015–16) *Tuition:* full-time $7260; part-time $605 per credit hour. *International tuition:* $7260 full-time. *Room and board:* room only: $3400 per academic year. *Required fees:* full-time $270; part-time $150 per credit.
Contact Dr. Kim A. Mitchell, Dean of the Graduate Program, Baccalaureate Nursing Program, Saint Francis Medical Center College of Nursing, 511 NE Greenleaf Street, Peoria, IL 61603.
Telephone: 309-655-2201. *Fax:* 309-624-8973.
E-mail: Kim.A.Mitchell@osfhealthcare.org.

MASTER'S DEGREE PROGRAM

Degree MSN
Available Programs Accelerated RN to Master's; Master's.
Concentrations Available Clinical nurse leader; nursing administration; nursing education. *Clinical nurse specialist programs in:* gerontology. *Nurse practitioner programs in:* adult-psychiatric mental health, family health, neonatal health, psychiatric/mental health.
Study Options Full-time and part-time.
Online Degree Options Yes (online only).
Program Entrance Requirements Clinical experience, computer literacy, minimum overall college GPA of 2.8, transcript of college record, CPR certification, written essay, immunizations, interview, 3 letters of recommendation, nursing research course, physical assessment course, professional liability insurance/malpractice insurance, prerequisite course work, resume, statistics course. *Application deadline:* Applications may be processed on a rolling basis for some programs. *Application fee:* $50.

Advanced Placement Credit given for nursing courses completed elsewhere dependent upon specific evaluations.
Degree Requirements 45 total credit hours, thesis or project.

POST-MASTER'S PROGRAM
Areas of Study Nursing education. *Clinical nurse specialist programs in:* gerontology. *Nurse practitioner programs in:* family health.

DOCTORAL DEGREE PROGRAM
Degree DNP
Available Programs Doctorate.
Areas of Study Clinical practice, nursing administration.
Online Degree Options Yes (online only).
Program Entrance Requirements Clinical experience, minimum overall college GPA of 3.2, 3 letters of recommendation, scholarly papers, statistics course, vita, writing sample. Application deadline: Applications may be processed on a rolling basis for some programs. Application fee: $50.
Degree Requirements 39 total credit hours, oral exam, residency.

St. John's College
Department of Nursing
Springfield, Illinois

http://www.stjohnscollegespringfield.edu/
Founded in 1886
DEGREE • BSN
Nursing Program Faculty 15 (13% with doctorates).
Baccalaureate Enrollment 81 **Women** 93% **Men** 7% **Part-time** 5%
Nursing Student Activities Student Nurses' Association.
Nursing Student Resources Academic advising; computer lab; daycare for children of students; interactive nursing skills videos; Internet; library services; resume preparation assistance; skills, simulation, or other laboratory.

BACCALAUREATE PROGRAMS

Degree BSN
Available Programs Generic Baccalaureate.
Study Options Full-time and part-time.
Program Entrance Requirements Transcript of college record, CPR certification, health exam, high school transcript, immunizations, 2 letters of recommendation, minimum GPA in nursing prerequisites of 2.4, professional liability insurance/malpractice insurance, prerequisite course work. Transfer students are accepted.
Advanced Placement Credit given for nursing courses completed elsewhere dependent upon specific evaluations.
Contact *Telephone:* 217-525-5628. *Fax:* 217-757-6870.

Saint Xavier University
School of Nursing
Chicago, Illinois

http://www.sxu.edu/academics/colleges_schools/son/
Founded in 1847
DEGREES • BSN • MSN • MSN/MBA
Nursing Program Faculty 35 (60% with doctorates).
Baccalaureate Enrollment 624 **Women** 84% **Men** 16% **Part-time** 13%
Graduate Enrollment 271 **Women** 91% **Men** 9% **Part-time** 51%
Distance Learning Courses Available.
Nursing Student Activities Nursing Honor Society, Sigma Theta Tau, Student Nurses' Association.
Nursing Student Resources Academic advising; academic or career counseling; assistance for students with disabilities; bookstore; campus computer network; career placement assistance; computer lab; computer-assisted instruction; e-mail services; employment services for current students; externships; housing assistance; interactive nursing skills videos; Internet; learning resource lab; library services; nursing audiovisuals; other; placement services for program completers; remedial services; resume preparation assistance; skills, simulation, or other laboratory; tutoring; unpaid internships.
Library Facilities 2,380 volumes in health, 1,400 volumes in nursing; 9,660 periodical subscriptions health-care related.

BACCALAUREATE PROGRAMS

Degree BSN

Available Programs Accelerated Baccalaureate for Second Degree; Generic Baccalaureate; LPN to RN Baccalaureate.

Site Options Chicago, IL.

Study Options Full-time.

Program Entrance Requirements Minimum overall college GPA of 2.75, transcript of college record, CPR certification, written essay, health exam, health insurance, high school biology, high school chemistry, high school foreign language, 3 years high school math, 4 years high school science, high school transcript, immunizations, minimum high school GPA of 2.75, minimum GPA in nursing prerequisites of 2.75, prerequisite course work. Transfer students are accepted. *Application deadline:* 5/1 (fall), 11/1 (spring). Applications may be processed on a rolling basis for some programs.

Advanced Placement Credit by examination available. Credit given for nursing courses completed elsewhere dependent upon specific evaluations.

Expenses (2014–15) *Tuition:* full-time $29,990; part-time $650 per credit hour. *International tuition:* $29,990 full-time. *Room and board:* $10,320; room only: $6140 per academic year. *Required fees:* full-time $1462; part-time $601 per term.

Financial Aid 98% of baccalaureate students in nursing programs received some form of financial aid in 2013–14. *Gift aid (need-based):* Federal Pell, FSEOG, state, private, college/university gift aid from institutional funds, United Negro College Fund, Federal Nursing. *Loans:* Federal Direct (Subsidized and Unsubsidized Stafford PLUS), Perkins. *Work-study:* Federal Work-Study, part-time campus jobs. *Financial aid application deadline (priority):* 3/1.

Contact Mr. Brian Hotzfield, Director, Undergraduate Admission, School of Nursing, Saint Xavier University, 3700 West 103rd Street, Chicago, IL 60655. *Telephone:* 773-298-3050. *Fax:* 773-298-3076. *E-mail:* admission@sxu.edu.

GRADUATE PROGRAMS

Expenses (2014–15) *Tuition:* full-time $10,560; part-time $880 per credit hour. *International tuition:* $10,560 full-time. *Room and board:* $11,280; room only: $8380 per academic year. *Required fees:* full-time $550; part-time $275 per term.

Financial Aid 66% of graduate students in nursing programs received some form of financial aid in 2013–14. Available to part-time students.

Contact Imelda Macias, Associate Director, Graduate Recruiting, School of Nursing, Saint Xavier University, 3700 West 103rd Street, Chicago, IL 60655. *Telephone:* 773-298-3057. *Fax:* 773-298-3951. *E-mail:* graduateadmission@sxu.edu.

MASTER'S DEGREE PROGRAM

Degrees MSN; MSN/MBA

Available Programs Master's.

Concentrations Available Clinical nurse leader; nursing administration. *Nurse practitioner programs in:* family health.

Site Options Chicago, IL.

Study Options Full-time and part-time.

Online Degree Options Yes.

Program Entrance Requirements Minimum overall college GPA of 3.0, transcript of college record, written essay, 2 letters of recommendation, prerequisite course work, GRE General Test or MAT. *Application deadline:* 7/1 (fall). Applications may be processed on a rolling basis for some programs.

Advanced Placement Credit given for nursing courses completed elsewhere dependent upon specific evaluations.

Degree Requirements 36 total credit hours, thesis or project.

POST-MASTER'S PROGRAM

Areas of Study Nursing education. *Nurse practitioner programs in:* family health.

Southern Illinois University Edwardsville
School of Nursing
Edwardsville, Illinois

http://www.siue.edu/nursing
Founded in 1957

DEGREES • BS • DNP • MS

Nursing Program Faculty 87 (38% with doctorates).

Baccalaureate Enrollment 713 **Women** 83% **Men** 17% **Part-time** 27%

Graduate Enrollment 263 **Women** 86% **Men** 14% **Part-time** 69%

Distance Learning Courses Available.

Nursing Student Activities Sigma Theta Tau, Student Nurses' Association, nursing club.

Nursing Student Resources Academic advising; academic or career counseling; assistance for students with disabilities; bookstore; campus computer network; career placement assistance; computer lab; computer-assisted instruction; daycare for children of students; e-mail services; employment services for current students; externships; housing assistance; interactive nursing skills videos; Internet; learning resource lab; library services; nursing audiovisuals; placement services for program completers; remedial services; resume preparation assistance; skills, simulation, or other laboratory; tutoring.

BACCALAUREATE PROGRAMS

Degree BS

Available Programs ADN to Baccalaureate; Accelerated Baccalaureate; Generic Baccalaureate.

Site Options Carbondale, IL.

Study Options Full-time.

Program Entrance Requirements Minimum overall college GPA of 2.5, transcript of college record, minimum GPA in nursing prerequisites of 2.7, prerequisite course work. Transfer students are accepted. *Application deadline:* 3/1 (fall).

Advanced Placement Credit given for nursing courses completed elsewhere dependent upon specific evaluations.

Contact *Telephone:* 618-650-3956. *Fax:* 618-650-3854.

GRADUATE PROGRAMS

Contact *Telephone:* 618-650-3956. *Fax:* 618-650-3854.

MASTER'S DEGREE PROGRAM

Degree MS

Available Programs Master's.

Concentrations Available Health-care administration; nurse anesthesia; nursing education. *Nurse practitioner programs in:* family health.

Site Options Springfield, IL.

Study Options Full-time and part-time.

Program Entrance Requirements Clinical experience, minimum overall college GPA of 3.0, transcript of college record, written essay, interview, 3 letters of recommendation, prerequisite course work, statistics course. *Application deadline:* 3/1 (fall), 6/1 (summer).

Advanced Placement Credit given for nursing courses completed elsewhere dependent upon specific evaluations.

Degree Requirements 35 total credit hours, thesis or project.

POST-MASTER'S PROGRAM

Areas of Study Health-care administration; nurse anesthesia; nursing education. *Nurse practitioner programs in:* family health.

DOCTORAL DEGREE PROGRAM

Degree DNP

Available Programs Doctorate.

Program Entrance Requirements Clinical experience, minimum overall college GPA of 3.0, interview by faculty committee, 3 letters of recommendation, MSN or equivalent, statistics course, vita, writing sample. Application deadline: 3/1 (fall).

Degree Requirements 36 total credit hours, written exam.

CONTINUING EDUCATION PROGRAM

Contact *Telephone:* 618-650-3908. *Fax:* 618-650-3854.

Trinity Christian College
Department of Nursing
Palos Heights, Illinois

http://www.trnty.edu/academics/nursing/nursing.html
Founded in 1959
DEGREE • BSN
Nursing Program Faculty 9
Baccalaureate Enrollment 200 **Women** 94.5% **Men** 5.5% **Part-time** 3%
Nursing Student Activities Student Nurses' Association.
Nursing Student Resources Academic advising; academic or career counseling; assistance for students with disabilities; bookstore; campus computer network; career placement assistance; computer lab; computer-assisted instruction; e-mail services; interactive nursing skills videos; Internet; learning resource lab; library services; nursing audiovisuals; resume preparation assistance; skills, simulation, or other laboratory; tutoring; unpaid internships.
Library Facilities 2,500 volumes in health, 500 volumes in nursing; 100 periodical subscriptions health-care related.

BACCALAUREATE PROGRAMS

Degree BSN
Available Programs ADN to Baccalaureate; Generic Baccalaureate.
Study Options Full-time.
Program Entrance Requirements Minimum overall college GPA of 2.5, transcript of college record, CPR certification, health exam, health insurance, high school biology, 3 years high school math, 2 years high school science, high school transcript, immunizations, minimum high school GPA of 2.0, minimum GPA in nursing prerequisites of 2.5, prerequisite course work. Transfer students are accepted. *Application deadline:* 8/15 (fall).
Advanced Placement Credit given for nursing courses completed elsewhere dependent upon specific evaluations.
Expenses (2014–15) *Tuition:* full-time $25,060. *Room and board:* $9390 per academic year. *Required fees:* full-time $1800.
Financial Aid 98% of baccalaureate students in nursing programs received some form of financial aid in 2013–14.
Contact Admissions Office, Department of Nursing, Trinity Christian College, 6601 West College Drive, Palos Heights, IL 60463. *Telephone:* 866-874-6463. *Fax:* 708-385-5665. *E-mail:* admissions@trnty.edu.

Trinity College of Nursing and Health Sciences
Trinity College of Nursing and Health Sciences
Rock Island, Illinois

http://www.trinitycollegeqc.edu/
Founded in 1994
DEGREE • BSN
Nursing Program Faculty 15 (20% with doctorates).
Baccalaureate Enrollment 76 **Women** 92% **Men** 8% **Part-time** 67%
Distance Learning Courses Available.
Nursing Student Activities Nursing Honor Society.
Nursing Student Resources Academic advising; academic or career counseling; assistance for students with disabilities; bookstore; campus computer network; career placement assistance; computer lab; computer-assisted instruction; daycare for children of students; e-mail services; interactive nursing skills videos; Internet; library services; nursing audio-visuals; placement services for program completers; remedial services; resume preparation assistance; skills, simulation, or other laboratory; tutoring.
Library Facilities 6,000 volumes in health, 3,400 volumes in nursing; 746 periodical subscriptions health-care related.

BACCALAUREATE PROGRAMS

Degree BSN
Available Programs ADN to Baccalaureate; Accelerated Baccalaureate; Accelerated Baccalaureate for Second Degree; Generic Baccalaureate; RN Baccalaureate.
Study Options Full-time.
Program Entrance Requirements Minimum overall college GPA of 2.75, transcript of college record, prerequisite course work. Transfer stu-

dents are accepted. *Application deadline:* 12/20 (fall). Applications may be processed on a rolling basis for some programs. *Application fee:* $50.
Advanced Placement Credit given for nursing courses completed elsewhere dependent upon specific evaluations.
Contact *Telephone:* 309-779-7708. *Fax:* 309-779-7798.

University of Illinois at Chicago
College of Nursing
Chicago, Illinois

http://www.nursing.uic.edu/
Founded in 1946
DEGREES • BSN • DNP • MS • PHD
Nursing Program Faculty 211 (50% with doctorates).
Baccalaureate Enrollment 421 **Women** 82% **Men** 18% **Part-time** 25%
Graduate Enrollment 924 **Women** 90% **Men** 10% **Part-time** 56%
Distance Learning Courses Available.
Nursing Student Activities Sigma Theta Tau, Student Nurses' Association.
Nursing Student Resources Academic advising; academic or career counseling; assistance for students with disabilities; bookstore; campus computer network; computer lab; computer-assisted instruction; daycare for children of students; e-mail services; employment services for current students; externships; Internet; learning resource lab; library services; nursing audiovisuals; remedial services; resume preparation assistance; skills, simulation, or other laboratory; tutoring.
Library Facilities 500,000 volumes in health; 5,100 periodical subscriptions health-care related.

BACCALAUREATE PROGRAMS

Degree BSN
Available Programs ADN to Baccalaureate; Baccalaureate for Second Degree; Generic Baccalaureate; RN Baccalaureate.
Site Options Urbana, Springfield, IL.
Study Options Full-time and part-time.
Online Degree Options Yes.
Program Entrance Requirements Minimum overall college GPA of 2.75, transcript of college record, written essay, immunizations, interview, 2 letters of recommendation, minimum GPA in nursing prerequisites of 2.5, prerequisite course work. Transfer students are accepted. *Application deadline:* 1/15 (fall).
Expenses (2015–16) *Tuition, state resident:* full-time $20,120. *Tuition, nonresident:* full-time $32,360. *Room and board:* $12,000; room only: $9000 per academic year. *Required fees:* full-time $3092.
Contact Michael Behlke, Recruitment and Admissions Coordinator, College of Nursing, University of Illinois at Chicago, 845 South Damen Avenue (MC 802), Chicago, IL 60612. *Telephone:* 312-996-9645. *Fax:* 312-996-8066. *E-mail:* mbehlke@uic.edu.

GRADUATE PROGRAMS

Expenses (2015–16) *Tuition, state resident:* full-time $22,250. *Tuition, nonresident:* full-time $34,720. *International tuition:* $34,720 full-time. *Room and board:* $12,000; room only: $9000 per academic year. *Required fees:* full-time $3092.
Financial Aid 79% of graduate students in nursing programs received some form of financial aid in 2014–15. 3 fellowships with full tuition reimbursements available were awarded; research assistantships with full tuition reimbursements available, teaching assistantships with full tuition reimbursements available, career-related internships or fieldwork, Federal Work-Study, institutionally sponsored loans, scholarships, traineeships, tuition waivers (full and partial), and unspecified assistantships also available. Aid available to part-time students. *Financial aid application deadline:* 3/1.
Contact Michael Spielman, Assistant Director of Recruitment and Admissions, College of Nursing, University of Illinois at Chicago, 845 South Damen Avenue (MC 802), Chicago, IL 60612. *Telephone:* 312-413-1550. *Fax:* 312-996-8066. *E-mail:* mspiel2@uic.edu.

MASTER'S DEGREE PROGRAM
Degree MS
Available Programs Master's; Master's for Non-Nursing College Graduates; Master's for Nurses with Non-Nursing Degrees.
Concentrations Available Clinical nurse leader.
Site Options Peoria, IL; Quad Cities, IL; Rockford, IL; Urbana, Springfield, IL.
Study Options Full-time and part-time.

Program Entrance Requirements Clinical experience, computer literacy, minimum overall college GPA of 3.0, transcript of college record, CPR certification, written essay, immunizations, interview, 3 letters of recommendation, nursing research course, physical assessment course, prerequisite course work, resume, statistics course, GRE General Test. *Application deadline:* 1/15 (fall).
Advanced Placement Credit given for nursing courses completed elsewhere dependent upon specific evaluations.

DOCTORAL DEGREE PROGRAM

Degree DNP
Available Programs Doctorate, Post-Baccalaureate Doctorate.
Areas of Study Advanced practice nursing, aging, clinical practice, community health, family health, gerontology, health policy, health-care systems, information systems, maternity-newborn, nursing administration, nursing policy, women's health.
Program Entrance Requirements Minimum overall college GPA of 3.0, interview, interview by faculty committee, 3 letters of recommendation, statistics course, vita, writing sample. Application deadline: 1/15 (fall).

Degree PhD
Available Programs Doctorate; Post-Baccalaureate Doctorate.
Areas of Study Advanced practice nursing, aging, bio-behavioral research, clinical practice, community health, faculty preparation, family health, forensic nursing, gerontology, health policy, health-care systems, individualized study, information systems, maternity-newborn, nursing administration, nursing policy, nursing research, nursing science, women's health.
Site Options Peoria, IL; Quad Cities, IL; Rockford, IL; Urbana, Springfield, IL.
Program Entrance Requirements Minimum overall college GPA of 3.0, interview by faculty committee, interview, 3 letters of recommendation, statistics course, vita, writing sample, GRE General Test. Application deadline: 12/1 (fall).
Degree Requirements 96 total credit hours, dissertation.

POSTDOCTORAL PROGRAM

Areas of Study Individualized study, information systems, nursing informatics, nursing interventions, nursing research, nursing science, vulnerable population.
Postdoctoral Program Contact Dr. Linda D. Scott, Associate Dean for Academic Affairs, College of Nursing, University of Illinois at Chicago, 845 South Damen Avenue (MC 802), Chicago, IL 60612. *Telephone:* 312-413-1505. *Fax:* 312-996-8066. *E-mail:* ldscott@uic.edu.

CONTINUING EDUCATION PROGRAM

Contact Dr. Lauren Diegel-Vacek, College of Nursing, University of Illinois at Chicago, 845 South Damen Avenue (MC 802), Chicago, IL 60612. *Telephone:* 312-413-5749. *E-mail:* ljvacek@uic.edu.

University of St. Francis
Leach College of Nursing
Joliet, Illinois

https://www.stfrancis.edu/academics/college-of-nursing
Founded in 1920
DEGREES • BSN • DNP • MSN
Nursing Program Faculty 43 (30% with doctorates).
Baccalaureate Enrollment 443 **Women** 89% **Men** 11% **Part-time** 26%
Graduate Enrollment 441 **Women** 91% **Men** 9% **Part-time** 81%
Distance Learning Courses Available.
Nursing Student Activities Nursing Honor Society, Sigma Theta Tau, Student Nurses' Association, nursing club.
Nursing Student Resources Academic advising; academic or career counseling; assistance for students with disabilities; bookstore; campus computer network; career placement assistance; computer lab; computer-assisted instruction; e-mail services; employment services for current students; externships; housing assistance; interactive nursing skills videos; Internet; learning resource lab; library services; nursing audiovisuals; remedial services; resume preparation assistance; skills, simulation, or other laboratory; tutoring.
Library Facilities 3,785 volumes in health, 3,175 volumes in nursing; 78 periodical subscriptions health-care related.

BACCALAUREATE PROGRAMS

Degree BSN
Available Programs Accelerated RN Baccalaureate; Generic Baccalaureate.
Study Options Full-time and part-time.
Online Degree Options Yes.
Program Entrance Requirements Minimum overall college GPA of 3.0, transcript of college record, high school biology, high school chemistry, 3 years high school math, 2 years high school science, high school transcript, minimum high school GPA of 2.5, minimum high school rank 50%, minimum GPA in nursing prerequisites of 2.75, prerequisite course work. Transfer students are accepted. *Application deadline:* 4/1 (fall), 11/1 (spring). Applications may be processed on a rolling basis for some programs.
Advanced Placement Credit by examination available. Credit given for nursing courses completed elsewhere dependent upon specific evaluations.
Expenses (2015–16) *Tuition:* full-time $29,630; part-time $825 per credit. *Room and board:* $9084 per academic year. *Required fees:* full-time $320; part-time $75 per term.
Financial Aid 86% of baccalaureate students in nursing programs received some form of financial aid in 2014–15. *Gift aid (need-based):* Federal Pell, FSEOG, state, private, college/university gift aid from institutional funds, Federal Nursing. *Loans:* Federal Direct (Subsidized and Unsubsidized Stafford PLUS), Perkins, alternative loans. *Work-study:* Federal Work-Study, part-time campus jobs. *Financial aid application deadline (priority):* 2/15.
Contact Cynthia Lambert, Director, Undergraduate Admissions, Leach College of Nursing, University of St. Francis, 500 Wilcox Street, Joliet, IL 60435. *Telephone:* 800-735-7500. *Fax:* 815-740-5078. *E-mail:* clambert@stfrancis.edu.

GRADUATE PROGRAMS

Expenses (2015–16) *Tuition:* part-time $760 per credit hour. *Required fees:* part-time $125 per term.
Financial Aid 73% of graduate students in nursing programs received some form of financial aid in 2014–15.
Contact Ms. Sandee Sloka, Director, Graduate/Degree Completion Admissions, Leach College of Nursing, University of St. Francis, 500 Wilcox Street, Joliet, IL 60435. *Telephone:* 800-735-7500. *Fax:* 815-740-3431. *E-mail:* ssloka@stfrancis.edu.

MASTER'S DEGREE PROGRAM

Degree MSN
Available Programs Master's; Master's for Nurses with Non-Nursing Degrees.
Concentrations Available Nursing administration; nursing education. *Nurse practitioner programs in:* family health, psychiatric/mental health.
Study Options Part-time.
Online Degree Options Yes.
Program Entrance Requirements Clinical experience, minimum overall college GPA of 3.0, transcript of college record, CPR certification, written essay, immunizations, interview, 2 letters of recommendation, nursing research course, physical assessment course, professional liability insurance/malpractice insurance, resume, statistics course. *Application deadline:* 3/1 (fall), 10/1 (spring). Applications may be processed on a rolling basis for some programs.
Advanced Placement Credit given for nursing courses completed elsewhere dependent upon specific evaluations.
Degree Requirements 47 total credit hours.

POST-MASTER'S PROGRAM

Areas of Study *Nurse practitioner programs in:* family health, psychiatric/mental health.

DOCTORAL DEGREE PROGRAM

Degree DNP
Available Programs Doctorate.
Areas of Study Nursing education.
Online Degree Options Yes (online only).
Program Entrance Requirements Minimum overall college GPA of 3.0, 2 letters of recommendation, MSN or equivalent, vita. Application deadline: 3/1 (fall), 10/1 (spring). Applications may be processed on a rolling basis for some programs.
Degree Requirements 40 total credit hours, residency.

Western Illinois University
School of Nursing
Macomb, Illinois

http://www.wiu.edu/nursing
Founded in 1899
DEGREE • BSN
Nursing Program Faculty 15 (40% with doctorates).
Baccalaureate Enrollment 74 **Women** 85% **Men** 15% **Part-time** 3%
Distance Learning Courses Available.
Nursing Student Activities Nursing Honor Society, Sigma Theta Tau, Student Nurses' Association.
Nursing Student Resources Academic advising; academic or career counseling; assistance for students with disabilities; bookstore; campus computer network; career placement assistance; computer lab; computer-assisted instruction; daycare for children of students; e-mail services; housing assistance; interactive nursing skills videos; Internet; learning resource lab; library services; nursing audiovisuals; resume preparation assistance; skills, simulation, or other laboratory; tutoring.

BACCALAUREATE PROGRAMS
Degree BSN
Available Programs Baccalaureate for Second Degree; Generic Baccalaureate; RN Baccalaureate.
Site Options Moline, IL.
Study Options Full-time.
Online Degree Options Yes.
Program Entrance Requirements Minimum overall college GPA of 3.0, transcript of college record, CPR certification, written essay, health exam, immunizations, 2 letters of recommendation, minimum high school GPA of 3.0, minimum GPA in nursing prerequisites of 3.0, professional liability insurance/malpractice insurance, prerequisite course work. Transfer students are accepted. *Application deadline:* 3/1 (fall). *Application fee:* $40.
Advanced Placement Credit given for nursing courses completed elsewhere dependent upon specific evaluations.
Expenses (2015–16) *Tuition, state resident:* full-time $16,320; part-time $294 per contact hour. *Tuition, nonresident:* full-time $16,320; part-time $294 per contact hour. *International tuition:* $25,000 full-time. *Room and board:* $7800; room only: $5750 per academic year. *Required fees:* full-time $3000; part-time $90 per credit; part-time $1500 per term.
Financial Aid *Gift aid (need-based):* Federal Pell, FSEOG, state, private, college/university gift aid from institutional funds. *Loans:* Federal Direct (Subsidized and Unsubsidized Stafford PLUS), Perkins, college/university. *Work-study:* Federal Work-Study, part-time campus jobs. *Financial aid application deadline (priority):* 2/15.
Contact Mr. Theo E. Schultz, Academic Advisor, School of Nursing, Western Illinois University, 1 University Circle, Macomb, IL 61455. *Telephone:* 309-298-2571. *Fax:* 309-298-3190. *E-mail:* t-schultz@wiu.ecu.

INDIANA

Anderson University
School of Nursing
Anderson, Indiana

http://www.anderson.edu/
Founded in 1917
DEGREES • BSN • MSN • MSN/MBA
Nursing Program Faculty 21 (10% with doctorates).
Baccalaureate Enrollment 138 **Women** 92% **Men** 8% **Part-time** 3%
Graduate Enrollment 27 **Women** 85% **Men** 15%
Distance Learning Courses Available.
Nursing Student Activities Sigma Theta Tau.
Nursing Student Resources Academic advising; academic or career counseling; assistance for students with disabilities; bookstore; campus computer network; career placement assistance; computer lab; computer-assisted instruction; e-mail services; employment services for current students; externships; housing assistance; interactive nursing skills videos; Internet; learning resource lab; library services; nursing audiovisuals;

paid internships; placement services for program completers; remedial services; resume preparation assistance; skills, simulation, or other laboratory; tutoring.
Library Facilities 570 volumes in health, 565 volumes in nursing; 54 periodical subscriptions health-care related.

BACCALAUREATE PROGRAMS
Degree BSN
Available Programs Generic Baccalaureate.
Study Options Full-time and part-time.
Program Entrance Requirements Minimum overall college GPA of 3.2, transcript of college record, CPR certification, health exam, high school biology, high school chemistry, 2 years high school math, 3 years high school science, high school transcript, immunizations, minimum high school GPA of 3.5, minimum high school rank 33%, minimum GPA in nursing prerequisites of 3.2, professional liability insurance/malpractice insurance, prerequisite course work. Transfer students are accepted. *Application deadline:* 5/31 (spring), 8/30 (summer).
Expenses (2015–16) *Tuition:* full-time $27,520; part-time $1116 per credit hour. *International tuition:* $27,520 full-time. *Room and board:* $9380 per academic year. *Required fees:* full-time $705; part-time $390 per term.
Financial Aid *Gift aid (need-based):* Federal Pell, FSEOG, state, private, college/university gift aid from institutional funds. *Loans:* Federal Direct (Subsidized and Unsubsidized Stafford PLUS), Perkins. *Work-study:* Federal Work-Study, part-time campus jobs. *Financial aid application deadline (priority):* 3/1.
Contact Dr. Lynn M. Schmidt, Associate Dean, School of Nursing, School of Nursing, Anderson University, 1100 East 5th Street, Anderson, IN 46012-3495. *Telephone:* 765-641-4388. *Fax:* 765-641-3095. *E-mail:* lmschmidt@anderson.edu.

GRADUATE PROGRAMS
Expenses (2015–16) *Tuition:* part-time $460 per credit hour.
Contact Dr. Lynn Schmidt, Associate Dean, Graduate Coordinator and Assistant Professor, School of Nursing, Anderson University, 1100 East 5th Street, Anderson, IN 46012-3495. *Telephone:* 765-641-4388. *Fax:* 765-641-3095. *E-mail:* lmschmidt@anderson.edu.

MASTER'S DEGREE PROGRAM
Degrees MSN; MSN/MBA
Available Programs Master's.
Concentrations Available Nursing administration; nursing education; nursing informatics.
Site Options Indianapolis, IN.
Study Options Full-time and part-time.
Program Entrance Requirements Clinical experience, minimum overall college GPA of 2.75, transcript of college record, CPR certification, written essay, immunizations, 3 letters of recommendation, professional liability insurance/malpractice insurance. *Application deadline:* Applications may be processed on a rolling basis for some programs. *Application fee:* $50.
Advanced Placement Credit given for nursing courses completed elsewhere dependent upon specific evaluations.
Degree Requirements 45 total credit hours, thesis or project.

POST-MASTER'S PROGRAM
Areas of Study Nursing administration; nursing education; nursing informatics.

Ball State University
School of Nursing
Muncie, Indiana

http://www.bsu.edu/nursing
Founded in 1918
DEGREES • BS • DNP • MS
Nursing Program Faculty 57 (33% with doctorates).
Baccalaureate Enrollment 401 **Women** 92% **Men** 8% **Part-time** 21%
Graduate Enrollment 336 **Women** 92% **Men** 8% **Part-time** 100%
Distance Learning Courses Available.
Nursing Student Activities Nursing Honor Society, Sigma Theta Tau, Student Nurses' Association.
Nursing Student Resources Academic advising; academic or career counseling; assistance for students with disabilities; bookstore; campus computer network; career placement assistance; computer lab; computer-

assisted instruction; e-mail services; employment services for current students; housing assistance; interactive nursing skills videos; Internet; learning resource lab; library services; nursing audiovisuals; placement services for program completers; remedial services; resume preparation assistance; skills, simulation, or other laboratory; tutoring.

Library Facilities 16,885 volumes in health, 9,221 volumes in nursing; 3,713 periodical subscriptions health-care related.

BACCALAUREATE PROGRAMS

Degree BS

Available Programs Accelerated RN Baccalaureate; Baccalaureate for Second Degree; Generic Baccalaureate; LPN to Baccalaureate.

Study Options Full-time and part-time.

Program Entrance Requirements Minimum overall college GPA of 3.0, transcript of college record, CPR certification, health exam, immunizations, minimum GPA in nursing prerequisites of 3.0, prerequisite course work. Transfer students are accepted. *Application deadline:* 8/29 (fall), 1/16 (spring).

Advanced Placement Credit given for nursing courses completed elsewhere dependent upon specific evaluations.

Expenses (2015–16) *Tuition, state resident:* full-time $3771; part-time $290 per credit hour. *Tuition, nonresident:* full-time $11,530; part-time $963 per credit hour. *International tuition:* $11,530 full-time. *Room and board:* $8820 per academic year. *Required fees:* full-time $662; part-time $662 per term.

Financial Aid *Gift aid (need-based):* Federal Pell, FSEOG, state, private, college/university gift aid from institutional funds. *Loans:* Federal Direct (Subsidized and Unsubsidized Stafford PLUS), Perkins. *Work-study:* Federal Work-Study, part-time campus jobs. *Financial aid application deadline (priority):* 3/10.

Contact Mrs. Jennifer Criss, Baccalaureate Compliance Coordinator, School of Nursing, Ball State University, CN 418, Muncie, IN 47306. *Telephone:* 765-285-5590. *Fax:* 765-285-2169. *E-mail:* jncriss@bsu.edu.

GRADUATE PROGRAMS

Expenses (2015–16) *Tuition, state resident:* part-time $386 per credit hour. *Tuition, nonresident:* part-time $673 per credit hour. *Room and board:* $8715 per academic year.

Financial Aid Unspecified assistantships available.

Contact Mrs. Shantelle Estes, Advisor, Graduate Programs, School of Nursing, Ball State University, CN 418, Muncie, IN 47306. *Telephone:* 765-285-9130. *Fax:* 765-285-2169. *E-mail:* smestes@bsu.edu.

MASTER'S DEGREE PROGRAM

Degree MS

Available Programs Master's; RN to Master's.

Concentrations Available Nursing administration; nursing education. *Nurse practitioner programs in:* family health.

Study Options Part-time.

Online Degree Options Yes (online only).

Program Entrance Requirements Computer literacy, minimum overall college GPA of 3.0, transcript of college record, CPR certification, written essay, immunizations, 3 letters of recommendation, nursing research course, physical assessment course, prerequisite course work. *Application deadline:* 2/9 (fall), 8/9 (spring). *Application fee:* $60.

Advanced Placement Credit given for nursing courses completed elsewhere dependent upon specific evaluations.

Degree Requirements 47 total credit hours.

POST-MASTER'S PROGRAM

Areas of Study Nursing education. *Nurse practitioner programs in:* family health.

DOCTORAL DEGREE PROGRAM

Degree DNP

Available Programs Doctorate.

Areas of Study Advanced practice nursing.

Online Degree Options Yes (online only).

Program Entrance Requirements Clinical experience, minimum overall college GPA of 3.2, interview by faculty committee, letters of recommendation, MSN or equivalent, statistics course, writing sample. Application deadline: 9/15 (spring). Application fee: $60.

Degree Requirements 40 total credit hours.

Bethel College
School of Nursing
Mishawaka, Indiana

http://www.bethelcollege.edu/
Founded in 1947

DEGREES • BSN • MSN

Nursing Program Faculty 37 (14% with doctorates).

Baccalaureate Enrollment 127 **Women** 92% **Men** 8% **Part-time** 34%

Graduate Enrollment 20 **Women** 95% **Men** 5% **Part-time** 100%

Distance Learning Courses Available.

Nursing Student Activities Sigma Theta Tau.

Nursing Student Resources Academic advising; academic or career counseling; assistance for students with disabilities; bookstore; campus computer network; career placement assistance; computer lab; computer-assisted instruction; e-mail services; employment services for current students; housing assistance; interactive nursing skills videos; Internet; learning resource lab; library services; nursing audiovisuals; remedial services; resume preparation assistance; skills, simulation, or other laboratory; tutoring.

Library Facilities 3,000 volumes in health, 2,050 volumes in nursing; 175 periodical subscriptions health-care related.

BACCALAUREATE PROGRAMS

Degree BSN

Available Programs ADN to Baccalaureate; Generic Baccalaureate; RN Baccalaureate.

Site Options St. Joseph, MI; Winona Lake, IN; Mishawaka, IN.

Study Options Full-time and part-time.

Program Entrance Requirements Minimum overall college GPA of 2.7, transcript of college record, CPR certification, written essay, health exam, health insurance, high school biology, high school chemistry, high school science, high school transcript, immunizations, 1 letter of recommendation, minimum high school GPA of 2.5, minimum GPA in nursing prerequisites of 2.7, prerequisite course work, RN licensure. Transfer students are accepted. *Application deadline:* 8/1 (fall). Applications may be processed on a rolling basis for some programs. *Application fee:* $25.

Advanced Placement Credit by examination available. Credit given for nursing courses completed elsewhere dependent upon specific evaluations.

Expenses (2015–16) *Tuition:* full-time $25,480; part-time $640 per credit hour. *International tuition:* $25,480 full-time. *Room and board:* $7160; room only: $3680 per academic year. *Required fees:* full-time $740.

Financial Aid 95% of baccalaureate students in nursing programs received some form of financial aid in 2014–15.

Contact Dr. Deborah R. Gillum, Dean of Nursing, School of Nursing, Bethel College, 1001 Bethel Circle, Mishawaka, IN 46545. *Telephone:* 574-807-7015. *Fax:* 574-257-2683. *E-mail:* gillumd@bethelcollege.edu.

GRADUATE PROGRAMS

Expenses (2015–16) *Tuition:* part-time $410 per credit hour.

Financial Aid 50% of graduate students in nursing programs received some form of financial aid in 2014–15.

Contact Dr. Rebecca Zellers, Coordinator of Graduate Nursing Programs, School of Nursing, Bethel College, 1001 Bethel Circle, Mishawaka, IN 46545. *Telephone:* 574-807-7809. *Fax:* 574-807-7955. *E-mail:* zellerr@bethelcollege.edu.

MASTER'S DEGREE PROGRAM

Degree MSN

Available Programs Master's.

Concentrations Available Nursing administration; nursing education.

Site Options Mishawaka, IN.

Study Options Full-time and part-time.

Program Entrance Requirements Clinical experience, computer literacy, minimum overall college GPA of 3.0, transcript of college record, CPR certification, immunizations, interview, 3 letters of recommendation, nursing research course, physical assessment course, prerequisite course work, statistics course. *Application deadline:* 8/1 (fall). Applications may be processed on a rolling basis for some programs. *Application fee:* $25.

Advanced Placement Credit given for nursing courses completed elsewhere dependent upon specific evaluations.

Degree Requirements 36 total credit hours, thesis or project.

POST-MASTER'S PROGRAM
Areas of Study Nursing administration; nursing education.

Goshen College
Department of Nursing
Goshen, Indiana

http://www.goshen.edu/
Founded in 1894

DEGREES • BSN • MSN
Nursing Program Faculty 12
Baccalaureate Enrollment 130 **Women** 95% **Men** 5%
Graduate Enrollment 44 **Women** 89% **Men** 11%
Nursing Student Activities Nursing Honor Society, Sigma Theta Tau, Student Nurses' Association.
Nursing Student Resources Academic advising; academic or career counseling; assistance for students with disabilities; bookstore; campus computer network; career placement assistance; computer lab; computer-assisted instruction; daycare for children of students; e-mail services; employment services for current students; externships; housing assistance; interactive nursing skills videos; Internet; learning resource lab; library services; nursing audiovisuals; placement services for program completers; remedial services; resume preparation assistance; skills, simulation, or other laboratory; tutoring.
Library Facilities 80 volumes in health, 80 volumes in nursing; 68 periodical subscriptions health-care related.

BACCALAUREATE PROGRAMS

Degree BSN
Available Programs Generic Baccalaureate; RN Baccalaureate.
Site Options Elkhart, IN.
Study Options Full-time and part-time.
Program Entrance Requirements Minimum overall college GPA of 2.7, transcript of college record, CPR certification, written essay, health exam, health insurance, high school chemistry, high school foreign language, 2 years high school math, high school science, high school transcript, immunizations, 2 letters of recommendation, minimum high school GPA of 2.7, minimum high school rank 50%. Transfer students are accepted. *Application deadline:* 8/15 (fall), 12/17 (winter), 3/1 (spring).
Advanced Placement Credit by examination available. Credit given for nursing courses completed elsewhere dependent upon specific evaluations.
Expenses (2014–15) *Tuition:* full-time $29,700; part-time $1235 per credit hour. *International tuition:* $29,700 full-time. *Room and board:* $9700; room only: $5200 per academic year. *Required fees:* full-time $500.
Financial Aid 98% of baccalaureate students in nursing programs received some form of financial aid in 2013–14. *Gift aid (need-based):* Federal Pell, FSEOG, state, private, college/university gift aid from institutional funds. *Loans:* Federal Nursing Student Loans, Federal Direct (Subsidized and Unsubsidized Stafford PLUS), Perkins. *Work-study:* Federal Work-Study, part-time campus jobs. *Financial aid application deadline (priority):* 3/1.
Contact Admissions, Department of Nursing, Goshen College, 1700 South Main Street, Goshen, IN 46526. *Telephone:* 574-535-7535. *Fax:* 574-535-7609. *E-mail:* admissions@goshen.edu.

GRADUATE PROGRAMS

Expenses (2014–15) *Tuition:* part-time $620 per credit hour. *International tuition:* $620 full-time. *Required fees:* full-time $130.
Financial Aid 25% of graduate students in nursing programs received some form of financial aid in 2013–14.
Contact Dr. Ruth Stoltzfus, Director, Master's in Nursing, Department of Nursing, Goshen College, 1700 South Main Street, Goshen, IN 46526. *Telephone:* 574-535-7973. *Fax:* 575-535-7259. *E-mail:* ruthas@goshen.edu.

MASTER'S DEGREE PROGRAM
Degree MSN
Available Programs Master's.
Concentrations Available Clinical nurse leader. *Nurse practitioner programs in:* family health.

Study Options Part-time.
Program Entrance Requirements Clinical experience, computer literacy, minimum overall college GPA of 3.0, transcript of college record, CPR certification, written essay, immunizations, interview, letters of recommendation, prerequisite course work, resume, statistics course. *Application deadline:* 3/15 (fall). *Application fee:* $50.
Degree Requirements 48 total credit hours.

Harrison College
RN to BSN Program
Indianapolis, Indiana

http://www.harrison.edu/academics/school-of-health-sciences/ctl/program_detail/id/1095/mid/1081
Founded in 1902

DEGREE • BSN

BACCALAUREATE PROGRAMS

Degree BSN
Available Programs RN Baccalaureate.
Contact Nursing Program, RN to BSN Program, Harrison College, 550 East Washington Street, Indianapolis, IN 46204. *Telephone:* 888-544-4422.

Huntington University
Department of Nursing
Huntington, Indiana

http://www.huntington.edu/nursing/
Founded in 1897

DEGREE • BSN
Nursing Program Faculty 4 (50% with doctorates).
Baccalaureate Enrollment 83 **Women** 93% **Men** 7%
Nursing Student Activities Student Nurses' Association.
Nursing Student Resources Academic advising; academic or career counseling; assistance for students with disabilities; bookstore; campus computer network; career placement assistance; computer lab; computer-assisted instruction; daycare for children of students; e-mail services; employment services for current students; externships; housing assistance; interactive nursing skills videos; Internet; learning resource lab; library services; nursing audiovisuals; other; remedial services; resume preparation assistance; skills, simulation, or other laboratory; tutoring; unpaid internships.
Library Facilities 400 volumes in health, 100 volumes in nursing; 114 periodical subscriptions health-care related.

BACCALAUREATE PROGRAMS

Degree BSN
Available Programs Generic Baccalaureate.
Study Options Full-time.
Program Entrance Requirements Minimum overall college GPA of 2.75, transcript of college record, CPR certification, health exam, high school biology, high school chemistry, 2 years high school math, 2 years high school science, high school transcript, immunizations, interview, minimum high school GPA of 2.0, minimum high school rank 0%, minimum GPA in nursing prerequisites of 3.0, professional liability insurance/malpractice insurance, prerequisite course work. Transfer students are accepted. *Application deadline:* 3/31 (fall). *Application fee:* $20.
Financial Aid *Gift aid (need-based):* Federal Pell, FSEOG, state, private, college/university gift aid from institutional funds. *Loans:* Federal Direct (Subsidized and Unsubsidized Stafford PLUS), Perkins. *Work-study:* Federal Work-Study. *Financial aid application deadline (priority):* 3/10.
Contact Dr. Margaret Winter, Director, Department of Nursing, Department of Nursing, Huntington University, 2303 College Avenue, Huntington, IN 46750. *Telephone:* 260-359-4360. *Fax:* 260-359-4133. *E-mail:* mwinter@huntington.edu.

Indiana State University

Department of Advanced Practice Nursing
Terre Haute, Indiana

https://www.indstate.edu/health/department/son
Founded in 1865

DEGREES • BS • DNP • MS

Nursing Program Faculty 58 (45% with doctorates).
Baccalaureate Enrollment 889 **Women** 86% **Men** 14% **Part-time** 28%
Graduate Enrollment 264 **Women** 90% **Men** 10% **Part-time** 99%
Distance Learning Courses Available.
Nursing Student Activities Sigma Theta Tau, Student Nurses' Association.
Nursing Student Resources Academic advising; academic or career counseling; assistance for students with disabilities; bookstore; campus computer network; career placement assistance; computer lab; computer-assisted instruction; daycare for children of students; e-mail services; employment services for current students; externships; housing assistance; interactive nursing skills videos; Internet; learning resource lab; library services; nursing audiovisuals; paid internships; placement services for program completers; remedial services; resume preparation assistance; skills, simulation, or other laboratory; tutoring; unpaid internships.
Library Facilities 12,000 volumes in health, 2,700 volumes in nursing; 9,100 periodical subscriptions health-care related.

BACCALAUREATE PROGRAMS

Degree BS
Available Programs Accelerated Baccalaureate for Second Degree; Generic Baccalaureate; LPN to Baccalaureate; RN Baccalaureate.
Study Options Full-time and part-time.
Online Degree Options Yes.
Program Entrance Requirements Minimum overall college GPA of 2.75, transcript of college record, CPR certification, health exam, high school biology, high school chemistry, high school foreign language, 3 years high school math, 3 years high school science, high school transcript, immunizations, minimum high school GPA of 3.0, minimum high school rank 40%, minimum GPA in nursing prerequisites of 2.75, prerequisite course work. Transfer students are accepted. *Application deadline:* 5/1 (fall), 11/1 (spring). *Application fee:* $25.
Advanced Placement Credit by examination available. Credit given for nursing courses completed elsewhere dependent upon specific evaluations.
Expenses (2015–16) *Tuition, state resident:* full-time $8380; part-time $304 per credit hour. *Tuition, nonresident:* full-time $18,508; part-time $656 per credit hour. *International tuition:* $18,508 full-time. *Room and board:* $9000; room only: $7000 per academic year. *Required fees:* full-time $500.
Financial Aid *Gift aid (need-based):* Federal Pell, FSEOG, state, private, college/university gift aid from institutional funds. *Loans:* Federal Direct (Subsidized and Unsubsidized Stafford PLUS), Perkins. *Work-study:* Federal Work-Study. *Financial aid application deadline:* 7/1(priority: 3/1).
Contact Office of Student Affairs, Department of Advanced Practice Nursing, Indiana State University, School of Nursing, 749 Chestnut Street, Terre Haute, IN 47809. *Telephone:* 812-237-2316. *Fax:* 812-237-8022.

GRADUATE PROGRAMS

Expenses (2015–16) *Tuition, state resident:* part-time $388 per credit hour. *Tuition, nonresident:* part-time $485 per credit hour.
Financial Aid Research assistantships, teaching assistantships, career-related internships or fieldwork and Federal Work-Study available.
Contact Dr. Erik Southard, Chairperson, Advanced Practice Nursing, Department of Advanced Practice Nursing, Indiana State University, Landsbaum Center for Health Education, 1433 No. 6 1/2 Street, Terre Haute, IN 47807. *Telephone:* 812-237-7916. *Fax:* 812-237-8939. *E-mail:* erik.southard@indstate.edu.

MASTER'S DEGREE PROGRAM

Degree MS
Available Programs Master's.
Concentrations Available Nursing education. *Nurse practitioner programs in:* family health.
Study Options Full-time and part-time.
Online Degree Options Yes (online only).
Program Entrance Requirements Clinical experience, minimum overall college GPA of 3.0, transcript of college record, CPR certification, written essay, immunizations, 3 letters of recommendation, prerequisite course work. *Application deadline:* 2/1 (fall), 9/1 (spring). *Application fee:* $35.
Advanced Placement Credit given for nursing courses completed elsewhere dependent upon specific evaluations.
Degree Requirements 48 total credit hours, thesis or project.

POST-MASTER'S PROGRAM

Areas of Study Nursing education. *Nurse practitioner programs in:* family health.

DOCTORAL DEGREE PROGRAM

Degree DNP
Available Programs Doctorate.
Areas of Study Advanced practice nursing, nursing administration, nursing education.
Online Degree Options Yes (online only).
Program Entrance Requirements Clinical experience, minimum overall college GPA of 3.0, 3 letters of recommendation, MSN or equivalent, statistics course, writing sample. Application deadline: Applications may be processed on a rolling basis for some programs. Application fee: $35.
Degree Requirements 39 total credit hours.

CONTINUING EDUCATION PROGRAM

Contact Ms. Esther Acree, Associate Professor and Program Director, Department of Advanced Practice Nursing, Indiana State University, 749 Chestnut Street, Terre Haute, IN 47809. *Telephone:* 812-237-2320. *E-mail:* esther.acree@indstate.edu.

Indiana University Bloomington

Department of Nursing–Bloomington Division
Bloomington, Indiana

Founded in 1820

DEGREE • BSN

Nursing Program Faculty 25 (3.5% with doctorates).
Baccalaureate Enrollment 187 **Women** 97% **Men** 3%
Distance Learning Courses Available.
Nursing Student Activities Nursing Honor Society, Sigma Theta Tau, Student Nurses' Association.
Nursing Student Resources Academic advising; academic or career counseling; assistance for students with disabilities; campus computer network; computer lab; computer-assisted instruction; e-mail services; employment services for current students; interactive nursing skills videos; Internet; learning resource lab; library services; nursing audiovisuals; remedial services; resume preparation assistance; skills, simulation, or other laboratory; tutoring.
Library Facilities 8,500 volumes in nursing; 1,000 periodical subscriptions health-care related.

BACCALAUREATE PROGRAMS

Degree BSN
Available Programs Baccalaureate for Second Degree; Generic Baccalaureate; RN Baccalaureate.
Site Options Columbus , IN; Bedford, IN; Bloomington , IN.
Study Options Full-time.
Program Entrance Requirements Minimum overall college GPA of 2.5, transcript of college record, CPR certification, written essay, health exam, health insurance, high school chemistry, 3 years high school math, high school transcript, immunizations, interview, minimum GPA in nursing prerequisites of 2.7, prerequisite course work. Transfer students are accepted. *Application deadline:* 3/15 (fall).
Advanced Placement Credit by examination available. Credit given for nursing courses completed elsewhere dependent upon specific evaluations.
Contact *Telephone:* 812-855-2592. *Fax:* 812-855-6986.

Indiana University East
School of Nursing
Richmond, Indiana

http://www.iue.edu/nursing/
Founded in 1971
DEGREE • BSN
Nursing Program Faculty 15 (7% with doctorates).
Baccalaureate Enrollment 201 **Women** 92.5% **Men** 7.5%
Nursing Student Activities Sigma Theta Tau, Student Nurses' Association.
Nursing Student Resources Academic advising; academic or career counseling; assistance for students with disabilities; bookstore; campus computer network; career placement assistance; computer lab; computer-assisted instruction; daycare for children of students; e-mail services; externships; interactive nursing skills videos; Internet; learning resource lab; library services; nursing audiovisuals; placement services for program completers; remedial services; resume preparation assistance; skills, simulation, or other laboratory; tutoring; unpaid internships.
Library Facilities 5,039 volumes in health, 3,418 volumes in nursing; 70 periodical subscriptions health-care related.

BACCALAUREATE PROGRAMS

Degree BSN
Available Programs ADN to Baccalaureate; Generic Baccalaureate; RN Baccalaureate.
Study Options Full-time.
Program Entrance Requirements Minimum overall college GPA of 2.7, transcript of college record, CPR certification, high school biology, high school chemistry, 3 years high school math, 3 years high school science, high school transcript, immunizations, minimum high school GPA of 2.0, minimum high school rank 50%, minimum GPA in nursing prerequisites of 2.0, prerequisite course work. Transfer students are accepted. *Application deadline:* 3/1 (fall).
Advanced Placement Credit by examination available. Credit given for nursing courses completed elsewhere dependent upon specific evaluations.
Contact *Telephone:* 765-973-8353. *Fax:* 765-973-8220.

Indiana University Kokomo
Indiana University School of Nursing
Kokomo, Indiana

Founded in 1945
DEGREE • BSN
Nursing Program Faculty 14 (43% with doctorates).
Baccalaureate Enrollment 235 **Women** 95% **Men** 5% **Part-time** 32%
Nursing Student Activities Sigma Theta Tau, Student Nurses' Association.
Nursing Student Resources Academic advising; academic or career counseling; assistance for students with disabilities; bookstore; campus computer network; career placement assistance; computer lab; computer-assisted instruction; daycare for children of students; e-mail services; employment services for current students; externships; interactive nursing skills videos; Internet; learning resource lab; library services; nursing audiovisuals; paid internships; remedial services; resume preparation assistance; skills, simulation, or other laboratory; tutoring.
Library Facilities 2,881 volumes in health, 1,513 volumes in nursing; 75 periodical subscriptions health-care related.

BACCALAUREATE PROGRAMS

Degree BSN
Available Programs Accelerated RN Baccalaureate; Generic Baccalaureate.
Site Options Peru, IN; Marion, IN; Logansport, IN.
Study Options Full-time.
Program Entrance Requirements Minimum overall college GPA of 2.5, transcript of college record, CPR certification, high school biology, high school chemistry, 4 years high school math, high school transcript, immunizations, minimum high school GPA of 2.0, minimum high school rank 50%, minimum GPA in nursing prerequisites of 2.7, prerequisite course work. Transfer students are accepted.
Contact *Telephone:* 765-455-9384. *Fax:* 765-455-9421.

CONTINUING EDUCATION PROGRAM
Contact *Telephone:* 765-455-9384. *Fax:* 765-455-9421.

Indiana University Northwest
School of Nursing
Gary, Indiana

http://www.iun.edu/nursing
Founded in 1959
DEGREE • BSN
Nursing Program Faculty 25 (20% with doctorates).
Baccalaureate Enrollment 220 **Women** 81% **Men** 19% **Part-time** 10%
Distance Learning Courses Available.
Nursing Student Activities Sigma Theta Tau, Student Nurses' Association.
Nursing Student Resources Academic advising; academic or career counseling; assistance for students with disabilities; bookstore; campus computer network; career placement assistance; computer lab; computer-assisted instruction; e-mail services; interactive nursing skills videos; Internet; learning resource lab; library services; nursing audiovisuals; placement services for program completers; remedial services; resume preparation assistance; skills, simulation, or other laboratory; tutoring.
Library Facilities 135,000 volumes in health, 6,100 volumes in nursing; 1,988 periodical subscriptions health-care related.

BACCALAUREATE PROGRAMS

Degree BSN
Available Programs Accelerated Baccalaureate for Second Degree; Generic Baccalaureate; RN Baccalaureate.
Study Options Full-time and part-time.
Online Degree Options Yes.
Program Entrance Requirements Minimum overall college GPA of 2.7, transcript of college record, CPR certification, health exam, health insurance, immunizations, minimum GPA in nursing prerequisites of 2.7, prerequisite course work. *Application deadline:* 4/1 (fall), 1/1 (summer).
Expenses (2015–16) *Tuition, state resident:* full-time $6262; part-time $209 per credit. *Tuition, nonresident:* full-time $17,490; part-time $583 per credit. *Required fees:* full-time $5000.
Financial Aid 75% of baccalaureate students in nursing programs received some form of financial aid in 2014–15.
Contact Ms. Anne Mitchell, Nursing Student Services Coordinator, School of Nursing, Indiana University Northwest, 3400 Broadway, Gary, IN 46408-1197. *Telephone:* 219-980-6611. *Fax:* 219-980-6578. *E-mail:* amitchel@iun.edu.

Indiana University–Purdue University Fort Wayne
Department of Nursing
Fort Wayne, Indiana

http://www.ipfw.edu/nursing
Founded in 1917
DEGREES • BS • DNP • MS
Nursing Program Faculty 54 (14% with doctorates).
Baccalaureate Enrollment 444 **Women** 89% **Men** 11% **Part-time** 30.7%
Graduate Enrollment 56 **Women** 95.5% **Men** 4.5% **Part-time** 97%
Distance Learning Courses Available.
Nursing Student Activities Sigma Theta Tau, nursing club.
Nursing Student Resources Academic advising; academic or career counseling; assistance for students with disabilities; bookstore; campus computer network; career placement assistance; computer lab; computer-assisted instruction; daycare for children of students; e-mail services; employment services for current students; housing assistance; interactive nursing skills videos; Internet; learning resource lab; library services; nursing audiovisuals; placement services for program completers; remedial services; resume preparation assistance; skills, simulation, or other laboratory; tutoring.
Library Facilities 1,100 volumes in health, 500 volumes in nursing; 120 periodical subscriptions health-care related.

BACCALAUREATE PROGRAMS

Degree BS
Available Programs Generic Baccalaureate; RN Baccalaureate.
Study Options Full-time and part-time.
Program Entrance Requirements Minimum overall college GPA of 2.5, transcript of college record, CPR certification, written essay, health exam, high school transcript, immunizations, minimum GPA in nursing prerequisites, professional liability insurance/malpractice insurance, prerequisite course work. Transfer students are accepted. *Application deadline:* 5/1 (fall), 12/1 (spring).
Advanced Placement Credit by examination available. Credit given for nursing courses completed elsewhere dependent upon specific evaluations.
Expenses (2015–16) *Tuition, state resident:* part-time $269 per credit hour. *Tuition, nonresident:* part-time $647 per credit hour. *Room and board:* $9000; room only: $6000 per academic year.
Financial Aid 70% of baccalaureate students in nursing programs received some form of financial aid in 2014–15.
Contact Ms. Joanne Bauman, Nursing Advisor, Department of Nursing, Indiana University–Purdue University Fort Wayne, 2101 East Coliseum Boulevard, Fort Wayne, IN 46805. *Telephone:* 260-481-6282. *Fax:* 260-481-6482. *E-mail:* baumanj@ipfw.edu.

GRADUATE PROGRAMS

Expenses (2015–16) *Tuition, state resident:* full-time $4329; part-time $361 per credit hour. *Tuition, nonresident:* full-time $4329; part-time $361 per credit hour. *International tuition:* $4329 full-time. *Room and board:* $6000 per academic year. *Required fees:* part-time $15 per credit.
Financial Aid 70% of graduate students in nursing programs received some form of financial aid in 2014–15.
Contact Dr. Deb Poling, Director of Graduate Nursing Programs, Department of Nursing, Indiana University–Purdue University Fort Wayne, 2101 East Coliseum Boulevard, Fort Wayne, IN 46805. *Telephone:* 260-481-6276. *Fax:* 260-481-6276. *E-mail:* polingd@ipfw.edu.

MASTER'S DEGREE PROGRAM

Degree MS
Available Programs Master's.
Concentrations Available *Clinical nurse specialist programs in:* adult-gerontology acute care, family health. *Nurse practitioner programs in:* adult health, family health, primary care.
Study Options Part-time.
Online Degree Options Yes (online only).
Program Entrance Requirements Computer literacy, minimum overall college GPA of 3.0, transcript of college record, CPR certification, immunizations, 3 letters of recommendation, nursing research course, physical assessment course, professional liability insurance/malpractice insurance, prerequisite course work, resume, statistics course. *Application deadline:* 3/1 (fall), 11/15 (spring), 4/1 (summer). *Application fee:* $40.
Degree Requirements 46 total credit hours, thesis or project.

DOCTORAL DEGREE PROGRAM

Degree DNP
Available Programs Doctorate.
Areas of Study Advanced practice nursing.
Online Degree Options Yes (online only).
Program Entrance Requirements Minimum overall college GPA of 3.0, 3 letters of recommendation, MSN or equivalent, statistics course, vita. Application deadline: 3/1 (spring). Application fee: $40.
Degree Requirements 54 total credit hours, residency.

Indiana University–Purdue University Indianapolis

School of Nursing
Indianapolis, Indiana

http://nursing.iu.edu
Founded in 1969

DEGREES • BSN • MSN • PHD
Nursing Program Faculty 194 (64% with doctorates).
Baccalaureate Enrollment 1,209 **Women** 89% **Men** 11% **Part-time** 22%
Graduate Enrollment 388 **Women** 89% **Men** 11% **Part-time** 82%
Distance Learning Courses Available.

Nursing Student Activities Sigma Theta Tau, Student Nurses' Association.
Nursing Student Resources Academic advising; academic or career counseling; assistance for students with disabilities; bookstore; campus computer network; computer lab; computer-assisted instruction; e-mail services; housing assistance; interactive nursing skills videos; Internet; learning resource lab; library services; nursing audiovisuals; remedial services; resume preparation assistance; skills, simulation, or other laboratory; tutoring.
Library Facilities 32,811 volumes in health, 9,179 volumes in nursing; 1,787 periodical subscriptions health-care related.

BACCALAUREATE PROGRAMS

Degree BSN
Available Programs ADN to Baccalaureate; Accelerated Baccalaureate for Second Degree; Generic Baccalaureate.
Site Options Columbus, IN; Bloomington, IN.
Study Options Full-time.
Online Degree Options Yes.
Program Entrance Requirements Minimum overall college GPA of 2.7, transcript of college record, CPR certification, health insurance, immunizations, minimum GPA in nursing prerequisites of 3.0, prerequisite course work. Transfer students are accepted. *Application deadline:* 3/15 (fall), 9/15 (spring).
Advanced Placement Credit by examination available.
Expenses (2015–16) *Tuition, state resident:* full-time $8010; part-time $267 per credit hour. *Tuition, nonresident:* full-time $28,740; part-time $958 per credit hour. *Room and board:* $18,898; room only: $5069 per academic year. *Required fees:* full-time $3332; part-time $87 per credit; part-time $361 per term.
Financial Aid 75% of baccalaureate students in nursing programs received some form of financial aid in 2014–15.
Contact Dr. Susan Hendricks, Associate Dean for Undergraduate Programs, School of Nursing, Indiana University–Purdue University Indianapolis, 1111 Middle Drive, Indianapolis, IN 46202. *Telephone:* 317-274-2806. *Fax:* 317-274-2996. *E-mail:* nursing@iu.edu.

GRADUATE PROGRAMS

Expenses (2015–16) *Tuition, state resident:* full-time $8048; part-time $503 per credit hour. *Tuition, nonresident:* full-time $22,960; part-time $1435 per credit hour. *Room and board:* $18,898; room only: $5069 per academic year. *Required fees:* full-time $2114; part-time $87 per credit; part-time $361 per term.
Financial Aid 75% of graduate students in nursing programs received some form of financial aid in 2014–15. Fellowships with full tuition reimbursements available, research assistantships with full tuition reimbursements available, teaching assistantships with full tuition reimbursements available, Federal Work-Study, institutionally sponsored loans, scholarships, and tuition waivers (full) available. Aid available to part-time students. *Financial aid application deadline:* 5/1.
Contact Dr. Patricia R. Ebright, Associate Dean for Graduate Programs, School of Nursing, Indiana University–Purdue University Indianapolis, 1111 Middle Drive, Indianapolis, IN 46202. *Telephone:* 317-274-3115. *Fax:* 317-274-2996. *E-mail:* nursing@iu.edu.

MASTER'S DEGREE PROGRAM

Degree MSN
Available Programs Master's; RN to Master's.
Concentrations Available Nursing administration; nursing education. *Clinical nurse specialist programs in:* adult-gerontology acute care, pediatric. *Nurse practitioner programs in:* adult-gerontology acute care, family health, pediatric primary care, psychiatric/mental health.
Study Options Full-time and part-time.
Online Degree Options Yes.
Program Entrance Requirements Clinical experience, computer literacy, minimum overall college GPA of 3.0, transcript of college record, CPR certification, written essay, immunizations, interview, 3 letters of recommendation, resume, statistics course. *Application deadline:* 1/15 (fall). *Application fee:* $60.
Advanced Placement Credit given for nursing courses completed elsewhere dependent upon specific evaluations.
Degree Requirements 42 total credit hours, thesis or project.

POST-MASTER'S PROGRAM

Areas of Study Nursing administration; nursing education; nursing informatics. *Clinical nurse specialist programs in:* adult-gerontology acute care, pediatric. *Nurse practitioner programs in:* adult-gerontology acute care, family health, pediatric primary care, psychiatric/mental health.

DOCTORAL DEGREE PROGRAM

Degree PhD

Available Programs Doctorate; Post-Baccalaureate Doctorate.

Areas of Study Aging, bio-behavioral research, faculty preparation, family health, health policy, health promotion/disease prevention, health-care systems, human health and illness, information systems, nursing administration, nursing education, nursing policy, nursing research, nursing science, oncology.

Program Entrance Requirements Minimum overall college GPA of 3.5, interview by faculty committee, 3 letters of recommendation, statistics course, vita, writing sample, GRE General Test. Application deadline: 1/15 (spring), 8/15 (summer).

Degree Requirements 90 total credit hours, dissertation, oral exam, written exam, residency.

POSTDOCTORAL PROGRAM

Areas of Study Adolescent health, cancer care, chronic illness, family health, health promotion/disease prevention, individualized study, nursing informatics, nursing research, nursing science.

Postdoctoral Program Contact Debbie Grew, Graduate Advisor, School of Nursing, Indiana University–Purdue University Indianapolis, 1111 Middle Drive, Indianapolis, IN 46202. *Telephone:* 317-274-2806. *Fax:* 317-274-2996. *E-mail:* nursing@iu.edu.

CONTINUING EDUCATION PROGRAM

Contact Lisa D. Wagnes, RN, Assistant Dean, Center for Professional Development and Lifelong Learning, School of Nursing, Indiana University–Purdue University Indianapolis, 1111 Middle Drive, Indianapolis, IN 46202. *Telephone:* 317-274-7779. *Fax:* 317-274-0012. *E-mail:* lwagnes@iu.edu.

Indiana University South Bend

Vera Z. Dwyer College of Health Sciences
South Bend, Indiana

http://www.iusb.edu/nursing/
Founded in 1922

DEGREES • BSN • MSN
Nursing Program Faculty 24 (30% with doctorates).
Baccalaureate Enrollment 213 **Women** 84% **Men** 16% **Part-time** 10%
Graduate Enrollment 45 **Women** 92% **Men** 8% **Part-time** 100%
Distance Learning Courses Available.
Nursing Student Activities Sigma Theta Tau, Student Nurses' Association.
Nursing Student Resources Academic advising; academic or career counseling; assistance for students with disabilities; bookstore; campus computer network; career placement assistance; computer lab; computer-assisted instruction; daycare for children of students; e-mail services; employment services for current students; externships; housing assistance; interactive nursing skills videos; Internet; learning resource lab; library services; nursing audiovisuals; placement services for program completers; resume preparation assistance; skills, simulation, or other laboratory; tutoring.
Library Facilities 4,300 volumes in health, 2,300 volumes in nursing; 145 periodical subscriptions health-care related.

BACCALAUREATE PROGRAMS

Degree BSN

Available Programs Accelerated Baccalaureate for Second Degree; Generic Baccalaureate; RN Baccalaureate.

Study Options Full-time and part-time.

Program Entrance Requirements Minimum overall college GPA of 2.5, transcript of college record, CPR certification, written essay, health exam, health insurance, high school biology, high school chemistry, high school transcript, immunizations, minimum high school GPA of 2.0, minimum high school rank 50%, minimum GPA in nursing prerequisites of 2.7, prerequisite course work. Transfer students are accepted. *Application deadline:* 3/1 (fall), 10/1 (spring), 2/1 (summer).

Advanced Placement Credit given for nursing courses completed elsewhere dependent upon specific evaluations.

Expenses (2015–16) *Tuition, state resident:* full-time $8400; part-time $213 per credit hour. *Tuition, nonresident:* full-time $21,000; part-time $593 per credit hour. *International tuition:* $21,000 full-time. *Required fees:* full-time $2700; part-time $336 per credit; part-time $886 per term.

Financial Aid 75% of baccalaureate students in nursing programs received some form of financial aid in 2014–15.

Contact Office of Student Services, Vera Z. Dwyer College of Health Sciences, Indiana University South Bend, 1700 Mishawaka Avenue, PO Box 7111, South Bend, IN 46634-7111. *Telephone:* 574-520-4571. *Fax:* 574-520-4461. *E-mail:* nursing@iusb.edu.

GRADUATE PROGRAMS

Expenses (2015–16) *Tuition, state resident:* full-time $6336; part-time $352 per credit hour. *Tuition, nonresident:* full-time $18,500; part-time $1026 per credit hour. *International tuition:* $18,500 full-time. *Required fees:* full-time $3800.

Financial Aid 50% of graduate students in nursing programs received some form of financial aid in 2014–15.

Contact Dr. Mario Ortiz, Director of Graduate Program in Nursing, Vera Z. Dwyer College of Health Sciences, Indiana University South Bend, 1700 Mishawaka Avenue, PO Box 7111, South Bend, IN 46634-7111. *Telephone:* 574-520-4207. *Fax:* 574-520-4461. *E-mail:* ortizmr@iusb.edu.

MASTER'S DEGREE PROGRAM

Degree MSN

Available Programs Master's.

Concentrations Available *Nurse practitioner programs in:* family health.

Study Options Part-time.

Program Entrance Requirements Clinical experience, computer literacy, minimum overall college GPA of 3.0, transcript of college record, CPR certification, written essay, immunizations, interview, 3 letters of recommendation, nursing research course, physical assessment course, statistics course. *Application deadline:* 4/1 (fall). *Application fee:* $40.

Advanced Placement Credit given for nursing courses completed elsewhere dependent upon specific evaluations.

Degree Requirements 42 total credit hours, thesis or project.

Indiana University Southeast

School of Nursing
New Albany, Indiana

http://www.ius.edu/nursing/
Founded in 1941

DEGREE • BSN
Nursing Program Faculty 23 (22% with doctorates).
Baccalaureate Enrollment 168 **Women** 91% **Men** 9%
Distance Learning Courses Available.
Nursing Student Activities Sigma Theta Tau, Student Nurses' Association.
Nursing Student Resources Academic advising; academic or career counseling; assistance for students with disabilities; bookstore; campus computer network; career placement assistance; computer lab; computer-assisted instruction; daycare for children of students; e-mail services; housing assistance; interactive nursing skills videos; Internet; learning resource lab; library services; nursing audiovisuals; remedial services; resume preparation assistance; skills, simulation, or other laboratory; tutoring.
Library Facilities 35 volumes in health, 15 volumes in nursing; 35 periodical subscriptions health-care related.

BACCALAUREATE PROGRAMS

Degree BSN

Available Programs Generic Baccalaureate; RN Baccalaureate.

Study Options Full-time.

Online Degree Options Yes.

Program Entrance Requirements Transcript of college record, CPR certification, immunizations, minimum GPA in nursing prerequisites of 2.5, prerequisite course work. Transfer students are accepted. *Application deadline:* 3/15 (spring). *Application fee:* $35.

Advanced Placement Credit given for nursing courses completed elsewhere dependent upon specific evaluations.

Expenses (2014–15) *Tuition, state resident:* full-time $12,473; part-time $208 per credit hour. *Tuition, nonresident:* full-time $17,490; part-time $583 per credit hour. *International tuition:* $17,490 full-time. *Room and board:* room only: $6764 per academic year. *Required fees:* full-time $1520; part-time $51 per credit.

Financial Aid 60% of baccalaureate students in nursing programs received some form of financial aid in 2013–14.

Contact Ms. Brenda Hackett, Nursing Advisor, School of Nursing, Indiana University Southeast, 4201 Grant Line Road, Life Sciences

Building, Room 276, New Albany, IN 47150-6405. *Telephone:* 812-941-2283. *Fax:* 812-941-2687. *E-mail:* bhackett@ius.edu.

Indiana Wesleyan University
School of Nursing
Marion, Indiana

http://www.indwes.edu/Academics/School-of-Nursing/
Founded in 1920
DEGREES • BSN • MSN
Nursing Program Faculty 210 (21% with doctorates).
Baccalaureate Enrollment 1,581 **Women** 93% **Men** 7% **Part-time** 9%
Graduate Enrollment 427 **Women** 95% **Men** 5% **Part-time** 10%
Distance Learning Courses Available.
Nursing Student Activities Nursing Honor Society, Sigma Theta Tau, Student Nurses' Association, nursing club.
Nursing Student Resources Academic advising; academic or career counseling; assistance for students with disabilities; bookstore; campus computer network; career placement assistance; computer lab; computer-assisted instruction; e-mail services; housing assistance; interactive nursing skills videos; Internet; learning resource lab; library services; nursing audiovisuals; remedial services; resume preparation assistance; skills, simulation, or other laboratory; tutoring.
Library Facilities 7,142 volumes in health, 5,672 volumes in nursing; 160 periodical subscriptions health-care related.

BACCALAUREATE PROGRAMS

Degree BSN
Available Programs Accelerated Baccalaureate for Second Degree; Generic Baccalaureate; RN Baccalaureate.
Site Options Lexington, KY; Merrillville, IN; Louisville, KY.
Study Options Full-time and part-time.
Program Entrance Requirements Minimum overall college GPA of 2.75, transcript of college record, CPR certification, written essay, health exam, health insurance, high school biology, high school chemistry, high school foreign language, 3 years high school math, 3 years high school science, high school transcript, immunizations, minimum high school GPA of 2.8, minimum GPA in nursing prerequisites of 2.75, prerequisite course work. Transfer students are accepted. *Application deadline:* 5/30 (fall), 12/1 (spring).
Advanced Placement Credit given for nursing courses completed elsewhere dependent upon specific evaluations.
Contact *Telephone:* 765-677-2268. *Fax:* 765-677-2284.

GRADUATE PROGRAMS

Contact *Telephone:* 765-677-2045. *Fax:* 765-677-2380.

MASTER'S DEGREE PROGRAM
Degree MSN
Available Programs Master's.
Concentrations Available Nursing administration; nursing education. *Nurse practitioner programs in:* family health.
Site Options Lexington, KY; Merrillville, IN; Louisville, KY.
Study Options Full-time and part-time.
Online Degree Options Yes.
Program Entrance Requirements Clinical experience, minimum overall college GPA of 3.0, transcript of college record, written essay, immunizations, interview, 3 letters of recommendation, nursing research course, physical assessment course, resume, statistics course.
Advanced Placement Credit given for nursing courses completed elsewhere dependent upon specific evaluations.
Degree Requirements 41 total credit hours, thesis or project.

POST-MASTER'S PROGRAM
Areas of Study Nursing administration; nursing education. *Nurse practitioner programs in:* family health.

Marian University
School of Nursing
Indianapolis, Indiana

http://www.marian.edu/Nursing/Pages/default.aspx
Founded in 1851
DEGREE • BSN
Nursing Program Faculty 35
Baccalaureate Enrollment 480 **Women** 95% **Men** 5% **Part-time** 10%
Distance Learning Courses Available.
Nursing Student Activities Nursing Honor Society, Sigma Theta Tau, Student Nurses' Association.
Nursing Student Resources Academic advising; academic or career counseling; assistance for students with disabilities; bookstore; campus computer network; career placement assistance; computer lab; computer-assisted instruction; e-mail services; employment services for current students; interactive nursing skills videos; Internet; learning resource lab; library services; nursing audiovisuals; remedial services; resume preparation assistance; skills, simulation, or other laboratory; tutoring; unpaid internships.
Library Facilities 3,250 volumes in health, 2,000 volumes in nursing; 116 periodical subscriptions health-care related.

BACCALAUREATE PROGRAMS

Degree BSN
Available Programs Accelerated Baccalaureate; Accelerated Baccalaureate for Second Degree; Accelerated RN Baccalaureate; Baccalaureate for Second Degree; Generic Baccalaureate; RN Baccalaureate.
Site Options Indianapolis, IN.
Study Options Full-time and part-time.
Online Degree Options Yes.
Program Entrance Requirements Minimum overall college GPA of 2.8, transcript of college record, CPR certification, health exam, health insurance, high school biology, high school chemistry, high school transcript, immunizations, minimum high school GPA of 2.3, minimum GPA in nursing prerequisites of 2.8, prerequisite course work. Transfer students are accepted. *Application deadline:* 7/15 (fall), 11/15 (winter), 12/15 (spring), 4/15 (summer). *Application fee:* $50.
Contact *Telephone:* 317-955-6157. *Fax:* 317-955-6135.

CONTINUING EDUCATION PROGRAM

Contact *Telephone:* 317-955-6145. *Fax:* 317-955-6135.

Purdue University
School of Nursing
West Lafayette, Indiana

http://www.nursing.purdue.edu/
Founded in 1869
DEGREES • BS • DNP • MS
Nursing Program Faculty 60 (15% with doctorates).
Baccalaureate Enrollment 552 **Women** 94% **Men** 6% **Part-time** .06%
Graduate Enrollment 48 **Women** 96% **Men** 4% **Part-time** 50%
Nursing Student Activities Sigma Theta Tau, Student Nurses' Association.
Nursing Student Resources Academic advising; academic or career counseling; assistance for students with disabilities; bookstore; campus computer network; career placement assistance; computer lab; computer-assisted instruction; e-mail services; interactive nursing skills videos; Internet; learning resource lab; library services; nursing audiovisuals; remedial services; resume preparation assistance; skills, simulation, or other laboratory; tutoring.
Library Facilities 200,000 volumes in health, 10,000 volumes in nursing; 1,000 periodical subscriptions health-care related.

BACCALAUREATE PROGRAMS

Degree BS
Available Programs ADN to Baccalaureate; Accelerated Baccalaureate for Second Degree; Baccalaureate for Second Degree; Generic Baccalaureate; RN Baccalaureate.
Site Options Indianapolis, IN.
Study Options Full-time and part-time.
Program Entrance Requirements Transcript of college record, CPR certification, health exam, health insurance, high school biology, high

school chemistry, high school foreign language, 3 years high school math, 3 years high school science, high school transcript, immunizations, letters of recommendation, minimum high school GPA of 3.0. Transfer students are accepted.

Advanced Placement Credit by examination available. Credit given for nursing courses completed elsewhere dependent upon specific evaluations.

Contact *Telephone:* 765-494-1776. *Fax:* 765-494-0544.

GRADUATE PROGRAMS

Contact *Telephone:* 765-494-4015. *Fax:* 765-496-1800.

MASTER'S DEGREE PROGRAM

Degree MS
Available Programs Master's.
Concentrations Available *Nurse practitioner programs in:* adult health, pediatric.
Study Options Full-time and part-time.
Program Entrance Requirements Clinical experience, computer literacy, minimum overall college GPA of 3.0, transcript of college record, CPR certification, written essay, interview, 3 letters of recommendation, professional liability insurance/malpractice insurance, prerequisite course work, resume, statistics course.
Advanced Placement Credit given for nursing courses completed elsewhere dependent upon specific evaluations.
Degree Requirements 46 total credit hours, thesis or project.

POST-MASTER'S PROGRAM

Areas of Study *Nurse practitioner programs in:* adult health, pediatric.

DOCTORAL DEGREE PROGRAM

Degree DNP
Available Programs Doctorate.
Areas of Study Advanced practice nursing, aging, biology of health and illness, clinical practice, critical care, ethics, gerontology, health policy, health promotion/disease prevention, health-care systems, illness and transition, individualized study, information systems, nursing administration, nursing education, nursing policy, nursing research, nursing science, oncology, urban health, women's health.
Program Entrance Requirements Clinical experience, minimum overall college GPA of 3.0, interview by faculty committee, interview, letters of recommendation, MSN or equivalent, statistics course, vita, writing sample.
Degree Requirements 83 total credit hours, oral exam, residency.

CONTINUING EDUCATION PROGRAM

Contact *Telephone:* 765-494-4030. *Fax:* 765-494-6339.

Purdue University Calumet
School of Nursing
Hammond, Indiana

---

http://webs.purduecal.edu/nursing/
Founded in 1951
DEGREES • BSN • MS
Nursing Program Faculty 45 (38% with doctorates).
Baccalaureate Enrollment 1,283 **Women** 90.1% **Men** 9.9% **Part-time** 75.4%
Graduate Enrollment 140 **Women** 93% **Men** 7% **Part-time** 97%
Distance Learning Courses Available.
Nursing Student Activities Sigma Theta Tau, Student Nurses' Association, nursing club.
Nursing Student Resources Academic advising; academic or career counseling; assistance for students with disabilities; bookstore; campus computer network; career placement assistance; computer lab; computer-assisted instruction; daycare for children of students; e-mail services; employment services for current students; externships; housing assistance; interactive nursing skills videos; Internet; learning resource lab; library services; nursing audiovisuals; other; paid internships; placement services for program completers; remedial services; resume preparation assistance; skills, simulation, or other laboratory; tutoring; unpaid internships.
Library Facilities 7,900 volumes in health, 1,140 volumes in nursing; 610 periodical subscriptions health-care related.

BACCALAUREATE PROGRAMS

Degree BSN
Available Programs Accelerated Baccalaureate for Second Degree; Generic Baccalaureate; LPN to Baccalaureate.
Study Options Full-time and part-time.
Online Degree Options Yes.
Program Entrance Requirements Minimum overall college GPA of 2.5, transcript of college record, CPR certification, health exam, high school biology, high school chemistry, 3 years high school math, 4 years high school science, high school transcript, immunizations, minimum GPA in nursing prerequisites of 2.0, prerequisite course work. Transfer students are accepted. *Application deadline:* 2/1 (fall).
Advanced Placement Credit by examination available. Credit given for nursing courses completed elsewhere dependent upon specific evaluations.
Expenses (2014–15) *Tuition, state resident:* full-time $6529; part-time $218 per credit hour. *Tuition, nonresident:* full-time $15,645; part-time $522 per credit hour. *International tuition:* $15,645 full-time. *Room and board:* room only: $8075 per academic year. *Required fees:* full-time $564; part-time $18 per credit.
Financial Aid 35% of baccalaureate students in nursing programs received some form of financial aid in 2013–14.
Contact Prof. Kathleen Ann Nix, Undergraduate Program Coordinator, School of Nursing, Purdue University Calumet, 2200 169th Street, Hammond, IN 46323-2094. *Telephone:* 219-989-2859. *Fax:* 219-989-2848. *E-mail:* nix@purduecal.edu.

GRADUATE PROGRAMS

Expenses (2014–15) *Tuition, state resident:* full-time $4971; part-time $276 per credit hour. *Tuition, nonresident:* full-time $10,948; part-time $608 per credit hour. *International tuition:* $10,948 full-time. *Room and board:* room only: $8075 per academic year. *Required fees:* full-time $349; part-time $18 per credit.
Financial Aid 50% of graduate students in nursing programs received some form of financial aid in 2013–14.
Contact Dr. Jane Walker, Graduate Program Coordinator, School of Nursing, Purdue University Calumet, 2200 169th Street, Hammond, IN 46323-2094. *Telephone:* 219-989-2815. *Fax:* 219-989-2848. *E-mail:* walkerj@calumet.purdue.edu.

MASTER'S DEGREE PROGRAM

Degree MS
Available Programs Master's.
Concentrations Available *Clinical nurse specialist programs in:* adult-gerontology acute care. *Nurse practitioner programs in:* family health.
Study Options Full-time and part-time.
Online Degree Options Yes.
Program Entrance Requirements Minimum overall college GPA of 3.0, transcript of college record, written essay, 3 letters of recommendation, physical assessment course, resume, statistics course. *Application deadline:* 2/15 (fall), 9/15 (spring), 2/15 (summer). *Application fee:* $55.
Advanced Placement Credit given for nursing courses completed elsewhere dependent upon specific evaluations.
Degree Requirements 47 total credit hours.

POST-MASTER'S PROGRAM

Areas of Study *Clinical nurse specialist programs in:* adult-gerontology acute care. *Nurse practitioner programs in:* family health.

Purdue University North Central
Department of Nursing
Westville, Indiana

---

https://www.pnc.edu/nu/
Founded in 1967
DEGREE • BS
Nursing Program Faculty 34 (35% with doctorates).
Baccalaureate Enrollment 150 **Women** 97% **Men** 3% **Part-time** 87%
Distance Learning Courses Available.
Nursing Student Activities Nursing Honor Society, Student Nurses' Association.
Nursing Student Resources Academic advising; academic or career counseling; assistance for students with disabilities; bookstore; campus computer network; career placement assistance; computer lab; computer-assisted instruction; daycare for children of students; e-mail services; interactive nursing skills videos; Internet; learning resource lab; library

services; nursing audiovisuals; placement services for program completers; resume preparation assistance; skills, simulation, or other laboratory; tutoring.
Library Facilities 1,100 volumes in health, 560 volumes in nursing; 229 periodical subscriptions health-care related.

BACCALAUREATE PROGRAMS

Degree BS
Available Programs ADN to Baccalaureate; Accelerated Baccalaureate; Accelerated Baccalaureate for Second Degree; Baccalaureate for Second Degree; LPN to Baccalaureate; RN Baccalaureate.
Site Options Valparaiso, IN.
Study Options Full-time and part-time.
Program Entrance Requirements Minimum overall college GPA of 2.5, transcript of college record, CPR certification, health exam, health insurance, high school biology, high school chemistry, 3 years high school math, 3 years high school science, high school transcript, immunizations, minimum high school GPA of 2.5, minimum high school rank 50%, minimum GPA in nursing prerequisites of 2.5, professional liability insurance/malpractice insurance, prerequisite course work. Transfer students are accepted. *Application deadline:* 1/16 (fall), 8/16 (spring).
Advanced Placement Credit by examination available. Credit given for nursing courses completed elsewhere dependent upon specific evaluations.
Contact *Telephone:* 219-785-5439. *Fax:* 219-785-5495.

Saint Joseph's College
St. Elizabeth School of Nursing
Rensselaer, Indiana

http://www.steson.org
Founded in 1889
DEGREE • BSN
Nursing Program Faculty 23 (4% with doctorates).
Baccalaureate Enrollment 192 **Women** 96% **Men** 4% **Part-time** 2%
Distance Learning Courses Available.
Nursing Student Activities Student Nurses' Association.
Nursing Student Resources Academic advising; assistance for students with disabilities; campus computer network; computer lab; computer-assisted instruction; e-mail services; interactive nursing skills videos; Internet; learning resource lab; library services; nursing audiovisuals; remedial services; resume preparation assistance; skills, simulation, or other laboratory; tutoring.
Library Facilities 900 volumes in health, 900 volumes in nursing; 50 periodical subscriptions health-care related.

BACCALAUREATE PROGRAMS

Degree BSN
Available Programs Accelerated Baccalaureate for Second Degree; Accelerated RN Baccalaureate; LPN to RN Baccalaureate; RN Baccalaureate.
Site Options Lafayette, IN.
Study Options Full-time and part-time.
Program Entrance Requirements Minimum overall college GPA of 2.0, transcript of college record, CPR certification, written essay, health exam, health insurance, high school biology, high school chemistry, 3 years high school math, 2 years high school science, high school transcript, immunizations, 3 letters of recommendation, TEAS-V admissions exam, minimum high school GPA of 2.0, minimum high school rank 51%. Transfer students are accepted. *Application deadline:* 5/1 (fall), 10/1 (spring). Applications may be processed on a rolling basis for some programs. *Application fee:* $25.
Advanced Placement Credit given for nursing courses completed elsewhere dependent upon specific evaluations.
Expenses (2015–16) *Tuition:* full-time $8960; part-time $525 per credit hour. *International tuition:* $8960 full-time. *Room and board:* $4450; room only: $2300 per academic year.
Financial Aid 95% of baccalaureate students in nursing programs received some form of financial aid in 2014–15.
Contact Anita K. Reed, Coordinator of Admissions, St. Elizabeth School of Nursing, Saint Joseph's College, 1508 Tippecanoe Street, Lafayette, IN 47904. *Telephone:* 765-423-6285. *Fax:* 765-423-6383.
E-mail: anita.reed@franciscanalliance.org.

Saint Mary's College
Department of Nursing
Notre Dame, Indiana

http://www.saintmarys.edu/nursing
Founded in 1844
DEGREES • BS • DNP
Nursing Program Faculty 26 (25% with doctorates).
Baccalaureate Enrollment 215 **Women** 100%
Graduate Enrollment 7
Distance Learning Courses Available.
Nursing Student Activities Nursing Honor Society, Sigma Theta Tau, Student Nurses' Association.
Nursing Student Resources Academic advising; academic or career counseling; assistance for students with disabilities; bookstore; campus computer network; career placement assistance; computer lab; computer-assisted instruction; daycare for children of students; e-mail services; employment services for current students; interactive nursing skills videos; Internet; learning resource lab; library services; nursing audiovisuals; placement services for program completers; remedial services; resume preparation assistance; skills, simulation, or other laboratory; tutoring.
Library Facilities 9,787 volumes in health, 5,149 volumes in nursing; 70 periodical subscriptions health-care related.

BACCALAUREATE PROGRAMS

Degree BS
Available Programs Generic Baccalaureate.
Site Options Goshen, IN; South Bend, IN.
Study Options Full-time.
Program Entrance Requirements Minimum overall college GPA of 2.5, transcript of college record, CPR certification, written essay, health exam, high school foreign language, 3 years high school math, 2 years high school science, high school transcript, immunizations, 2 letters of recommendation, minimum GPA in nursing prerequisites of 2.80. Transfer students are accepted. *Application deadline:* Applications may be processed on a rolling basis for some programs. *Application fee:* $30.
Advanced Placement Credit given for nursing courses completed elsewhere dependent upon specific evaluations.
Expenses (2015–16) *Tuition:* full-time $36,600; part-time $1440 per credit. *Room and board:* $9000; room only: $4700 per academic year. *Required fees:* full-time $1160.
Financial Aid 75% of baccalaureate students in nursing programs received some form of financial aid in 2014–15.
Contact Ms. April Lane, Advisor, Nursing, Department of Nursing, Saint Mary's College, 1 Havican Hall, Notre Dame, IN 46556. *Telephone:* 574-284-4790. *Fax:* 574-284-4810. *E-mail:* alane@saintmarys.edu.

GRADUATE PROGRAMS

Expenses (2015–16) *Tuition:* full-time $10,024.
Contact Ms. April Lane, Advisor, Nursing, Department of Nursing, Saint Mary's College, 1 Havican hall, Notre Dame, IN 46556. *Telephone:* 574-284-4790. *Fax:* 574-284-4810. *E-mail:* alane@saintmarys.edu.

DOCTORAL DEGREE PROGRAM
Degree DNP
Available Programs Post-Baccalaureate Doctorate.
Areas of Study Family health.
Program Entrance Requirements Clinical experience, minimum overall college GPA of 3.0, interview by faculty committee, interview, letters of recommendation, statistics course, vita, writing sample. Application deadline: Applications may be processed on a rolling basis for some programs. Application fee: $65.
Degree Requirements 77 total credit hours, oral exam.

University of Evansville
Department of Nursing
Evansville, Indiana

http://www.evansville.edu/majors/nursing/
Founded in 1854
DEGREE • BSN
Nursing Program Faculty 11 (28% with doctorates).
Baccalaureate Enrollment 188 **Women** 86% **Men** 14% **Part-time** 20%

Distance Learning Courses Available.

Nursing Student Activities Sigma Theta Tau, Student Nurses' Association.

Nursing Student Resources Academic advising; academic or career counseling; assistance for students with disabilities; bookstore; campus computer network; career placement assistance; computer lab; computer-assisted instruction; e-mail services; employment services for current students; externships; housing assistance; interactive nursing skills videos; Internet; learning resource lab; library services; nursing audiovisuals; paid internships; placement services for program completers; remedial services; resume preparation assistance; skills, simulation, or other laboratory; tutoring; unpaid internships.

Library Facilities 11,000 volumes in nursing; 155 periodical subscriptions health-care related.

BACCALAUREATE PROGRAMS

Degree BSN

Available Programs Generic Baccalaureate; RN Baccalaureate.

Site Options Henderson, KY.

Study Options Full-time and part-time.

Program Entrance Requirements CPR certification, health exam, health insurance, high school chemistry, 3 years high school math, 2 years high school science, high school transcript, immunizations, minimum high school rank 67%, professional liability insurance/malpractice insurance. Transfer students are accepted. *Application deadline:* Applications may be processed on a rolling basis for some programs. *Application fee:* $35.

Advanced Placement Credit given for nursing courses completed elsewhere dependent upon specific evaluations.

Contact *Telephone:* 812-488-2414. *Fax:* 812-488-2717.

University of Indianapolis
School of Nursing
Indianapolis, Indiana

http://www.uindy.edu/

Founded in 1902

DEGREES • BSN • DNP • MSN

Nursing Program Faculty 39 (52% with doctorates).

Baccalaureate Enrollment 498 **Women** 92.4% **Men** 7.6% **Part-time** 53.4%

Graduate Enrollment 335 **Women** 95.3% **Men** 4.7% **Part-time** 98%

Distance Learning Courses Available.

Nursing Student Activities Nursing Honor Society, Sigma Theta Tau, Student Nurses' Association.

Nursing Student Resources Academic advising; academic or career counseling; assistance for students with disabilities; bookstore; campus computer network; career placement assistance; computer lab; computer-assisted instruction; e-mail services; employment services for current students; externships; housing assistance; interactive nursing skills videos; Internet; learning resource lab; library services; nursing audiovisuals; other; paid internships; placement services for program completers; remedial services; resume preparation assistance; skills, simulation, or other laboratory; tutoring; unpaid internships.

Library Facilities 15,600 volumes in health, 360 volumes in nursing; 600 periodical subscriptions health-care related.

BACCALAUREATE PROGRAMS

Degree BSN

Available Programs Accelerated Baccalaureate for Second Degree; Generic Baccalaureate; RN Baccalaureate.

Site Options Indianapolis, IN.

Study Options Full-time and part-time.

Online Degree Options Yes.

Program Entrance Requirements Minimum overall college GPA of 2.82, transcript of college record, CPR certification, health exam, health insurance, high school biology, high school chemistry, 2 years high school math, 2 years high school science, high school transcript, immunizations, minimum GPA in nursing prerequisites of 2.0, prerequisite course work. Transfer students are accepted. *Application deadline:* 4/15 (fall), 10/15 (winter). *Application fee:* $25.

Advanced Placement Credit by examination available. Credit given for nursing courses completed elsewhere dependent upon specific evaluations.

Expenses (2015–16) *Tuition:* full-time $27,010; part-time $1080 per credit hour. *International tuition:* $27,010 full-time. *Required fees:* full-time $500; part-time $180 per term.

Financial Aid 70% of baccalaureate students in nursing programs received some form of financial aid in 2014–15. *Gift aid (need-based):* Federal Pell, FSEOG, state, private, college/university gift aid from institutional funds. *Loans:* Federal Direct (Subsidized and Unsubsidized Stafford PLUS), Perkins. *Work-study:* Federal Work-Study, part-time campus jobs. *Financial aid application deadline (priority):* 3/10.

Contact Mrs. Cheryl Conces, Undergraduate Program Director, School of Nursing, University of Indianapolis, 1400 East Hanna Avenue, Indianapolis, IN 46227-3697. *Telephone:* 317-788-3206. *Fax:* 317-788-6208. *E-mail:* cconces@uindy.edu.

GRADUATE PROGRAMS

Expenses (2015–16) *Tuition:* full-time $8304; part-time $692 per credit hour. *International tuition:* $8304 full-time. *Required fees:* full-time $500; part-time $50 per term.

Financial Aid 60% of graduate students in nursing programs received some form of financial aid in 2014–15.

Contact Dr. Norma Hall, Director, Graduate Program, School of Nursing, University of Indianapolis, 1400 East Hanna Avenue, Indianapolis, IN 46227-3697. *Telephone:* 317-788-3206. *Fax:* 317-788-6208. *E-mail:* hallne@uindy.edu.

MASTER'S DEGREE PROGRAM

Degree MSN

Available Programs Master's.

Concentrations Available Nursing administration; nursing education. *Nurse practitioner programs in:* adult health, family health, gerontology, neonatal health, women's health.

Site Options Indianapolis, IN.

Study Options Full-time and part-time.

Online Degree Options Yes.

Program Entrance Requirements Clinical experience, minimum overall college GPA of 3.0, transcript of college record, CPR certification, written essay, immunizations, interview, 3 letters of recommendation, nursing research course, professional liability insurance/malpractice insurance, prerequisite course work, resume, statistics course. *Application deadline:* 4/15 (fall). Applications may be processed on a rolling basis for some programs. *Application fee:* $60.

Degree Requirements 39 total credit hours, thesis or project, comprehensive exam.

POST-MASTER'S PROGRAM

Areas of Study Nursing administration; nursing education. *Nurse practitioner programs in:* adult health, family health, gerontology, neonatal health, women's health.

DOCTORAL DEGREE PROGRAM

Degree DNP

Available Programs Doctorate.

Areas of Study Health-care systems.

Site Options Indianapolis, IN.

Online Degree Options Yes (online only).

Program Entrance Requirements Clinical experience, minimum overall college GPA of 3.25, interview by faculty committee, 3 letters of recommendation, MSN or equivalent, statistics course, vita, writing sample. Application deadline: 4/15 (fall), 10/15 (winter). Applications may be processed on a rolling basis for some programs. Application fee: $60.

Degree Requirements 35 total credit hours.

University of Saint Francis
Department of Nursing
Fort Wayne, Indiana

http://nursing.sf.edu/

Founded in 1890

DEGREES • BSN • MSN

Nursing Program Faculty 35 (5% with doctorates).

Baccalaureate Enrollment 254 **Women** 91% **Men** 9% **Part-time** 4%

Graduate Enrollment 103 **Women** 90% **Men** 10% **Part-time** 56%

Distance Learning Courses Available.

Nursing Student Activities Nursing Honor Society, Sigma Theta Tau, Student Nurses' Association.

Nursing Student Resources Academic advising; academic or career counseling; assistance for students with disabilities; bookstore; campus computer network; career placement assistance; computer lab; computer-assisted instruction; e-mail services; employment services for current students; externships; housing assistance; interactive nursing skills videos; Internet; learning resource lab; library services; nursing audiovisuals; paid internships; remedial services; resume preparation assistance; skills, simulation, or other laboratory; tutoring; unpaid internships.

Library Facilities 6,233 volumes in health, 3,376 volumes in nursing; 2,468 periodical subscriptions health-care related.

BACCALAUREATE PROGRAMS

Degree BSN

Available Programs ADN to Baccalaureate; Generic Baccalaureate; RN Baccalaureate.

Study Options Full-time and part-time.

Online Degree Options Yes.

Program Entrance Requirements Minimum overall college GPA of 2.7, transcript of college record, CPR certification, health exam, high school biology, high school chemistry, 1 year of high school math, high school transcript, immunizations, minimum high school GPA of 2.7, minimum GPA in nursing prerequisites of 2.7, prerequisite course work. Transfer students are accepted. *Application deadline:* 7/31 (fall), 11/18 (spring). Applications may be processed on a rolling basis for some programs.

Advanced Placement Credit given for nursing courses completed elsewhere dependent upon specific evaluations.

Expenses (2015–16) *Tuition:* full-time $26,250; part-time $830 per credit hour. *International tuition:* $26,250 full-time. *Room and board:* $9276 per academic year. *Required fees:* full-time $550; part-time $25 per term.

Financial Aid 96% of baccalaureate students in nursing programs received some form of financial aid in 2014–15.

Contact Megan Winegarden, BSN Program Director, Department of Nursing, University of Saint Francis, 2701 Spring Street, Fort Wayne, IN 46808. *Telephone:* 260-399-7700 Ext. 8513. *Fax:* 260-399-8167. *E-mail:* mwinegarden@sf.edu.

GRADUATE PROGRAMS

Expenses (2015–16) *Tuition:* part-time $870 per credit hour. *Required fees:* part-time $24 per credit; part-time $275 per term.

Financial Aid 96% of graduate students in nursing programs received some form of financial aid in 2014–15. Federal Work-Study, scholarships, and unspecified assistantships available. Aid available to part-time students. *Financial aid application deadline:* 3/10.

Contact Wendy Clark, MSN Program Director, Department of Nursing, University of Saint Francis, 2701 Spring Street, Fort Wayne, IN 46808. *Telephone:* 260-399-7700 Ext. 8534. *Fax:* 260-399-8167. *E-mail:* wclark@sf.edu.

MASTER'S DEGREE PROGRAM

Degree MSN

Available Programs Master's; Master's for Nurses with Non-Nursing Degrees; RN to Master's.

Concentrations Available *Nurse practitioner programs in:* family health.

Study Options Full-time and part-time.

Program Entrance Requirements Computer literacy, minimum overall college GPA of 3.2, transcript of college record, CPR certification, written essay, immunizations, interview, 3 letters of recommendation, nursing research course, physical assessment course, resume, statistics course, GRE (if undergraduate GPA is less than 3.0). *Application deadline:* 7/28 (fall), 4/14 (summer).

Advanced Placement Credit given for nursing courses completed elsewhere dependent upon specific evaluations.

Degree Requirements 48 total credit hours.

POST-MASTER'S PROGRAM

Areas of Study *Nurse practitioner programs in:* family health.

University of Southern Indiana
College of Nursing and Health Professions
Evansville, Indiana

http://www.usi.edu/health
Founded in 1965
DEGREES • BSN • DNP • MSN
Nursing Program Faculty 63 (63% with doctorates).
Baccalaureate Enrollment 580 Women 90% Men 10% Part-time 36%
Graduate Enrollment 427 Women 87% Men 13% Part-time 72%
Distance Learning Courses Available.
Nursing Student Activities Sigma Theta Tau, Student Nurses' Association.
Nursing Student Resources Academic advising; academic or career counseling; assistance for students with disabilities; bookstore; campus computer network; career placement assistance; computer lab; computer-assisted instruction; daycare for children of students; e-mail services; employment services for current students; housing assistance; interactive nursing skills videos; Internet; learning resource lab; library services; nursing audiovisuals; placement services for program completers; remedial services; resume preparation assistance; skills, simulation, or other laboratory; tutoring; unpaid internships.
Library Facilities 9,200 volumes in health, 1,500 volumes in nursing; 2,000 periodical subscriptions health-care related.

BACCALAUREATE PROGRAMS

Degree BSN
Available Programs Generic Baccalaureate; RN Baccalaureate.
Study Options Full-time.
Online Degree Options Yes.
Program Entrance Requirements Minimum overall college GPA of 3.0, transcript of college record, CPR certification, written essay, health exam, health insurance, high school transcript, immunizations, minimum GPA in nursing prerequisites of 2.0, professional liability insurance/malpractice insurance, prerequisite course work. Transfer students are accepted. *Application deadline:* 8/1 (fall).
Advanced Placement Credit given for nursing courses completed elsewhere dependent upon specific evaluations.
Expenses (2015–16) *Tuition, state resident:* full-time $6837; part-time $228 per credit hour. *Tuition, nonresident:* full-time $16,619; part-time $554 per credit hour. *International tuition:* $17,450 full-time. *Room and board:* $4138; room only: $2182 per academic year. *Required fees:* full-time $1560; part-time $52 per credit.
Financial Aid 71% of baccalaureate students in nursing programs received some form of financial aid in 2014–15. *Gift aid (need-based):* Federal Pell, FSEOG, state, private, college/university gift aid from institutional funds, Federal Nursing. *Loans:* Federal Direct (Subsidized and Unsubsidized Stafford PLUS). *Work-study:* Federal Work-Study. *Financial aid application deadline:* Continuous.
Contact Dr. Sarah Stevens, Director of CNHP Advising Center, College of Nursing and Health Professions, University of Southern Indiana, 8600 University Boulevard, Evansville, IN 47712. *Telephone:* 812-461-5238. *Fax:* 812-465-7092. *E-mail:* sestevens@usi.edu.

GRADUATE PROGRAMS

Expenses (2015–16) *Tuition, state resident:* full-time $8110; part-time $338 per credit hour. *Tuition, nonresident:* full-time $8110; part-time $338 per credit hour. *International tuition:* $17,450 full-time. *Room and board:* $4138; room only: $2182 per academic year. *Required fees:* full-time $3415; part-time $142 per credit.
Financial Aid 69% of graduate students in nursing programs received some form of financial aid in 2014–15. Federal Work-Study, scholarships, tuition waivers (full and partial), and unspecified assistantships available. *Financial aid application deadline:* 3/1.
Contact Dr. Mellisa Hall, Chair, College of Nursing and Health Professions, University of Southern Indiana, 8600 University Boulevard, Evansville, IN 47712. *Telephone:* 812-465-1168. *Fax:* 812-465-7092. *E-mail:* mhall@usi.edu.

MASTER'S DEGREE PROGRAM

Degree MSN
Available Programs Master's.
Concentrations Available Nursing administration; nursing education. *Clinical nurse specialist programs in:* adult health. *Nurse practitioner programs in:* acute care, family health, primary care, psychiatric/mental health.
Study Options Full-time and part-time.

Online Degree Options Yes (online only).

Program Entrance Requirements Computer literacy, minimum overall college GPA of 3.0, transcript of college record, CPR certification, written essay, immunizations, 2 letters of recommendation, professional liability insurance/malpractice insurance, resume, statistics course. *Application deadline:* 2/1 (fall). *Application fee:* $25.

Advanced Placement Credit given for nursing courses completed elsewhere dependent upon specific evaluations.

Degree Requirements 42 total credit hours.

POST-MASTER'S PROGRAM

Areas of Study Nursing administration; nursing education. *Clinical nurse specialist programs in:* adult health. *Nurse practitioner programs in:* acute care, family health, primary care, psychiatric/mental health.

DOCTORAL DEGREE PROGRAM

Degree DNP

Available Programs Doctorate.

Areas of Study Clinical practice, nursing administration.

Program Entrance Requirements Clinical experience, minimum overall college GPA of 3.0, 3 letters of recommendation, MSN or equivalent, vita, writing sample. Application deadline: 1/15 (fall). Application fee: $25.

Degree Requirements 78 total credit hours.

CONTINUING EDUCATION PROGRAM

Contact Peggy Graul, Coordinator of Continuing Education for Nursing and Health Professions, College of Nursing and Health Professions, University of Southern Indiana, 8600 University Boulevard, Evansville, IN 47712. *Telephone:* 812-465-1161. *Fax:* 812-465-7092. *E-mail:* pgraul@usi.edu.

Valparaiso University
College of Nursing and Health Professions
Valparaiso, Indiana

http://www.valpo.edu/nursing
Founded in 1859
DEGREES • BSN • DNP • MSN • MSN/MHA
Nursing Program Faculty 20 (75% with doctorates).
Baccalaureate Enrollment 393 **Women** 89% **Men** 11% **Part-time** 1%
Graduate Enrollment 84 **Women** 86% **Men** 14% **Part-time** 27%
Distance Learning Courses Available.
Nursing Student Activities Sigma Theta Tau, Student Nurses' Association.
Nursing Student Resources Academic advising; academic or career counseling; assistance for students with disabilities; bookstore; campus computer network; career placement assistance; computer lab; computer-assisted instruction; e-mail services; employment services for current students; externships; housing assistance; interactive nursing skills videos; Internet; learning resource lab; library services; nursing audiovisuals; placement services for program completers; remedial services; resume preparation assistance; skills, simulation, or other laboratory; tutoring; unpaid internships.
Library Facilities 11,900 volumes in health, 1,950 volumes in nursing; 9,025 periodical subscriptions health-care related.

BACCALAUREATE PROGRAMS

Degree BSN

Available Programs Accelerated Baccalaureate; Generic Baccalaureate; RN Baccalaureate.

Study Options Full-time and part-time.

Program Entrance Requirements Minimum overall college GPA of 3.0, transcript of college record, CPR certification, written essay, high school biology, high school chemistry, 2 years high school math, 4 years high school science, high school transcript, immunizations, minimum high school GPA of 2.0, minimum GPA in nursing prerequisites of 2.5, professional liability insurance/malpractice insurance. Transfer students are accepted. *Application deadline:* Applications may be processed on a rolling basis for some programs.

Advanced Placement Credit by examination available. Credit given for nursing courses completed elsewhere dependent upon specific evaluations.

Expenses (2015–16) *Tuition:* full-time $17,515; part-time $1565 per semester. *International tuition:* $17,515 full-time. *Room and board:* $11,020; room only: $7300 per academic year. *Required fees:* full-time $1130; part-time $102 per term.

Financial Aid *Gift aid (need-based):* Federal Pell, FSEOG, state, private, college/university gift aid from institutional funds. *Loans:* Federal Direct (Subsidized and Unsubsidized Stafford PLUS), Perkins, college/university, private loans. *Work-study:* Federal Work-Study, part-time campus jobs. *Financial aid application deadline (priority):* 3/1.

Contact Admissions Counselor, College of Nursing and Health Professions, Valparaiso University, Office of Admission, Duesenberg Welcome Center, Valparaiso, IN 46383. *Telephone:* 219-464-5011. *Fax:* 219-464-6888. *E-mail:* admitinfo@valpo.edu.

GRADUATE PROGRAMS

Expenses (2015–16) *Tuition:* full-time $14,700; part-time $700 per credit. *International tuition:* $14,700 full-time. *Room and board:* $10,000 per academic year. *Required fees:* full-time $428; part-time $107 per term.

Contact Dr. Julie Koch, Assistant Dean for Graduate Nursing Programs, College of Nursing and Health Professions, Valparaiso University, 836 LaPorte Avenue, Valparaiso, IN 46383-6493. *Telephone:* 219-464-5291. *Fax:* 219-464-5425. *E-mail:* julie.koch@valpo.edu.

MASTER'S DEGREE PROGRAM

Degrees MSN; MSN/MHA

Available Programs Master's; RN to Master's.

Concentrations Available Nursing education.

Study Options Full-time and part-time.

Program Entrance Requirements Minimum overall college GPA of 3.0, transcript of college record, CPR certification, written essay, immunizations, 2 letters of recommendation, nursing research course, physical assessment course, statistics course. *Application deadline:* Applications may be processed on a rolling basis for some programs. *Application fee:* $30.

Advanced Placement Credit given for nursing courses completed elsewhere dependent upon specific evaluations.

Degree Requirements 30 total credit hours.

DOCTORAL DEGREE PROGRAM

Degree DNP

Available Programs Doctorate; Post-Baccalaureate Doctorate.

Areas of Study Advanced practice nursing, family health.

Program Entrance Requirements Minimum overall college GPA of 3.0, interview, 3 letters of recommendation, MSN or equivalent, statistics course, vita, writing sample. Application deadline: 4/15 (fall). Application fee: $30.

Degree Requirements 70 total credit hours.

CONTINUING EDUCATION PROGRAM

Contact Dr. Lindsay Munden, Assistant Professor, College of Nursing and Health Professions, Valparaiso University, 836 LaPorte Avenue, Valparaiso, IN 46383-6493. *Telephone:* 219-464-5287. *Fax:* 219-464-5425. *E-mail:* lindsay.munden@valpo.edu.

Vincennes University
Department of Nursing
Vincennes, Indiana

Founded in 1801
DEGREE • BSN

BACCALAUREATE PROGRAMS

Degree BSN

Available Programs RN Baccalaureate.

Contact *Telephone:* 812-888-8888.

IOWA

Allen College
Graduate Programs
Waterloo, Iowa

http://www.allencollege.edu/
Founded in 1989
DEGREES • BSN • DNP • MSN
Nursing Program Faculty 54 (31% with doctorates).
Baccalaureate Enrollment 298 **Women** 93% **Men** 7% **Part-time** 34%
Graduate Enrollment 220 **Women** 90% **Men** 10% **Part-time** 80%
Distance Learning Courses Available.
Nursing Student Activities Sigma Theta Tau, Student Nurses' Association, nursing club.
Nursing Student Resources Academic advising; academic or career counseling; campus computer network; career placement assistance; computer lab; computer-assisted instruction; e-mail services; externships; housing assistance; interactive nursing skills videos; Internet; library services; nursing audiovisuals; other; paid internships; placement services for program completers; resume preparation assistance; skills, simulation, or other laboratory; tutoring.
Library Facilities 12,635 volumes in health, 11,735 volumes in nursing; 218 periodical subscriptions health-care related.

BACCALAUREATE PROGRAMS

Degree BSN
Available Programs ADN to Baccalaureate; Accelerated Baccalaureate; Accelerated Baccalaureate for Second Degree; Accelerated RN Baccalaureate; Baccalaureate for Second Degree; Generic Baccalaureate; LPN to Baccalaureate; RN Baccalaureate.
Study Options Full-time and part-time.
Online Degree Options Yes.
Program Entrance Requirements Minimum overall college GPA of 2.7, transcript of college record, CPR certification, health exam, immunizations, 1 letter of recommendation, minimum GPA in nursing prerequisites of 2.9, prerequisite course work. Transfer students are accepted. *Application deadline:* 2/1 (fall), 6/1 (spring), 6/1 (summer). Applications may be processed on a rolling basis for some programs. *Application fee:* $50.
Advanced Placement Credit given for nursing courses completed elsewhere dependent upon specific evaluations.
Expenses (2015–16) *Tuition:* full-time $16,072; part-time $574 per credit hour. *International tuition:* $16,072 full-time. *Room and board:* $7281; room only: $3640 per academic year. *Required fees:* full-time $1301; part-time $77 per credit.
Contact Andrea Schmit, Admissions Counselor, Graduate Programs, Allen College, 1825 Logan Avenue, Waterloo, IA 50703. *Telephone:* 319-226-2014. *Fax:* 319-226-2010.
E-mail: Admissions@AllenCollege.edu.

GRADUATE PROGRAMS

Expenses (2015–16) *Tuition:* full-time $15,560; part-time $778 per credit hour. *International tuition:* $15,560 full-time. *Room and board:* $7281; room only: $3640 per academic year. *Required fees:* full-time $1240; part-time $77 per credit.
Financial Aid Institutionally sponsored loans, scholarships, and traineeships available.
Contact Lisa Fickenscher, Admissions Counselor, Graduate Programs, Allen College, 1825 Logan Avenue, Waterloo, IA 50703. *Telephone:* 319-226-2014. *Fax:* 319-226-2010.
E-mail: Admissions@AllenCollege.edu.

MASTER'S DEGREE PROGRAM
Degree MSN
Available Programs Master's; Master's for Nurses with Non-Nursing Degrees.
Concentrations Available Nursing administration; nursing education. *Nurse practitioner programs in:* adult health, adult-gerontology acute care, community health, family health, psychiatric/mental health.
Study Options Full-time and part-time.
Online Degree Options Yes.
Program Entrance Requirements Clinical experience, computer literacy, minimum overall college GPA of 3.0, transcript of college record, CPR certification, written essay, immunizations, interview, 3 letters of recommendation, nursing research course, professional liability insurance/malpractice insurance, prerequisite course work, resume, statistics course. *Application deadline:* 2/1 (fall), 9/1 (spring). Applications may be processed on a rolling basis for some programs. *Application fee:* $50.
Advanced Placement Credit given for nursing courses completed elsewhere dependent upon specific evaluations.
Degree Requirements 44 total credit hours, thesis or project.

POST-MASTER'S PROGRAM
Areas of Study Nursing administration; nursing education. *Nurse practitioner programs in:* adult health, adult-gerontology acute care, community health, family health, psychiatric/mental health.

DOCTORAL DEGREE PROGRAM
Degree DNP
Available Programs Doctorate.
Online Degree Options Yes (online only).
Program Entrance Requirements Clinical experience, minimum overall college GPA of 3.25, interview by faculty committee, 3 letters of recommendation, MSN or equivalent, statistics course, vita, writing sample. Application deadline: Applications may be processed on a rolling basis for some programs. Application fee: $50.
Degree Requirements 33 total credit hours.

POSTDOCTORAL PROGRAM
Postdoctoral Program Contact Dr. Diane Young, Department Chair, MSN Program, Graduate Programs, Allen College, 1825 Logan Avenue, Waterloo, IA 50703. *Telephone:* 319-226-2047. *Fax:* 319-226-2070. *E-mail:* youngdm@ihs.org.

CONTINUING EDUCATION PROGRAM

Contact Dina Dowden, Continuing Education Coordinator, Graduate Programs, Allen College, 1825 Logan Avenue, Waterloo, IA 50703. *Telephone:* 319-226-2017. *Fax:* 319-226-2051. *E-mail:* Dina.Dowden@AllenCollege.edu.

Briar Cliff University
Department of Nursing
Sioux City, Iowa

http://www.briarcliff.edu/
Founded in 1930
DEGREES • BSN • DNP • MSN
Nursing Program Faculty 9 (33% with doctorates).
Baccalaureate Enrollment 125 **Women** 90% **Men** 10% **Part-time** 25%
Graduate Enrollment 50 **Women** 95% **Men** 5% **Part-time** 75%
Distance Learning Courses Available.
Nursing Student Activities Sigma Theta Tau, Student Nurses' Association, nursing club.
Nursing Student Resources Academic advising; academic or career counseling; assistance for students with disabilities; bookstore; campus computer network; career placement assistance; computer lab; computer-assisted instruction; e-mail services; employment services for current students; externships; interactive nursing skills videos; Internet; learning resource lab; library services; nursing audiovisuals; placement services for program completers; remedial services; resume preparation assistance; skills, simulation, or other laboratory; tutoring.
Library Facilities 7,954 volumes in health, 266 volumes in nursing; 4,102 periodical subscriptions health-care related.

BACCALAUREATE PROGRAMS

Degree BSN
Available Programs ADN to Baccalaureate; Generic Baccalaureate; LPN to Baccalaureate; RN Baccalaureate.
Study Options Full-time and part-time.
Program Entrance Requirements Minimum overall college GPA of 2.75, transcript of college record, CPR certification, written essay, health exam, high school foreign language, high school transcript, immunizations, minimum GPA in nursing prerequisites of 2.75, prerequisite course work. Transfer students are accepted. *Application deadline:* 8/15 (fall), 12/1 (winter), 12/1 (spring), 4/1 (summer). Applications may be processed on a rolling basis for some programs. *Application fee:* $25.
Advanced Placement Credit given for nursing courses completed elsewhere dependent upon specific evaluations.
Contact *Telephone:* 712-279-1662. *Fax:* 712-279-5299.

GRADUATE PROGRAMS

Contact *Telephone:* 712-279-1662. *Fax:* 712-279-5299.

MASTER'S DEGREE PROGRAM

Degree MSN
Available Programs Master's.
Concentrations Available Nursing education.
Study Options Part-time.
Online Degree Options Yes (online only).
Program Entrance Requirements Clinical experience, computer literacy, minimum overall college GPA of 3.0, transcript of college record, CPR certification, written essay, immunizations, 2 letters of recommendation, nursing research course, physical assessment course, resume, statistics course. *Application deadline:* 7/15 (fall). Applications may be processed on a rolling basis for some programs. *Application fee:* $25.
Advanced Placement Credit given for nursing courses completed elsewhere dependent upon specific evaluations.
Degree Requirements 44 total credit hours, thesis or project, comprehensive exam.

DOCTORAL DEGREE PROGRAM

Degree DNP
Available Programs Doctorate.
Areas of Study Advanced practice nursing, family health, gerontology.
Online Degree Options Yes (online only).
Program Entrance Requirements Clinical experience, minimum overall college GPA of 3.00, 2 letters of recommendation, statistics course, vita, writing sample. Application deadline: 7/15 (fall). Application fee: $25.
Degree Requirements 79 total credit hours, oral exam.

CONTINUING EDUCATION PROGRAM

Contact *Telephone:* 712-279-1662. *Fax:* 712-279-5299.

Clarke University
Department of Nursing and Health
Dubuque, Iowa

http://www.clarke.edu/nursing
Founded in 1843
DEGREES • BSN • DNP
Nursing Program Faculty 24 (25% with doctorates).
Baccalaureate Enrollment 177 **Women** 92% **Men** 8% **Part-time** 5%
Graduate Enrollment 65 **Women** 99% **Men** 1% **Part-time** 35%
Nursing Student Activities Sigma Theta Tau, Student Nurses' Association.
Nursing Student Resources Academic advising; academic or career counseling; assistance for students with disabilities; bookstore; campus computer network; career placement assistance; computer lab; computer-assisted instruction; e-mail services; employment services for current students; externships; housing assistance; interactive nursing skills videos; Internet; learning resource lab; library services; nursing audiovisuals; paid internships; placement services for program completers; remedial services; resume preparation assistance; skills, simulation, or other laboratory; tutoring; unpaid internships.
Library Facilities 6,700 volumes in health, 3,100 volumes in nursing; 62 periodical subscriptions health-care related.

BACCALAUREATE PROGRAMS

Degree BSN
Available Programs Generic Baccalaureate; RN Baccalaureate.
Site Options Dubuque, IA.
Study Options Full-time and part-time.
Program Entrance Requirements Minimum overall college GPA of 3.0, transcript of college record, CPR certification, written essay, health exam, health insurance, high school chemistry, high school foreign language, high school math, high school transcript, immunizations, interview, 2 letters of recommendation, minimum high school GPA of 2.0, minimum GPA in nursing prerequisites of 2.0, professional liability insurance/malpractice insurance, prerequisite course work. Transfer students are accepted. *Application deadline:* Applications may be processed on a rolling basis for some programs.
Advanced Placement Credit given for nursing courses completed elsewhere dependent upon specific evaluations.

Expenses (2015–16) *Tuition:* full-time $29,000. *International tuition:* $29,000 full-time. *Room and board:* $9000; room only: $4300 per academic year. *Required fees:* full-time $1340.
Financial Aid 83% of baccalaureate students in nursing programs received some form of financial aid in 2014–15. *Gift aid (need-based):* Federal Pell, FSEOG, state, private, college/university gift aid from institutional funds. *Loans:* Federal Nursing Student Loans, Federal Direct (Subsidized and Unsubsidized Stafford PLUS), Perkins, college/university, private loans. *Work-study:* Federal Work-Study. *Financial aid application deadline (priority):* 4/15.
Contact Emily Kruse, Director of Admissions, Department of Nursing and Health, Clarke University, 1550 Clarke Drive, Dubuque, IA 52001. *Telephone:* 563-588-6436. *Fax:* 563-588-8666.
E-mail: emily.kruse@clarke.edu.

GRADUATE PROGRAMS

Expenses (2015–16) *Tuition:* full-time $20,800; part-time $800 per credit hour. *Required fees:* full-time $2080.
Financial Aid 75% of graduate students in nursing programs received some form of financial aid in 2014–15. Career-related internships or fieldwork available. Aid available to part-time students.
Contact Ms. Kara Schroeder, Academic Program Coordinator, Department of Nursing and Health, Clarke University, 1550 Clarke Drive, Dubuque, IA 52001. *Telephone:* 563-588-6595. *Fax:* 563-588-6789. *E-mail:* kara.schroeder@clarke.edu.

MASTER'S DEGREE PROGRAM

Program Entrance Requirements GRE General Test or MAT. *Application deadline:* Applications may be processed on a rolling basis for some programs.

DOCTORAL DEGREE PROGRAM

Degree DNP
Available Programs Doctorate; Post-Baccalaureate Doctorate.
Areas of Study Family health.
Program Entrance Requirements Clinical experience, minimum overall college GPA of 3.0, interview by faculty committee, interview, letters of recommendation, vita, writing sample. Application deadline: 2/1 (fall). Applications may be processed on a rolling basis for some programs. Application fee: $35.
Degree Requirements 81 total credit hours, written exam.

CONTINUING EDUCATION PROGRAM

Contact Dr. Jan L. Lee, Chairperson of Department of Nursing and Health, Department of Nursing and Health, Clarke University, 1550 Clarke Drive, Dubuque, IA 52001. *Telephone:* 563-588-6339. *Fax:* 563-588-8684. *E-mail:* jan.lee@clarke.edu.

Coe College
Department of Nursing
Cedar Rapids, Iowa

http://www.coe.edu/
Founded in 1851
DEGREE • BSN
Nursing Program Faculty 7 (86% with doctorates).
Baccalaureate Enrollment 50 **Women** 85% **Men** 15%
Nursing Student Activities Student Nurses' Association.
Nursing Student Resources Academic advising; academic or career counseling; assistance for students with disabilities; bookstore; campus computer network; career placement assistance; computer lab; e-mail services; employment services for current students; housing assistance; Internet; learning resource lab; library services; nursing audiovisuals; remedial services; resume preparation assistance; skills, simulation, or other laboratory; tutoring; unpaid internships.
Library Facilities 2,929 volumes in health, 492 volumes in nursing; 34 periodical subscriptions health-care related.

BACCALAUREATE PROGRAMS

Degree BSN
Available Programs Generic Baccalaureate.
Study Options Full-time and part-time.
Program Entrance Requirements Minimum overall college GPA of 2.7, transcript of college record, CPR certification, written essay, health exam, health insurance, high school chemistry, high school transcript, immunizations, minimum high school GPA of 2.0, minimum GPA in

nursing prerequisites of 2.7, prerequisite course work. Transfer students are accepted. *Application deadline:* 12/1 (fall). Applications may be processed on a rolling basis for some programs. *Application fee:* $50.
Advanced Placement Credit given for nursing courses completed elsewhere dependent upon specific evaluations.
Contact *Telephone:* 319-399-8046. *Fax:* 319-399-8816.

Dordt College
Nursing Program
Sioux Center, Iowa

Founded in 1955
DEGREE • BSN
Nursing Program Faculty 3

BACCALAUREATE PROGRAMS

Degree BSN
Available Programs Generic Baccalaureate.
Contact *Telephone:* 712-722-6000.

Grand View University
Division of Nursing
Des Moines, Iowa

http://www.grandview.edu
Founded in 1896
DEGREES • BSN • MS
Nursing Program Faculty 18 (33% with doctorates).
Baccalaureate Enrollment 200 **Women** 90% **Men** 10% **Part-time** 5%
Graduate Enrollment 6 **Women** 83% **Men** 17% **Part-time** 100%
Distance Learning Courses Available.
Nursing Student Activities Sigma Theta Tau, Student Nurses' Association.
Nursing Student Resources Academic advising; academic or career counseling; assistance for students with disabilities; bookstore; campus computer network; career placement assistance; computer lab; computer-assisted instruction; e-mail services; employment services for current students; externships; housing assistance; interactive nursing skills videos; Internet; learning resource lab; library services; nursing audiovisuals; placement services for program completers; remedial services; resume preparation assistance; skills, simulation, or other laboratory; tutoring; unpaid internships.
Library Facilities 5,672 volumes in health, 4,061 volumes in nursing; 370 periodical subscriptions health-care related.

BACCALAUREATE PROGRAMS

Degree BSN
Available Programs Generic Baccalaureate; RN Baccalaureate.
Study Options Full-time and part-time.
Program Entrance Requirements Minimum overall college GPA of 2.75, transcript of college record, CPR certification, health exam, health insurance, high school chemistry, high school transcript, immunizations, 3 letters of recommendation, minimum GPA in nursing prerequisites of 2.75, prerequisite course work. Transfer students are accepted. *Application deadline:* 2/1 (fall), 10/1 (spring). Applications may be processed on a rolling basis for some programs.
Advanced Placement Credit by examination available. Credit given for nursing courses completed elsewhere dependent upon specific evaluations.
Contact *Telephone:* 515-263-2859. *Fax:* 515-263-6077.

GRADUATE PROGRAMS

Contact *Telephone:* 515-263-2859. *Fax:* 515-263-6077.

MASTER'S DEGREE PROGRAM
Degree MS
Available Programs Master's.
Concentrations Available Clinical nurse leader.
Study Options Part-time.
Program Entrance Requirements Clinical experience, computer literacy, minimum overall college GPA of 3.0, transcript of college record, CPR certification, written essay, immunizations, interview, 3 letters of recommendation, nursing research course, physical assessment course,

professional liability insurance/malpractice insurance, prerequisite course work, resume, statistics course. *Application deadline:* 7/1 (fall). Applications may be processed on a rolling basis for some programs.
Degree Requirements 40 total credit hours, thesis or project.

CONTINUING EDUCATION PROGRAM
Contact *Telephone:* 515-263-2869. *Fax:* 515-263-6700.

Iowa Wesleyan College
Division of Nursing
Mount Pleasant, Iowa

http://www.iwc.edu/
Founded in 1842
DEGREE • BSN
Nursing Program Faculty 7 (29% with doctorates).
Baccalaureate Enrollment 80 **Women** 92% **Men** 8% **Part-time** 2%
Distance Learning Courses Available.
Nursing Student Activities Student Nurses' Association.
Nursing Student Resources Academic advising; academic or career counseling; assistance for students with disabilities; bookstore; campus computer network; career placement assistance; computer lab; computer-assisted instruction; e-mail services; employment services for current students; interactive nursing skills videos; Internet; learning resource lab; library services; nursing audiovisuals; remedial services; resume preparation assistance; skills, simulation, or other laboratory; tutoring; unpaid internships.
Library Facilities 500 volumes in health, 300 volumes in nursing; 40 periodical subscriptions health-care related.

BACCALAUREATE PROGRAMS

Degree BSN
Available Programs ADN to Baccalaureate; Baccalaureate for Second Degree; Generic Baccalaureate; LPN to Baccalaureate; LPN to RN Baccalaureate; RN Baccalaureate.
Study Options Full-time and part-time.
Program Entrance Requirements Minimum overall college GPA of 2.25, transcript of college record, CPR certification, health exam, health insurance, high school transcript, immunizations, interview, minimum high school GPA of 2.25, minimum high school rank 50%, minimum GPA in nursing prerequisites of 2.25, professional liability insurance/malpractice insurance, prerequisite course work. Transfer students are accepted. *Application deadline:* 8/1 (fall). Applications may be processed on a rolling basis for some programs.
Contact *Telephone:* 800-582-2383 Ext. 6231. *Fax:* 319-385-6296.

Luther College
Department of Nursing
Decorah, Iowa

http://www.nursing.luther.edu/
Founded in 1861
DEGREE • BA
Nursing Program Faculty 15 (20% with doctorates).
Baccalaureate Enrollment 96 **Women** 96% **Men** 4%
Nursing Student Activities Student Nurses' Association.
Nursing Student Resources Academic advising; academic or career counseling; assistance for students with disabilities; bookstore; campus computer network; career placement assistance; computer lab; computer-assisted instruction; e-mail services; employment services for current students; externships; Internet; learning resource lab; library services; nursing audiovisuals; paid internships; placement services for program completers; remedial services; resume preparation assistance; skills, simulation, or other laboratory; tutoring; unpaid internships.
Library Facilities 4,324 volumes in health, 3,337 volumes in nursing; 35 periodical subscriptions health-care related.

BACCALAUREATE PROGRAMS

Degree BA
Available Programs Generic Baccalaureate.
Site Options Rochester, MN.
Study Options Full-time.

Program Entrance Requirements Minimum overall college GPA of 2.75, health exam, 3 years high school math, 2 years high school science, high school transcript, minimum high school rank 50%, minimum GPA in nursing prerequisites of 2.75, prerequisite course work. Transfer students are accepted. *Application deadline:* Applications may be processed on a rolling basis for some programs.

Advanced Placement Credit given for nursing courses completed elsewhere dependent upon specific evaluations.

Expenses (2015–16) *Tuition:* full-time $38,940. *International tuition:* $38,940 full-time. *Room and board:* $7920; room only: $3570 per academic year. *Required fees:* full-time $250.

Financial Aid 100% of baccalaureate students in nursing programs received some form of financial aid in 2014–15. *Gift aid (need-based):* Federal Pell, FSEOG, state, private, college/university gift aid from institutional funds. *Loans:* Federal Direct (Subsidized and Unsubsidized Stafford PLUS), Perkins, college/university. *Work-study:* Federal Work-Study, part-time campus jobs. *Financial aid application deadline (priority):* 3/1.

Contact Ms. Tracy Elsbernd, Administrative Assistant, Department of Nursing, Luther College, 700 College Drive, Decorah, IA 52101. *Telephone:* 563-387-1057. *Fax:* 563-387-2149. *E-mail:* elsbtr01@luther.edu.

CONTINUING EDUCATION PROGRAM

Contact Ms. Tracy Elsbernd, Administrative Assistant, Department of Nursing, Luther College, 700 College Drive, Decorah, IA 52101. *Telephone:* 563-387-1057. *Fax:* 563-387-2149. *E-mail:* elsbtr01@luther.edu.

See display below and full description on page 500.

Mercy College of Health Sciences
Division of Nursing
Des Moines, Iowa

http://www.mchs.edu/
Founded in 1995
DEGREE • BSN
Nursing Program Faculty 22 (2% with doctorates).

Baccalaureate Enrollment 76 **Women** 98% **Men** 2% **Part-time** 98%
Nursing Student Activities Sigma Theta Tau, Student Nurses' Association.

Nursing Student Resources Academic advising; academic or career counseling; assistance for students with disabilities; campus computer network; career placement assistance; computer lab; computer-assisted instruction; daycare for children of students; e-mail services; employment services for current students; interactive nursing skills videos; Internet; learning resource lab; library services; nursing audiovisuals; placement services for program completers; skills, simulation, or other laboratory.

BACCALAUREATE PROGRAMS

Degree BSN
Available Programs ADN to Baccalaureate.
Study Options Full-time and part-time.
Program Entrance Requirements Minimum overall college GPA of 2.7, transcript of college record, CPR certification, health exam, high school biology, high school chemistry, high school transcript, immunizations, minimum GPA in nursing prerequisites of 2.7, prerequisite course work, RN licensure. Transfer students are accepted. *Application deadline:* Applications may be processed on a rolling basis for some programs. *Application fee:* $25.

Advanced Placement Credit given for nursing courses completed elsewhere dependent upon specific evaluations.

Contact *Telephone:* 515-643-3180. *Fax:* 515-643-6698.

Morningside College
Department of Nursing Education
Sioux City, Iowa

http://www.morningside.edu/academics/undergraduate-programs/nursing/
Founded in 1894
DEGREES • BSN • MSN
Nursing Program Faculty 18 (33% with doctorates).
Baccalaureate Enrollment 90 **Women** 87% **Men** 13%
Graduate Enrollment 41 **Women** 88% **Men** 12% **Part-time** 80%

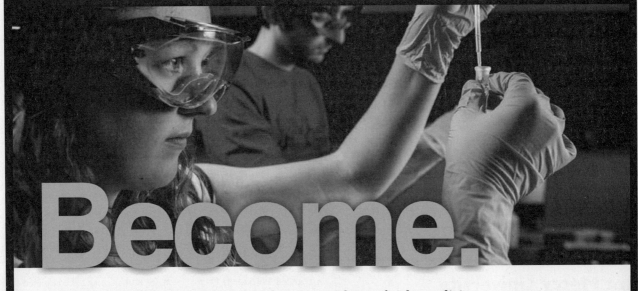

Become.

At Luther College, rigorous academics within a faith tradition of debate and dialogue help students discover their life's meaning—**and what they will become.**

LUTHER COLLEGE

www.luther.edu | admissions@luther.edu | 800-4LUTHER

Distance Learning Courses Available.

Nursing Student Activities Sigma Theta Tau, Student Nurses' Association.

Nursing Student Resources Academic advising; academic or career counseling; assistance for students with disabilities; bookstore; campus computer network; computer-assisted instruction; e-mail services; employment services for current students; externships; housing assistance; interactive nursing skills videos; Internet; learning resource lab; library services; nursing audiovisuals; remedial services; resume preparation assistance; skills, simulation, or other laboratory; tutoring; unpaid internships.

BACCALAUREATE PROGRAMS

Degree BSN

Available Programs Baccalaureate for Second Degree; Generic Baccalaureate; International Nurse to Baccalaureate; LPN to Baccalaureate.

Study Options Full-time and part-time.

Program Entrance Requirements Minimum overall college GPA of 2.75, transcript of college record, CPR certification, immunizations, interview, minimum GPA in nursing prerequisites of 2.0, prerequisite course work. Transfer students are accepted. *Application deadline:* 8/15 (fall).

Advanced Placement Credit given for nursing courses completed elsewhere dependent upon specific evaluations.

Expenses (2015–16) *Tuition:* full-time $26,680. *International tuition:* $26,680 full-time. *Room and board:* $8710; room only: $4600 per academic year. *Required fees:* full-time $670.

Financial Aid *Gift aid (need-based):* Federal Pell, FSEOG, state, college/university gift aid from institutional funds. *Loans:* Federal Direct (Subsidized and Unsubsidized Stafford PLUS), Perkins, college/university, private loans. *Work-study:* Federal Work-Study, part-time campus jobs. *Financial aid application deadline (priority):* 3/1.

Contact Dr. Mary B. Kovarna, Professor and Chair, Department of Nursing Education, Morningside College, Nylen School of Nursing, 1501 Morningside Avenue, Sioux City, IA 51106-1751. *Telephone:* 712-274-5156. *Fax:* 712-274-5559. *E-mail:* kovarna@morningside.edu.

GRADUATE PROGRAMS

Expenses (2015–16) *Tuition:* part-time $275 per credit.

Contact Dr. Jacklyn Barber, EdD, Dean of the Nylen School of Nursing, Department of Nursing Education, Morningside College, Nylen School of Nursing, 1501 Morningside Avenue, Sioux City, IA 51106. *Telephone:* 712-274-5297. *Fax:* 712-274-5559. *E-mail:* barber@morningside.edu.

MASTER'S DEGREE PROGRAM

Degree MSN

Available Programs Master's.

Concentrations Available Clinical nurse leader. *Nurse practitioner programs in:* adult-gerontology acute care, family health.

Study Options Full-time and part-time.

Online Degree Options Yes (online only).

Program Entrance Requirements Minimum overall college GPA of 3.0, transcript of college record, CPR certification, written essay, 3 letters of recommendation, resume. *Application deadline:* Applications may be processed on a rolling basis for some programs. *Application fee:* $25.

Advanced Placement Credit given for nursing courses completed elsewhere dependent upon specific evaluations.

Degree Requirements Thesis or project.

POST-MASTER'S PROGRAM

Areas of Study Clinical nurse leader. *Nurse practitioner programs in:* adult-gerontology acute care, family health.

Mount Mercy University

Department of Nursing
Cedar Rapids, Iowa

http://www.mtmercy.edu/
Founded in 1928

DEGREES • BSN • MSN

Nursing Program Faculty 46 (9% with doctorates).
Baccalaureate Enrollment 355 **Women** 97% **Men** 3% **Part-time** 35%
Graduate Enrollment 55 **Women** 99% **Men** 1% **Part-time** 2%

Distance Learning Courses Available.

Nursing Student Activities Sigma Theta Tau, Student Nurses' Association.

Nursing Student Resources Academic advising; academic or career counseling; assistance for students with disabilities; bookstore; campus computer network; career placement assistance; computer lab; computer-assisted instruction; e-mail services; employment services for current students; externships; housing assistance; interactive nursing skills videos; Internet; learning resource lab; library services; nursing audiovisuals; paid internships; placement services for program completers; remedial services; resume preparation assistance; skills, simulation, or other laboratory; tutoring; unpaid internships.

Library Facilities 5,400 volumes in health, 1,475 volumes in nursing; 130 periodical subscriptions health-care related.

BACCALAUREATE PROGRAMS

Degree BSN

Available Programs ADN to Baccalaureate; Generic Baccalaureate.

Study Options Full-time and part-time.

Online Degree Options Yes.

Program Entrance Requirements Minimum overall college GPA of 2.7, transcript of college record, CPR certification, health exam, health insurance, high school chemistry, 2 years high school math, 2 years high school science, high school transcript, immunizations, minimum high school rank 75%, minimum GPA in nursing prerequisites of 2.7, prerequisite course work. Transfer students are accepted. *Application deadline:* 5/31 (fall), 10/1 (winter), 10/1 (spring), 4/1 (summer).

Advanced Placement Credit by examination available. Credit given for nursing courses completed elsewhere dependent upon specific evaluations.

Expenses (2015–16) *Tuition:* full-time $28,226; part-time $768 per credit hour. *International tuition:* $28,226 full-time. *Room and board:* $2500; room only: $2100 per academic year. *Required fees:* full-time $400.

Financial Aid 96% of baccalaureate students in nursing programs received some form of financial aid in 2014–15.

Contact Dr. Mary P. Tarbox, Professor and Chair, Department of Nursing, Mount Mercy University, 1330 Elmhurst Drive NE, Cedar Rapids, IA 52402. *Telephone:* 800-248-4504 Ext. 6460. *Fax:* 319-368-6479. *E-mail:* mtarbox@mtmercy.edu.

GRADUATE PROGRAMS

Expenses (2015–16) *Tuition:* full-time $13,680; part-time $570 per credit hour. *International tuition:* $13,680 full-time. *Required fees:* full-time $100.

Financial Aid 50% of graduate students in nursing programs received some form of financial aid in 2014–15.

Contact Dr. Mary P. Tarbox, Chair, Department of Nursing, Mount Mercy University, 1330 Elmhurst Drive NE, Cedar Rapids, IA 52402. *Telephone:* 319-368-6471. *Fax:* 319-368-6479. *E-mail:* mtarbox@mtmercy.edu.

MASTER'S DEGREE PROGRAM

Degree MSN

Available Programs Master's.

Concentrations Available Nursing administration; nursing education. *Clinical nurse specialist programs in:* community health, public health.

Study Options Full-time and part-time.

Program Entrance Requirements Clinical experience, minimum overall college GPA of 3.0, transcript of college record, CPR certification, immunizations, 2 letters of recommendation, statistics course. *Application deadline:* Applications may be processed on a rolling basis for some programs.

Advanced Placement Credit given for nursing courses completed elsewhere dependent upon specific evaluations.

Degree Requirements 36 total credit hours, thesis or project.

CONTINUING EDUCATION PROGRAM

Contact Dr. Mary P. Tarbox, EdD, Department Chair, Department of Nursing, Mount Mercy University, 1330 Elmhurst Drive NE, Cedar Rapids, IA 52402. *Telephone:* 319-368-6471. *Fax:* 319-368-6479. *E-mail:* mtarbox@mtmercy.edu.

See display on next page and full description on page 504.

Northwestern College

Nursing Program
Orange City, Iowa

http://www.nwciowa.edu/nursing
Founded in 1882

DEGREE • BSN

Nursing Program Faculty 8 (12% with doctorates).
Baccalaureate Enrollment 58 **Women** 93% **Men** 7% **Part-time** 3%
Nursing Student Activities Nursing Honor Society, Sigma Theta Tau, Student Nurses' Association, nursing club.
Nursing Student Resources Academic advising; assistance for students with disabilities; bookstore; campus computer network; career placement assistance; computer lab; e-mail services; housing assistance; interactive nursing skills videos; Internet; learning resource lab; library services; nursing audiovisuals; placement services for program completers; remedial services; resume preparation assistance; skills, simulation, or other laboratory; tutoring.

BACCALAUREATE PROGRAMS

Degree BSN
Available Programs Generic Baccalaureate.
Study Options Full-time.
Program Entrance Requirements Transcript of college record, CPR certification, written essay, health exam, immunizations, minimum GPA in nursing prerequisites of 2.7, prerequisite course work. Transfer students are accepted. *Application deadline:* 4/10 (spring). *Application fee:* $550.
Advanced Placement Credit given for nursing courses completed elsewhere dependent upon specific evaluations.
Contact *Telephone:* 712-707-7086.

St. Ambrose University

Program in Nursing (BSN)
Davenport, Iowa

http://www.sau.edu/
Founded in 1882

DEGREES • BSN • MSN

Nursing Program Faculty 17 (35% with doctorates).
Baccalaureate Enrollment 266 **Women** 96% **Men** 4% **Part-time** 38%
Graduate Enrollment 14 **Women** 100% **Part-time** 100%
Nursing Student Activities Student Nurses' Association.
Nursing Student Resources Academic advising; academic or career counseling; assistance for students with disabilities; bookstore; campus computer network; career placement assistance; computer lab; e-mail services; employment services for current students; housing assistance; interactive nursing skills videos; Internet; learning resource lab; library services; nursing audiovisuals; resume preparation assistance; skills, simulation, or other laboratory; tutoring; unpaid internships.
Library Facilities 1,793 volumes in health, 674 volumes in nursing; 157 periodical subscriptions health-care related.

BACCALAUREATE PROGRAMS

Degree BSN
Available Programs Generic Baccalaureate; RN Baccalaureate.
Study Options Full-time and part-time.
Program Entrance Requirements Minimum overall college GPA of 3.0, transcript of college record, CPR certification, health exam, health insurance, high school biology, high school chemistry, high school foreign language, 3 years high school math, high school transcript, immunizations, minimum GPA in nursing prerequisites of 3.0, prerequisite course work. Transfer students are accepted. *Application deadline:* 4/1 (fall), 10/25 (winter), 11/30 (spring), 4/15 (summer). Applications may be processed on a rolling basis for some programs. *Application fee:* $25.
Advanced Placement Credit by examination available. Credit given for nursing courses completed elsewhere dependent upon specific evaluations.
Contact *Telephone:* 563-333-6076.

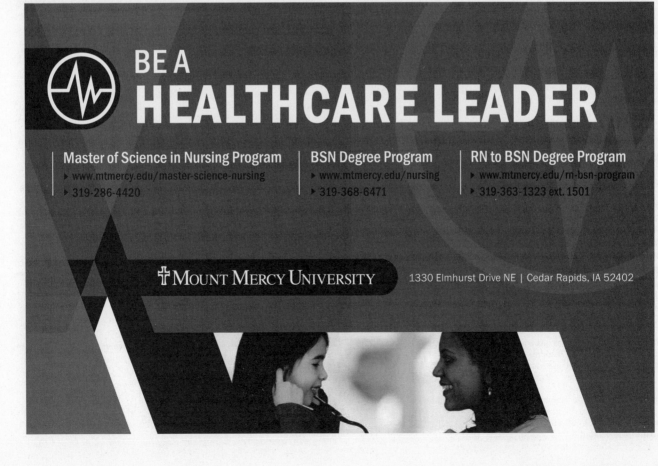

BE A
HEALTHCARE LEADER

Master of Science in Nursing Program
▸ www.mtmercy.edu/master-science-nursing
▸ 319-286-4420

BSN Degree Program
▸ www.mtmercy.edu/nursing
▸ 319-368-6471

RN to BSN Degree Program
▸ www.mtmercy.edu/rn-bsn-program
▸ 319-363-1323 ext. 1501

✝ MOUNT MERCY UNIVERSITY   1330 Elmhurst Drive NE | Cedar Rapids, IA 52402

GRADUATE PROGRAMS

Contact *Telephone:* 563-333-6069. *Fax:* 563-333-6063.

MASTER'S DEGREE PROGRAM
Degree MSN
Available Programs Master's.
Concentrations Available Health-care administration; nursing administration.
Study Options Part-time.
Program Entrance Requirements Clinical experience, minimum overall college GPA of 3.0, transcript of college record, CPR certification, immunizations, 3 letters of recommendation, physical assessment course, resume, statistics course. *Application deadline:* 4/15 (fall). Applications may be processed on a rolling basis for some programs. *Application fee:* $25.
Advanced Placement Credit given for nursing courses completed elsewhere dependent upon specific evaluations.
Degree Requirements 37 total credit hours, thesis or project.

CONTINUING EDUCATION PROGRAM

Contact *Telephone:* 563-333-6076. *Fax:* 563-333-6063.

University of Dubuque
School of Professional Programs
Dubuque, Iowa

http://www.dbq.edu/
Founded in 1852
DEGREE • BSN
Nursing Program Faculty 8 (1% with doctorates).
Baccalaureate Enrollment 58 **Women** 86% **Men** 14%
Nursing Student Activities Student Nurses' Association.
Nursing Student Resources Academic advising; academic or career counseling; assistance for students with disabilities; bookstore; campus computer network; career placement assistance; computer lab; daycare for children of students; e-mail services; employment services for current students; interactive nursing skills videos; Internet; learning resource lab; library services; nursing audiovisuals; resume preparation assistance; skills, simulation, or other laboratory; tutoring; unpaid internships.

BACCALAUREATE PROGRAMS

Degree BSN
Available Programs RN Baccalaureate.
Study Options Full-time.
Program Entrance Requirements Transcript of college record, CPR certification, health exam, health insurance, immunizations, 2 letters of recommendation, minimum GPA in nursing prerequisites of 2.75, professional liability insurance/malpractice insurance, prerequisite course work. Transfer students are accepted.
Contact *Telephone:* 563-589-3000.

The University of Iowa
College of Nursing
Iowa City, Iowa

http://www.nursing.uiowa.edu/
Founded in 1847
DEGREES • BSN • MSN • MSN/MBA • MSN/MPH • PHD
Nursing Program Faculty 67 (63% with doctorates).
Baccalaureate Enrollment 618 **Women** 93% **Men** 7% **Part-time** 25%
Graduate Enrollment 258 **Women** 89% **Men** 11% **Part-time** 50%
Nursing Student Activities Sigma Theta Tau, Student Nurses' Association.
Nursing Student Resources Academic advising; academic or career counseling; assistance for students with disabilities; campus computer network; career placement assistance; computer lab; computer-assisted instruction; e-mail services; employment services for current students; Internet; learning resource lab; nursing audiovisuals; placement services for program completers; resume preparation assistance; skills, simulation, or other laboratory; tutoring.
Library Facilities 273,469 volumes in health; 2,500 periodical subscriptions health-care related.

BACCALAUREATE PROGRAMS

Degree BSN
Available Programs Generic Baccalaureate; RN Baccalaureate.
Study Options Full-time and part-time.
Program Entrance Requirements Minimum overall college GPA of 2.7, transcript of college record, CPR certification, written essay, health exam, health insurance, high school biology, high school chemistry, high school foreign language, 3 years high school math, 3 years high school science, high school transcript, immunizations, minimum GPA in nursing prerequisites of 2.7, professional liability insurance/malpractice insurance, prerequisite course work. Transfer students are accepted.
Advanced Placement Credit given for nursing courses completed elsewhere dependent upon specific evaluations.
Contact *Telephone:* 319-335-7016. *Fax:* 319-384-4423.

GRADUATE PROGRAMS

Contact *Telephone:* 319-335-7021. *Fax:* 319-335-9990.

MASTER'S DEGREE PROGRAM
Degrees MSN; MSN/MBA; MSN/MPH
Available Programs Accelerated RN to Master's; Master's; Master's for Nurses with Non-Nursing Degrees.
Concentrations Available Nurse anesthesia; nursing administration; nursing education; nursing informatics. *Clinical nurse specialist programs in:* adult health, community health, gerontology, occupational health, psychiatric/mental health. *Nurse practitioner programs in:* adult health, family health, gerontology, neonatal health, pediatric, psychiatric/mental health.
Study Options Full-time and part-time.
Program Entrance Requirements Computer literacy, minimum overall college GPA of 3.0, transcript of college record, written essay, immunizations, 3 letters of recommendation, nursing research course, physical assessment course, professional liability insurance/malpractice insurance, prerequisite course work, resume, statistics course.
Advanced Placement Credit given for nursing courses completed elsewhere dependent upon specific evaluations.
Degree Requirements 33 total credit hours, thesis or project.

POST-MASTER'S PROGRAM
Areas of Study Nursing informatics. *Clinical nurse specialist programs in:* adult health, psychiatric/mental health. *Nurse practitioner programs in:* adult health, family health, gerontology, pediatric, psychiatric/mental health.

DOCTORAL DEGREE PROGRAM
Degree PhD
Available Programs Doctorate; Post-Baccalaureate Doctorate.
Areas of Study Aging, family health, gerontology, individualized study, information systems, nursing administration.
Program Entrance Requirements Minimum overall college GPA of 3.0, interview, 3 letters of recommendation, statistics course, vita, GRE General Test.
Degree Requirements 60 total credit hours, dissertation, oral exam, written exam, residency.

POSTDOCTORAL PROGRAM
Areas of Study Family health, nursing informatics, nursing interventions, outcomes.
Postdoctoral Program Contact *Telephone:* 319-335-7021. *Fax:* 319-335-9990.

CONTINUING EDUCATION PROGRAM

Contact *Telephone:* 319-335-7075. *Fax:* 319-335-9990.

Upper Iowa University
RN-BSN Nursing Program
Fayette, Iowa

http://www.uiu.edu/nursing/
Founded in 1857
DEGREE • BSN
Nursing Program Faculty 10

BACCALAUREATE PROGRAMS

Degree BSN

Available Programs RN Baccalaureate.
Site Options Cedar Rapids, IA; West Des Moines, IA.
Program Entrance Requirements Minimum overall college GPA of 2.5, transcript of college record, CPR certification, health exam, high school transcript, RN licensure. Transfer students are accepted.
Contact *Telephone:* 563-425-5357.

William Penn University
Nursing Division
Oskaloosa, Iowa

http://www.wmpenn.edu
Founded in 1873
DEGREE • BSN
Nursing Program Faculty 4 (1% with doctorates).
Baccalaureate Enrollment 39 **Women** 96% **Men** 4% **Part-time** 50%
Nursing Student Activities Nursing Honor Society.
Nursing Student Resources Academic advising; academic or career counseling; assistance for students with disabilities; bookstore; computer lab; computer-assisted instruction; e-mail services; employment services for current students; externships; housing assistance; interactive nursing skills videos; Internet; library services; nursing audiovisuals; remedial services; resume preparation assistance; skills, simulation, or other laboratory; tutoring; unpaid internships.
Library Facilities 884 volumes in health, 82 volumes in nursing; 6 periodical subscriptions health-care related.

BACCALAUREATE PROGRAMS
Degree BSN
Available Programs ADN to Baccalaureate.
Site Options Ottumwa, IA; Clive, IA; Creston, IA.
Study Options Full-time and part-time.
Program Entrance Requirements Transcript of college record, CPR certification, health exam, health insurance, immunizations, minimum high school GPA of 2.5, professional liability insurance/malpractice insurance, RN licensure. Transfer students are accepted. *Application deadline:* 8/25 (fall), 1/12 (spring). Applications may be processed on a rolling basis for some programs.
Advanced Placement Credit given for nursing courses completed elsewhere dependent upon specific evaluations.
Expenses (2015–16) *Tuition:* part-time $450 per credit hour. *Room and board:* $3800; room only: $2050 per academic year.
Contact Dr. Brenda Lee Krogh Duree, Nursing Director, Nursing Division, William Penn University, 201 Trueblood Avenue, Oskaloosa, IA 52577. *Telephone:* 641-673-1064. *Fax:* 641-673-2139. *E-mail:* kroghdureeb@wmpenn.edu.

KANSAS

Baker University
School of Nursing
Topeka, Kansas

http://www.bakeru.edu/
Founded in 1858
DEGREES • BSN • MSN
Nursing Program Faculty 19 (39% with doctorates).
Baccalaureate Enrollment 168 **Women** 91% **Men** 9% **Part-time** 5%
Graduate Enrollment 12
Nursing Student Activities Sigma Theta Tau, Student Nurses' Association.
Nursing Student Resources Academic advising; academic or career counseling; assistance for students with disabilities; bookstore; campus computer network; computer lab; computer-assisted instruction; e-mail services; Internet; learning resource lab; library services; nursing audiovisuals; resume preparation assistance; skills, simulation, or other laboratory; tutoring.
Library Facilities 5,000 volumes in health, 2,716 volumes in nursing; 414 periodical subscriptions health-care related.

BACCALAUREATE PROGRAMS
Degree BSN
Available Programs Generic Baccalaureate; LPN to Baccalaureate.
Site Options Topeka, KS.
Study Options Full-time and part-time.
Program Entrance Requirements Transcript of college record, CPR certification, written essay, health exam, health insurance, high school transcript, immunizations, interview, 2 letters of recommendation, minimum GPA in nursing prerequisites of 2.7, professional liability insurance/malpractice insurance, prerequisite course work. Transfer students are accepted. *Application deadline:* 12/15 (fall), 7/31 (spring).
Advanced Placement Credit given for nursing courses completed elsewhere dependent upon specific evaluations.
Expenses (2015–16) *Tuition:* full-time $17,800; part-time $590 per credit hour. *International tuition:* $17,800 full-time. *Required fees:* full-time $950; part-time $650 per term.
Financial Aid 80% of baccalaureate students in nursing programs received some form of financial aid in 2014–15.
Contact Ms. Cara Bonfiglio, Student Affairs Specialist, School of Nursing, Baker University, 1500 SW 10th Street, Topeka, KS 66604-1353. *Telephone:* 785-354-5850. *Fax:* 785-354-5832. *E-mail:* cbonfig@stormontvail.org.

GRADUATE PROGRAMS
Expenses (2015–16) *Tuition:* full-time $4800; part-time $400 per credit hour. *International tuition:* $4800 full-time. *Required fees:* full-time $300; part-time $30 per credit.
Contact Dr. Carol Moore, Associate Dean Graduate Programs, School of Nursing, Baker University, 1500 SW 10th Street, Topeka, KS 66604. *Telephone:* 785-354-5837. *E-mail:* carmoore@stormontvail.org.

MASTER'S DEGREE PROGRAM
Degree MSN
Available Programs Master's.
Concentrations Available Health-care administration; nursing education.
Study Options Full-time and part-time.
Online Degree Options Yes (online only).
Program Entrance Requirements Clinical experience, computer literacy, minimum overall college GPA of 3.0, transcript of college record, CPR certification, written essay, immunizations, nursing research course, physical assessment course, statistics course. *Application deadline:* 7/15 (fall), 12/1 (spring), 5/15 (summer). Applications may be processed on a rolling basis for some programs.
Advanced Placement Credit given for nursing courses completed elsewhere dependent upon specific evaluations.
Degree Requirements 37 total credit hours, thesis or project.

Benedictine College
Department of Nursing
Atchison, Kansas

http://www.benedictine.edu/
Founded in 1859
DEGREE • BSN
Nursing Program Faculty 8 (25% with doctorates).
Baccalaureate Enrollment 50 **Women** 100%
Nursing Student Activities Student Nurses' Association.
Nursing Student Resources Academic advising; academic or career counseling; bookstore; campus computer network; career placement assistance; computer lab; e-mail services; employment services for current students; Internet; learning resource lab; library services; nursing audiovisuals; resume preparation assistance; skills, simulation, or other laboratory; tutoring.

BACCALAUREATE PROGRAMS
Degree BSN
Available Programs Generic Baccalaureate.
Study Options Full-time.
Program Entrance Requirements Minimum overall college GPA of 2.75, transcript of college record, CPR certification, written essay, health exam, health insurance, immunizations, 2 letters of recommendation, minimum GPA in nursing prerequisites of 2.75, prerequisite course work. Transfer students are accepted. *Application deadline:* 1/15 (fall). *Application fee:* $40.

Advanced Placement Credit given for nursing courses completed elsewhere dependent upon specific evaluations.
Expenses (2015–16) *Tuition:* full-time $29,950. *Room and board:* $9165 per academic year. *Required fees:* full-time $500.
Financial Aid 100% of baccalaureate students in nursing programs received some form of financial aid in 2014–15.
Contact Lynne Connelly, Director of Nursing, Department of Nursing, Benedictine College, 1020 North 2nd Street, Atchison, KS 66002. *Telephone:* 913-360-7560. *Fax:* 913-360-7645. *E-mail:* lconnelly@benedictine.edu.

Bethel College
Department of Nursing
North Newton, Kansas

http://www.bethelks.edu/
Founded in 1887

DEGREE • BSN
Nursing Program Faculty 8
Baccalaureate Enrollment 42 **Women** 75% **Men** 25% **Part-time** 1%
Distance Learning Courses Available.
Nursing Student Activities Nursing Honor Society, Sigma Theta Tau, Student Nurses' Association.
Nursing Student Resources Academic advising; academic or career counseling; assistance for students with disabilities; bookstore; campus computer network; computer lab; e-mail services; employment services for current students; housing assistance; Internet; learning resource lab; library services; nursing audiovisuals; resume preparation assistance; skills, simulation, or other laboratory; tutoring.
Library Facilities 5,690 volumes in health, 3,150 volumes in nursing; 445 periodical subscriptions health-care related.

BACCALAUREATE PROGRAMS

Degree BSN
Available Programs Generic Baccalaureate; LPN to Baccalaureate; RN Baccalaureate.
Study Options Full-time and part-time.
Online Degree Options Yes.
Program Entrance Requirements Minimum overall college GPA of 3.0, transcript of college record, CPR certification, written essay, health exam, health insurance, high school transcript, immunizations, interview, 2 letters of recommendation, minimum high school GPA of 2.75, minimum GPA in nursing prerequisites of 2.0, prerequisite course work. Transfer students are accepted. *Application deadline:* 2/1 (fall).
Advanced Placement Credit given for nursing courses completed elsewhere dependent upon specific evaluations.
Contact *Telephone:* 316-283-5295 Ext. 377. *Fax:* 316-284-5286.

Emporia State University
Newman Division of Nursing
Emporia, Kansas

http://www.emporia.edu/nursing
Founded in 1863

DEGREE • BSN
Nursing Program Faculty 12 (25% with doctorates).
Baccalaureate Enrollment 126 **Women** 94% **Men** 6%
Nursing Student Activities Sigma Theta Tau, Student Nurses' Association.
Nursing Student Resources Academic advising; academic or career counseling; assistance for students with disabilities; bookstore; campus computer network; career placement assistance; computer lab; computer-assisted instruction; daycare for children of students; e-mail services; employment services for current students; housing assistance; interactive nursing skills videos; Internet; learning resource lab; library services; nursing audiovisuals; placement services for program completers; remedial services; resume preparation assistance; skills, simulation, or other laboratory; tutoring.
Library Facilities 53,197 volumes in health, 2,200 volumes in nursing; 186 periodical subscriptions health-care related.

BACCALAUREATE PROGRAMS

Degree BSN

Available Programs ADN to Baccalaureate; Generic Baccalaureate; LPN to Baccalaureate; RN Baccalaureate.
Study Options Full-time.
Program Entrance Requirements Transcript of college record, written essay, minimum GPA in nursing prerequisites of 2.5, prerequisite course work. Transfer students are accepted. *Application deadline:* 5/1 (fall). *Application fee:* $25.
Advanced Placement Credit given for nursing courses completed elsewhere dependent upon specific evaluations.
Financial Aid 90% of baccalaureate students in nursing programs received some form of financial aid in 2013–14. *Gift aid (need-based):* Federal Pell, FSEOG, state, private, college/university gift aid from institutional funds, Jones Foundation Grants. *Loans:* Federal Direct (Subsidized and Unsubsidized Stafford PLUS), Perkins, alternative loans, Alaska Loans. *Work-study:* Federal Work-Study, part-time campus jobs. *Financial aid application deadline (priority):* 3/15.
Contact Linda Adams Welding, Chair/Nursing Director, Newman Division of Nursing, Emporia State University, 1127 Chestnut Street, Emporia, KS 66801. *Telephone:* 620-343-6800. *Fax:* 620-341-7871. *E-mail:* ladamswe@emporia.edu.

Fort Hays State University
Department of Nursing
Hays, Kansas

http://www.fhsu.edu/nursing/
Founded in 1902

DEGREES • BSN • MSN
Nursing Program Faculty 26 (23% with doctorates).
Baccalaureate Enrollment 241 **Women** 90% **Men** 10% **Part-time** 2%
Graduate Enrollment 118 **Women** 88% **Men** 12% **Part-time** 12%
Distance Learning Courses Available.
Nursing Student Activities Sigma Theta Tau, Student Nurses' Association, nursing club.
Nursing Student Resources Academic advising; academic or career counseling; assistance for students with disabilities; bookstore; campus computer network; career placement assistance; computer lab; computer-assisted instruction; daycare for children of students; e-mail services; employment services for current students; housing assistance; interactive nursing skills videos; Internet; learning resource lab; library services; nursing audiovisuals; paid internships; placement services for program completers; remedial services; resume preparation assistance; skills, simulation, or other laboratory; tutoring.
Library Facilities 2,234 volumes in health, 454 volumes in nursing; 193 periodical subscriptions health-care related.

BACCALAUREATE PROGRAMS

Degree BSN
Available Programs Generic Baccalaureate; RN Baccalaureate.
Study Options Full-time and part-time.
Online Degree Options Yes.
Program Entrance Requirements Minimum overall college GPA of 2.75, transcript of college record, CPR certification, written essay, health exam, health insurance, high school transcript, immunizations, interview, 2 letters of recommendation, minimum GPA in nursing prerequisites of 2.75, professional liability insurance/malpractice insurance, prerequisite course work, RN licensure. Transfer students are accepted. *Application deadline:* 3/1 (fall), 10/1 (spring). Applications may be processed on a rolling basis for some programs. *Application fee:* $30.
Advanced Placement Credit by examination available. Credit given for nursing courses completed elsewhere dependent upon specific evaluations.
Expenses (2015–16) *Tuition, area resident:* full-time $4654; part-time $155 per credit hour. *Tuition, state resident:* full-time $6441; part-time $214 per credit hour. *Tuition, nonresident:* full-time $13,657; part-time $455 per credit hour. *Room and board:* $7477; room only: $3652 per academic year. *Required fees:* full-time $1080; part-time $36 per credit.
Financial Aid 80% of baccalaureate students in nursing programs received some form of financial aid in 2014–15. *Gift aid (need-based):* Federal Pell, FSEOG, state, private, college/university gift aid from institutional funds. *Loans:* Federal Direct (Subsidized and Unsubsidized Stafford PLUS), college/university. *Work-study:* Federal Work-Study, part-time campus jobs. *Financial aid application deadline (priority):* 3/1.
Contact Mrs. Carolyn Insley, Coordinator of BSN Program, Department of Nursing, Fort Hays State University, 600 Park Street, Stroup Hall,

Room 147, Hays, KS 67601-4099. *Telephone:* 785-628-4514. *Fax:* 785-628-4080. *E-mail:* cinsley@fhsu.edu.

GRADUATE PROGRAMS

Expenses (2015–16) *Tuition, area resident:* full-time $1927; part-time $214 per credit hour. *Tuition, state resident:* full-time $2728; part-time $303 per credit hour. *Tuition, nonresident:* full-time $4888; part-time $543 per credit hour. *International tuition:* $20,061 full-time. *Room and board:* $7477; room only: $3652 per academic year. *Required fees:* full-time $1080; part-time $36 per credit.

Financial Aid 80% of graduate students in nursing programs received some form of financial aid in 2014–15. 1 teaching assistantship (averaging $5,000 per year) was awarded; research assistantships.

Contact Mrs. Christine L. Hober, Associate Professor, Department of Nursing, Fort Hays State University, 600 Park Street, Stroup Hall, Room 127, Hays, KS 67601-4099. *Telephone:* 785-628-4511. *Fax:* 785-628-4080. *E-mail:* chober@fhsu.edu.

MASTER'S DEGREE PROGRAM

Degree MSN

Available Programs Master's.

Concentrations Available Nursing administration; nursing education. *Nurse practitioner programs in:* family health.

Study Options Full-time and part-time.

Program Entrance Requirements Clinical experience, computer literacy, minimum overall college GPA of 3.0, transcript of college record, CPR certification, written essay, immunizations, 2 letters of recommendation, physical assessment course, professional liability insurance/malpractice insurance, prerequisite course work, statistics course, GRE General Test or MAT. *Application deadline:* 7/1 (fall), 10/1 (spring), 3/1 (summer). *Application fee:* $40.

Advanced Placement Credit given for nursing courses completed elsewhere dependent upon specific evaluations.

Degree Requirements 36 total credit hours, thesis or project, comprehensive exam.

POST-MASTER'S PROGRAM

Areas of Study Nursing administration; nursing education.

Kansas Wesleyan University
Department of Nursing Education
Salina, Kansas

http://www.kwu.edu/academics/academic-departments/nursing
Founded in 1886

DEGREE • BSN

Nursing Program Faculty 8 (13% with doctorates).

Baccalaureate Enrollment 68 **Women** 91% **Men** 9% **Part-time** 2%

Nursing Student Activities Nursing club.

Nursing Student Resources Academic advising; academic or career counseling; assistance for students with disabilities; bookstore; campus computer network; career placement assistance; computer lab; computer-assisted instruction; e-mail services; employment services for current students; housing assistance; Internet; learning resource lab; library services; nursing audiovisuals; resume preparation assistance; skills, simulation, or other laboratory; tutoring.

Library Facilities 15,921 volumes in health, 8,700 volumes in nursing; 1,123 periodical subscriptions health-care related.

BACCALAUREATE PROGRAMS

Degree BSN

Available Programs ADN to Baccalaureate; Generic Baccalaureate; RN Baccalaureate.

Study Options Full-time and part-time.

Program Entrance Requirements Minimum overall college GPA of 2.6, transcript of college record, health exam, high school transcript, immunizations, minimum GPA in nursing prerequisites of 2.6, prerequisite course work. Transfer students are accepted. *Application deadline:* Applications may be processed on a rolling basis for some programs.

Advanced Placement Credit by examination available. Credit given for nursing courses completed elsewhere dependent upon specific evaluations.

Contact *Telephone:* 785-827-5541 Ext. 2311. *Fax:* 785-827-0927.

MidAmerica Nazarene University
Division of Nursing
Olathe, Kansas

http://www.mnu.edu/
Founded in 1966

DEGREES • BSN • MSN

Nursing Program Faculty 18 (39% with doctorates).

Baccalaureate Enrollment 366 **Women** 87% **Men** 13% **Part-time** 36%

Graduate Enrollment 103 **Women** 94% **Men** 6% **Part-time** 85%

Distance Learning Courses Available.

Nursing Student Activities Nursing Honor Society, Student Nurses' Association, nursing club.

Nursing Student Resources Academic advising; assistance for students with disabilities; bookstore; campus computer network; computer lab; e-mail services; interactive nursing skills videos; Internet; learning resource lab; library services; nursing audiovisuals; resume preparation assistance; skills, simulation, or other laboratory; tutoring; unpaid internships.

Library Facilities 1,903 volumes in health, 547 volumes in nursing; 115 periodical subscriptions health-care related.

BACCALAUREATE PROGRAMS

Degree BSN

Available Programs Accelerated Baccalaureate; Accelerated RN Baccalaureate; RN Baccalaureate.

Site Options Liberty, MO; North Kansas City, MO.

Study Options Full-time.

Online Degree Options Yes.

Program Entrance Requirements Minimum overall college GPA of 2.6, transcript of college record, CPR certification, health insurance, high school transcript, immunizations, 2 letters of recommendation, minimum GPA in nursing prerequisites of 3.6, prerequisite course work. Transfer students are accepted. *Application deadline:* 10/1 (fall), 2/1 (spring).

Advanced Placement Credit by examination available. Credit given for nursing courses completed elsewhere dependent upon specific evaluations.

Expenses (2014–15) *Tuition:* full-time $24,270; part-time $800 per credit hour. *Room and board:* $2965 per academic year.

Financial Aid 80% of baccalaureate students in nursing programs received some form of financial aid in 2013–14.

Contact Dr. Susan G. Larson, Dean, School of Nursing and Health Science, Division of Nursing, MidAmerica Nazarene University, 2030 East College Way, Olathe, KS 66062-1899. *Telephone:* 913-971-3698. *Fax:* 913-971-3408. *E-mail:* slarson@mnu.edu.

GRADUATE PROGRAMS

Expenses (2014–15) *Tuition:* part-time $445 per credit hour.

Financial Aid 50% of graduate students in nursing programs received some form of financial aid in 2013–14.

Contact Dr. Karen D. Wiegman, Associate Dean, Graduate Studies in Nursing, Division of Nursing, MidAmerica Nazarene University, 2030 East College Way, Olathe, KS 66062-1899. *Telephone:* 913-971-3081. *E-mail:* kdwiegman@mnu.edu.

MASTER'S DEGREE PROGRAM

Degree MSN

Available Programs Master's; RN to Master's.

Concentrations Available Health-care administration; nursing education.

Site Options Liberty, MO; North Kansas City, MO.

Study Options Full-time and part-time.

Online Degree Options Yes.

Program Entrance Requirements Minimum overall college GPA of 3.0, transcript of college record, prerequisite course work, statistics course. *Application deadline:* Applications may be processed on a rolling basis for some programs.

Advanced Placement Credit by examination available. Credit given for nursing courses completed elsewhere dependent upon specific evaluations.

Degree Requirements 39 total credit hours, thesis or project.

Newman University
Division of Nursing
Wichita, Kansas

http://www.newmanu.edu/
Founded in 1933

DEGREES • BSN • MS

Nursing Program Faculty 15 (7% with doctorates).
Baccalaureate Enrollment 100 **Women** 89% **Men** 11%
Graduate Enrollment 47 **Women** 49% **Men** 51%
Distance Learning Courses Available.
Nursing Student Activities Sigma Theta Tau, nursing club.
Nursing Student Resources Academic advising; academic or career counseling; assistance for students with disabilities; bookstore; campus computer network; computer lab; computer-assisted instruction; e-mail services; Internet; learning resource lab; library services; nursing audiovisuals; remedial services; resume preparation assistance; skills, simulation, or other laboratory; tutoring.
Library Facilities 1,528 volumes in health, 938 volumes in nursing; 144 periodical subscriptions health-care related.

BACCALAUREATE PROGRAMS

Degree BSN

Available Programs Generic Baccalaureate; LPN to Baccalaureate; RN Baccalaureate.
Study Options Full-time and part-time.
Online Degree Options Yes.
Program Entrance Requirements Minimum overall college GPA of 2.85, transcript of college record, CPR certification, written essay, health exam, health insurance, immunizations, interview, 2 letters of recommendation, minimum GPA in nursing prerequisites of 2.85, professional liability insurance/malpractice insurance, prerequisite course work. Transfer students are accepted. *Application deadline:* Applications may be processed on a rolling basis for some programs.
Advanced Placement Credit given for nursing courses completed elsewhere dependent upon specific evaluations.
Expenses (2015–16) *Tuition:* full-time $24,920; part-time $831 per credit hour. *International tuition:* $24,920 full-time. *Room and board:* $3670; room only: $1875 per academic year. *Required fees:* full-time $1265; part-time $17 per credit; part-time $378 per term.
Financial Aid 99% of baccalaureate students in nursing programs received some form of financial aid in 2014–15.
Contact Prof. Teresa S. Vetter, RN, Director of Nursing, Division of Nursing, Newman University, 3100 McCormick Avenue, Wichita, KS 67213-2097. *Telephone:* 316-942-4291 Ext. 2134. *Fax:* 316-942-4483. *E-mail:* vettert@newmanu.edu.

GRADUATE PROGRAMS

Expenses (2015–16) *Tuition:* full-time $27,480; part-time $916 per credit hour. *International tuition:* $27,480 full-time. *Room and board:* $4360; room only: $2565 per academic year. *Required fees:* full-time $1930; part-time $17 per credit; part-time $710 per term.
Financial Aid 98% of graduate students in nursing programs received some form of financial aid in 2014–15. *Application deadline:* 8/15.
Contact Ms. Sharon Niemann, Director, Master of Science in Nurse Anesthesia Program, Division of Nursing, Newman University, 3100 McCormick Avenue, Wichita, KS 67213-2097. *Telephone:* 316-942-4291 Ext. 2272. *Fax:* 316-942-4483. *E-mail:* niemanns@newmanu.edu.

MASTER'S DEGREE PROGRAM

Degree MS

Available Programs Master's.
Concentrations Available Nurse anesthesia.
Study Options Full-time.
Program Entrance Requirements Clinical experience, minimum overall college GPA of 3.45, transcript of college record, CPR certification, interview, 3 letters of recommendation, nursing research course, resume, statistics course, MAT. *Application deadline:* 8/1 (fall). *Application fee:* $25.
Degree Requirements 60 total credit hours, thesis or project.

Ottawa University–Kansas City
Nursing Program
Overland Park, Kansas

http://www.ottawa.edu/home
DEGREE • BSN

BACCALAUREATE PROGRAMS

Degree BSN

Available Programs RN Baccalaureate.
Program Entrance Requirements *Application deadline:* Applications may be processed on a rolling basis for some programs.
Contact Kathy Kump, Director, Nursing Program, Ottawa University–Kansas City, 4370 West 109th Street, Suite 200, Overland Park, KS 66211. *Telephone:* 913-266-8607. *E-mail:* kathy.kump@ottawa.edu.

Pittsburg State University
Department of Nursing
Pittsburg, Kansas

http://www.pittstate.edu/nurs
Founded in 1903

DEGREES • BSN • DNP • MSN

Nursing Program Faculty 18 (44% with doctorates).
Baccalaureate Enrollment 202 **Women** 90% **Men** 10%
Graduate Enrollment 34 **Women** 85% **Men** 15%
Distance Learning Courses Available.
Nursing Student Activities Nursing Honor Society, Sigma Theta Tau, Student Nurses' Association, nursing club.
Nursing Student Resources Academic advising; academic or career counseling; assistance for students with disabilities; bookstore; campus computer network; career placement assistance; computer lab; computer-assisted instruction; daycare for children of students; e-mail services; employment services for current students; externships; housing assistance; interactive nursing skills videos; Internet; learning resource lab; library services; nursing audiovisuals; placement services for program completers; remedial services; resume preparation assistance; skills, simulation, or other laboratory; tutoring; unpaid internships.
Library Facilities 45,044 volumes in nursing.

BACCALAUREATE PROGRAMS

Degree BSN

Available Programs Generic Baccalaureate; RN Baccalaureate.
Study Options Full-time.
Online Degree Options Yes.
Program Entrance Requirements Minimum overall college GPA of 2.5, transcript of college record, CPR certification, immunizations, 3 letters of recommendation, minimum GPA in nursing prerequisites of 2.5, professional liability insurance/malpractice insurance, prerequisite course work. Transfer students are accepted. *Application deadline:* 12/15 (fall). *Application fee:* $30.
Advanced Placement Credit by examination available. Credit given for nursing courses completed elsewhere dependent upon specific evaluations.
Expenses (2015–16) *Tuition, state resident:* full-time $3254; part-time $230 per credit hour. *Tuition, nonresident:* full-time $8489; part-time $578 per credit hour. *International tuition:* $16,978 full-time. *Room and board:* $6734 per academic year.
Financial Aid 95% of baccalaureate students in nursing programs received some form of financial aid in 2014–15. *Gift aid (need-based):* Federal Pell, FSEOG, state, private, college/university gift aid from institutional funds. *Loans:* Federal Nursing Student Loans, Federal Direct (Subsidized and Unsubsidized Stafford PLUS), Perkins, college/university. *Work-study:* Federal Work-Study, part-time campus jobs. *Financial aid application deadline (priority):* 3/1.
Contact Dr. Barbara Ruth McClaskey, Coordinator of Bachelor of Science in Nursing Program, Department of Nursing, Pittsburg State University, 1701 South Broadway, Pittsburg, KS 66762. *Telephone:* 620-235-4437. *Fax:* 620-235-4449. *E-mail:* bmcclaskey@pittstate.edu.

GRADUATE PROGRAMS

Expenses (2015–16) *Tuition, state resident:* full-time $3644; part-time $305 per credit hour. *Tuition, nonresident:* full-time $8524; part-time

$711 per credit hour. *International tuition:* $17,048 full-time. *Required fees:* full-time $425.

Financial Aid 90% of graduate students in nursing programs received some form of financial aid in 2014–15.

Contact Dr. Mary Carol Pomatto, Master of Science Coordinator, Department of Nursing, Pittsburg State University, 1701 South Broadway, Pittsburg, KS 66762. *Telephone:* 620-235-4431. *Fax:* 620-235-4449. *E-mail:* mpomatto@pittstate.edu.

MASTER'S DEGREE PROGRAM
Degree MSN

Available Programs Master's.

Concentrations Available Nursing administration; nursing education. *Nurse practitioner programs in:* family health.

Study Options Full-time and part-time.

Program Entrance Requirements Clinical experience, computer literacy, minimum overall college GPA of 3.0, transcript of college record, CPR certification, written essay, immunizations, 3 letters of recommendation, nursing research course, physical assessment course, professional liability insurance/malpractice insurance, prerequisite course work, resume, statistics course, GRE General Test. *Application deadline:* 3/15 (fall). *Application fee:* $55.

Advanced Placement Credit given for nursing courses completed elsewhere dependent upon specific evaluations.

Degree Requirements 47 total credit hours, thesis or project, comprehensive exam.

DOCTORAL DEGREE PROGRAM
Degree DNP

Available Programs Doctorate.

Areas of Study Family health, nursing education.

Program Entrance Requirements Clinical experience, minimum overall college GPA of 3.5, interview, 3 letters of recommendation, MSN or equivalent, statistics course, vita, writing sample. Application deadline: 11/9 (fall), 3/15 (spring). Application fee: $55.

Degree Requirements 32 total credit hours, written exam, residency.

CONTINUING EDUCATION PROGRAM

Contact Dr. Kristi L. Frisbee, Coordinator of Continuing Nursing Education, Department of Nursing, Pittsburg State University, 1701 South Broadway, McPherson Hall, Room 121, Pittsburg, KS 66762. *Telephone:* 620-235-4434. *Fax:* 620-235-4449. *E-mail:* kfrisbee@pittstate.edu.

Tabor College
Department of Nursing
Hillsboro, Kansas

http://www.tabor.edu/
Founded in 1908
DEGREES • BSN • MSN
Nursing Program Faculty 12 (25% with doctorates).
Baccalaureate Enrollment 100 **Women** 90% **Men** 10% **Part-time** 100%
Graduate Enrollment 14
Distance Learning Courses Available.
Nursing Student Activities Sigma Theta Tau.
Nursing Student Resources Academic advising; academic or career counseling; bookstore; campus computer network; computer lab; e-mail services; Internet; learning resource lab; library services; nursing audiovisuals; remedial services; resume preparation assistance; skills, simulation, or other laboratory; tutoring.
Library Facilities 240 volumes in health, 140 volumes in nursing; 600 periodical subscriptions health-care related.

BACCALAUREATE PROGRAMS

Degree BSN
Available Programs ADN to Baccalaureate; Accelerated RN Baccalaureate.
Site Options Wichita, KS; Colby, KS; Larned, KS.
Study Options Full-time and part-time.
Online Degree Options Yes (online only).
Program Entrance Requirements Minimum overall college GPA of 2.0, transcript of college record, CPR certification, immunizations, professional liability insurance/malpractice insurance, RN licensure.

Transfer students are accepted. *Application deadline:* Applications may be processed on a rolling basis for some programs.
Advanced Placement Credit by examination available. Credit given for nursing courses completed elsewhere dependent upon specific evaluations.
Financial Aid 75% of baccalaureate students in nursing programs received some form of financial aid in 2014–15.
Contact Aubrey Smith, Education Consultant, Department of Nursing, Tabor College, 7348 West 21st Street, Suite 117, Wichita, KS 67205. *Telephone:* 316-729-6333. *Fax:* 316-773-5436.
E-mail: aubreys@tabor.edu.

GRADUATE PROGRAMS

Contact Aubrey Smith, Education Consultant, Department of Nursing, Tabor College, 7348 W 21st Street, Suite 117, Wichita, KS 67205. *Telephone:* 316-729-6333. *E-mail:* aubreys@tabor.edu.

MASTER'S DEGREE PROGRAM
Degree MSN
Available Programs Master's.
Concentrations Available Health-care administration; nursing education; nursing informatics.
Study Options Full-time and part-time.
Online Degree Options Yes (online only).
Program Entrance Requirements Minimum overall college GPA of 3.0, transcript of college record, CPR certification, written essay, immunizations, letters of recommendation, professional liability insurance/malpractice insurance, statistics course. *Application deadline:* Applications may be processed on a rolling basis for some programs.
Advanced Placement Credit given for nursing courses completed elsewhere dependent upon specific evaluations.
Degree Requirements 36 total credit hours, thesis or project.

The University of Kansas
School of Nursing
Kansas City, Kansas

http://www.nursing.kumc.edu
Founded in 1866
DEGREES • BSN • MS • MS/MHSA • MS/MPH • PHD
Nursing Program Faculty 74 (58% with doctorates).
Baccalaureate Enrollment 260 **Women** 88% **Men** 12% **Part-time** 10%
Graduate Enrollment 411 **Women** 93% **Men** 7% **Part-time** 93%
Distance Learning Courses Available.
Nursing Student Activities Nursing Honor Society, Sigma Theta Tau, Student Nurses' Association, nursing club.
Nursing Student Resources Academic advising; academic or career counseling; assistance for students with disabilities; bookstore; campus computer network; computer lab; computer-assisted instruction; e-mail services; employment services for current students; interactive nursing skills videos; Internet; learning resource lab; library services; nursing audiovisuals; remedial services; resume preparation assistance; skills, simulation, or other laboratory.
Library Facilities 180,000 volumes in health, 5,050 volumes in nursing; 6,500 periodical subscriptions health-care related.

BACCALAUREATE PROGRAMS

Degree BSN
Available Programs ADN to Baccalaureate; Generic Baccalaureate; RN Baccalaureate.
Study Options Full-time and part-time.
Program Entrance Requirements Minimum overall college GPA of 2.5, transcript of college record, CPR certification, written essay, health exam, health insurance, immunizations, 3 letters of recommendation, minimum GPA in nursing prerequisites of 2.5, prerequisite course work. Transfer students are accepted. *Application deadline:* 10/15 (fall). *Application fee:* $60.
Advanced Placement Credit given for nursing courses completed elsewhere dependent upon specific evaluations.
Contact *Telephone:* 913-588-1619. *Fax:* 913-588-1615.

GRADUATE PROGRAMS

Contact *Telephone:* 913-588-1619. *Fax:* 913-588-1615.

MASTER'S DEGREE PROGRAM
Degrees MS; MS/MHSA; MS/MPH

Available Programs Master's; RN to Master's.
Concentrations Available Health-care administration; nurse-midwifery; nursing administration; nursing informatics. *Clinical nurse specialist programs in:* adult health, gerontology. *Nurse practitioner programs in:* adult health, family health, gerontology, psychiatric/mental health.
Site Options Garden City, KS.
Study Options Full-time and part-time.
Online Degree Options Yes.
Program Entrance Requirements Clinical experience, minimum overall college GPA of 3.0, transcript of college record, CPR certification, immunizations, interview, 3 letters of recommendation, physical assessment course, resume, statistics course. *Application deadline:* 4/1 (fall), 9/1 (spring). *Application fee:* $60.
Degree Requirements 37 total credit hours, thesis or project, comprehensive exam.

POST-MASTER'S PROGRAM

Areas of Study Health-care administration; nurse-midwifery; nursing administration; nursing informatics. *Clinical nurse specialist programs in:* adult health, gerontology. *Nurse practitioner programs in:* adult health, family health, gerontology, psychiatric/mental health.

DOCTORAL DEGREE PROGRAM

Degree PhD
Available Programs Doctorate; Post-Baccalaureate Doctorate.
Areas of Study Nursing research.
Online Degree Options Yes.
Program Entrance Requirements Clinical experience, minimum overall college GPA of 3.5, interview by faculty committee, interview, 3 letters of recommendation, statistics course, vita, writing sample, GRE General Test (for PhD only). Application deadline: 12/1 (summer). Application fee: $60.
Degree Requirements 65 total credit hours, dissertation, oral exam, written exam, residency.

POSTDOCTORAL PROGRAM

Areas of Study Gerontology, nursing research, outcomes, self-care.
Postdoctoral Program Contact *Telephone:* 913-588-1692.

CONTINUING EDUCATION PROGRAM

Contact *Telephone:* 913-588-4488. *Fax:* 913-588-4486.

University of Saint Mary
Bachelor of Science in Nursing Program
Leavenworth, Kansas

http://www.stmary.edu/acad_nursing/default.asp
Founded in 1923
DEGREES • BSN • MSN
Nursing Program Faculty 45 (9% with doctorates).
Baccalaureate Enrollment 306 **Women** 91% **Men** 9% **Part-time** 9%
Graduate Enrollment 29
Distance Learning Courses Available.
Nursing Student Activities Nursing Honor Society, Student Nurses' Association.
Nursing Student Resources Academic advising; academic or career counseling; assistance for students with disabilities; bookstore; campus computer network; e-mail services; employment services for current students; Internet; learning resource lab; library services; nursing audiovisuals; resume preparation assistance; skills, simulation, or other laboratory; tutoring.

BACCALAUREATE PROGRAMS

Degree BSN
Available Programs Accelerated Baccalaureate; Generic Baccalaureate; RN Baccalaureate.
Study Options Full-time.
Online Degree Options Yes.
Program Entrance Requirements Minimum overall college GPA of 2.5, transcript of college record, CPR certification, written essay, health exam, health insurance, immunizations, 2 letters of recommendation, minimum GPA in nursing prerequisites of 2.5, prerequisite course work. Transfer students are accepted. *Application deadline:* 3/15 (fall). Applications may be processed on a rolling basis for some programs.
Expenses (2014–15) *Tuition:* full-time $23,000.

Contact Emily Jefferies, Program Coordinator, Bachelor of Science in Nursing Program, University of Saint Mary, 4100 South 4th Street, Leavenworth, KS 66048. *Telephone:* 913-758-4381. *Fax:* 913-758-4356. *E-mail:* emily.jefferies@stmary.edu.

GRADUATE PROGRAMS

Expenses (2014–15) *Tuition:* part-time $550 per credit hour.
Contact Dr. Linda King, MSN Program Director, Bachelor of Science in Nursing Program, University of Saint Mary, 4100 South 4th Street, Leavenworth, KS 66048. *Telephone:* 913-758-6298. *Fax:* 913-758-4356. *E-mail:* linda.king@stmary.edu.

MASTER'S DEGREE PROGRAM

Degree MSN
Available Programs Master's.
Concentrations Available Nursing administration; nursing education.
Study Options Full-time and part-time.
Online Degree Options Yes (online only).
Program Entrance Requirements Minimum overall college GPA of 3.0, transcript of college record, written essay, 3 letters of recommendation, resume. *Application deadline:* Applications may be processed on a rolling basis for some programs.
Degree Requirements 35 total credit hours, thesis or project.

Washburn University
School of Nursing
Topeka, Kansas

http://www.washburn.edu/academics/college-schools/nursing/index.html
Founded in 1865
DEGREES • BSN • MSN
Nursing Program Faculty 29 (24% with doctorates).
Baccalaureate Enrollment 315 **Women** 89% **Men** 11% **Part-time** 1%
Graduate Enrollment 51 **Women** 90% **Men** 10% **Part-time** 70%
Nursing Student Activities Sigma Theta Tau, Student Nurses' Association, nursing club.
Nursing Student Resources Academic advising; academic or career counseling; assistance for students with disabilities; bookstore; campus computer network; career placement assistance; computer lab; computer-assisted instruction; e-mail services; employment services for current students; interactive nursing skills videos; Internet; learning resource lab; library services; nursing audiovisuals; remedial services; resume preparation assistance; skills, simulation, or other laboratory; tutoring; unpaid internships.
Library Facilities 12,880 volumes in health, 1,612 volumes in nursing; 84 periodical subscriptions health-care related.

BACCALAUREATE PROGRAMS

Degree BSN
Available Programs ADN to Baccalaureate; Baccalaureate for Second Degree; Generic Baccalaureate; LPN to Baccalaureate; RN Baccalaureate.
Study Options Full-time.
Program Entrance Requirements Minimum overall college GPA of 2.7, transcript of college record, CPR certification, written essay, health exam, health insurance, immunizations, interview, 2 letters of recommendation, minimum GPA in nursing prerequisites of 2.0, professional liability insurance/malpractice insurance, prerequisite course work. Transfer students are accepted.
Advanced Placement Credit by examination available. Credit given for nursing courses completed elsewhere dependent upon specific evaluations.
Contact *Telephone:* 785-231-1032 Ext. 1525. *Fax:* 785-231-1032.

GRADUATE PROGRAMS

Contact *Telephone:* 785-231-1010 Ext. 1533. *Fax:* 785-213-1032.

MASTER'S DEGREE PROGRAM

Degree MSN
Available Programs Master's.
Concentrations Available Nursing administration. *Nurse practitioner programs in:* adult health, family health.
Study Options Full-time and part-time.
Program Entrance Requirements Computer literacy, transcript of college record, CPR certification, written essay, immunizations, 2 letters

of recommendation, nursing research course, physical assessment course, professional liability insurance/malpractice insurance, prerequisite course work, resume, statistics course. *Application deadline:* 3/15 (fall). *Application fee:* $35.

Degree Requirements 42 total credit hours, thesis or project.

POST-MASTER'S PROGRAM

Areas of Study Nursing education.

CONTINUING EDUCATION PROGRAM

Contact *Telephone:* 785-231-1010 Ext. 1526. *Fax:* 785-231-1032.

Wichita State University
School of Nursing
Wichita, Kansas

http://www.wichita.edu/nursing
Founded in 1895

DEGREES • BSN • DNP

Nursing Program Faculty 53 (25% with doctorates).
Baccalaureate Enrollment 251 **Women** 90% **Men** 10% **Part-time** 1%
Graduate Enrollment 150 **Women** 94% **Men** 6% **Part-time** 66%
Distance Learning Courses Available.
Nursing Student Activities Sigma Theta Tau, Student Nurses' Association.
Nursing Student Resources Academic advising; academic or career counseling; assistance for students with disabilities; bookstore; campus computer network; career placement assistance; computer lab; computer-assisted instruction; daycare for children of students; e-mail services; employment services for current students; housing assistance; interactive nursing skills videos; Internet; learning resource lab; library services; nursing audiovisuals; resume preparation assistance; skills, simulation, or other laboratory; tutoring.
Library Facilities 31,320 volumes in health, 2,746 volumes in nursing; 406 periodical subscriptions health-care related.

BACCALAUREATE PROGRAMS

Degree BSN

Available Programs ADN to Baccalaureate; Accelerated Baccalaureate; Accelerated Baccalaureate for Second Degree; Generic Baccalaureate; LPN to RN Baccalaureate; RN Baccalaureate.
Site Options Derby, KS.
Study Options Full-time.
Online Degree Options Yes.
Program Entrance Requirements Minimum overall college GPA of 2.75, transcript of college record, CPR certification, written essay, health exam, health insurance, immunizations, minimum GPA in nursing prerequisites of 3.0, professional liability insurance/malpractice insurance, prerequisite course work. Transfer students are accepted. *Application deadline:* 2/1 (fall), 9/1 (spring).
Advanced Placement Credit given for nursing courses completed elsewhere dependent upon specific evaluations.
Expenses (2014–15) *Tuition, state resident:* full-time $5300. *Tuition, nonresident:* full-time $6000. *Room and board:* $15,000; room only: $11,000 per academic year. *Required fees:* full-time $1000.
Financial Aid 80% of baccalaureate students in nursing programs received some form of financial aid in 2013–14.
Contact Ms. Christina Rexroad, Undergraduate Administrative Assistant, School of Nursing, Wichita State University, 1845 Fairmount Street, Wichita, KS 67260-0041. *Telephone:* 316-978-5801. *Fax:* 316-978-3094. *E-mail:* nursing.undergraduate@wichita.edu.

GRADUATE PROGRAMS

Expenses (2014–15) *Tuition, state resident:* part-time $264 per credit hour. *Tuition, nonresident:* full-time $649; part-time $649 per credit hour. *Required fees:* full-time $157; part-time $62 per credit; part-time $79 per term.
Financial Aid 80% of graduate students in nursing programs received some form of financial aid in 2013–14.
Contact Dr. Alicia Huckstadt, Director, Graduate Program, School of Nursing, Wichita State University, 1845 Fairmount Street, Wichita, KS 67260-0041. *Telephone:* 316-978-3610. *Fax:* 316-978-3094. *E-mail:* alicia.huckstadt@wichita.edu.

MASTER'S DEGREE PROGRAM

Program Entrance Requirements *Application deadline:* Applications may be processed on a rolling basis for some programs. *Application fee:* $35.

DOCTORAL DEGREE PROGRAM

Degree DNP
Available Programs Doctorate; Post-Baccalaureate Doctorate.
Areas of Study Advanced practice nursing, clinical practice, critical care, faculty preparation, family health, health policy, health promotion/disease prevention, health-care systems, human health and illness, nursing administration, nursing education, nursing policy, nursing research, nursing science.
Online Degree Options Yes.
Program Entrance Requirements Clinical experience, minimum overall college GPA of 3.0, interview, 3 letters of recommendation, statistics course, vita. Application deadline: 5/1 (fall), 10/15 (spring). Application fee: $35.
Degree Requirements 74 total credit hours, written exam, residency.

KENTUCKY

Bellarmine University
Donna and Allan Lansing School of Nursing and Health Sciences
Louisville, Kentucky

http://www.bellarmine.edu/
Founded in 1950

DEGREES • BSN • DNP • MSN • MSN/MBA

Nursing Program Faculty 85 (15% with doctorates).
Baccalaureate Enrollment 210 **Women** 88.8% **Men** 11.2% **Part-time** 18%
Graduate Enrollment 79 **Women** 92.8% **Men** 7.2% **Part-time** 89.6%
Nursing Student Activities Sigma Theta Tau, Student Nurses' Association.
Nursing Student Resources Academic advising; academic or career counseling; assistance for students with disabilities; bookstore; campus computer network; career placement assistance; computer lab; computer-assisted instruction; e-mail services; employment services for current students; externships; housing assistance; interactive nursing skills videos; Internet; learning resource lab; library services; nursing audiovisuals; paid internships; placement services for program completers; remedial services; resume preparation assistance; skills, simulation, or other laboratory; tutoring; unpaid internships.
Library Facilities 4,670 volumes in health, 1,644 volumes in nursing; 93 periodical subscriptions health-care related.

BACCALAUREATE PROGRAMS

Degree BSN

Available Programs Accelerated Baccalaureate for Second Degree; Generic Baccalaureate; RN Baccalaureate.
Study Options Full-time and part-time.
Program Entrance Requirements Minimum overall college GPA of 2.5, transcript of college record, CPR certification, written essay, health exam, health insurance, high school biology, high school chemistry, 2 years high school math, 2 years high school science, high school transcript, immunizations, interview, minimum high school GPA of 2.75, minimum GPA in nursing prerequisites of 2.75, prerequisite course work. Transfer students are accepted. *Application deadline:* 8/15 (fall), 1/3 (winter), 1/3 (spring), 5/3 (summer). Applications may be processed on a rolling basis for some programs. *Application fee:* $25.
Advanced Placement Credit by examination available. Credit given for nursing courses completed elsewhere dependent upon specific evaluations.
Contact *Telephone:* 502-452-8279. *Fax:* 502-452-8058.

GRADUATE PROGRAMS

Contact *Telephone:* 502-452-8364. *Fax:* 502-452-8058.

MASTER'S DEGREE PROGRAM

Degrees MSN; MSN/MBA

Available Programs Master's; Master's for Nurses with Non-Nursing Degrees; RN to Master's.

Concentrations Available Nursing administration; nursing education.

Study Options Part-time.

Program Entrance Requirements Minimum overall college GPA of 2.75, transcript of college record, professional liability insurance/malpractice insurance, GRE General Test. *Application deadline:* 8/20 (fall), 1/5 (winter), 1/5 (spring), 5/1 (summer). Applications may be processed on a rolling basis for some programs. *Application fee:* $25.

Advanced Placement Credit given for nursing courses completed elsewhere dependent upon specific evaluations.

Degree Requirements 38 total credit hours, thesis or project.

POST-MASTER'S PROGRAM

Areas of Study *Nurse practitioner programs in:* family health.

DOCTORAL DEGREE PROGRAM

Degree DNP

Available Programs Doctorate for Nurses with Non-Nursing Degrees.

Areas of Study Advanced practice nursing, family health.

Program Entrance Requirements Minimum overall college GPA of 3.5, interview by faculty committee, 3 letters of recommendation, MSN or equivalent, vita, GRE General Test. Application deadline: 8/15 (fall), 1/5 (spring), 5/3 (summer). Application fee: $25.

Degree Requirements Residency.

CONTINUING EDUCATION PROGRAM

Contact *Telephone:* 502-452-8161. *Fax:* 502-452-8203.

Berea College
Department of Nursing
Berea, Kentucky

http://www.berea.edu/nur/
Founded in 1855

DEGREE • BSN

Nursing Program Faculty 9 (55% with doctorates).

Baccalaureate Enrollment 21 **Women** 76% **Men** 24%

Nursing Student Activities Nursing Honor Society, Student Nurses' Association.

Nursing Student Resources Academic advising; academic or career counseling; assistance for students with disabilities; bookstore; campus computer network; career placement assistance; computer lab; computer-assisted instruction; daycare for children of students; e-mail services; employment services for current students; externships; housing assistance; interactive nursing skills videos; Internet; learning resource lab; library services; nursing audiovisuals; paid internships; placement services for program completers; remedial services; resume preparation assistance; skills, simulation, or other laboratory; tutoring; unpaid internships.

Library Facilities 8,937 volumes in health, 7,130 volumes in nursing; 3,460 periodical subscriptions health-care related.

BACCALAUREATE PROGRAMS

Degree BSN

Available Programs Generic Baccalaureate.

Study Options Full-time.

Program Entrance Requirements Minimum high school GPA, minimum GPA in nursing prerequisites of 3.0, prerequisite course work. Transfer students are accepted.

Expenses (2015–16) *Room and board:* $1520; room only: $750 per academic year.

Financial Aid *Gift aid (need-based):* Federal Pell, FSEOG, state, private, college/university gift aid from institutional funds. *Loans:* Federal Direct (Subsidized and Unsubsidized Stafford PLUS), Perkins, college/university. *Work-study:* Federal Work-Study, part-time campus jobs. *Financial aid application deadline:* 3/1(priority: 1/31).

Contact Luke Hodson, Director of Admissions/Operations, Department of Nursing, Berea College, CPO 2220, Berea, KY 40404. *Telephone:* 859-985-3503. *E-mail:* luke_hodson@berea.edu.

Eastern Kentucky University
Department of Baccalaureate and Graduate Nursing
Richmond, Kentucky

http://www.bsn-gn.eku.edu/
Founded in 1906

DEGREES • BSN • MSN

Nursing Program Faculty 42 (40% with doctorates).

Baccalaureate Enrollment 500

Graduate Enrollment 200

Distance Learning Courses Available.

Nursing Student Activities Sigma Theta Tau, Student Nurses' Association.

Nursing Student Resources Academic advising; academic or career counseling; assistance for students with disabilities; bookstore; campus computer network; computer lab; computer-assisted instruction; e-mail services; housing assistance; interactive nursing skills videos; Internet; learning resource lab; library services; nursing audiovisuals; skills, simulation, or other laboratory.

BACCALAUREATE PROGRAMS

Degree BSN

Available Programs Accelerated RN Baccalaureate; Baccalaureate for Second Degree; Generic Baccalaureate; RN Baccalaureate.

Site Options Hazard, KY; Corbin, KY; Danville, KY.

Study Options Full-time and part-time.

Program Entrance Requirements Minimum overall college GPA of 2.5, CPR certification, immunizations, professional liability insurance/malpractice insurance, prerequisite course work. Transfer students are accepted.

Advanced Placement Credit given for nursing courses completed elsewhere dependent upon specific evaluations.

Contact *Telephone:* 859-622-1827. *Fax:* 859-622-1972.

GRADUATE PROGRAMS

Contact *Telephone:* 859-622-1838. *Fax:* 859-622-1972.

MASTER'S DEGREE PROGRAM

Degree MSN

Available Programs Master's.

Concentrations Available Nursing education. *Clinical nurse specialist programs in:* public health. *Nurse practitioner programs in:* family health, psychiatric/mental health.

Site Options Hazard, KY; Corbin, KY; Danville, KY.

Study Options Full-time and part-time.

Program Entrance Requirements Minimum overall college GPA of 2.75, transcript of college record, written essay, 3 letters of recommendation, statistics course.

Advanced Placement Credit given for nursing courses completed elsewhere dependent upon specific evaluations.

Degree Requirements 48 total credit hours, thesis or project, comprehensive exam.

Frontier Nursing University
Nursing Degree Programs
Hyden, Kentucky

http://www.frontier.edu/
Founded in 1939

DEGREES • DNP • MSN

Nursing Program Faculty 104 (71% with doctorates).

Graduate Enrollment 1,513 **Women** 95% **Men** 5% **Part-time** 27%

Distance Learning Courses Available.

Nursing Student Activities Nursing Honor Society, Sigma Theta Tau.

Nursing Student Resources Academic advising; academic or career counseling; assistance for students with disabilities; bookstore; campus computer network; computer lab; computer-assisted instruction; e-mail services; interactive nursing skills videos; Internet; learning resource lab; library services; nursing audiovisuals; resume preparation assistance; skills, simulation, or other laboratory.

Library Facilities 400 volumes in health, 250 volumes in nursing; 2,375 periodical subscriptions health-care related.

GRADUATE PROGRAMS

Expenses (2015–16) *Tuition:* full-time $15,047; part-time $535 per credit hour. *International tuition:* $15,047 full-time. *Required fees:* full-time $1000.

Contact Doctorate and Master in Nursing Programs, Nursing Degree Programs, Frontier Nursing University, PO Box 528, 195 School Street, Hyden, KY 41749. *Telephone:* 606-672-2312. *E-mail:* fsmfn@ midwives.org.

MASTER'S DEGREE PROGRAM

Degree MSN

Available Programs Accelerated AD/RN to Master's; Master's for Nurses with Non-Nursing Degrees.

Concentrations Available Nurse-midwifery. *Nurse practitioner programs in:* family health, women's health.

Study Options Full-time and part-time.

Online Degree Options Yes (online only).

Program Entrance Requirements Clinical experience, minimum overall college GPA of 3.0, transcript of college record, written essay, immunizations, 3 letters of recommendation, physical assessment course, prerequisite course work, resume, statistics course. *Application deadline:* 4/20 (fall), 7/20 (winter), 10/30 (spring), 2/1 (summer). *Application fee:* $100.

Advanced Placement Credit given for nursing courses completed elsewhere dependent upon specific evaluations.

Degree Requirements 64 total credit hours.

POST-MASTER'S PROGRAM

Areas of Study Nurse-midwifery. *Nurse practitioner programs in:* family health, women's health.

DOCTORAL DEGREE PROGRAM

Degree DNP

Available Programs Doctorate.

Areas of Study Advanced practice nursing, family health, maternity-newborn, women's health.

Online Degree Options Yes (online only).

Program Entrance Requirements Minimum overall college GPA of 3.0, 3 letters of recommendation, MSN or equivalent, statistics course, vita. Application deadline: 5/18 (fall), 8/17 (winter), 12/2 (spring), 2/16 (summer). Application fee: $100.

Degree Requirements 33 total credit hours.

See display below and full description on page 494.

Kentucky Christian University
School of Nursing
Grayson, Kentucky

http://www.kcu.edu/yancey-nursing
Founded in 1919

DEGREE • BSN

Nursing Program Faculty 6 (20% with doctorates).

Baccalaureate Enrollment 63 **Women** 90% **Men** 10%

Nursing Student Activities Student Nurses' Association.

Nursing Student Resources Academic advising; assistance for students with disabilities; bookstore; campus computer network; computer lab; e-mail services; housing assistance; interactive nursing skills videos; Internet; learning resource lab; library services; nursing audiovisuals; other; remedial services; skills, simulation, or other laboratory.

Library Facilities 400 volumes in health, 300 volumes in nursing; 200 periodical subscriptions health-care related.

BACCALAUREATE PROGRAMS

Degree BSN

Available Programs Generic Baccalaureate.

Study Options Full-time.

Program Entrance Requirements Transcript of college record, written essay, health exam, health insurance, high school transcript, immunizations, minimum GPA in nursing prerequisites of 2.5, prerequisite course work. Transfer students are accepted.

Contact *Telephone:* 606-474-3255. *Fax:* 606-474-3342.

CONTINUING EDUCATION PROGRAM

Contact *Telephone:* 606-474-3271. *Fax:* 606-474-3342.

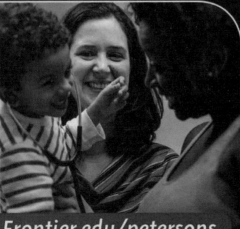

Sometimes your career chooses you...

Answer the call.

Become a Nurse-Midwife or Nurse Practitioner

 FRONTIER NURSING UNIVERSITY

Frontier.edu/petersons

Ranked #1 Nurse-Midwifery Program in the U.S.

 BEST GRAD SCHOOLS U.S.News NURSING NURSE MIDWIFERY 2016

Kentucky State University
School of Nursing
Frankfort, Kentucky

http://www.kysu.edu/
Founded in 1886
DEGREE • BSN
Nursing Program Faculty 18 (11% with doctorates).
Baccalaureate Enrollment 25
Nursing Student Activities Student Nurses' Association.
Nursing Student Resources Academic advising; academic or career counseling; assistance for students with disabilities; bookstore; campus computer network; career placement assistance; computer lab; computer-assisted instruction; e-mail services; externships; housing assistance; interactive nursing skills videos; Internet; learning resource lab; library services; nursing audiovisuals; other; placement services for program completers; remedial services; resume preparation assistance; skills, simulation, or other laboratory; tutoring.

BACCALAUREATE PROGRAMS

Degree BSN
Available Programs ADN to Baccalaureate.
Program Entrance Requirements Transfer students are accepted.
Contact *Telephone:* 502-597-6963. *Fax:* 502-597-5818.

Lindsey Wilson College
Nursing Division
Columbia, Kentucky

http://www.lindsey.edu/academics/undergraduate-programs/bachelor-of-science/nursing.aspx
Founded in 1903
DEGREE • BSN

BACCALAUREATE PROGRAMS

Degree BSN
Available Programs RN Baccalaureate.
Contact Division of Nursing, Nursing Division, Lindsey Wilson College, 210 Lindsey Wilson Street, Columbia, KY 42728. *Telephone:* 270-384-7352. *E-mail:* nursing@lindsey.edu.

Midway University
Program in Nursing (Baccalaureate)
Midway, Kentucky

http://www.midway.edu/
Founded in 1847
DEGREE • BSN
Nursing Program Faculty 3 (67% with doctorates).
Baccalaureate Enrollment 28 **Women** 90% **Men** 10% **Part-time** 20%
Distance Learning Courses Available.
Nursing Student Activities Sigma Theta Tau, Student Nurses' Association.
Nursing Student Resources Academic advising; academic or career counseling; assistance for students with disabilities; bookstore; campus computer network; career placement assistance; computer lab; computer-assisted instruction; e-mail services; externships; interactive nursing skills videos; Internet; learning resource lab; library services; nursing audiovisuals; placement services for program completers; remedial services; resume preparation assistance; skills, simulation, or other laboratory; tutoring; unpaid internships.
Library Facilities 1,200 volumes in health, 800 volumes in nursing; 102 periodical subscriptions health-care related.

BACCALAUREATE PROGRAMS

Degree BSN
Available Programs ADN to Baccalaureate; Accelerated RN Baccalaureate; RN Baccalaureate.
Study Options Full-time and part-time.
Online Degree Options Yes.
Program Entrance Requirements Minimum overall college GPA of 2.5, CPR certification, health insurance, immunizations, interview, 3 letters of recommendation, minimum GPA in nursing prerequisites of 2.5, prerequisite course work, RN licensure. Transfer students are accepted. *Application deadline:* 3/15 (fall), 3/15 (winter), 10/15 (spring), 3/15 (summer). Applications may be processed on a rolling basis for some programs. *Application fee:* $30.
Advanced Placement Credit given for nursing courses completed elsewhere dependent upon specific evaluations.
Expenses (2015–16) *Tuition:* part-time $395 per credit hour. *Room and board:* $8000 per academic year.
Contact Dr. Barbara R. Kitchen, Dean, School of Health Sciences, Program in Nursing (Baccalaureate), Midway University, 512 East Stephens Street, Midway, KY 40347. *Telephone:* 859-846-5335. *Fax:* 859-846-5876. *E-mail:* bkitchen@midway.edu.

CONTINUING EDUCATION PROGRAM

Contact Dr. Barbara R. Kitchen, Dean, School of Health Sciences, Program in Nursing (Baccalaureate), Midway University, 512 East Stephens Street, Midway, KY 40347. *Telephone:* 859-846-5335. *Fax:* 859-846-5876. *E-mail:* bkitchen@midway.edu.

Morehead State University
Department of Nursing
Morehead, Kentucky

http://www.moreheadstate.edu/nursing
Founded in 1922
DEGREE • BSN
Nursing Program Faculty 46 (17% with doctorates).
Baccalaureate Enrollment 282 **Women** 91% **Men** 9% **Part-time** 51%
Distance Learning Courses Available.
Nursing Student Activities Student Nurses' Association.
Nursing Student Resources Academic advising; academic or career counseling; assistance for students with disabilities; bookstore; campus computer network; career placement assistance; computer lab; computer-assisted instruction; e-mail services; interactive nursing skills videos; Internet; learning resource lab; library services; nursing audiovisuals; remedial services; resume preparation assistance; skills, simulation, or other laboratory; tutoring.
Library Facilities 500,000 volumes in health, 860 volumes in nursing; 286 periodical subscriptions health-care related.

BACCALAUREATE PROGRAMS

Degree BSN
Available Programs ADN to Baccalaureate; Generic Baccalaureate; RN Baccalaureate.
Site Options Ashland, KY; Prestonsburg, KY; Mt. Sterling, KY.
Study Options Full-time.
Online Degree Options Yes.
Program Entrance Requirements Minimum overall college GPA of 2.0, transcript of college record, CPR certification, health insurance, immunizations, minimum GPA in nursing prerequisites of 3.0, prerequisite course work. Transfer students are accepted. *Application deadline:* 3/15 (fall).
Advanced Placement Credit by examination available. Credit given for nursing courses completed elsewhere dependent upon specific evaluations.
Expenses (2015–16) *Tuition, state resident:* full-time $8098; part-time $338 per credit hour. *Tuition, nonresident:* full-time $20,246; part-time $844 per credit hour. *International tuition:* $20,246 full-time. *Room and board:* $8300; room only: $4500 per academic year. *Required fees:* full-time $350.
Financial Aid 85% of baccalaureate students in nursing programs received some form of financial aid in 2014–15. *Gift aid (need-based):* Federal Pell, FSEOG, state, private, college/university gift aid from institutional funds. *Loans:* Federal Direct (Subsidized and Unsubsidized Stafford PLUS), Perkins, college/university. *Work-study:* Federal Work-Study, part-time campus jobs. *Financial aid application deadline (priority):* 3/15.
Contact Ms. Carla June Aagaard, Academic Counseling Coordinator, Department of Nursing, Morehead State University, 316 West 2nd Street, CHER 201, Morehead, KY 40351. *Telephone:* 606-783-2641. *Fax:* 606-783-9211. *E-mail:* c.aagaard@moreheadstate.edu.

Murray State University
Program in Nursing
Murray, Kentucky

http://www.murraystate.edu/
Founded in 1922

DEGREES • BSN • MSN

Nursing Program Faculty 16 (47% with doctorates).

Baccalaureate Enrollment 206 **Women** 94% **Men** 6%

Graduate Enrollment 48 **Women** 85% **Men** 15%

Distance Learning Courses Available.

Nursing Student Activities Sigma Theta Tau, Student Nurses' Association.

Nursing Student Resources Academic advising; academic or career counseling; assistance for students with disabilities; bookstore; campus computer network; career placement assistance; computer lab; computer-assisted instruction; daycare for children of students; e-mail services; employment services for current students; externships; housing assistance; interactive nursing skills videos; Internet; learning resource lab; library services; nursing audiovisuals; placement services for program completers; remedial services; resume preparation assistance; skills, simulation, or other laboratory; tutoring; unpaid internships.

Library Facilities 4,060 volumes in health, 2,160 volumes in nursing; 124 periodical subscriptions health-care related.

BACCALAUREATE PROGRAMS

Degree BSN

Available Programs Generic Baccalaureate; RN Baccalaureate.

Site Options Hopkinsville, KY; Paducah, KY; Madisonville, KY.

Study Options Full-time.

Program Entrance Requirements Transcript of college record, CPR certification, immunizations, minimum GPA in nursing prerequisites of 2.5, professional liability insurance/malpractice insurance, prerequisite course work. Transfer students are accepted. *Application deadline:* 5/1 (fall), 11/22 (spring).

Advanced Placement Credit by examination available. Credit given for nursing courses completed elsewhere dependent upon specific evaluations.

Contact *Telephone:* 270-809-2193. *Fax:* 270-809-6662.

GRADUATE PROGRAMS

Contact *Telephone:* 270-809-6671. *Fax:* 270-809-6662.

MASTER'S DEGREE PROGRAM

Degree MSN

Available Programs Master's.

Concentrations Available Nurse anesthesia. *Clinical nurse specialist programs in:* adult health, critical care, medical-surgical. *Nurse practitioner programs in:* family health.

Site Options Hopkinsville, KY; Paducah, KY; Madisonville, KY.

Study Options Full-time and part-time.

Program Entrance Requirements Clinical experience, minimum overall college GPA of 3.0, transcript of college record, CPR certification, immunizations, interview, 3 letters of recommendation, nursing research course, physical assessment course, professional liability insurance/malpractice insurance, prerequisite course work, statistics course, GRE General Test. *Application deadline:* 11/1 (fall).

Advanced Placement Credit given for nursing courses completed elsewhere dependent upon specific evaluations.

Degree Requirements 46 total credit hours.

POST-MASTER'S PROGRAM

Areas of Study Nurse anesthesia. *Clinical nurse specialist programs in:* adult health, critical care, medical-surgical. *Nurse practitioner programs in:* family health.

CONTINUING EDUCATION PROGRAM

Contact *Telephone:* 270-809-6674. *Fax:* 270-809-6662.

Northern Kentucky University
Department of Nursing
Highland Heights, Kentucky

http://www.nku.edu/
Founded in 1968

DEGREES • BSN • DNP • MSN

Nursing Program Faculty 100 (35% with doctorates).

Baccalaureate Enrollment 472 **Women** 93% **Men** 7% **Part-time** 17%

Graduate Enrollment 275 **Women** 95% **Men** 5% **Part-time** 90%

Distance Learning Courses Available.

Nursing Student Activities Sigma Theta Tau, Student Nurses' Association.

Nursing Student Resources Academic advising; academic or career counseling; assistance for students with disabilities; bookstore; campus computer network; career placement assistance; computer lab; computer-assisted instruction; daycare for children of students; e-mail services; employment services for current students; housing assistance; interactive nursing skills videos; Internet; learning resource lab; library services; nursing audiovisuals; resume preparation assistance; skills, simulation, or other laboratory; tutoring.

Library Facilities 6,380 volumes in health, 3,500 volumes in nursing; 100 periodical subscriptions health-care related.

BACCALAUREATE PROGRAMS

Degree BSN

Available Programs Accelerated Baccalaureate for Second Degree; Generic Baccalaureate; RN Baccalaureate.

Study Options Full-time.

Program Entrance Requirements Minimum overall college GPA of 2.5, transcript of college record, CPR certification, health exam, health insurance, high school biology, high school chemistry, 3 years high school math, high school transcript, immunizations, minimum GPA in nursing prerequisites of 3.0, prerequisite course work. Transfer students are accepted. *Application deadline:* 1/15 (fall), 8/15 (spring). *Application fee:* $40.

Advanced Placement Credit by examination available. Credit given for nursing courses completed elsewhere dependent upon specific evaluations.

Expenses (2015–16) *Tuition, state resident:* full-time $4368; part-time $364 per credit hour. *Tuition, nonresident:* full-time $8736; part-time $728 per credit hour. *International tuition:* $8736 full-time. *Room and board:* $8000; room only: $4400 per academic year. *Required fees:* full-time $400.

Contact Dr. Mary Kishman, Chair, Department of Nursing, Northern Kentucky University, Nunn Drive, AHC 303, Highland Heights, KY 41099. *Telephone:* 859-572-5248. *Fax:* 859-572-6098. *E-mail:* kishmanm1@nku.edu.

GRADUATE PROGRAMS

Expenses (2015–16) *Tuition, state resident:* part-time $597 per credit hour. *Tuition, nonresident:* part-time $597 per credit hour. *Required fees:* part-time $40 per credit.

Contact Dr. Adrianne J Lane, Chief Nurse Administrator and Chair of Advanced Nursing Studies, Department of Nursing, Northern Kentucky University, HC 206, Highland Heights, KY 41099. *Telephone:* 859-572-7918. *Fax:* 859-572-1934. *E-mail:* lanea6@nku.edu.

MASTER'S DEGREE PROGRAM

Degree MSN

Available Programs Master's.

Concentrations Available Nursing administration; nursing education; nursing informatics. *Nurse practitioner programs in:* adult health, adult-gerontology acute care, family health, pediatric primary care, primary care.

Study Options Part-time.

Online Degree Options Yes (online only).

Program Entrance Requirements Clinical experience, minimum overall college GPA of 3.0, transcript of college record, CPR certification, written essay, immunizations, 2 letters of recommendation, professional liability insurance/malpractice insurance, prerequisite course work, resume, statistics course. *Application deadline:* 2/15 (fall), 10/15 (spring). *Application fee:* $40.

Advanced Placement Credit given for nursing courses completed elsewhere dependent upon specific evaluations.

Degree Requirements 42 total credit hours, thesis or project.

POST-MASTER'S PROGRAM

Areas of Study *Nurse practitioner programs in:* adult health, adult-gerontology acute care, adult-psychiatric mental health, family health, pediatric primary care, primary care.

DOCTORAL DEGREE PROGRAM

Degree DNP

Available Programs Doctorate.

Online Degree Options Yes.

Program Entrance Requirements Minimum overall college GPA of 3.0, interview, 3 letters of recommendation, MSN or equivalent, statistics course, vita, writing sample. Application deadline: 4/1 (fall). Application fee: $40.

Degree Requirements 36 total credit hours, dissertation.

CONTINUING EDUCATION PROGRAM

Contact Dr. Kimberly McErlane, Director of Nursing and Interprofessional Research Center, Department of Nursing, Northern Kentucky University, NKU, HC 354, Highland Heights, KY 41099. *Telephone:* 859-572-6324. *Fax:* 859-572-1934. *E-mail:* mcerlanek1@nku.edu.

Spalding University
School of Nursing
Louisville, Kentucky

http://www.spalding.edu/nursing
Founded in 1814

DEGREES • BSN • DNP • MSN

Nursing Program Faculty 44 (18% with doctorates).
Baccalaureate Enrollment 110 **Women** 95% **Men** 5%
Graduate Enrollment 92 **Women** 99.5% **Men** .5% **Part-time** 48%
Nursing Student Activities Sigma Theta Tau, Student Nurses' Association.
Nursing Student Resources Academic advising; academic or career counseling; assistance for students with disabilities; bookstore; campus computer network; career placement assistance; computer lab; computer-assisted instruction; e-mail services; employment services for current students; interactive nursing skills videos; Internet; learning resource lab; library services; nursing audiovisuals; remedial services; resume preparation assistance; skills, simulation, or other laboratory; tutoring.
Library Facilities 2,875 volumes in health, 1,125 volumes in nursing; 367 periodical subscriptions health-care related.

BACCALAUREATE PROGRAMS

Degree BSN

Available Programs Accelerated Baccalaureate for Second Degree; Baccalaureate for Second Degree; Generic Baccalaureate; RN Baccalaureate.
Study Options Full-time.
Program Entrance Requirements Minimum overall college GPA of 2.5, transcript of college record, CPR certification, health exam, health insurance, high school transcript, immunizations, minimum GPA in nursing prerequisites of 3.0, professional liability insurance/malpractice insurance, prerequisite course work. Transfer students are accepted. *Application deadline:* Applications may be processed on a rolling basis for some programs.
Advanced Placement Credit given for nursing courses completed elsewhere dependent upon specific evaluations.
Expenses (2014–15) *Room and board:* $8400; room only: $5600 per academic year.
Financial Aid 95% of baccalaureate students in nursing programs received some form of financial aid in 2013–14.
Contact Mrs. Jacqui McMillian-Bohler, Director, Baccalaureate Program in Nursing, School of Nursing, Spalding University, 901 South Fourth Street, Louisville, KY 40203. *Telephone:* 502-873-4295. *E-mail:* jmcmillian-bohler@spalding.edu.

GRADUATE PROGRAMS

Financial Aid Career-related internships or fieldwork, scholarships, and traineeships available.
Contact Dr. Pamela King, Director, Master's Programs, School of Nursing, Spalding University, 901 South Fourth Street, Louisville, KY 40203-2188. *Telephone:* 502-873-4292. *E-mail:* pking@spalding.edu.

MASTER'S DEGREE PROGRAM

Degree MSN

Available Programs Master's; RN to Master's.
Concentrations Available *Nurse practitioner programs in:* family health, pediatric.
Study Options Full-time and part-time.
Program Entrance Requirements Computer literacy, minimum overall college GPA of 3.0, transcript of college record, CPR certification, written essay, immunizations, interview, 2 letters of recommendation, nursing research course, physical assessment course, professional liability insurance/malpractice insurance, prerequisite course work, resume, statistics course, GRE General Test. *Application deadline:* Applications may be processed on a rolling basis for some programs.
Advanced Placement Credit given for nursing courses completed elsewhere dependent upon specific evaluations.
Degree Requirements 49 total credit hours.

POST-MASTER'S PROGRAM

Areas of Study *Nurse practitioner programs in:* family health, pediatric.

DOCTORAL DEGREE PROGRAM

Degree DNP

Available Programs Doctorate.
Program Entrance Requirements Minimum overall college GPA of 3.0, 3 letters of recommendation, MSN or equivalent, vita. Application deadline: Applications may be processed on a rolling basis for some programs.
Degree Requirements 36 total credit hours.

CONTINUING EDUCATION PROGRAM

Contact Dr. Patricia Spurr, Continuing Education Administrator, School of Nursing, Spalding University, 901 South Fourth Street, 901 South 4th Street, Louisville, KY 40203-2188. *Telephone:* 502-585-7125. *Fax:* 502-588-7175. *E-mail:* pspurr@spalding.edu.

Sullivan University
RN to BSN Program
Louisville, Kentucky

Founded in 1864

DEGREE • BSN

Nursing Program Faculty 16 (80% with doctorates).
Baccalaureate Enrollment 9 **Women** 95% **Men** 5%
Nursing Student Activities Nursing club.
Nursing Student Resources Academic advising; academic or career counseling; assistance for students with disabilities; bookstore; campus computer network; career placement assistance; computer lab; computer-assisted instruction; e-mail services; employment services for current students; Internet; library services; nursing audiovisuals; placement services for program completers; resume preparation assistance; tutoring.
Library Facilities 1,162 volumes in health, 25 volumes in nursing; 1,500 periodical subscriptions health-care related.

BACCALAUREATE PROGRAMS

Degree BSN

Available Programs Accelerated RN Baccalaureate.
Study Options Full-time.
Online Degree Options Yes.
Program Entrance Requirements Minimum overall college GPA of 2.5, transcript of college record, CPR certification, health exam, health insurance, immunizations, minimum GPA in nursing prerequisites of 2.5, professional liability insurance/malpractice insurance, prerequisite course work, RN licensure. *Application deadline:* 9/27 (fall), 1/3 (winter), 3/27 (spring), 6/26 (summer). *Application fee:* $50.
Advanced Placement Credit given for nursing courses completed elsewhere dependent upon specific evaluations.
Expenses (2014–15) *Tuition:* part-time $320 per credit hour. *International tuition:* $337 full-time.
Financial Aid 60% of baccalaureate students in nursing programs received some form of financial aid in 2013–14.
Contact Mr. Ryan T. Davisson, Associate Director of Admissions, RN to BSN Program, Sullivan University, 3101 Bardstown Road, Nolan Building, Louisville, KY 40205. *Telephone:* 502-456-6504. *Fax:* 502-456-0032. *E-mail:* rdavisson@sullivan.edu.

Thomas More College
Program in Nursing
Crestview Hills, Kentucky

http://www.thomasmore.edu/
Founded in 1921
DEGREE • BSN
Nursing Program Faculty 10 (.2% with doctorates).
Baccalaureate Enrollment 160 **Women** 86% **Men** 14%
Nursing Student Activities Student Nurses' Association.
Nursing Student Resources Academic advising; academic or career counseling; assistance for students with disabilities; bookstore; campus computer network; career placement assistance; computer lab; computer-assisted instruction; e-mail services; employment services for current students; interactive nursing skills videos; Internet; learning resource lab; library services; nursing audiovisuals; other; placement services for program completers; remedial services; resume preparation assistance; skills, simulation, or other laboratory; tutoring.
Library Facilities 450 volumes in health, 200 volumes in nursing; 50 periodical subscriptions health-care related.

BACCALAUREATE PROGRAMS

Degree BSN
Available Programs Accelerated RN Baccalaureate; Generic Baccalaureate.
Study Options Full-time.
Program Entrance Requirements Transcript of college record, CPR certification, health exam, health insurance, high school transcript, immunizations, minimum GPA in nursing prerequisites of 2.75, professional liability insurance/malpractice insurance, prerequisite course work. Transfer students are accepted. *Application deadline:* Applications may be processed on a rolling basis for some programs.
Advanced Placement Credit given for nursing courses completed elsewhere dependent upon specific evaluations.
Expenses (2015–16) *Tuition:* full-time $17,268; part-time $605 per credit hour. *Required fees:* full-time $1400; part-time $70 per credit.
Financial Aid 90% of baccalaureate students in nursing programs received some form of financial aid in 2014–15.
Contact Dr. Lisa Spangler Torok, Chair, Program in Nursing, Thomas More College, 333 Thomas More Parkway, Crestview Hills, KY 41017. *Telephone:* 859-344-3413. *Fax:* 859-344-3537. *E-mail:* torokl@thomasmore.edu.

Union College
School of Nursing & Health Sciences
Barbourville, Kentucky

Founded in 1879
DEGREE • BSN

BACCALAUREATE PROGRAMS

Degree BSN
Available Programs Generic Baccalaureate.
Study Options Full-time and part-time.
Contact *Telephone:* 606-546-1212.

University of Kentucky
College of Nursing
Lexington, Kentucky

http://www.uknursing.uky.edu/
Founded in 1865
DEGREES • BSN • MSN • PHD
Nursing Program Faculty 65 (54% with doctorates).
Baccalaureate Enrollment 260 **Women** 97% **Men** 3% **Part-time** 14%
Graduate Enrollment 221 **Women** 92% **Men** 8% **Part-time** 35%
Nursing Student Activities Sigma Theta Tau, Student Nurses' Association.
Nursing Student Resources Academic advising; academic or career counseling; assistance for students with disabilities; bookstore; campus computer network; career placement assistance; computer lab; computer-assisted instruction; e-mail services; interactive nursing skills videos; Internet; learning resource lab; library services; nursing audiovisuals; skills, simulation, or other laboratory.
Library Facilities 105,793 volumes in health; 3,347 periodical subscriptions health-care related.

BACCALAUREATE PROGRAMS

Degree BSN
Available Programs Baccalaureate for Second Degree; Generic Baccalaureate; RN Baccalaureate.
Study Options Full-time and part-time.
Program Entrance Requirements Minimum overall college GPA of 2.5, transcript of college record, CPR certification, written essay, high school transcript, immunizations, minimum GPA in nursing prerequisites of 2.5, prerequisite course work. Transfer students are accepted.
Advanced Placement Credit by examination available. Credit given for nursing courses completed elsewhere dependent upon specific evaluations.
Contact *Telephone:* 859-323-5108. *Fax:* 859-323-1057.

GRADUATE PROGRAMS

Contact *Telephone:* 859-323-5108. *Fax:* 859-323-1057.

MASTER'S DEGREE PROGRAM
Degree MSN
Available Programs Master's; RN to Master's.
Concentrations Available Nurse case management; nursing administration. *Clinical nurse specialist programs in:* acute care, adult health, community health, critical care, gerontology, medical-surgical, oncology, parent-child, pediatric, perinatal, psychiatric/mental health, public health, women's health. *Nurse practitioner programs in:* acute care, adult health, family health, gerontology, pediatric, psychiatric/mental health.
Site Options Morehead, KY.
Study Options Full-time and part-time.
Program Entrance Requirements Clinical experience, minimum overall college GPA of 2.75, transcript of college record, written essay, interview, 3 letters of recommendation, physical assessment course, statistics course.
Advanced Placement Credit given for nursing courses completed elsewhere dependent upon specific evaluations.
Degree Requirements 40 total credit hours, comprehensive exam.

POST-MASTER'S PROGRAM
Areas of Study Nurse case management. *Nurse practitioner programs in:* acute care, adult health, family health, gerontology, pediatric, psychiatric/mental health.

DOCTORAL DEGREE PROGRAM
Degree PhD
Available Programs Doctorate.
Areas of Study Nursing research.
Program Entrance Requirements Minimum overall college GPA of 3.3, interview, 3 letters of recommendation, MSN or equivalent, statistics course, writing sample, GRE General Test.
Degree Requirements 63 total credit hours, dissertation, oral exam, written exam, residency.

CONTINUING EDUCATION PROGRAM

Contact *Telephone:* 859-323-3851. *Fax:* 859-323-1057.

University of Louisville
School of Nursing
Louisville, Kentucky

http://www.louisville.edu/nursing
Founded in 1798
DEGREES • BSN • MSN • PHD
Nursing Program Faculty 81 (42% with doctorates).
Baccalaureate Enrollment 491 **Women** 86% **Men** 14% **Part-time** 4%
Graduate Enrollment 98 **Women** 81% **Men** 19% **Part-time** 29%
Distance Learning Courses Available.
Nursing Student Activities Sigma Theta Tau, Student Nurses' Association.
Nursing Student Resources Academic advising; academic or career counseling; assistance for students with disabilities; bookstore; campus computer network; career placement assistance; computer lab; computer-assisted instruction; e-mail services; employment services for current stu-

dents; housing assistance; interactive nursing skills videos; Internet; learning resource lab; library services; nursing audiovisuals; skills, simulation, or other laboratory; tutoring.
Library Facilities 253,595 volumes in health, 2,806 volumes in nursing; 4,329 periodical subscriptions health-care related.

BACCALAUREATE PROGRAMS

Degree BSN
Available Programs Generic Baccalaureate; RN Baccalaureate.
Site Options Owensboro, KY.
Study Options Full-time.
Online Degree Options Yes.
Program Entrance Requirements Minimum overall college GPA of 2.8, transcript of college record, CPR certification, written essay, health insurance, high school foreign language, 3 years high school math, 3 years high school science, high school transcript, immunizations, minimum high school GPA of 2.8, minimum GPA in nursing prerequisites of 2.8, professional liability insurance/malpractice insurance, prerequisite course work. Transfer students are accepted. *Application deadline:* 5/1 (fall), 9/15 (spring). *Application fee:* $50.
Advanced Placement Credit by examination available. Credit given for nursing courses completed elsewhere dependent upon specific evaluations.
Expenses (2015–16) *Tuition, state resident:* full-time $10,542; part-time $440 per credit hour. *Tuition, nonresident:* full-time $24,848; part-time $1350 per credit hour. *International tuition:* $24,848 full-time. *Required fees:* full-time $2940.
Financial Aid 100% of baccalaureate students in nursing programs received some form of financial aid in 2014–15. *Gift aid (need-based):* Federal Pell, FSEOG, state, private, college/university gift aid from institutional funds. *Loans:* Federal Nursing Student Loans, Federal Direct (Subsidized and Unsubsidized Stafford PLUS), Perkins. *Work-study:* Federal Work-Study. *Financial aid application deadline (priority):* 3/15.
Contact Trish Hart, Director of Student Services, School of Nursing, University of Louisville, 555 South Floyd Street, Louisville, KY 40202. *Telephone:* 502-852-8298. *Fax:* 502-852-8783. *E-mail:* trish.hart@louisville.edu.

GRADUATE PROGRAMS

Expenses (2015–16) *Tuition, state resident:* full-time $11,664; part-time $649 per credit hour. *Tuition, nonresident:* full-time $24,274; part-time $1350 per credit hour. *International tuition:* $36,000 full-time. *Room and board:* $8000; room only: $7000 per academic year. *Required fees:* full-time $3000.
Financial Aid 100% of graduate students in nursing programs received some form of financial aid in 2014–15. Fellowships with full tuition reimbursements available, research assistantships with full tuition reimbursements available, teaching assistantships with full tuition reimbursements available, institutionally sponsored loans, scholarships, traineeships, and unspecified assistantships available. Aid available to part-time students. *Financial aid application deadline:* 4/15.
Contact Dr. Lee Ridner, Associate Dean for Graduate Programs, School of Nursing, University of Louisville, 555 South Floyd Street, Louisville, KY 40292. *Telephone:* 502-852-8387. *Fax:* 502-852-8783. *E-mail:* slridn01@louisville.edu.

MASTER'S DEGREE PROGRAM

Degree MSN
Available Programs Accelerated Master's for Non-Nursing College Graduates.
Concentrations Available Nursing education.
Study Options Full-time.
Program Entrance Requirements Clinical experience, minimum overall college GPA of 3.0, transcript of college record, CPR certification, written essay, immunizations, 2 letters of recommendation, professional liability insurance/malpractice insurance, GRE General Test. *Application deadline:* 4/1 (fall). *Application fee:* $60.
Advanced Placement Credit given for nursing courses completed elsewhere dependent upon specific evaluations.
Degree Requirements 65 total credit hours.

DOCTORAL DEGREE PROGRAM

Degree PhD
Available Programs Doctorate; Post-Baccalaureate Doctorate.
Areas of Study Faculty preparation, health policy, individualized study, nursing research, nursing science.
Program Entrance Requirements Minimum overall college GPA of 3.0, interview by faculty committee, 3 letters of recommendation, vita,

writing sample, GRE General Test. *Application deadline:* 2/1 (fall). *Application fee:* $60.
Degree Requirements 40 total credit hours, dissertation, written exam.

POSTDOCTORAL PROGRAM

Postdoctoral Program Contact Dr. Rosalie Mainous, Associate Dean for Graduate Academic Affairs, School of Nursing, University of Louisville, 555 South Floyd Street, Louisville, KY 40292. *Telephone:* 502-852-8387. *Fax:* 502-852-8783.
E-mail: rosalie.mainous@louisville.edu.

CONTINUING EDUCATION PROGRAM

Contact Dr. Deborah Thomas, Director, School of Nursing, University of Louisville, 555 South Floyd Street, K-3019, Louisville, KY 40292. *Telephone:* 502-852-8392. *Fax:* 502-852-8783.
E-mail: dvthom01@louisville.edu.

University of Pikeville
RN to BSN Completion Program
Pikeville, Kentucky

Founded in 1889
DEGREE • BSN

BACCALAUREATE PROGRAMS

Degree BSN
Available Programs RN Baccalaureate.
Contact *Telephone:* 616-218-5750.

Western Kentucky University
School of Nursing
Bowling Green, Kentucky

http://www.wku.edu/nursing/
Founded in 1906
DEGREES • BSN • DNP • MSN
Nursing Program Faculty 51 (40% with doctorates).
Baccalaureate Enrollment 790 **Women** 93% **Men** 7% **Part-time** 30%
Graduate Enrollment 198 **Women** 96% **Men** 4% **Part-time** 75%
Distance Learning Courses Available.
Nursing Student Activities Nursing Honor Society, Sigma Theta Tau, Student Nurses' Association.
Nursing Student Resources Academic advising; academic or career counseling; assistance for students with disabilities; bookstore; campus computer network; career placement assistance; computer lab; computer-assisted instruction; e-mail services; employment services for current students; externships; housing assistance; interactive nursing skills videos; Internet; learning resource lab; library services; nursing audiovisuals; paid internships; placement services for program completers; remedial services; resume preparation assistance; skills, simulation, or other laboratory; tutoring; unpaid internships.
Library Facilities 17,880 volumes in health, 1,697 volumes in nursing; 217 periodical subscriptions health-care related.

BACCALAUREATE PROGRAMS

Degree BSN
Available Programs ADN to Baccalaureate; Baccalaureate for Second Degree; Generic Baccalaureate; RN Baccalaureate.
Study Options Full-time.
Program Entrance Requirements Minimum overall college GPA of 2.75, transcript of college record, CPR certification, health exam, health insurance, high school transcript, immunizations, minimum GPA in nursing prerequisites of 3.0, professional liability insurance/malpractice insurance, prerequisite course work. Transfer students are accepted. *Application deadline:* 1/15 (fall), 7/15 (spring).
Advanced Placement Credit by examination available. Credit given for nursing courses completed elsewhere dependent upon specific evaluations.
Expenses (2015–16) *Tuition, state resident:* full-time $9482. *Tuition, nonresident:* full-time $24,132. *International tuition:* $24,780 full-time. *Room and board:* $6530; room only: $4170 per academic year. *Required fees:* full-time $800.

Financial Aid 80% of baccalaureate students in nursing programs received some form of financial aid in 2014–15.
Contact Dr. Sherry Lovan, Program Coordinator, School of Nursing, Western Kentucky University, MCHC 2204, #11036, Bowling Green, KY 42101-3576. *Telephone:* 270-745-4379. *Fax:* 270-745-3392. *E-mail:* sherry.lovan@wku.edu.

GRADUATE PROGRAMS

Expenses (2015–16) *Tuition, state resident:* part-time $652 per credit hour. *Tuition, nonresident:* part-time $833 per credit hour.
Financial Aid 50% of graduate students in nursing programs received some form of financial aid in 2014–15. Research assistantships with partial tuition reimbursements available, teaching assistantships with partial tuition reimbursements available, Federal Work-Study, institutionally sponsored loans, traineeships, tuition waivers (partial), and unspecified assistantships available. Aid available to part-time students. *Financial aid application deadline:* 4/1.
Contact Dr. Beverly C. Siegrist, Professor, School of Nursing, Western Kentucky University, MCHC 3340, #11036, Bowling Green, KY 42101. *Telephone:* 270-745-3490. *Fax:* 270-745-3392. *E-mail:* beverly.siegrist@wku.edu.

MASTER'S DEGREE PROGRAM

Degree MSN
Available Programs Accelerated Master's for Nurses with Non-Nursing Degrees; Master's.
Concentrations Available Nursing administration; nursing education. *Nurse practitioner programs in:* psychiatric/mental health.
Study Options Full-time and part-time.
Online Degree Options Yes.
Program Entrance Requirements Clinical experience, computer literacy, minimum overall college GPA of 2.75, transcript of college record, CPR certification, written essay, immunizations, interview, 3 letters of recommendation, nursing research course, physical assessment course, professional liability insurance/malpractice insurance, statistics course, GRE General Test. *Application deadline:* Applications may be processed on a rolling basis for some programs. *Application fee:* $60.
Advanced Placement Credit given for nursing courses completed elsewhere dependent upon specific evaluations.
Degree Requirements 45 total credit hours, thesis or project, comprehensive exam.

POST-MASTER'S PROGRAM

Areas of Study Nursing administration; nursing education. *Nurse practitioner programs in:* family health, psychiatric/mental health.

DOCTORAL DEGREE PROGRAM

Degree DNP
Available Programs Doctorate; Post-Baccalaureate Doctorate.
Areas of Study Advanced practice nursing, nursing policy.
Program Entrance Requirements Clinical experience, minimum overall college GPA of 3.25, interview by faculty committee, statistics course, writing sample. Application deadline: Applications may be processed on a rolling basis for some programs. Application fee: $100.
Degree Requirements 76 total credit hours, written exam, residency.

CONTINUING EDUCATION PROGRAM

Contact Ms. Kim Vickous, School of Nursing, Western Kentucky University, MCHC 2220, #11036, Bowling Green, KY 42101-3576. *Telephone:* 270-745-3876. *Fax:* 270-745-3392. *E-mail:* kim.vickous@wku.edu.

LOUISIANA

Dillard University
Division of Nursing
New Orleans, Louisiana

http://www.dillard.edu/index.php?option=com_content&view =article&id=106&Itemid=91
Founded in 1869
DEGREE • BSN
Nursing Program Faculty 13 (31% with doctorates).

Baccalaureate Enrollment 100 **Women** 98% **Men** 2%
Nursing Student Activities Nursing Honor Society, Sigma Theta Tau, Student Nurses' Association.
Nursing Student Resources Academic advising; academic or career counseling; assistance for students with disabilities; bookstore; campus computer network; career placement assistance; computer lab; computer-assisted instruction; e-mail services; externships; interactive nursing skills videos; Internet; learning resource lab; library services; nursing audiovisuals; paid internships; placement services for program completers; remedial services; resume preparation assistance; skills, simulation, or other laboratory; tutoring.
Library Facilities 21 periodical subscriptions health-care related.

BACCALAUREATE PROGRAMS

Degree BSN
Available Programs Generic Baccalaureate; LPN to RN Baccalaureate; RN Baccalaureate.
Study Options Full-time.
Program Entrance Requirements Minimum overall college GPA of 2.7, transcript of college record, CPR certification, health exam, health insurance, high school transcript, immunizations, interview, minimum GPA in nursing prerequisites of 2.7, professional liability insurance/malpractice insurance, prerequisite course work. Transfer students are accepted. *Application deadline:* 3/1 (fall).
Advanced Placement Credit by examination available.
Expenses (2015–16) *Tuition:* full-time $15,308; part-time $171 per credit hour. *Room and board:* $5408 per academic year. *Required fees:* full-time $1600; part-time $800 per term.
Contact Dr. Sharon Hutchinson, School of Nursing, Division of Nursing, Dillard University, 2601 Gentilly Boulevard, New Orleans, LA 70122. *Telephone:* 504-816-4717. *Fax:* 504-816-4137. *E-mail:* shutchinson@dillard.edu.

CONTINUING EDUCATION PROGRAM

Contact Dr. Charlotte Hurst, Coordinator, Continuing Education, Division of Nursing, Dillard University, 2601 Gentilly Boulevard, PSB 102, New Orleans, LA 70122. *Telephone:* 504-816-4717. *Fax:* 504-816-4861. *E-mail:* churst@dillard.edu.

Grambling State University
School of Nursing
Grambling, Louisiana

http://www.gram.edu/
Founded in 1901
DEGREES • BSN • MSN
Nursing Program Faculty 23 (20% with doctorates).
Baccalaureate Enrollment 600 **Women** 85% **Men** 15% **Part-time** 5%
Graduate Enrollment 41 **Women** 86% **Men** 14%
Distance Learning Courses Available.
Nursing Student Activities Student Nurses' Association.
Nursing Student Resources Academic advising; academic or career counseling; assistance for students with disabilities; bookstore; campus computer network; career placement assistance; computer lab; computer-assisted instruction; e-mail services; employment services for current students; interactive nursing skills videos; Internet; learning resource lab; library services; nursing audiovisuals; skills, simulation, or other laboratory; tutoring.
Library Facilities 10,000 volumes in health, 5,000 volumes in nursing; 65 periodical subscriptions health-care related.

BACCALAUREATE PROGRAMS

Degree BSN
Available Programs Generic Baccalaureate; LPN to RN Baccalaureate; RN Baccalaureate.
Study Options Full-time.
Program Entrance Requirements Transcript of college record, CPR certification, health exam, high school foreign language, 3 years high school math, 3 years high school science, high school transcript, immunizations, minimum high school GPA of 2.0, minimum GPA in nursing prerequisites of 2.75, professional liability insurance/malpractice insurance, prerequisite course work. Transfer students are accepted. *Application deadline:* 6/1 (fall), 12/1 (spring). *Application fee:* $20.
Advanced Placement Credit given for nursing courses completed elsewhere dependent upon specific evaluations.
Contact *Telephone:* 318-274-2528. *Fax:* 318-274-3491.

GRADUATE PROGRAMS

Contact *Telephone:* 318-274-2897. *Fax:* 318-274-3491.

MASTER'S DEGREE PROGRAM
Degree MSN
Available Programs Master's.
Concentrations Available Nursing education. *Clinical nurse specialist programs in:* adult health, maternity-newborn, pediatric. *Nurse practitioner programs in:* family health, pediatric.
Study Options Full-time and part-time.
Program Entrance Requirements Clinical experience, minimum overall college GPA of 3.0, transcript of college record, CPR certification, immunizations, interview, 3 letters of recommendation, physical assessment course, professional liability insurance/malpractice insurance, prerequisite course work, statistics course, GRE. *Application deadline:* 6/1 (fall). *Application fee:* $20.
Advanced Placement Credit given for nursing courses completed elsewhere dependent upon specific evaluations.
Degree Requirements 49 total credit hours, thesis or project, comprehensive exam.

POST-MASTER'S PROGRAM
Areas of Study *Nurse practitioner programs in:* family health.

Louisiana College
Department of Nursing
Pineville, Louisiana

http://www.lacollege.edu/
Founded in 1906
DEGREE • BSN
Nursing Program Faculty 6 (17% with doctorates).
Baccalaureate Enrollment 100
Nursing Student Activities Sigma Theta Tau, Student Nurses' Association.
Nursing Student Resources Academic advising; academic or career counseling; assistance for students with disabilities; bookstore; campus computer network; career placement assistance; computer lab; computer-assisted instruction; e-mail services; employment services for current students; externships; Internet; learning resource lab; library services; nursing audiovisuals; skills, simulation, or other laboratory; tutoring; unpaid internships.
Library Facilities 3,426 volumes in health, 500 volumes in nursing; 142 periodical subscriptions health-care related.

BACCALAUREATE PROGRAMS

Degree BSN
Available Programs Generic Baccalaureate.
Study Options Full-time.
Program Entrance Requirements Minimum overall college GPA of 2.6, transcript of college record, CPR certification, health exam, health insurance, immunizations, interview, minimum high school GPA of 2.0, minimum high school rank 50%, minimum GPA in nursing prerequisites of 2.6, professional liability insurance/malpractice insurance, prerequisite course work. Transfer students are accepted.
Advanced Placement Credit given for nursing courses completed elsewhere dependent upon specific evaluations.
Contact *Telephone:* 318-487-7127. *Fax:* 318-487-7488.

Louisiana State University at Alexandria
Nursing Program
Alexandria, Louisiana

Founded in 1960
DEGREE • BSN

BACCALAUREATE PROGRAMS

Degree BSN
Available Programs RN Baccalaureate.
Program Entrance Requirements Minimum overall college GPA of 2.5, RN licensure.
Contact *Telephone:* 318-473-6417.

Louisiana State University Health Sciences Center
School of Nursing
New Orleans, Louisiana

https://nursing.lsuhsc.edu/
Founded in 1931
DEGREES • BSN • DNP
Nursing Program Faculty 78 (43% with doctorates).
Baccalaureate Enrollment 739 **Women** 87% **Men** 13% **Part-time** 28%
Graduate Enrollment 278 **Women** 76% **Men** 24% **Part-time** 44%
Nursing Student Activities Nursing Honor Society, Sigma Theta Tau, Student Nurses' Association.
Nursing Student Resources Academic advising; academic or career counseling; assistance for students with disabilities; bookstore; campus computer network; computer lab; computer-assisted instruction; e-mail services; housing assistance; interactive nursing skills videos; Internet; learning resource lab; library services; nursing audiovisuals; skills, simulation, or other laboratory; tutoring.
Library Facilities 215,833 volumes in health, 9,490 volumes in nursing; 5,389 periodical subscriptions health-care related.

BACCALAUREATE PROGRAMS

Degree BSN
Available Programs Accelerated Baccalaureate for Second Degree; Generic Baccalaureate; RN Baccalaureate.
Study Options Full-time and part-time.
Program Entrance Requirements Minimum overall college GPA of 2.0, transcript of college record, written essay, interview, minimum GPA in nursing prerequisites of 2.8, prerequisite course work. Transfer students are accepted. *Application deadline:* 1/15 (fall), 8/15 (spring). *Application fee:* $50.
Financial Aid 79% of baccalaureate students in nursing programs received some form of financial aid in 2013–14.
Contact Dr. Catherine Lopez, Assistant Dean for Student Services, School of Nursing, Louisiana State University Health Sciences Center, 1900 Gravier Street, New Orleans, LA 70112. *Telephone:* 504-568-4180. *Fax:* 504-568-5853. *E-mail:* clopez@lsuhsc.edu.

GRADUATE PROGRAMS

Financial Aid 66% of graduate students in nursing programs received some form of financial aid in 2013–14. Federal Work-Study, institutionally sponsored loans, scholarships, and traineeships available.
Contact Dr. Catherine Lopez, Assistant Dean for Student Services, School of Nursing, Louisiana State University Health Sciences Center, 1900 Gravier Street, New Orleans, LA 70112. *Telephone:* 504-568-4180. *Fax:* 504-568-5853. *E-mail:* clopez@lsuhsc.edu.

MASTER'S DEGREE PROGRAM
Program Entrance Requirements GRE General Test, MAT. *Application deadline:* 2/1 (fall), 9/1 (spring), 1/15 (summer). *Application fee:* $100.

DOCTORAL DEGREE PROGRAM
Degree DNP
Available Programs Doctorate.
Areas of Study Advanced practice nursing, clinical practice, community health, gerontology, maternity-newborn, nursing administration.
Program Entrance Requirements Clinical experience, minimum overall college GPA of 3.5, interview, 3 letters of recommendation, MSN or equivalent, scholarly papers, vita, writing sample, GRE General Test. Application deadline: 2/1 (fall), 9/1 (spring). Application fee: $50.
Degree Requirements 54 total credit hours, dissertation, oral exam.

POSTDOCTORAL PROGRAM
Postdoctoral Program Contact Dr. Anita Hufft, Associate Dean, School of Nursing, Louisiana State University Health Sciences Center, 1900 Gravier Street, New Orleans, LA 70112. *Telephone:* 504-568-4107. *Fax:* 504-568-5853. *E-mail:* ahufft@lsuhsc.edu.

CONTINUING EDUCATION PROGRAM
Contact Ms. Alicia Dean, RN, Coordinator of Continuing Nursing Education, School of Nursing, Louisiana State University Health Sciences Center, 1900 Gravier Street, New Orleans, LA 70112. *Telephone:* 504-568-4202. *E-mail:* adean2@lsuhsc.edu.

Loyola University New Orleans
School of Nursing
New Orleans, Louisiana

http://www.css.loyno.edu/nursing
Founded in 1912
DEGREES • BSN • DNP • MSN
Nursing Program Faculty 32 (69% with doctorates).
Baccalaureate Enrollment 15 **Women** 98% **Men** 2% **Part-time** 100%
Graduate Enrollment 574 **Women** 93% **Men** 7% **Part-time** 73%
Distance Learning Courses Available.
Nursing Student Activities Sigma Theta Tau.
Nursing Student Resources Academic advising; academic or career counseling; assistance for students with disabilities; bookstore; campus computer network; career placement assistance; computer lab; computer-assisted instruction; e-mail services; interactive nursing skills videos; Internet; learning resource lab; library services; nursing audiovisuals; skills, simulation, or other laboratory; tutoring.
Library Facilities 6,881 volumes in health, 913 volumes in nursing; 6,716 periodical subscriptions health-care related.

BACCALAUREATE PROGRAMS

Degree BSN
Available Programs RN Baccalaureate.
Study Options Full-time and part-time.
Online Degree Options Yes (online only).
Program Entrance Requirements Minimum overall college GPA of 2.5, transcript of college record, written essay, immunizations, minimum GPA in nursing prerequisites of 2.0, professional liability insurance/malpractice insurance, RN licensure. Transfer students are accepted. *Application deadline:* Applications may be processed on a rolling basis for some programs. *Application fee:* $40.
Advanced Placement Credit by examination available. Credit given for nursing courses completed elsewhere dependent upon specific evaluations.
Expenses (2014–15) *Tuition:* part-time $506 per credit hour.
Financial Aid 98% of baccalaureate students in nursing programs received some form of financial aid in 2013–14.
Contact Mrs. Valerie Garcia, Administrative Assistant, School of Nursing, Loyola University New Orleans, 6363 St. Charles Avenue, Campus Box 45, New Orleans, LA 70118. *Telephone:* 504-865-3250. *Fax:* 504-865-3254. *E-mail:* vgarcia@gmail.com.

GRADUATE PROGRAMS

Expenses (2014–15) *Tuition:* part-time $818 per credit hour.
Financial Aid 82% of graduate students in nursing programs received some form of financial aid in 2013–14. Traineeships and Incumbent Workers Training Program grants available. *Financial aid application deadline:* 5/1.
Contact Ms. Shauna Crowden, Office Manager, School of Nursing, Loyola University New Orleans, 6363 St. Charles Avenue, Campus Box 45, New Orleans, LA 70118. *Telephone:* 504-865-2643. *Fax:* 504-865-3254. *E-mail:* nursing@loyno.edu.

MASTER'S DEGREE PROGRAM
Degree MSN
Available Programs Master's; Master's for Nurses with Non-Nursing Degrees.
Concentrations Available Health-care administration; nurse case management.
Study Options Full-time and part-time.
Online Degree Options Yes.
Program Entrance Requirements Clinical experience, minimum overall college GPA of 3.0, transcript of college record, CPR certification, written essay, immunizations, interview, 3 letters of recommendation, nursing research course, professional liability insurance/malpractice insurance, prerequisite course work, statistics course. *Application deadline:* Applications may be processed on a rolling basis for some programs. *Application fee:* $40.
Advanced Placement Credit given for nursing courses completed elsewhere dependent upon specific evaluations.
Degree Requirements 36 total credit hours, thesis or project.

POST-MASTER'S PROGRAM
Areas of Study *Nurse practitioner programs in:* adult health, family health.

DOCTORAL DEGREE PROGRAM
Degree DNP
Available Programs Doctorate; Post-Baccalaureate Doctorate.
Areas of Study Advanced practice nursing, clinical practice, faculty preparation, family health, nursing administration.
Online Degree Options Yes (online only).
Program Entrance Requirements Clinical experience, minimum overall college GPA of 3.2, interview by faculty committee, interview, 3 letters of recommendation, MSN or equivalent, statistics course, vita, writing sample. Application deadline: 11/15 (fall), 2/1 (spring). Application fee: $75.
Degree Requirements 78 total credit hours, dissertation, written exam, residency.

McNeese State University
College of Nursing
Lake Charles, Louisiana

http://www.mcneese.edu/
Founded in 1939
DEGREES • BSN • MSN
Nursing Program Faculty 59 (23% with doctorates).
Baccalaureate Enrollment 1,031 **Women** 83% **Men** 17% **Part-time** 11%
Graduate Enrollment 132 **Women** 78% **Men** 22% **Part-time** 88%
Distance Learning Courses Available.
Nursing Student Activities Sigma Theta Tau, Student Nurses' Association.
Nursing Student Resources Academic advising; academic or career counseling; assistance for students with disabilities; bookstore; campus computer network; career placement assistance; computer lab; computer-assisted instruction; daycare for children of students; e-mail services; employment services for current students; housing assistance; interactive nursing skills videos; Internet; learning resource lab; library services; nursing audiovisuals; placement services for program completers; resume preparation assistance; skills, simulation, or other laboratory; tutoring.
Library Facilities 41,000 volumes in health, 27,500 volumes in nursing; 120 periodical subscriptions health-care related.

BACCALAUREATE PROGRAMS

Degree BSN
Available Programs ADN to Baccalaureate; Generic Baccalaureate; LPN to Baccalaureate; LPN to RN Baccalaureate.
Study Options Full-time and part-time.
Program Entrance Requirements Minimum overall college GPA of 2.7, transcript of college record, CPR certification, health exam, health insurance, high school transcript, immunizations, minimum high school GPA of 2.5, minimum GPA in nursing prerequisites of 2.7, prerequisite course work. Transfer students are accepted. *Application deadline:* 10/15 (fall), 3/24 (spring). *Application fee:* $30.
Advanced Placement Credit by examination available. Credit given for nursing courses completed elsewhere dependent upon specific evaluations.
Expenses (2015–16) *Tuition, state resident:* full-time $2769; part-time $841 per course. *Tuition, nonresident:* full-time $7862; part-time $841 per course. *Room and board:* $580; room only: $275 per academic year. *Required fees:* full-time $60.
Financial Aid 89% of baccalaureate students in nursing programs received some form of financial aid in 2014–15. *Gift aid (need-based):* Federal Pell, FSEOG, state. *Loans:* Federal Direct (Subsidized Stafford), Perkins. *Work-study:* Federal Work-Study, part-time campus jobs. *Financial aid application deadline (priority):* 5/1.
Contact Dr. Peggy L. Wolfe, Dean and Professor, College of Nursing, McNeese State University, PO Box 90415, Lake Charles, LA 70609-0415. *Telephone:* 337-475-5820. *Fax:* 337-475-5924. *E-mail:* pwolfe@mail.mcneese.edu.

GRADUATE PROGRAMS

Expenses (2015–16) *Tuition, state resident:* full-time $3009; part-time $934 per course. *Tuition, nonresident:* full-time $8102.
Contact Dr. Peggy Wolfe, Dean, College of Nursing, McNeese State University, PO Box 90415, Lake Charles, LA 70609-0415. *Telephone:* 337-475-5820. *Fax:* 337-475-5702. *E-mail:* pwolfe@mcneese.edu.

MASTER'S DEGREE PROGRAM
Degree MSN

Available Programs Master's.

Concentrations Available Nursing administration; nursing education. *Nurse practitioner programs in:* family health, psychiatric/mental health.

Site Options Baton Rouge, LA; Lafayette, LA; Lake Charles, LA.

Study Options Full-time and part-time.

Online Degree Options Yes (online only).

Program Entrance Requirements Minimum overall college GPA of 2.7, transcript of college record, written essay, immunizations, 2 letters of recommendation, physical assessment course, statistics course, GRE. *Application deadline:* 5/15 (fall), 11/1 (spring). *Application fee:* $20.

Advanced Placement Credit given for nursing courses completed elsewhere dependent upon specific evaluations.

Degree Requirements 46 total credit hours, thesis or project.

POST-MASTER'S PROGRAM

Areas of Study *Nurse practitioner programs in:* family health, psychiatric/mental health.

CONTINUING EDUCATION PROGRAM

Contact Dr. Rhonda LeJeune Johnson, Continuing Education Coordinator, College of Nursing, McNeese State University, PO Box 90415, Lake Charles, LA 70609-0415. *Telephone:* 337-475-5929. *Fax:* 337-475-5924. *E-mail:* MSUconCE@mcneese.edu.

Nicholls State University
Department of Nursing
Thibodaux, Louisiana

http://www.nicholls.edu/nursing/
Founded in 1948

DEGREE • BSN
Nursing Program Faculty 19 (21% with doctorates).

BACCALAUREATE PROGRAMS

Degree BSN

Available Programs Generic Baccalaureate; LPN to Baccalaureate; RN Baccalaureate.

Program Entrance Requirements Minimum overall college GPA of 2.75, transcript of college record, minimum GPA in nursing prerequisites of 2.0, prerequisite course work. Transfer students are accepted.

Contact *Telephone:* 985-448-4696. *Fax:* 985-448-4932.

CONTINUING EDUCATION PROGRAM

Contact *Telephone:* 985-448-4696. *Fax:* 985-448-4932.

Northwestern State University of Louisiana
College of Nursing and School of Allied Health
Shreveport, Louisiana

http://www.nsula.edu/nursing
Founded in 1884

DEGREES • BSN • DNP • MSN
Nursing Program Faculty 73 (16% with doctorates).
Baccalaureate Enrollment 1,196 **Women** 85% **Men** 15% **Part-time** 40%
Graduate Enrollment 252 **Women** 87% **Men** 13% **Part-time** 94%
Distance Learning Courses Available.
Nursing Student Activities Sigma Theta Tau, Student Nurses' Association.
Nursing Student Resources Academic advising; academic or career counseling; assistance for students with disabilities; bookstore; campus computer network; computer lab; computer-assisted instruction; e-mail services; employment services for current students; interactive nursing skills videos; Internet; learning resource lab; library services; nursing audiovisuals; remedial services; resume preparation assistance; skills, simulation, or other laboratory; tutoring.
Library Facilities 4,443 volumes in health, 3,047 volumes in nursing; 1,360 periodical subscriptions health-care related.

BACCALAUREATE PROGRAMS

Degree BSN

Available Programs ADN to Baccalaureate; Generic Baccalaureate; LPN to Baccalaureate; RN Baccalaureate.

Site Options Alexandria, LA.

Study Options Full-time and part-time.

Online Degree Options Yes.

Program Entrance Requirements Minimum overall college GPA of 2.0, transcript of college record, CPR certification, health exam, health insurance, high school transcript, immunizations, minimum GPA in nursing prerequisites of 2.7, prerequisite course work. Transfer students are accepted. *Application deadline:* 5/15 (fall), 8/15 (spring). *Application fee:* $20.

Advanced Placement Credit by examination available. Credit given for nursing courses completed elsewhere dependent upon specific evaluations.

Expenses (2014–15) *Tuition, state resident:* full-time $7401. *Tuition, nonresident:* full-time $23,493. *Room and board:* $15,766; room only: $10,741 per academic year. *Required fees:* full-time $3273.

Financial Aid 80% of baccalaureate students in nursing programs received some form of financial aid in 2013–14.

Contact Ms. Linda Copple, Program Director, BSN Program, College of Nursing and School of Allied Health, Northwestern State University of Louisiana, 1800 Line Avenue, Shreveport, LA 71101. *Telephone:* 318-677-3100. *Fax:* 318-677-3127. *E-mail:* copplel@nsula.edu.

GRADUATE PROGRAMS

Expenses (2014–15) *Tuition, state resident:* full-time $8754. *Tuition, nonresident:* full-time $24,846. *Required fees:* full-time $3096.

Financial Aid 25% of graduate students in nursing programs received some form of financial aid in 2013–14. Career-related internships or fieldwork and Federal Work-Study available. Aid available to part-time students. *Financial aid application deadline:* 5/1.

Contact Dr. Connie Mott, Coordinator, Graduate Studies and Research in Nursing, College of Nursing and School of Allied Health, Northwestern State University of Louisiana, 1800 Line Avenue, Shreveport, LA 71101. *Telephone:* 318-677-3100. *Fax:* 318-677-3127. *E-mail:* roppoloc@nsula.edu.

MASTER'S DEGREE PROGRAM

Degree MSN

Available Programs Master's.

Concentrations Available Nursing administration; nursing education. *Nurse practitioner programs in:* adult-gerontology acute care, family health, pediatric primary care, women's health.

Site Options Alexandria, LA.

Study Options Full-time and part-time.

Program Entrance Requirements Clinical experience, minimum overall college GPA of 3.0, transcript of college record, CPR certification, immunizations, 2 letters of recommendation, professional liability insurance/malpractice insurance, GRE General Test. *Application deadline:* 6/1 (fall). *Application fee:* $20.

Advanced Placement Credit given for nursing courses completed elsewhere dependent upon specific evaluations.

Degree Requirements 39 total credit hours, thesis or project, comprehensive exam.

POST-MASTER'S PROGRAM

Areas of Study *Nurse practitioner programs in:* adult-gerontology acute care, family health, pediatric primary care, women's health.

DOCTORAL DEGREE PROGRAM

Degree DNP

Available Programs Doctorate.

Areas of Study Clinical practice.

Online Degree Options Yes (online only).

Program Entrance Requirements Clinical experience, minimum overall college GPA of 3.0, interview by faculty committee, interview, 3 letters of recommendation, MSN or equivalent, vita, writing sample. Application deadline: 5/15 (fall). Application fee: $20.

Degree Requirements 38 total credit hours.

CONTINUING EDUCATION PROGRAM

Contact Ms. Heather Hayter, Lead Nurse Planner, College of Nursing and School of Allied Health, Northwestern State University of Louisiana, 1800 Line Avenue, Shreveport, LA 71101. *Telephone:* 318-677-3105. *Fax:* 318-677-3127. *E-mail:* hayterh@nsula.edu.

Our Lady of Holy Cross College
Division of Nursing
New Orleans, Louisiana

http://www.olhcc.edu/
Founded in 1916
DEGREE • BSN
Nursing Program Faculty 16 (32% with doctorates).
Baccalaureate Enrollment 168 **Women** 90% **Men** 10% **Part-time** 11%
Nursing Student Activities Sigma Theta Tau, Student Nurses' Association, nursing club.
Nursing Student Resources Academic advising; academic or career counseling; assistance for students with disabilities; bookstore; campus computer network; career placement assistance; computer lab; computer-assisted instruction; e-mail services; interactive nursing skills videos; Internet; learning resource lab; library services; nursing audiovisuals; remedial services; resume preparation assistance; skills, simulation, or other laboratory; tutoring.
Library Facilities 5,000 volumes in health, 3,100 volumes in nursing; 103 periodical subscriptions health-care related.

BACCALAUREATE PROGRAMS
Degree BSN
Available Programs Generic Baccalaureate.
Study Options Full-time.
Program Entrance Requirements Minimum overall college GPA of 2.5, transcript of college record, CPR certification, written essay, health exam, health insurance, high school transcript, immunizations, 3 letters of recommendation, minimum high school GPA of 2.0, minimum GPA in nursing prerequisites of 2.5, professional liability insurance/malpractice insurance, prerequisite course work. Transfer students are accepted.
Advanced Placement Credit by examination available. Credit given for nursing courses completed elsewhere dependent upon specific evaluations.
Contact *Telephone:* 504-398-2215. *Fax:* 504-391-2421.

Our Lady of the Lake College
Division of Nursing
Baton Rouge, Louisiana

http://www.ollusa.edu/s/1190/start2012.aspx
Founded in 1990
DEGREES • BSN • MSN
Nursing Program Faculty 38 (21% with doctorates).
Baccalaureate Enrollment 265 **Women** 85% **Men** 15% **Part-time** 19%
Graduate Enrollment 87 **Women** 45% **Men** 55%
Distance Learning Courses Available.
Nursing Student Activities Nursing Honor Society, Student Nurses' Association.
Nursing Student Resources Academic advising; academic or career counseling; assistance for students with disabilities; bookstore; campus computer network; career placement assistance; computer lab; computer-assisted instruction; e-mail services; employment services for current students; interactive nursing skills videos; Internet; learning resource lab; library services; nursing audiovisuals; paid internships; remedial services; resume preparation assistance; skills, simulation, or other laboratory; tutoring.
Library Facilities 10,000 volumes in health, 1,000 volumes in nursing; 200 periodical subscriptions health-care related.

BACCALAUREATE PROGRAMS
Degree BSN
Available Programs ADN to Baccalaureate; Accelerated Baccalaureate for Second Degree; Generic Baccalaureate; LPN to Baccalaureate; RN Baccalaureate.
Study Options Full-time.
Online Degree Options Yes.
Program Entrance Requirements Minimum overall college GPA of 2.0, transcript of college record, CPR certification, written essay, health exam, health insurance, immunizations, minimum GPA in nursing prerequisites of 2.75, professional liability insurance/malpractice insurance, prerequisite course work. Transfer students are accepted. *Application deadline:* 1/15 (fall), 7/15 (spring). *Application fee:* $35.

Advanced Placement Credit given for nursing courses completed elsewhere dependent upon specific evaluations.
Contact *Telephone:* 225-768-1793. *Fax:* 225-768-1760.

GRADUATE PROGRAMS
Contact *Telephone:* 225-768-1779. *Fax:* 225-768-1760.

MASTER'S DEGREE PROGRAM
Degree MSN
Available Programs Master's.
Concentrations Available Nurse anesthesia; nursing administration; nursing education.
Study Options Full-time.
Program Entrance Requirements Clinical experience, minimum overall college GPA of 3.3, transcript of college record, interview, 3 letters of recommendation, nursing research course, physical assessment course, statistics course. *Application deadline:* 12/1 (fall), 7/15 (spring). *Application fee:* $35.
Advanced Placement Credit given for nursing courses completed elsewhere dependent upon specific evaluations.
Degree Requirements 80 total credit hours, thesis or project.

CONTINUING EDUCATION PROGRAM
Contact *Telephone:* 225-768-1708. *Fax:* 225-214-1940.

Southeastern Louisiana University
School of Nursing
Hammond, Louisiana

http://www.selu.edu/acad_research/depts/nurs
Founded in 1925
DEGREES • BS • DNP • MSN
Nursing Program Faculty 65 (30% with doctorates).
Baccalaureate Enrollment 1,383 **Women** 86.5% **Men** 13.5% **Part-time** 14%
Graduate Enrollment 175 **Women** 89.7% **Men** 10.3% **Part-time** 76.6%
Distance Learning Courses Available.
Nursing Student Activities Nursing Honor Society, Sigma Theta Tau, Student Nurses' Association.
Nursing Student Resources Academic advising; academic or career counseling; assistance for students with disabilities; bookstore; campus computer network; career placement assistance; computer lab; computer-assisted instruction; e-mail services; employment services for current students; interactive nursing skills videos; Internet; learning resource lab; library services; nursing audiovisuals; other; resume preparation assistance; skills, simulation, or other laboratory; tutoring.
Library Facilities 23,099 volumes in health, 3,609 volumes in nursing; 175 periodical subscriptions health-care related.

BACCALAUREATE PROGRAMS
Degree BS
Available Programs Accelerated Baccalaureate for Second Degree; Generic Baccalaureate; LPN to RN Baccalaureate; RN Baccalaureate.
Site Options Baton Rouge, LA.
Study Options Full-time and part-time.
Online Degree Options Yes.
Program Entrance Requirements Minimum overall college GPA of 2.0, CPR certification, health exam, high school biology, high school chemistry, 4 years high school math, 4 years high school science, high school transcript, immunizations, minimum high school GPA of 2.0, minimum GPA in nursing prerequisites of 3.0, prerequisite course work. Transfer students are accepted. *Application deadline:* 7/15 (fall), 12/1 (spring), 5/1 (summer). Applications may be processed on a rolling basis for some programs. *Application fee:* $20.
Advanced Placement Credit given for nursing courses completed elsewhere dependent upon specific evaluations.
Expenses (2015–16) *Tuition, area resident:* full-time $5278. *Tuition, state resident:* full-time $5278; part-time $303 per credit hour. *Tuition, nonresident:* full-time $17,756; part-time $796 per credit hour. *International tuition:* $17,756 full-time. *Room and board:* $7370; room only: $4660 per academic year. *Required fees:* full-time $2002.
Financial Aid 54% of baccalaureate students in nursing programs received some form of financial aid in 2014–15. *Gift aid (need-based):*

Federal Pell, FSEOG, state, private, college/university gift aid from institutional funds. *Loans:* Federal Direct (Subsidized and Unsubsidized Stafford PLUS), Perkins, college/university. *Work-study:* Federal Work-Study, part-time campus jobs. *Financial aid application deadline (priority):* 5/1.

Contact Dr. Eileen Creel, Department Head, School of Nursing, Southeastern Louisiana University, SLU 10835, Hammond, LA 70402. *Telephone:* 985-549-2156. *Fax:* 985-549-2869. *E-mail:* nursing@selu.edu.

GRADUATE PROGRAMS

Expenses (2015–16) *Tuition, state resident:* full-time $6107; part-time $436 per credit hour. *Tuition, nonresident:* full-time $18,584; part-time $1129 per credit hour. *International tuition:* $18,584 full-time. *Room and board:* $7370; room only: $4660 per academic year. *Required fees:* full-time $1737.

Financial Aid Federal Work-Study, institutionally sponsored loans, scholarships, traineeships, and unspecified assistantships available.

Contact Dr. Ann Carruth, Dean of Nursing, School of Nursing, Southeastern Louisiana University, SLU 10448, Hammond, LA 70402. *Telephone:* 985-549-2156. *Fax:* 985-549-2869. *E-mail:* nursing@selu.edu.

MASTER'S DEGREE PROGRAM

Degree MSN

Available Programs Master's.

Concentrations Available Nursing administration. *Nurse practitioner programs in:* family health, psychiatric/mental health.

Site Options Lake Charles, LA; Lafayette, LA.

Study Options Full-time and part-time.

Online Degree Options Yes.

Program Entrance Requirements Clinical experience, minimum overall college GPA of 2.7, transcript of college record, written essay, immunizations, letters of recommendation, physical assessment course, prerequisite course work, resume, statistics course, GRE (verbal and quantitative). *Application deadline:* 7/15 (fall), 12/1 (spring), 5/1 (summer). Applications may be processed on a rolling basis for some programs. *Application fee:* $20.

Advanced Placement Credit given for nursing courses completed elsewhere dependent upon specific evaluations.

Degree Requirements 39 total credit hours, thesis or project.

POST-MASTER'S PROGRAM

Areas of Study *Nurse practitioner programs in:* family health, psychiatric/mental health.

DOCTORAL DEGREE PROGRAM

Degree DNP

Available Programs Doctorate.

Site Options Lafayette, LA.

Program Entrance Requirements Minimum overall college GPA of 3.3, interview, 3 letters of recommendation, MSN or equivalent, vita. Application deadline: 7/15 (fall), 12/1 (spring), 5/1 (summer). Applications may be processed on a rolling basis for some programs. Application fee: $20.

Degree Requirements 39 total credit hours.

Southern University and Agricultural and Mechanical College

School of Nursing
Baton Rouge, Louisiana

http://www.subr.edu/
Founded in 1880
DEGREES • BSN • MSN • PHD
Nursing Program Faculty 36 (3% with doctorates).
Baccalaureate Enrollment 1,020 **Women** 91% **Men** 9% **Part-time** 12%
Nursing Student Activities Nursing Honor Society, Student Nurses' Association, nursing club.
Nursing Student Resources Academic advising; academic or career counseling; assistance for students with disabilities; bookstore; campus computer network; computer lab; computer-assisted instruction; e-mail services; interactive nursing skills videos; Internet; learning resource lab;

library services; nursing audiovisuals; resume preparation assistance; skills, simulation, or other laboratory; tutoring.
Library Facilities 4,220 volumes in health, 716 volumes in nursing; 114 periodical subscriptions health-care related.

BACCALAUREATE PROGRAMS

Degree BSN

Available Programs Generic Baccalaureate.

Study Options Full-time and part-time.

Program Entrance Requirements Minimum overall college GPA of 2.6, CPR certification, health exam, immunizations, minimum GPA in nursing prerequisites, prerequisite course work. Transfer students are accepted.

Contact *Telephone:* 225-771-3416. *Fax:* 225-771-2651.

GRADUATE PROGRAMS

Contact *Telephone:* 225-771-2663. *Fax:* 225-771-3547.

MASTER'S DEGREE PROGRAM

Degree MSN

Available Programs Master's.

Concentrations Available Health-care administration; nursing education. *Clinical nurse specialist programs in:* family health. *Nurse practitioner programs in:* family health.

Study Options Full-time and part-time.

Program Entrance Requirements Minimum overall college GPA of 3.0, transcript of college record, 3 letters of recommendation, physical assessment course, statistics course, GRE General Test.

Degree Requirements 46 total credit hours, thesis or project, comprehensive exam.

POST-MASTER'S PROGRAM

Areas of Study *Nurse practitioner programs in:* family health.

DOCTORAL DEGREE PROGRAM

Degree PhD

Areas of Study Advanced practice nursing, nursing education, nursing research, women's health.

Program Entrance Requirements Clinical experience, minimum overall college GPA of 3.2, interview by faculty committee, 3 letters of recommendation, MSN or equivalent, scholarly papers, statistics course, vita, writing sample, GRE General Test.

Degree Requirements 60 total credit hours, dissertation, written exam.

University of Louisiana at Lafayette

College of Nursing
Lafayette, Louisiana

http://www.nursing.louisiana.edu/
Founded in 1898
DEGREES • BSN • MSN
Nursing Program Faculty 47 (13% with doctorates).
Baccalaureate Enrollment 1,354 **Women** 83% **Men** 17% **Part-time** 10%
Distance Learning Courses Available.
Nursing Student Activities Nursing Honor Society, Sigma Theta Tau, Student Nurses' Association.
Nursing Student Resources Academic advising; academic or career counseling; assistance for students with disabilities; bookstore; campus computer network; career placement assistance; computer lab; computer-assisted instruction; daycare for children of students; e-mail services; employment services for current students; externships; housing assistance; interactive nursing skills videos; Internet; learning resource lab; library services; nursing audiovisuals; other; paid internships; placement services for program completers; remedial services; resume preparation assistance; skills, simulation, or other laboratory; tutoring; unpaid internships.
Library Facilities 6,883 volumes in health, 4,593 volumes in nursing; 184 periodical subscriptions health-care related.

BACCALAUREATE PROGRAMS

Degree BSN

Available Programs ADN to Baccalaureate; Accelerated Baccalaureate for Second Degree; Generic Baccalaureate; LPN to Baccalaureate.

Study Options Full-time and part-time.
Online Degree Options Yes.
Program Entrance Requirements Minimum overall college GPA of 2.8, transcript of college record, CPR certification, health exam, health insurance, high school biology, high school chemistry, high school foreign language, 2 years high school math, 3 years high school science, high school transcript, immunizations, minimum high school GPA of 2.0, minimum high school rank 25%, minimum GPA in nursing prerequisites of 2.0, prerequisite course work. Transfer students are accepted. *Application deadline:* 4/1 (fall), 11/2 (spring).
Advanced Placement Credit by examination available. Credit given for nursing courses completed elsewhere dependent upon specific evaluations.
Contact *Telephone:* 337-482-5604. *Fax:* 337-482-5700.

GRADUATE PROGRAMS

Contact *Telephone:* 337-482-5639. *Fax:* 337-482-5650.

MASTER'S DEGREE PROGRAM
Degree MSN
Available Programs Master's; RN to Master's.
Concentrations Available Health-care administration; nursing administration; nursing education. *Clinical nurse specialist programs in:* adult health, psychiatric/mental health. *Nurse practitioner programs in:* adult health, psychiatric/mental health.
Site Options Hammond, LA; Baton Rouge, LA; Lake Charles, LA.
Study Options Full-time and part-time.
Online Degree Options Yes (online only).
Program Entrance Requirements Minimum overall college GPA of 2.75, transcript of college record, immunizations, 3 letters of recommendation, physical assessment course, statistics course, GRE General Test. *Application deadline:* Applications may be processed on a rolling basis for some programs. *Application fee:* $25.
Advanced Placement Credit given for nursing courses completed elsewhere dependent upon specific evaluations.
Degree Requirements 38 total credit hours, thesis or project.

POST-MASTER'S PROGRAM
Areas of Study *Clinical nurse specialist programs in:* adult health, psychiatric/mental health. *Nurse practitioner programs in:* adult health, psychiatric/mental health.

CONTINUING EDUCATION PROGRAM
Contact *Telephone:* 337-482-5648. *Fax:* 337-482-5053.

University of Louisiana at Monroe
Nursing
Monroe, Louisiana

http://www.ulm.edu/nursing
Founded in 1931
DEGREE • BS
Nursing Program Faculty 29 (2% with doctorates).
Baccalaureate Enrollment 237 **Women** 85% **Men** 15% **Part-time** 20%
Distance Learning Courses Available.
Nursing Student Activities Sigma Theta Tau, Student Nurses' Association.
Nursing Student Resources Academic advising; academic or career counseling; assistance for students with disabilities; bookstore; campus computer network; computer lab; computer-assisted instruction; daycare for children of students; e-mail services; employment services for current students; interactive nursing skills videos; Internet; learning resource lab; library services; nursing audiovisuals; placement services for program completers; remedial services; resume preparation assistance; skills, simulation, or other laboratory; tutoring.
Library Facilities 20,924 volumes in health, 3,000 volumes in nursing; 425 periodical subscriptions health-care related.

BACCALAUREATE PROGRAMS
Degree BS
Available Programs ADN to Baccalaureate; Generic Baccalaureate; LPN to Baccalaureate; RN Baccalaureate.
Study Options Full-time and part-time.
Online Degree Options Yes (online only).

Program Entrance Requirements Transcript of college record, CPR certification, health exam, health insurance, high school transcript, immunizations, minimum high school GPA of 2.0, minimum high school rank 50%, minimum GPA in nursing prerequisites of 2.8, professional liability insurance/malpractice insurance, prerequisite course work. Transfer students are accepted. *Application deadline:* 3/1 (fall), 9/1 (spring). *Application fee:* $50.
Advanced Placement Credit given for nursing courses completed elsewhere dependent upon specific evaluations.
Contact *Telephone:* 318-342-1640. *Fax:* 318-342-1567.

CONTINUING EDUCATION PROGRAM
Contact *Telephone:* 318-342-1640. *Fax:* 318-342-1567.

University of Phoenix–New Orleans Learning Center
College of Nursing
Metairie, Louisiana

Founded in 1976
DEGREE • BSN
Nursing Program Faculty 2 (50% with doctorates).
Baccalaureate Enrollment 9
Nursing Student Activities Sigma Theta Tau.
Nursing Student Resources Academic advising; academic or career counseling; assistance for students with disabilities; bookstore; campus computer network; computer lab; computer-assisted instruction; e-mail services; interactive nursing skills videos; Internet; learning resource lab; library services; nursing audiovisuals; remedial services; tutoring.
Library Facilities 1,300 periodical subscriptions health-care related.

BACCALAUREATE PROGRAMS
Degree BSN
Available Programs Accelerated Baccalaureate; LPN to Baccalaureate.
Study Options Full-time.
Program Entrance Requirements Transcript of college record, CPR certification, immunizations, 1 letter of recommendation, RN licensure. Transfer students are accepted. *Application deadline:* Applications may be processed on a rolling basis for some programs.
Advanced Placement Credit by examination available. Credit given for nursing courses completed elsewhere dependent upon specific evaluations.
Contact *Telephone:* 504-461-8852.

MAINE

Husson University
School of Nursing
Bangor, Maine

http://www.husson.edu/
Founded in 1898
DEGREES • BSN • MSN
Nursing Program Faculty 13 (15% with doctorates).
Baccalaureate Enrollment 291 **Women** 93% **Men** 7%
Graduate Enrollment 49 **Women** 92% **Men** 8% **Part-time** 26%
Distance Learning Courses Available.
Nursing Student Activities Sigma Theta Tau, Student Nurses' Association, nursing club.
Nursing Student Resources Academic advising; academic or career counseling; assistance for students with disabilities; bookstore; campus computer network; career placement assistance; computer lab; computer-assisted instruction; e-mail services; employment services for current students; externships; interactive nursing skills videos; Internet; learning resource lab; library services; nursing audiovisuals; remedial services; resume preparation assistance; skills, simulation, or other laboratory; tutoring; unpaid internships.
Library Facilities 3,450 volumes in health, 1,100 volumes in nursing; 183 periodical subscriptions health-care related.

BACCALAUREATE PROGRAMS

Degree BSN

Available Programs Generic Baccalaureate.

Study Options Full-time and part-time.

Program Entrance Requirements Minimum overall college GPA of 3.0, transcript of college record, written essay, health exam, health insurance, high school biology, high school chemistry, 2 years high school math, 2 years high school science, high school transcript, immunizations, 2 letters of recommendation, minimum high school GPA of 3.0, minimum GPA in nursing prerequisites of 3.0, prerequisite course work. Transfer students are accepted. *Application deadline:* Applications may be processed on a rolling basis for some programs. *Application fee:* $25.

Advanced Placement Credit by examination available. Credit given for nursing courses completed elsewhere dependent upon specific evaluations.

Contact *Telephone:* 207-941-7058. *Fax:* 207-941-7198.

GRADUATE PROGRAMS

Contact *Telephone:* 207-941-7166. *Fax:* 207-941-7198.

MASTER'S DEGREE PROGRAM

Degree MSN

Available Programs Master's; Master's for Nurses with Non-Nursing Degrees.

Concentrations Available Nursing education. *Clinical nurse specialist programs in:* psychiatric/mental health. *Nurse practitioner programs in:* family health.

Site Options South Portland, ME; Presque Isle, ME.

Study Options Full-time and part-time.

Program Entrance Requirements Clinical experience, minimum overall college GPA of 3.0, transcript of college record, CPR certification, written essay, immunizations, interview, 3 letters of recommendation, physical assessment course, prerequisite course work, statistics course. *Application deadline:* Applications may be processed on a rolling basis for some programs. *Application fee:* $25.

Advanced Placement Credit by examination available. Credit given for nursing courses completed elsewhere dependent upon specific evaluations.

Degree Requirements 44 total credit hours, thesis or project.

POST-MASTER'S PROGRAM

Areas of Study Nursing education. *Clinical nurse specialist programs in:* psychiatric/mental health. *Nurse practitioner programs in:* family health, psychiatric/mental health.

Saint Joseph's College of Maine
Master of Science in Nursing Program
Standish, Maine

http://www.sjcme.edu/
Founded in 1912

DEGREES • BSN • MSN • MSN/MHA

Nursing Program Faculty 65 (8% with doctorates).

Baccalaureate Enrollment 558 **Women** 95% **Men** 5% **Part-time** 48%

Graduate Enrollment 343 **Women** 93% **Men** 7% **Part-time** 100%

Distance Learning Courses Available.

Nursing Student Activities Sigma Theta Tau, Student Nurses' Association.

Nursing Student Resources Academic advising; academic or career counseling; assistance for students with disabilities; bookstore; campus computer network; computer lab; computer-assisted instruction; e-mail services; interactive nursing skills videos; Internet; learning resource lab; library services; nursing audiovisuals; remedial services; resume preparation assistance; skills, simulation, or other laboratory; tutoring.

Library Facilities 4,114 volumes in health, 409 volumes in nursing; 108 periodical subscriptions health-care related.

BACCALAUREATE PROGRAMS

Degree BSN

Available Programs Generic Baccalaureate; RN Baccalaureate.

Study Options Full-time and part-time.

Program Entrance Requirements Minimum overall college GPA of 2.0, transcript of college record, written essay, health exam, health insurance, high school biology, high school chemistry, 3 years high school math, 2 years high school science, high school transcript, immuni-

zations, 1 letter of recommendation, minimum high school GPA of 2.0. *Application deadline:* 5/1 (spring). *Application fee:* $250.

Advanced Placement Credit given for nursing courses completed elsewhere dependent upon specific evaluations.

Contact *Telephone:* 207-893-7830. *Fax:* 207-892-7423.

GRADUATE PROGRAMS

Contact *Telephone:* 207-893-7956. *Fax:* 207-893-7520.

MASTER'S DEGREE PROGRAM

Degrees MSN; MSN/MHA

Available Programs Master's; Master's for Nurses with Non-Nursing Degrees; RN to Master's.

Concentrations Available Nursing administration; nursing education.

Study Options Full-time and part-time.

Online Degree Options Yes (online only).

Program Entrance Requirements Clinical experience, computer literacy, minimum overall college GPA of 3.0, transcript of college record, prerequisite course work, resume, MAT. *Application deadline:* Applications may be processed on a rolling basis for some programs.

Advanced Placement Credit given for nursing courses completed elsewhere dependent upon specific evaluations.

Degree Requirements 42 total credit hours, thesis or project.

CONTINUING EDUCATION PROGRAM

Contact *Telephone:* 207-893-7956. *Fax:* 207-893-7520.

University of Maine
School of Nursing
Orono, Maine

https://umaine.edu/
Founded in 1865

DEGREES • BSN • MSN

Nursing Program Faculty 20 (40% with doctorates).

Baccalaureate Enrollment 407 **Women** 90% **Men** 10% **Part-time** .5%

Graduate Enrollment 27 **Women** 99% **Men** 1% **Part-time** 50%

Distance Learning Courses Available.

Nursing Student Activities Sigma Theta Tau, Student Nurses' Association.

Nursing Student Resources Academic advising; academic or career counseling; assistance for students with disabilities; bookstore; campus computer network; computer lab; daycare for children of students; e-mail services; employment services for current students; housing assistance; interactive nursing skills videos; Internet; learning resource lab; library services; nursing audiovisuals; skills, simulation, or other laboratory; tutoring.

Library Facilities 20,600 volumes in health, 2,100 volumes in nursing; 3,750 periodical subscriptions health-care related.

BACCALAUREATE PROGRAMS

Degree BSN

Available Programs Generic Baccalaureate; RN Baccalaureate.

Site Options Presque Isle, ME; Augusta, ME; Portland, ME.

Study Options Full-time and part-time.

Program Entrance Requirements Minimum overall college GPA of 2.75, transcript of college record, CPR certification, written essay, health exam, high school biology, high school chemistry, high school foreign language, 3 years high school math, 3 years high school science, high school transcript, immunizations, interview, minimum high school rank 30%. Transfer students are accepted.

Advanced Placement Credit by examination available. Credit given for nursing courses completed elsewhere dependent upon specific evaluations.

Contact *Telephone:* 207-581-2588. *Fax:* 207-581-2585.

GRADUATE PROGRAMS

Contact *Telephone:* 207-581-2605. *Fax:* 207-581-2585.

MASTER'S DEGREE PROGRAM

Degree MSN

Available Programs Master's; RN to Master's.

Concentrations Available Health-care administration; nursing education. *Nurse practitioner programs in:* family health.

Study Options Full-time and part-time.

Program Entrance Requirements Clinical experience, minimum overall college GPA of 3.0, transcript of college record, CPR certification, written essay, immunizations, interview, 3 letters of recommendation, nursing research course, physical assessment course, statistics course, GRE General Test.
Advanced Placement Credit given for nursing courses completed elsewhere dependent upon specific evaluations.
Degree Requirements 47 total credit hours, thesis or project.

University of Maine at Augusta
Nursing Programs
Augusta, Maine

http://www.uma.edu/
Founded in 1965
DEGREE • BSN

BACCALAUREATE PROGRAMS

Degree BSN
Available Programs RN Baccalaureate.
Contact Dr. Lynne King, Academic Coordinator, Nursing Programs, University of Maine at Augusta, 46 University Drive, Augusta, ME 04330-9410. *Telephone:* 207-621-3236. *E-mail:* lking@maine.edu.

University of Maine at Fort Kent
Department of Nursing
Fort Kent, Maine

http://www.umfk.edu/
Founded in 1878
DEGREE • BSN
Nursing Program Faculty 8 (50% with doctorates).
Baccalaureate Enrollment 525 **Women** 90% **Men** 10% **Part-time** 63%
Distance Learning Courses Available.
Nursing Student Activities Nursing Honor Society, Student Nurses' Association, nursing club.
Nursing Student Resources Academic advising; academic or career counseling; assistance for students with disabilities; bookstore; campus computer network; career placement assistance; computer lab; computer-assisted instruction; e-mail services; employment services for current students; externships; housing assistance; interactive nursing skills videos; Internet; learning resource lab; library services; nursing audiovisuals; paid internships; placement services for program completers; remedial services; resume preparation assistance; skills, simulation, or other laboratory; tutoring; unpaid internships.
Library Facilities 3,386 volumes in health, 2,425 volumes in nursing; 73 periodical subscriptions health-care related.

BACCALAUREATE PROGRAMS

Degree BSN
Available Programs Accelerated Baccalaureate; Generic Baccalaureate; RN Baccalaureate.
Site Options Augusta , ME.
Study Options Full-time and part-time.
Online Degree Options Yes.
Program Entrance Requirements Minimum overall college GPA of 2.5, CPR certification, written essay, health exam, health insurance, high school chemistry, high school foreign language, high school math, high school transcript, immunizations, minimum GPA in nursing prerequisites of 2.5, prerequisite course work. Transfer students are accepted. *Application deadline:* 8/15 (fall), 1/10 (spring). *Application fee:* $40.
Advanced Placement Credit given for nursing courses completed elsewhere dependent upon specific evaluations.
Expenses (2015–16) *Tuition, state resident:* full-time $3300; part-time $220 per credit hour. *Tuition, nonresident:* full-time $4950; part-time $330 per credit hour. *International tuition:* $4950 full-time. *Room and board:* $7910; room only: $4250 per academic year. *Required fees:* full-time $375; part-time $25 per credit.
Financial Aid 93% of baccalaureate students in nursing programs received some form of financial aid in 2014–15.
Contact Ms. Diane Griffin, Chair of Admission, Advisement, and Advancement Committee, Department of Nursing, University of Maine at Fort Kent, 23 University Drive, Fort Kent, ME 04743-1292.

Telephone: 207-834-8622. *Fax:* 207-834-7577.
E-mail: dgriffin@maine.edu.

University of New England
Department of Nursing
Biddeford, Maine

http://www.une.edu/
Founded in 1831
DEGREE • BSN
Nursing Program Faculty 16 (26% with doctorates).
Baccalaureate Enrollment 133 **Women** 73% **Men** 27%
Nursing Student Activities Nursing Honor Society, Sigma Theta Tau, Student Nurses' Association, nursing club.
Nursing Student Resources Academic advising; academic or career counseling; assistance for students with disabilities; bookstore; campus computer network; career placement assistance; computer lab; computer-assisted instruction; e-mail services; employment services for current students; housing assistance; interactive nursing skills videos; Internet; learning resource lab; library services; nursing audiovisuals; placement services for program completers; remedial services; resume preparation assistance; skills, simulation, or other laboratory; tutoring; unpaid internships.
Library Facilities 10,000 volumes in health, 5,500 volumes in nursing; 1,300 periodical subscriptions health-care related.

BACCALAUREATE PROGRAMS

Degree BSN
Available Programs Accelerated RN Baccalaureate; Generic Baccalaureate; RN Baccalaureate.
Study Options Full-time and part-time.
Program Entrance Requirements Minimum overall college GPA of 3.0, transcript of college record, CPR certification, health exam, health insurance, high school biology, high school chemistry, 2 years high school math, 2 years high school science, high school transcript, immunizations, minimum high school GPA of 3.0, professional liability insurance/malpractice insurance. Transfer students are accepted. *Application deadline:* 2/15 (fall). *Application fee:* $100.
Advanced Placement Credit by examination available. Credit given for nursing courses completed elsewhere dependent upon specific evaluations.
Contact *Telephone:* 207-602-2297.

CONTINUING EDUCATION PROGRAM

Contact *Telephone:* 207-602-2050. *Fax:* 207-602-5973.

University of Southern Maine
School of Nursing
Portland, Maine

http://www.usm.maine.edu/nursing
Founded in 1878
DEGREES • BS • DNP • MS
Nursing Program Faculty 76 (18% with doctorates).
Baccalaureate Enrollment 360 **Women** 87% **Men** 13% **Part-time** 20%
Graduate Enrollment 106 **Women** 84% **Men** 16% **Part-time** 44%
Distance Learning Courses Available.
Nursing Student Activities Sigma Theta Tau, Student Nurses' Association.
Nursing Student Resources Academic advising; academic or career counseling; assistance for students with disabilities; bookstore; campus computer network; computer lab; computer-assisted instruction; e-mail services; interactive nursing skills videos; Internet; learning resource lab; library services; nursing audiovisuals; remedial services; resume preparation assistance; skills, simulation, or other laboratory; tutoring.
Library Facilities 18,042 volumes in health, 622 volumes in nursing; 230 periodical subscriptions health-care related.

BACCALAUREATE PROGRAMS

Degree BS
Available Programs ADN to Baccalaureate; Accelerated Baccalaureate for Second Degree; Generic Baccalaureate; RN Baccalaureate.
Site Options Lewiston, ME.

Study Options Full-time and part-time.

Program Entrance Requirements Minimum overall college GPA of 3.0, transcript of college record, written essay, high school biology, high school chemistry, 3 years high school math, 2 years high school science, high school transcript, immunizations, 2 letters of recommendation, minimum high school GPA of 3.0. Transfer students are accepted. *Application deadline:* 1/15 (fall), 10/1 (summer). *Application fee:* $40.

Advanced Placement Credit by examination available. Credit given for nursing courses completed elsewhere dependent upon specific evaluations.

Expenses (2015–16) *Tuition, state resident:* full-time $7590; part-time $253 per credit. *Tuition, nonresident:* full-time $19,950; part-time $665 per credit. *International tuition:* $19,950 full-time. *Room and board:* $9820; room only: $4600 per academic year. *Required fees:* full-time $1330; part-time $28 per credit; part-time $245 per term.

Contact Ms. Brenda D. Webster, Coordinator of Nursing Student Services, School of Nursing, University of Southern Maine, PO Box 9300, Portland, ME 04104-9300. *Telephone:* 207-780-4802. *Fax:* 207-780-4973. *E-mail:* brenda@maine.edu.

GRADUATE PROGRAMS

Expenses (2015–16) *Tuition, state resident:* full-time $6840; part-time $380 per credit. *Tuition, nonresident:* full-time $18,468; part-time $1026 per credit. *International tuition:* $18,468 full-time. *Room and board:* $9820; room only: $4600 per academic year. *Required fees:* full-time $867; part-time $28 per credit; part-time $363 per term.

Financial Aid Research assistantships, teaching assistantships, career-related internships or fieldwork, Federal Work-Study, scholarships, traineeships, tuition waivers (full and partial), and unspecified assistantships available.

Contact Ms. Brenda D. Webster, Coordinator of Nursing Student Services, School of Nursing, University of Southern Maine, PO Box 9300, Portland, ME 04104-9300. *Telephone:* 207-780-4802. *Fax:* 207-780-4973. *E-mail:* bwebster@usm.maine.edu.

MASTER'S DEGREE PROGRAM

Degree MS

Available Programs Master's; Master's for Non-Nursing College Graduates; Master's for Nurses with Non-Nursing Degrees; RN to Master's.

Concentrations Available Nursing education. *Nurse practitioner programs in:* family health, psychiatric/mental health.

Study Options Full-time and part-time.

Program Entrance Requirements Minimum overall college GPA of 3.0, transcript of college record, written essay, 2 letters of recommendation, physical assessment course, prerequisite course work, statistics course, GRE General Test or MAT. *Application deadline:* 4/1 (fall), 10/1 (spring), 11/1 (summer). *Application fee:* $65.

Advanced Placement Credit given for nursing courses completed elsewhere dependent upon specific evaluations.

Degree Requirements 53 total credit hours.

POST-MASTER'S PROGRAM

Areas of Study *Nurse practitioner programs in:* family health, psychiatric/mental health.

DOCTORAL DEGREE PROGRAM

Degree DNP

Available Programs Doctorate.

Areas of Study Clinical practice, ethics, health policy, health-care systems, nursing policy.

Program Entrance Requirements Clinical experience, minimum overall college GPA of 3.25, interview by faculty committee, 3 letters of recommendation, MSN or equivalent, statistics course, vita, writing sample, GRE. Application deadline: 3/15 (fall). Application fee: $65.

Degree Requirements 43 total credit hours, residency.

CONTINUING EDUCATION PROGRAM

Contact Professional Development Programs, School of Nursing, University of Southern Maine, USM Professional Development Programs, PO Box 9300, Portland, ME 04104-9300. *Telephone:* 207-780-5900. *E-mail:* usmpdp@maine.edu.

MARYLAND

Bowie State University
Department of Nursing
Bowie, Maryland

http://www.bowiestate.edu/academics/departments/nursing
Founded in 1865
DEGREES • BSN • MSN
Nursing Program Faculty 20 (35% with doctorates).
Baccalaureate Enrollment 225 **Women** 88% **Men** 12% **Part-time** 25%
Graduate Enrollment 43 **Women** 87% **Men** 13% **Part-time** 5%
Distance Learning Courses Available.
Nursing Student Activities Nursing Honor Society, Student Nurses' Association.
Nursing Student Resources Academic advising; academic or career counseling; assistance for students with disabilities; bookstore; campus computer network; computer lab; computer-assisted instruction; housing assistance; interactive nursing skills videos; Internet; library services; nursing audiovisuals; skills, simulation, or other laboratory; tutoring.

BACCALAUREATE PROGRAMS

Degree BSN

Available Programs Accelerated Baccalaureate; Generic Baccalaureate; RN Baccalaureate.

Study Options Full-time.

Program Entrance Requirements Minimum overall college GPA of 2.75, transcript of college record, health exam, health insurance, high school biology, high school chemistry, 4 years high school math, 4 years high school science, high school transcript, immunizations, minimum high school GPA of 3.0, minimum GPA in nursing prerequisites of 2.75, prerequisite course work. Transfer students are accepted. *Application deadline:* 3/31 (fall).

Advanced Placement Credit given for nursing courses completed elsewhere dependent upon specific evaluations.

Contact *Telephone:* 301-860-3202. *Fax:* 301-860-3222.

GRADUATE PROGRAMS

Contact *Telephone:* 301-860-3202. *Fax:* 301-860-3222.

MASTER'S DEGREE PROGRAM

Degree MSN

Available Programs Master's.

Concentrations Available Nursing education. *Nurse practitioner programs in:* family health.

Study Options Full-time and part-time.

Program Entrance Requirements Clinical experience, minimum overall college GPA of 2.5, CPR certification, written essay, immunizations, 3 letters of recommendation, physical assessment course, professional liability insurance/malpractice insurance, resume, statistics course. *Application deadline:* 11/30 (fall), 4/30 (spring). Applications may be processed on a rolling basis for some programs.

Advanced Placement Credit by examination available. Credit given for nursing courses completed elsewhere dependent upon specific evaluations.

Degree Requirements 45 total credit hours, comprehensive exam.

Coppin State University
Helene Fuld School of Nursing
Baltimore, Maryland

http://www.coppin.edu/nursing
Founded in 1900
DEGREES • BSN • MSN
Nursing Program Faculty 45 (18% with doctorates).
Baccalaureate Enrollment 529 **Women** 91% **Men** 9% **Part-time** 33%
Graduate Enrollment 32 **Women** 94% **Men** 6% **Part-time** 22%
Distance Learning Courses Available.
Nursing Student Activities Nursing Honor Society, Sigma Theta Tau, Student Nurses' Association.
Nursing Student Resources Academic advising; academic or career counseling; assistance for students with disabilities; bookstore; campus computer network; career placement assistance; computer lab; computer-

assisted instruction; e-mail services; externships; interactive nursing skills videos; Internet; learning resource lab; library services; nursing audiovisuals; other; placement services for program completers; remedial services; resume preparation assistance; skills, simulation, or other laboratory; tutoring; unpaid internships.
Library Facilities 1,339 volumes in health, 1,298 volumes in nursing; 132 periodical subscriptions health-care related.

BACCALAUREATE PROGRAMS

Degree BSN
Available Programs Accelerated RN Baccalaureate; Baccalaureate for Second Degree; Generic Baccalaureate; RN Baccalaureate.
Site Options Baltimore, MD.
Study Options Full-time and part-time.
Program Entrance Requirements Written essay, health exam, high school biology, high school chemistry, high school foreign language, 3 years high school math, 2 years high school science, high school transcript, immunizations, 3 letters of recommendation, minimum high school GPA of 2.5, minimum GPA in nursing prerequisites of 2.5. Transfer students are accepted.
Contact *Telephone:* 410-951-3988. *Fax:* 410-400-5978.

GRADUATE PROGRAMS

Contact *Telephone:* 410-951-3988. *Fax:* 410-400-5978.

MASTER'S DEGREE PROGRAM

Degree MSN
Available Programs Master's.
Concentrations Available *Nurse practitioner programs in:* family health.
Site Options Baltimore, MD.
Study Options Full-time and part-time.
Program Entrance Requirements Clinical experience, computer literacy, minimum overall college GPA of 3.0, transcript of college record, CPR certification, written essay, immunizations, interview, 3 letters of recommendation, nursing research course, physical assessment course, statistics course.
Advanced Placement Credit given for nursing courses completed elsewhere dependent upon specific evaluations.
Degree Requirements 48 total credit hours, thesis or project, comprehensive exam.

POST-MASTER'S PROGRAM

Areas of Study *Nurse practitioner programs in:* family health.

Frostburg State University
Nursing Department
Frostburg, Maryland

Founded in 1898
DEGREE • BSN

BACCALAUREATE PROGRAMS

Degree BSN
Available Programs RN Baccalaureate.
Study Options Part-time.
Online Degree Options Yes (online only).
Program Entrance Requirements Prerequisite course work, RN licensure. *Application deadline:* 4/1 (summer).
Contact *Telephone:* 301-687-4141.

Hood College
BSN Completion Program
Frederick, Maryland

http://www.hood.edu
Founded in 1893
DEGREE • BSN
Nursing Program Faculty 5 (40% with doctorates).
Baccalaureate Enrollment 17 **Women** 100% **Part-time** 100%
Nursing Student Resources Academic advising; academic or career counseling; assistance for students with disabilities; bookstore; campus computer network; career placement assistance; computer lab; computer-

assisted instruction; e-mail services; externships; interactive nursing skills videos; Internet; learning resource lab; library services; nursing audiovisuals; remedial services; resume preparation assistance; skills, simulation, or other laboratory; tutoring; unpaid internships.
Library Facilities 690 volumes in health, 71 volumes in nursing; 6,588 periodical subscriptions health-care related.

BACCALAUREATE PROGRAMS

Degree BSN
Available Programs Generic Baccalaureate; RN Baccalaureate.
Study Options Full-time and part-time.
Program Entrance Requirements Transcript of college record, prerequisite course work, RN licensure. Transfer students are accepted. *Application deadline:* 8/15 (fall). Applications may be processed on a rolling basis for some programs.
Expenses (2014–15) *Tuition:* full-time $45,730; part-time $975 per credit hour. *International tuition:* $45,730 full-time. *Room and board:* $11,610; room only: $6080 per academic year. *Required fees:* full-time $500; part-time $160 per term.
Financial Aid 70% of baccalaureate students in nursing programs received some form of financial aid in 2013–14. *Gift aid (need-based):* Federal Pell, FSEOG, state, private, college/university gift aid from institutional funds. *Loans:* Federal Direct (Subsidized and Unsubsidized Stafford PLUS), Perkins. *Work-study:* Federal Work-Study, part-time campus jobs. *Financial aid application deadline:* Continuous.
Contact Ms. Cheryl Banks, Associate Director of Admissions, BSN Completion Program, Hood College, 401 Rosemont Avenue, Frederick, MD 21701. *Telephone:* 301-696-3354. *E-mail:* banks@hood.edu.

Johns Hopkins University
School of Nursing
Baltimore, Maryland

http://www.nursing.jhu.edu
Founded in 1876
DEGREES • DNP • MSN • MSN/MBA • MSN/MPH • MSN/PHD • PHD
Nursing Program Faculty 180 (36% with doctorates).
Graduate Enrollment 449 **Women** 90% **Men** 10% **Part-time** 30%
Distance Learning Courses Available.
Nursing Student Activities Nursing Honor Society, Sigma Theta Tau, Student Nurses' Association, nursing club.
Nursing Student Resources Academic advising; academic or career counseling; assistance for students with disabilities; bookstore; campus computer network; career placement assistance; computer lab; computer-assisted instruction; e-mail services; employment services for current students; housing assistance; Internet; learning resource lab; library services; nursing audiovisuals; resume preparation assistance; skills, simulation, or other laboratory; tutoring.

GRADUATE PROGRAMS

Expenses (2015–16) *Tuition:* full-time $36,216; part-time $1509 per credit hour. *International tuition:* $36,216 full-time. *Required fees:* part-time $158 per term.
Financial Aid 58% of graduate students in nursing programs received some form of financial aid in 2014–15. Fellowships with partial tuition reimbursements available, research assistantships with full tuition reimbursements available, teaching assistantships with full tuition reimbursements available, career-related internships or fieldwork, Federal Work-Study, scholarships, traineeships, and tuition waivers (partial) available. Aid available to part-time students. *Financial aid application deadline:* 3/1.
Contact Ms. Cathy Wilson, Office of Admissions, School of Nursing, Johns Hopkins University, 525 North Wolfe Street, Baltimore, MD 21205-2110. *Telephone:* 410-955-7548. *E-mail:* jhuson@jhu.edu.

MASTER'S DEGREE PROGRAM

Degrees MSN; MSN/MBA; MSN/MPH; MSN/PhD
Available Programs Master's; Master's for Nurses with Non-Nursing Degrees.
Concentrations Available Health-care administration; nurse case management. *Clinical nurse specialist programs in:* acute care, adult health, adult-gerontology acute care. *Nurse practitioner programs in:* acute care, adult health, adult-gerontology acute care, community health, family health, gerontology, pediatric, pediatric primary care, primary care, women's health.

Study Options Full-time and part-time.
Online Degree Options Yes.
Program Entrance Requirements Computer literacy, minimum overall college GPA of 3.0, transcript of college record, CPR certification, written essay, immunizations, 3 letters of recommendation, prerequisite course work, resume, statistics course.*Application fee:* $75.
Advanced Placement Credit given for nursing courses completed elsewhere dependent upon specific evaluations.
Degree Requirements 36 total credit hours, comprehensive exam.

POST-MASTER'S PROGRAM
Areas of Study Nursing education. *Clinical nurse specialist programs in:* acute care, adult health, adult-gerontology acute care. *Nurse practitioner programs in:* acute care, adult health, adult-gerontology acute care, adult-psychiatric mental health, family health, gerontology, pediatric, pediatric primary care, primary care, psychiatric/mental health.

DOCTORAL DEGREE PROGRAM
Degree DNP
Available Programs Doctorate.
Areas of Study Health-care systems.
Program Entrance Requirements Minimum overall college GPA of 3.0, clinical experience, interview by faculty committee, 3 letters of recommendation, MSN or equivalent, vita, writing sample. Application deadline: 1/1 (summer). Application fee: $100.
Degree Requirements 40 total credit hours, Capstone project.

Degree PhD
Available Programs Doctorate.
Areas of Study Advanced practice nursing, aging, bio-behavioral research, biology of health and illness, clinical practice, clinical research, community health, critical care, ethics, faculty preparation, family health, forensic nursing, gerontology, health policy, health promotion/disease prevention, health-care systems, human health and illness, illness and transition, individualized study, information systems, nursing research, nursing science, palliative care, urban health, women's health.
Program Entrance Requirements Minimum overall college GPA of 3.0, interview, 3 letters of recommendation, MSN or equivalent, statistics course, vita, writing sample, GRE (for PhD). Application deadline: 1/15 (fall). Application fee: $100.

Degree Requirements 56 total credit hours, dissertation, oral exam, written exam.

POSTDOCTORAL PROGRAM
Areas of Study Health promotion/disease prevention, individualized study, nursing research, vulnerable population.
Postdoctoral Program Contact Ms. Cathy Wilson, Office of Admissions, School of Nursing, Johns Hopkins University, 525 North Wolfe Street, Baltimore, MD 21205-2110. *Telephone:* 410-955-7548. *E-mail:* jhuson@jhu.edu.

CONTINUING EDUCATION PROGRAM
Contact Ms. Kristine Vliet, Executive Director, Professional Programs, School of Nursing, Johns Hopkins University, 525 North Wolfe Street, Baltimore, MD 21205-2110. *Telephone:* 410-955-4766.
E-mail: son-professionalprgm@jhu.edu.

See display below and full description on page 498.

Morgan State University
Bachelor of Science in Nursing
Baltimore, Maryland

http://www.morgan.edu/school_of_community_health_and_policy/programs/nursing.html
Founded in 1867
DEGREE • BS

BACCALAUREATE PROGRAMS
Degree BS
Available Programs Generic Baccalaureate; RN Baccalaureate.
Contact Nursing Program, Bachelor of Science in Nursing, Morgan State University, 1700 East Cold Spring Lane, Jenkins Behavioral Center, Baltimore, MD 21251. *Telephone:* 443-885-4144.
E-mail: shelia.richburg@morgan.edu.

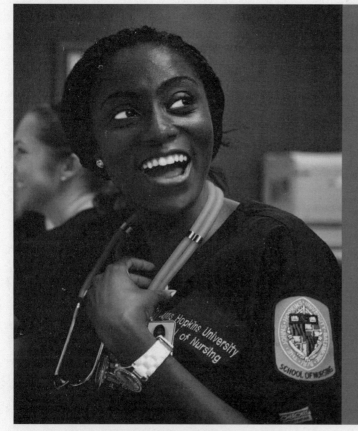

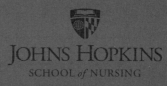

YOUR NEW ADVENTURE STARTS AT JOHNS HOPKINS

Discover the people, places, and possibilities of nursing while earning a master's degree in five semesters. Explore the new Master of Science in Nursing (MSN) Entry into Nursing program, specifically designed for non-nursing bachelor's degree graduates and career changers.

Learn more at **nursing.jhu.edu/nursingcareer**

For information on all program offerings call 410-955-7548.

JOHNS HOPKINS
SCHOOL *of* NURSING

Notre Dame of Maryland University
Department of Nursing
Baltimore, Maryland

http://www.ndm.edu/academics/departments-and-programs/nursing/
Founded in 1873

DEGREE • BS
Nursing Program Faculty 5 (60% with doctorates).
Nursing Student Resources Library services.

BACCALAUREATE PROGRAMS

Degree BS
Available Programs Accelerated RN Baccalaureate; RN Baccalaureate.
Site Options Frederick, MD; Aberdeen, MD.
Study Options Full-time and part-time.
Program Entrance Requirements Minimum overall college GPA of 2.5, transcript of college record, interview, minimum GPA in nursing prerequisites of 2.0, prerequisite course work, RN licensure. Transfer students are accepted.
Advanced Placement Credit by examination available. Credit given for nursing courses completed elsewhere dependent upon specific evaluations.
Contact *Telephone:* 410-532-5500.

Salisbury University
Department of Nursing
Salisbury, Maryland

https://www.salisbury.edu/nursing
Founded in 1925

DEGREES • BS • DNP • MS
Nursing Program Faculty 48 (40% with doctorates).
Baccalaureate Enrollment 538 **Women** 90% **Men** 10% **Part-time** 4.3%
Graduate Enrollment 29 **Women** 90% **Men** 10% **Part-time** 24.1%
Distance Learning Courses Available.
Nursing Student Activities Nursing Honor Society, Sigma Theta Tau, Student Nurses' Association.
Nursing Student Resources Academic advising; academic or career counseling; assistance for students with disabilities; bookstore; campus computer network; career placement assistance; computer lab; computer-assisted instruction; e-mail services; employment services for current students; externships; housing assistance; interactive nursing skills videos; Internet; learning resource lab; library services; nursing audiovisuals; paid internships; placement services for program completers; remedial services; resume preparation assistance; skills, simulation, or other laboratory; tutoring; unpaid internships.
Library Facilities 8,386 volumes in health, 882 volumes in nursing; 6,120 periodical subscriptions health-care related.

BACCALAUREATE PROGRAMS

Degree BS
Available Programs ADN to Baccalaureate; Accelerated Baccalaureate for Second Degree; Generic Baccalaureate; RN Baccalaureate.
Study Options Full-time and part-time.
Program Entrance Requirements Minimum overall college GPA of 3.0, transcript of college record, CPR certification, health exam, high school biology, high school chemistry, 2 years high school math, high school transcript, immunizations, minimum GPA in nursing prerequisites of 3.0, prerequisite course work. Transfer students are accepted. *Application deadline:* 2/1 (fall). *Application fee:* $50.
Expenses (2015–16) *Tuition, state resident:* full-time $6712; part-time $276 per credit. *Tuition, nonresident:* full-time $15,058; part-time $623 per credit. *International tuition:* $15,058 full-time. *Room and board:* $11,010; room only: $6360 per academic year. *Required fees:* full-time $2374; part-time $78 per credit.
Financial Aid 83% of baccalaureate students in nursing programs received some form of financial aid in 2014–15.
Contact Dr. Jeffrey Willey, Chair and Assistant Professor, Department of Nursing, Department of Nursing, Salisbury University, 1101 Camden Avenue, Salisbury, MD 21801. *Telephone:* 410-543-6344. *Fax:* 410-548-3313. *E-mail:* jawilley@salisbury.edu.

GRADUATE PROGRAMS

Expenses (2015–16) *Tuition, state resident:* part-time $620 per credit. *Tuition, nonresident:* part-time $787 per credit.
Financial Aid 73% of graduate students in nursing programs received some form of financial aid in 2014–15. Career-related internships or fieldwork, institutionally sponsored loans, scholarships, and unspecified assistantships available. Aid available to part-time students. *Financial aid application deadline:* 3/1.
Contact Dr. Lisa Seldomridge, Director, Graduate and Second Degree Programs, Department of Nursing, Salisbury University, 1101 Camden Avenue, Salisbury, MD 21801. *Telephone:* 410-543-6413. *Fax:* 410-548-3313. *E-mail:* laseldomridge@salisbury.edu.

MASTER'S DEGREE PROGRAM
Degree MS
Available Programs Master's; RN to Master's.
Concentrations Available Health-care administration; nursing education.
Study Options Full-time and part-time.
Program Entrance Requirements Minimum overall college GPA of 3.0, transcript of college record, CPR certification, written essay, immunizations, interview, 2 letters of recommendation, nursing research course, physical assessment course, professional liability insurance/malpractice insurance, prerequisite course work, resume, statistics course. *Application deadline:* 5/15 (fall). Applications may be processed on a rolling basis for some programs. *Application fee:* $65.
Advanced Placement Credit given for nursing courses completed elsewhere dependent upon specific evaluations.
Degree Requirements 35 total credit hours, thesis or project.

POST-MASTER'S PROGRAM
Areas of Study Health-care administration; nursing education.

DOCTORAL DEGREE PROGRAM
Degree DNP
Available Programs Doctorate.
Areas of Study Advanced practice nursing, biology of health and illness, clinical practice, community health, family health, gerontology, health policy, health promotion/disease prevention, health-care systems, individualized study, information systems, nursing policy, women's health.
Program Entrance Requirements Clinical experience, minimum overall college GPA of 3.5, interview, 3 letters of recommendation, MSN or equivalent, statistics course, vita, writing sample, GRE. Application deadline: 5/15 (fall). Applications may be processed on a rolling basis for some programs. Application fee: $65.
Degree Requirements 38 total credit hours.

POSTDOCTORAL PROGRAM
Areas of Study Family health.
Postdoctoral Program Contact Dr. Lisa A. Seldomridge, Director, Graduate and Second Degree Programs, Department of Nursing, Salisbury University, 1101 Camden Avenue, Salisbury, MD 21801-6860. *Telephone:* 410-543-6413. *Fax:* 410-548-3313. *E-mail:* laseldomridge@salisbury.edu.

Stevenson University
Nursing Division
Stevenson, Maryland

http://www.stevenson.edu/academics/undergraduate-programs/nursing/
Founded in 1952

DEGREES • BS • MS
Nursing Program Faculty 27 (48% with doctorates).
Baccalaureate Enrollment 477 **Women** 93% **Men** 7%
Graduate Enrollment 130 **Women** 95% **Men** 5% **Part-time** 100%
Distance Learning Courses Available.
Nursing Student Activities Sigma Theta Tau, Student Nurses' Association, nursing club.
Nursing Student Resources Academic advising; academic or career counseling; assistance for students with disabilities; bookstore; campus computer network; career placement assistance; computer lab; computer-assisted instruction; e-mail services; employment services for current students; externships; interactive nursing skills videos; Internet; learning resource lab; library services; nursing audiovisuals; placement services

for program completers; remedial services; resume preparation assistance; skills, simulation, or other laboratory; tutoring.
Library Facilities 3,309 volumes in health, 402 volumes in nursing; 4,166 periodical subscriptions health-care related.

BACCALAUREATE PROGRAMS

Degree BS
Available Programs ADN to Baccalaureate; Accelerated RN Baccalaureate; Baccalaureate for Second Degree; Generic Baccalaureate; RN Baccalaureate.
Site Options Baltimore, MD; southern state, MD; Eastern shore, MD.
Study Options Full-time and part-time.
Online Degree Options Yes (online only).
Program Entrance Requirements Minimum overall college GPA of 3.0, transcript of college record, written essay, health exam, health insurance, high school biology, high school chemistry, 2 years high school math, high school transcript, immunizations, interview, minimum high school GPA of 3.0, minimum GPA in nursing prerequisites of 3.0. Transfer students are accepted. *Application deadline:* 2/1 (spring). *Application fee:* $40.
Advanced Placement Credit by examination available. Credit given for nursing courses completed elsewhere dependent upon specific evaluations.
Expenses (2015–16) *Tuition:* full-time $28,864; part-time $730 per credit. *Room and board:* room only: $8718 per academic year. *Required fees:* full-time $2134; part-time $75 per term.
Financial Aid *Gift aid (need-based):* Federal Pell, FSEOG, state, private, college/university gift aid from institutional funds. *Loans:* Federal Direct (Subsidized and Unsubsidized Stafford PLUS), Perkins. *Work-study:* Federal Work-Study. *Financial aid application deadline (priority):* 2/15.
Contact Mrs. Ellen R. Clayton, RN, Interim Department Chair, Nursing, Nursing Division, Stevenson University, 1525 Greenspring Valley Road, Stevenson, MD 21153-0641. *Telephone:* 443-334-2558. *Fax:* 443-334-2558. *E-mail:* eclayton@stevenson.edu.

GRADUATE PROGRAMS

Expenses (2015–16) *Tuition:* part-time $625 per credit. *Required fees:* part-time $125 per term.
Contact Dr. Judith Feustle, Associate Dean, GPS Nursing, Nursing Division, Stevenson University, Garrison Hall, 100 Campus Circle, Owings MIlls, MD 21117. *Telephone:* 443-352-4292. *Fax:* 443-394-0538. *E-mail:* jfeustle@stevenson.edu.

MASTER'S DEGREE PROGRAM
Degree MS
Available Programs Accelerated Master's; Accelerated RN to Master's; RN to Master's.
Concentrations Available Health-care administration; nursing administration; nursing education.
Site Options Baltimore, MD; southern state, MD; Eastern shore, MD.
Study Options Part-time.
Online Degree Options Yes (online only).
Program Entrance Requirements Computer literacy, minimum overall college GPA of 3.0, transcript of college record, immunizations, letters of recommendation, nursing research course. *Application deadline:* Applications may be processed on a rolling basis for some programs.
Advanced Placement Credit given for nursing courses completed elsewhere dependent upon specific evaluations.
Degree Requirements 36 total credit hours, thesis or project.

Towson University
Department of Nursing
Towson, Maryland

http://www.towson.edu/nursing
Founded in 1866
DEGREES • BS • MS
Nursing Program Faculty 80 (15% with doctorates).
Baccalaureate Enrollment 375 **Women** 87% **Men** 13% **Part-time** 3%
Graduate Enrollment 100 **Women** 95% **Men** 5% **Part-time** 60%
Distance Learning Courses Available.
Nursing Student Activities Sigma Theta Tau, Student Nurses' Association.
Nursing Student Resources Academic advising; academic or career counseling; assistance for students with disabilities; bookstore; campus computer network; career placement assistance; computer lab; computer-

assisted instruction; daycare for children of students; e-mail services; housing assistance; interactive nursing skills videos; Internet; learning resource lab; library services; nursing audiovisuals; remedial services; resume preparation assistance; skills, simulation, or other laboratory; tutoring.
Library Facilities 16,457 volumes in health, 1,460 volumes in nursing; 721 periodical subscriptions health-care related.

BACCALAUREATE PROGRAMS

Degree BS
Available Programs ADN to Baccalaureate; Generic Baccalaureate; RN Baccalaureate.
Site Options Hagerstown, MD.
Study Options Full-time and part-time.
Program Entrance Requirements Minimum overall college GPA of 3.0, transcript of college record, CPR certification, health exam, health insurance, immunizations, professional liability insurance/malpractice insurance, prerequisite course work. Transfer students are accepted. *Application deadline:* 1/15 (fall), 8/15 (spring). *Application fee:* $200.
Advanced Placement Credit given for nursing courses completed elsewhere dependent upon specific evaluations.
Expenses (2014–15) *Tuition, state resident:* full-time $3002; part-time $260 per unit. *Tuition, nonresident:* full-time $8841; part-time $740 per unit. *Required fees:* full-time $540; part-time $111 per credit.
Financial Aid 30% of baccalaureate students in nursing programs received some form of financial aid in 2013–14.
Contact Ms. Brook R. Necker, Admissions and Retention Coordinator, Department of Nursing, Towson University, 8000 York Road, Towson, MD 21252-0001. *Telephone:* 410-704-4170.
E-mail: bnecker@towson.edu.

GRADUATE PROGRAMS

Expenses (2014–15) *Tuition, state resident:* part-time $365 per unit. *Tuition, nonresident:* part-time $755 per unit. *Required fees:* part-time $103 per credit.
Financial Aid 15% of graduate students in nursing programs received some form of financial aid in 2013–14.
Contact Dr. Kathleen Ogle, Graduate Program Director, Department of Nursing, Towson University, 8000 York Road, Towson, MD 21252-0001. *Telephone:* 410-704-4389. *Fax:* 410-704-4325.
E-mail: kogle@towson.edu.

MASTER'S DEGREE PROGRAM
Degree MS
Available Programs Master's.
Concentrations Available Health-care administration; nursing education.
Site Options Hagerstown, MD.
Study Options Full-time and part-time.
Program Entrance Requirements Minimum overall college GPA of 3.0, transcript of college record, CPR certification, written essay, immunizations, nursing research course, physical assessment course, resume, statistics course. *Application deadline:* 8/1 (fall), 12/1 (spring), 5/1 (summer). Applications may be processed on a rolling basis for some programs. *Application fee:* $50.
Advanced Placement Credit given for nursing courses completed elsewhere dependent upon specific evaluations.
Degree Requirements 36 total credit hours.

POST-MASTER'S PROGRAM
Areas of Study Health-care administration; nursing education.

University of Maryland, Baltimore
Nursing Programs
Baltimore, Maryland

http://www.nursing.umaryland.edu/
Founded in 1807
DEGREES • BSN • DNP • MS • MS/MBA • MS/MPH • PHD
Nursing Program Faculty 153 (63% with doctorates).
Baccalaureate Enrollment 776 **Women** 86% **Men** 14% **Part-time** 28.99%
Graduate Enrollment 943 **Women** 89% **Men** 11% **Part-time** 60.76%
Distance Learning Courses Available.

Nursing Student Activities Nursing Honor Society, Sigma Theta Tau, Student Nurses' Association.

Nursing Student Resources Academic advising; academic or career counseling; assistance for students with disabilities; bookstore; campus computer network; career placement assistance; computer lab; computer-assisted instruction; e-mail services; employment services for current students; interactive nursing skills videos; Internet; learning resource lab; library services; nursing audiovisuals; remedial services; resume preparation assistance; skills, simulation, or other laboratory; tutoring.

Library Facilities 360,000 volumes in health, 60 volumes in nursing; 2,400 periodical subscriptions health-care related.

BACCALAUREATE PROGRAMS

Degree BSN
Available Programs ADN to Baccalaureate; Generic Baccalaureate; RN Baccalaureate.
Site Options Rockville-Shady Grove, MD; Laurel, MD.
Study Options Full-time and part-time.
Online Degree Options Yes.
Program Entrance Requirements Minimum overall college GPA of 3.0, transcript of college record, CPR certification, written essay, health exam, health insurance, immunizations, 2 letters of recommendation, prerequisite course work. Transfer students are accepted. *Application deadline:* 2/1 (fall), 9/1 (spring). *Application fee:* $75.
Advanced Placement Credit by examination available.
Expenses (2015–16) *Tuition, state resident:* full-time $8329; part-time $365 per credit. *Tuition, nonresident:* full-time $30,965; part-time $806 per credit. *International tuition:* $30,965 full-time. *Required fees:* full-time $3506; part-time $146 per credit.
Contact Ms. Marchelle Payne-Gassaway, Director of Admissions, Nursing Programs, University of Maryland, Baltimore, 655 West Lombard Street, Room 102, Baltimore, MD 21201-1579. *Telephone:* 410-706-0501. *Fax:* 410-706-7238.
E-mail: gassaway@son.umaryland.edu.

GRADUATE PROGRAMS

Expenses (2015–16) *Tuition, state resident:* full-time $12,276; part-time $682 per credit. *Tuition, nonresident:* full-time $22,518; part-time $1251 per credit. *International tuition:* $22,518 full-time. *Required fees:* full-time $3926; part-time $218 per credit.
Contact Ms. Marchelle Payne-Gassaway, Director of Admissions, Nursing Programs, University of Maryland, Baltimore, 655 West Lombard Street, Room 102, Baltimore, MD 21201-1579. *Telephone:* 410-706-0501. *Fax:* 410-706-7238.
E-mail: gassaway@son.umaryland.edu.

MASTER'S DEGREE PROGRAM

Degrees MS; MS/MBA; MS/MPH
Available Programs Master's; RN to Master's.
Concentrations Available Clinical nurse leader; health-care administration; nursing informatics. *Clinical nurse specialist programs in:* community health.
Study Options Full-time and part-time.
Online Degree Options Yes.
Program Entrance Requirements Computer literacy, minimum overall college GPA of 3.0, transcript of college record, CPR certification, written essay, immunizations, interview, 1 letter of recommendation, nursing research course, prerequisite course work, resume. *Application deadline:* 2/1 (fall), 9/1 (spring). Applications may be processed on a rolling basis for some programs. *Application fee:* $75.
Advanced Placement Credit given for nursing courses completed elsewhere dependent upon specific evaluations.
Degree Requirements 38 total credit hours, comprehensive exam.

DOCTORAL DEGREE PROGRAM

Degree DNP
Available Programs Doctorate; Post-Baccalaureate Doctorate.
Areas of Study Advanced practice nursing, aging, bio-behavioral research, biology of health and illness, clinical practice, clinical research, critical care, family health, gerontology, health policy, health promotion/disease prevention, health-care systems, human health and illness, illness and transition, maternity-newborn, nurse case management, nursing administration, nursing education, nursing policy, nursing research, nursing science, palliative care.
Program Entrance Requirements Clinical experience, minimum overall college GPA of 3.0, interview by faculty committee, interview, 3 letters of recommendation, MSN or equivalent, vita, writing sample. Application deadline: 11/1 (fall). Application fee: $75.
Degree Requirements 79 total credit hours.

Degree PhD
Available Programs Doctorate, Post-Baccalaureate Doctorate.
Areas of Study Addiction/substance abuse, aging, bio-behavioral research, biology of health and illness, critical care, gerontology, health promotion/disease prevention, illness and transition, maternity-newborn, nursing administration, nursing research, nursing science, oncology.
Program Entrance Requirements Minimum overall college GPA of 3.5, interview, interview by faculty committee, 3 letters of recommendation, statistics course, vita. Application deadline: 2/16 (fall). Application fee: $75.
Degree Requirements 60 total credit hours, dissertation, oral exam, residency, written exam; 18 additional credits for BSN-PhD.

CONTINUING EDUCATION PROGRAM

Contact Patricia D. Franklin, Assistant Professor and Director of Professional Education, Nursing Programs, University of Maryland, Baltimore, 655 West Lombard Street, Room 311H, Baltimore, MD 21201-1579. *Telephone:* 410-706-7630.
E-mail: franklin@son.umaryland.edu.

MASSACHUSETTS

American International College
Division of Nursing
Springfield, Massachusetts

http://www.aic.edu/academics/hs/nursing
Founded in 1885
DEGREES • BSN • MSN
Nursing Program Faculty 15 (33% with doctorates).
Baccalaureate Enrollment 366 **Women** 88% **Men** 12% **Part-time** 8%
Graduate Enrollment 53 **Women** 94% **Men** 6% **Part-time** 4%
Distance Learning Courses Available.
Nursing Student Activities Nursing Honor Society, Sigma Theta Tau, Student Nurses' Association.
Nursing Student Resources Academic advising; academic or career counseling; assistance for students with disabilities; bookstore; campus computer network; career placement assistance; computer lab; e-mail services; employment services for current students; externships; housing assistance; interactive nursing skills videos; Internet; learning resource lab; library services; nursing audiovisuals; other; placement services for program completers; remedial services; resume preparation assistance; skills, simulation, or other laboratory; tutoring; unpaid internships.
Library Facilities 2,155 volumes in health, 235 volumes in nursing; 67 periodical subscriptions health-care related.

BACCALAUREATE PROGRAMS

Degree BSN
Available Programs ADN to Baccalaureate; Accelerated Baccalaureate for Second Degree; Baccalaureate for Second Degree; Generic Baccalaureate; RN Baccalaureate.
Study Options Full-time and part-time.
Program Entrance Requirements Minimum overall college GPA of 2.5, transcript of college record, health exam, health insurance, high school biology, high school chemistry, 3 years high school math, 2 years high school science, high school transcript, immunizations, minimum high school GPA of 2.5, minimum GPA in nursing prerequisites of 2.5, professional liability insurance/malpractice insurance, prerequisite course work. Transfer students are accepted. *Application deadline:* 2/15 (fall). Applications may be processed on a rolling basis for some programs. *Application fee:* $25.
Advanced Placement Credit by examination available. Credit given for nursing courses completed elsewhere dependent upon specific evaluations.
Expenses (2015–16) *Tuition:* full-time $31,870; part-time $660 per credit. *International tuition:* $31,870 full-time. *Room and board:* $12,900; room only: $6660 per academic year. *Required fees:* full-time $1193; part-time $596 per term.
Financial Aid 100% of baccalaureate students in nursing programs received some form of financial aid in 2014–15.
Contact Mr. Jonathan Scully, Director of Undergraduate Admissions, Division of Nursing, American International College, 1000 State Street,

Springfield, MA 01109. *Telephone:* 413-205-3270. *Fax:* 413-205-3275. *E-mail:* jonathan.scully@aic.edu.

GRADUATE PROGRAMS

Expenses (2015–16) *Tuition:* full-time $7800; part-time $650 per credit. *International tuition:* $7800 full-time. *Room and board:* $12,900; room only: $6660 per academic year. *Required fees:* full-time $60; part-time $30 per term.
Financial Aid 54% of graduate students in nursing programs received some form of financial aid in 2014–15.
Contact Ms. Kerry Barnes, Director of Graduate Admissions, Division of Nursing, American International College, 1000 State Street, Springfield, MA 01109. *Telephone:* 413-205-3703. *Fax:* 413-205-3201. *E-mail:* kerry.barnes@aic.edu.

MASTER'S DEGREE PROGRAM

Degree MSN
Available Programs Accelerated Master's; Accelerated Master's for Nurses with Non-Nursing Degrees; Accelerated RN to Master's; Master's; Master's for Nurses with Non-Nursing Degrees; RN to Master's.
Concentrations Available Nursing administration; nursing education. *Nurse practitioner programs in:* family health.
Study Options Full-time and part-time.
Online Degree Options Yes (online only).
Program Entrance Requirements Clinical experience, minimum overall college GPA of 3.0, transcript of college record, CPR certification, written essay, immunizations, 2 letters of recommendation, professional liability insurance/malpractice insurance, prerequisite course work, resume. *Application deadline:* 9/1 (fall), 1/5 (spring). Applications may be processed on a rolling basis for some programs. *Application fee:* $50.
Advanced Placement Credit given for nursing courses completed elsewhere dependent upon specific evaluations.
Degree Requirements 36 total credit hours, thesis or project.

Anna Maria College
Department of Nursing
Paxton, Massachusetts

http://www.annamaria.edu/
Founded in 1946
DEGREE • BSN
Nursing Program Faculty 6 (16% with doctorates).
Baccalaureate Enrollment 32 **Women** 94% **Men** 6% **Part-time** 100%
Nursing Student Activities Sigma Theta Tau.
Nursing Student Resources Academic advising; academic or career counseling; assistance for students with disabilities; bookstore; campus computer network; career placement assistance; computer lab; e-mail services; employment services for current students; Internet; learning resource lab; library services; nursing audiovisuals; placement services for program completers; remedial services; resume preparation assistance; skills, simulation, or other laboratory; tutoring; unpaid internships.
Library Facilities 3,000 volumes in health, 400 volumes in nursing; 22 periodical subscriptions health-care related.

BACCALAUREATE PROGRAMS

Degree BSN
Available Programs ADN to Baccalaureate; RN Baccalaureate.
Study Options Part-time.
Program Entrance Requirements Minimum overall college GPA of 2.5, transcript of college record, interview, 1 letter of recommendation, minimum high school GPA of 2.5, minimum GPA in nursing prerequisites of 2.5, RN licensure. Transfer students are accepted. *Application deadline:* Applications may be processed on a rolling basis for some programs. *Application fee:* $40.
Advanced Placement Credit by examination available. Credit given for nursing courses completed elsewhere dependent upon specific evaluations.
Contact *Telephone:* 508-829-3316 Ext. 316. *Fax:* 508-849-3343 Ext. 371.

CONTINUING EDUCATION PROGRAM

Contact *Telephone:* 508-849-3316 Ext. 316. *Fax:* 508-849-3343 Ext. 371.

Becker College
Nursing Programs
Worcester, Massachusetts

http://www.becker.edu/academics/departments-programs/health-sciences/nursing
Founded in 1784
DEGREE • BSN
Nursing Program Faculty 30 (14% with doctorates).
Baccalaureate Enrollment 88 **Women** 92% **Men** 8% **Part-time** 20%
Nursing Student Activities Student Nurses' Association, nursing club.
Nursing Student Resources Academic advising; academic or career counseling; assistance for students with disabilities; bookstore; campus computer network; career placement assistance; computer lab; e-mail services; employment services for current students; externships; interactive nursing skills videos; Internet; learning resource lab; library services; nursing audiovisuals; other; placement services for program completers; remedial services; resume preparation assistance; skills, simulation, or other laboratory; tutoring; unpaid internships.
Library Facilities 3,073 volumes in health, 547 volumes in nursing; 2,268 periodical subscriptions health-care related.

BACCALAUREATE PROGRAMS

Degree BSN
Available Programs ADN to Baccalaureate; Generic Baccalaureate; RN Baccalaureate.
Study Options Full-time.
Program Entrance Requirements Minimum overall college GPA, transcript of college record, health exam, health insurance, high school biology, high school transcript, letters of recommendation, minimum high school GPA, minimum GPA in nursing prerequisites, prerequisite course work. Transfer students are accepted. *Application deadline:* 2/15 (fall), 1/5 (spring).
Advanced Placement Credit by examination available.
Expenses (2014–15) *Tuition:* full-time $32,870; part-time $1305 per credit. *Room and board:* $12,000 per academic year. *Required fees:* full-time $2000.
Financial Aid 100% of baccalaureate students in nursing programs received some form of financial aid in 2013–14. *Gift aid (need-based):* Federal Pell, FSEOG, state, private, college/university gift aid from institutional funds. *Loans:* Federal Direct (Subsidized and Unsubsidized Stafford PLUS), state, alternative loans. *Work-study:* Federal Work-Study. *Financial aid application deadline (priority):* 3/15.
Contact Linda Esper, Director and Professor of Nursing, Nursing Programs, Becker College, 61 Sever Street, Worcester, MA 01609. *Telephone:* 508-373-9727. *Fax:* 508-849-5385. *E-mail:* linda.esper@becker.edu.

CONTINUING EDUCATION PROGRAM

Contact Mr. Robert Outerbridge, Director of Enrollment Management, Center for Accelerated and Professional Studies, Nursing Programs, Becker College, 61 Sever Street, Weller 300, Worcester, MA 01609. *Telephone:* 508-373-9510. *Fax:* 508-791-9241. *E-mail:* robert.outerbridge@becker.edu.

Boston College
William F. Connell School of Nursing
Chestnut Hill, Massachusetts

http://www.bc.edu/nursing
Founded in 1863
DEGREES • BS • MS • MS/MA • MS/MBA • MS/PHD • PHD
Nursing Program Faculty 105 (42% with doctorates).
Baccalaureate Enrollment 411 **Women** 94% **Men** 6%
Graduate Enrollment 267 **Women** 89% **Men** 11% **Part-time** 27%
Nursing Student Activities Nursing Honor Society, Sigma Theta Tau, Student Nurses' Association.
Nursing Student Resources Academic advising; academic or career counseling; assistance for students with disabilities; bookstore; campus computer network; career placement assistance; computer lab; computer-assisted instruction; e-mail services; employment services for current students; externships; housing assistance; interactive nursing skills videos; Internet; learning resource lab; library services; nursing audiovisuals; other; placement services for program completers; remedial services;

resume preparation assistance; skills, simulation, or other laboratory; tutoring; unpaid internships.

Library Facilities 65,000 volumes in health, 20,000 volumes in nursing; 5,395 periodical subscriptions health-care related.

BACCALAUREATE PROGRAMS

Degree BS

Available Programs Generic Baccalaureate.

Study Options Full-time.

Program Entrance Requirements Transcript of college record, written essay, health exam, health insurance, high school biology, high school chemistry, high school foreign language, 4 years high school math, 4 years high school science, high school transcript, immunizations, 2 letters of recommendation. Transfer students are accepted. *Application deadline:* 1/1 (fall), 11/1 (winter). *Application fee:* $70.

Advanced Placement Credit given for nursing courses completed elsewhere dependent upon specific evaluations.

Expenses (2015–16) *Tuition:* full-time $48,540. *International tuition:* $48,540 full-time. *Room and board:* $13,496; room only: $8390 per academic year. *Required fees:* full-time $1266.

Financial Aid 82% of baccalaureate students in nursing programs received some form of financial aid in 2014–15.

Contact Office of Undergraduate Admissions, William F. Connell School of Nursing, Boston College, 140 Commonwealth Avenue, Devlin Hall 208, Chestnut Hill, MA 02467-3812. *Telephone:* 617-552-3100. *Fax:* 617-552-0798.

GRADUATE PROGRAMS

Expenses (2015–16) *Tuition:* part-time $1248 per credit hour. *International tuition:* $1248 full-time. *Required fees:* full-time $90; part-time $60 per credit.

Financial Aid 84% of graduate students in nursing programs received some form of financial aid in 2014–15. 8 fellowships with full tuition reimbursements available (averaging $23,112 per year), 24 teaching assistantships (averaging $4,900 per year) were awarded; research assistantships, scholarships, tuition waivers (partial), and unspecified assistantships also available. Aid available to part-time students. *Financial aid application deadline:* 3/1.

Contact Ms. Marybeth Crowley, Graduate Programs and Admissions Specialist, William F. Connell School of Nursing, Boston College, 140 Commonwealth Avenue, Maloney Hall, Chestnut Hill, MA 02467-3812. *Telephone:* 617-552-4928. *Fax:* 617-552-2121. *E-mail:* csongrad@bc.edu.

MASTER'S DEGREE PROGRAM

Degrees MS; MS/MA; MS/MBA, MS/PHD

Available Programs Accelerated Master's for Non-Nursing College Graduates; Master's; RN to Master's.

Concentrations Available Nurse anesthesia. *Nurse practitioner programs in:* adult-gerontology primary care, family health, pediatric primary care, psychiatric/mental health, women's health.

Study Options Full-time and part-time.

Program Entrance Requirements Minimum overall college GPA of 3.3, transcript of college record, CPR certification, written essay, immunizations, 2 letters of recommendation, professional liability insurance/malpractice insurance, resume, statistics course. *Application deadline:* 3/15 (fall), 9/30 (spring). *Application fee:* $40.

Advanced Placement Credit given for nursing courses completed elsewhere dependent upon specific evaluations.

Degree Requirements 45 total credit hours, comprehensive exam.

POST-MASTER'S PROGRAM

Areas of Study Nurse anesthesia. *Nurse practitioner programs in:* family health, pediatric primary care, psychiatric/mental health, women's health.

DOCTORAL DEGREE PROGRAM

Degree PhD

Available Programs Doctorate; Post-Baccalaureate Doctorate.

Areas of Study Aging, bio-behavioral research, clinical research, ethics, family health, gerontology, health promotion/disease prevention, health-care systems, human health and illness, illness and transition, individualized study, nursing research, nursing science, oncology, urban health.

Program Entrance Requirements Minimum overall college GPA of 3.5, interview by faculty committee, interview, 3 letters of recommendation, MSN or equivalent, statistics course, vita, writing sample, GRE General Test. Application deadline: 1/15 (fall). Application fee: $40.

Degree Requirements 46 total credit hours, dissertation, oral exam, written exam.

CONTINUING EDUCATION PROGRAM

Contact Dr. Jean Weyman, Assistant Dean, Continuing Education, William F. Connell School of Nursing, Boston College, 140 Commonwealth Avenue, Maloney Hall, Chestnut Hill, MA 02467-3812. *Telephone:* 617-552-4256. *Fax:* 617-552-0745. *E-mail:* jean.weyman@bc.edu.

Curry College
Division of Nursing
Milton, Massachusetts

http://www.curry.edu/
Founded in 1879

DEGREES • BS • MSN

Nursing Program Faculty 48 (33% with doctorates).

Baccalaureate Enrollment 611 **Women** 92% **Men** 8% **Part-time** 48%

Graduate Enrollment 31 **Women** 97% **Men** 3% **Part-time** 100%

Nursing Student Activities Sigma Theta Tau, Student Nurses' Association.

Nursing Student Resources Academic advising; academic or career counseling; assistance for students with disabilities; bookstore; campus computer network; career placement assistance; computer lab; computer-assisted instruction; daycare for children of students; e-mail services; employment services for current students; housing assistance; interactive nursing skills videos; Internet; learning resource lab; library services; nursing audiovisuals; placement services for program completers; remedial services; resume preparation assistance; skills, simulation, or other laboratory; tutoring.

Library Facilities 5,867 volumes in health, 4,589 volumes in nursing; 162 periodical subscriptions health-care related.

BACCALAUREATE PROGRAMS

Degree BS

Available Programs Accelerated Baccalaureate for Second Degree; Generic Baccalaureate; RN Baccalaureate; RPN to Baccalaureate.

Site Options Boston, MA; Plymouth, MA.

Study Options Full-time.

Program Entrance Requirements Written essay, health exam, health insurance, high school biology, high school chemistry, high school foreign language, 4 years high school math, 4 years high school science, high school transcript, immunizations, 1 letter of recommendation, minimum high school GPA of 2.75, minimum GPA in nursing prerequisites of 3.0. Transfer students are accepted. *Application deadline:* 4/1 (fall). Applications may be processed on a rolling basis for some programs. *Application fee:* $50.

Advanced Placement Credit by examination available. Credit given for nursing courses completed elsewhere dependent upon specific evaluations.

Contact *Telephone:* 800-669-0686. *Fax:* 617-333-2114.

GRADUATE PROGRAMS

Contact *Telephone:* 617-333-2243. *Fax:* 617-333-6680.

MASTER'S DEGREE PROGRAM

Degree MSN

Available Programs Master's; RN to Master's.

Concentrations Available Clinical nurse leader.

Site Options Boston, MA.

Program Entrance Requirements Minimum overall college GPA of 3.0, transcript of college record, written essay, immunizations, 2 letters of recommendation, nursing research course, physical assessment course, resume, statistics course. *Application deadline:* Applications may be processed on a rolling basis for some programs. *Application fee:* $50.

Degree Requirements 37 total credit hours, thesis or project.

Elms College
School of Nursing
Chicopee, Massachusetts

http://www.elms.edu/
Founded in 1928

DEGREES • BS • DNP • MSN • MSN/MBA

Nursing Program Faculty 18 (61% with doctorates).

Baccalaureate Enrollment 240 **Women** 87% **Men** 13% **Part-time** 35%

Graduate Enrollment 42 **Women** 97% **Men** 3% **Part-time** 50%

Distance Learning Courses Available.

Nursing Student Activities Nursing Honor Society, Sigma Theta Tau, Student Nurses' Association.

Nursing Student Resources Academic advising; academic or career counseling; assistance for students with disabilities; bookstore; campus computer network; career placement assistance; computer lab; computer-assisted instruction; e-mail services; employment services for current students; externships; interactive nursing skills videos; Internet; learning resource lab; library services; nursing audiovisuals; resume preparation assistance; skills, simulation, or other laboratory; tutoring.

Library Facilities 3,832 volumes in health, 3,000 volumes in nursing; 130 periodical subscriptions health-care related.

BACCALAUREATE PROGRAMS

Degree BS

Available Programs Accelerated Baccalaureate; Generic Baccalaureate; RN Baccalaureate.

Site Options Gardner, MA; Pittsfield, MA; Worcester, MA.

Study Options Full-time and part-time.

Program Entrance Requirements Minimum overall college GPA of 2.5, transcript of college record, CPR certification, written essay, health exam, health insurance, high school biology, high school chemistry, high school transcript, immunizations, interview, 2 letters of recommendation, minimum high school GPA of 3.3, minimum high school rank 25%, minimum GPA in nursing prerequisites of 2.5, professional liability insurance/malpractice insurance. Transfer students are accepted. *Application deadline:* Applications may be processed on a rolling basis for some programs. *Application fee:* $30.

Advanced Placement Credit given for nursing courses completed elsewhere dependent upon specific evaluations.

Expenses (2015–16) *Tuition:* full-time $30,768; part-time $624 per credit. *International tuition:* $30,768 full-time. *Room and board:* $11,708 per academic year. *Required fees:* full-time $1512.

Financial Aid *Gift aid (need-based):* Federal Pell, FSEOG, state, private, college/university gift aid from institutional funds. *Loans:* Federal Direct (Subsidized and Unsubsidized Stafford PLUS), Perkins. *Work-study:* Federal Work-Study. *Financial aid application deadline (priority):* 3/1.

Contact Dr. Kathleen B. Scoble, Director and Chair, School of Nursing, Elms College, 291 Springfield Street, Chicopee, MA 01013. *Telephone:* 413-265-2237. *Fax:* 413-265-2335. *E-mail:* scoblek@elms.edu.

GRADUATE PROGRAMS

Expenses (2015–16) *Tuition:* part-time $720 per credit.

Contact Dr. Cynthia Dakin, Director of Graduate Program, School of Nursing, Elms College, 291 Springfield Street, Chicopee, MA 01013. *Telephone:* 413-265-2455. *E-mail:* dakinc@elms.edu.

MASTER'S DEGREE PROGRAM

Degrees MSN; MSN/MBA

Available Programs Master's; RN to Master's.

Concentrations Available Nursing administration; nursing education.

Study Options Full-time and part-time.

Program Entrance Requirements Minimum overall college GPA of 3.0, transcript of college record, CPR certification, written essay, immunizations, interview, 2 letters of recommendation, professional liability insurance/malpractice insurance, resume. *Application deadline:* Applications may be processed on a rolling basis for some programs. *Application fee:* $30.

Degree Requirements 36 total credit hours, thesis or project.

DOCTORAL DEGREE PROGRAM

Degree DNP

Available Programs Doctorate.

Areas of Study Family health, gerontology.

Site Options Pittsfield, MA.

Program Entrance Requirements Minimum overall college GPA of 3.0, interview by faculty committee, interview, 3 letters of recommendation, statistics course. Application deadline: 5/15 (spring). Application fee: $50.

Degree Requirements 81 total credit hours.

Emmanuel College

Department of Nursing
Boston, Massachusetts

http://www.emmanuel.edu/graduate-professional-programs/academics/nursing.html

Founded in 1919

DEGREES • BS • MS

Nursing Program Faculty 19 (37% with doctorates).

Baccalaureate Enrollment 78 **Women** 95% **Men** 5% **Part-time** 99%

Graduate Enrollment 43 **Women** 98% **Men** 2% **Part-time** 53%

Distance Learning Courses Available.

Nursing Student Activities Sigma Theta Tau.

Nursing Student Resources Academic advising; academic or career counseling; assistance for students with disabilities; bookstore; campus computer network; computer lab; computer-assisted instruction; e-mail services; interactive nursing skills videos; Internet; library services; nursing audiovisuals; resume preparation assistance; skills, simulation, or other laboratory; tutoring.

Library Facilities 2,522 volumes in health, 713 volumes in nursing; 7,625 periodical subscriptions health-care related.

BACCALAUREATE PROGRAMS

Degree BS

Available Programs RN Baccalaureate.

Site Options Boston, MA.

Study Options Full-time and part-time.

Program Entrance Requirements Minimum overall college GPA of 2.0, transcript of college record, written essay, interview, 2 letters of recommendation, prerequisite course work, RN licensure. Transfer students are accepted. *Application deadline:* Applications may be processed on a rolling basis for some programs.

Advanced Placement Credit by examination available. Credit given for nursing courses completed elsewhere dependent upon specific evaluations.

Expenses (2015–16) *Tuition:* part-time $1816 per course.

Financial Aid *Gift aid (need-based):* Federal Pell, FSEOG, state, private, college/university gift aid from institutional funds. *Loans:* Federal Direct (Subsidized and Unsubsidized Stafford PLUS), Perkins, state. *Work-study:* Federal Work-Study, part-time campus jobs. *Financial aid application deadline (priority):* 2/15.

Contact Dr. Mary Diane Arathuzik, RN, Chair and Associate Professor, Department of Nursing, Emmanuel College, 400 The Fenway, Boston, MA 02115. *Telephone:* 617-735-9845. *Fax:* 617-507-0434. *E-mail:* arathuzi@emmanuel.edu.

GRADUATE PROGRAMS

Expenses (2015–16) *Tuition:* part-time $2581 per course.

Contact Dr. Mary Diane Arathuzik, RN, Chair and Associate Professor of Nursing, Department of Nursing, Emmanuel College, 400 The Fenway, Boston, MA 02115. *Telephone:* 617-735-9845. *Fax:* 617-507-0434. *E-mail:* arathuzi@emmanuel.edu.

MASTER'S DEGREE PROGRAM

Degree MS

Available Programs Master's.

Concentrations Available Nursing administration; nursing education.

Site Options Boston, MA.

Study Options Full-time and part-time.

Program Entrance Requirements Clinical experience, minimum overall college GPA of 3.0, transcript of college record, written essay, 2 letters of recommendation, resume. *Application deadline:* 4/30 (fall).

Advanced Placement Credit given for nursing courses completed elsewhere dependent upon specific evaluations.

Degree Requirements 36 total credit hours, comprehensive exam.

See display on next page and full description on page 492.

Endicott College

Major in Nursing
Beverly, Massachusetts

http://www.endicott.edu/
Founded in 1939
DEGREES • BS • MSN
Nursing Program Faculty 27 (25% with doctorates).
Baccalaureate Enrollment 170 **Women** 95% **Men** 5% **Part-time** 20%
Graduate Enrollment 25 **Women** 97% **Men** 3%
Distance Learning Courses Available.
Nursing Student Activities Nursing Honor Society, Sigma Theta Tau, Student Nurses' Association.
Nursing Student Resources Academic advising; academic or career counseling; assistance for students with disabilities; bookstore; campus computer network; career placement assistance; computer lab; computer-assisted instruction; e-mail services; externships; interactive nursing skills videos; Internet; learning resource lab; library services; nursing audiovisuals; resume preparation assistance; skills, simulation, or other laboratory; tutoring; unpaid internships.
Library Facilities 2,828 volumes in health, 624 volumes in nursing; 55 periodical subscriptions health-care related.

BACCALAUREATE PROGRAMS

Degree BS
Available Programs Generic Baccalaureate; RN Baccalaureate.
Site Options Beverly, MA.
Study Options Full-time.
Program Entrance Requirements Minimum overall college GPA of 2.5, transcript of college record, written essay, health exam, health insurance, high school biology, high school chemistry, 3 years high school math, 2 years high school science, high school transcript, immunizations, 1 letter of recommendation, minimum high school GPA of 2.5, minimum high school rank 50%, minimum GPA in nursing prerequisites of 2.5. Transfer students are accepted.
Advanced Placement Credit given for nursing courses completed elsewhere dependent upon specific evaluations.
Contact *Telephone:* 978-232-2005. *Fax:* 978-232-2500.

GRADUATE PROGRAMS

MASTER'S DEGREE PROGRAM
Degree MSN
Available Programs Master's.
Concentrations Available Nursing administration; nursing education.
Site Options Beverly, MA.
Study Options Full-time and part-time.
Program Entrance Requirements Clinical experience, transcript of college record, written essay, letters of recommendation, statistics course.
Advanced Placement Credit given for nursing courses completed elsewhere dependent upon specific evaluations.
Degree Requirements 33 total credit hours, thesis or project.

CONTINUING EDUCATION PROGRAM

Contact *Telephone:* 978-232-2328. *Fax:* 978-232-3100.

Fitchburg State University

Department of Nursing
Fitchburg, Massachusetts

http://www.fitchburgstate.edu/academics/academic-departments/department-homepage-nursing/
Founded in 1894
DEGREES • BS • MS
Nursing Program Faculty 18 (28% with doctorates).
Baccalaureate Enrollment 450 **Part-time** 22%
Graduate Enrollment 32 **Women** 97% **Men** 3% **Part-time** 100%
Distance Learning Courses Available.
Nursing Student Activities Sigma Theta Tau, Student Nurses' Association.
Nursing Student Resources Academic advising; academic or career counseling; assistance for students with disabilities; bookstore; campus computer network; career placement assistance; computer lab; computer-assisted instruction; e-mail services; employment services for current students; housing assistance; interactive nursing skills videos; Internet; learning resource lab; library services; nursing audiovisuals; remedial

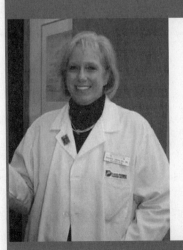

Where an RN becomes a transformational leader

This is the Emmanuel College Nursing Program

- After 30 years of educating Boston's best nurses, our BSN, MSN and graduate certificate programs are preparing leaders in the field.

- Two distinct tracks within the MSN and graduate certificate programs: Nursing Education or Nursing Management/Administration.

- Flexible schedule – classes meet once every other week in the evening.

- Small classes led by expert faculty, who also provide academic advising.

- Experiential learning opportunities offered right in the Longwood Medical and Academic Area.

- BSN and MSN programs accredited by the Commission on Collegiate Nursing Education (CCNE).

LEARN MORE

617-735-9700 | emmanuel.edu/PETERSONS
400 The Fenway, Boston, MA 02115

EMMANUEL COLLEGE
Graduate and Professional Programs

services; resume preparation assistance; skills, simulation, or other laboratory; tutoring; unpaid internships.

Library Facilities 13,451 volumes in health, 11,923 volumes in nursing; 7,605 periodical subscriptions health-care related.

BACCALAUREATE PROGRAMS

Degree BS

Available Programs Accelerated LPN to Baccalaureate; Generic Baccalaureate; RN Baccalaureate.

Study Options Full-time.

Online Degree Options Yes.

Program Entrance Requirements Transcript of college record, written essay, health insurance, high school biology, high school chemistry, high school foreign language, 4 years high school math, 3 years high school science, high school transcript, immunizations, minimum high school GPA of 3.0, minimum GPA in nursing prerequisites of 2.5. Transfer students are accepted. *Application deadline:* 1/1 (fall). Applications may be processed on a rolling basis for some programs. *Application fee:* $25.

Expenses (2015–16) *Tuition, state resident:* full-time $970; part-time $40 per credit. *Tuition, nonresident:* full-time $7050; part-time $294 per credit. *Room and board:* $9130; room only: $6000 per academic year. *Required fees:* part-time $374 per credit; part-time $4483 per term.

Financial Aid 76% of baccalaureate students in nursing programs received some form of financial aid in 2014–15.

Contact Mr. Sean Ganas, Director of Admissions, Department of Nursing, Fitchburg State University, 160 Pearl Street, Fitchburg, MA 01420-2697. *Telephone:* 978-665-3140. *Fax:* 978-665-4540. *E-mail:* sganas@fitchburgstate.edu.

GRADUATE PROGRAMS

Expenses (2015–16) *Tuition, state resident:* part-time $167 per credit. *Tuition, nonresident:* part-time $167 per credit.

Financial Aid 20% of graduate students in nursing programs received some form of financial aid in 2014–15.

Contact Dr. Robert Dumas, Chairperson, Forensic Nursing Program, Department of Nursing, Fitchburg State University, 160 Pearl Street, Fitchburg, MA 01420-2697. *Telephone:* 978-665-3026. *Fax:* 978-665-4501. *E-mail:* rdumas@fitchburgstate.edu.

MASTER'S DEGREE PROGRAM

Degree MS

Available Programs Master's.

Study Options Part-time.

Online Degree Options Yes (online only).

Program Entrance Requirements Clinical experience, computer literacy, minimum overall college GPA of 2.8, transcript of college record, written essay, immunizations, 3 letters of recommendation, nursing research course, physical assessment course, prerequisite course work, resume, statistics course. *Application deadline:* Applications may be processed on a rolling basis for some programs. *Application fee:* $25.

Degree Requirements 39 total credit hours, thesis or project.

Framingham State University

Department of Nursing
Framingham, Massachusetts

http://www.framingham.edu/nursing
Founded in 1839

DEGREES • BS • MSN

Nursing Program Faculty 8 (75% with doctorates).

Baccalaureate Enrollment 74 **Women** 85% **Men** 15% **Part-time** 90%

Graduate Enrollment 58 **Women** 98% **Men** 2% **Part-time** 100%

Nursing Student Activities Sigma Theta Tau.

Nursing Student Resources Academic advising; academic or career counseling; assistance for students with disabilities; bookstore; campus computer network; career placement assistance; computer lab; computer-assisted instruction; daycare for children of students; e-mail services; employment services for current students; housing assistance; interactive nursing skills videos; Internet; learning resource lab; library services; nursing audiovisuals; placement services for program completers; remedial services; resume preparation assistance; skills, simulation, or other laboratory; tutoring.

Library Facilities 5,338 volumes in health, 5,338 volumes in nursing; 1,200 periodical subscriptions health-care related.

BACCALAUREATE PROGRAMS

Degree BS

Available Programs ADN to Baccalaureate.

Study Options Full-time and part-time.

Program Entrance Requirements Minimum overall college GPA of 3.0, transcript of college record, written essay, RN licensure. Transfer students are accepted. *Application deadline:* Applications may be processed on a rolling basis for some programs. *Application fee:* $50.

Advanced Placement Credit by examination available. Credit given for nursing courses completed elsewhere dependent upon specific evaluations.

Contact *Telephone:* 508-626-4713. *Fax:* 508-626-4746.

GRADUATE PROGRAMS

Contact *Telephone:* 508-626-4713. *Fax:* 508-626-4746.

MASTER'S DEGREE PROGRAM

Degree MSN

Available Programs Master's.

Concentrations Available Nursing administration; nursing education.

Study Options Part-time.

Program Entrance Requirements Minimum overall college GPA of 3.0, transcript of college record, written essay, interview, 3 letters of recommendation, nursing research course, resume, statistics course. *Application deadline:* 6/1 (fall). Applications may be processed on a rolling basis for some programs. *Application fee:* $50.

Degree Requirements 36 total credit hours, thesis or project.

CONTINUING EDUCATION PROGRAM

Contact *Telephone:* 508-626-4713. *Fax:* 508-626-4746.

Labouré College

Bachelor of Science in Nursing Program
Boston, Massachusetts

Founded in 1971

DEGREE • BSN

BACCALAUREATE PROGRAMS

Degree BSN

Available Programs Generic Baccalaureate.

Contact *Telephone:* 617-202-3149.

MCPHS University

School of Nursing
Boston, Massachusetts

http://www.mcphs.edu/
Founded in 1823

DEGREE • BSN

Nursing Program Faculty 16 (44% with doctorates).

Baccalaureate Enrollment 358 **Women** 66.3% **Men** 33.7%

Distance Learning Courses Available.

Nursing Student Activities Nursing Honor Society, Sigma Theta Tau, Student Nurses' Association, nursing club.

Nursing Student Resources Academic advising; academic or career counseling; assistance for students with disabilities; bookstore; campus computer network; career placement assistance; computer lab; computer-assisted instruction; e-mail services; employment services for current students; housing assistance; interactive nursing skills videos; Internet; learning resource lab; library services; nursing audiovisuals; remedial services; resume preparation assistance; skills, simulation, or other laboratory; tutoring.

Library Facilities 17,400 volumes in health, 1,200 volumes in nursing; 10,000 periodical subscriptions health-care related.

BACCALAUREATE PROGRAMS

Degree BSN

Available Programs Accelerated Baccalaureate; Accelerated Baccalaureate for Second Degree.

Site Options Manchester , NH; Worcester , MA.

Study Options Full-time.

Program Entrance Requirements Minimum overall college GPA of 2.5, written essay, high school biology, high school chemistry, 3 years high school math, 2 years high school science, high school transcript, 2 letters of recommendation, prerequisite course work. Transfer students are accepted. *Application deadline:* 2/1 (fall), 10/1 (spring). *Application fee:* $70.
Contact *Telephone:* 800-225-5506.

CONTINUING EDUCATION PROGRAM

Contact *Telephone:* 617-735-1080.

MGH Institute of Health Professions
School of Nursing
Boston, Massachusetts

http://www.mghihp.edu/academics/nursing/
Founded in 1977
DEGREES • BSN • DNP • MS
Nursing Program Faculty 63 (71% with doctorates).
Baccalaureate Enrollment 199 **Women** 83% **Men** 17% **Part-time** 3%
Graduate Enrollment 376 **Women** 89% **Men** 11% **Part-time** 17%
Distance Learning Courses Available.
Nursing Student Activities Nursing Honor Society, Sigma Theta Tau, Student Nurses' Association, nursing club.
Nursing Student Resources Academic advising; academic or career counseling; assistance for students with disabilities; bookstore; campus computer network; career placement assistance; computer lab; computer-assisted instruction; daycare for children of students; e-mail services; employment services for current students; interactive nursing skills videos; Internet; learning resource lab; library services; nursing audiovisuals; remedial services; resume preparation assistance; skills, simulation, or other laboratory; tutoring.
Library Facilities 10,000 volumes in health, 8,000 volumes in nursing; 2,500 periodical subscriptions health-care related.

BACCALAUREATE PROGRAMS

Degree BSN
Available Programs Accelerated Baccalaureate.
Site Options Boston, MA.
Study Options Full-time.
Program Entrance Requirements Transcript of college record, written essay, health insurance, immunizations, 3 letters of recommendation, minimum GPA in nursing prerequisites of 3.0, prerequisite course work. Transfer students are accepted. *Application deadline:* 7/1 (spring), 11/1 (summer). *Application fee:* $100.
Advanced Placement Credit by examination available. Credit given for nursing courses completed elsewhere dependent upon specific evaluations.
Expenses (2015–16) *Tuition:* full-time $53,200. *International tuition:* $53,200 full-time. *Required fees:* full-time $3250.
Contact Admissions, School of Nursing, MGH Institute of Health Professions, 36 1st Avenue, Boston, MA 02129. *Telephone:* 617-726-3140. *Fax:* 617-726-8010. *E-mail:* admissions@mghihp.edu.

GRADUATE PROGRAMS

Expenses (2015–16) *Tuition:* full-time $52,650; part-time $1170 per credit. *International tuition:* $52,650 full-time. *Required fees:* full-time $3250.
Financial Aid 4 research assistantships (averaging $1,200 per year), 17 teaching assistantships (averaging $1,200 per year) were awarded; career-related internships or fieldwork, scholarships, traineeships, and unspecified assistantships also available.
Contact Office of Admissions, School of Nursing, MGH Institute of Health Professions, 36 1st Avenue, Building 39, Boston, MA 02129. *Telephone:* 617-726-3140. *Fax:* 617-726-8010.
E-mail: admissions@mghihp.edu.

MASTER'S DEGREE PROGRAM

Degree MS
Available Programs Master's; Master's for Non-Nursing College Graduates; Master's for Nurses with Non-Nursing Degrees; RN to Master's.
Concentrations Available Clinical nurse leader; health-care administration; nursing administration; nursing education. *Nurse practitioner programs in:* acute care, adult health, adult-gerontology acute care, adult-

psychiatric mental health, family health, gerontology, pediatric, primary care, psychiatric/mental health, women's health.
Site Options Boston, MA.
Study Options Full-time and part-time.
Program Entrance Requirements Minimum overall college GPA of 3.0, transcript of college record, CPR certification, written essay, immunizations, 3 letters of recommendation, professional liability insurance/malpractice insurance, prerequisite course work, resume, statistics course, GRE General Test. *Application deadline:* 1/1 (fall). *Application fee:* $100.
Advanced Placement Credit by examination available. Credit given for nursing courses completed elsewhere dependent upon specific evaluations.
Degree Requirements 93 total credit hours, thesis or project.

POST-MASTER'S PROGRAM

Areas of Study Clinical nurse leader; health-care administration. *Nurse practitioner programs in:* acute care, adult health, adult-gerontology acute care, adult-psychiatric mental health, gerontology, pediatric, primary care, psychiatric/mental health, women's health.

DOCTORAL DEGREE PROGRAM

Degree DNP
Available Programs Doctorate; Doctorate for Nurses with Non-Nursing Degrees; Post-Baccalaureate Doctorate.
Areas of Study Nurse executive, nursing administration.
Site Options Boston, MA.
Online Degree Options Yes.
Program Entrance Requirements Minimum overall college GPA of 3.0, interview by faculty committee, 3 letters of recommendation, MSN or equivalent, vita. Application deadline: 6/1 (fall), 11/30 (spring). Applications may be processed on a rolling basis for some programs. Application fee: $100.
Degree Requirements 43 total credit hours.

Northeastern University
School of Nursing
Boston, Massachusetts

http://www.northeastern.edu/bouve/nursing/index.html
Founded in 1898
DEGREES • BSN • MS • MS/MBA • PHD
Nursing Program Faculty 169 (28% with doctorates).
Baccalaureate Enrollment 545 **Women** 92% **Men** 8% **Part-time** 2%
Graduate Enrollment 590 **Women** 78% **Men** 22% **Part-time** 29%
Distance Learning Courses Available.
Nursing Student Activities Sigma Theta Tau, Student Nurses' Association.
Nursing Student Resources Academic advising; academic or career counseling; assistance for students with disabilities; bookstore; campus computer network; career placement assistance; computer lab; computer-assisted instruction; e-mail services; employment services for current students; housing assistance; Internet; learning resource lab; library services; placement services for program completers; resume preparation assistance; skills, simulation, or other laboratory; tutoring.

BACCALAUREATE PROGRAMS

Degree BSN
Available Programs Accelerated Baccalaureate for Second Degree; Generic Baccalaureate; RN Baccalaureate.
Study Options Full-time.
Program Entrance Requirements Health insurance, high school foreign language, 4 years high school science, high school transcript, immunizations. Transfer students are accepted. *Application deadline:* 1/15 (fall). *Application fee:* $75.
Expenses (2015–16) *Tuition:* full-time $44,620. *International tuition:* $44,620 full-time. *Room and board:* $15,000 per academic year. *Required fees:* full-time $910.
Financial Aid *Gift aid (need-based):* Federal Pell, FSEOG, state, private, college/university gift aid from institutional funds. *Loans:* Federal Nursing Student Loans, Federal Direct (Subsidized and Unsubsidized Stafford PLUS), Perkins, state, college/university. *Work-study:* Federal Work-Study. *Financial aid application deadline (priority):* 2/15.
Contact Undergraduate Admissions, School of Nursing, Northeastern University, 360 Huntington Avenue, 200 Kerr Hall, Boston, MA 02115.

Telephone: 617-373-2200. *Fax:* 617-373-8780.
E-mail: admissions@neu.edu.

GRADUATE PROGRAMS

Financial Aid Fellowships, research assistantships, teaching assistantships, career-related internships or fieldwork, institutionally sponsored loans, scholarships, traineeships, tuition waivers (full and partial), and unspecified assistantships available.
Contact *Telephone:* 617-373-3501. *E-mail:* bouvegrad@neu.edu.

MASTER'S DEGREE PROGRAM

Degrees MS; MS/MBA
Available Programs Master's; Master's for Non-Nursing College Graduates.
Concentrations Available Nurse anesthesia; nursing administration; nursing informatics. *Nurse practitioner programs in:* adult-gerontology acute care, family health, neonatal health, pediatric, pediatric primary care, primary care, psychiatric/mental health.
Study Options Full-time and part-time.
Program Entrance Requirements Minimum overall college GPA of 3.0, transcript of college record, written essay, 3 letters of recommendation, statistics course, GRE General Test. *Application deadline:* 3/15 (fall). *Application fee:* $75.
Degree Requirements 43 total credit hours.

POST-MASTER'S PROGRAM

Areas of Study Nurse anesthesia. *Nurse practitioner programs in:* adult-gerontology acute care, neonatal health, pediatric, pediatric primary care, psychiatric/mental health.

DOCTORAL DEGREE PROGRAM

Degree PhD
Available Programs Post-Baccalaureate Doctorate.
Areas of Study Addiction/substance abuse, nursing education, nursing research, oncology, urban health, women's health.
Site Options San Antonio, TX.
Program Entrance Requirements Minimum overall college GPA of 3.5, interview, 3 letters of recommendation, MSN or equivalent, statistics course. Application deadline: 4/15 (fall).
Degree Requirements Dissertation.

CONTINUING EDUCATION PROGRAM

Contact Bouve College of Health Sciences, School of Nursing, Northeastern University, 360 Huntington Avenue, 123 Behrakis Health Sciences Building, Boston, MA 02115. *Telephone:* 617-373-2708. *E-mail:* bouvegrad@neu.edu.

Regis College
School of Nursing, Science and Health Professions
Weston, Massachusetts

http://www.regiscollege.edu/grad
Founded in 1927
DEGREES • BSN • DNP • MSN
Nursing Program Faculty 36 (75% with doctorates).
Baccalaureate Enrollment 78
Graduate Enrollment 650 **Women** 90% **Men** 10%
Nursing Student Activities Sigma Theta Tau, Student Nurses' Association, nursing club.
Nursing Student Resources Academic advising; academic or career counseling; assistance for students with disabilities; bookstore; campus computer network; career placement assistance; computer lab; e-mail services; Internet; learning resource lab; library services; nursing audiovisuals; resume preparation assistance; skills, simulation, or other laboratory; tutoring.
Library Facilities 6,300 volumes in health, 4,700 volumes in nursing; 228 periodical subscriptions health-care related.

BACCALAUREATE PROGRAMS

Degree BSN
Available Programs ADN to Baccalaureate; Accelerated Baccalaureate; Accelerated Baccalaureate for Second Degree; Accelerated RN Baccalaureate; Baccalaureate for Second Degree; Generic Baccalaureate; RN Baccalaureate.

Site Options Newton, MA; Medford, MA; Boston, MA.
Study Options Full-time.
Program Entrance Requirements Written essay, health exam, health insurance, high school foreign language, 3 years high school math, 2 years high school science, high school transcript, immunizations, 2 letters of recommendation, minimum high school GPA of 3.0, minimum high school rank 40%, minimum GPA in nursing prerequisites. Transfer students are accepted. *Application deadline:* Applications may be processed on a rolling basis for some programs. *Application fee:* $50.
Advanced Placement Credit by examination available. Credit given for nursing courses completed elsewhere dependent upon specific evaluations.
Contact Dr. Penelope Glynn, Dean, School of Nursing and Health Sciences, School of Nursing, Science and Health Professions, Regis College, 235 Wellesley Street, Weston, MA 02493. *Telephone:* 781-768-7090. *Fax:* 781-768-7071. *E-mail:* penelope.glynn@regiscollege.edu.

GRADUATE PROGRAMS

Financial Aid Research assistantships, Federal Work-Study, scholarships, traineeships, and unspecified assistantships available.
Contact Ms. Shelagh Tomaino, Director of Graduate Admission, School of Nursing, Science and Health Professions, Regis College, 235 Wellesley Street, Weston, MA 02493. *Telephone:* 781-768-7330. *Fax:* 781-768-7071. *E-mail:* shelagh.tomaino@regiscollege.edu.

MASTER'S DEGREE PROGRAM

Degree MSN
Available Programs Accelerated AD/RN to Master's; Accelerated Master's; Accelerated Master's for Non-Nursing College Graduates; Accelerated Master's for Nurses with Non-Nursing Degrees; Accelerated RN to Master's; Master's; Master's for Non-Nursing College Graduates; Master's for Nurses with Non-Nursing Degrees; RN to Master's.
Concentrations Available Clinical nurse leader; health-care administration; nurse case management; nursing administration; nursing education; nursing informatics. *Clinical nurse specialist programs in:* adult-gerontology acute care. *Nurse practitioner programs in:* adult health, family health, gerontology, pediatric, primary care, psychiatric/mental health, women's health.
Site Options Newton, MA; Medford, MA; Boston, MA.
Study Options Full-time and part-time.
Program Entrance Requirements Computer literacy, minimum overall college GPA of 3.0, transcript of college record, CPR certification, written essay, immunizations, interview, 2 letters of recommendation, physical assessment course, professional liability insurance/malpractice insurance, prerequisite course work, resume, statistics course, GRE General Test or MAT. *Application deadline:* Applications may be processed on a rolling basis for some programs. *Application fee:* $75.
Advanced Placement Credit by examination available. Credit given for nursing courses completed elsewhere dependent upon specific evaluations.
Degree Requirements 44 total credit hours, thesis or project.

POST-MASTER'S PROGRAM

Areas of Study Clinical nurse leader; health-care administration; nurse case management; nursing administration; nursing education. *Nurse practitioner programs in:* adult health, family health, gerontology, pediatric, primary care, psychiatric/mental health, women's health.

DOCTORAL DEGREE PROGRAM

Degree DNP
Available Programs Doctorate; Post-Baccalaureate Doctorate.
Areas of Study Gerontology, health policy, nursing administration, nursing education, nursing policy.
Program Entrance Requirements Clinical experience, minimum overall college GPA of 3.5, interview by faculty committee, interview, 2 letters of recommendation, MSN or equivalent, statistics course, vita, writing sample, MAT or GRE if GPA from master's lower than 3.5. Application deadline: Applications may be processed on a rolling basis for some programs. Application fee: $75.
Degree Requirements 50 total credit hours.

CONTINUING EDUCATION PROGRAM

Contact Dr. Claudia Pouravelis, Associate Dean of Graduate Affairs, School of Nursing, Science and Health Professions, Regis College, 235 Wellesley Street, Weston, MA 02493. *Telephone:* 781-768-7058. *Fax:* 781-768-8218. *E-mail:* claudia.pouravelis@regiscollege.edu.

Salem State University
Program in Nursing
Salem, Massachusetts

http://www.salemstate.edu/
Founded in 1854

DEGREES • BSN • MSN • MSN/MBA

Nursing Program Faculty 110 (30% with doctorates).
Distance Learning Courses Available.
Nursing Student Activities Nursing Honor Society, Sigma Theta Tau, Student Nurses' Association.
Nursing Student Resources Academic advising; academic or career counseling; assistance for students with disabilities; bookstore; campus computer network; computer lab; computer-assisted instruction; daycare for children of students; e-mail services; employment services for current students; externships; housing assistance; interactive nursing skills videos; Internet; learning resource lab; library services; nursing audiovisuals; paid internships; remedial services; resume preparation assistance; skills, simulation, or other laboratory; tutoring.
Library Facilities 2,000 volumes in health, 1,600 volumes in nursing; 50 periodical subscriptions health-care related.

BACCALAUREATE PROGRAMS

Degree BSN
Available Programs ADN to Baccalaureate; Accelerated Baccalaureate for Second Degree; Accelerated RN Baccalaureate; Generic Baccalaureate; International Nurse to Baccalaureate; LPN to Baccalaureate; LPN to RN Baccalaureate.
Study Options Full-time and part-time.
Program Entrance Requirements Minimum overall college GPA of 3.5, transcript of college record, CPR certification, health exam, health insurance, high school biology, high school chemistry, 3 years high school math, 2 years high school science, high school transcript, immunizations, interview, minimum high school GPA of 3.5, professional liability insurance/malpractice insurance. Transfer students are accepted. *Application deadline:* 12/1 (fall), 11/1 (spring), 2/1 (summer). Applications may be processed on a rolling basis for some programs. *Application fee:* $40.
Advanced Placement Credit by examination available. Credit given for nursing courses completed elsewhere dependent upon specific evaluations.
Expenses (2015–16) *Tuition, state resident:* full-time $910; part-time $38 per credit. *Tuition, nonresident:* full-time $7050; part-time $293 per credit. *International tuition:* $7050 full-time. *Room and board:* $8000; room only: $3500 per academic year. *Required fees:* part-time $385 per credit; part-time $4500 per term.
Financial Aid 60% of baccalaureate students in nursing programs received some form of financial aid in 2014–15.
Contact Dr. Mary Dunn, Assistant Dean of Admissions, Program in Nursing, Salem State University, 352 Lafayette Street, Salem, MA 01970. *Telephone:* 978-542-6200. *E-mail:* admissions@salemstate.edu.

GRADUATE PROGRAMS

Expenses (2015–16) *Tuition, state resident:* full-time $1260; part-time $140 per credit. *Tuition, nonresident:* full-time $2070; part-time $230 per credit. *International tuition:* $2070 full-time. *Room and board:* $8000; room only: $5000 per academic year. *Required fees:* part-time $243 per credit; part-time $4374 per term.
Financial Aid 30% of graduate students in nursing programs received some form of financial aid in 2014–15. Career-related internships or fieldwork, Federal Work-Study, scholarships, and unspecified assistantships available. Aid available to part-time students. *Financial aid application deadline:* 5/1.
Contact Dr. Joanne Carlson, Coordinator, Graduate Program, Program in Nursing, Salem State University, 352 Lafayette Street, Salem, MA 01970. *Telephone:* 978-542-6983. *Fax:* 978-542-2016. *E-mail:* jcarlson@salemstate.edu.

MASTER'S DEGREE PROGRAM

Degrees MSN; MSN/MBA
Available Programs Master's; RN to Master's.
Concentrations Available Clinical nurse leader; nursing administration; nursing education. *Clinical nurse specialist programs in:* community health, public health, rehabilitation. *Nurse practitioner programs in:* women's health.

Study Options Full-time and part-time.
Program Entrance Requirements Clinical experience, computer literacy, minimum overall college GPA of 3.0, transcript of college record, CPR certification, written essay, immunizations, interview, 3 letters of recommendation, professional liability insurance/malpractice insurance, resume, statistics course, GRE or MAT. *Application deadline:* 3/1 (fall), 10/1 (winter), 10/1 (spring), 3/1 (summer). Applications may be processed on a rolling basis for some programs. *Application fee:* $50.
Advanced Placement Credit given for nursing courses completed elsewhere dependent upon specific evaluations.
Degree Requirements 39 total credit hours, thesis or project.

CONTINUING EDUCATION PROGRAM

Contact Prof. Tammi Magazzu, Coordinator, Program in Nursing, Salem State University, 352 Lafayette Street, Salem, MA 01970. *Telephone:* 978-542-7017. *Fax:* 978-542-2016. *E-mail:* tmagazzu@salemstate.edu.

Simmons College
School of Nursing and Health Sciences
Boston, Massachusetts

http://www.simmons.edu/snhs/
Founded in 1899

DEGREES • BS • DNP • MS

Nursing Program Faculty 10 (90% with doctorates).
Baccalaureate Enrollment 500 **Women** 100% **Part-time** 18%
Graduate Enrollment 1,223 **Women** 91.5% **Men** 8.5% **Part-time** 72.8%
Distance Learning Courses Available.
Nursing Student Activities Nursing Honor Society, Sigma Theta Tau, Student Nurses' Association, nursing club.
Nursing Student Resources Academic advising; academic or career counseling; assistance for students with disabilities; bookstore; campus computer network; career placement assistance; computer lab; computer-assisted instruction; e-mail services; employment services for current students; housing assistance; interactive nursing skills videos; Internet; learning resource lab; library services; nursing audiovisuals; placement services for program completers; remedial services; resume preparation assistance; skills, simulation, or other laboratory; tutoring; unpaid internships.
Library Facilities 3,068 volumes in health, 2,200 volumes in nursing; 583 periodical subscriptions health-care related.

BACCALAUREATE PROGRAMS

Degree BS
Available Programs ADN to Baccalaureate; Accelerated Baccalaureate; Accelerated Baccalaureate for Second Degree; Baccalaureate for Second Degree; Generic Baccalaureate; LPN to Baccalaureate; RN Baccalaureate.
Site Options Weymouth (South Shore Hospital), MA.
Study Options Full-time and part-time.
Program Entrance Requirements Transcript of college record, written essay, health exam, health insurance, high school biology, high school chemistry, high school foreign language, 4 years high school math, 3 years high school science, high school transcript, immunizations, 2 letters of recommendation, minimum GPA in nursing prerequisites of 3.0, prerequisite course work. Transfer students are accepted. *Application deadline:* 2/1 (fall), 11/1 (spring). *Application fee:* $55.
Advanced Placement Credit given for nursing courses completed elsewhere dependent upon specific evaluations.
Expenses (2015–16) *Tuition:* full-time $39,880; part-time $1247 per credit. *International tuition:* $39,880 full-time. *Room and board:* $14,040 per academic year. *Required fees:* full-time $1060; part-time $260 per term.
Financial Aid *Gift aid (need-based):* Federal Pell, FSEOG, state, private, college/university gift aid from institutional funds. *Loans:* Federal Direct (Subsidized and Unsubsidized Stafford PLUS), Perkins, college/university. *Work-study:* Federal Work-Study. *Financial aid application deadline (priority):* 3/1.
Contact Ellen Johnson, Director of Undergraduate Admission, School of Nursing and Health Sciences, Simmons College, 300 The Fenway, Boston, MA 02115. *Telephone:* 617-521-2515. *Fax:* 617-521-3190. *E-mail:* ugadm@simmons.edu.

GRADUATE PROGRAMS

Expenses (2015–16) *Tuition:* part-time $1274 per credit. *Room and board:* $16,516 per academic year. *Required fees:* part-time $100 per term.
Contact Mr. Brett Dimarzo, Director of Graduate Admission, School of Nursing and Health Sciences, Simmons College, 300 The Fenway, Boston, MA 02115. *Telephone:* 617-521-2605. *Fax:* 617-521-2651. *E-mail:* brett.dimarzo@simmons.edu.

MASTER'S DEGREE PROGRAM
Degree MS
Available Programs Accelerated Master's; Accelerated Master's for Non-Nursing College Graduates; Master's; RN to Master's.
Concentrations Available *Nurse practitioner programs in:* family health, primary care.
Site Options Weymouth (South Shore Hospital), MA; Boston (Longwood Medical Area), MA.
Study Options Full-time and part-time.
Online Degree Options Yes.
Program Entrance Requirements Clinical experience, computer literacy, minimum overall college GPA of 3.0, transcript of college record, written essay, 3 letters of recommendation, physical assessment course, prerequisite course work, resume, statistics course. *Application deadline:* 2/5 (fall), 1/10 (summer). *Application fee:* $50.
Degree Requirements 48 total credit hours.

DOCTORAL DEGREE PROGRAM
Degree DNP
Available Programs Doctorate; Post-Baccalaureate Doctorate.
Areas of Study Clinical practice.
Program Entrance Requirements Clinical experience, minimum overall college GPA of 3.0, 3 letters of recommendation, MSN or equivalent, statistics course, vita, writing sample. Application deadline: 6/1 (fall), 10/1 (spring). Application fee: $50.
Degree Requirements 36 total credit hours.

University of Massachusetts Amherst
College of Nursing
Amherst, Massachusetts

http://www.umass.edu/nursing
Founded in 1863
DEGREES • BS • MS • PHD
Nursing Program Faculty 85 (60% with doctorates).
Baccalaureate Enrollment 509 **Women** 90% **Men** 10% **Part-time** 1%
Graduate Enrollment 237 **Women** 91% **Men** 9% **Part-time** 79%
Distance Learning Courses Available.
Nursing Student Activities Sigma Theta Tau, Student Nurses' Association.
Nursing Student Resources Academic advising; academic or career counseling; bookstore; campus computer network; career placement assistance; computer lab; computer-assisted instruction; e-mail services; employment services for current students; housing assistance; interactive nursing skills videos; Internet; learning resource lab; library services; nursing audiovisuals; resume preparation assistance; skills, simulation, or other laboratory; tutoring; unpaid internships.
Library Facilities 354,775 volumes in health, 47,634 volumes in nursing; 3,772 periodical subscriptions health-care related.

BACCALAUREATE PROGRAMS
Degree BS
Available Programs Accelerated Baccalaureate for Second Degree; Accelerated RN Baccalaureate; Generic Baccalaureate.
Site Options Springfield, MA.
Study Options Full-time.
Online Degree Options Yes.
Program Entrance Requirements Minimum overall college GPA of 3.0, transcript of college record, CPR certification, written essay, health exam, health insurance, high school foreign language, 3 years high school math, 3 years high school science, high school transcript, immunizations, 1 letter of recommendation, minimum high school GPA of 3.5, minimum GPA in nursing prerequisites of 2.5, professional liability insurance/malpractice insurance, prerequisite course work. *Application deadline:* 1/15 (fall). *Application fee:* $70.

Advanced Placement Credit given for nursing courses completed elsewhere dependent upon specific evaluations.
Financial Aid 86% of baccalaureate students in nursing programs received some form of financial aid in 2013–14.
Contact Ms. Elizabeth Theroux, Academic Secretary, Undergraduate Nursing Education, College of Nursing, University of Massachusetts Amherst, 026 Skinner Hall, 651 North Pleasant Street, Amherst, MA 01003-9304. *Telephone:* 413-545-5096. *Fax:* 413-577-2550. *E-mail:* etheroux@acad.umass.edu.

GRADUATE PROGRAMS

Financial Aid 38% of graduate students in nursing programs received some form of financial aid in 2013–14. Fellowships with full and partial tuition reimbursements available, research assistantships with full and partial tuition reimbursements available, teaching assistantships with full and partial tuition reimbursements available, career-related internships or fieldwork, Federal Work-Study, scholarships, traineeships, tuition waivers (full and partial), and unspecified assistantships available. Aid available to part-time students. *Financial aid application deadline:* 12/15.
Contact Ms. Karen Ayotte, Academic Services Graduate Program Assistant, College of Nursing, University of Massachusetts Amherst, 125 Skinner Hall, 651 North Pleasant Street, Amherst, MA 01003-9299. *Telephone:* 413-545-1302. *Fax:* 413-577-2550. *E-mail:* kayotte@nursing.umass.edu.

MASTER'S DEGREE PROGRAM
Degree MS
Available Programs Master's.
Concentrations Available Clinical nurse leader.
Study Options Full-time and part-time.
Online Degree Options Yes (online only).
Program Entrance Requirements Minimum overall college GPA of 3.0, transcript of college record, CPR certification, written essay, immunizations, 2 letters of recommendation, physical assessment course, professional liability insurance/malpractice insurance, prerequisite course work, statistics course. *Application deadline:* 12/15 (fall). Applications may be processed on a rolling basis for some programs. *Application fee:* $65.
Advanced Placement Credit given for nursing courses completed elsewhere dependent upon specific evaluations.
Degree Requirements 37 total credit hours.

DOCTORAL DEGREE PROGRAM
Degree PhD
Available Programs Doctorate; Post-Baccalaureate Doctorate.
Areas of Study Faculty preparation, health promotion/disease prevention, health-care systems, individualized study, nursing education, nursing research, nursing science.
Program Entrance Requirements Minimum overall college GPA of 3.2, interview, 2 letters of recommendation, MSN or equivalent, scholarly papers, statistics course, vita, writing sample. Application deadline: 12/15 (fall). Applications may be processed on a rolling basis for some programs. Application fee: $65.
Degree Requirements 57 total credit hours, dissertation, oral exam, written exam, residency.

CONTINUING EDUCATION PROGRAM
Contact Ms. Karen Ayotte, Academic Services Graduate Program Assistant, College of Nursing, University of Massachusetts Amherst, 022 Skinner Hall, 651 North Pleasant Street, Amherst, MA 01003-9299. *Telephone:* 413-545-1302. *Fax:* 413-577-2550. *E-mail:* kayotte@nursing.umass.edu.

University of Massachusetts Boston
College of Nursing and Health Sciences
Boston, Massachusetts

http://www.umb.edu
Founded in 1964
DEGREES • BS • DNP • MS • PHD
Nursing Program Faculty 161 (30% with doctorates).
Baccalaureate Enrollment 1,180 **Women** 86% **Men** 14% **Part-time** 46%

Graduate Enrollment 264 **Women** 91% **Men** 9% **Part-time** 73%
Distance Learning Courses Available.
Nursing Student Activities Nursing Honor Society, Sigma Theta Tau, Student Nurses' Association.
Nursing Student Resources Academic advising; academic or career counseling; assistance for students with disabilities; bookstore; campus computer network; career placement assistance; computer lab; computer-assisted instruction; daycare for children of students; e-mail services; employment services for current students; housing assistance; interactive nursing skills videos; Internet; learning resource lab; library services; nursing audiovisuals; other; paid internships; remedial services; resume preparation assistance; skills, simulation, or other laboratory; tutoring.
Library Facilities 3,700 volumes in health, 603 volumes in nursing; 4,815 periodical subscriptions health-care related.

BACCALAUREATE PROGRAMS

Degree BS
Available Programs Accelerated Baccalaureate for Second Degree; Generic Baccalaureate; RN Baccalaureate.
Site Options West Barnstable, MA.
Study Options Full-time.
Online Degree Options Yes.
Program Entrance Requirements Minimum overall college GPA of 3.0, transcript of college record, written essay, health insurance, 3 years high school math, high school transcript, immunizations, 2 letters of recommendation, minimum high school GPA of 3.0. Transfer students are accepted. *Application deadline:* 12/1 (fall), 12/1 (spring), 12/1 (summer). *Application fee:* $60.
Advanced Placement Credit given for nursing courses completed elsewhere dependent upon specific evaluations.
Expenses (2015–16) *Tuition, state resident:* full-time $12,682; part-time $529 per credit. *Tuition, nonresident:* full-time $29,920; part-time $1247 per credit. *International tuition:* $30,230 full-time. *Required fees:* full-time $1025; part-time $500 per term.
Financial Aid 70% of baccalaureate students in nursing programs received some form of financial aid in 2014–15.
Contact Mr. Jon Hutton, Director of Enrollment Information Services, College of Nursing and Health Sciences, University of Massachusetts Boston, 100 Morrissey Boulevard, Boston, MA 02125. *Telephone:* 617-287-6000. *Fax:* 617-287-5999.
E-mail: enrollment.information@umb.edu.

GRADUATE PROGRAMS

Expenses (2015–16) *Tuition, state resident:* full-time $16,115; part-time $672 per credit. *Tuition, nonresident:* full-time $31,115; part-time $1297 per credit. *International tuition:* $31,425 full-time. *Required fees:* full-time $1425; part-time $700 per term.
Financial Aid 40% of graduate students in nursing programs received some form of financial aid in 2014–15. Research assistantships with full tuition reimbursements available, teaching assistantships with full tuition reimbursements available, career-related internships or fieldwork, Federal Work-Study, and unspecified assistantships available. Aid available to part-time students. *Financial aid application deadline:* 3/1.
Contact Mr. Jon Hutton, Director of Enrollment Information Services, College of Nursing and Health Sciences, University of Massachusetts Boston, 100 Morrissey Boulevard, Boston, MA 02125. *Telephone:* 617-287-6000. *Fax:* 617-287-6040.
E-mail: enrollment.information@umb.edu.

MASTER'S DEGREE PROGRAM

Degree MS
Available Programs Master's.
Concentrations Available *Clinical nurse specialist programs in:* adult-gerontology acute care, family health. *Nurse practitioner programs in:* adult-gerontology acute care, family health.
Study Options Full-time and part-time.
Program Entrance Requirements Clinical experience, minimum overall college GPA of 3.0, transcript of college record, written essay, immunizations, 3 letters of recommendation, physical assessment course, statistics course. *Application deadline:* 3/15 (fall), 10/15 (spring). *Application fee:* $100.
Advanced Placement Credit given for nursing courses completed elsewhere dependent upon specific evaluations.
Degree Requirements 48 total credit hours, thesis or project.

POST-MASTER'S PROGRAM

Areas of Study Nursing education. *Clinical nurse specialist programs in:* adult-gerontology acute care, family health. *Nurse practitioner programs in:* adult-gerontology acute care, family health.

DOCTORAL DEGREE PROGRAM

Degree DNP
Available Programs Doctorate.
Areas of Study Advanced practice nursing.
Online Degree Options Yes (online only).
Program Entrance Requirements Minimum overall college GPA of 3.2, clinical experience, 3 letters of recommendation, MSN or equivalent, statistics course, vita, writing sample. Application deadline: 5/1 (fall), 12/1 (winter). Application fee: $60.
Degree Requirements 39 total credit hours, Capstone project, residency.

Degree PhD
Available Programs Doctorate; Post-Baccalaureate Doctorate.
Areas of Study Health policy, health promotion/disease prevention.
Program Entrance Requirements Clinical experience, minimum overall college GPA of 3.3, interview by faculty committee, interview, 3 letters of recommendation, MSN or equivalent, statistics course, vita, writing sample, GRE General Test. Application deadline: 1/15 (fall). Applications may be processed on a rolling basis for some programs. Application fee: $100.
Degree Requirements 60 total credit hours, dissertation, oral exam, written exam, residency.

POSTDOCTORAL PROGRAM

Areas of Study Cancer care, nursing research.
Postdoctoral Program Contact Dr. Haeok Lee, PhD Program Director, College of Nursing and Health Sciences, University of Massachusetts Boston, College of Nursing and Health Sciences, 100 Morrissey Boulevard, Boston, MA 02125. *Telephone:* 617-287-5071. *E-mail:* haeok.lee@umb.edu.

CONTINUING EDUCATION PROGRAM

Contact Ms. Wanda Willard, Director of Credit Programs, College of Nursing and Health Sciences, University of Massachusetts Boston, 100 Morrissey Boulevard, Wheatley Building, 2nd Floor, Boston, MA 02125-3393. *Telephone:* 617-287-7874. *Fax:* 617-287-7922. *E-mail:* wanda.willard@umb.edu.

University of Massachusetts Dartmouth
College of Nursing
North Dartmouth, Massachusetts

http://www.umassd.edu/nursing
Founded in 1895
DEGREES • BS • DNP • MS • PHD
Nursing Program Faculty 68 (19% with doctorates).
Baccalaureate Enrollment 612 **Women** 88.4% **Men** 11.6% **Part-time** 28.3%
Graduate Enrollment 122 **Women** 92.6% **Men** 7.4% **Part-time** 100%
Distance Learning Courses Available.
Nursing Student Activities Sigma Theta Tau, Student Nurses' Association, nursing club.
Nursing Student Resources Academic advising; academic or career counseling; assistance for students with disabilities; bookstore; campus computer network; career placement assistance; computer lab; computer-assisted instruction; e-mail services; employment services for current students; externships; housing assistance; interactive nursing skills videos; Internet; learning resource lab; library services; nursing audiovisuals; placement services for program completers; resume preparation assistance; skills, simulation, or other laboratory; tutoring; unpaid internships.
Library Facilities 3,998 volumes in health, 1,355 volumes in nursing; 7,900 periodical subscriptions health-care related.

BACCALAUREATE PROGRAMS

Degree BS
Available Programs Generic Baccalaureate; RN Baccalaureate.
Study Options Full-time and part-time.
Online Degree Options Yes.
Program Entrance Requirements Transcript of college record, written essay, high school biology, high school chemistry, high school foreign language, 3 years high school math, 3 years high school science, high school transcript, 1 letter of recommendation, minimum high school GPA of 3.0. Transfer students are accepted. *Application deadline:* 2/1 (fall).

Applications may be processed on a rolling basis for some programs. *Application fee:* $60.

Advanced Placement Credit by examination available. Credit given for nursing courses completed elsewhere dependent upon specific evaluations.

Expenses (2015–16) *Tuition, state resident:* full-time $1417; part-time $59 per credit hour. *Tuition, nonresident:* full-time $8099; part-time $337 per credit hour. *International tuition:* $8099 full-time. *Room and board:* $11,622; room only: $7609 per academic year. *Required fees:* part-time $474 per credit.

Financial Aid *Gift aid (need-based):* Federal Pell, FSEOG, state, private, college/university gift aid from institutional funds. *Loans:* Federal Nursing Student Loans, Federal Direct (Subsidized and Unsubsidized Stafford PLUS), Perkins, state. *Work-study:* Federal Work-Study, part-time campus jobs. *Financial aid application deadline (priority):* 3/1.

Contact Admissions Office, College of Nursing, University of Massachusetts Dartmouth, 285 Old Westport Road, North Dartmouth, MA 02747. *Telephone:* 508-999-8605. *Fax:* 508-999-8755. *E-mail:* admissions@umassd.edu.

GRADUATE PROGRAMS

Expenses (2015–16) *Tuition, state resident:* full-time $2071; part-time $86 per credit hour. *Tuition, nonresident:* full-time $8099; part-time $337 per credit hour. *International tuition:* $8099 full-time. *Room and board:* $11,622; room only: $7609 per academic year.

Financial Aid 1 fellowship (averaging $24,000 per year), 3 teaching assistantships (averaging $4,333 per year) were awarded; Federal Work-Study and unspecified assistantships also available.

Contact Dr. Janet Sobczak, Director of Master's Programs, College of Nursing, University of Massachusetts Dartmouth, 285 Old Westport Road, North Dartmouth, MA 02747-2300. *Telephone:* 508-910-6487. *E-mail:* vvital@umassd.edu.

MASTER'S DEGREE PROGRAM

Degree MS

Available Programs Master's; RN to Master's.

Concentrations Available Nursing administration; nursing education. *Clinical nurse specialist programs in:* adult health, community health.

Study Options Full-time and part-time.

Program Entrance Requirements Clinical experience, minimum overall college GPA of 3.0, transcript of college record, written essay, 3 letters of recommendation, resume, GRE (if fewer than 45 credits at baccalaureate degree granting school). *Application deadline:* 3/15 (fall). *Application fee:* $60.

Advanced Placement Credit given for nursing courses completed elsewhere dependent upon specific evaluations.

Degree Requirements 39 total credit hours, thesis or project.

DOCTORAL DEGREE PROGRAM

Degree DNP

Available Programs Doctorate.

Areas of Study Gerontology, human health and illness, nursing education.

Program Entrance Requirements Minimum overall college GPA of 3.3, clinical experience, 3 letters of recommendation. Application deadline: 3/15 (fall). Application fee: $60.

Degree Requirements 63 total credit hours, Capstone project, residency.

Degree PhD

Available Programs Doctorate.

Areas of Study Human health and illness, nursing education.

Program Entrance Requirements Clinical experience, minimum overall college GPA of 3.3, 3 letters of recommendation, vita, writing sample, GRE (for PHD, if fewer than 45 credits at baccalaureate degree granting school for DNP). Application deadline: 2/15 (fall). Application fee: $60.

Degree Requirements 52 total credit hours, dissertation.

CONTINUING EDUCATION PROGRAM

Contact University Extension, College of Nursing, University of Massachusetts Dartmouth, 285 Old Westport Road, North Dartmouth, MA 02747-2300. *Telephone:* 508-999-9202. *E-mail:* extension@umassd.edu.

University of Massachusetts Lowell

School of Nursing
Lowell, Massachusetts

http://www.uml.edu/SHE/Nursing/default.aspx
Founded in 1894

DEGREES • BS • DNP • MS • PHD

Nursing Program Faculty 50 (47% with doctorates).

Baccalaureate Enrollment 433 **Women** 92% **Men** 8% **Part-time** 14%

Graduate Enrollment 133 **Women** 92% **Men** 8% **Part-time** 72%

Distance Learning Courses Available.

Nursing Student Activities Nursing Honor Society, Sigma Theta Tau, Student Nurses' Association, nursing club.

Nursing Student Resources Academic advising; academic or career counseling; assistance for students with disabilities; bookstore; campus computer network; career placement assistance; computer lab; computer-assisted instruction; e-mail services; employment services for current students; housing assistance; interactive nursing skills videos; Internet; learning resource lab; library services; nursing audiovisuals; other; placement services for program completers; resume preparation assistance; skills, simulation, or other laboratory; tutoring; unpaid internships.

Library Facilities 29,100 volumes in health, 4,465 volumes in nursing; 350 periodical subscriptions health-care related.

BACCALAUREATE PROGRAMS

Degree BS

Available Programs Generic Baccalaureate; RN Baccalaureate.

Study Options Full-time.

Program Entrance Requirements Minimum overall college GPA of 2.7, transcript of college record, CPR certification, health exam, health insurance, high school chemistry, high school foreign language, 3 years high school math, 3 years high school science, high school transcript, immunizations, minimum high school GPA of 3.25, minimum GPA in nursing prerequisites of 2.7, professional liability insurance/malpractice insurance. *Application deadline:* 11/1 (fall), 1/1 (winter). Applications may be processed on a rolling basis for some programs. *Application fee:* $60.

Advanced Placement Credit by examination available.

Expenses (2015–16) *Tuition, state resident:* full-time $1454. *Tuition, nonresident:* full-time $8567. *Room and board:* $11,670; room only: $7710 per academic year.

Contact Office of Undergraduate Admissions, School of Nursing, University of Massachusetts Lowell, 883 Broadway Street, Suite 110, Lowell, MA 01854-3931. *Telephone:* 978-934-3931. *E-mail:* admissions@uml.edu.

GRADUATE PROGRAMS

Expenses (2015–16) *Tuition, state resident:* full-time $1637. *Tuition, nonresident:* full-time $6425. *Room and board:* $11,670; room only: $7710 per academic year.

Financial Aid 37 fellowships, 10 teaching assistantships were awarded; research assistantships, career-related internships or fieldwork, Federal Work-Study, institutionally sponsored loans, scholarships, and traineeships also available.

Contact Dr. Barbara Mawn, PhD and Graduate Program Director, School of Nursing, University of Massachusetts Lowell, 113 Wilder Street, Suite 200, Lowell, MA 01854-5126. *Telephone:* 978-934-4845. *Fax:* 978-934-2015. *E-mail:* barbara_mawn@uml.edu.

MASTER'S DEGREE PROGRAM

Degree MS

Available Programs Master's.

Concentrations Available *Nurse practitioner programs in:* family health, gerontology.

Study Options Full-time and part-time.

Program Entrance Requirements Computer literacy, minimum overall college GPA of 3.0, transcript of college record, CPR certification, written essay, immunizations, interview, 3 letters of recommendation, statistics course, GRE General Test. *Application deadline:* Applications may be processed on a rolling basis for some programs. *Application fee:* $60.

Advanced Placement Credit given for nursing courses completed elsewhere dependent upon specific evaluations.

Degree Requirements 42 total credit hours, thesis or project.

DOCTORAL DEGREE PROGRAM

Degree DNP
Available Programs Doctorate.
Areas of Study Advanced practice nursing.
Program Entrance Requirements Minimum overall college GPA of 3.0, interview, interview by faculty committee, letters of recommendation, MSN or equivalent, statistics course, vita. Application deadline: 11/1 (fall), 4/1 (spring). Applications may be processed on a rolling basis for some programs. Application fee: $50.
Degree Requirements 33 total credit hours, scholarly project.

Degree PhD
Available Programs Doctorate.
Areas of Study Health promotion/disease prevention.
Program Entrance Requirements Minimum overall college GPA of 3.4, interview by faculty committee, interview, 3 letters of recommendation, MSN or equivalent, scholarly papers, statistics course, writing sample, GRE General Test. Application deadline: Applications may be processed on a rolling basis for some programs. Application fee: $60.
Degree Requirements 48 total credit hours, dissertation, oral exam, written exam.

University of Massachusetts Medical School

Graduate School of Nursing
Worcester, Massachusetts

http://www.umassmed.edu/gsn/
Founded in 1962
DEGREES • MS • PHD
Nursing Program Faculty 51 (40% with doctorates).
Graduate Enrollment 174 **Women** 87% **Men** 13% **Part-time** 4%
Distance Learning Courses Available.
Nursing Student Activities Sigma Theta Tau, Student Nurses' Association.
Nursing Student Resources Academic advising; academic or career counseling; assistance for students with disabilities; bookstore; campus computer network; computer lab; computer-assisted instruction; e-mail services; interactive nursing skills videos; Internet; learning resource lab; library services; nursing audiovisuals; skills, simulation, or other laboratory; unpaid internships.
Library Facilities 207,500 volumes in health, 1,173 volumes in nursing; 5,400 periodical subscriptions health-care related.

GRADUATE PROGRAMS

Contact *Telephone:* 508-856-5756. *Fax:* 508-856-5756.

MASTER'S DEGREE PROGRAM

Degree MS
Available Programs Accelerated Master's for Non-Nursing College Graduates; Master's.
Concentrations Available Nursing education. *Nurse practitioner programs in:* acute care, family health, gerontology, primary care.
Site Options Shrewsbury, MA; Worcester, MA.
Study Options Full-time and part-time.
Program Entrance Requirements Clinical experience, computer literacy, minimum overall college GPA of 3.0, transcript of college record, CPR certification, written essay, immunizations, interview, 3 letters of recommendation, physical assessment course, prerequisite course work, resume, statistics course, GRE General Test. *Application deadline:* 3/15 (fall). Applications may be processed on a rolling basis for some programs.
Advanced Placement Credit given for nursing courses completed elsewhere dependent upon specific evaluations.
Degree Requirements 42 total credit hours.

POST-MASTER'S PROGRAM

Areas of Study Nursing education. *Nurse practitioner programs in:* acute care, gerontology, primary care.

DOCTORAL DEGREE PROGRAM

Degree PhD
Available Programs Doctorate.
Areas of Study Advanced practice nursing, bio-behavioral research, clinical practice, critical care, family health, health promotion/disease prevention, human health and illness, illness and transition, nursing research, nursing science, oncology.
Site Options Worcester, MA.
Program Entrance Requirements Minimum overall college GPA of 3.0, interview by faculty committee, interview, 3 letters of recommendation, MSN or equivalent, scholarly papers, statistics course, vita, writing sample, GRE General Test. Application deadline: 3/15 (fall). Applications may be processed on a rolling basis for some programs.
Degree Requirements 57 total credit hours, dissertation, oral exam, written exam.

CONTINUING EDUCATION PROGRAM

Contact *Telephone:* 508-856-3488. *Fax:* 508-856-6552.

Westfield State University

Nursing Program
Westfield, Massachusetts

http://www.westfield.ma.edu//academics/nursing-program
Founded in 1838
DEGREE • BSN

BACCALAUREATE PROGRAMS

Degree BSN
Available Programs Generic Baccalaureate.
Contact Nursing Degree Program, Nursing Program, Westfield State University, 577 Western Avenue, Westfield, MA 01086. *Telephone:* 413-572-5300.

Worcester State University

Department of Nursing
Worcester, Massachusetts

http://www.worcester.edu/Nursing
Founded in 1874
DEGREES • BS • MS
Nursing Program Faculty 38 (50% with doctorates).
Baccalaureate Enrollment 512 **Women** 88% **Men** 12% **Part-time** 16%
Graduate Enrollment 115 **Women** 91% **Men** 9% **Part-time** 99%
Distance Learning Courses Available.
Nursing Student Activities Nursing Honor Society, Sigma Theta Tau, Student Nurses' Association, nursing club.
Nursing Student Resources Academic advising; academic or career counseling; assistance for students with disabilities; bookstore; campus computer network; career placement assistance; computer lab; computer-assisted instruction; e-mail services; employment services for current students; externships; housing assistance; interactive nursing skills videos; Internet; learning resource lab; library services; nursing audiovisuals; paid internships; remedial services; resume preparation assistance; skills, simulation, or other laboratory; tutoring; unpaid internships.
Library Facilities 1,794 volumes in health, 651 volumes in nursing; 7,456 periodical subscriptions health-care related.

BACCALAUREATE PROGRAMS

Degree BS
Available Programs ADN to Baccalaureate; Generic Baccalaureate; LPN to Baccalaureate; LPN to RN Baccalaureate; RN Baccalaureate.
Site Options Worcester, MA.
Study Options Full-time.
Program Entrance Requirements Transcript of college record, high school foreign language, 3 years high school math, 3 years high school science, high school transcript, minimum high school GPA of 3.0. *Application deadline:* 1/15 (fall). Applications may be processed on a rolling basis for some programs. *Application fee:* $50.
Advanced Placement Credit by examination available.
Expenses (2015–16) *Tuition, state resident:* full-time $970; part-time $40 per credit hour. *Tuition, nonresident:* full-time $7050; part-time $61 per credit hour. *Room and board:* $11,890; room only: $8370 per academic year. *Required fees:* part-time $329 per credit; part-time $3944 per term.
Contact Mr. Joseph Dicarlo, Director, Admissions, Department of Nursing, Worcester State University, 486 Chandler Street, Worcester, MA

01602. *Telephone:* 508-929-8040. *Fax:* 508-929-8183. *E-mail:* Joseph.Dicarlo@worcester.edu.

GRADUATE PROGRAMS

Expenses (2015–16) *Tuition, state resident:* part-time $150 per credit hour. *Required fees:* part-time $138 per credit.
Contact Dr. Stephanie Chalupka, Associate Dean for Nursing, Department of Nursing, Worcester State University, 486 Chandler Street, Worcester, MA 01602. *Telephone:* 508-929-8129. *Fax:* 508-929-8168. *E-mail:* schalupka@worcester.edu.

MASTER'S DEGREE PROGRAM
Degree MS
Available Programs Master's; Master's for Nurses with Non-Nursing Degrees; RN to Master's.
Concentrations Available Nursing education. *Clinical nurse specialist programs in:* public/community health.
Study Options Full-time and part-time.
Program Entrance Requirements Clinical experience, computer literacy, minimum overall college GPA of 3.0, transcript of college record, CPR certification, written essay, immunizations, 2 letters of recommendation, nursing research course, professional liability insurance/malpractice insurance, prerequisite course work, resume, statistics course. *Application deadline:* 6/15 (fall), 11/1 (spring), 4/1 (summer). Applications may be processed on a rolling basis for some programs. *Application fee:* $50.
Degree Requirements 36 total credit hours, thesis or project.

POST-MASTER'S PROGRAM
Areas of Study Nursing education. *Clinical nurse specialist programs in:* public/community health.

CONTINUING EDUCATION PROGRAM

Contact Ms. Gina Fleury, RN, Clinical Resource Coordinator, Department of Nursing, Worcester State University, 486 Chandler Street, Worcester, MA 01602. *Telephone:* 508-929-8683. *E-mail:* gfleury@worcester.edu.

MICHIGAN

Andrews University
Department of Nursing
Berrien Springs, Michigan

http://www.andrews.edu/
Founded in 1874
DEGREES • BS • DNP
Nursing Program Faculty 11 (50% with doctorates).
Baccalaureate Enrollment 104
Graduate Enrollment 14
Distance Learning Courses Available.
Nursing Student Activities Nursing Honor Society, Sigma Theta Tau, Student Nurses' Association.
Nursing Student Resources Academic advising; academic or career counseling; assistance for students with disabilities; bookstore; campus computer network; career placement assistance; computer lab; computer-assisted instruction; daycare for children of students; e-mail services; employment services for current students; externships; housing assistance; interactive nursing skills videos; Internet; learning resource lab; library services; nursing audiovisuals; paid internships; placement services for program completers; remedial services; resume preparation assistance; skills, simulation, or other laboratory; tutoring; unpaid internships.
Library Facilities 77,000 volumes in health, 500 volumes in nursing; 700 periodical subscriptions health-care related.

BACCALAUREATE PROGRAMS

Degree BS
Available Programs ADN to Baccalaureate; Generic Baccalaureate.
Study Options Full-time.
Online Degree Options Yes.

Program Entrance Requirements Minimum overall college GPA of 3.0, transcript of college record, health exam, high school transcript, immunizations, minimum GPA in nursing prerequisites of 3.0. Transfer students are accepted. *Application deadline:* 5/15 (fall).
Contact Dr. Frances Johnson, Director of Undergraduate Programs, Department of Nursing, Andrews University, Berrien Springs, MI 49104. *Telephone:* 269-471-3192. *Fax:* 269-471-3454. *E-mail:* francesj@andrews.edu.

GRADUATE PROGRAMS

Financial Aid Institutionally sponsored loans available.
Contact Dr. Jochebed B. Ade-Oshifogun, Director of Graduate Program, Department of Nursing, Andrews University, 8475 University Boulevard, Berrien Springs, MI 49104. *Telephone:* 269-471-3363. *Fax:* 269-471-3454. *E-mail:* jochebed@andrews.edu.

MASTER'S DEGREE PROGRAM
Program Entrance Requirements GRE.

DOCTORAL DEGREE PROGRAM
Degree DNP
Available Programs Doctorate; Post-Baccalaureate Doctorate.
Areas of Study Advanced practice nursing, family health, nursing education.
Online Degree Options Yes (online only).
Program Entrance Requirements Clinical experience, minimum overall college GPA of 3.25, letters of recommendation, statistics course, vita, writing sample. Application deadline: 4/15 (summer).
Degree Requirements 40 total credit hours, written exam.

Baker College
School of Nursing
Flint, Michigan

http://www.baker.edu/programs-degrees/interests/school-of-nursing/
Founded in 1911
DEGREE • BSN

BACCALAUREATE PROGRAMS

Degree BSN
Available Programs ADN to Baccalaureate; Accelerated Baccalaureate; Generic Baccalaureate.
Contact School of Nursing, School of Nursing, Baker College, 1050 West Bristol Road, Flint, MI 48507. *Telephone:* 810-766-4000.

Calvin College
Department of Nursing
Grand Rapids, Michigan

http://www.calvin.edu/academic/nursing
Founded in 1876
DEGREE • BSN
Nursing Program Faculty 20 (20% with doctorates).
Baccalaureate Enrollment 120 **Women** 95% **Men** 5%
Nursing Student Activities Sigma Theta Tau, Student Nurses' Association, nursing club.
Nursing Student Resources Academic advising; academic or career counseling; assistance for students with disabilities; bookstore; campus computer network; career placement assistance; computer lab; computer-assisted instruction; e-mail services; employment services for current students; externships; housing assistance; interactive nursing skills videos; Internet; learning resource lab; library services; nursing audiovisuals; paid internships; placement services for program completers; remedial services; resume preparation assistance; skills, simulation, or other laboratory; tutoring.

BACCALAUREATE PROGRAMS

Degree BSN
Available Programs Generic Baccalaureate.
Site Options Grand Rapids, MI.
Study Options Full-time.

Program Entrance Requirements Minimum overall college GPA of 2.5, transcript of college record, CPR certification, health exam, health insurance, immunizations, 2 letters of recommendation, minimum GPA in nursing prerequisites of 2.5, professional liability insurance/malpractice insurance, prerequisite course work. Transfer students are accepted.
Contact *Telephone:* 616-526-6268. *Fax:* 616-526-8567.

Davenport University
Division of Nursing
Grand Rapids, Michigan

Founded in 1866
DEGREE • BSN
Nursing Program Faculty 40
Baccalaureate Enrollment 215 Women 94% Men 6% Part-time 17%
Distance Learning Courses Available.
Nursing Student Activities Student Nurses' Association.
Nursing Student Resources Academic advising; academic or career counseling; assistance for students with disabilities; bookstore; campus computer network; career placement assistance; computer lab; computer-assisted instruction; e-mail services; employment services for current students; externships; housing assistance; interactive nursing skills videos; Internet; learning resource lab; library services; nursing audiovisuals; placement services for program completers; remedial services; resume preparation assistance; skills, simulation, or other laboratory; tutoring.
Library Facilities 100 volumes in health, 50 volumes in nursing; 20 periodical subscriptions health-care related.

BACCALAUREATE PROGRAMS

Degree BSN
Available Programs ADN to Baccalaureate; Generic Baccalaureate; RN Baccalaureate.
Site Options Midland, MI; Warren, MI.
Study Options Full-time and part-time.
Online Degree Options Yes.
Program Entrance Requirements Minimum overall college GPA of 3.5, transcript of college record, CPR certification, written essay, health exam, health insurance, high school biology, high school chemistry, 2 years high school math, 3 years high school science, high school transcript, immunizations, 2 letters of recommendation, minimum high school GPA of 3.5, minimum GPA in nursing prerequisites. Transfer students are accepted. *Application deadline:* 1/31 (fall).
Advanced Placement Credit by examination available. Credit given for nursing courses completed elsewhere dependent upon specific evaluations.
Contact *Telephone:* 616-451-3511. *Fax:* 616-732-1145.

Davenport University
Bachelor of Science in Nursing Program
Kalamazoo, Michigan

Founded in 1977
DEGREE • BSN

BACCALAUREATE PROGRAMS

Degree BSN
Available Programs Generic Baccalaureate; RN Baccalaureate.
Contact *Telephone:* 616-871-3977. *Fax:* 616-554-5225.

Eastern Michigan University
School of Nursing
Ypsilanti, Michigan

http://www.emich.edu/nursing
Founded in 1849
DEGREES • BSN • MSN
Nursing Program Faculty 94 (35% with doctorates).

Baccalaureate Enrollment 518 Women 83% Men 17% Part-time 46%
Graduate Enrollment 26 Women 85% Men 15% Part-time 77%
Distance Learning Courses Available.
Nursing Student Activities Sigma Theta Tau, Student Nurses' Association.
Nursing Student Resources Academic advising; academic or career counseling; assistance for students with disabilities; bookstore; campus computer network; career placement assistance; computer lab; computer-assisted instruction; daycare for children of students; e-mail services; employment services for current students; housing assistance; interactive nursing skills videos; Internet; learning resource lab; library services; nursing audiovisuals; placement services for program completers; remedial services; resume preparation assistance; skills, simulation, or other laboratory; tutoring.
Library Facilities 29,975 volumes in health, 3,246 volumes in nursing; 6,975 periodical subscriptions health-care related.

BACCALAUREATE PROGRAMS

Degree BSN
Available Programs ADN to Baccalaureate; Baccalaureate for Second Degree; Generic Baccalaureate; RN Baccalaureate.
Site Options Jackson, MI; Dearborn-Beaumont Hosp, MI; Detroit, MI; Livonia, MI; Ann Arbor, MI.
Study Options Full-time and part-time.
Online Degree Options Yes.
Program Entrance Requirements Transcript of college record, CPR certification, health exam, health insurance, immunizations, minimum GPA in nursing prerequisites of 3.0, prerequisite course work, RN licensure. Transfer students are accepted. *Application deadline:* 5/15 (fall). *Application fee:* $30.
Advanced Placement Credit by examination available. Credit given for nursing courses completed elsewhere dependent upon specific evaluations.
Expenses (2015–16) *Tuition, state resident:* full-time $7110; part-time $296 per credit hour. *Tuition, nonresident:* full-time $20,946; part-time $873 per credit hour. *International tuition:* $20,946 full-time. *Room and board:* $8708; room only: $4610 per academic year. *Required fees:* full-time $3086; part-time $181 per credit.
Contact Ms. Nancy Higgins, BSN Program Coordinator, School of Nursing, Eastern Michigan University, 323 Marshall Building, Ypsilanti, MI 48197. *Telephone:* 734-487-2334. *Fax:* 734-487-6946.
E-mail: nancy.higgins@emich.edu.

GRADUATE PROGRAMS

Expenses (2015–16) *Tuition, state resident:* full-time $10,746; part-time $597 per credit hour. *Tuition, nonresident:* full-time $19,800; part-time $1100 per credit hour. *International tuition:* $19,800 full-time. *Room and board:* $8708; room only: $4610 per academic year.
Contact Roberta Towne, Graduate Programs Coordinator, School of Nursing, Eastern Michigan University, 311 Marshall Building, Ypsilanti, MI 48197. *Telephone:* 734-487-2340. *Fax:* 734-487-6946.
E-mail: rtowne1@emich.edu.

MASTER'S DEGREE PROGRAM
Degree MSN
Available Programs Master's; Master's for Nurses with Non-Nursing Degrees.
Concentrations Available Nursing education. *Clinical nurse specialist programs in:* adult-gerontology acute care. *Nurse practitioner programs in:* adult-gerontology acute care, primary care.
Site Options Livonia, MI; Ann Arbor, MI.
Study Options Part-time.
Program Entrance Requirements Clinical experience, minimum overall college GPA of 3.0, transcript of college record, CPR certification, written essay, immunizations, 2 letters of recommendation, physical assessment course, statistics course. *Application deadline:* 4/8 (winter).
Advanced Placement Credit by examination available. Credit given for nursing courses completed elsewhere dependent upon specific evaluations.
Degree Requirements 43 total credit hours.

POST-MASTER'S PROGRAM
Areas of Study Nursing education.

Ferris State University
School of Nursing
Big Rapids, Michigan

http://www.ferris.edu/
Founded in 1884
DEGREES • BSN • MSN • MSN/MBA
Nursing Program Faculty 24 (20% with doctorates).
Baccalaureate Enrollment 675 **Women** 89% **Men** 11% **Part-time** 79%
Graduate Enrollment 96 **Women** 89% **Men** 11% **Part-time** 100%
Distance Learning Courses Available.
Nursing Student Activities Sigma Theta Tau, Student Nurses' Association, nursing club.
Nursing Student Resources Academic advising; academic or career counseling; assistance for students with disabilities; bookstore; campus computer network; computer lab; computer-assisted instruction; daycare for children of students; e-mail services; employment services for current students; housing assistance; interactive nursing skills videos; Internet; library services; nursing audiovisuals; remedial services; resume preparation assistance; skills, simulation, or other laboratory; tutoring.
Library Facilities 12,177 volumes in health, 785 volumes in nursing; 515 periodical subscriptions health-care related.

BACCALAUREATE PROGRAMS

Degree BSN
Available Programs Generic Baccalaureate; RN Baccalaureate.
Site Options Traverse City, MI; Greenville, MI; Grand Rapids, MI.
Study Options Full-time.
Online Degree Options Yes.
Program Entrance Requirements Minimum overall college GPA of 2.7, transcript of college record, immunizations, minimum GPA in nursing prerequisites of 2.7, prerequisite course work. Transfer students are accepted. *Application deadline:* 3/15 (fall), 3/15 (spring), 3/15 (summer). Applications may be processed on a rolling basis for some programs.
Advanced Placement Credit by examination available. Credit given for nursing courses completed elsewhere dependent upon specific evaluations.
Expenses (2015–16) *Tuition, state resident:* full-time $10,444. *Tuition, nonresident:* full-time $15,680. *International tuition:* $16,772 full-time.
Financial Aid *Gift aid (need-based):* Federal Pell, FSEOG, state, private, college/university gift aid from institutional funds. *Loans:* Federal Nursing Student Loans, Federal Direct (Subsidized and Unsubsidized Stafford PLUS), Perkins, college/university, alternative loans. *Work-study:* Federal Work-Study, part-time campus jobs. *Financial aid application deadline (priority):* 2/15.
Contact Dr. Susan J. Owens, Chair, School of Nursing, School of Nursing, Ferris State University, 200 Ferris Drive, VFS 400-A, Big Rapids, MI 49307. *Telephone:* 231-591-2267. *Fax:* 231-591-2325. *E-mail:* SusanOwens@ferris.edu.

GRADUATE PROGRAMS

Expenses (2015–16) *Tuition, state resident:* part-time $512 per credit hour. *Tuition, nonresident:* part-time $768 per credit hour.
Contact Dr. Sharon Colley, MSN Program Coordinator, School of Nursing, Ferris State University, 200 Ferris Drive, VFS 304, Big Rapids, MI 49307. *Telephone:* 231-591-2288. *Fax:* 231-591-2325. *E-mail:* SharonColley@ferris.edu.

MASTER'S DEGREE PROGRAM
Degrees MSN; MSN/MBA
Available Programs Accelerated AD/RN to Master's; Accelerated RN to Master's; Master's; RN to Master's.
Concentrations Available Nursing administration; nursing education; nursing informatics.
Study Options Full-time and part-time.
Online Degree Options Yes (online only).
Program Entrance Requirements Clinical experience, minimum overall college GPA of 3.0, transcript of college record, written essay, immunizations, 3 letters of recommendation, resume. *Application deadline:* 8/1 (fall), 12/1 (winter), 12/2 (spring).
Advanced Placement Credit given for nursing courses completed elsewhere dependent upon specific evaluations.
Degree Requirements 37 total credit hours, thesis or project, comprehensive exam.

Finlandia University
College of Professional Studies
Hancock, Michigan

http://www.finlandia.edu/
Founded in 1896
DEGREE • BSN
Nursing Program Faculty 11 (10% with doctorates).
Baccalaureate Enrollment 70 **Women** 80% **Men** 20% **Part-time** 12%
Distance Learning Courses Available.
Nursing Student Activities Student Nurses' Association, nursing club.
Nursing Student Resources Academic advising; academic or career counseling; assistance for students with disabilities; bookstore; campus computer network; career placement assistance; computer lab; computer-assisted instruction; e-mail services; externships; interactive nursing skills videos; Internet; learning resource lab; library services; nursing audiovisuals; placement services for program completers; remedial services; resume preparation assistance; skills, simulation, or other laboratory; tutoring.
Library Facilities 4,601 volumes in health, 2,316 volumes in nursing; 97 periodical subscriptions health-care related.

BACCALAUREATE PROGRAMS

Degree BSN
Available Programs Generic Baccalaureate; RN Baccalaureate.
Study Options Full-time.
Online Degree Options Yes.
Program Entrance Requirements Minimum overall college GPA of 2.5, transcript of college record, CPR certification, health exam, health insurance, high school biology, high school chemistry, 1 year of high school math, 2 years high school science, high school transcript, immunizations, minimum high school GPA of 2.5, minimum GPA in nursing prerequisites of 2.7, prerequisite course work. Transfer students are accepted. *Application deadline:* Applications may be processed on a rolling basis for some programs.
Advanced Placement Credit given for nursing courses completed elsewhere dependent upon specific evaluations.
Financial Aid 98% of baccalaureate students in nursing programs received some form of financial aid in 2013–14. *Gift aid (need-based):* Federal Pell, FSEOG, state, private, college/university gift aid from institutional funds. *Loans:* Federal Direct (Subsidized and Unsubsidized Stafford PLUS), private loans. *Work-study:* Federal Work-Study. *Financial aid application deadline (priority):* 3/1.
Contact Travis Hanson, Admissions Office, College of Professional Studies, Finlandia University, 601 Quincy Street, Hancock, MI 49930. *Telephone:* 906-487-7352. *E-mail:* travis.hanson@finlandia.edu.

Grand Valley State University
Kirkhof College of Nursing
Allendale, Michigan

http://www.gvsu.edu/kcon
Founded in 1960
DEGREES • BSN • DNP • MSN
Nursing Program Faculty 109 (32% with doctorates).
Baccalaureate Enrollment 468 **Women** 88% **Men** 12% **Part-time** 21%
Graduate Enrollment 113 **Women** 88% **Men** 12% **Part-time** 50%
Distance Learning Courses Available.
Nursing Student Activities Sigma Theta Tau, Student Nurses' Association.
Nursing Student Resources Academic advising; academic or career counseling; assistance for students with disabilities; bookstore; campus computer network; career placement assistance; computer lab; computer-assisted instruction; daycare for children of students; e-mail services; employment services for current students; housing assistance; interactive nursing skills videos; Internet; learning resource lab; library services; nursing audiovisuals; remedial services; resume preparation assistance; skills, simulation, or other laboratory; tutoring.
Library Facilities 19,510 volumes in health, 1,468 volumes in nursing; 4,578 periodical subscriptions health-care related.

BACCALAUREATE PROGRAMS

Degree BSN

Available Programs ADN to Baccalaureate; Accelerated Baccalaureate for Second Degree; Generic Baccalaureate; RN Baccalaureate.
Site Options Grand Rapids, MI.
Study Options Full-time and part-time.
Program Entrance Requirements Minimum overall college GPA of 3.0, transcript of college record, CPR certification, health exam, immunizations, interview, minimum GPA in nursing prerequisites of 3.0, prerequisite course work. Transfer students are accepted. *Application deadline:* 1/31 (fall), 8/31 (winter).
Advanced Placement Credit given for nursing courses completed elsewhere dependent upon specific evaluations.
Expenses (2014–15) *Tuition, state resident:* full-time $10,752; part-time $448 per credit hour. *Tuition, nonresident:* full-time $15,408; part-time $642 per credit hour. *Room and board:* $8200; room only: $6400 per academic year.
Financial Aid 77% of baccalaureate students in nursing programs received some form of financial aid in 2013–14. *Gift aid (need-based):* Federal Pell, FSEOG, state, private, college/university gift aid from institutional funds. *Loans:* Federal Nursing Student Loans, Federal Direct (Subsidized and Unsubsidized Stafford PLUS), Perkins. *Work-study:* Federal Work-Study, part-time campus jobs. *Financial aid application deadline (priority):* 3/1.
Contact Ms. Kristin Norton, Director of Student Services, Kirkhof College of Nursing, Grand Valley State University, Cook-DeVos Center for Health Sciences, 301 Michigan Street NE, Room 322, Grand Rapids, MI 49503-3314. *Telephone:* 616-331-5637. *Fax:* 616-331-2510. *E-mail:* nortonkr@gvsu.edu.

GRADUATE PROGRAMS

Expenses (2014–15) *Tuition, state resident:* part-time $614 per credit hour. *Tuition, nonresident:* part-time $804 per credit hour. *Room and board:* $8200; room only: $6600 per academic year.
Financial Aid 80% of graduate students in nursing programs received some form of financial aid in 2013–14. 31 fellowships (averaging $11,141 per year), 25 research assistantships with full and partial tuition reimbursements available (averaging $7,339 per year) were awarded; career-related internships or fieldwork, Federal Work-Study, institutionally sponsored loans, and traineeships also available. *Financial aid application deadline:* 2/15.
Contact Ms. Linda Buck, Student Services Coordinator, Kirkhof College of Nursing, Grand Valley State University, Cook-DeVos Center for Health Sciences, 301 Michigan Street NE, Room 318, Grand Rapids, MI 49503-3314. *Telephone:* 616-331-5785. *Fax:* 616-331-2510. *E-mail:* buckli@gvsu.edu.

MASTER'S DEGREE PROGRAM

Degree MSN
Available Programs Master's.
Concentrations Available Clinical nurse leader.
Site Options Grand Rapids, MI.
Study Options Full-time.
Program Entrance Requirements Minimum overall college GPA of 3.0, transcript of college record, CPR certification, written essay, immunizations, interview, resume, GRE. *Application deadline:* 2/1 (fall). *Application fee:* $30.
Advanced Placement Credit given for nursing courses completed elsewhere dependent upon specific evaluations.
Degree Requirements 44 total credit hours, thesis or project.

DOCTORAL DEGREE PROGRAM

Degree DNP
Available Programs Post-Baccalaureate Doctorate.
Areas of Study Advanced practice nursing, nursing administration.
Site Options Grand Rapids, MI.
Program Entrance Requirements Minimum overall college GPA of 3.0, interview, vita, writing sample. Application deadline: 2/1 (fall). Application fee: $30.
Degree Requirements Dissertation.

CONTINUING EDUCATION PROGRAM

Contact Ms. Tamara Mohr, Academic Community Liaison, Kirkhof College of Nursing, Grand Valley State University, Cook-DeVos Center for Health Sciences, 301 Michigan Street NE, Room 310, Grand Rapids, MI 49503-3314. *Telephone:* 616-331-5763. *Fax:* 616-331-2510. *E-mail:* mohrt@gvsu.edu.

Hope College
Department of Nursing
Holland, Michigan

http://www.hope.edu
Founded in 1866
DEGREE • BSN
Nursing Program Faculty 16 (19% with doctorates).
Baccalaureate Enrollment 132 **Women** 95.4% **Men** 4.6%
Nursing Student Activities Sigma Theta Tau, Student Nurses' Association.
Nursing Student Resources Academic advising; academic or career counseling; assistance for students with disabilities; bookstore; campus computer network; career placement assistance; computer lab; computer-assisted instruction; e-mail services; employment services for current students; housing assistance; interactive nursing skills videos; Internet; learning resource lab; library services; nursing audiovisuals; remedial services; resume preparation assistance; skills, simulation, or other laboratory; tutoring; unpaid internships.
Library Facilities 6,920 volumes in health, 418 volumes in nursing; 9,991 periodical subscriptions health-care related.

BACCALAUREATE PROGRAMS

Degree BSN
Available Programs Generic Baccalaureate.
Site Options Cutlerville, MI; Grand Rapids, MI; Holland , MI.
Study Options Full-time and part-time.
Program Entrance Requirements Minimum overall college GPA of 3.2, transcript of college record, written essay, 2 letters of recommendation, prerequisite course work. Transfer students are accepted. *Application deadline:* 10/1 (fall), 2/1 (winter).
Expenses (2015–16) *Tuition:* full-time $30,370; part-time $475 per contact hour. *Room and board:* $9390; room only: $4310 per academic year.
Financial Aid 97% of baccalaureate students in nursing programs received some form of financial aid in 2014–15. *Gift aid (need-based):* Federal Pell, FSEOG, state, private, college/university gift aid from institutional funds. *Loans:* Federal Direct (Subsidized and Unsubsidized Stafford PLUS), Perkins. *Work-study:* Federal Work-Study, part-time campus jobs. *Financial aid application deadline (priority):* 3/1.
Contact Ms. Jill Trujillo, Nursing Contact, Department of Nursing, Hope College, 35 East 12th Street, Holland, MI 49422-9000. *Telephone:* 616-395-7420. *Fax:* 616-395-7163. *E-mail:* nursing@hope.edu.

Lake Superior State University
Department of Nursing
Sault Sainte Marie, Michigan

http://www.lssu.edu/nursing/
Founded in 1946
DEGREE • BSN
Nursing Program Faculty 25 (10% with doctorates).
Baccalaureate Enrollment 142 **Women** 85% **Men** 15%
Distance Learning Courses Available.
Nursing Student Activities Sigma Theta Tau, Student Nurses' Association.
Nursing Student Resources Academic advising; academic or career counseling; assistance for students with disabilities; bookstore; campus computer network; career placement assistance; computer lab; computer-assisted instruction; daycare for children of students; e-mail services; employment services for current students; housing assistance; interactive nursing skills videos; Internet; learning resource lab; library services; nursing audiovisuals; placement services for program completers; remedial services; resume preparation assistance; skills, simulation, or other laboratory; tutoring.
Library Facilities 5,246 volumes in health, 942 volumes in nursing; 1,196 periodical subscriptions health-care related.

BACCALAUREATE PROGRAMS

Degree BSN
Available Programs ADN to Baccalaureate; Generic Baccalaureate; LPN to Baccalaureate; LPN to RN Baccalaureate; RN Baccalaureate; RPN to Baccalaureate.
Site Options Escanaba, MI; Petoskey, MI.

Study Options Full-time.

Program Entrance Requirements Minimum overall college GPA of 2.7, transcript of college record, CPR certification, health exam, health insurance, high school biology, high school chemistry, high school transcript, immunizations, minimum high school GPA of 2.0, minimum GPA in nursing prerequisites of 2.7, professional liability insurance/malpractice insurance, prerequisite course work. Transfer students are accepted. *Application deadline:* 3/1 (fall), 11/1 (spring).

Expenses (2015–16) *Tuition, state resident:* full-time $5196; part-time $433 per credit hour. *Tuition, nonresident:* full-time $5196; part-time $433 per credit hour. *International tuition:* $7800 full-time. *Room and board:* $9290 per academic year. *Required fees:* full-time $1600.

Financial Aid 90% of baccalaureate students in nursing programs received some form of financial aid in 2014–15.

Contact Mr. Ronald S. Hutchins, Academic Dean of Nursing and Health Sciences, Department of Nursing, Lake Superior State University, 650 West Easterday Avenue, Sault Sainte Marie, MI 49783. *Telephone:* 906-635-2446. *Fax:* 906-635-2266. *E-mail:* rhutchins@lssu.edu.

Madonna University
College of Nursing and Health
Livonia, Michigan

http://www.madonna.edu/
Founded in 1947

DEGREES • BSN • DNP • MSN • MSN/MBA
Nursing Program Faculty 77 (35% with doctorates).
Baccalaureate Enrollment 427 **Women** 87% **Men** 13% **Part-time** 32%
Graduate Enrollment 240 **Women** 88% **Men** 12% **Part-time** 98%
Distance Learning Courses Available.
Nursing Student Activities Sigma Theta Tau, Student Nurses' Association.
Nursing Student Resources Academic advising; academic or career counseling; assistance for students with disabilities; bookstore; campus computer network; career placement assistance; computer lab; computer-assisted instruction; e-mail services; employment services for current students; interactive nursing skills videos; Internet; learning resource lab; library services; nursing audiovisuals; placement services for program completers; remedial services; resume preparation assistance; skills, simulation, or other laboratory; tutoring; unpaid internships.
Library Facilities 3,632 volumes in health; 2,778 periodical subscriptions health-care related.

BACCALAUREATE PROGRAMS

Degree BSN
Available Programs ADN to Baccalaureate; Generic Baccalaureate; LPN to Baccalaureate; RN Baccalaureate.
Study Options Full-time and part-time.
Program Entrance Requirements Minimum overall college GPA of 3.0, transcript of college record, CPR certification, written essay, health exam, high school biology, high school chemistry, 1 year of high school math, high school transcript, immunizations, minimum high school GPA of 3.0, minimum GPA in nursing prerequisites of 3.0, professional liability insurance/malpractice insurance, prerequisite course work. Transfer students are accepted. *Application deadline:* 1/31 (fall), 7/31 (winter). Applications may be processed on a rolling basis for some programs. *Application fee:* $25.
Advanced Placement Credit by examination available.
Expenses (2015–16) *Tuition:* full-time $16,440; part-time $685 per credit hour. *International tuition:* $19,200 full-time. *Room and board:* $4140 per academic year.
Contact Ms. Colleen Kibin, Nursing Admissions Officer, College of Nursing and Health, Madonna University, 36600 Schoolcraft Road, Livonia, MI 48150-1173. *Telephone:* 734-793-5768. *E-mail:* ckibin@madonna.edu.

GRADUATE PROGRAMS

Expenses (2015–16) *Tuition:* full-time $18,240; part-time $760 per credit hour. *Room and board:* $4430 per academic year. *Required fees:* full-time $210; part-time $50 per credit.
Contact Mr. Sandro Faber-Bermudez, Admissions Officer, Graduate Nursing program, College of Nursing and Health, Madonna University, 36600 Schoolcraft Road, Livonia, MI 48150-1173. *Telephone:* 734-432-5407. *Fax:* 734-432-5463. *E-mail:* sfaber-bermudez@madonna.edu.

MASTER'S DEGREE PROGRAM

Degrees MSN; MSN/MBA
Available Programs Master's.
Concentrations Available Nursing administration. *Nurse practitioner programs in:* adult-gerontology acute care, primary care.
Study Options Full-time and part-time.
Program Entrance Requirements Clinical experience, computer literacy, minimum overall college GPA of 3.0, transcript of college record, CPR certification, written essay, immunizations, interview, 2 letters of recommendation, nursing research course, physical assessment course, professional liability insurance/malpractice insurance, prerequisite course work, resume, statistics course. *Application deadline:* 2/1 (fall), 2/1 (winter), 2/1 (spring), 2/1 (summer). *Application fee:* $25.
Advanced Placement Credit given for nursing courses completed elsewhere dependent upon specific evaluations.
Degree Requirements 50 total credit hours, thesis or project.

POST-MASTER'S PROGRAM

Areas of Study Nursing administration. *Nurse practitioner programs in:* adult-gerontology acute care, primary care.

DOCTORAL DEGREE PROGRAM

Degree DNP
Available Programs Doctorate.
Areas of Study Individualized study, nursing administration.
Program Entrance Requirements Clinical experience, minimum overall college GPA of 3.0, interview by faculty committee, interview, 3 letters of recommendation, MSN or equivalent, statistics course, vita, writing sample. Application deadline: 3/1 (fall). Application fee: $25.
Degree Requirements 38 total credit hours, written exam.

Michigan State University
College of Nursing
East Lansing, Michigan

http://www.nursing.msu.edu/
Founded in 1855

DEGREES • BSN • DNP • MSN • PHD
Nursing Program Faculty 93 (47% with doctorates).
Baccalaureate Enrollment 454 **Women** 88.9% **Men** 11.1% **Part-time** 13.7%
Graduate Enrollment 209 **Women** 86.1% **Men** 13.9% **Part-time** 52.2%
Distance Learning Courses Available.
Nursing Student Activities Sigma Theta Tau, Student Nurses' Association.
Nursing Student Resources Academic advising; academic or career counseling; assistance for students with disabilities; bookstore; campus computer network; career placement assistance; computer lab; computer-assisted instruction; daycare for children of students; e-mail services; employment services for current students; externships; housing assistance; interactive nursing skills videos; Internet; learning resource lab; library services; nursing audiovisuals; placement services for program completers; remedial services; resume preparation assistance; skills, simulation, or other laboratory; tutoring.
Library Facilities 250,754 volumes in health, 9,377 volumes in nursing; 9,313 periodical subscriptions health-care related.

BACCALAUREATE PROGRAMS

Degree BSN
Available Programs Accelerated Baccalaureate for Second Degree; Generic Baccalaureate; RN Baccalaureate.
Site Options Detroit, MI.
Study Options Full-time.
Online Degree Options Yes.
Program Entrance Requirements Minimum overall college GPA of 2.75, transcript of college record, written essay, 2 letters of recommendation, minimum GPA in nursing prerequisites of 2.0, prerequisite course work. Transfer students are accepted. *Application deadline:* 5/1 (fall), 12/1 (spring), 12/1 (summer).
Advanced Placement Credit given for nursing courses completed elsewhere dependent upon specific evaluations.
Expenses (2015–16) *Tuition, state resident:* full-time $15,105; part-time $504 per credit hour. *Tuition, nonresident:* full-time $37,508; part-time $1250 per credit hour. *International tuition:* $37,508 full-time. *Room and board:* $9524 per academic year. *Required fees:* full-time $56.

Financial Aid 67% of baccalaureate students in nursing programs received some form of financial aid in 2014–15. *Gift aid (need-based):* Federal Pell, FSEOG, state, private, college/university gift aid from institutional funds, United Negro College Fund. *Loans:* Federal Direct (Subsidized and Unsubsidized Stafford PLUS), Perkins, college/university. *Work-study:* Federal Work-Study. *Financial aid application deadline:* Continuous.

Contact Office of Student Support Services, College of Nursing, Michigan State University, Bott Building for Nursing Education and Research, 1355 Bogue Street, Room C120, East Lansing, MI 48824. *Telephone:* 517-353-4827. *Fax:* 517-432-8251. *E-mail:* nurse@hc.msu.edu.

GRADUATE PROGRAMS

Expenses (2015–16) *Tuition, state resident:* part-time $672 per credit hour. *Tuition, nonresident:* part-time $1320 per credit hour. *Room and board:* $9444 per academic year.

Financial Aid 56% of graduate students in nursing programs received some form of financial aid in 2014–15. 1 research assistantship with tuition reimbursement available (averaging $6,110 per year), 2 teaching assistantships with tuition reimbursements available (averaging $7,076 per year) were awarded.

Contact Nikki O'Brien, Program Advisor, College of Nursing, Michigan State University, Bott Building for Nursing Education and Research, 1355 Bogue Street, Room C120, East Lansing, MI 48824. *Telephone:* 517-353-4827. *Fax:* 517-432-8251. *E-mail:* obrienni@msu.edu.

MASTER'S DEGREE PROGRAM

Degree MSN

Available Programs Master's.

Concentrations Available Nurse anesthesia. *Clinical nurse specialist programs in:* adult health, gerontology. *Nurse practitioner programs in:* adult health, family health, gerontology.

Study Options Full-time and part-time.

Online Degree Options Yes.

Program Entrance Requirements Clinical experience, minimum overall college GPA of 3.0, transcript of college record, CPR certification, written essay, immunizations, interview, 3 letters of recommendation, prerequisite course work, resume, statistics course. *Application deadline:* 2/1 (fall), 3/15 (spring). Applications may be processed on a rolling basis for some programs.

Advanced Placement Credit given for nursing courses completed elsewhere dependent upon specific evaluations.

Degree Requirements Thesis or project.

DOCTORAL DEGREE PROGRAM

Degree DNP

Available Programs Doctorate.

Areas of Study Advanced practice nursing.

Program Entrance Requirements Minimum overall college GPA of 3.0, clinical experience, interview by faculty committee, MSN or equivalent, statistics course, vita, writing sample. Application deadline: 5/1 (spring).

Degree Requirements 36 total credit hours, scholarly/synthesis project, oral presentation of project.

Degree PhD

Available Programs Doctorate; Post-Baccalaureate Doctorate.

Areas of Study Family health, gerontology, health promotion/disease prevention, human health and illness, individualized study, maternity-newborn, nursing research, oncology, women's health.

Program Entrance Requirements Minimum overall college GPA of 3.0, interview by faculty committee, interview, 3 letters of recommendation, statistics course, vita, writing sample. Application deadline: 12/1 (fall). Applications may be processed on a rolling basis for some programs.

Degree Requirements 72 total credit hours, dissertation, written exam, residency.

POSTDOCTORAL PROGRAM

Areas of Study Cancer care, family health, gerontology, health promotion/disease prevention, individualized study, women's health.

Postdoctoral Program Contact Barbara Smith, Associate Dean for Research, College of Nursing, Michigan State University, Bott Building for Nursing Education and Research, 1355 Bogue Street, Room C200, East Lansing, MI 48824. *Telephone:* 517-432-9159. *Fax:* 404-651-4871. *E-mail:* barbara.smith@hc.msu.edu.

CONTINUING EDUCATION PROGRAM

Contact Kathy Forrest, Instructor and Coordinator Professional Programs, College of Nursing, Michigan State University, Life Sciences Building, 1355 Bogue Street, Room A112, East Lansing, MI 48824. *Telephone:* 517-432-0393. *Fax:* 517-432-8131. *E-mail:* kathy.forrest@hc.msu.edu.

Northern Michigan University
College of Nursing and Allied Health Science
Marquette, Michigan

http://www.nmu.edu/nursing/
Founded in 1899

DEGREES • BSN • DNP

Nursing Program Faculty 28 (34% with doctorates).
Baccalaureate Enrollment 208 **Women** 84% **Men** 16%
Graduate Enrollment 19 **Women** 81% **Men** 19% **Part-time** 100%
Distance Learning Courses Available.
Nursing Student Activities Sigma Theta Tau, Student Nurses' Association.
Nursing Student Resources Academic advising; academic or career counseling; assistance for students with disabilities; bookstore; campus computer network; career placement assistance; computer lab; computer-assisted instruction; e-mail services; employment services for current students; housing assistance; interactive nursing skills videos; Internet; learning resource lab; library services; nursing audiovisuals; other; paid internships; placement services for program completers; remedial services; resume preparation assistance; skills, simulation, or other laboratory; tutoring.
Library Facilities 32,879 volumes in health, 1,291 volumes in nursing; 5,000 periodical subscriptions health-care related.

BACCALAUREATE PROGRAMS

Degree BSN

Available Programs ADN to Baccalaureate; Generic Baccalaureate; LPN to RN Baccalaureate; RN Baccalaureate.

Study Options Full-time.

Program Entrance Requirements Minimum overall college GPA of 2.75, transcript of college record, CPR certification, health exam, high school transcript, immunizations, minimum GPA in nursing prerequisites of 2.0, prerequisite course work. Transfer students are accepted. *Application deadline:* 2/1 (fall), 10/1 (winter).

Advanced Placement Credit given for nursing courses completed elsewhere dependent upon specific evaluations.

Expenses (2015–16) *Tuition, state resident:* full-time $10,453; part-time $383 per credit. *Tuition, nonresident:* full-time $15,854; part-time $632 per credit. *Room and board:* $9286; room only: $4572 per academic year. *Required fees:* full-time $63; part-time $32 per term.

Contact Dr. Nanci K. Gasiewicz, Associate Dean and Director, College of Nursing and Allied Health Science, Northern Michigan University, 1401 Presque Isle Avenue, 2301 New Science Facility, Marquette, MI 49855. *Telephone:* 906-227-2834. *Fax:* 906-227-1658. *E-mail:* ngasiewi@nmu.edu.

GRADUATE PROGRAMS

Expenses (2015–16) *Tuition, state resident:* part-time $645 per credit. *Tuition, nonresident:* part-time $645 per credit. *Required fees:* part-time $13 per credit.

Financial Aid Career-related internships or fieldwork, Federal Work-Study, institutionally sponsored loans, and unspecified assistantships available.

Contact Dr. Melissa M. Romero, Graduate Program Coordinator, College of Nursing and Allied Health Science, Northern Michigan University, 1401 Presque Isle Avenue, 2131 New Science Facility, Marquette, MI 49855. *Telephone:* 906-227-2488. *Fax:* 906-227-1658. *E-mail:* mromero@nmu.edu.

MASTER'S DEGREE PROGRAM

Program Entrance Requirements GRE General Test. *Application deadline:* 2/1 (fall).

DOCTORAL DEGREE PROGRAM

Degree DNP

Available Programs Doctorate; Post-Baccalaureate Doctorate.

Areas of Study Family health.

Program Entrance Requirements Minimum overall college GPA of 3.0, interview by faculty committee, 2 letters of recommendation, statistics course, vita, writing sample. Application deadline: 4/1 (fall).
Degree Requirements 77 total credit hours, written exam, residency.

CONTINUING EDUCATION PROGRAM

Contact Dr. Robert Winn, Associate Provost Graduate Education, College of Nursing and Allied Health Science, Northern Michigan University, 1401 Presque Isle Avenue, 401 Cohodas Hall, Marquette, MI 49855. *Telephone:* 906-227-2300. *Fax:* 906-227-2315. *E-mail:* rwinn@nmu.edu.

Oakland University
School of Nursing
Rochester, Michigan

http://www.oakland.edu/
Founded in 1957

DEGREES • BSN • DNP • MSN
Nursing Program Faculty 44 (50% with doctorates).
Baccalaureate Enrollment 462 Women 89% Men 11% Part-time 29%
Graduate Enrollment 123 Women 79% Men 21% Part-time 35%
Distance Learning Courses Available.
Nursing Student Activities Nursing Honor Society, Sigma Theta Tau, Student Nurses' Association.
Nursing Student Resources Academic advising; academic or career counseling; assistance for students with disabilities; bookstore; campus computer network; career placement assistance; computer lab; computer-assisted instruction; e-mail services; employment services for current students; externships; housing assistance; interactive nursing skills videos; Internet; learning resource lab; library services; nursing audiovisuals; paid internships; placement services for program completers; remedial services; resume preparation assistance; skills, simulation, or other laboratory; tutoring; unpaid internships.
Library Facilities 12,652 volumes in health, 2,780 volumes in nursing; 375 periodical subscriptions health-care related.

BACCALAUREATE PROGRAMS
Degree BSN
Available Programs ADN to Baccalaureate; Accelerated Baccalaureate for Second Degree; Generic Baccalaureate.
Site Options Mount Clemens, MI; Auburn Hills, MI.
Study Options Full-time.
Program Entrance Requirements Minimum overall college GPA of 3.2, transcript of college record, high school biology, high school chemistry, 4 years high school math, 3 years high school science, high school transcript, minimum high school GPA of 3.2, minimum GPA in nursing prerequisites of 3.2, prerequisite course work. Transfer students are accepted. *Application deadline:* 5/15 (fall), 8/15 (winter).
Expenses (2014–15) *Tuition, area resident:* part-time $355 per credit hour. *Tuition, state resident:* part-time $410 per credit hour. *Tuition, nonresident:* part-time $800 per credit hour.
Financial Aid 75% of baccalaureate students in nursing programs received some form of financial aid in 2013–14.
Contact Dr. Sarah Newton, Undergraduate Program Director, School of Nursing, Oakland University, 3004 Human Health Building, Rochester, MI 48309-4401. *Telephone:* 248-364-8771. *E-mail:* newton@oakland.edu.

GRADUATE PROGRAMS
Financial Aid 60% of graduate students in nursing programs received some form of financial aid in 2013–14. Federal Work-Study, institutionally sponsored loans, and tuition waivers (full) available. *Financial aid application deadline:* 3/1.
Contact Patrina Carper, Academic Adviser, School of Nursing, Oakland University, 3032 Human Health Building, Rochester, MI 48309-4401. *Telephone:* 248-364-8766. *Fax:* 248-364-8783. *E-mail:* carper@oakland.edu.

MASTER'S DEGREE PROGRAM
Degree MSN
Available Programs Master's.
Concentrations Available Nurse anesthesia; nursing education. *Nurse practitioner programs in:* adult health, family health, gerontology.
Site Options Mount Clemens, MI; Auburn Hills, MI.
Study Options Full-time and part-time.

Program Entrance Requirements Clinical experience, minimum overall college GPA of 3.0, transcript of college record, CPR certification, written essay, immunizations, interview, 2 letters of recommendation, nursing research course, physical assessment course, GRE General Test. *Application deadline:* 4/1 (spring).
Advanced Placement Credit given for nursing courses completed elsewhere dependent upon specific evaluations.
Degree Requirements 48 total credit hours, thesis or project.

POST-MASTER'S PROGRAM
Areas of Study Nurse anesthesia; nursing education. *Nurse practitioner programs in:* adult health, family health, gerontology.

DOCTORAL DEGREE PROGRAM
Degree DNP
Available Programs Doctorate; Doctorate for Nurses with Non-Nursing Degrees.
Areas of Study Advanced practice nursing, aging, clinical nurse leader, clinical practice, clinical research, family health, forensic nursing, gerontology, health policy, health promotion/disease prevention, health-care systems, human health and illness, individualized study, information systems, nursing education, nursing policy, nursing research, nursing science.
Program Entrance Requirements Clinical experience, minimum overall college GPA of 3.0, 2 letters of recommendation, MSN or equivalent. *Application deadline:* 7/15 (summer).
Degree Requirements 38 total credit hours.

CONTINUING EDUCATION PROGRAM
Contact Dr. Kristina White, Director, Center for Professional Development, School of Nursing, Oakland University, 3033 Human Health Building, Rochester, MI 48309-4401. *Telephone:* 248-364-8755. *Fax:* 248-364-8783. *E-mail:* white2@oakland.edu.

Rochester College
School of Nursing
Rochester Hills, Michigan

http://www.rc.edu/academics/undergraduate/school-of-nursing/
Founded in 1959

DEGREE • BSN
Baccalaureate Enrollment 62
Nursing Student Activities Student Nurses' Association.
Nursing Student Resources Academic advising; academic or career counseling; assistance for students with disabilities; bookstore; campus computer network; career placement assistance; computer lab; computer-assisted instruction; e-mail services; housing assistance; interactive nursing skills videos; Internet; learning resource lab; library services; nursing audiovisuals; remedial services; resume preparation assistance; skills, simulation, or other laboratory; tutoring.

BACCALAUREATE PROGRAMS
Degree BSN
Available Programs Generic Baccalaureate; RN Baccalaureate.
Study Options Full-time.
Program Entrance Requirements Minimum overall college GPA of 3.2, transcript of college record, interview, minimum GPA in nursing prerequisites of 3.0, prerequisite course work. Transfer students are accepted. *Application deadline:* 6/1 (fall).
Contact Ms. Susan Griffin, School of Nursing Coordinator, School of Nursing, Rochester College, 800 West Avon Road, Rochester Hills, MI 48307. *Telephone:* 248-218-2280. *E-mail:* sgriffin@rc.edu.

Saginaw Valley State University
College of Health and Human Services
University Center, Michigan

http://www.svsu.edu/collegeofhealthhumanservices
Founded in 1963

DEGREES • BSN • DNP • MSN
Nursing Program Faculty 19 (70% with doctorates).
Baccalaureate Enrollment 450 Women 80% Men 20%

Graduate Enrollment 51 **Women** 92% **Men** 8% **Part-time** 100%
Distance Learning Courses Available.
Nursing Student Activities Sigma Theta Tau, Student Nurses' Association.
Nursing Student Resources Academic advising; academic or career counseling; assistance for students with disabilities; bookstore; campus computer network; career placement assistance; computer lab; computer-assisted instruction; e-mail services; employment services for current students; externships; interactive nursing skills videos; Internet; learning resource lab; library services; nursing audiovisuals; remedial services; resume preparation assistance; skills, simulation, or other laboratory; tutoring; unpaid internships.

BACCALAUREATE PROGRAMS

Degree BSN
Available Programs ADN to Baccalaureate; Baccalaureate for Second Degree; Generic Baccalaureate; RN Baccalaureate.
Study Options Full-time.
Program Entrance Requirements Minimum overall college GPA of 2.8, transcript of college record, CPR certification, health exam, immunizations, minimum GPA in nursing prerequisites of 2.8, professional liability insurance/malpractice insurance, prerequisite course work. Transfer students are accepted. *Application deadline:* 4/15 (fall), 10/15 (winter).
Advanced Placement Credit given for nursing courses completed elsewhere dependent upon specific evaluations.
Financial Aid *Gift aid (need-based):* Federal Pell, FSEOG, state, private, college/university gift aid from institutional funds. *Loans:* Federal Direct (Subsidized and Unsubsidized Stafford PLUS), CitiAssist Loans, Chase Select loans, Charter One TruFit Student Loans, Discover Private Educational Loans. *Work-study:* Federal Work-Study, part-time campus jobs. *Financial aid application deadline:* Continuous.
Contact Dr. Rebecca Toth, Nursing Department Chair, College of Health and Human Services, Saginaw Valley State University, 7400 Bay Road, H228, University Center, MI 48710-0001. *Telephone:* 989-964-4542. *Fax:* 989-964-4925. *E-mail:* rstoth@svsu.edu.

GRADUATE PROGRAMS

Financial Aid Federal Work-Study and scholarships available.
Contact Dr. Karen Brown-Fackler, Nursing Graduate Programs Coordinator, College of Health and Human Services, Saginaw Valley State University, 7400 Bay Road, H219, University Center, MI 48710-0001. *Telephone:* 989-964-2185. *Fax:* 989-964-4925. *E-mail:* kmbrown4@svsu.edu.

MASTER'S DEGREE PROGRAM
Degree MSN
Available Programs Accelerated AD/RN to Master's; Master's; RN to Master's.
Concentrations Available Clinical nurse leader; nursing administration; nursing education. *Clinical nurse specialist programs in:* family health. *Nurse practitioner programs in:* family health.
Study Options Part-time.
Program Entrance Requirements Clinical experience, minimum overall college GPA of 3.0, transcript of college record, CPR certification, written essay, immunizations, interview, 3 letters of recommendation, professional liability insurance/malpractice insurance, resume, statistics course. *Application deadline:* Applications may be processed on a rolling basis for some programs.
Advanced Placement Credit given for nursing courses completed elsewhere dependent upon specific evaluations.
Degree Requirements 39 total credit hours, thesis or project.

POST-MASTER'S PROGRAM
Areas of Study Nursing administration; nursing education. *Nurse practitioner programs in:* family health.

DOCTORAL DEGREE PROGRAM
Degree DNP
Available Programs Doctorate; Post-Baccalaureate Doctorate.
Areas of Study Family health.
Program Entrance Requirements Clinical experience, minimum overall college GPA of 3.0, interview, letters of recommendation, statistics course, vita, GRE. Application deadline: Applications may be processed on a rolling basis for some programs.
Degree Requirements Dissertation.

CONTINUING EDUCATION PROGRAM

Contact CE Coordinator, College of Health and Human Services, Saginaw Valley State University, 7400 Bay Road, University Center, MI

48710-0001. *Telephone:* 989-964-4595. *Fax:* 989-964-4925. *E-mail:* nursing@svsu.edu.

Siena Heights University
Nursing Program
Adrian, Michigan

http://www.sienaheights.edu/
Founded in 1919
DEGREE • BSN
Nursing Program Faculty 8 (10% with doctorates).
Baccalaureate Enrollment 78 **Women** 87% **Men** 13% **Part-time** 60%
Distance Learning Courses Available.
Nursing Student Activities Student Nurses' Association.
Nursing Student Resources Academic advising; academic or career counseling; assistance for students with disabilities; bookstore; campus computer network; career placement assistance; computer lab; computer-assisted instruction; e-mail services; interactive nursing skills videos; Internet; learning resource lab; library services; nursing audiovisuals; skills, simulation, or other laboratory; tutoring.
Library Facilities 200 volumes in health, 80 volumes in nursing; 150 periodical subscriptions health-care related.

BACCALAUREATE PROGRAMS

Degree BSN
Available Programs Generic Baccalaureate; RN Baccalaureate.
Site Options Monroe, MI.
Study Options Full-time.
Online Degree Options Yes.
Program Entrance Requirements Minimum overall college GPA of 3.0, transcript of college record, CPR certification, health exam, health insurance, high school transcript, immunizations, minimum GPA in nursing prerequisites of 3.0, professional liability insurance/malpractice insurance, prerequisite course work. Transfer students are accepted. *Application deadline:* 10/1 (fall).
Expenses (2014–15) *Tuition:* full-time $22,000; part-time $480 per credit hour. *Room and board:* $9300; room only: $5000 per academic year. *Required fees:* full-time $1000.
Financial Aid 90% of baccalaureate students in nursing programs received some form of financial aid in 2013–14.
Contact Mrs. Trudy Mohre, Director of Admissions, Nursing Program, Siena Heights University, 1247 East Siena Heights Drive, Adrian, MI 49221. *Telephone:* 517-264-7180. *E-mail:* tmohre@sienaheighs.edu.

Spring Arbor University
Program in Nursing
Spring Arbor, Michigan

http://www.arbor.edu/bsn
Founded in 1873
DEGREES • BSN • MSN • MSN/MBA
Nursing Program Faculty 19 (26% with doctorates).
Baccalaureate Enrollment 217 **Women** 89% **Men** 11%
Graduate Enrollment 80 **Women** 92% **Men** 8%
Distance Learning Courses Available.
Nursing Student Resources Academic advising; academic or career counseling; assistance for students with disabilities; bookstore; campus computer network; career placement assistance; computer lab; computer-assisted instruction; e-mail services; Internet; library services; nursing audiovisuals; other; tutoring.
Library Facilities 1,000 volumes in health, 350 volumes in nursing; 52 periodical subscriptions health-care related.

BACCALAUREATE PROGRAMS

Degree BSN
Available Programs ADN to Baccalaureate.
Site Options Battle Creek, MI; Gaylord, MI; Jackson, MI; Flint, MI; Traverse City, MI; Southfield, MI; Grand Rapids, MI; Lambertville, MI; Lansing, MI; Kalamazoo, MI.
Program Entrance Requirements Minimum overall college GPA of 2.5, transcript of college record, written essay, high school biology, high school chemistry, 1 year of high school math, 2 years high school science, high school transcript, minimum GPA in nursing prerequisites of

2.5, RN licensure. Transfer students are accepted. *Application deadline:* Applications may be processed on a rolling basis for some programs. **Contact** *Telephone:* 517-750-6579. *Fax:* 517-750-6602.

GRADUATE PROGRAMS

Contact *Telephone:* 800-968-0011 Ext. 1703. *Fax:* 517-750-6799.

MASTER'S DEGREE PROGRAM
Degrees MSN; MSN/MBA
Available Programs Master's.
Concentrations Available Nursing education. *Nurse practitioner programs in:* adult health, gerontology.
Study Options Full-time.
Online Degree Options Yes (online only).
Program Entrance Requirements Minimum overall college GPA of 3.0, transcript of college record, written essay, interview, 2 letters of recommendation, nursing research course, prerequisite course work, statistics course. *Application deadline:* 7/1 (fall), 1/5 (spring). *Application fee:* $30.
Degree Requirements 54 total credit hours, thesis or project.

University of Detroit Mercy
McAuley School of Nursing
Detroit, Michigan

http://www.udmercy.edu/healthprof/nursing/
Founded in 1877
DEGREES • BSN • MSN
Nursing Program Faculty 80
Baccalaureate Enrollment 933 **Women** 88% **Men** 12% **Part-time** 46%
Graduate Enrollment 132 **Women** 95% **Men** 5% **Part-time** 96%
Distance Learning Courses Available.
Nursing Student Activities Sigma Theta Tau, Student Nurses' Association.
Nursing Student Resources Academic advising; academic or career counseling; bookstore; campus computer network; career placement assistance; computer lab; computer-assisted instruction; e-mail services; Internet; learning resource lab; library services; nursing audiovisuals; other; paid internships; placement services for program completers; remedial services; resume preparation assistance; skills, simulation, or other laboratory; tutoring.
Library Facilities 32,330 volumes in health, 3,404 volumes in nursing; 2,670 periodical subscriptions health-care related.

BACCALAUREATE PROGRAMS

Degree BSN
Available Programs Accelerated Baccalaureate for Second Degree; Generic Baccalaureate; RN Baccalaureate.
Site Options Dearborn, MI; Grand Rapids, MI; Wayne, MI.
Study Options Full-time and part-time.
Program Entrance Requirements Minimum overall college GPA of 2.5, transcript of college record, CPR certification, health exam, health insurance, high school biology, high school chemistry, 2 years high school math, 2 years high school science, high school transcript, immunizations, minimum high school GPA of 2.5, minimum GPA in nursing prerequisites of 2.5, prerequisite course work. Transfer students are accepted.
Advanced Placement Credit given for nursing courses completed elsewhere dependent upon specific evaluations.
Contact *Telephone:* 313-993-1245. *Fax:* 313-993-3325.

GRADUATE PROGRAMS

Contact *Telephone:* 313-993-6423. *Fax:* 313-993-6175.

MASTER'S DEGREE PROGRAM
Degree MSN
Available Programs Accelerated AD/RN to Master's; Master's; Master's for Nurses with Non-Nursing Degrees.
Concentrations Available Nursing administration; nursing education. *Nurse practitioner programs in:* family health.
Study Options Full-time and part-time.
Program Entrance Requirements Clinical experience, minimum overall college GPA of 3.0, transcript of college record, CPR certification, immunizations, interview, 3 letters of recommendation, resume.
Degree Requirements 50 total credit hours.

POST-MASTER'S PROGRAM
Areas of Study Nursing administration; nursing education. *Nurse practitioner programs in:* family health.

University of Michigan
School of Nursing
Ann Arbor, Michigan

http://www.nursing.umich.edu/
Founded in 1817
DEGREES • BSN • MS • MSN/MBA • MSN/MPH • PHD
Nursing Program Faculty 130 (66% with doctorates).
Baccalaureate Enrollment 618 **Women** 90% **Men** 10% **Part-time** 13%
Graduate Enrollment 240 **Women** 95% **Men** 5% **Part-time** 40%
Distance Learning Courses Available.
Nursing Student Activities Nursing Honor Society, Sigma Theta Tau, Student Nurses' Association, nursing club.
Nursing Student Resources Academic advising; academic or career counseling; assistance for students with disabilities; bookstore; campus computer network; career placement assistance; computer lab; computer-assisted instruction; daycare for children of students; e-mail services; employment services for current students; externships; housing assistance; interactive nursing skills videos; Internet; learning resource lab; library services; nursing audiovisuals; paid internships; placement services for program completers; remedial services; resume preparation assistance; skills, simulation, or other laboratory; tutoring; unpaid internships.
Library Facilities 1.2 million volumes in nursing.

BACCALAUREATE PROGRAMS

Degree BSN
Available Programs Accelerated Baccalaureate for Second Degree; Generic Baccalaureate; RN Baccalaureate.
Site Options Kalamazoo, MI; Traverse City, MI.
Study Options Full-time and part-time.
Program Entrance Requirements Minimum overall college GPA of 3.0, transcript of college record, written essay, high school chemistry, 2 years high school math, 2 years high school science, high school transcript, minimum high school GPA of 3.0, prerequisite course work. Transfer students are accepted. *Application deadline:* 2/1 (fall). Applications may be processed on a rolling basis for some programs. *Application fee:* $80.
Advanced Placement Credit given for nursing courses completed elsewhere dependent upon specific evaluations.
Contact *Telephone:* 734-647-1443. *Fax:* 734-936-0740.

GRADUATE PROGRAMS

Contact *Telephone:* 734-764-7188. *Fax:* 734-647-1419.

MASTER'S DEGREE PROGRAM
Degrees MS; MSN/MBA; MSN/MPH
Available Programs Accelerated RN to Master's; Master's; RN to Master's.
Concentrations Available Health-care administration; nurse-midwifery; nursing administration; nursing informatics. *Clinical nurse specialist programs in:* community health, gerontology, home health care, medical-surgical, occupational health, psychiatric/mental health. *Nurse practitioner programs in:* acute care, adult health, family health, gerontology, pediatric, primary care, psychiatric/mental health.
Study Options Full-time and part-time.
Program Entrance Requirements Computer literacy, minimum overall college GPA of 3.0, transcript of college record, written essay, interview, 3 letters of recommendation, resume. *Application deadline:* 2/1 (fall). Applications may be processed on a rolling basis for some programs. *Application fee:* $80.
Advanced Placement Credit given for nursing courses completed elsewhere dependent upon specific evaluations.
Degree Requirements 37 total credit hours, thesis or project.

POST-MASTER'S PROGRAM
Areas of Study Health-care administration; nurse-midwifery; nursing administration; nursing informatics. *Clinical nurse specialist programs in:* community health, gerontology, home health care, medical-surgical, occupational health, psychiatric/mental health, women's health. *Nurse practitioner programs in:* acute care, adult health, family health, geron-

tology, pediatric, primary care, psychiatric/mental health, women's health.

DOCTORAL DEGREE PROGRAM

Degree PhD

Available Programs Doctorate; Post-Baccalaureate Doctorate.

Areas of Study Advanced practice nursing, aging, bio-behavioral research, biology of health and illness, community health, critical care, ethics, family health, gerontology, health policy, health promotion/disease prevention, health-care systems, individualized study, information systems, neuro-behavior, nursing administration, nursing policy, nursing research, nursing science, women's health.

Program Entrance Requirements Minimum overall college GPA of 3.0, interview, 3 letters of recommendation, scholarly papers, vita, writing sample. Application deadline: 12/11 (fall). Application fee: $80.

Degree Requirements 50 total credit hours, dissertation, oral exam, written exam, residency.

POSTDOCTORAL PROGRAM

Areas of Study Addiction/substance abuse, aging, chronic illness, community health, family health, gerontology, health promotion/disease prevention, individualized study, information systems, neuro-behavior, nursing interventions, nursing research, nursing science, vulnerable population, women's health.

Postdoctoral Program Contact *Telephone:* 734-764-9454. *Fax:* 734-763-6668.

University of Michigan–Flint
Department of Nursing
Flint, Michigan

http://www.umflint.edu/nursing
Founded in 1956

DEGREES • BSN • DNP • MSN

Nursing Program Faculty 109 (26% with doctorates).

Baccalaureate Enrollment 1,310 **Women** 83.52% **Men** 16.48% **Part-time** 65.11%

Graduate Enrollment 212 **Women** 87.26% **Men** 12.74% **Part-time** 38.2%

Distance Learning Courses Available.

Nursing Student Activities Nursing Honor Society, Sigma Theta Tau, Student Nurses' Association, nursing club.

Nursing Student Resources Academic advising; academic or career counseling; assistance for students with disabilities; bookstore; campus computer network; career placement assistance; computer lab; computer-assisted instruction; daycare for children of students; e-mail services; employment services for current students; externships; housing assistance; interactive nursing skills videos; Internet; library services; nursing audiovisuals; remedial services; resume preparation assistance; skills, simulation, or other laboratory; tutoring.

Library Facilities 17,761 volumes in health, 1,528 volumes in nursing; 205 periodical subscriptions health-care related.

BACCALAUREATE PROGRAMS

Degree BSN

Available Programs Accelerated Baccalaureate for Second Degree; RN Baccalaureate; RPN to Baccalaureate.

Site Options Port Huron, MI; Alpena, MI; Lansing, MI; Detroit, MI; Flint, MI.

Study Options Full-time.

Online Degree Options Yes.

Program Entrance Requirements Minimum overall college GPA of 3.0, transcript of college record, CPR certification, written essay, health exam, health insurance, immunizations, 2 letters of recommendation, minimum high school GPA of 3.0, minimum GPA in nursing prerequisites of 3.0, prerequisite course work. Transfer students are accepted. *Application deadline:* 8/22 (fall), 12/14 (winter), 4/18 (spring), 6/14 (summer). *Application fee:* $30.

Advanced Placement Credit by examination available. Credit given for nursing courses completed elsewhere dependent upon specific evaluations.

Expenses (2015–16) *Tuition, state resident:* full-time $11,262; part-time $469 per credit hour. *Tuition, nonresident:* full-time $22,512; part-time $938 per credit hour. *International tuition:* $22,512 full-time. *Room and board:* $8178; room only: $5178 per academic year. *Required fees:* full-time $562; part-time $232 per term.

Contact Ms. Laura Martin, Senior Secretary, Department of Nursing, University of Michigan–Flint, Department of Nursing, 2180 William S. White, School of Health Professions and Studies, Flint, MI 48502-1950. *Telephone:* 810-762-3420. *Fax:* 810-766-6851. *E-mail:* lamart@umflint.edu.

GRADUATE PROGRAMS

Expenses (2015–16) *Tuition, state resident:* full-time $8492; part-time $531 per credit hour. *Tuition, nonresident:* full-time $12,728; part-time $796 per credit hour. *International tuition:* $12,728 full-time. *Room and board:* $8178; room only: $5178 per academic year. *Required fees:* full-time $632; part-time $267 per term.

Contact Ms. Laura Martin, Senior Secretary, Department of Nursing, University of Michigan–Flint, Department of Nursing, 2180 William S. White, School of Health Professions and Studies, Flint, MI 48502-1950. *Telephone:* 810-762-3420. *Fax:* 810-766-6851. *E-mail:* lamart@umflint.edu.

MASTER'S DEGREE PROGRAM

Degree MSN

Available Programs Accelerated RN to Master's; RN to Master's.

Site Options Flint, MI.

Study Options Full-time and part-time.

Online Degree Options Yes.

Program Entrance Requirements Minimum overall college GPA of 3.2, transcript of college record, prerequisite course work, statistics course. *Application deadline:* 6/1 (winter). *Application fee:* $55.

Advanced Placement Credit by examination available. Credit given for nursing courses completed elsewhere dependent upon specific evaluations.

Degree Requirements 48 total credit hours.

POST-MASTER'S PROGRAM

Areas of Study *Clinical nurse specialist programs in:* psychiatric/mental health.

DOCTORAL DEGREE PROGRAM

Degree DNP

Available Programs Doctorate.

Areas of Study Advanced practice nursing, family health, gerontology.

Site Options Flint, MI.

Online Degree Options Yes (online only).

Program Entrance Requirements Clinical experience, minimum overall college GPA of 3.2, interview, 3 letters of recommendation, statistics course, vita, writing sample. Application deadline: 8/1 (fall), 11/15 (winter), 2/15 (spring), 2/15 (summer). Applications may be processed on a rolling basis for some programs. Application fee: $55.

Degree Requirements 78 total credit hours.

Wayne State University
College of Nursing
Detroit, Michigan

http://www.nursing.wayne.edu/
Founded in 1868

DEGREES • BSN • MSN • PHD

Nursing Program Faculty 72 (63% with doctorates).

Baccalaureate Enrollment 308 **Women** 79% **Men** 21% **Part-time** 37%

Graduate Enrollment 270 **Women** 93% **Men** 7% **Part-time** 53%

Distance Learning Courses Available.

Nursing Student Activities Nursing Honor Society, Sigma Theta Tau, Student Nurses' Association, nursing club.

Nursing Student Resources Academic advising; academic or career counseling; assistance for students with disabilities; bookstore; campus computer network; career placement assistance; computer lab; computer-assisted instruction; e-mail services; employment services for current students; housing assistance; interactive nursing skills videos; Internet; learning resource lab; library services; nursing audiovisuals; placement services for program completers; resume preparation assistance; skills, simulation, or other laboratory; tutoring.

Library Facilities 156,000 volumes in health, 6,600 volumes in nursing; 5,000 periodical subscriptions health-care related.

BACCALAUREATE PROGRAMS

Degree BSN

Available Programs Accelerated Baccalaureate for Second Degree; Generic Baccalaureate; RN Baccalaureate.

Study Options Full-time and part-time.

Program Entrance Requirements Minimum overall college GPA of 2.0, transcript of college record, interview, minimum GPA in nursing prerequisites of 2.5, prerequisite course work. Transfer students are accepted. *Application deadline:* 3/31 (fall). *Application fee:* $50.

Expenses (2015–16) *Tuition, state resident:* full-time $10,416; part-time $347 per credit hour. *Tuition, nonresident:* full-time $23,856; part-time $795 per credit hour. *International tuition:* $23,856 full-time. *Room and board:* $9874 per academic year. *Required fees:* full-time $904.

Financial Aid 95% of baccalaureate students in nursing programs received some form of financial aid in 2014–15.

Contact Office of Student Affairs, College of Nursing, Wayne State University, 5557 Cass Avenue, Detroit, MI 48202. *Telephone:* 313-577-4082. *Fax:* 313-577-6949.

GRADUATE PROGRAMS

Expenses (2015–16) *Tuition, state resident:* full-time $19,324; part-time $805 per credit hour. *Tuition, nonresident:* full-time $35,114; part-time $1463 per credit hour. *International tuition:* $35,114 full-time. *Room and board:* $9874 per academic year. *Required fees:* full-time $1201; part-time $791 per term.

Financial Aid 81% of graduate students in nursing programs received some form of financial aid in 2014–15. 43 fellowships with tuition reimbursements available, 5 teaching assistantships with tuition reimbursements available (averaging $26,209 per year) were awarded; research assistantships with tuition reimbursements available, institutionally sponsored loans, scholarships, traineeships, and unspecified assistantships also available. Aid available to part-time students. *Financial aid application deadline:* 3/31.

Contact Office of Student Affairs, College of Nursing, Wayne State University, 5557 Cass Avenue, Detroit, MI 48202. *Telephone:* 313-577-4082. *Fax:* 313-577-6949.

MASTER'S DEGREE PROGRAM

Degree MSN

Available Programs Master's.

Concentrations Available Nurse-midwifery. *Nurse practitioner programs in:* gerontology, neonatal health, pediatric, psychiatric/mental health.

Study Options Full-time and part-time.

Program Entrance Requirements Minimum overall college GPA of 3.0, transcript of college record, written essay, 3 letters of recommendation, resume. *Application deadline:* 7/1 (fall), 11/1 (winter), 4/1 (spring), 4/1 (summer).

Advanced Placement Credit given for nursing courses completed elsewhere dependent upon specific evaluations.

Degree Requirements 47 total credit hours.

POST-MASTER'S PROGRAM

Areas of Study Nurse-midwifery; nursing education. *Nurse practitioner programs in:* gerontology, pediatric, pediatric primary care, psychiatric/mental health.

DOCTORAL DEGREE PROGRAM

Degree PhD

Available Programs Doctorate; Post-Baccalaureate Doctorate.

Program Entrance Requirements Clinical experience, minimum overall college GPA of 3.0, interview by faculty committee, interview, 2 letters of recommendation, vita, writing sample, GRE General Test (for applicants without a master's degree). Application deadline: 1/15 (fall). Applications may be processed on a rolling basis for some programs. Application fee: $50.

Degree Requirements 90 total credit hours, dissertation, residency.

POSTDOCTORAL PROGRAM

Postdoctoral Program Contact Mr. Dennis Ross, Academic Services Officer, College of Nursing, Wayne State University, 5557 Cass Avenue, Detroit, MI 48202. *Telephone:* 313-577-4082. *Fax:* 313-577-6949. *E-mail:* nursinginfo@wayne.edu.

Western Michigan University
College of Health and Human Services
Kalamazoo, Michigan

Founded in 1903

DEGREES • BSN • MSN

Nursing Program Faculty 38 (26% with doctorates).

Baccalaureate Enrollment 383 **Women** 85% **Men** 15% **Part-time** 21%

Graduate Enrollment 7 **Women** 85% **Men** 15% **Part-time** 100%

Nursing Student Activities Sigma Theta Tau, Student Nurses' Association.

Nursing Student Resources Academic advising; academic or career counseling; assistance for students with disabilities; bookstore; campus computer network; career placement assistance; computer lab; computer-assisted instruction; daycare for children of students; e-mail services; employment services for current students; externships; housing assistance; interactive nursing skills videos; Internet; learning resource lab; library services; nursing audiovisuals; placement services for program completers; remedial services; resume preparation assistance; skills, simulation, or other laboratory.

Library Facilities 766 volumes in nursing; 362 periodical subscriptions health-care related.

BACCALAUREATE PROGRAMS

Degree BSN

Available Programs ADN to Baccalaureate; Generic Baccalaureate.

Site Options St. Joseph, MI.

Study Options Full-time and part-time.

Program Entrance Requirements Minimum overall college GPA of 3.0, transcript of college record, CPR certification, high school biology, high school chemistry, 3 years high school math, 3 years high school science, high school transcript, immunizations, minimum high school GPA of 3.0, minimum GPA in nursing prerequisites of 3.0, prerequisite course work. Transfer students are accepted. *Application deadline:* Applications may be processed on a rolling basis for some programs. *Application fee:* $35.

Advanced Placement Credit given for nursing courses completed elsewhere dependent upon specific evaluations.

Contact *Telephone:* 269-387-8150. *Fax:* 269-387-8170.

GRADUATE PROGRAMS

Contact *Telephone:* 269-387-8162.

MASTER'S DEGREE PROGRAM

Degree MSN

Available Programs Master's.

Concentrations Available Nursing administration; nursing education.

Site Options St. Joseph, MI.

Study Options Part-time.

Program Entrance Requirements Minimum overall college GPA of 3.4, transcript of college record, interview, 3 letters of recommendation, resume. *Application deadline:* Applications may be processed on a rolling basis for some programs. *Application fee:* $40.

Degree Requirements 36 total credit hours, thesis or project, comprehensive exam.

CONTINUING EDUCATION PROGRAM

Contact *Telephone:* 269-387-8150.

MINNESOTA

Augsburg College
Program in Nursing
Minneapolis, Minnesota

http://www.augsburg.edu/nursing

Founded in 1869

DEGREES • BS • MA

Nursing Program Faculty 12 (85% with doctorates).

Baccalaureate Enrollment 225 **Women** 85% **Men** 15% **Part-time** 59%

Graduate Enrollment 95 **Women** 82% **Men** 18% **Part-time** 50%

Nursing Student Resources Academic advising; academic or career counseling; assistance for students with disabilities; bookstore; campus computer network; computer lab; computer-assisted instruction; e-mail services; Internet; library services; tutoring.
Library Facilities 2,500 volumes in health, 200 volumes in nursing; 70 periodical subscriptions health-care related.

BACCALAUREATE PROGRAMS

Degree BS
Available Programs ADN to Baccalaureate.
Site Options Rochester, MN; Minneapolis/St. Paul, MN.
Study Options Full-time and part-time.
Program Entrance Requirements Minimum overall college GPA of 2.5, transcript of college record, CPR certification, written essay, high school transcript, immunizations, letters of recommendation, prerequisite course work, RN licensure. Transfer students are accepted.
Contact Admissions Counselor, Program in Nursing, Augsburg College, 2211 Riverside Avenue South, CB 65, Minneapolis, MN 55454. *Telephone:* 612-330-1101. *Fax:* 612-330-1784.
E-mail: wecinfo@augsburg.edu.

GRADUATE PROGRAMS

Contact Graduate Admissions Counselor, Program in Nursing, Augsburg College, 2211 Riverside Avenue South, CB 65, Minneapolis, MN 55454. *Telephone:* 612-330-1101. *Fax:* 612-330-1784.
E-mail: manursing@augsburg.edu.

MASTER'S DEGREE PROGRAM

Degree MA
Available Programs Master's.
Concentrations Available *Clinical nurse specialist programs in:* community health.
Site Options Rochester, MN; Minneapolis/St. Paul, MN.
Study Options Full-time and part-time.
Program Entrance Requirements Computer literacy, minimum overall college GPA of 3.0, transcript of college record, written essay, immunizations, 3 letters of recommendation, prerequisite course work, statistics course.
Advanced Placement Credit given for nursing courses completed elsewhere dependent upon specific evaluations.
Degree Requirements 44 total credit hours, thesis or project.

DOCTORAL DEGREE PROGRAM

Site Options Minneapolis/St. Paul, MN.

Bemidji State University
Department of Nursing
Bemidji, Minnesota

http://www.bemidjistate.edu/academics/departments/nursing/
Founded in 1919

DEGREE • BS
Nursing Program Faculty 5 (60% with doctorates).
Baccalaureate Enrollment 62 **Women** 95% **Men** 5% **Part-time** 68%
Distance Learning Courses Available.
Nursing Student Resources Academic advising; academic or career counseling; assistance for students with disabilities; bookstore; campus computer network; career placement assistance; computer lab; computer-assisted instruction; daycare for children of students; e-mail services; employment services for current students; housing assistance; Internet; library services; nursing audiovisuals; remedial services; tutoring.
Library Facilities 9,000 volumes in health, 1,000 volumes in nursing; 300 periodical subscriptions health-care related.

BACCALAUREATE PROGRAMS

Degree BS
Available Programs Generic Baccalaureate; RN Baccalaureate.
Study Options Full-time and part-time.
Program Entrance Requirements Minimum overall college GPA, transcript of college record, immunizations, professional liability insurance/malpractice insurance, RN licensure. Transfer students are accepted.
Contact *Telephone:* 218-755-3892. *Fax:* 218-755-4402.

CONTINUING EDUCATION PROGRAM

Contact *Telephone:* 218-755-3892. *Fax:* 218-755-4402.

Bethel University
Department of Nursing
St. Paul, Minnesota

http://cas.bethel.edu/academics/departments/nursing/
Founded in 1871

DEGREES • BSN • MA
Nursing Program Faculty 36 (40% with doctorates).
Baccalaureate Enrollment 283 **Women** 93.6% **Men** 6.4%
Graduate Enrollment 66 **Women** 97% **Men** 3%
Distance Learning Courses Available.
Nursing Student Activities Sigma Theta Tau, nursing club.
Nursing Student Resources Academic advising; academic or career counseling; assistance for students with disabilities; bookstore; campus computer network; career placement assistance; computer lab; computer-assisted instruction; daycare for children of students; e-mail services; employment services for current students; interactive nursing skills videos; Internet; learning resource lab; library services; nursing audiovisuals; paid internships; placement services for program completers; remedial services; resume preparation assistance; skills, simulation, or other laboratory; tutoring.
Library Facilities 4,900 volumes in nursing; 1,006 periodical subscriptions health-care related.

BACCALAUREATE PROGRAMS

Degree BSN
Available Programs Generic Baccalaureate; RN Baccalaureate.
Site Options Brooklyn Park, MN.
Study Options Full-time and part-time.
Program Entrance Requirements Minimum overall college GPA of 2.5, transcript of college record, CPR certification, written essay, health exam, health insurance, high school transcript, immunizations, interview, 2 letters of recommendation, minimum GPA in nursing prerequisites of 2.5, professional liability insurance/malpractice insurance, prerequisite course work. Transfer students are accepted. *Application deadline:* 9/15 (fall).
Advanced Placement Credit given for nursing courses completed elsewhere dependent upon specific evaluations.
Contact *Telephone:* 651-638-6455. *Fax:* 651-635-1965.

GRADUATE PROGRAMS

Contact *Telephone:* 651-635-8080. *Fax:* 651-635-1965.

MASTER'S DEGREE PROGRAM

Degree MA
Available Programs Master's.
Concentrations Available Nursing administration; nursing education.
Study Options Full-time and part-time.
Program Entrance Requirements Clinical experience, computer literacy, minimum overall college GPA of 3.0, transcript of college record, written essay, immunizations, interview, 3 letters of recommendation, professional liability insurance/malpractice insurance, resume, statistics course, MAT. *Application deadline:* Applications may be processed on a rolling basis for some programs. *Application fee:* $25.
Advanced Placement Credit given for nursing courses completed elsewhere dependent upon specific evaluations.
Degree Requirements 43 total credit hours, thesis or project.

Capella University
Nursing Programs
Minneapolis, Minnesota

Founded in 1993
DEGREES • BSN • DNP • MSN

BACCALAUREATE PROGRAMS

Degree BSN
Available Programs RN Baccalaureate.
Program Entrance Requirements RN licensure. *Application fee:* $50.
Contact *Telephone:* 866-283-7921. *Fax:* 612-337-5396.

GRADUATE PROGRAMS

Contact *Telephone:* 866-283-7921. *Fax:* 612-337-5396.

MASTER'S DEGREE PROGRAM

Degree MSN
Available Programs Accelerated RN to Master's; Master's.
Concentrations Available Nursing administration; nursing education. *Clinical nurse specialist programs in:* gerontology.
Program Entrance Requirements Minimum overall college GPA of 3.0.*Application fee:* $50.

DOCTORAL DEGREE PROGRAM

Degree DNP
Available Programs Doctorate.
Areas of Study Nursing administration.
Program Entrance Requirements Minimum overall college GPA of 3.0. Application fee: $50.

College of Saint Benedict
Department of Nursing
Saint Joseph, Minnesota

http://www.csbsju.edu/nursing/
Founded in 1887

DEGREE • BS

Nursing Program Faculty 17 (50% with doctorates).
Baccalaureate Enrollment 162 **Women** 90% **Men** 10% **Part-time** 1%
Nursing Student Activities Nursing Honor Society, Sigma Theta Tau, Student Nurses' Association, nursing club.
Nursing Student Resources Academic advising; academic or career counseling; assistance for students with disabilities; bookstore; campus computer network; career placement assistance; computer lab; computer-assisted instruction; e-mail services; employment services for current students; interactive nursing skills videos; Internet; learning resource lab; library services; nursing audiovisuals; paid internships; placement services for program completers; remedial services; resume preparation assistance; skills, simulation, or other laboratory; tutoring; unpaid internships.
Library Facilities 7,300 volumes in health, 700 volumes in nursing; 335 periodical subscriptions health-care related.

BACCALAUREATE PROGRAMS

Degree BS
Available Programs Generic Baccalaureate.
Study Options Full-time.
Program Entrance Requirements Transcript of college record, CPR certification, health exam, health insurance, immunizations, minimum GPA in nursing prerequisites of 2.75, professional liability insurance/malpractice insurance, prerequisite course work. *Application deadline:* 5/1 (fall).
Advanced Placement Credit given for nursing courses completed elsewhere dependent upon specific evaluations.
Contact *Telephone:* 320-363-5223. *Fax:* 320-363-6099.

The College of St. Scholastica
Department of Nursing
Duluth, Minnesota

http://www.css.edu
Founded in 1912

DEGREES • BS • DNP

Nursing Program Faculty 35 (45% with doctorates).
Baccalaureate Enrollment 712 **Women** 86.24% **Men** 13.76% **Part-time** 43%
Graduate Enrollment 138 **Women** 86.24% **Men** 13.76% **Part-time** 26.8%
Distance Learning Courses Available.
Nursing Student Activities Sigma Theta Tau, Student Nurses' Association.
Nursing Student Resources Academic advising; academic or career counseling; assistance for students with disabilities; bookstore; campus computer network; career placement assistance; computer lab; computer-assisted instruction; e-mail services; interactive nursing skills videos; Internet; learning resource lab; library services; nursing audiovisuals; paid internships; placement services for program completers; remedial services; resume preparation assistance; skills, simulation, or other laboratory; tutoring; unpaid internships.
Library Facilities 6,549 volumes in health, 1,568 volumes in nursing; 174 periodical subscriptions health-care related.

BACCALAUREATE PROGRAMS

Degree BS
Available Programs ADN to Baccalaureate; Accelerated Baccalaureate for Second Degree; Generic Baccalaureate.
Site Options Duluth, MN; St. Cloud, MN.
Study Options Full-time.
Online Degree Options Yes.
Program Entrance Requirements Minimum overall college GPA of 3.0, transcript of college record, CPR certification, health exam, health insurance, high school transcript, immunizations, minimum GPA in nursing prerequisites of 2.0, prerequisite course work. Transfer students are accepted. *Application deadline:* 9/20 (fall).
Expenses (2015–16) *Tuition:* full-time $33,784; part-time $1056 per credit. *Room and board:* $8932; room only: $5540 per academic year. *Required fees:* full-time $525; part-time $25 per term.
Financial Aid *Gift aid (need-based):* Federal Pell, FSEOG, state, private, college/university gift aid from institutional funds. *Loans:* Federal Nursing Student Loans, Federal Direct (Subsidized and Unsubsidized Stafford PLUS), Perkins, state. *Work-study:* Federal Work-Study, part-time campus jobs. *Financial aid application deadline (priority):* 3/1.
Contact Ms. Paula Byrne, Chair, Department of Traditional Undergraduate Nursing, Department of Nursing, The College of St. Scholastica, 1200 Kenwood Avenue, Duluth, MN 55811. *Telephone:* 218-723-6020. *Fax:* 218-733-2221. *E-mail:* pbyrne@css.edu.

GRADUATE PROGRAMS

Expenses (2015–16) *Tuition:* part-time $800 per credit. *International tuition:* $800 full-time. *Room and board:* $16,713 per academic year. *Required fees:* part-time $400 per term.
Financial Aid Scholarships available.
Contact Dr. Carolyn Robinson, Chair, Graduate Nursing Department, Department of Nursing, The College of St. Scholastica, 1200 Kenwood Avenue, Duluth, MN 55811. *Telephone:* 218-723-6590. *Fax:* 218-733-2221. *E-mail:* crobinson1@css.edu.

MASTER'S DEGREE PROGRAM

Program Entrance Requirements GRE General Test. *Application deadline:* 3/1 (spring). *Application fee:* $50.

DOCTORAL DEGREE PROGRAM

Degree DNP
Available Programs Doctorate; Post-Baccalaureate Doctorate.
Areas of Study Advanced practice nursing, gerontology, health policy, nursing administration, nursing education, nursing policy.
Site Options Duluth, MN; St. Cloud, MN.
Program Entrance Requirements Clinical experience, minimum overall college GPA of 3.0, interview by faculty committee, 3 letters of recommendation, vita, writing sample. Application deadline: 3/1 (spring). Application fee: $50.
Degree Requirements 83 total credit hours, dissertation.

POSTDOCTORAL PROGRAM

Postdoctoral Program Contact Dr. Carleen A. Maynard, Chair, Graduate Nursing Department, Department of Nursing, The College of St. Scholastica, 1200 Kenwood Avenue, Duluth, MN 55811. *Telephone:* 218-723-6452. *Fax:* 218-733-2295. *E-mail:* cmaynard@css.edu.

Concordia College
Department of Nursing
Moorhead, Minnesota

http://www.cord.edu/Academics/Nursing/index.php
Founded in 1891

DEGREES • BA • MS

Nursing Program Faculty 6 (33% with doctorates).
Baccalaureate Enrollment 75
Graduate Enrollment 2 **Women** 100%
Nursing Student Activities Sigma Theta Tau, Student Nurses' Association.

Nursing Student Resources Academic advising; academic or career counseling; assistance for students with disabilities; bookstore; campus computer network; career placement assistance; computer lab; computer-assisted instruction; e-mail services; employment services for current students; externships; housing assistance; interactive nursing skills videos; Internet; learning resource lab; library services; nursing audiovisuals; paid internships; placement services for program completers; remedial services; resume preparation assistance; skills, simulation, or other laboratory; tutoring; unpaid internships.

Library Facilities 2,135 volumes in health, 837 volumes in nursing; 81 periodical subscriptions health-care related.

BACCALAUREATE PROGRAMS

Degree BA

Available Programs Accelerated Baccalaureate for Second Degree; Generic Baccalaureate.

Study Options Full-time.

Program Entrance Requirements Minimum overall college GPA of 2.9, transcript of college record, CPR certification, health exam, health insurance, immunizations, interview, 2 letters of recommendation, minimum GPA in nursing prerequisites of 2.7, professional liability insurance/malpractice insurance, prerequisite course work. Transfer students are accepted.

Advanced Placement Credit by examination available. Credit given for nursing courses completed elsewhere dependent upon specific evaluations.

Contact *Telephone:* 218-299-3879. *Fax:* 218-299-4309.

GRADUATE PROGRAMS

Contact *Telephone:* 218-299-3879. *Fax:* 218-299-4309.

MASTER'S DEGREE PROGRAM

Degree MS

Available Programs Master's.

Concentrations Available Nursing education.

Study Options Full-time and part-time.

Program Entrance Requirements Computer literacy, minimum overall college GPA of 3.0, transcript of college record, written essay, interview, 3 letters of recommendation.

Advanced Placement Credit given for nursing courses completed elsewhere dependent upon specific evaluations.

Degree Requirements 36 total credit hours, thesis or project, comprehensive exam.

Crown College
Nursing Department
St. Bonifacius, Minnesota

http://www.crown.edu/
Founded in 1916

DEGREE • BSN

Nursing Program Faculty 6

Baccalaureate Enrollment 20 **Women** 100%

Distance Learning Courses Available.

Nursing Student Activities Student Nurses' Association.

Nursing Student Resources Academic advising; academic or career counseling; assistance for students with disabilities; bookstore; campus computer network; computer lab; computer-assisted instruction; e-mail services; employment services for current students; housing assistance; interactive nursing skills videos; Internet; learning resource lab; library services; nursing audiovisuals; remedial services; resume preparation assistance; skills, simulation, or other laboratory; tutoring; unpaid internships.

BACCALAUREATE PROGRAMS

Degree BSN

Available Programs Generic Baccalaureate.

Site Options Owatonna, MN.

Study Options Full-time.

Program Entrance Requirements CPR certification, written essay, health exam, immunizations, 2 letters of recommendation, minimum high school GPA, minimum GPA in nursing prerequisites of 2.5, prerequisite

course work. Transfer students are accepted. *Application deadline:* 2/1 (spring).

Contact *Telephone:* 952-446-4482.

Globe University–Woodbury
Bachelor of Science in Nursing
Woodbury, Minnesota

http://www.globeuniversity.edu/
Founded in 1885

DEGREE • BS

Nursing Program Faculty 16

Baccalaureate Enrollment 135

Nursing Student Activities Student Nurses' Association.

Nursing Student Resources Academic advising; academic or career counseling; assistance for students with disabilities; bookstore; campus computer network; career placement assistance; computer lab; computer-assisted instruction; e-mail services; employment services for current students; interactive nursing skills videos; Internet; learning resource lab; library services; nursing audiovisuals; placement services for program completers; remedial services; resume preparation assistance; skills, simulation, or other laboratory; tutoring; unpaid internships.

BACCALAUREATE PROGRAMS

Degree BS

Available Programs Generic Baccalaureate.

Study Options Full-time and part-time.

Program Entrance Requirements Minimum overall college GPA of 2.75, transcript of college record, CPR certification, written essay, health exam, high school biology, high school chemistry, 2 years high school science, high school transcript, immunizations, interview, 2 letters of recommendation, minimum high school GPA of 2.75, minimum high school rank 60%, minimum GPA in nursing prerequisites of 2.75, prerequisite course work. Transfer students are accepted. *Application deadline:* Applications may be processed on a rolling basis for some programs. *Application fee:* $50.

Advanced Placement Credit given for nursing courses completed elsewhere dependent upon specific evaluations.

Contact *Telephone:* 612-798-3762.

Gustavus Adolphus College
Department of Nursing
St. Peter, Minnesota

http://www.gustavus.edu/
Founded in 1862

DEGREE • BA

Nursing Program Faculty 9 (20% with doctorates).

Baccalaureate Enrollment 76 **Women** 92% **Men** 8%

Nursing Student Activities Sigma Theta Tau, Student Nurses' Association.

Nursing Student Resources Academic advising; academic or career counseling; assistance for students with disabilities; bookstore; campus computer network; career placement assistance; computer lab; computer-assisted instruction; e-mail services; employment services for current students; housing assistance; interactive nursing skills videos; Internet; learning resource lab; library services; nursing audiovisuals; paid internships; remedial services; resume preparation assistance; skills, simulation, or other laboratory; tutoring; unpaid internships.

BACCALAUREATE PROGRAMS

Degree BA

Available Programs Generic Baccalaureate.

Study Options Full-time.

Program Entrance Requirements Minimum overall college GPA of 2.7, transcript of college record, written essay, high school transcript, immunizations, interview, minimum GPA in nursing prerequisites, prerequisite course work. Transfer students are accepted.

Contact *Telephone:* 507-933-6126. *Fax:* 507-933-6153.

Herzing University
Nursing Program
Minneapolis, Minnesota

http://www.herzing.edu/minneapolis
Founded in 1961
DEGREE • BSN
Nursing Program Faculty 4 (.5% with doctorates).
Baccalaureate Enrollment 71 **Women** 90% **Men** 10%
Nursing Student Activities Student Nurses' Association.
Nursing Student Resources Academic advising; academic or career counseling; campus computer network; career placement assistance; computer lab; computer-assisted instruction; e-mail services; employment services for current students; externships; interactive nursing skills videos; Internet; learning resource lab; library services; nursing audiovisuals; remedial services; resume preparation assistance; skills, simulation, or other laboratory; tutoring; unpaid internships.
Library Facilities 100 volumes in health, 50 volumes in nursing; 150 periodical subscriptions health-care related.

BACCALAUREATE PROGRAMS

Degree BSN
Available Programs Generic Baccalaureate; LPN to Baccalaureate.
Study Options Full-time.
Program Entrance Requirements Minimum overall college GPA of 2.5, CPR certification, health exam, immunizations, minimum high school GPA of 2.0. *Application deadline:* 6/5 (summer). Applications may be processed on a rolling basis for some programs. *Application fee:* $125.
Expenses (2015–16) *Tuition:* full-time $10,666; part-time $3522 per semester.
Financial Aid 90% of baccalaureate students in nursing programs received some form of financial aid in 2014–15.
Contact Nursing Information, Nursing Program, Herzing University, 5700 West Broadway, Crystal, MN 55428. *Telephone:* 763-535-3000. *Fax:* 763-535-9205. *E-mail:* mpl-info@herzing.edu.

Metropolitan State University
College of Health, Community and Professional Studies
St. Paul, Minnesota

http://www.metrostate.edu/msweb/explore/chcps/departments /nursing/
Founded in 1971
DEGREES • BSN • DNP • MSN
Nursing Program Faculty 16 (69% with doctorates).
Baccalaureate Enrollment 310 **Women** 89% **Men** 11% **Part-time** 50%
Graduate Enrollment 45 **Women** 95% **Men** 5% **Part-time** 20%
Distance Learning Courses Available.
Nursing Student Activities Student Nurses' Association.
Nursing Student Resources Academic advising; academic or career counseling; assistance for students with disabilities; bookstore; campus computer network; career placement assistance; computer lab; computer-assisted instruction; e-mail services; interactive nursing skills videos; Internet; learning resource lab; library services; nursing audiovisuals; remedial services; skills, simulation, or other laboratory; unpaid internships.

BACCALAUREATE PROGRAMS

Degree BSN
Available Programs Generic Baccalaureate; RN Baccalaureate.
Site Options Minneapolis, MN.
Study Options Full-time.
Program Entrance Requirements Transcript of college record, immunizations, minimum GPA in nursing prerequisites of 2.75, prerequisite course work. Transfer students are accepted. *Application deadline:* 2/1 (fall). *Application fee:* $20.
Advanced Placement Credit given for nursing courses completed elsewhere dependent upon specific evaluations.
Financial Aid 25% of baccalaureate students in nursing programs received some form of financial aid in 2013–14. *Gift aid (need-based):* Federal Pell, FSEOG, state, private, college/university gift aid from institutional funds. *Loans:* Federal Direct (Subsidized and Unsubsidized Stafford PLUS), state. *Work-study:* Federal Work-Study, part-time campus jobs. *Financial aid application deadline (priority):* 5/1.
Contact Sandi Gerick, Director of Advising, College of Health, Community and Professional Studies, Metropolitan State University, 700 East Seventh Street, St. Paul, MN 55106-5000. *Telephone:* 651-793-1379. *Fax:* 651-793-1382. *E-mail:* sandi.gerick@metrostate.edu.

GRADUATE PROGRAMS

Financial Aid 10% of graduate students in nursing programs received some form of financial aid in 2013–14. Fellowships, career-related internships or fieldwork, Federal Work-Study, institutionally sponsored loans, and traineeships available.
Contact Ms. Lynn Iverson-Eyestone, Academic Advisor, College of Health, Community and Professional Studies, Metropolitan State University, 700 East Seventh Street, St. Paul, MN 55106-5000. *Telephone:* 651-793-1356. *Fax:* 651-793-1382. *E-mail:* lynn.iversoneyestone@metropolitanstate.edu.

MASTER'S DEGREE PROGRAM

Degree MSN
Available Programs Master's for Nurses with Non-Nursing Degrees; RN to Master's.
Concentrations Available Nursing administration; nursing education.
Study Options Full-time and part-time.
Online Degree Options Yes.
Program Entrance Requirements Computer literacy, minimum overall college GPA of 3.0, transcript of college record, written essay, immunizations, interview, 2 letters of recommendation, statistics course, GRE General Test. *Application deadline:* 1/31 (fall). *Application fee:* $20.
Advanced Placement Credit given for nursing courses completed elsewhere dependent upon specific evaluations.
Degree Requirements 41 total credit hours, thesis or project.

POST-MASTER'S PROGRAM

Areas of Study Nursing administration; nursing education.

DOCTORAL DEGREE PROGRAM

Degree DNP
Available Programs Doctorate.
Areas of Study Advanced practice nursing.
Program Entrance Requirements Minimum overall college GPA of 3.0, 3 letters of recommendation, writing sample. Application deadline: 1/15 (fall). Application fee: $40.
Degree Requirements Oral exam, written exam.

Minnesota State University Mankato
School of Nursing
Mankato, Minnesota

http://www.mnsu.edu/nursing/
Founded in 1868
DEGREES • BS • DNP • MSN • MSN/MS
Nursing Program Faculty 48 (21% with doctorates).
Baccalaureate Enrollment 292 **Women** 90% **Men** 10% **Part-time** 1%
Graduate Enrollment 60 **Women** 96% **Men** 4% **Part-time** 48%
Distance Learning Courses Available.
Nursing Student Activities Nursing Honor Society, Sigma Theta Tau, Student Nurses' Association.
Nursing Student Resources Academic advising; academic or career counseling; assistance for students with disabilities; bookstore; campus computer network; career placement assistance; computer lab; computer-assisted instruction; daycare for children of students; e-mail services; employment services for current students; Internet; learning resource lab; library services; nursing audiovisuals; paid internships; placement services for program completers; resume preparation assistance; skills, simulation, or other laboratory; tutoring.
Library Facilities 35,852 volumes in health, 1,500 volumes in nursing; 156 periodical subscriptions health-care related.

BACCALAUREATE PROGRAMS

Degree BS
Available Programs Accelerated Baccalaureate for Second Degree; Generic Baccalaureate; RN Baccalaureate.
Study Options Full-time and part-time.

Program Entrance Requirements Minimum overall college GPA of 2.5, transcript of college record, health exam, health insurance, minimum GPA in nursing prerequisites of 2.0, prerequisite course work. Transfer students are accepted.
Advanced Placement Credit by examination available. Credit given for nursing courses completed elsewhere dependent upon specific evaluations.
Contact *Telephone:* 507-389-6828. *Fax:* 507-389-6516.

GRADUATE PROGRAMS

Contact *Telephone:* 507-389-1317. *Fax:* 507-389-6516.

MASTER'S DEGREE PROGRAM
Degrees MSN; MSN/MS
Available Programs Accelerated RN to Master's; Master's; Master's for Nurses with Non-Nursing Degrees; RN to Master's.
Concentrations Available Nursing education. *Clinical nurse specialist programs in:* adult health, family health, pediatric. *Nurse practitioner programs in:* family health.
Study Options Full-time and part-time.
Program Entrance Requirements Clinical experience, computer literacy, minimum overall college GPA of 3.0, transcript of college record, CPR certification, written essay, immunizations, 3 letters of recommendation, nursing research course, professional liability insurance/malpractice insurance, prerequisite course work, resume, statistics course.
Advanced Placement Credit given for nursing courses completed elsewhere dependent upon specific evaluations.
Degree Requirements 53 total credit hours, thesis or project.

POST-MASTER'S PROGRAM
Areas of Study Nursing education. *Clinical nurse specialist programs in:* family health. *Nurse practitioner programs in:* family health.

DOCTORAL DEGREE PROGRAM
Degree DNP
Available Programs Doctorate.
Degree Requirements 36 total credit hours.

CONTINUING EDUCATION PROGRAM

Contact *Telephone:* 507-389-5194. *Fax:* 507-389-6516.

Minnesota State University Moorhead
School of Nursing and Healthcare Leadership
Moorhead, Minnesota

http://www.mnstate.edu/snhl/
Founded in 1885
DEGREES • BSN • MS • MSN/MHA
Nursing Program Faculty 11 (36% with doctorates).
Baccalaureate Enrollment 212 **Women** 95% **Men** 5% **Part-time** 90%
Graduate Enrollment 43 **Women** 97% **Men** 3% **Part-time** 90%
Distance Learning Courses Available.
Nursing Student Activities Sigma Theta Tau.
Nursing Student Resources Academic advising; academic or career counseling; assistance for students with disabilities; bookstore; campus computer network; career placement assistance; computer lab; computer-assisted instruction; daycare for children of students; e-mail services; employment services for current students; Internet; library services; nursing audiovisuals; placement services for program completers; remedial services; resume preparation assistance; tutoring; unpaid internships.
Library Facilities 5,560 volumes in health, 824 volumes in nursing; 50 periodical subscriptions health-care related.

BACCALAUREATE PROGRAMS

Degree BSN
Available Programs ADN to Baccalaureate; RN Baccalaureate.
Study Options Full-time and part-time.
Online Degree Options Yes (online only).
Program Entrance Requirements Minimum overall college GPA of 2.75, transcript of college record, CPR certification, written essay, high school transcript, immunizations, 2 letters of recommendation, prerequisite course work, RN licensure. Transfer students are accepted. *Application deadline:* 3/15 (fall), 10/15 (spring).

Expenses (2015–16) *Tuition, state resident:* full-time $6120; part-time $255 per credit. *Tuition, nonresident:* full-time $12,360; part-time $515 per credit.
Financial Aid *Gift aid (need-based):* Federal Pell, FSEOG, state, private, college/university gift aid from institutional funds, TEACH Grants. *Loans:* Federal Direct (Subsidized and Unsubsidized Stafford PLUS), Perkins, state, private loans. *Work-study:* Federal Work-Study, part-time campus jobs. *Financial aid application deadline (priority):* 2/15.
Contact Dr. Barbara Matthees, Professor, School of Nursing and Healthcare Leadership, Minnesota State University Moorhead, 1104 7th Avenue South, Moorhead, MN 56563. *Telephone:* 218-477-2695. *Fax:* 218-477-5990. *E-mail:* matthees@mnstate.edu.

GRADUATE PROGRAMS

Expenses (2015–16) *Tuition, state resident:* full-time $8730; part-time $485 per credit. *Tuition, nonresident:* full-time $16,470; part-time $915 per credit.
Contact Dr. Barbara Matthees, Professor, School of Nursing and Healthcare Leadership, Minnesota State University Moorhead, 1104 7th Avenue South, Moorhead, MN 56563. *Telephone:* 218-477-2695. *Fax:* 218-477-5990. *E-mail:* matthees@mnstate.edu.

MASTER'S DEGREE PROGRAM
Degrees MS; MSN/MHA
Available Programs Master's.
Concentrations Available Health-care administration; nursing administration; nursing education.
Study Options Full-time and part-time.
Online Degree Options Yes (online only).
Program Entrance Requirements Computer literacy, minimum overall college GPA of 3.0, transcript of college record, CPR certification, written essay, interview, 3 letters of recommendation, professional liability insurance/malpractice insurance, resume, statistics course. *Application deadline:* Applications may be processed on a rolling basis for some programs.
Advanced Placement Credit given for nursing courses completed elsewhere dependent upon specific evaluations.
Degree Requirements 45 total credit hours, thesis or project.

Rasmussen College Bloomington
School of Nursing
Bloomington, Minnesota

http://www.rasmussen.edu/locations/minnesota/
Founded in 1904
DEGREE • BSN

BACCALAUREATE PROGRAMS

Degree BSN
Available Programs RN Baccalaureate.
Program Entrance Requirements *Application deadline:* Applications may be processed on a rolling basis for some programs.
Contact Joan K. Rich, Vice President of Nursing, School of Nursing, Rasmussen College Bloomington, 8300 Norman Center Drive, Suite 300, Bloomington, MN 55435. *Telephone:* 952-830-3881. *E-mail:* joan.rich@rasmussen.edu.

St. Catherine University
Department of Nursing
St. Paul, Minnesota

https://www2.stkate.edu/nursing-ba/home
Founded in 1905
DEGREES • BS • DNP • MS
Nursing Program Faculty 58 (52% with doctorates).
Baccalaureate Enrollment 294 **Women** 97% **Men** 3% **Part-time** 41%
Graduate Enrollment 210 **Women** 93% **Men** 7% **Part-time** 6%
Distance Learning Courses Available.
Nursing Student Activities Sigma Theta Tau, Student Nurses' Association.
Nursing Student Resources Academic advising; academic or career counseling; assistance for students with disabilities; bookstore; campus computer network; career placement assistance; computer lab; computer-

assisted instruction; daycare for children of students; e-mail services; employment services for current students; housing assistance; interactive nursing skills videos; Internet; learning resource lab; library services; nursing audiovisuals; paid internships; remedial services; resume preparation assistance; skills, simulation, or other laboratory; tutoring; unpaid internships.

Library Facilities 9,650 volumes in health, 1,120 volumes in nursing; 6,035 periodical subscriptions health-care related.

BACCALAUREATE PROGRAMS

Degree BS

Available Programs ADN to Baccalaureate; Generic Baccalaureate; RN Baccalaureate.

Site Options St. Louis Park, MN; Minneapolis, MN; St. Paul, MN.

Study Options Full-time.

Program Entrance Requirements Minimum overall college GPA of 3.0, transcript of college record, CPR certification, health insurance, immunizations, minimum GPA in nursing prerequisites of 3.0, prerequisite course work. Transfer students are accepted. *Application deadline:* 10/15 (fall).

Expenses (2015–16) *Tuition:* part-time $1164 per credit. *Room and board:* $8750; room only: $5150 per academic year. *Required fees:* part-time $747 per term.

Financial Aid *Gift aid (need-based):* Federal Pell, FSEOG, state, private, college/university gift aid from institutional funds. *Loans:* Federal Nursing Student Loans, Federal Direct (Subsidized and Unsubsidized Stafford PLUS), Perkins, state, alternative loans. *Work-study:* Federal Work-Study, part-time campus jobs. *Financial aid application deadline (priority):* 4/15.

Contact Dr. Dianne Nelson, Baccalaureate Program Director, Department of Nursing, St. Catherine University, 2004 Randolph Avenue, St. Paul, MN 55105. *Telephone:* 651-690-6967. *Fax:* 651-690-6941. *E-mail:* denelson@stkate.edu.

GRADUATE PROGRAMS

Expenses (2015–16) *Tuition:* part-time $948 per credit. *Required fees:* part-time $45 per term.

Contact Dr. Suzan Ulrich, Assistant Dean for Graduate Nursing, Department of Nursing, St. Catherine University, 2004 Randolph Avenue, #4250, St. Paul, MN 55105. *Telephone:* 651-690-6580. *Fax:* 651-690-6941. *E-mail:* sculrich@stkate.edu.

MASTER'S DEGREE PROGRAM

Degree MS

Available Programs Master's; Master's for Non-Nursing College Graduates.

Concentrations Available Nursing education. *Nurse practitioner programs in:* adult health, gerontology, pediatric primary care.

Study Options Full-time.

Program Entrance Requirements Clinical experience, minimum overall college GPA of 3.0, transcript of college record, CPR certification, written essay, immunizations, interview, 3 letters of recommendation, resume, statistics course. *Application deadline:* 12/1 (fall). *Application fee:* $100.

Advanced Placement Credit given for nursing courses completed elsewhere dependent upon specific evaluations.

Degree Requirements 39 total credit hours, thesis or project, comprehensive exam.

POST-MASTER'S PROGRAM

Areas of Study Nursing education. *Nurse practitioner programs in:* adult health, gerontology, pediatric primary care.

DOCTORAL DEGREE PROGRAM

Degree DNP

Available Programs Doctorate.

Areas of Study Advanced practice nursing, ethics, health policy, healthcare systems, nursing education, nursing policy.

Program Entrance Requirements Minimum overall college GPA of 3.0, interview by faculty committee, interview, 3 letters of recommendation, MSN or equivalent, statistics course, vita, writing sample. Application deadline: 1/15 (winter).

Degree Requirements 33 total credit hours.

St. Cloud State University
Department of Nursing Science
St. Cloud, Minnesota

Founded in 1869

DEGREE • BS

Nursing Program Faculty 12 (25% with doctorates).

Baccalaureate Enrollment 111

Nursing Student Activities Nursing club.

Nursing Student Resources Academic advising; academic or career counseling; assistance for students with disabilities; bookstore; campus computer network; career placement assistance; computer lab; computer-assisted instruction; daycare for children of students; e-mail services; interactive nursing skills videos; Internet; learning resource lab; library services; nursing audiovisuals; remedial services; resume preparation assistance; skills, simulation, or other laboratory; tutoring; unpaid internships.

Library Facilities 18,000 volumes in health, 750 volumes in nursing; 100 periodical subscriptions health-care related.

BACCALAUREATE PROGRAMS

Degree BS

Available Programs Generic Baccalaureate.

Study Options Full-time.

Program Entrance Requirements Minimum overall college GPA of 2.75, transcript of college record, CPR certification, health exam, immunizations, 2 letters of recommendation, minimum GPA in nursing prerequisites of 2.75, prerequisite course work.

Contact *Telephone:* 320-308-1749.

Saint Mary's University of Minnesota
B.S. in Nursing
Winona, Minnesota

http://www.smumn.edu/degree-completion-home/areas-of-study/bs-in-nursing

Founded in 1912

DEGREES • BS • MS

Nursing Program Faculty 13 (70% with doctorates).

Baccalaureate Enrollment 32 **Women** 75% **Men** 25% **Part-time** 97%

Graduate Enrollment 157 **Women** 57% **Men** 43%

Distance Learning Courses Available.

Nursing Student Resources Academic advising; academic or career counseling; assistance for students with disabilities; bookstore; campus computer network; computer lab; e-mail services; Internet; library services.

BACCALAUREATE PROGRAMS

Degree BS

Available Programs RN Baccalaureate.

Site Options Minneapolis, MN.

Study Options Full-time and part-time.

Online Degree Options Yes (online only).

Program Entrance Requirements Minimum overall college GPA of 2.5, transcript of college record, written essay, interview, letters of recommendation, RN licensure. Transfer students are accepted. *Application deadline:* Applications may be processed on a rolling basis for some programs. *Application fee:* $25.

Expenses (2015–16) *Tuition:* full-time $15,120; part-time $420 per credit.

Financial Aid 35% of baccalaureate students in nursing programs received some form of financial aid in 2014–15. *Gift aid (need-based):* Federal Pell, FSEOG, state, college/university gift aid from institutional funds. *Loans:* Federal Direct (Subsidized and Unsubsidized Stafford PLUS), Perkins, state. *Work-study:* Federal Work-Study, part-time campus jobs. *Financial aid application deadline (priority):* 3/15.

Contact Saint Mary's University of Minnesota Online Processing Center, B.S. in Nursing, Saint Mary's University of Minnesota, 1415 West 22nd Street, Suite 500, Oak Brook, IL 60523. *Telephone:* 877-308-9954. *E-mail:* tc-admission@smumn.edu.

GRADUATE PROGRAMS

Expenses (2015–16) *Tuition:* full-time $13,440; part-time $560 per credit.

Financial Aid 74% of graduate students in nursing programs received some form of financial aid in 2014–15.

Contact Merri L. Moody, APRN, CRNA, DNP, Program Director, B.S. in Nursing, Saint Mary's University of Minnesota, 2500 Park Avenue, Minneapolis, MN 55404. *Telephone:* 612-728-5133. *E-mail:* mmoody@ smumn.edu.

MASTER'S DEGREE PROGRAM

Degree MS

Available Programs Master's.

Concentrations Available Nurse anesthesia.

Site Options Minneapolis, MN.

Study Options Full-time.

Program Entrance Requirements Clinical experience, minimum overall college GPA of 3.2, transcript of college record, written essay, immunizations, prerequisite course work, resume. *Application deadline:* 4/1 (summer). *Application fee:* $25.

Degree Requirements 64 total credit hours, thesis or project, comprehensive exam.

St. Olaf College

Nursing Program
Northfield, Minnesota

http://www.stolaf.edu/depts/nursing/
Founded in 1874

DEGREE • BA

Nursing Program Faculty 5 (60% with doctorates).

Baccalaureate Enrollment 47 **Women** 94% **Men** 6%

Nursing Student Activities Sigma Theta Tau, Student Nurses' Association.

Nursing Student Resources Academic advising; academic or career counseling; assistance for students with disabilities; bookstore; campus computer network; career placement assistance; computer lab; computer-assisted instruction; e-mail services; employment services for current students; externships; interactive nursing skills videos; Internet; learning resource lab; library services; nursing audiovisuals; paid internships; remedial services; resume preparation assistance; skills, simulation, or other laboratory; tutoring; unpaid internships.

Library Facilities 7,090 volumes in health, 1,366 volumes in nursing; 2,892 periodical subscriptions health-care related.

BACCALAUREATE PROGRAMS

Degree BA

Available Programs Generic Baccalaureate.

Study Options Full-time.

Program Entrance Requirements Minimum overall college GPA of 2.85, transcript of college record, CPR certification, written essay, health exam, health insurance, immunizations, interview, minimum GPA in nursing prerequisites of 2.7, prerequisite course work. Transfer students are accepted. *Application deadline:* 11/15 (fall). Applications may be processed on a rolling basis for some programs.

Advanced Placement Credit given for nursing courses completed elsewhere dependent upon specific evaluations.

Expenses (2015–16) *Tuition:* full-time $42,940; part-time $5370 per course. *Room and board:* $9790; room only: $4720 per academic year. *Required fees:* full-time $1535.

Financial Aid 100% of baccalaureate students in nursing programs received some form of financial aid in 2014–15.

Contact Chair, Department of Nursing, Nursing Program, St. Olaf College, Department of Nursing, 1520 St. Olaf Avenue, Northfield, MN 55057-1098. *Telephone:* 507-786-3265. *Fax:* 507-786-3733. *E-mail:* neal@stolaf.edu.

Southwest Minnesota State University

Nursing Department
Marshall, Minnesota

http://www.smsu.edu/academics/departments/nursing/
Founded in 1963

DEGREE • BSN

Nursing Program Faculty 3 (66% with doctorates).

Baccalaureate Enrollment 85 **Women** 93% **Men** 7% **Part-time** 82%

Distance Learning Courses Available.

Nursing Student Resources Academic advising; academic or career counseling; assistance for students with disabilities; bookstore; campus computer network; computer lab; computer-assisted instruction; e-mail services; library services; nursing audiovisuals; resume preparation assistance; skills, simulation, or other laboratory; tutoring.

Library Facilities 4,450 volumes in health, 103 volumes in nursing; 1,300 periodical subscriptions health-care related.

BACCALAUREATE PROGRAMS

Degree BSN

Available Programs ADN to Baccalaureate.

Study Options Full-time and part-time.

Online Degree Options Yes (online only).

Program Entrance Requirements Transcript of college record, CPR certification, health exam, immunizations, minimum GPA in nursing prerequisites of 2.75, RN licensure. Transfer students are accepted. *Application deadline:* 3/1 (fall), 10/1 (spring). Applications may be processed on a rolling basis for some programs. *Application fee:* $20.

Contact Ms. Laurie Jo Johansen, Director of Nursing, Nursing Department, Southwest Minnesota State University, 1501 State Street, Marshall, MN 56258. *Telephone:* 507-537-7590. *Fax:* 507-537-6815. *E-mail:* laurie.johansen@smsu.edu.

University of Minnesota, Twin Cities Campus

School of Nursing
Minneapolis, Minnesota

http://www.nursing.umn.edu/
Founded in 1851

DEGREES • BSN • DNP • PHD

Nursing Program Faculty 85 (90% with doctorates).

Baccalaureate Enrollment 392 **Women** 87% **Men** 13% **Part-time** 8%

Graduate Enrollment 512 **Women** 88% **Men** 12% **Part-time** 44%

Distance Learning Courses Available.

Nursing Student Activities Nursing Honor Society, Sigma Theta Tau, Student Nurses' Association, nursing club.

Nursing Student Resources Academic advising; academic or career counseling; assistance for students with disabilities; bookstore; campus computer network; computer lab; computer-assisted instruction; daycare for children of students; e-mail services; employment services for current students; housing assistance; Internet; learning resource lab; library services; skills, simulation, or other laboratory.

Library Facilities 4,000 volumes in health, 1,500 volumes in nursing; 4,800 periodical subscriptions health-care related.

BACCALAUREATE PROGRAMS

Degree BSN

Available Programs Generic Baccalaureate.

Site Options Rochester, MN.

Study Options Full-time.

Program Entrance Requirements Minimum overall college GPA of 2.8, transcript of college record, CPR certification, written essay, health exam, health insurance, immunizations, minimum GPA in nursing prerequisites of 2.8, prerequisite course work. Transfer students are accepted. *Application deadline:* 2/1 (fall). *Application fee:* $60.

Contact *Telephone:* 612-625-7980. *Fax:* 612-625-7727.

GRADUATE PROGRAMS

Contact *Telephone:* 612-625-7980. *Fax:* 612-625-7727.

MASTER'S DEGREE PROGRAM
Program Entrance Requirements GRE General Test.

DOCTORAL DEGREE PROGRAM
Degree DNP

Available Programs Doctorate, Doctorate for Nurses with Non-Nursing Degrees, Post-Baccalaureate Doctorate.

Areas of Study Advanced practice nursing, community health, gerontology, information systems, maternity-newborn, women's health.

Program Entrance Requirements Minimum overall college GPA of 3.0, interview, interview by faculty committee, 2 letters of recommendation, writing sample, vita. Application deadline: 3/1 (fall). Applications may be processed on a rolling basis for some programs. Application fee: $60.

Degree Requirements 30-60 total credit hours, project and thesis presentation.

Degree PhD

Available Programs Doctorate; Doctorate for Nurses with Non-Nursing Degrees; Post-Baccalaureate Doctorate.

Program Entrance Requirements Minimum overall college GPA of 3.0, interview by faculty committee, interview, 2 letters of recommendation, vita, writing sample, GRE General Test. Application deadline: 3/1 (fall). Applications may be processed on a rolling basis for some programs. Application fee: $60.

Degree Requirements 60 total credit hours, dissertation, oral exam, written exam.

CONTINUING EDUCATION PROGRAM

Contact *Telephone:* 612-625-7980. *Fax:* 612-625-7727.

University of Northwestern–St. Paul
School of Nursing
St. Paul, Minnesota

https://www.unwsp.edu/
Founded in 1902

DEGREE • BSN
Nursing Program Faculty 11
Baccalaureate Enrollment 41
Nursing Student Activities Student Nurses' Association.
Nursing Student Resources Academic advising; academic or career counseling; assistance for students with disabilities; bookstore; campus computer network; career placement assistance; computer lab; computer-assisted instruction; e-mail services; employment services for current students; interactive nursing skills videos; Internet; learning resource lab; library services; nursing audiovisuals; remedial services; resume preparation assistance; skills, simulation, or other laboratory; tutoring.
Library Facilities 175 volumes in health, 155 volumes in nursing; 5 periodical subscriptions health-care related.

BACCALAUREATE PROGRAMS

Degree BSN

Available Programs Accelerated Baccalaureate for Second Degree; Accelerated RN Baccalaureate.
Study Options Full-time.
Program Entrance Requirements Transcript of college record, CPR certification, written essay, health exam, health insurance, immunizations, interview, 2 letters of recommendation, minimum GPA in nursing prerequisites of 2.75, prerequisite course work. Transfer students are accepted. *Application deadline:* Applications may be processed on a rolling basis for some programs.
Contact Leane Gondek, Coordinator of Nursing Operations, School of Nursing, University of Northwestern–St. Paul, 3003 Snelling Avenue North, St Paul, MN 55113. *Telephone:* 651-628-3456. *E-mail:* nursing@unwsp.edu.

Walden University
Nursing Programs
Minneapolis, Minnesota

http://www.waldenu.edu/colleges-schools/school-of-nursing
Founded in 1970

DEGREES • BSN • DNP • MSN • PHD
Nursing Program Faculty 541 (83% with doctorates).
Baccalaureate Enrollment 1,769 **Women** 90% **Men** 10% **Part-time** 83%
Graduate Enrollment 8,956 **Women** 92% **Men** 8% **Part-time** 49%
Distance Learning Courses Available.
Nursing Student Activities Nursing Honor Society.
Nursing Student Resources Academic advising; academic or career counseling; assistance for students with disabilities; bookstore; e-mail services; library services; nursing audiovisuals; remedial services; resume preparation assistance; tutoring.
Library Facilities 6,956 periodical subscriptions health-care related.

BACCALAUREATE PROGRAMS

Degree BSN

Available Programs RN Baccalaureate.
Study Options Full-time and part-time.
Online Degree Options Yes (online only).
Program Entrance Requirements Transcript of college record, high school transcript, prerequisite course work, RN licensure. Transfer students are accepted. *Application deadline:* Applications may be processed on a rolling basis for some programs.
Expenses (2014–15) *Tuition:* full-time $11,520; part-time $310 per credit hour. *International tuition:* $11,520 full-time. *Required fees:* full-time $360; part-time $120 per term.
Contact Dr. Karen Ouzts, Program Director, Nursing Programs, Walden University, 100 Washington Avenue South, Suite 900, Minneapolis, MN 55401. *Telephone:* 720-383-1356. *E-mail:* karen.ouzts@waldenu.edu.

GRADUATE PROGRAMS

Expenses (2014–15) *Tuition:* part-time $625 per credit hour. *Required fees:* part-time $120 per term.
Contact Dr. Vincent Hall, Program Director, Nursing Programs, Walden University, 100 Washington Avenue South, Suite 900, Minneapolis, MN 55401. *E-mail:* vincent.hall@waldenu.edu.

MASTER'S DEGREE PROGRAM
Degree MSN

Available Programs Master's; RN to Master's.
Concentrations Available Nursing administration; nursing education; nursing informatics. *Nurse practitioner programs in:* adult-gerontology acute care, family health, gerontology.
Study Options Full-time and part-time.
Online Degree Options Yes (online only).
Program Entrance Requirements Minimum overall college GPA of 2.5, transcript of college record. *Application deadline:* Applications may be processed on a rolling basis for some programs.
Degree Requirements 56 total credit hours, thesis or project.

POST-MASTER'S PROGRAM
Areas of Study Nursing administration; nursing education; nursing informatics.

DOCTORAL DEGREE PROGRAM
Degree DNP

Available Programs Doctorate.
Areas of Study Health policy.
Online Degree Options Yes (online only).
Program Entrance Requirements Minimum overall college GPA of 3.0, MSN or equivalent. Application deadline: Applications may be processed on a rolling basis for some programs.
Degree Requirements 53 total credit hours.

Degree PhD

Available Programs Doctorate.
Areas of Study Nursing administration, nursing education, nursing policy.
Online Degree Options Yes (online only).

Program Entrance Requirements Minimum overall college GPA of 3.0, MSN or equivalent. Application deadline: Applications are processed on a rolling basis.

Degree Requirements 78 total credit hours, dissertation.

Winona State University
College of Nursing and Health Sciences
Winona, Minnesota

http://www.winona.edu/nursing/
Founded in 1858

DEGREES • BS • DNP • MS

Nursing Program Faculty 39 (46% with doctorates).

Baccalaureate Enrollment 400 **Women** 94% **Men** 6% **Part-time** 13%

Graduate Enrollment 110 **Women** 89% **Men** 11% **Part-time** 65%

Distance Learning Courses Available.

Nursing Student Activities Sigma Theta Tau, Student Nurses' Association, nursing club.

Nursing Student Resources Academic advising; academic or career counseling; assistance for students with disabilities; bookstore; campus computer network; career placement assistance; computer lab; computer-assisted instruction; daycare for children of students; e-mail services; employment services for current students; externships; housing assistance; Internet; learning resource lab; library services; nursing audiovisuals; paid internships; placement services for program completers; remedial services; resume preparation assistance; skills, simulation, or other laboratory; tutoring.

Library Facilities 6,132 volumes in health, 3,920 volumes in nursing; 413 periodical subscriptions health-care related.

BACCALAUREATE PROGRAMS

Degree BS

Available Programs Generic Baccalaureate; RN Baccalaureate.

Site Options Rochester, MN.

Study Options Full-time and part-time.

Program Entrance Requirements Minimum overall college GPA of 3.0, transcript of college record, CPR certification, health exam, health insurance, immunizations, minimum GPA in nursing prerequisites of 3.3, professional liability insurance/malpractice insurance, prerequisite course work. Transfer students are accepted. *Application deadline:* 11/1 (fall), 1/31 (spring).

Contact *Telephone:* 507-457-5120. *Fax:* 507-457-5550.

GRADUATE PROGRAMS

Contact *Telephone:* 507-285-7135. *Fax:* 507-292-5127.

MASTER'S DEGREE PROGRAM

Degree MS

Available Programs Master's; Master's for Nurses with Non-Nursing Degrees; RN to Master's.

Concentrations Available Nursing administration; nursing education. *Clinical nurse specialist programs in:* adult health. *Nurse practitioner programs in:* adult health, family health.

Site Options Rochester, MN.

Study Options Full-time and part-time.

Program Entrance Requirements Clinical experience, computer literacy, minimum overall college GPA of 3.0, transcript of college record, CPR certification, written essay, immunizations, interview, 3 letters of recommendation, nursing research course, physical assessment course, professional liability insurance/malpractice insurance, statistics course, GRE (if GPA less than 3.0). *Application deadline:* 12/1 (fall). *Application fee:* $20.

Advanced Placement Credit given for nursing courses completed elsewhere dependent upon specific evaluations.

Degree Requirements 43 total credit hours, thesis or project.

POST-MASTER'S PROGRAM

Areas of Study Nursing administration; nursing education. *Clinical nurse specialist programs in:* adult health. *Nurse practitioner programs in:* adult health, family health.

DOCTORAL DEGREE PROGRAM

Degree DNP

Available Programs Doctorate.

Areas of Study Advanced practice nursing, faculty preparation, nursing administration.

Site Options Rochester, MN.

Online Degree Options Yes (online only).

Program Entrance Requirements Clinical experience, minimum overall college GPA of 3.0, 2 letters of recommendation, MSN or equivalent, statistics course, vita, writing sample. Application deadline: 3/15 (spring). Application fee: $20.

Degree Requirements 36 total credit hours, oral exam.

MISSISSIPPI

Alcorn State University
School of Nursing
Natchez, Mississippi

http://www.alcorn.edu/academics/schools/son/index.aspx
Founded in 1871

DEGREES • BSN • MSN

Nursing Program Faculty 21 (29% with doctorates).

Baccalaureate Enrollment 63 **Women** 88.8% **Men** 11.2% **Part-time** 7.9%

Graduate Enrollment 53 **Women** 89.3% **Men** 10.7% **Part-time** 78.6%

Distance Learning Courses Available.

Nursing Student Activities Nursing Honor Society, Sigma Theta Tau, Student Nurses' Association.

Nursing Student Resources Academic advising; campus computer network; computer lab; housing assistance; learning resource lab; library services; nursing audiovisuals; paid internships; skills, simulation, or other laboratory.

Library Facilities 2,082 volumes in health, 1,385 volumes in nursing; 30 periodical subscriptions health-care related.

BACCALAUREATE PROGRAMS

Degree BSN

Available Programs Generic Baccalaureate; LPN to RN Baccalaureate; RN Baccalaureate.

Study Options Full-time.

Online Degree Options Yes.

Program Entrance Requirements Minimum overall college GPA of 2.5, transcript of college record, health exam, immunizations, minimum high school GPA of 2.5, professional liability insurance/malpractice insurance, prerequisite course work. Transfer students are accepted. *Application deadline:* 12/19 (fall).

Contact *Telephone:* 601-304-4305. *Fax:* 601-304-4398.

GRADUATE PROGRAMS

Contact *Telephone:* 601-304-4303. *Fax:* 601-304-4398.

MASTER'S DEGREE PROGRAM

Degree MSN

Available Programs Master's.

Concentrations Available Nursing education. *Nurse practitioner programs in:* family health.

Study Options Full-time and part-time.

Online Degree Options Yes.

Program Entrance Requirements Computer literacy, minimum overall college GPA of 3.0, transcript of college record, written essay, 2 letters of recommendation, statistics course. *Application deadline:* 7/15 (fall). *Application fee:* $10.

Advanced Placement Credit given for nursing courses completed elsewhere dependent upon specific evaluations.

Degree Requirements 43 total credit hours, thesis or project.

POST-MASTER'S PROGRAM

Areas of Study Nursing education. *Nurse practitioner programs in:* family health.

Delta State University

School of Nursing
Cleveland, Mississippi

http://nursing.deltastate.edu/
Founded in 1924
DEGREES • BSN • DNP • MSN
Nursing Program Faculty 17 (50% with doctorates).
Baccalaureate Enrollment 160 Women 80% Men 20% Part-time 7%
Graduate Enrollment 53 Women 80% Men 20% Part-time 22%
Distance Learning Courses Available.
Nursing Student Activities Sigma Theta Tau, Student Nurses' Association.
Nursing Student Resources Academic advising; academic or career counseling; assistance for students with disabilities; bookstore; campus computer network; career placement assistance; computer lab; computer-assisted instruction; daycare for children of students; e-mail services; externships; housing assistance; interactive nursing skills videos; Internet; learning resource lab; library services; nursing audiovisuals; other; remedial services; resume preparation assistance; skills, simulation, or other laboratory; tutoring.
Library Facilities 5,000 volumes in health, 1,000 volumes in nursing; 120 periodical subscriptions health-care related.

BACCALAUREATE PROGRAMS

Degree BSN
Available Programs ADN to Baccalaureate; Generic Baccalaureate.
Study Options Full-time and part-time.
Program Entrance Requirements Transcript of college record, CPR certification, health exam, health insurance, immunizations, 3 letters of recommendation, minimum GPA in nursing prerequisites of 2.5, professional liability insurance/malpractice insurance, prerequisite course work. Transfer students are accepted. *Application deadline:* 3/1 (fall).
Advanced Placement Credit given for nursing courses completed elsewhere dependent upon specific evaluations.
Expenses (2015–16) *Tuition, state resident:* full-time $3006. *International tuition:* $3006 full-time. *Room and board:* $4000 per academic year.
Financial Aid *Gift aid (need-based):* Federal Pell, FSEOG, state, private, college/university gift aid from institutional funds. *Loans:* Federal Direct (Subsidized and Unsubsidized Stafford PLUS), Perkins. *Work-study:* Federal Work-Study, part-time campus jobs. *Financial aid application deadline (priority):* 3/1.
Contact Dr. Vicki L. Bingham, Chair of Academic Programs, School of Nursing, Delta State University, PO Box 3343, Cleveland, MS 38733. *Telephone:* 662-846-4255. *Fax:* 662-846-4267. *E-mail:* vbingham@deltastate.edu.

GRADUATE PROGRAMS

Expenses (2015–16) *Tuition, state resident:* full-time $3006. *Tuition, nonresident:* full-time $3006. *Room and board:* $4000 per academic year.
Financial Aid Research assistantships, career-related internships or fieldwork, Federal Work-Study, and institutionally sponsored loans available.
Contact Dr. Vicki L. Bingham, Chair of Academic Programs, School of Nursing, Delta State University, PO Box 3343, Cleveland, MS 38733. *Telephone:* 662-846-4255. *Fax:* 662-846-4267. *E-mail:* vbingham@deltastate.edu.

MASTER'S DEGREE PROGRAM

Degree MSN
Available Programs Master's; Master's for Nurses with Non-Nursing Degrees.
Concentrations Available Nursing administration; nursing education. *Nurse practitioner programs in:* family health, gerontology, psychiatric/mental health.
Study Options Full-time and part-time.
Online Degree Options Yes (online only).
Program Entrance Requirements Clinical experience, computer literacy, minimum overall college GPA of 3.0, transcript of college record, CPR certification, written essay, immunizations, interview, 3 letters of recommendation, nursing research course, physical assessment course, professional liability insurance/malpractice insurance, prerequisite course work, resume, statistics course, GRE General Test. *Application deadline:* 2/1 (fall).

Advanced Placement Credit given for nursing courses completed elsewhere dependent upon specific evaluations.
Degree Requirements 44 total credit hours, thesis or project, comprehensive exam.

POST-MASTER'S PROGRAM

Areas of Study Nursing administration; nursing education. *Nurse practitioner programs in:* family health, gerontology, psychiatric/mental health.

DOCTORAL DEGREE PROGRAM

Degree DNP
Available Programs Doctorate; Post-Baccalaureate Doctorate.
Areas of Study Advanced practice nursing, family health.
Online Degree Options Yes (online only).
Program Entrance Requirements Clinical experience, minimum overall college GPA of 3.2, interview, 3 letters of recommendation, statistics course, vita, writing sample. Application deadline: 4/1 (fall).
Degree Requirements 31 total credit hours.

Mississippi College

School of Nursing
Clinton, Mississippi

http://www.mc.edu/
Founded in 1826
DEGREE • BSN
Nursing Program Faculty 21 (19% with doctorates).
Baccalaureate Enrollment 153 Women 82% Men 18% Part-time 7%
Distance Learning Courses Available.
Nursing Student Activities Sigma Theta Tau, Student Nurses' Association, nursing club.
Nursing Student Resources Academic advising; academic or career counseling; assistance for students with disabilities; bookstore; campus computer network; career placement assistance; computer lab; computer-assisted instruction; e-mail services; employment services for current students; externships; housing assistance; interactive nursing skills videos; Internet; learning resource lab; library services; nursing audiovisuals; paid internships; placement services for program completers; remedial services; resume preparation assistance; skills, simulation, or other laboratory; tutoring; unpaid internships.
Library Facilities 43,000 volumes in health, 8,000 volumes in nursing; 290 periodical subscriptions health-care related.

BACCALAUREATE PROGRAMS

Degree BSN
Available Programs Generic Baccalaureate; RN Baccalaureate.
Study Options Full-time and part-time.
Program Entrance Requirements Minimum overall college GPA of 2.5, transcript of college record, CPR certification, health exam, high school biology, high school chemistry, high school transcript, immunizations, 2 letters of recommendation, minimum GPA in nursing prerequisites of 2.5, professional liability insurance/malpractice insurance, prerequisite course work. Transfer students are accepted. *Application deadline:* 2/1 (fall), 9/1 (spring), 4/1 (summer).
Advanced Placement Credit given for nursing courses completed elsewhere dependent upon specific evaluations.
Expenses (2014–15) *Tuition:* full-time $14,670; part-time $459 per credit hour. *International tuition:* $14,670 full-time. *Room and board:* $8425 per academic year. *Required fees:* full-time $705; part-time $179 per term.
Financial Aid 95% of baccalaureate students in nursing programs received some form of financial aid in 2013–14. *Gift aid (need-based):* Federal Pell, FSEOG, state, private, college/university gift aid from institutional funds, Federal Nursing. *Loans:* Federal Nursing Student Loans, Federal Direct (Subsidized and Unsubsidized Stafford PLUS), Perkins, college/university. *Work-study:* Federal Work-Study. *Financial aid application deadline (priority):* 3/1.
Contact Dr. Mary Jean Padgett, Dean, School of Nursing, Mississippi College, Box 4037, 200 South Capitol Street, Clinton, MS 39058. *Telephone:* 601-925-3278. *Fax:* 601-925-3379. *E-mail:* padgett@mc.edu.

Mississippi University for Women
College of Nursing and Speech Language Pathology
Columbus, Mississippi

http://www.muw.edu/nursing
Founded in 1884

DEGREES • BSN • DNP • MSN

Nursing Program Faculty 44 (44% with doctorates).
Baccalaureate Enrollment 491 **Women** 82% **Men** 18% **Part-time** 1%
Graduate Enrollment 45 **Women** 85% **Men** 15% **Part-time** 1%
Distance Learning Courses Available.
Nursing Student Activities Sigma Theta Tau, Student Nurses' Association.
Nursing Student Resources Academic advising; academic or career counseling; assistance for students with disabilities; bookstore; campus computer network; career placement assistance; computer lab; computer-assisted instruction; daycare for children of students; e-mail services; employment services for current students; externships; housing assistance; interactive nursing skills videos; Internet; learning resource lab; library services; nursing audiovisuals; paid internships; placement services for program completers; remedial services; resume preparation assistance; skills, simulation, or other laboratory; tutoring; unpaid internships.
Library Facilities 27,522 volumes in health, 23,610 volumes in nursing; 242 periodical subscriptions health-care related.

BACCALAUREATE PROGRAMS

Degree BSN
Available Programs ADN to Baccalaureate; Generic Baccalaureate.
Site Options Tupelo, MS.
Study Options Full-time.
Online Degree Options Yes.
Program Entrance Requirements Minimum overall college GPA of 2.75, transcript of college record, CPR certification, health exam, health insurance, immunizations, minimum GPA in nursing prerequisites of 2.75, professional liability insurance/malpractice insurance, prerequisite course work. Transfer students are accepted. *Application deadline:* 1/20 (fall).
Advanced Placement Credit given for nursing courses completed elsewhere dependent upon specific evaluations.
Expenses (2015–16) *Tuition, state resident:* full-time $5780; part-time $241 per credit hour. *Tuition, nonresident:* full-time $15,847; part-time $461 per credit hour. *Room and board:* $3296 per academic year. *Required fees:* full-time $800.
Financial Aid 90% of baccalaureate students in nursing programs received some form of financial aid in 2014–15.
Contact Dr. Tammie McCoy, Baccalaureate Nursing Department Chair, College of Nursing and Speech Language Pathology, Mississippi University for Women, 1100 College Street, MUW-910, Columbus, MS 39701-5800. *Telephone:* 662-329-7301. *Fax:* 662-329-8559. *E-mail:* tmmccoy@muw.edu.

GRADUATE PROGRAMS

Expenses (2015–16) *Tuition, area resident:* full-time $5680; part-time $316 per credit hour. *Tuition, state resident:* full-time $5680; part-time $321 per credit hour. *Tuition, nonresident:* full-time $15,847; part-time $881 per credit hour. *Room and board:* $3296 per academic year. *Required fees:* full-time $800.
Financial Aid 80% of graduate students in nursing programs received some form of financial aid in 2014–15. Fellowships, Federal Work-Study, institutionally sponsored loans, and traineeships available. *Financial aid application deadline:* 4/1.
Contact Dr. Johnnie Sue Wijewardane, Graduate Nursing Program Department Chair, College of Nursing and Speech Language Pathology, Mississippi University for Women, 1100 College Street, MUW-910, Columbus, MS 39701-5800. *Telephone:* 662-329-7323. *Fax:* 662-329-7372. *E-mail:* jswijewardane@muw.edu.

MASTER'S DEGREE PROGRAM

Degree MSN
Available Programs Master's.
Concentrations Available *Nurse practitioner programs in:* family health.
Study Options Full-time.
Program Entrance Requirements Clinical experience, computer literacy, minimum overall college GPA of 3.0, transcript of college record, CPR certification, written essay, immunizations, interview, 3 letters of recommendation, nursing research course, physical assessment course, professional liability insurance/malpractice insurance, prerequisite course work, resume, statistics course, GRE General Test. *Application deadline:* 2/1 (fall). *Application fee:* $25.
Advanced Placement Credit given for nursing courses completed elsewhere dependent upon specific evaluations.
Degree Requirements 39 total credit hours, thesis or project, comprehensive exam.

POST-MASTER'S PROGRAM

Areas of Study *Nurse practitioner programs in:* family health.

DOCTORAL DEGREE PROGRAM

Degree DNP
Available Programs Doctorate; Post-Baccalaureate Doctorate.
Areas of Study Advanced practice nursing.
Program Entrance Requirements Clinical experience, minimum overall college GPA of 3.0, interview, letters of recommendation, MSN or equivalent, statistics course, vita, writing sample. Application deadline: 2/1 (fall). Application fee: $25.
Degree Requirements 44 total credit hours, oral exam, written exam, residency.

University of Mississippi Medical Center
School of Nursing
Jackson, Mississippi

http://www.umc.edu/son/
Founded in 1955

DEGREES • BSN • DNP • MSN

Nursing Program Faculty 69 (64% with doctorates).
Baccalaureate Enrollment 406 **Women** 86.5% **Men** 13.5% **Part-time** 9%
Graduate Enrollment 411 **Women** 91% **Men** 9% **Part-time** 41%
Distance Learning Courses Available.
Nursing Student Activities Nursing Honor Society, Sigma Theta Tau, Student Nurses' Association, nursing club.
Nursing Student Resources Academic advising; academic or career counseling; assistance for students with disabilities; bookstore; campus computer network; career placement assistance; computer lab; computer-assisted instruction; e-mail services; employment services for current students; externships; interactive nursing skills videos; Internet; learning resource lab; library services; nursing audiovisuals; remedial services; skills, simulation, or other laboratory; tutoring; unpaid internships.
Library Facilities 72,557 volumes in health, 8,170 volumes in nursing; 4,180 periodical subscriptions health-care related.

BACCALAUREATE PROGRAMS

Degree BSN
Available Programs ADN to Baccalaureate; Accelerated Baccalaureate for Second Degree; Generic Baccalaureate.
Site Options Oxford, MS.
Study Options Full-time and part-time.
Program Entrance Requirements Minimum overall college GPA of 2.5, transcript of college record, CPR certification, health exam, health insurance, immunizations, minimum GPA in nursing prerequisites of 2.5, professional liability insurance/malpractice insurance, prerequisite course work. Transfer students are accepted. *Application deadline:* 1/15 (summer). *Application fee:* $25.
Advanced Placement Credit given for nursing courses completed elsewhere dependent upon specific evaluations.
Expenses (2014–15) *Tuition, state resident:* full-time $6996; part-time $292 per credit hour. *Tuition, nonresident:* full-time $19,044; part-time $794 per credit hour. *International tuition:* $19,044 full-time. *Required fees:* full-time $800.
Financial Aid 78% of baccalaureate students in nursing programs received some form of financial aid in 2013–14.
Contact Dr. Marcia Rachel, Associate Dean for Academic Affairs, School of Nursing, University of Mississippi Medical Center, 2500 North State Street, Jackson, MS 39216-4505. *Telephone:* 601-984-6228. *Fax:* 601-815-4067. *E-mail:* mrachel@umc.edu.

GRADUATE PROGRAMS

Expenses (2014–15) *Tuition, state resident:* full-time $6996; part-time $389 per credit hour. *Tuition, nonresident:* full-time $19,044; part-time $1058 per credit hour. *International tuition:* $19,044 full-time.

Financial Aid 80% of graduate students in nursing programs received some form of financial aid in 2013–14. Institutionally sponsored loans and scholarships available. Aid available to part-time students. *Financial aid application deadline:* 4/1.

Contact Dr. Marcia Rachel, Associate Dean for Academic Affairs, School of Nursing, University of Mississippi Medical Center, 2500 North State Street, Jackson, MS 39216-4505. *Telephone:* 601-984-6228. *Fax:* 601-815-4067. *E-mail:* mrachel@umc.edu.

MASTER'S DEGREE PROGRAM

Degree MSN

Available Programs Master's; RN to Master's.

Concentrations Available Nursing administration; nursing education. *Nurse practitioner programs in:* adult-gerontology acute care, family health, gerontology, psychiatric/mental health.

Study Options Full-time and part-time.

Program Entrance Requirements Computer literacy, minimum overall college GPA of 3.0, transcript of college record, CPR certification, immunizations, 3 letters of recommendation, professional liability insurance/malpractice insurance, resume, statistics course, GRE. *Application deadline:* 3/31 (fall), 10/15 (spring), 2/15 (summer). Applications may be processed on a rolling basis for some programs. *Application fee:* $25.

Advanced Placement Credit given for nursing courses completed elsewhere dependent upon specific evaluations.

Degree Requirements 46 total credit hours, comprehensive exam.

POST-MASTER'S PROGRAM

Areas of Study Nursing administration; nursing education. *Nurse practitioner programs in:* adult-gerontology acute care, family health, gerontology, psychiatric/mental health.

DOCTORAL DEGREE PROGRAM

Degree DNP

Available Programs Doctorate; Post-Baccalaureate Doctorate.

Areas of Study Advanced practice nursing, nursing administration.

Program Entrance Requirements Minimum overall college GPA of 3.0, interview by faculty committee, interview, MSN or equivalent, statistics course, vita, GRE. Application deadline: 3/31 (fall). Application fee: $25.

Degree Requirements 60 total credit hours, dissertation, oral exam, written exam, residency.

CONTINUING EDUCATION PROGRAM

Contact Dr. P. Renee Williams, Director of Continuing Education, School of Nursing, University of Mississippi Medical Center, 2500 North State Street, Jackson, MS 39216-4505. *Telephone:* 601-984-6227. *Fax:* 601-984-6214. *E-mail:* rwilliams@umc.edu.

University of Southern Mississippi
College of Nursing
Hattiesburg, Mississippi

http://www.usm.edu/nursing/
Founded in 1910

DEGREES • BSN • MSN • PHD

Nursing Program Faculty 43 (72% with doctorates).

Baccalaureate Enrollment 413 **Women** 80% **Men** 20% **Part-time** 2%

Graduate Enrollment 196 **Women** 73% **Men** 27% **Part-time** 25%

Distance Learning Courses Available.

Nursing Student Activities Nursing Honor Society, Sigma Theta Tau, Student Nurses' Association, nursing club.

Nursing Student Resources Academic advising; academic or career counseling; assistance for students with disabilities; bookstore; campus computer network; career placement assistance; computer lab; computer-assisted instruction; e-mail services; employment services for current students; externships; housing assistance; interactive nursing skills videos; Internet; learning resource lab; library services; nursing audiovisuals; placement services for program completers; remedial services; resume preparation assistance; skills, simulation, or other laboratory; tutoring.

Library Facilities 13,932 volumes in health, 7,202 volumes in nursing; 2,042 periodical subscriptions health-care related.

BACCALAUREATE PROGRAMS

Degree BSN

Available Programs Generic Baccalaureate.

Site Options Long Beach, MS.

Study Options Full-time and part-time.

Program Entrance Requirements Minimum overall college GPA of 2.5, transcript of college record, written essay, health insurance, high school transcript, immunizations, minimum GPA in nursing prerequisites of 2.5, professional liability insurance/malpractice insurance, prerequisite course work. Transfer students are accepted. *Application deadline:* 2/1 (fall), 9/1 (spring).

Expenses (2015–16) *Tuition, state resident:* full-time $7224; part-time $301 per credit hour. *Tuition, nonresident:* full-time $16,194; part-time $370 per credit hour. *Room and board:* $8622 per academic year. *Required fees:* full-time $560.

Financial Aid 89% of baccalaureate students in nursing programs received some form of financial aid in 2014–15.

Contact Cindy Sheffield, Assistant to the Dean for Academic/Advisement Records, College of Nursing, University of Southern Mississippi, 118 College Drive, Box 5095, Hattiesburg, MS 39406-5095. *Telephone:* 601-266-5454. *Fax:* 601-266-5711. *E-mail:* cynthia.sheffield@usm.edu.

GRADUATE PROGRAMS

Expenses (2015–16) *Tuition, state resident:* part-time $402 per credit hour. *Tuition, nonresident:* part-time $493 per credit hour.

Financial Aid 80% of graduate students in nursing programs received some form of financial aid in 2014–15. Research assistantships with full tuition reimbursements available, teaching assistantships, Federal Work-Study, institutionally sponsored loans, scholarships, traineeships, and unspecified assistantships available. *Financial aid application deadline:* 3/15.

Contact Ms. Cynthia Sheffield, Assistant to the Dean for Academic/Advisement Records, College of Nursing, University of Southern Mississippi, 118 College Drive, Box 5095, Hattiesburg, MS 39406-5095. *Telephone:* 601-266-5454. *Fax:* 601-266-5711. *E-mail:* Cynthia.Sheffield@usm.edu.

MASTER'S DEGREE PROGRAM

Degree MSN

Available Programs Master's.

Concentrations Available Nurse anesthesia. *Nurse practitioner programs in:* family health, psychiatric/mental health.

Site Options Long Beach, MS.

Study Options Full-time and part-time.

Program Entrance Requirements Minimum overall college GPA of 3.0, transcript of college record, CPR certification, immunizations, 3 letters of recommendation, professional liability insurance/malpractice insurance, statistics course, GRE General Test. *Application deadline:* 3/1 (fall), 9/1 (spring).

Degree Requirements 45 total credit hours, thesis or project, comprehensive exam.

POST-MASTER'S PROGRAM

Areas of Study Nurse anesthesia. *Nurse practitioner programs in:* family health, psychiatric/mental health.

DOCTORAL DEGREE PROGRAM

Degree PhD

Available Programs Doctorate; Post-Baccalaureate Doctorate.

Program Entrance Requirements Clinical experience, minimum overall college GPA of 3.5, interview by faculty committee, 3 letters of recommendation, MSN or equivalent, statistics course, vita, writing sample, GRE General Test. Application deadline: 3/1 (fall).

Degree Requirements 72 total credit hours, dissertation, written exam.

William Carey University
School of Nursing
Hattiesburg, Mississippi

http://www.wmcarey.edu/
Founded in 1906

DEGREES • BSN • MSN • PHD

Nursing Program Faculty 25 (40% with doctorates).

Baccalaureate Enrollment 214 **Women** 85% **Men** 15% **Part-time** 26%

Graduate Enrollment 91 **Women** 89% **Men** 11% **Part-time** 45%

Distance Learning Courses Available.
Nursing Student Activities Sigma Theta Tau, Student Nurses' Association.
Nursing Student Resources Academic advising; academic or career counseling; assistance for students with disabilities; bookstore; campus computer network; computer lab; computer-assisted instruction; e-mail services; interactive nursing skills videos; Internet; learning resource lab; library services; nursing audiovisuals; resume preparation assistance; skills, simulation, or other laboratory; tutoring.
Library Facilities 450 volumes in health, 450 volumes in nursing; 50 periodical subscriptions health-care related.

BACCALAUREATE PROGRAMS

Degree BSN
Available Programs ADN to Baccalaureate; Generic Baccalaureate.
Site Options Biloxi, MS; New Orleans, LA.
Study Options Full-time and part-time.
Program Entrance Requirements Minimum overall college GPA of 2.75, transcript of college record, CPR certification, health exam, high school transcript, immunizations, minimum GPA in nursing prerequisites, professional liability insurance/malpractice insurance, prerequisite course work. Transfer students are accepted. *Application deadline:* 2/22 (fall), 8/10 (spring). *Application fee:* $40.
Advanced Placement Credit given for nursing courses completed elsewhere dependent upon specific evaluations.
Contact *Telephone:* 601-318-6478. *Fax:* 601-318-6446.

GRADUATE PROGRAMS

Contact *Telephone:* 601-318-6478.

MASTER'S DEGREE PROGRAM
Degree MSN
Available Programs Master's.
Concentrations Available Nursing education.
Site Options Biloxi, MS.
Study Options Full-time and part-time.
Program Entrance Requirements Computer literacy, minimum overall college GPA of 3.0, transcript of college record, CPR certification, written essay, immunizations, 2 letters of recommendation, nursing research course, professional liability insurance/malpractice insurance, prerequisite course work, resume. *Application deadline:* 8/15 (fall), 2/15 (spring). Applications may be processed on a rolling basis for some programs. *Application fee:* $30.
Advanced Placement Credit given for nursing courses completed elsewhere dependent upon specific evaluations.
Degree Requirements 35 total credit hours, thesis or project.

DOCTORAL DEGREE PROGRAM
Degree PhD
Available Programs Doctorate.
Areas of Study Nursing education.
Program Entrance Requirements Minimum overall college GPA of 3.5, 3 letters of recommendation, MSN or equivalent, statistics course, vita, writing sample. Application deadline: 6/22 (fall). Applications may be processed on a rolling basis for some programs. Application fee: $390.
Degree Requirements 56 total credit hours, dissertation, written exam.

MISSOURI

Avila University
School of Nursing
Kansas City, Missouri

http://www.avila.edu/nursing
Founded in 1916
DEGREE • BSN
Nursing Program Faculty 17 (6% with doctorates).
Baccalaureate Enrollment 114 Women 88% Men 12% Part-time 2%
Distance Learning Courses Available.
Nursing Student Activities Student Nurses' Association.
Nursing Student Resources Academic advising; academic or career counseling; assistance for students with disabilities; bookstore; campus computer network; career placement assistance; computer lab; computer-assisted instruction; e-mail services; employment services for current students; interactive nursing skills videos; Internet; learning resource lab; library services; nursing audiovisuals; remedial services; resume preparation assistance; skills, simulation, or other laboratory; tutoring.
Library Facilities 250 volumes in health, 200 volumes in nursing; 500 periodical subscriptions health-care related.

BACCALAUREATE PROGRAMS

Degree BSN
Available Programs Generic Baccalaureate; RN Baccalaureate.
Study Options Full-time.
Program Entrance Requirements Minimum overall college GPA of 2.75, transcript of college record, CPR certification, written essay, health insurance, immunizations, interview, minimum GPA in nursing prerequisites of 2.0, prerequisite course work. Transfer students are accepted. *Application deadline:* 1/10 (fall). *Application fee:* $45.
Advanced Placement Credit given for nursing courses completed elsewhere dependent upon specific evaluations.
Expenses (2015–16) *Tuition:* full-time $12,750; part-time $665 per credit. *International tuition:* $12,750 full-time. *Room and board:* $7500 per academic year. *Required fees:* full-time $2050; part-time $38 per credit.
Financial Aid 97% of baccalaureate students in nursing programs received some form of financial aid in 2014–15.
Contact Office of Admissions, School of Nursing, Avila University, 11901 Wornall Road, Kansas City, MO 64145-1698. *Telephone:* 816-501-2400. *Fax:* 816-501-2453. *E-mail:* admissions@avila.edu.

Central Methodist University
College of Liberal Arts and Sciences
Fayette, Missouri

http://www.centralmethodist.edu/
Founded in 1854
DEGREES • BSN • MSN
Nursing Program Faculty 30 (26% with doctorates).
Baccalaureate Enrollment 325 Women 92% Men 8%
Graduate Enrollment 33 Women 96% Men 4%
Distance Learning Courses Available.
Nursing Student Activities Sigma Theta Tau, Student Nurses' Association.
Nursing Student Resources Academic advising; academic or career counseling; assistance for students with disabilities; bookstore; campus computer network; computer lab; computer-assisted instruction; e-mail services; interactive nursing skills videos; Internet; learning resource lab; library services; nursing audiovisuals; resume preparation assistance; skills, simulation, or other laboratory; tutoring.

BACCALAUREATE PROGRAMS

Degree BSN
Available Programs ADN to Baccalaureate; Accelerated Baccalaureate for Second Degree; Generic Baccalaureate.
Site Options Columbia, MO; St. Louis, MO; Rolla, MO.
Study Options Full-time.
Online Degree Options Yes.
Program Entrance Requirements Minimum overall college GPA, transcript of college record, CPR certification, written essay, health insurance, high school transcript, immunizations, minimum GPA in nursing prerequisites, prerequisite course work. Transfer students are accepted. *Application deadline:* 4/1 (fall), 1/1 (spring). Applications may be processed on a rolling basis for some programs.
Advanced Placement Credit by examination available. Credit given for nursing courses completed elsewhere dependent upon specific evaluations.
Contact *Telephone:* 660-248-6359.

GRADUATE PROGRAMS

Contact *Telephone:* 660-248-6639. *Fax:* 660-248-6243.

MASTER'S DEGREE PROGRAM
Degree MSN
Available Programs Master's.
Concentrations Available Clinical nurse leader; nursing education.
Study Options Full-time and part-time.
Online Degree Options Yes (online only).

Program Entrance Requirements Clinical experience, computer literacy, minimum overall college GPA of 3.0, transcript of college record, CPR certification, written essay, immunizations, nursing research course, professional liability insurance/malpractice insurance, prerequisite course work, statistics course. *Application deadline:* Applications may be processed on a rolling basis for some programs.
Advanced Placement Credit given for nursing courses completed elsewhere dependent upon specific evaluations.
Degree Requirements 34 total credit hours, thesis or project.

Chamberlain College of Nursing
Chamberlain College of Nursing
St. Louis, Missouri

http://www.chamberlain.edu/
Founded in 1889
DEGREE • BSN
Nursing Program Faculty 80 (21% with doctorates).
Distance Learning Courses Available.
Nursing Student Activities Student Nurses' Association.
Nursing Student Resources Academic advising; academic or career counseling; assistance for students with disabilities; bookstore; campus computer network; career placement assistance; computer lab; computer-assisted instruction; e-mail services; employment services for current students; housing assistance; Internet; learning resource lab; library services; nursing audiovisuals; placement services for program completers; skills, simulation, or other laboratory; tutoring.
Library Facilities 3,287 volumes in health, 957 volumes in nursing; 182 periodical subscriptions health-care related.

BACCALAUREATE PROGRAMS
Degree BSN
Available Programs ADN to Baccalaureate; Accelerated RN Baccalaureate; Generic Baccalaureate; LPN to RN Baccalaureate; RN Baccalaureate.
Site Options Columbus, OH; Phoenix, AZ; Addison, IL.
Study Options Full-time.
Online Degree Options Yes (online only).
Program Entrance Requirements Minimum overall college GPA of 2.75, transcript of college record, written essay, health exam, health insurance, high school biology, high school chemistry, 3 years high school math, 3 years high school science, high school transcript, immunizations, interview, minimum high school GPA of 2.75, minimum high school rank 33%. Transfer students are accepted.
Advanced Placement Credit by examination available. Credit given for nursing courses completed elsewhere dependent upon specific evaluations.
Contact *Telephone:* 800-942-4310 Ext. 1. *Fax:* 314-768-3044.

College of the Ozarks
Armstrong McDonald School of Nursing
Point Lookout, Missouri

http://www.cofo.edu/
Founded in 1906
DEGREE • BSN
Nursing Program Faculty 9 (33% with doctorates).
Baccalaureate Enrollment 61 **Women** 70% **Men** 30%
Nursing Student Activities Nursing club.
Nursing Student Resources Academic advising; academic or career counseling; assistance for students with disabilities; bookstore; campus computer network; career placement assistance; computer lab; computer-assisted instruction; daycare for children of students; e-mail services; employment services for current students; externships; housing assistance; interactive nursing skills videos; Internet; learning resource lab; library services; nursing audiovisuals; paid internships; placement services for program completers; remedial services; resume preparation assistance; skills, simulation, or other laboratory; tutoring; unpaid internships.
Library Facilities 1,400 volumes in health, 560 volumes in nursing; 40 periodical subscriptions health-care related.

BACCALAUREATE PROGRAMS
Degree BSN
Available Programs Generic Baccalaureate.
Study Options Full-time and part-time.
Program Entrance Requirements Minimum overall college GPA of 2.5, transcript of college record, written essay, health exam, 2 years high school math, high school transcript, immunizations, interview, 2 letters of recommendation, minimum high school GPA of 3.0, minimum high school rank 51%, minimum GPA in nursing prerequisites of 2.5, professional liability insurance/malpractice insurance, prerequisite course work. Transfer students are accepted. *Application deadline:* 3/1 (spring).
Expenses (2015–16) *Room and board:* $6500; room only: $3250 per academic year.
Financial Aid 100% of baccalaureate students in nursing programs received some form of financial aid in 2014–15. *Gift aid (need-based):* Federal Pell, FSEOG, state, private, college/university gift aid from institutional funds. *Work-study:* Federal Work-Study, part-time campus jobs. *Financial aid application deadline (priority):* 2/15.
Contact Mrs. Deborah J. Lyon, Office Manager, Armstrong McDonald School of Nursing, College of the Ozarks, PO Box 17, Point Lookout, MO 65726. *Telephone:* 417-690-2421. *Fax:* 417-690-2422. *E-mail:* dlyon@cofo.edu.

Cox College
Department of Nursing
Springfield, Missouri

http://coxcollege.edu/
Founded in 1994
DEGREES • BSN • MSN
Nursing Program Faculty 61 (10% with doctorates).
Baccalaureate Enrollment 240 **Women** 87% **Men** 13% **Part-time** 80%
Graduate Enrollment 83 **Women** 92% **Men** 8%
Distance Learning Courses Available.
Nursing Student Activities Nursing Honor Society, Student Nurses' Association, nursing club.
Nursing Student Resources Academic advising; academic or career counseling; assistance for students with disabilities; bookstore; campus computer network; career placement assistance; computer lab; computer-assisted instruction; daycare for children of students; e-mail services; employment services for current students; externships; housing assistance; interactive nursing skills videos; Internet; learning resource lab; library services; nursing audiovisuals; placement services for program completers; remedial services; resume preparation assistance; skills, simulation, or other laboratory; tutoring.
Library Facilities 5,500 volumes in health, 1,900 volumes in nursing; 250 periodical subscriptions health-care related.

BACCALAUREATE PROGRAMS
Degree BSN
Available Programs ADN to Baccalaureate; Accelerated Baccalaureate; Accelerated Baccalaureate for Second Degree; Baccalaureate for Second Degree; Generic Baccalaureate; LPN to Baccalaureate; LPN to RN Baccalaureate; RN Baccalaureate.
Site Options Springfield, MO.
Study Options Full-time.
Online Degree Options Yes (online only).
Program Entrance Requirements Minimum overall college GPA of 3.0, transcript of college record, CPR certification, high school transcript, immunizations, interview, minimum high school GPA of 3.0, minimum GPA in nursing prerequisites of 3.0, professional liability insurance/malpractice insurance, prerequisite course work, RN licensure. Transfer students are accepted. *Application deadline:* 1/15 (fall), 8/15 (spring). *Application fee:* $45.
Advanced Placement Credit given for nursing courses completed elsewhere dependent upon specific evaluations.
Contact *Telephone:* 417-269-3401. *Fax:* 417-269-3586.

GRADUATE PROGRAMS
Contact *Telephone:* 417-269-3401.

MASTER'S DEGREE PROGRAM
Degree MSN
Available Programs Master's; RN to Master's.
Concentrations Available Clinical nurse leader; nursing education. *Clinical nurse specialist programs in:* family health.

Site Options Springfield, MO.
Study Options Full-time and part-time.
Online Degree Options Yes (online only).
Program Entrance Requirements Clinical experience, computer literacy, minimum overall college GPA of 3.0, transcript of college record, CPR certification, written essay, immunizations, interview, letters of recommendation, resume. *Application deadline:* 3/1 (fall). *Application fee:* $45.
Degree Requirements 42 total credit hours, thesis or project.

CONTINUING EDUCATION PROGRAM

Contact *Telephone:* 417-269-5062.

Culver-Stockton College
Blessing–Rieman College of Nursing
Canton, Missouri

http://www.culver.edu/

See description of programs under Blessing–Rieman College of Nursing (Quincy, Illinois).

Goldfarb School of Nursing at Barnes-Jewish College
Goldfarb School of Nursing at Barnes-Jewish College
St. Louis, Missouri

Founded in 1902
DEGREES • BSN • MSN • PHD
Nursing Program Faculty 56 (39% with doctorates).
Baccalaureate Enrollment 631 **Women** 88% **Men** 12% **Part-time** 11%
Graduate Enrollment 89 **Women** 93% **Men** 7% **Part-time** 34%
Distance Learning Courses Available.
Nursing Student Activities Sigma Theta Tau, Student Nurses' Association.
Nursing Student Resources Academic advising; academic or career counseling; assistance for students with disabilities; bookstore; campus computer network; career placement assistance; computer lab; computer-assisted instruction; e-mail services; employment services for current students; housing assistance; interactive nursing skills videos; Internet; learning resource lab; library services; nursing audiovisuals; remedial services; resume preparation assistance; skills, simulation, or other laboratory; tutoring.
Library Facilities 1,100 volumes in health, 700 volumes in nursing; 15,000 periodical subscriptions health-care related.

BACCALAUREATE PROGRAMS

Degree BSN
Available Programs ADN to Baccalaureate; Accelerated Baccalaureate; Accelerated Baccalaureate for Second Degree; Generic Baccalaureate; RN Baccalaureate.
Site Options Town and Country, MO.
Study Options Full-time.
Program Entrance Requirements Minimum overall college GPA of 3.0, transcript of college record, CPR certification, health exam, high school biology, high school transcript, immunizations, minimum high school GPA of 3.0, minimum GPA in nursing prerequisites of 3.0, prerequisite course work. Transfer students are accepted. *Application deadline:* 8/15 (fall), 12/15 (spring), 4/1 (summer). Applications may be processed on a rolling basis for some programs. *Application fee:* $50.
Advanced Placement Credit by examination available. Credit given for nursing courses completed elsewhere dependent upon specific evaluations.
Expenses (2015–16) *Tuition:* full-time $28,865; part-time $733 per credit. *Required fees:* full-time $1398.
Financial Aid 81% of baccalaureate students in nursing programs received some form of financial aid in 2014–15.
Contact Karen Sartorius, Enrollment Coordinator, Goldfarb School of Nursing at Barnes-Jewish College, 4483 Duncan, MS #90-36-697, St. Louis, MO 63110-1091. *Telephone:* 314-454-7057. *Fax:* 314-362-9250. *E-mail:* ksartorius@bjc.org.

GRADUATE PROGRAMS

Expenses (2015–16) *Tuition:* full-time $14,598; part-time $795 per credit. *Required fees:* full-time $45; part-time $15 per term.
Contact Ms. Karen Sartorius, Admissions Specialist, Goldfarb School of Nursing at Barnes-Jewish College, 4483 Duncan, MS #90-36-697, St. Louis, MO 63110-1091. *Telephone:* 314-454-7057. *Fax:* 314-362-9250. *E-mail:* ksartorius@bjc.org.

MASTER'S DEGREE PROGRAM
Degree MSN
Available Programs Master's.
Concentrations Available Health-care administration; nurse anesthesia; nursing administration; nursing education. *Nurse practitioner programs in:* adult health, adult-gerontology acute care.
Study Options Full-time and part-time.
Program Entrance Requirements Clinical experience, computer literacy, minimum overall college GPA of 3.0, transcript of college record, CPR certification, immunizations, 2 letters of recommendation, nursing research course, physical assessment course, resume, statistics course. *Application deadline:* 8/20 (fall), 12/15 (spring), 4/15 (summer). Applications may be processed on a rolling basis for some programs. *Application fee:* $50.
Advanced Placement Credit given for nursing courses completed elsewhere dependent upon specific evaluations.
Degree Requirements 45 total credit hours, thesis or project.

POST-MASTER'S PROGRAM
Areas of Study Health-care administration; nursing administration; nursing education. *Nurse practitioner programs in:* adult health, adult-gerontology acute care.

DOCTORAL DEGREE PROGRAM
Degree PhD
Available Programs Doctorate.
Areas of Study Clinical practice, nursing administration, nursing education.
Program Entrance Requirements Minimum overall college GPA of 3.0, interview by faculty committee, interview, 3 letters of recommendation, MSN or equivalent, statistics course, vita, writing sample. Application deadline: 7/15 (fall). Applications may be processed on a rolling basis for some programs. Application fee: $50.
Degree Requirements 111 total credit hours, dissertation, oral exam, written exam, residency.

Graceland University
School of Nursing
Independence, Missouri

http://www.graceland.edu/nursing
Founded in 1895
DEGREES • BSN • DNP • MSN
Nursing Program Faculty 22 (45% with doctorates).
Baccalaureate Enrollment 167 **Women** 93% **Men** 7%
Graduate Enrollment 505 **Women** 88% **Men** 12%
Distance Learning Courses Available.
Nursing Student Activities Nursing Honor Society, Sigma Theta Tau, Student Nurses' Association, nursing club.
Nursing Student Resources Academic advising; academic or career counseling; assistance for students with disabilities; bookstore; campus computer network; computer lab; computer-assisted instruction; e-mail services; housing assistance; interactive nursing skills videos; Internet; learning resource lab; library services; nursing audiovisuals; skills, simulation, or other laboratory; tutoring.
Library Facilities 4,195 volumes in health, 2,234 volumes in nursing; 561 periodical subscriptions health-care related.

BACCALAUREATE PROGRAMS

Degree BSN
Available Programs ADN to Baccalaureate; Accelerated Baccalaureate; RN Baccalaureate.
Site Options Independence, MO.
Study Options Full-time.
Program Entrance Requirements Minimum overall college GPA of 2.75, transcript of college record, written essay, health exam, health insurance, immunizations, interview, 2 letters of recommendation,

minimum GPA in nursing prerequisites of 2.0, prerequisite course work. Transfer students are accepted. *Application deadline:* 11/30 (fall).

Advanced Placement Credit given for nursing courses completed elsewhere dependent upon specific evaluations.

Financial Aid *Gift aid (need-based):* Federal Pell, FSEOG, state, private, college/university gift aid from institutional funds. *Loans:* Federal Direct (Subsidized and Unsubsidized Stafford PLUS), Perkins, state, college/university. *Work-study:* Federal Work-Study, part-time campus jobs. *Financial aid application deadline:* Continuous.

Contact Ms. Laurie Hale, Admissions Counselor, School of Nursing, Graceland University, 1401 West Truman Road, Independence, MO 64050-3434. *Telephone:* 800-423-4675. *Fax:* 816-833-2990. *E-mail:* lhale@graceland.edu.

GRADUATE PROGRAMS

Contact Mr. Loren Spicer, Admissions Representative, School of Nursing, Graceland University, 1401 West Truman Road, Independence, MO 64050-3434. *Telephone:* 816-423-4718. *Fax:* 816-833-2990. *E-mail:* lspicer@graceland.edu.

MASTER'S DEGREE PROGRAM

Degree MSN

Available Programs Master's; RN to Master's.

Concentrations Available Nursing education. *Nurse practitioner programs in:* family health.

Site Options Independence, MO.

Study Options Full-time and part-time.

Program Entrance Requirements Clinical experience, minimum overall college GPA of 3.0, transcript of college record, 3 letters of recommendation. *Application deadline:* 6/1 (fall), 10/1 (winter), 2/1 (spring). *Application fee:* $50.

Advanced Placement Credit given for nursing courses completed elsewhere dependent upon specific evaluations.

Degree Requirements 47 total credit hours, thesis or project, comprehensive exam.

POST-MASTER'S PROGRAM

Areas of Study Nursing education. *Nurse practitioner programs in:* family health.

DOCTORAL DEGREE PROGRAM

Degree DNP

Available Programs Doctorate.

Areas of Study Ethics, health policy, health-care systems, information systems, nursing policy, nursing science.

Site Options Independence, MO.

Online Degree Options Yes (online only).

Program Entrance Requirements Minimum overall college GPA of 3.2, 3 letters of recommendation, MSN or equivalent, writing sample. Application deadline: 5/15 (fall). Application fee: $50.

Degree Requirements 31 total credit hours.

Hannibal-LaGrange University
Division of Nursing and Allied Health
Hannibal, Missouri

http://www.hlg.edu/index.php
Founded in 1858

DEGREE • BSN

BACCALAUREATE PROGRAMS

Degree BSN

Available Programs RN Baccalaureate.

Online Degree Options Yes (online only).

Program Entrance Requirements Minimum overall college GPA of 2.5, RN licensure.

Contact Donna White, MSN, RN, RN-BSN Program Coordinator, Division of Nursing and Allied Health, Hannibal-LaGrange University, 2800 Palmyra Road, Hannibal, MO 63401. *Telephone:* 573-629-4147. *E-mail:* nursing@hlg.edu.

Lincoln University
Department of Nursing
Jefferson City, Missouri

http://www.lincolnu.edu/web/dept.-of-nursing-science/nursing-science
Founded in 1866

DEGREE • BSN

Distance Learning Courses Available.

Nursing Student Resources Academic advising; academic or career counseling; assistance for students with disabilities; bookstore; campus computer network; computer lab; e-mail services; Internet; library services; remedial services; tutoring.

BACCALAUREATE PROGRAMS

Degree BSN

Available Programs RN Baccalaureate.

Contact *Telephone:* 573-681-5421.

Maryville University of Saint Louis
The Catherine McAuley School of Nursing, College of Health Professions
St. Louis, Missouri

https://www.maryville.edu/hp/
Founded in 1872

DEGREES • BSN • DNP • MSN

Nursing Program Faculty 204 (42% with doctorates).

Baccalaureate Enrollment 496 **Women** 92% **Men** 8% **Part-time** 52%

Graduate Enrollment 2,592 **Women** 90% **Men** 10% **Part-time** 98%

Distance Learning Courses Available.

Nursing Student Activities Sigma Theta Tau, Student Nurses' Association, nursing club.

Nursing Student Resources Academic advising; academic or career counseling; assistance for students with disabilities; bookstore; campus computer network; career placement assistance; computer lab; computer-assisted instruction; e-mail services; externships; interactive nursing skills videos; Internet; learning resource lab; library services; nursing audiovisuals; paid internships; remedial services; resume preparation assistance; skills, simulation, or other laboratory; tutoring.

Library Facilities 8,680 volumes in health, 1,464 volumes in nursing; 4,315 periodical subscriptions health-care related.

BACCALAUREATE PROGRAMS

Degree BSN

Available Programs Accelerated Baccalaureate; Accelerated RN Baccalaureate; Generic Baccalaureate; LPN to Baccalaureate; RN Baccalaureate.

Study Options Full-time and part-time.

Program Entrance Requirements Minimum overall college GPA of 3.0, transcript of college record, health exam, high school transcript, immunizations, minimum high school GPA of 3.0, minimum GPA in nursing prerequisites of 3.0. Transfer students are accepted. *Application deadline:* 12/15 (fall). Applications may be processed on a rolling basis for some programs.

Advanced Placement Credit given for nursing courses completed elsewhere dependent upon specific evaluations.

Expenses (2015–16) *Tuition:* full-time $25,558; part-time $766 per credit hour. *Room and board:* $10,240 per academic year. *Required fees:* full-time $1400; part-time $310 per term.

Financial Aid 80% of baccalaureate students in nursing programs received some form of financial aid in 2014–15. *Gift aid (need-based):* Federal Pell, FSEOG, state, private, college/university gift aid from institutional funds, Academic Competitiveness Grants, National SMART Grants, TEACH Grants. *Loans:* Federal Direct (Subsidized and Unsubsidized Stafford PLUS), Perkins, private loans. *Work-study:* Federal Work-Study, part-time campus jobs. *Financial aid application deadline (priority):* 3/1.

Contact Dr. Elizabeth Buck, Director, The Catherine McAuley School of Nursing, College of Health Professions, Maryville University of Saint Louis, 650 Maryville University Drive, St. Louis, MO 63141-7299. *Telephone:* 314-529-9453. *Fax:* 314-529-9495. *E-mail:* ebuck@maryville.edu.

GRADUATE PROGRAMS

Expenses (2015–16) *Tuition:* full-time $25,558; part-time $781 per credit hour. *Required fees:* full-time $1400; part-time $310 per term.
Financial Aid 73% of graduate students in nursing programs received some form of financial aid in 2014–15.
Contact Dr. Elizabeth Buck, Director, The Catherine McAuley School of Nursing, College of Health Professions, Maryville University of Saint Louis, 650 Maryville University Drive, St. Louis, MO 63141-7299. *Telephone:* 314-529-9453. *Fax:* 314-529-9495.
E-mail: ebuck@maryville.edu.

MASTER'S DEGREE PROGRAM

Degree MSN
Available Programs Master's.
Concentrations Available *Nurse practitioner programs in:* acute care, adult health, family health, gerontology.
Study Options Full-time and part-time.
Program Entrance Requirements Minimum overall college GPA of 3.0, transcript of college record, written essay, 3 letters of recommendation, resume, statistics course. *Application deadline:* Applications may be processed on a rolling basis for some programs.
Advanced Placement Credit by examination available. Credit given for nursing courses completed elsewhere dependent upon specific evaluations.
Degree Requirements 42 total credit hours, thesis or project.

POST-MASTER'S PROGRAM

Areas of Study *Nurse practitioner programs in:* acute care, adult health, family health, gerontology, pediatric primary care.

DOCTORAL DEGREE PROGRAM

Degree DNP
Available Programs Doctorate; Post-Baccalaureate Doctorate.
Areas of Study Clinical practice.
Online Degree Options Yes (online only).
Program Entrance Requirements Minimum overall college GPA of 3.25, 3 letters of recommendation, MSN or equivalent, vita, writing sample. Application deadline: Applications may be processed on a rolling basis for some programs.
Degree Requirements 30 total credit hours.

Missouri Southern State University

Department of Nursing
Joplin, Missouri

http://www.mssu.edu
Founded in 1937
DEGREES • BSN • MSN
Nursing Program Faculty 10 (10% with doctorates).
Baccalaureate Enrollment 107 **Women** 79.44% **Men** 20.56%
Graduate Enrollment 49 **Women** 96% **Men** 4% **Part-time** 31%
Distance Learning Courses Available.
Nursing Student Activities Nursing Honor Society, Student Nurses' Association.
Nursing Student Resources Academic advising; academic or career counseling; assistance for students with disabilities; bookstore; campus computer network; career placement assistance; computer lab; computer-assisted instruction; daycare for children of students; e-mail services; employment services for current students; housing assistance; interactive nursing skills videos; Internet; learning resource lab; library services; nursing audiovisuals; remedial services; resume preparation assistance; skills, simulation, or other laboratory; tutoring.
Library Facilities 4,872 volumes in health, 4,470 volumes in nursing; 4,412 periodical subscriptions health-care related.

BACCALAUREATE PROGRAMS

Degree BSN
Available Programs ADN to Baccalaureate; Baccalaureate for Second Degree; Generic Baccalaureate; LPN to Baccalaureate; RN Baccalaureate.
Study Options Full-time.
Program Entrance Requirements Transcript of college record, CPR certification, health exam, health insurance, immunizations, minimum GPA in nursing prerequisites of 2.5, professional liability insurance/mal-practice insurance, prerequisite course work, RN licensure. Transfer students are accepted. *Application deadline:* 1/31 (fall). *Application fee:* $50.
Advanced Placement Credit by examination available. Credit given for nursing courses completed elsewhere dependent upon specific evaluations.
Contact *Telephone:* 417-625-9322. *Fax:* 417-625-3186.

GRADUATE PROGRAMS

Contact *Telephone:* 417-625-9322. *Fax:* 417-625-3186.

MASTER'S DEGREE PROGRAM

Degree MSN
Available Programs Master's.
Concentrations Available Nursing education. *Clinical nurse specialist programs in:* family health.
Study Options Full-time and part-time.
Program Entrance Requirements Minimum overall college GPA of 3.0, transcript of college record, resume. *Application deadline:* 12/1 (fall). *Application fee:* $35.
Degree Requirements 42 total credit hours.

Missouri State University

Department of Nursing
Springfield, Missouri

http://www.missouristate.edu/nursing
Founded in 1905
DEGREES • BSN • DNP • MSN
Nursing Program Faculty 23 (39% with doctorates).
Baccalaureate Enrollment 231 **Women** 90% **Men** 10% **Part-time** 30%
Graduate Enrollment 47 **Women** 97% **Men** 3% **Part-time** 30%
Distance Learning Courses Available.
Nursing Student Activities Sigma Theta Tau, Student Nurses' Association.
Nursing Student Resources Academic advising; academic or career counseling; assistance for students with disabilities; bookstore; campus computer network; career placement assistance; computer lab; computer-assisted instruction; daycare for children of students; e-mail services; employment services for current students; externships; housing assistance; interactive nursing skills videos; Internet; learning resource lab; library services; nursing audiovisuals; paid internships; placement services for program completers; remedial services; resume preparation assistance; skills, simulation, or other laboratory; tutoring; unpaid internships.
Library Facilities 10,500 volumes in health, 3,516 volumes in nursing; 370 periodical subscriptions health-care related.

BACCALAUREATE PROGRAMS

Degree BSN
Available Programs ADN to Baccalaureate; Accelerated RN Baccalaureate; Generic Baccalaureate; RN Baccalaureate.
Study Options Full-time.
Online Degree Options Yes.
Program Entrance Requirements Minimum overall college GPA of 2.75, transcript of college record, CPR certification, written essay, health insurance, immunizations, prerequisite course work. Transfer students are accepted. *Application deadline:* 1/31 (summer). *Application fee:* $50.
Advanced Placement Credit given for nursing courses completed elsewhere dependent upon specific evaluations.
Expenses (2014–15) *Tuition, state resident:* full-time $7008; part-time $204 per credit hour. *Tuition, nonresident:* full-time $13,668; part-time $426 per credit hour. *International tuition:* $13,668 full-time. *Room and board:* $7678 per academic year. *Required fees:* full-time $888; part-time $361 per term.
Financial Aid 65% of baccalaureate students in nursing programs received some form of financial aid in 2013–14.
Contact Dr. Kathryn L. Hope, Head, Department of Nursing, Department of Nursing, Missouri State University, 901 South National Avenue, Springfield, MO 65897. *Telephone:* 417-836-5310. *Fax:* 417-836-5484. *E-mail:* kathrynhope@missouristate.edu.

GRADUATE PROGRAMS

Expenses (2014–15) *Tuition, state resident:* full-time $5388; part-time $250 per credit hour. *Tuition, nonresident:* full-time $9906; part-time

$501 per credit hour. *International tuition:* $9906 full-time. *Room and board:* $7678 per academic year. *Required fees:* full-time $888.

Financial Aid 25% of graduate students in nursing programs received some form of financial aid in 2013–14. Research assistantships, Federal Work-Study, institutionally sponsored loans, scholarships, and unspecified assistantships available. *Financial aid application deadline:* 3/31.

Contact Dr. Kathryn L. Hope, Head, Department of Nursing, Department of Nursing, Missouri State University, 901 South National Avenue, Springfield, MO 65897. *Telephone:* 417-836-5310. *Fax:* 417-836-5484. *E-mail:* kathrynhope@missouristate.edu.

MASTER'S DEGREE PROGRAM

Degree MSN

Available Programs Accelerated AD/RN to Master's; Master's; RN to Master's.

Concentrations Available Nursing education.

Study Options Full-time and part-time.

Online Degree Options Yes (online only).

Program Entrance Requirements Computer literacy, minimum overall college GPA of 3.0, transcript of college record, CPR certification, immunizations, interview, nursing research course, physical assessment course, professional liability insurance/malpractice insurance, prerequisite course work, statistics course, GRE General Test. *Application deadline:* 8/1 (fall), 12/1 (winter), 12/1 (spring), 5/1 (summer). *Application fee:* $50.

Advanced Placement Credit given for nursing courses completed elsewhere dependent upon specific evaluations.

Degree Requirements 39 total credit hours, thesis or project, comprehensive exam.

POST-MASTER'S PROGRAM

Areas of Study Nursing education.

DOCTORAL DEGREE PROGRAM

Degree DNP

Available Programs Doctorate; Post-Baccalaureate Doctorate.

Areas of Study Advanced practice nursing, health-care systems.

Online Degree Options Yes.

Program Entrance Requirements Clinical experience, minimum overall college GPA of 3.25, interview by faculty committee, interview, statistics course, vita, writing sample. Application deadline: 12/1 (summer). Application fee: $50.

Degree Requirements 82 total credit hours, oral exam.

CONTINUING EDUCATION PROGRAM

Contact Virginia Cordova, Program Coordinator, Department of Nursing, Missouri State University, 901 South National Avenue, Department of Continuing Education, Springfield, MO 65897. *Telephone:* 417-836-6660. *Fax:* 417-836-7674. *E-mail:* virginiacordova@missouristate.edu.

Missouri Valley College
School of Nursing and Health Sciences
Marshall, Missouri

http://www.moval.edu/snhs/nursing/
Founded in 1889

DEGREE • BSN

Nursing Program Faculty 7 (3% with doctorates).

Baccalaureate Enrollment 10 **Women** 100%

Distance Learning Courses Available.

Nursing Student Activities Sigma Theta Tau, Student Nurses' Association.

Nursing Student Resources Academic advising; academic or career counseling; assistance for students with disabilities; bookstore; campus computer network; computer lab; computer-assisted instruction; daycare for children of students; e-mail services; employment services for current students; housing assistance; interactive nursing skills videos; Internet; learning resource lab; library services; nursing audiovisuals; remedial services; resume preparation assistance; skills, simulation, or other laboratory; tutoring.

Library Facilities 513 volumes in health, 246 volumes in nursing; 1,215 periodical subscriptions health-care related.

BACCALAUREATE PROGRAMS

Degree BSN

Available Programs Generic Baccalaureate.

Study Options Full-time.

Online Degree Options Yes (online only).

Program Entrance Requirements Minimum overall college GPA of 2.75, transcript of college record, CPR certification, health exam, immunizations, interview, 3 letters of recommendation, minimum GPA in nursing prerequisites of 3.0, professional liability insurance/malpractice insurance, prerequisite course work. Transfer students are accepted. *Application deadline:* 4/1 (spring). *Application fee:* $25.

Advanced Placement Credit given for nursing courses completed elsewhere dependent upon specific evaluations.

Expenses (2015–16) *Tuition:* full-time $19,750; part-time $350 per credit hour. *International tuition:* $19,750 full-time. *Room and board:* $8400; room only: $3950 per academic year. *Required fees:* full-time $2500; part-time $800 per term.

Financial Aid 100% of baccalaureate students in nursing programs received some form of financial aid in 2014–15. *Gift aid (need-based):* Federal Pell, FSEOG, state, private, college/university gift aid from institutional funds. *Loans:* Federal Direct (Subsidized and Unsubsidized Stafford PLUS), Perkins. *Work-study:* Federal Work-Study, part-time campus jobs. *Financial aid application deadline (priority):* 3/15.

Contact Dr. Peggy A. Van Dyke, RN, Dean, School of Nursing, School of Nursing and Health Sciences, Missouri Valley College, 500 East College, Marshall, MO 65340. *Telephone:* 660-831-0832. *Fax:* 660-831-0832. *E-mail:* vandykep@yahoo.com.

Missouri Western State University
Department of Nursing
St. Joseph, Missouri

http://www.missouriwestern.edu/nursing
Founded in 1915

DEGREES • BSN • MSN

Nursing Program Faculty 35 (23% with doctorates).

Baccalaureate Enrollment 200 **Women** 86% **Men** 14% **Part-time** 7%

Graduate Enrollment 17 **Women** 100% **Part-time** 100%

Distance Learning Courses Available.

Nursing Student Activities Sigma Theta Tau, Student Nurses' Association.

Nursing Student Resources Academic advising; academic or career counseling; assistance for students with disabilities; bookstore; campus computer network; career placement assistance; computer lab; computer-assisted instruction; e-mail services; employment services for current students; interactive nursing skills videos; Internet; learning resource lab; library services; nursing audiovisuals; placement services for program completers; remedial services; resume preparation assistance; skills, simulation, or other laboratory; tutoring; unpaid internships.

Library Facilities 29 periodical subscriptions health-care related.

BACCALAUREATE PROGRAMS

Degree BSN

Available Programs ADN to Baccalaureate; Generic Baccalaureate.

Site Options Kansas City, MO.

Study Options Full-time.

Program Entrance Requirements Minimum overall college GPA of 2.7, transcript of college record, CPR certification, written essay, health insurance, high school transcript, immunizations, minimum GPA in nursing prerequisites of 2.7, prerequisite course work. Transfer students are accepted. *Application deadline:* 1/15 (fall), 7/31 (spring). *Application fee:* $45.

Advanced Placement Credit by examination available. Credit given for nursing courses completed elsewhere dependent upon specific evaluations.

Contact *Telephone:* 816-271-4415. *Fax:* 816-271-5849.

GRADUATE PROGRAMS

Contact *Telephone:* 816-271-4415. *Fax:* 816-271-5849.

MASTER'S DEGREE PROGRAM

Degree MSN

Available Programs Master's.

Concentrations Available Health-care administration.

Study Options Part-time.

Program Entrance Requirements Minimum overall college GPA of 2.75, transcript of college record, written essay, interview, nursing

research course, prerequisite course work, statistics course. *Application deadline:* 7/15 (fall), 10/15 (spring). *Application fee:* $30.
Degree Requirements 36 total credit hours, thesis or project.

CONTINUING EDUCATION PROGRAM

Contact *Telephone:* 816-271-4415. *Fax:* 816-271-5849.

Research College of Nursing
College of Nursing
Kansas City, Missouri

http://www.researchcollege.edu/
Founded in 1980
DEGREES • BSN • MSN
Nursing Program Faculty 36 (16% with doctorates).
Baccalaureate Enrollment 292 **Women** 91% **Men** 9%
Graduate Enrollment 152 **Women** 89% **Men** 11%
Distance Learning Courses Available.
Nursing Student Activities Sigma Theta Tau, Student Nurses' Association.
Nursing Student Resources Academic advising; academic or career counseling; bookstore; campus computer network; career placement assistance; computer lab; computer-assisted instruction; daycare for children of students; e-mail services; housing assistance; Internet; learning resource lab; library services; resume preparation assistance; skills, simulation, or other laboratory; tutoring.

BACCALAUREATE PROGRAMS

Degree BSN
Available Programs Accelerated Baccalaureate; Accelerated Baccalaureate for Second Degree; Baccalaureate for Second Degree; Generic Baccalaureate.
Study Options Full-time.
Program Entrance Requirements Transcript of college record, high school chemistry, 3 years high school math, 2 years high school science, high school transcript, minimum high school rank 50%, minimum GPA in nursing prerequisites of 2.7. Transfer students are accepted. *Application deadline:* 2/15 (spring). *Application fee:* $45.
Advanced Placement Credit given for nursing courses completed elsewhere dependent upon specific evaluations.
Expenses (2015–16) *Tuition:* full-time $34,000; part-time $1134 per credit hour. *International tuition:* $34,000 full-time. *Room and board:* $9255; room only: $5755 per academic year. *Required fees:* full-time $850; part-time $100 per credit.
Financial Aid 97% of baccalaureate students in nursing programs received some form of financial aid in 2014–15.
Contact Ms. Leslie Ann Burry, Director of Admission, College of Nursing, Research College of Nursing, 2525 East Meyer Boulevard, Kansas City, MO 64132-1199. *Telephone:* 816-995-2820. *Fax:* 816-995-2813. *E-mail:* leslie.burry@researchcollege.edu.

GRADUATE PROGRAMS

Expenses (2015–16) *Tuition:* part-time $500 per credit hour. *Room and board:* room only: $5000 per academic year. *Required fees:* part-time $25 per credit.
Financial Aid 10% of graduate students in nursing programs received some form of financial aid in 2014–15.
Contact Ms. Leslie Ann Burry, Director of Admission, College of Nursing, Research College of Nursing, 2525 East Meyer Boulevard, Kansas City, MO 64132-1199. *Telephone:* 816-995-2820. *Fax:* 816-995-2813. *E-mail:* leslie.burry@researchcollege.edu.

MASTER'S DEGREE PROGRAM
Degree MSN
Available Programs Master's; RN to Master's.
Concentrations Available Clinical nurse leader; nursing administration; nursing education. *Nurse practitioner programs in:* adult health, family health.
Study Options Part-time.
Online Degree Options Yes.
Program Entrance Requirements Minimum overall college GPA of 3.0, transcript of college record, written essay, interview, 3 letters of recommendation, physical assessment course, resume, statistics course. *Application deadline:* 2/15 (fall). *Application fee:* $60.
Advanced Placement Credit given for nursing courses completed elsewhere dependent upon specific evaluations.

Degree Requirements 45 total credit hours, thesis or project.

POST-MASTER'S PROGRAM
Areas of Study Clinical nurse leader; nursing administration; nursing education. *Nurse practitioner programs in:* adult health, family health.

Saint Louis University
School of Nursing
St. Louis, Missouri

http://www.nursing.slu.edu
Founded in 1818
DEGREES • BSN • DNP • MSN • PHD
Nursing Program Faculty 125 (35% with doctorates).
Baccalaureate Enrollment 605 **Women** 91% **Men** 9% **Part-time** 11%
Graduate Enrollment 450 **Women** 85% **Men** 15% **Part-time** 38%
Distance Learning Courses Available.
Nursing Student Activities Nursing Honor Society, Sigma Theta Tau, Student Nurses' Association.
Nursing Student Resources Academic advising; academic or career counseling; assistance for students with disabilities; bookstore; campus computer network; career placement assistance; computer lab; computer-assisted instruction; e-mail services; employment services for current students; housing assistance; interactive nursing skills videos; Internet; learning resource lab; library services; nursing audiovisuals; remedial services; resume preparation assistance; skills, simulation, or other laboratory; tutoring; unpaid internships.
Library Facilities 275,000 volumes in health, 4,800 volumes in nursing; 8,429 periodical subscriptions health-care related.

BACCALAUREATE PROGRAMS

Degree BSN
Available Programs ADN to Baccalaureate; Accelerated Baccalaureate; Accelerated Baccalaureate for Second Degree; Accelerated RN Baccalaureate; Baccalaureate for Second Degree; Generic Baccalaureate; RN Baccalaureate; RPN to Baccalaureate.
Site Options St. Louis, MO.
Study Options Full-time and part-time.
Online Degree Options Yes.
Program Entrance Requirements Minimum overall college GPA of 3.4, transcript of college record, health exam, high school biology, high school chemistry, high school transcript, immunizations, minimum high school GPA of 3.2. Transfer students are accepted. *Application deadline:* 12/1 (fall).
Advanced Placement Credit by examination available. Credit given for nursing courses completed elsewhere dependent upon specific evaluations.
Expenses (2015–16) *Tuition:* full-time $38,700. *International tuition:* $38,700 full-time. *Room and board:* $10,336 per academic year. *Required fees:* full-time $526.
Contact Mr. Scott Ragsdale, Recruitment Specialist, School of Nursing, Saint Louis University, 3525 Caroline Street, St. Louis, MO 63104. *Telephone:* 314-977-8995. *Fax:* 314-977-8949. *E-mail:* sragsda2@slu.edu.

GRADUATE PROGRAMS

Expenses (2015–16) *Tuition:* part-time $1050 per credit hour. *International tuition:* $1050 full-time. *Required fees:* full-time $669; part-time $30 per credit; part-time $384 per term.
Financial Aid 2 research assistantships (averaging $10,250 per year), 5 teaching assistantships (averaging $11,000 per year) were awarded; Federal Work-Study, scholarships, traineeships, tuition waivers, and unspecified assistantships also available.
Contact Dr. Joanne Thanavaro, Associate Dean for Graduate Education, School of Nursing, Saint Louis University, 3525 Caroline Street, St. Louis, MO 63104. *Telephone:* 314-977-8908. *Fax:* 314-977-8949. *E-mail:* jthanava@slu.edu.

MASTER'S DEGREE PROGRAM
Degree MSN
Available Programs Accelerated Master's; Accelerated Master's for Non-Nursing College Graduates; Accelerated Master's for Nurses with Non-Nursing Degrees; Master's; Master's for Non-Nursing College Graduates; Master's for Nurses with Non-Nursing Degrees.
Concentrations Available Clinical nurse leader; nursing education. *Nurse practitioner programs in:* acute care, adult-gerontology acute care,

family health, pediatric primary care, primary care, psychiatric/mental health.
Site Options St. Louis, MO.
Study Options Full-time and part-time.
Online Degree Options Yes (online only).
Program Entrance Requirements Minimum overall college GPA of 3.25, transcript of college record, CPR certification, immunizations, 3 letters of recommendation, resume. *Application deadline:* 3/1 (fall), 8/1 (spring). *Application fee:* $55.
Advanced Placement Credit given for nursing courses completed elsewhere dependent upon specific evaluations.
Degree Requirements 41 total credit hours, comprehensive exam.

POST-MASTER'S PROGRAM

Areas of Study Clinical nurse leader; nursing education. *Nurse practitioner programs in:* acute care, adult-gerontology acute care, family health, pediatric primary care, primary care, psychiatric/mental health.

DOCTORAL DEGREE PROGRAM

Degree DNP
Available Programs Doctorate.
Areas of Study Advanced practice nursing.
Online Degree Options Yes (online only).
Program Entrance Requirements Minimum overall college GPA of 3.25, 3 letters of recommendation, MSN or equivalent, statistics course, vita, writing sample. Application deadline: 3/15 (fall). Applications may be processed on a rolling basis for some programs. Application fee: $40.
Degree Requirements 28 total credit hours, dissertation.

Degree PhD
Available Programs Doctorate; Post-Baccalaureate Doctorate.
Areas of Study Advanced practice nursing, clinical practice, nursing education, nursing research.
Site Options St. Louis, MO.
Program Entrance Requirements Minimum overall college GPA of 3.25, 3 letters of recommendation, MSN or equivalent, statistics course, vita, writing sample, GRE General Test. Application deadline: 6/1 (fall), 11/1 (spring). Applications may be processed on a rolling basis for some programs. Application fee: $55.
Degree Requirements 69 total credit hours, dissertation, oral exam, written exam, residency.

CONTINUING EDUCATION PROGRAM

Contact Mrs. Cathi Slinkard, Continuing Education Director, School of Nursing, Saint Louis University, 3525 Caroline Street, St. Louis, MO 63104. *Telephone:* 314-977-1909. *Fax:* 314-977-8949.
E-mail: cslinkar@slu.edu.

Saint Luke's College of Health Sciences
Nursing College
Kansas City, Missouri

http://www.saintlukescollege.edu/
Founded in 1903
DEGREE • BSN
Nursing Program Faculty 17 (18% with doctorates).
Baccalaureate Enrollment 115 **Women** 95% **Men** 5% **Part-time** 12%
Nursing Student Activities Student Nurses' Association.
Nursing Student Resources Academic advising; assistance for students with disabilities; bookstore; campus computer network; career placement assistance; computer lab; computer-assisted instruction; e-mail services; employment services for current students; interactive nursing skills videos; Internet; learning resource lab; library services; nursing audiovisuals; paid internships; skills, simulation, or other laboratory; tutoring.

BACCALAUREATE PROGRAMS

Degree BSN
Available Programs Generic Baccalaureate.
Site Options Kansas City, MO.
Study Options Full-time and part-time.
Program Entrance Requirements Transcript of college record, CPR certification, written essay, health exam, health insurance, high school transcript, immunizations, interview, 3 letters of recommendation,

minimum GPA in nursing prerequisites of 2.7, prerequisite course work. Transfer students are accepted.
Advanced Placement Credit given for nursing courses completed elsewhere dependent upon specific evaluations.
Contact *Telephone:* 816-932-2367.

Southeast Missouri State University
Department of Nursing
Cape Girardeau, Missouri

http://www.semo.edu/nursing
Founded in 1873
DEGREES • BSN • MSN
Nursing Program Faculty 26 (35% with doctorates).
Baccalaureate Enrollment 200 **Women** 95% **Men** 5% **Part-time** 5%
Graduate Enrollment 23 **Women** 99% **Men** 1%
Nursing Student Activities Nursing Honor Society, Sigma Theta Tau, Student Nurses' Association.
Nursing Student Resources Academic advising; academic or career counseling; assistance for students with disabilities; bookstore; campus computer network; career placement assistance; computer lab; computer-assisted instruction; e-mail services; employment services for current students; housing assistance; Internet; learning resource lab; library services; nursing audiovisuals; placement services for program completers; remedial services; resume preparation assistance; skills, simulation, or other laboratory; tutoring.
Library Facilities 450,750 volumes in health, 16,145 volumes in nursing; 75 periodical subscriptions health-care related.

BACCALAUREATE PROGRAMS

Degree BSN
Available Programs Generic Baccalaureate; RN Baccalaureate.
Study Options Full-time.
Online Degree Options Yes.
Program Entrance Requirements Minimum overall college GPA of 2.8, transcript of college record, CPR certification, health insurance, immunizations, professional liability insurance/malpractice insurance, prerequisite course work. Transfer students are accepted. *Application deadline:* 3/1 (fall), 10/1 (spring).
Expenses (2015–16) *Tuition, state resident:* full-time $7400; part-time $231 per credit hour. *Tuition, nonresident:* full-time $13,088; part-time $409 per credit hour. *International tuition:* $13,088 full-time. *Room and board:* $8300; room only: $5500 per academic year. *Required fees:* full-time $640; part-time $10 per credit; part-time $320 per term.
Contact Dr. Kathy Ham, Director of Undergraduate Studies, Department of Nursing, Southeast Missouri State University, One University Plaza, Mail Stop 8300, Cape Girardeau, MO 63701-4799. *Telephone:* 573-651-6732. *Fax:* 573-651-2142. *E-mail:* kham@semo.edu.

GRADUATE PROGRAMS

Expenses (2015–16) *Tuition, state resident:* full-time $2628; part-time $292 per credit hour. *Tuition, nonresident:* full-time $4644; part-time $394 per credit hour. *International tuition:* $4644 full-time. *Required fees:* full-time $306; part-time $17 per credit; part-time $153 per term.
Financial Aid 6 teaching assistantships (averaging $7,907 per year) were awarded; career-related internships or fieldwork, Federal Work-Study, scholarships, traineeships, tuition waivers (full), and unspecified assistantships also available.
Contact Dr. Elaine Jackson, Director, Graduate Studies, Department of Nursing, Southeast Missouri State University, One University Plaza, Mail Stop 8300, Cape Girardeau, MO 63701-4799. *Telephone:* 573-651-2871. *Fax:* 573-651-2142. *E-mail:* ejackson@semo.edu.

MASTER'S DEGREE PROGRAM

Degree MSN
Available Programs Master's.
Concentrations Available Nursing education. *Nurse practitioner programs in:* family health.
Study Options Full-time.
Program Entrance Requirements Clinical experience, minimum overall college GPA of 3.25, transcript of college record, CPR certification, written essay, immunizations, physical assessment course, profes-

sional liability insurance/malpractice insurance, prerequisite course work, resume, statistics course. *Application deadline:* 4/1 (fall).
Degree Requirements 44 total credit hours, comprehensive exam.

POST-MASTER'S PROGRAM
Areas of Study *Nurse practitioner programs in:* family health.

Southwest Baptist University
College of Nursing
Bolivar, Missouri

http://www.sbuniv.edu/collegeofnursing
Founded in 1878
DEGREES • BSN • MSN
Nursing Program Faculty 12 (25% with doctorates).
Baccalaureate Enrollment 143 **Women** 87.5% **Men** 12.5% **Part-time** 82.5%
Graduate Enrollment 31 **Women** 96.8% **Men** 3.2% **Part-time** 74.1%
Distance Learning Courses Available.
Nursing Student Activities Nursing Honor Society, Student Nurses' Association.
Nursing Student Resources Academic advising; bookstore; campus computer network; computer lab; computer-assisted instruction; e-mail services; interactive nursing skills videos; Internet; learning resource lab; library services; nursing audiovisuals; skills, simulation, or other laboratory.
Library Facilities 4,042 volumes in health, 3,602 volumes in nursing; 41,500 periodical subscriptions health-care related.

BACCALAUREATE PROGRAMS

Degree BSN
Available Programs RN Baccalaureate.
Site Options Springfield, MO.
Study Options Full-time and part-time.
Program Entrance Requirements Minimum overall college GPA of 2.5, transcript of college record, CPR certification, high school transcript, immunizations, letters of recommendation, minimum GPA in nursing prerequisites of 2.5, professional liability insurance/malpractice insurance, prerequisite course work, RN licensure. Transfer students are accepted. *Application deadline:* 8/15 (fall), 1/1 (winter), 1/15 (spring), 6/1 (summer). Applications may be processed on a rolling basis for some programs.
Advanced Placement Credit given for nursing courses completed elsewhere dependent upon specific evaluations.
Contact *Telephone:* 417-820-5060. *Fax:* 417-887-4847.

GRADUATE PROGRAMS

Contact *Telephone:* 417-820-5058. *Fax:* 417-887-4847.

MASTER'S DEGREE PROGRAM
Degree MSN
Available Programs Master's.
Concentrations Available Nursing administration; nursing education.
Site Options Springfield, MO.
Study Options Full-time and part-time.
Online Degree Options Yes.
Program Entrance Requirements Computer literacy, minimum overall college GPA of 3.0, transcript of college record, CPR certification, written essay, immunizations, letters of recommendation, nursing research course, physical assessment course, professional liability insurance/malpractice insurance, statistics course. *Application deadline:* 7/15 (fall), 1/1 (spring). Applications may be processed on a rolling basis for some programs. *Application fee:* $30.
Advanced Placement Credit given for nursing courses completed elsewhere dependent upon specific evaluations.
Degree Requirements 36 total credit hours, thesis or project, comprehensive exam.

Truman State University
Program in Nursing
Kirksville, Missouri

http://nursing.truman.edu/
Founded in 1867
DEGREE • BSN
Nursing Program Faculty 11 (18% with doctorates).
Baccalaureate Enrollment 172 **Women** 94% **Men** 6% **Part-time** 1%
Nursing Student Activities Nursing Honor Society, Sigma Theta Tau, Student Nurses' Association, nursing club.
Nursing Student Resources Academic advising; academic or career counseling; assistance for students with disabilities; bookstore; campus computer network; career placement assistance; computer lab; computer-assisted instruction; e-mail services; employment services for current students; externships; interactive nursing skills videos; Internet; learning resource lab; library services; nursing audiovisuals; paid internships; remedial services; resume preparation assistance; skills, simulation, or other laboratory; tutoring; unpaid internships.
Library Facilities 6,923 volumes in health, 1,654 volumes in nursing; 900 periodical subscriptions health-care related.

BACCALAUREATE PROGRAMS

Degree BSN
Available Programs Generic Baccalaureate.
Study Options Full-time.
Program Entrance Requirements Minimum overall college GPA of 2.75, transcript of college record, written essay, high school biology, high school chemistry, high school foreign language, 3 years high school math, 3 years high school science, high school transcript, immunizations, minimum high school GPA of 3.3, minimum GPA in nursing prerequisites of 3.0. Transfer students are accepted.
Contact *Telephone:* 660-785-4557. *Fax:* 660-785-7424.

University of Central Missouri
Department of Nursing
Warrensburg, Missouri

http://www.ucmo.edu/nursing
Founded in 1871
DEGREES • BS • MSN
Nursing Program Faculty 17 (35% with doctorates).
Baccalaureate Enrollment 156 **Women** 90% **Men** 10%
Graduate Enrollment 166 **Women** 95% **Men** 5% **Part-time** 99%
Distance Learning Courses Available.
Nursing Student Activities Nursing club.
Nursing Student Resources Academic advising; academic or career counseling; assistance for students with disabilities; bookstore; campus computer network; career placement assistance; computer lab; computer-assisted instruction; daycare for children of students; e-mail services; employment services for current students; externships; housing assistance; interactive nursing skills videos; Internet; learning resource lab; library services; nursing audiovisuals; placement services for program completers; remedial services; resume preparation assistance; skills, simulation, or other laboratory; tutoring.
Library Facilities 17,000 volumes in health, 1,000 volumes in nursing; 300 periodical subscriptions health-care related.

BACCALAUREATE PROGRAMS

Degree BS
Available Programs ADN to Baccalaureate; Generic Baccalaureate; RN Baccalaureate.
Site Options Lee's Summit, MO; Warrensburg, MO.
Study Options Full-time.
Online Degree Options Yes.
Program Entrance Requirements Minimum overall college GPA of 2.75, minimum GPA in nursing prerequisites of 2.0, prerequisite course work. Transfer students are accepted. *Application deadline:* 1/1 (fall), 7/1 (spring). *Application fee:* $30.
Advanced Placement Credit by examination available. Credit given for nursing courses completed elsewhere dependent upon specific evaluations.
Expenses (2015–16) *Tuition, state resident:* full-time $6446; part-time $215 per credit hour. *Tuition, nonresident:* full-time $12,891; part-time

$430 per credit hour. *Room and board:* $6644; room only: $5186 per academic year. *Required fees:* part-time $438 per term.

Financial Aid 90% of baccalaureate students in nursing programs received some form of financial aid in 2014–15.

Contact Dr. Julie Clawson, Chair, Department of Nursing, Department of Nursing, University of Central Missouri, UHC 106, Warrensburg, MO 64093. *Telephone:* 660-543-4775. *Fax:* 660-543-8304. *E-mail:* clawson@ucmo.edu.

GRADUATE PROGRAMS

Expenses (2015–16) *Tuition, state resident:* part-time $278 per credit hour. *Tuition, nonresident:* part-time $557 per credit hour. *Room and board:* $6644; room only: $5186 per academic year. *Required fees:* part-time $175 per term.

Financial Aid 70% of graduate students in nursing programs received some form of financial aid in 2014–15.

Contact Ms. Tina Church-Hockett, Director of the Graduate School and International Admissions, Department of Nursing, University of Central Missouri, WDE 1800, Warrensburg, MO 64093. *Telephone:* 660-543-4621. *E-mail:* church@ucmo.edu.

MASTER'S DEGREE PROGRAM

Degree MSN

Available Programs Master's.

Concentrations Available Nursing education. *Nurse practitioner programs in:* family health.

Site Options Lee's Summit, MO; Warrensburg, MO.

Study Options Part-time.

Online Degree Options Yes (online only).

Program Entrance Requirements Clinical experience, minimum overall college GPA of 3.0, transcript of college record, CPR certification, immunizations, professional liability insurance/malpractice insurance. *Application deadline:* 2/15 (fall), 9/15 (spring), 2/15 (summer).

Advanced Placement Credit given for nursing courses completed elsewhere dependent upon specific evaluations.

Degree Requirements 33 total credit hours, thesis or project.

University of Missouri
Sinclair School of Nursing
Columbia, Missouri

http://www.nursing.missouri.edu/
Founded in 1839

DEGREES • BSN • MSN • MSN/PHD • PHD

Baccalaureate Enrollment 380 **Women** 90% **Men** 10% **Part-time** 31%

Graduate Enrollment 200 **Women** 95% **Men** 5% **Part-time** 77%

Distance Learning Courses Available.

Nursing Student Activities Nursing Honor Society, Sigma Theta Tau, Student Nurses' Association, nursing club.

Nursing Student Resources Academic advising; academic or career counseling; assistance for students with disabilities; bookstore; campus computer network; career placement assistance; computer lab; computer-assisted instruction; daycare for children of students; e-mail services; employment services for current students; externships; housing assistance; interactive nursing skills videos; Internet; learning resource lab; library services; nursing audiovisuals; paid internships; remedial services; resume preparation assistance; skills, simulation, or other laboratory; tutoring; unpaid internships.

Library Facilities 114,580 volumes in health, 6,416 volumes in nursing.

BACCALAUREATE PROGRAMS

Degree BSN

Available Programs ADN to Baccalaureate; Accelerated Baccalaureate; Accelerated Baccalaureate for Second Degree; Generic Baccalaureate; RN Baccalaureate.

Study Options Full-time and part-time.

Online Degree Options Yes.

Program Entrance Requirements Minimum overall college GPA of 2.5, transcript of college record, CPR certification, high school biology, high school chemistry, 4 years high school math, 3 years high school science, high school transcript, immunizations, interview, minimum GPA in nursing prerequisites of 2.5, prerequisite course work. Transfer students are accepted.

Advanced Placement Credit by examination available. Credit given for nursing courses completed elsewhere dependent upon specific evaluations.

Contact *Telephone:* 573-882-0277. *Fax:* 573-884-4544.

GRADUATE PROGRAMS

Contact *Telephone:* 573-882-0277.

MASTER'S DEGREE PROGRAM

Degrees MSN; MSN/PhD

Available Programs Master's.

Concentrations Available Nursing administration; nursing education. *Clinical nurse specialist programs in:* acute care, adult health, cardiovascular, community health, critical care, home health care, maternity-newborn, oncology, palliative care, pediatric, public health, rehabilitation, school health, women's health. *Nurse practitioner programs in:* family health, gerontology, pediatric, primary care, psychiatric/mental health.

Study Options Full-time and part-time.

Online Degree Options Yes (online only).

Program Entrance Requirements Computer literacy, minimum overall college GPA of 3.0, transcript of college record, CPR certification, immunizations, interview, 2 letters of recommendation, nursing research course, prerequisite course work, statistics course, GRE General Test.

Advanced Placement Credit given for nursing courses completed elsewhere dependent upon specific evaluations.

Degree Requirements 43 total credit hours, comprehensive exam.

POST-MASTER'S PROGRAM

Areas of Study Nursing administration; nursing education. *Clinical nurse specialist programs in:* acute care, adult health, cardiovascular, community health, critical care, home health care, maternity-newborn, oncology, palliative care, pediatric, public health, rehabilitation, school health, women's health. *Nurse practitioner programs in:* family health, gerontology, pediatric, primary care, psychiatric/mental health.

DOCTORAL DEGREE PROGRAM

Degree PhD

Available Programs Doctorate; Post-Baccalaureate Doctorate.

Areas of Study Aging, family health, gerontology, health promotion/disease prevention, health-care systems, human health and illness, nursing research, oncology, women's health.

Program Entrance Requirements Minimum overall college GPA of 3.5, interview by faculty committee, 3 letters of recommendation, vita, writing sample.

Degree Requirements 72 total credit hours, dissertation, oral exam, written exam, residency.

CONTINUING EDUCATION PROGRAM

Contact *Telephone:* 573-882-0215. *Fax:* 573-884-4544.

University of Missouri–Kansas City
School of Nursing and Health Studies
Kansas City, Missouri

http://www.umkc.edu/nursing
Founded in 1929

DEGREES • BSN • DNP • MSN • PHD

Nursing Program Faculty 99 (44% with doctorates).

Baccalaureate Enrollment 569 **Women** 85% **Men** 15% **Part-time** 40%

Graduate Enrollment 389 **Women** 88% **Men** 12% **Part-time** 87%

Distance Learning Courses Available.

Nursing Student Activities Sigma Theta Tau, Student Nurses' Association.

Nursing Student Resources Academic advising; academic or career counseling; assistance for students with disabilities; bookstore; campus computer network; career placement assistance; computer lab; computer-assisted instruction; e-mail services; employment services for current students; housing assistance; interactive nursing skills videos; Internet; learning resource lab; library services; nursing audiovisuals; other; paid internships; placement services for program completers; remedial services; resume preparation assistance; skills, simulation, or other laboratory; tutoring.

Library Facilities 118,853 volumes in health; 32,569 periodical subscriptions health-care related.

BACCALAUREATE PROGRAMS

Degree BSN
Available Programs Accelerated Baccalaureate for Second Degree; Generic Baccalaureate; RN Baccalaureate.
Study Options Full-time.
Online Degree Options Yes.
Program Entrance Requirements Transcript of college record, CPR certification, written essay, health insurance, immunizations, 1 letter of recommendation, minimum GPA in nursing prerequisites of 2.75, prerequisite course work. Transfer students are accepted. *Application deadline:* 1/31 (fall). *Application fee:* $55.
Expenses (2014–15) *Tuition, state resident:* full-time $6482; part-time $270 per credit hour. *Tuition, nonresident:* full-time $23,412; part-time $976 per credit hour. *International tuition:* $23,412 full-time. *Room and board:* $9284; room only: $8015 per academic year. *Required fees:* full-time $1980; part-time $67 per credit; part-time $439 per term.
Financial Aid 30% of baccalaureate students in nursing programs received some form of financial aid in 2013–14. *Gift aid (need-based):* Federal Pell, FSEOG, state, private, college/university gift aid from institutional funds, United Negro College Fund, Federal Nursing. *Loans:* Federal Nursing Student Loans, Federal Direct (Subsidized and Unsubsidized Stafford PLUS), Perkins, state, college/university. *Work-study:* Federal Work-Study. *Financial aid application deadline (priority):* 3/1.
Contact Mrs. Judy A. Jellison, Director, Nursing Student Services, School of Nursing and Health Studies, University of Missouri–Kansas City, 2464 Charlotte Street, Kansas City, MO 64108. *Telephone:* 816-235-1740. *Fax:* 816-235-6593. *E-mail:* jellisonj@umkc.edu.

GRADUATE PROGRAMS

Expenses (2014–15) *Tuition, state resident:* full-time $8220; part-time $343 per credit hour. *Tuition, nonresident:* full-time $8220; part-time $343 per credit hour. *International tuition:* $8220 full-time. *Room and board:* $9284; room only: $8015 per academic year. *Required fees:* full-time $512; part-time $14 per credit; part-time $226 per term.
Financial Aid 56% of graduate students in nursing programs received some form of financial aid in 2013–14. 3 teaching assistantships with partial tuition reimbursements available (averaging $9,233 per year) were awarded; fellowships, research assistantships, career-related internships or fieldwork, Federal Work-Study, institutionally sponsored loans, and tuition waivers (full and partial) also available. Aid available to part-time students. *Financial aid application deadline:* 3/1.
Contact Mrs. Judy A. Jellison, Director, Nursing Student Services, School of Nursing and Health Studies, University of Missouri–Kansas City, 2464 Charlotte Street, Kansas City, MO 64108. *Telephone:* 816-235-1740. *Fax:* 816-235-6593. *E-mail:* jellisonj@umkc.edu.

MASTER'S DEGREE PROGRAM
Degree MSN
Available Programs Master's.
Concentrations Available Nursing education. *Nurse practitioner programs in:* neonatal health, psychiatric/mental health.
Study Options Full-time and part-time.
Program Entrance Requirements Clinical experience, computer literacy, minimum overall college GPA of 3.2, transcript of college record, CPR certification, written essay, immunizations, 3 letters of recommendation, physical assessment course, prerequisite course work, resume, statistics course. *Application deadline:* 12/1 (fall), 12/1 (summer). *Application fee:* $60.
Degree Requirements 43 total credit hours.

POST-MASTER'S PROGRAM
Areas of Study *Nurse practitioner programs in:* neonatal health, psychiatric/mental health, women's health.

DOCTORAL DEGREE PROGRAM
Degree DNP
Available Programs Doctorate, Post-Baccalaureate Doctorate.
Areas of Study Family health, gerontology, nurse anesthesia, pediatric, women's health.
Online Degree Options Yes (varies by program).
Program Entrance Requirements Minimum overall college GPA of 3.5 for individualized clinical project, 3.2 for all others. Application deadline: 2/1 (individualized clinical project), 12/15 (all others).
Degree Requirements 73-74 total credit hours, depending on program chosen; 31 credit hours for individualized clinical project.

Degree PhD
Available Programs Doctorate; Doctorate for Nurses with Non-Nursing Degrees; Post-Baccalaureate Doctorate.
Areas of Study Biology of health and illness, community health, family health, health promotion/disease prevention, human health and illness, individualized study, nursing education, nursing policy, nursing research, nursing science, women's health.
Site Options St. Joseph, MO.
Online Degree Options Yes (online only).
Program Entrance Requirements Minimum overall college GPA of 3.5, interview by faculty committee, interview, 3 letters of recommendation, MSN or equivalent, vita, writing sample, GRE. Application deadline: 2/1 (summer). Application fee: $60.
Degree Requirements 61 total credit hours, dissertation, oral exam, written exam, residency.

CONTINUING EDUCATION PROGRAM

Contact Jodi M. Baker, Continuing Education Coordinator, School of Nursing and Health Studies, University of Missouri–Kansas City, 2464 Charlotte Street, Kansas City, MO 64108. *Telephone:* 816-235-6463. *Fax:* 816-235-1701. *E-mail:* bakerjm@umkc.edu.

University of Missouri–St. Louis
College of Nursing
St. Louis, Missouri

http://www.umsl.edu/divisions/nursing/
Founded in 1963
DEGREES • BSN • DNP • MSN • PHD
Nursing Program Faculty 89 (28% with doctorates).
Baccalaureate Enrollment 840 **Women** 88% **Men** 12% **Part-time** 35%
Graduate Enrollment 245 **Women** 95% **Men** 5% **Part-time** 93%
Distance Learning Courses Available.
Nursing Student Activities Nursing Honor Society, Sigma Theta Tau, Student Nurses' Association.
Nursing Student Resources Academic advising; academic or career counseling; assistance for students with disabilities; bookstore; campus computer network; career placement assistance; computer lab; computer-assisted instruction; daycare for children of students; e-mail services; employment services for current students; externships; interactive nursing skills videos; Internet; learning resource lab; library services; nursing audiovisuals; remedial services; resume preparation assistance; skills, simulation, or other laboratory; tutoring; unpaid internships.
Library Facilities 88,762 volumes in health, 17,937 volumes in nursing; 8,515 periodical subscriptions health-care related.

BACCALAUREATE PROGRAMS

Degree BSN
Available Programs Accelerated Baccalaureate; Accelerated Baccalaureate for Second Degree; Generic Baccalaureate; RN Baccalaureate.
Site Options St. Charles, MO; St. Louis, MO.
Study Options Full-time and part-time.
Online Degree Options Yes.
Program Entrance Requirements Minimum overall college GPA of 2.5, transcript of college record, CPR certification, health exam, health insurance, high school foreign language, 4 years high school math, 3 years high school science, high school transcript, immunizations, minimum high school GPA of 2.8, minimum GPA in nursing prerequisites, prerequisite course work. Transfer students are accepted. *Application deadline:* 2/1 (fall), 10/1 (spring), 9/15 (summer). *Application fee:* $35.
Expenses (2015–16) *Tuition, state resident:* full-time $10,065; part-time $336 per credit hour. *Tuition, nonresident:* full-time $25,512; part-time $850 per credit hour. *International tuition:* $25,512 full-time. *Room and board:* $9052; room only: $5280 per academic year. *Required fees:* part-time $196 per credit.
Financial Aid *Gift aid (need-based):* Federal Pell, FSEOG, state, private, college/university gift aid from institutional funds, United Negro College Fund, Federal Nursing, TEACH Grants. *Loans:* Federal Nursing Student Loans, Federal Direct (Subsidized and Unsubsidized Stafford PLUS), Perkins, state. *Work-study:* Federal Work-Study. *Financial aid application deadline (priority):* 3/1.
Contact Student Services, College of Nursing, University of Missouri–St. Louis, One University Boulevard, Nursing Administration Building, St. Louis, MO 63121-4400. *Telephone:* 314-516-6066. *Fax:* 314-516-7519. *E-mail:* nursing@umsl.edu.

GRADUATE PROGRAMS

Expenses (2015–16) *Tuition, state resident:* full-time $10,459; part-time $436 per credit hour. *Tuition, nonresident:* full-time $25,176; part-time $1049 per credit hour. *International tuition:* $25,176 full-time. *Room and board:* $9052; room only: $5280 per academic year.
Financial Aid 1 research assistantship (averaging $10,800 per year) was awarded.
Contact Student Services, College of Nursing, University of Missouri–St. Louis, One University Boulevard, Nursing Administration Building, St. Louis, MO 63121-4400. *Telephone:* 314-516-6066. *Fax:* 314-516-7519. *E-mail:* nursing@umsl.edu.

MASTER'S DEGREE PROGRAM
Degree MSN
Available Programs Master's.
Concentrations Available Nursing education. *Nurse practitioner programs in:* adult-gerontology acute care, family health, pediatric, psychiatric/mental health, women's health.
Site Options Park Hills, MO; St. Charles, MO.
Study Options Part-time.
Program Entrance Requirements Clinical experience, minimum overall college GPA of 3.0, transcript of college record, CPR certification, written essay, immunizations, 2 letters of recommendation, physical assessment course, prerequisite course work, resume, statistics course. *Application deadline:* 2/15 (fall). *Application fee:* $50.
Degree Requirements 43 total credit hours.

POST-MASTER'S PROGRAM
Areas of Study Nursing education. *Nurse practitioner programs in:* adult-gerontology acute care, family health, pediatric primary care, psychiatric/mental health, women's health.

DOCTORAL DEGREE PROGRAM
Degree DNP
Available Programs Doctorate; Post-Baccalaureate Doctorate.
Areas of Study Advanced practice nursing.
Program Entrance Requirements Minimum overall college GPA of 3.3, interview by faculty committee, 2 letters of recommendation, statistics course, writing sample, GRE. Application deadline: 4/1 (fall). Application fee: $50.
Degree Requirements 57 total credit hours.

Degree PhD
Available Programs Doctorate, Post-Baccalaureate Doctorate.
Areas of Study Nursing research.
Program Entrance Requirements Minimum overall college GPA of 3.2, interview by faculty committee, 2 letters of recommendation, statistics course, vita, writing sample. Application deadline: 4/1 (fall). Application fee: $50.
Degree Requirements 65 total credit hours, dissertation.

Webster University
Department of Nursing
St. Louis, Missouri

http://www.webster.edu/arts-and-sciences/academics/nursing/nursing.html
Founded in 1915
DEGREES • BSN • MSN
Nursing Program Faculty 12 (72% with doctorates).
Baccalaureate Enrollment 150 **Women** 93% **Men** 7% **Part-time** 90%
Graduate Enrollment 75 **Women** 90% **Men** 10% **Part-time** 100%
Nursing Student Activities Nursing Honor Society, Sigma Theta Tau.
Nursing Student Resources Academic advising; academic or career counseling; assistance for students with disabilities; bookstore; campus computer network; career placement assistance; computer lab; e-mail services; employment services for current students; Internet; learning resource lab; library services; nursing audiovisuals; placement services for program completers; remedial services; resume preparation assistance; skills, simulation, or other laboratory; tutoring.
Library Facilities 7,030 volumes in health, 3,114 volumes in nursing; 108 periodical subscriptions health-care related.

BACCALAUREATE PROGRAMS
Degree BSN
Available Programs ADN to Baccalaureate; RN Baccalaureate.

Site Options Kansas City, MO.
Program Entrance Requirements Minimum overall college GPA of 2.5, transcript of college record, immunizations, interview, prerequisite course work, RN licensure. Transfer students are accepted.
Contact *Telephone:* 314-968-7483. *Fax:* 314-963-6101.

GRADUATE PROGRAMS
Contact *Telephone:* 314-968-7483. *Fax:* 314-963-6101.

MASTER'S DEGREE PROGRAM
Degree MSN
Available Programs Master's; RN to Master's.
Concentrations Available Nursing administration; nursing education. *Clinical nurse specialist programs in:* family health.
Site Options Kansas City, MO.
Study Options Part-time.
Program Entrance Requirements Clinical experience, computer literacy, minimum overall college GPA of 3.0, transcript of college record, written essay, immunizations, interview, 3 letters of recommendation, nursing research course, physical assessment course, resume, statistics course.
Advanced Placement Credit given for nursing courses completed elsewhere dependent upon specific evaluations.
Degree Requirements 36 total credit hours, thesis or project.

William Jewell College
Department of Nursing
Liberty, Missouri

http://www.jewell.edu/
Founded in 1849
DEGREE • BS
Nursing Program Faculty 36 (25% with doctorates).
Baccalaureate Enrollment 210 **Women** 89% **Men** 11%
Distance Learning Courses Available.
Nursing Student Activities Nursing Honor Society, Sigma Theta Tau, Student Nurses' Association.
Nursing Student Resources Academic advising; academic or career counseling; assistance for students with disabilities; bookstore; campus computer network; career placement assistance; computer lab; computer-assisted instruction; e-mail services; employment services for current students; externships; housing assistance; interactive nursing skills videos; Internet; learning resource lab; library services; nursing audiovisuals; paid internships; placement services for program completers; resume preparation assistance; skills, simulation, or other laboratory; tutoring; unpaid internships.
Library Facilities 3,093 volumes in health, 1,440 volumes in nursing; 23,579 periodical subscriptions health-care related.

BACCALAUREATE PROGRAMS
Degree BS
Available Programs Accelerated Baccalaureate; Accelerated Baccalaureate for Second Degree; Generic Baccalaureate; RN Baccalaureate.
Study Options Full-time.
Online Degree Options Yes (online only).
Program Entrance Requirements Minimum overall college GPA of 2.7, transcript of college record, CPR certification, written essay, health insurance, high school transcript, immunizations, interview, 2 letters of recommendation, minimum high school GPA of 3.0, minimum GPA in nursing prerequisites of 2.7, professional liability insurance/malpractice insurance, prerequisite course work. Transfer students are accepted. *Application deadline:* 6/1 (fall), 12/1 (winter), 12/1 (spring), 3/1 (summer). Applications may be processed on a rolling basis for some programs. *Application fee:* $25.
Advanced Placement Credit given for nursing courses completed elsewhere dependent upon specific evaluations.
Expenses (2015–16) *Tuition:* full-time $31,730; part-time $480 per credit hour. *Room and board:* $8880; room only: $4950 per academic year. *Required fees:* full-time $2000; part-time $125 per term.
Financial Aid 95% of baccalaureate students in nursing programs received some form of financial aid in 2014–15.
Contact Ms. Katie A. Stiles, Nursing Admissions Counselor, Department of Nursing, William Jewell College, 500 College Hill, Box 2002, Liberty, MO 64068. *Telephone:* 816-415-5072. *Fax:* 816-415-5024.
E-mail: stilesk@william.jewell.edu.

MONTANA

Carroll College
Department of Nursing
Helena, Montana

http://www.carroll.edu/academics/majors/nursing/
Founded in 1909

DEGREE • BS

Nursing Program Faculty 18 (5% with doctorates).
Baccalaureate Enrollment 125 **Women** 94% **Men** 6% **Part-time** 2%
Nursing Student Activities Nursing Honor Society, Sigma Theta Tau, Student Nurses' Association, nursing club.
Nursing Student Resources Academic advising; academic or career counseling; assistance for students with disabilities; bookstore; campus computer network; career placement assistance; computer lab; computer-assisted instruction; e-mail services; employment services for current students; externships; housing assistance; interactive nursing skills videos; Internet; learning resource lab; library services; nursing audiovisuals; paid internships; placement services for program completers; remedial services; resume preparation assistance; skills, simulation, or other laboratory; tutoring; unpaid internships.
Library Facilities 1,000 volumes in health, 150 volumes in nursing; 9,000 periodical subscriptions health-care related.

BACCALAUREATE PROGRAMS

Degree BS
Available Programs Generic Baccalaureate.
Study Options Full-time.
Program Entrance Requirements Minimum overall college GPA of 2.75, transcript of college record, health insurance, high school transcript, immunizations, minimum GPA in nursing prerequisites of 2.75, prerequisite course work. Transfer students are accepted. *Application deadline:* 3/1 (spring).
Expenses (2015–16) *Tuition:* full-time $30,104; part-time $1254 per credit. *International tuition:* $30,104 full-time. *Room and board:* $4688; room only: $4530 per academic year. *Required fees:* full-time $1600; part-time $800 per term.
Financial Aid 99% of baccalaureate students in nursing programs received some form of financial aid in 2014–15.
Contact Ms. Cynthia Thornquist, Director of Admissions and Enrollment, Department of Nursing, Carroll College, 1601 North Benton Avenue, Helena, MT 59625. *Telephone:* 406-447-4384. *Fax:* 406-447-4533. *E-mail:* cthornqu@carroll.edu.

Montana State University
College of Nursing
Bozeman, Montana

http://www.montana.edu/nursing
Founded in 1893

DEGREES • BSN • DNP • MN

Nursing Program Faculty 103 (30% with doctorates).
Baccalaureate Enrollment 934 **Women** 87% **Men** 13% **Part-time** 17.6%
Graduate Enrollment 70 **Women** 95% **Men** 5% **Part-time** 34.1%
Distance Learning Courses Available.
Nursing Student Activities Sigma Theta Tau, Student Nurses' Association.
Nursing Student Resources Academic advising; academic or career counseling; assistance for students with disabilities; bookstore; campus computer network; career placement assistance; computer lab; computer-assisted instruction; daycare for children of students; e-mail services; employment services for current students; housing assistance; Internet; library services; nursing audiovisuals; paid internships; placement services for program completers; remedial services; resume preparation assistance; skills, simulation, or other laboratory; tutoring; unpaid internships.
Library Facilities 30,350 volumes in health, 2,172 volumes in nursing; 1,910 periodical subscriptions health-care related.

BACCALAUREATE PROGRAMS

Degree BSN

Available Programs Accelerated Baccalaureate for Second Degree; Baccalaureate for Second Degree; Generic Baccalaureate; LPN to Baccalaureate.
Site Options Billings, MT; Great Falls, MT; Missoula, MT.
Study Options Full-time and part-time.
Program Entrance Requirements Minimum overall college GPA of 2.75, transcript of college record, CPR certification, health insurance, high school transcript, immunizations, minimum high school GPA of 2.5, minimum high school rank 50%, minimum GPA in nursing prerequisites of 2.75. Transfer students are accepted. *Application deadline:* 8/1 (fall), 1/1 (spring), 5/1 (summer). Applications may be processed on a rolling basis for some programs. *Application fee:* $30.
Advanced Placement Credit by examination available. Credit given for nursing courses completed elsewhere dependent upon specific evaluations.
Financial Aid *Gift aid (need-based):* Federal Pell, FSEOG, state, private, college/university gift aid from institutional funds, Federal Nursing. *Loans:* Federal Nursing Student Loans, Federal Direct (Subsidized and Unsubsidized Stafford PLUS), Perkins, college/university. *Work-study:* Federal Work-Study, part-time campus jobs. *Financial aid application deadline (priority):* 3/1.
Contact Dr. Teresa Seright, Associate Dean, College of Nursing, Montana State University, 111 Sherrick Hall, PO Box 173560, Bozeman, MT 59717-3560. *Telephone:* 406-994-5726. *Fax:* 406-994-6020. *E-mail:* teresa.seright@montana.edu.

GRADUATE PROGRAMS

Financial Aid 8 teaching assistantships (averaging $7,050 per year) were awarded; scholarships, traineeships, and tuition waivers (partial) also available.
Contact Ms. Kate Hallowell, Graduate Program Assistant, College of Nursing, Montana State University, 122 Sherrick Hall, PO Box 173560, Bozeman, MT 59717-3560. *Telephone:* 406-994-3500. *Fax:* 406-994-6020. *E-mail:* khallowell@montana.edu.

MASTER'S DEGREE PROGRAM

Degree MN
Available Programs Master's.
Concentrations Available Clinical nurse leader.
Study Options Full-time and part-time.
Program Entrance Requirements Computer literacy, minimum overall college GPA of 3.0, transcript of college record, CPR certification, written essay, immunizations, interview, 3 letters of recommendation, nursing research course, physical assessment course, prerequisite course work, statistics course, GRE General Test. *Application deadline:* 2/15 (fall). *Application fee:* $60.
Advanced Placement Credit given for nursing courses completed elsewhere dependent upon specific evaluations.
Degree Requirements 34 total credit hours, thesis or project, comprehensive exam.

POST-MASTER'S PROGRAM

Areas of Study Nursing education.

DOCTORAL DEGREE PROGRAM

Degree DNP
Available Programs Doctorate; Post-Baccalaureate Doctorate.
Areas of Study Advanced practice nursing.
Program Entrance Requirements Minimum overall college GPA of 3.0, interview by faculty committee, 3 letters of recommendation, statistics course, vita, writing sample. Application deadline: 2/15 (fall). Application fee: $60.
Degree Requirements 65 total credit hours.

Montana State University–Northern
College of Nursing
Havre, Montana

http://www.msun.edu/academics/nursing
Founded in 1929

DEGREE • BSN

Nursing Program Faculty 12 (8% with doctorates).
Baccalaureate Enrollment 53 **Women** 96% **Men** 4% **Part-time** 92%
Distance Learning Courses Available.
Nursing Student Activities Nursing club.

Nursing Student Resources Academic advising; academic or career counseling; assistance for students with disabilities; bookstore; campus computer network; career placement assistance; computer lab; computer-assisted instruction; e-mail services; employment services for current students; housing assistance; interactive nursing skills videos; Internet; learning resource lab; library services; nursing audiovisuals; remedial services; resume preparation assistance; skills, simulation, or other laboratory; tutoring.

Library Facilities 2,600 volumes in health, 1,300 volumes in nursing; 40 periodical subscriptions health-care related.

BACCALAUREATE PROGRAMS

Degree BSN

Available Programs ADN to Baccalaureate; RN Baccalaureate.

Site Options Great Falls, MT; Lewistown, MT.

Study Options Full-time and part-time.

Online Degree Options Yes (online only).

Program Entrance Requirements Minimum overall college GPA of 2.25, transcript of college record, CPR certification, health exam, health insurance, immunizations, professional liability insurance/malpractice insurance, prerequisite course work, RN licensure. Transfer students are accepted. *Application deadline:* 8/1 (fall), 1/10 (winter), 5/2 (summer). Applications may be processed on a rolling basis for some programs. *Application fee:* $30.

Advanced Placement Credit given for nursing courses completed elsewhere dependent upon specific evaluations.

Contact *Telephone:* 406-265-4196 Ext. 4196. *Fax:* 406-265-3772.

Montana Tech of The University of Montana
Bachelor of Science in Registered Nursing
Butte, Montana

http://www.mtech.edu/academics/clsps/nursing/
Founded in 1895
DEGREE • BS

BACCALAUREATE PROGRAMS

Degree BS

Available Programs RN Baccalaureate.

Contact Nursing Department, Bachelor of Science in Registered Nursing, Montana Tech of The University of Montana, 1300 West Park Street, Butte, MT 59701. *Telephone:* 406-496-4390.

Salish Kootenai College
Nursing Department
Pablo, Montana

Founded in 1977
DEGREE • BS
Nursing Program Faculty 7
Nursing Student Activities Nursing club.
Nursing Student Resources Academic advising; academic or career counseling; bookstore; computer lab; daycare for children of students; employment services for current students; Internet; library services.

BACCALAUREATE PROGRAMS

Degree BS

Available Programs RN Baccalaureate.

Study Options Full-time and part-time.

Program Entrance Requirements Transcript of college record, CPR certification, health exam, health insurance, high school biology, high school chemistry, 2 years high school math, 2 years high school science, high school transcript, immunizations, minimum high school GPA of 2.5, professional liability insurance/malpractice insurance, prerequisite course work, RN licensure.

Contact *Telephone:* 406-275-4800.

NEBRASKA

Bryan College of Health Sciences
School of Nursing
Lincoln, Nebraska

http://www.bryanhealth.com/collegeofhealthsciences
DEGREES • BSN • EDD • MSN
Nursing Program Faculty 30 (7% with doctorates).
Baccalaureate Enrollment 488 **Women** 91.8% **Men** 8.2% **Part-time** 50.6%
Graduate Enrollment 79 **Women** 63.3% **Men** 36.7% **Part-time** 13.9%
Distance Learning Courses Available.
Nursing Student Activities Sigma Theta Tau, Student Nurses' Association.
Nursing Student Resources Academic advising; academic or career counseling; assistance for students with disabilities; campus computer network; career placement assistance; computer lab; computer-assisted instruction; e-mail services; employment services for current students; housing assistance; interactive nursing skills videos; Internet; learning resource lab; library services; nursing audiovisuals; other; remedial services; resume preparation assistance; skills, simulation, or other laboratory; tutoring.
Library Facilities 2,500 volumes in health, 2,000 volumes in nursing; 6,000 periodical subscriptions health-care related.

BACCALAUREATE PROGRAMS

Degree BSN

Available Programs Generic Baccalaureate; RN Baccalaureate.

Study Options Full-time.

Program Entrance Requirements Minimum overall college GPA of 2.5, transcript of college record, CPR certification, written essay, health insurance, high school chemistry, high school foreign language, 3 years high school math, 3 years high school science, high school transcript, immunizations, interview, 2 letters of recommendation, minimum high school GPA of 2.75, minimum GPA in nursing prerequisites of 2.5, professional liability insurance/malpractice insurance. Transfer students are accepted. *Application deadline:* 1/15 (fall), 6/1 (spring). *Application fee:* $50.

Advanced Placement Credit given for nursing courses completed elsewhere dependent upon specific evaluations.

Expenses (2015–16) *Tuition:* full-time $12,360; part-time $515 per credit hour. *Required fees:* full-time $720; part-time $360 per credit.

Contact Kelli Backman, Director of Enrollment, School of Nursing, Bryan College of Health Sciences, 5035 Everett Street, Lincoln, NE 68505. *Telephone:* 402-481-8698. *Fax:* 402-481-8421. *E-mail:* kelli.backman@bryanhealth.org.

GRADUATE PROGRAMS

Expenses (2015–16) *Tuition:* part-time $485 per credit hour. *Required fees:* part-time $30 per credit.

Financial Aid 100% of graduate students in nursing programs received some form of financial aid in 2014–15.

Contact Dr. Marcia Kube, RN, Dean of Graduate Nursing and Health Professions, School of Nursing, Bryan College of Health Sciences, 5035 Everett Street, Lincoln, NE 68506. *Telephone:* 402-481-8845. *Fax:* 402-481-8404. *E-mail:* marcia.kube@bryanhealth.org.

MASTER'S DEGREE PROGRAM
Degree MSN

Available Programs Master's.

Concentrations Available Nursing administration; nursing education.

Study Options Full-time and part-time.

Program Entrance Requirements Minimum overall college GPA of 3.0, transcript of college record, written essay, immunizations, 2 letters of recommendation, prerequisite course work. *Application deadline:* 5/30 (fall), 10/31 (spring). *Application fee:* $75.

Degree Requirements 36 total credit hours, thesis or project.

DOCTORAL DEGREE PROGRAM
Degree EdD

Available Programs Doctorate.

Areas of Study Nursing education.

Program Entrance Requirements Minimum overall college GPA of 3.0, interview by faculty committee, 2 letters of recommendation, MSN or equivalent, writing sample. Application deadline: 5/30 (fall), 10/31 (spring). Application fee: $75.

Degree Requirements 54 total credit hours, dissertation.

Clarkson College
Master of Science in Nursing Program
Omaha, Nebraska

http://www.clarksoncollege.edu/academics/nursing/
Founded in 1888
DEGREES • BSN • MSN
Nursing Program Faculty 42 (6% with doctorates).
Baccalaureate Enrollment 500 **Women** 90% **Men** 10% **Part-time** 15%
Graduate Enrollment 200 **Women** 90% **Men** 10% **Part-time** 50%
Distance Learning Courses Available.
Nursing Student Activities Sigma Theta Tau, Student Nurses' Association.
Nursing Student Resources Academic advising; academic or career counseling; assistance for students with disabilities; bookstore; campus computer network; career placement assistance; computer lab; computer-assisted instruction; daycare for children of students; e-mail services; employment services for current students; interactive nursing skills videos; Internet; learning resource lab; library services; nursing audiovisuals; placement services for program completers; resume preparation assistance; skills, simulation, or other laboratory; tutoring.
Library Facilities 7,500 volumes in health, 2,200 volumes in nursing; 600 periodical subscriptions health-care related.

BACCALAUREATE PROGRAMS

Degree BSN
Available Programs ADN to Baccalaureate; Accelerated RN Baccalaureate; Baccalaureate for Second Degree; Generic Baccalaureate; LPN to Baccalaureate; LPN to RN Baccalaureate; RN Baccalaureate.
Study Options Full-time and part-time.
Online Degree Options Yes.
Program Entrance Requirements Minimum overall college GPA of 2.5, transcript of college record, CPR certification, written essay, health exam, health insurance, 2 years high school math, 2 years high school science, high school transcript, immunizations, minimum high school GPA of 2.5, minimum high school rank 50%. Transfer students are accepted. *Application fee:* $35.
Advanced Placement Credit given for nursing courses completed elsewhere dependent upon specific evaluations.
Contact *Telephone:* 402-552-3100. *Fax:* 402-552-6057.

GRADUATE PROGRAMS

Contact *Telephone:* 800-647-5500. *Fax:* 402-552-6057.

MASTER'S DEGREE PROGRAM
Degree MSN
Available Programs Master's; RN to Master's.
Concentrations Available Health-care administration; nurse anesthesia; nursing administration; nursing education. *Nurse practitioner programs in:* adult health, family health.
Study Options Full-time and part-time.
Online Degree Options Yes (online only).
Program Entrance Requirements Clinical experience, minimum overall college GPA of 3.0, transcript of college record, written essay, 2 letters of recommendation, resume. *Application deadline:* 7/1 (fall), 11/15 (spring), 4/1 (summer). *Application fee:* $35.
Advanced Placement Credit given for nursing courses completed elsewhere dependent upon specific evaluations.
Degree Requirements 46 total credit hours, thesis or project.

POST-MASTER'S PROGRAM
Areas of Study Health-care administration; nurse anesthesia; nursing administration; nursing education. *Nurse practitioner programs in:* adult health, family health.

CONTINUING EDUCATION PROGRAM

Contact *Telephone:* 402-552-3100. *Fax:* 402-552-6057.

College of Saint Mary
Division of Health Care Professions
Omaha, Nebraska

http://www.csm.edu/
Founded in 1923
DEGREES • BSN • MSN
Nursing Program Faculty 18 (6% with doctorates).
Baccalaureate Enrollment 45 **Women** 100% **Part-time** 65%
Graduate Enrollment 20 **Women** 100% **Part-time** 50%
Distance Learning Courses Available.
Nursing Student Activities Nursing Honor Society, Sigma Theta Tau, Student Nurses' Association, nursing club.
Nursing Student Resources Academic advising; academic or career counseling; assistance for students with disabilities; bookstore; campus computer network; career placement assistance; computer lab; computer-assisted instruction; daycare for children of students; e-mail services; employment services for current students; housing assistance; interactive nursing skills videos; Internet; learning resource lab; library services; nursing audiovisuals; other; placement services for program completers; remedial services; resume preparation assistance; skills, simulation, or other laboratory; tutoring; unpaid internships.
Library Facilities 30 volumes in health, 30 volumes in nursing; 100 periodical subscriptions health-care related.

BACCALAUREATE PROGRAMS

Degree BSN
Available Programs ADN to Baccalaureate; Generic Baccalaureate; LPN to Baccalaureate.
Study Options Full-time and part-time.
Program Entrance Requirements Minimum overall college GPA of 2.75, transcript of college record, CPR certification, health exam, health insurance, high school biology, high school chemistry, high school foreign language, high school transcript, immunizations, minimum high school GPA of 3.0, minimum GPA in nursing prerequisites of 2.75. Transfer students are accepted.
Contact *Telephone:* 402-399-2400.

GRADUATE PROGRAMS

Contact *Telephone:* 402-399-2400.

MASTER'S DEGREE PROGRAM
Degree MSN
Available Programs Master's.
Concentrations Available Nursing education.
Study Options Full-time and part-time.
Program Entrance Requirements Computer literacy, minimum overall college GPA of 3.0, transcript of college record, CPR certification, immunizations, prerequisite course work. *Application deadline:* Applications may be processed on a rolling basis for some programs.
Degree Requirements Thesis or project.

Creighton University
College of Nursing
Omaha, Nebraska

http://www.creighton.edu/nursing/
Founded in 1878
DEGREES • BSN • DNP • MSN
Nursing Program Faculty 47 (53% with doctorates).
Baccalaureate Enrollment 482 **Women** 90% **Men** 10% **Part-time** 4.35%
Graduate Enrollment 347 **Women** 92% **Men** 8% **Part-time** 37.75%
Distance Learning Courses Available.
Nursing Student Activities Nursing Honor Society, Sigma Theta Tau, Student Nurses' Association, nursing club.
Nursing Student Resources Academic advising; academic or career counseling; assistance for students with disabilities; bookstore; campus computer network; career placement assistance; computer lab; computer-assisted instruction; daycare for children of students; e-mail services; employment services for current students; Internet; learning resource lab; library services; nursing audiovisuals; remedial services; resume preparation assistance; skills, simulation, or other laboratory; tutoring; unpaid internships.

Library Facilities 31,370 volumes in health, 2,012 volumes in nursing; 9,369 periodical subscriptions health-care related.

BACCALAUREATE PROGRAMS

Degree BSN

Available Programs Accelerated Baccalaureate for Second Degree; Generic Baccalaureate.

Site Options Hastings, NE.

Study Options Full-time and part-time.

Program Entrance Requirements Minimum overall college GPA of 2.0, transcript of college record, CPR certification, written essay, health exam, health insurance, high school chemistry, high school foreign language, 3 years high school math, 2 years high school science, high school transcript, immunizations, 1 letter of recommendation, minimum high school GPA of 3.0, minimum high school rank 50%, professional liability insurance/malpractice insurance, prerequisite course work. Transfer students are accepted. *Application deadline:* 5/1 (fall). Applications may be processed on a rolling basis for some programs. *Application fee:* $50.

Advanced Placement Credit given for nursing courses completed elsewhere dependent upon specific evaluations.

Expenses (2015–16) *Tuition:* full-time $34,810; part-time $1090 per credit hour. *Room and board:* $10,294; room only: $5850 per academic year. *Required fees:* full-time $2337.

Financial Aid 97% of baccalaureate students in nursing programs received some form of financial aid in 2014–15. *Gift aid (need-based):* Federal Pell, FSEOG, state, private, college/university gift aid from institutional funds. *Loans:* Federal Nursing Student Loans, Federal Direct (Subsidized and Unsubsidized Stafford PLUS), Perkins. *Work-study:* Federal Work-Study. *Financial aid application deadline (priority):* 3/1.

Contact Jan Schnack, Student Affairs Specialist, College of Nursing, Creighton University, 2500 California Plaza, Omaha, NE 68178. *Telephone:* 402-280-3107. *Fax:* 402-280-2045. *E-mail:* jschnack@creighton.edu.

GRADUATE PROGRAMS

Expenses (2015–16) *Tuition:* part-time $800 per credit hour. *Room and board:* $12,708; room only: $10,380 per academic year. *Required fees:* part-time $258 per term.

Financial Aid 82% of graduate students in nursing programs received some form of financial aid in 2014–15. Career-related internships or fieldwork, Federal Work-Study, institutionally sponsored loans, and traineeships available.

Contact Shannon Cox, Enrollment Specialist, College of Nursing, Creighton University, 2500 California Plaza, Omaha, NE 68178. *Telephone:* 402-280-2067. *Fax:* 402-280-2045. *E-mail:* shannoncox@creighton.edu.

MASTER'S DEGREE PROGRAM

Degree MSN

Available Programs Master's.

Concentrations Available Clinical nurse leader; nursing administration.

Site Options Hastings, NE.

Study Options Full-time and part-time.

Online Degree Options Yes (online only).

Program Entrance Requirements Clinical experience, minimum overall college GPA of 3.0, transcript of college record, CPR certification, written essay, immunizations, 3 letters of recommendation, physical assessment course, prerequisite course work, resume, statistics course. *Application deadline:* 7/15 (fall), 11/15 (spring), 4/15 (summer). Applications may be processed on a rolling basis for some programs. *Application fee:* $50.

Advanced Placement Credit given for nursing courses completed elsewhere dependent upon specific evaluations.

Degree Requirements 46 total credit hours, thesis or project.

POST-MASTER'S PROGRAM

Areas of Study Nursing administration. *Nurse practitioner programs in:* acute care, adult health, adult-gerontology acute care, family health, neonatal health, pediatric.

DOCTORAL DEGREE PROGRAM

Degree DNP

Available Programs Doctorate; Post-Baccalaureate Doctorate.

Areas of Study Advanced practice nursing.

Site Options Hastings, NE.

Online Degree Options Yes (online only).

Program Entrance Requirements Clinical experience, minimum overall college GPA of 3.0, 3 letters of recommendation, statistics course, vita. Application deadline: 7/15 (fall), 11/15 (spring), 4/15 (summer). Applications may be processed on a rolling basis for some programs. Application fee: $50.

Degree Requirements 75 total credit hours, residency.

CONTINUING EDUCATION PROGRAM

Contact Sally O'Neill, Associate Vice Provost Health Sciences Continuing Education, College of Nursing, Creighton University, 601 North 30th, Suite 2130, Omaha, NE 68131. *Telephone:* 402-280-1830. *E-mail:* sallyoneill@creighton.edu.

Doane College

Nursing Program
Crete, Nebraska

http://www.doane.edu/nursing
Founded in 1872

DEGREE • BSN

BACCALAUREATE PROGRAMS

Degree BSN

Available Programs RN Baccalaureate.

Contact RN to BSN Program, Nursing Program, Doane College, 303 North 52nd Street, Lincoln, NE 68504. *Telephone:* 888-803-6263.

Midland University

Department of Nursing
Fremont, Nebraska

http://www.midlandu.edu/
Founded in 1883

DEGREE • BSN

Nursing Program Faculty 12 (25% with doctorates).

Baccalaureate Enrollment 130 **Women** 93% **Men** 7% **Part-time** 9%

Distance Learning Courses Available.

Nursing Student Activities Sigma Theta Tau, Student Nurses' Association.

Nursing Student Resources Academic advising; academic or career counseling; assistance for students with disabilities; bookstore; campus computer network; career placement assistance; computer lab; computer-assisted instruction; e-mail services; employment services for current students; housing assistance; interactive nursing skills videos; Internet; learning resource lab; library services; nursing audiovisuals; paid internships; placement services for program completers; remedial services; resume preparation assistance; skills, simulation, or other laboratory; tutoring; unpaid internships.

Library Facilities 4,700 volumes in health, 2,000 volumes in nursing; 550 periodical subscriptions health-care related.

BACCALAUREATE PROGRAMS

Degree BSN

Available Programs ADN to Baccalaureate; Generic Baccalaureate; LPN to RN Baccalaureate; RN Baccalaureate.

Site Options Columbus, NE.

Study Options Full-time and part-time.

Program Entrance Requirements Minimum overall college GPA of 2.5, transcript of college record, CPR certification, written essay, health exam, high school transcript, immunizations, interview, 2 letters of recommendation, minimum GPA in nursing prerequisites of 2.5, prerequisite course work. Transfer students are accepted. *Application deadline:* 3/1 (spring). Applications may be processed on a rolling basis for some programs.

Advanced Placement Credit given for nursing courses completed elsewhere dependent upon specific evaluations.

Contact *Telephone:* 402-941-6505. *Fax:* 402-941-6513.

Nebraska Methodist College
Department of Nursing
Omaha, Nebraska

http://www.methodistcollege.edu/
Founded in 1891
DEGREES • BSN • DNP • MSN
Nursing Program Faculty 35 (34% with doctorates).
Baccalaureate Enrollment 536 **Women** 92% **Men** 8% **Part-time** 46%
Graduate Enrollment 148 **Women** 95% **Men** 5% **Part-time** 26%
Distance Learning Courses Available.
Nursing Student Activities Nursing Honor Society, Sigma Theta Tau, Student Nurses' Association.
Nursing Student Resources Academic advising; academic or career counseling; assistance for students with disabilities; bookstore; campus computer network; career placement assistance; computer lab; computer-assisted instruction; e-mail services; employment services for current students; interactive nursing skills videos; Internet; learning resource lab; library services; nursing audiovisuals; remedial services; resume preparation assistance; skills, simulation, or other laboratory; tutoring.
Library Facilities 8,000 volumes in health, 4,500 volumes in nursing; 13,600 periodical subscriptions health-care related.

BACCALAUREATE PROGRAMS

Degree BSN
Available Programs Accelerated Baccalaureate for Second Degree; Accelerated RN Baccalaureate; Generic Baccalaureate; LPN to Baccalaureate; LPN to RN Baccalaureate; RN Baccalaureate.
Study Options Full-time and part-time.
Program Entrance Requirements Minimum overall college GPA of 2.5, transcript of college record, written essay, high school biology, high school chemistry, 2 years high school math, 2 years high school science, high school transcript, immunizations, interview, minimum high school GPA of 2.5, minimum GPA in nursing prerequisites of 2.5. Transfer students are accepted. *Application deadline:* Applications may be processed on a rolling basis for some programs. *Application fee:* $25.
Advanced Placement Credit given for nursing courses completed elsewhere dependent upon specific evaluations.
Expenses (2014–15) *Tuition:* full-time $16,230; part-time $541 per credit hour. *Room and board:* room only: $7174 per academic year. *Required fees:* full-time $630.
Financial Aid 96% of baccalaureate students in nursing programs received some form of financial aid in 2013–14. *Gift aid (need-based):* Federal Pell, FSEOG, state, private, college/university gift aid from institutional funds, Federal Nursing. *Loans:* Federal Nursing Student Loans, Federal Direct (Subsidized and Unsubsidized Stafford PLUS), Perkins, college/university, private loans. *Work-study:* Federal Work-Study. *Financial aid application deadline (priority):* 4/1.
Contact Megan Maryott, Director, Enrollment Services, Department of Nursing, Nebraska Methodist College, 720 North 87th Street, Omaha, NE 68114-2852. *Telephone:* 402-354-7200. *Fax:* 402-354-7020. *E-mail:* admissions@methodistcollege.edu.

GRADUATE PROGRAMS

Expenses (2014–15) *Tuition:* full-time $12,564; part-time $698 per credit hour. *Room and board:* room only: $7174 per academic year. *Required fees:* full-time $450.
Financial Aid 82% of graduate students in nursing programs received some form of financial aid in 2013–14.
Contact Megan Maryott, Director, Enrollment Services, Department of Nursing, Nebraska Methodist College, 720 North 87th Street, Omaha, NE 68114-2852. *Telephone:* 402-354-7200. *Fax:* 402-354-7020. *E-mail:* admissions@methodistcollege.edu.

MASTER'S DEGREE PROGRAM
Degree MSN
Available Programs Master's; Master's for Nurses with Non-Nursing Degrees; RN to Master's.
Concentrations Available Nursing administration; nursing education.
Study Options Full-time and part-time.
Online Degree Options Yes (online only).
Program Entrance Requirements Computer literacy, minimum overall college GPA of 3.0, transcript of college record, CPR certification, written essay, immunizations, interview, 2 letters of recommendation, nursing research course, physical assessment course, prerequisite course work, resume, statistics course. *Application deadline:* Applications may be processed on a rolling basis for some programs. *Application fee:* $25.

Advanced Placement Credit given for nursing courses completed elsewhere dependent upon specific evaluations.
Degree Requirements 36 total credit hours, thesis or project.

POST-MASTER'S PROGRAM
Areas of Study Nursing administration; nursing education.

DOCTORAL DEGREE PROGRAM
Degree DNP
Available Programs Doctorate.
Areas of Study Advanced practice nursing, family health.
Online Degree Options Yes (online only).
Program Entrance Requirements Clinical experience, minimum overall college GPA of 3.0, interview by faculty committee, interview, 3 letters of recommendation, statistics course, vita, writing sample. Application deadline: Applications may be processed on a rolling basis for some programs. Application fee: $25.
Degree Requirements 75 total credit hours, dissertation, written exam, residency.

CONTINUING EDUCATION PROGRAM

Contact Phyllis Zimmermann, Director, Continuing Education, Department of Nursing, Nebraska Methodist College, 720 North 87th Street, Omaha, NE 68114-2852. *Telephone:* 402-354-7109. *Fax:* 402-354-7055. *E-mail:* phyllis.zimmermann@methodistcollege.edu.

Nebraska Wesleyan University
Department of Nursing
Lincoln, Nebraska

http://www.nebrwesleyan.edu/
Founded in 1887
DEGREES • BSN • MSN • MSN/MBA
Nursing Program Faculty 38 (30% with doctorates).
Baccalaureate Enrollment 199 **Women** 90% **Men** 10% **Part-time** 30%
Graduate Enrollment 89 **Women** 91% **Men** 9% **Part-time** 20%
Distance Learning Courses Available.
Nursing Student Activities Nursing Honor Society, Sigma Theta Tau, Student Nurses' Association, nursing club.
Nursing Student Resources Academic advising; academic or career counseling; assistance for students with disabilities; bookstore; campus computer network; career placement assistance; computer lab; e-mail services; Internet; library services; nursing audiovisuals; resume preparation assistance; skills, simulation, or other laboratory; unpaid internships.
Library Facilities 5,000 volumes in health, 3,700 volumes in nursing; 470 periodical subscriptions health-care related.

BACCALAUREATE PROGRAMS

Degree BSN
Available Programs ADN to Baccalaureate; Generic Baccalaureate; International Nurse to Baccalaureate.
Site Options Council Bluffs, IA; Lincoln, NE; Omaha, NE.
Study Options Full-time.
Program Entrance Requirements Minimum overall college GPA of 2.0, CPR certification, written essay, health exam, health insurance, high school chemistry, high school transcript, immunizations, interview, 2 letters of recommendation, prerequisite course work. Transfer students are accepted. *Application deadline:* 3/15 (fall). *Application fee:* $100.
Advanced Placement Credit given for nursing courses completed elsewhere dependent upon specific evaluations.
Expenses (2015–16) *Tuition:* full-time $29,300; part-time $1075 per credit hour. *International tuition:* $29,300 full-time. *Room and board:* $8500; room only: $5000 per academic year. *Required fees:* full-time $850; part-time $400 per credit.
Financial Aid 64% of baccalaureate students in nursing programs received some form of financial aid in 2014–15.
Contact Ms. Kellie Long, Assistant Professor, Nursing and Pre-licensure BSN Program Coordinator, Department of Nursing, Nebraska Wesleyan University, 5000 St. Paul Avenue, Lincoln, NE 68504. *Telephone:* 800-541-3818. *E-mail:* klong2@nebrwesleyan.edu.

GRADUATE PROGRAMS

Expenses (2015–16) *Tuition:* part-time $395 per credit. *International tuition:* $395 full-time. *Required fees:* full-time $30.
Financial Aid 60% of graduate students in nursing programs received some form of financial aid in 2014–15.

Contact Dr. Molly M. Fitzke, Nursing Program Coordinator, Department of Nursing, Nebraska Wesleyan University, 5000 St. Paul Avenue, Lincoln, NE 68504. *Telephone:* 402-465-2334. *Fax:* 402-465-2179. *E-mail:* mfitzke@nebrwesleyan.edu.

MASTER'S DEGREE PROGRAM

Degrees MSN; MSN/MBA
Available Programs Accelerated AD/RN to Master's; Accelerated Master's; Accelerated RN to Master's; Master's; RN to Master's.
Concentrations Available Nursing administration; nursing education.
Site Options Lincoln, NE; Omaha, NE.
Study Options Full-time and part-time.
Program Entrance Requirements Clinical experience, computer literacy, minimum overall college GPA of 3.0, transcript of college record, written essay, immunizations, 2 letters of recommendation, nursing research course, resume. *Application deadline:* 8/1 (fall), 12/10 (spring). Applications may be processed on a rolling basis for some programs. *Application fee:* $100.
Advanced Placement Credit by examination available. Credit given for nursing courses completed elsewhere dependent upon specific evaluations.
Degree Requirements 40 total credit hours, thesis or project.

POST-MASTER'S PROGRAM

Areas of Study Nursing administration; nursing education.

Union College
Division of Nursing
Lincoln, Nebraska

http://www.ucollege.edu/nursing
Founded in 1891
DEGREE • BSN
Nursing Program Faculty 14
Baccalaureate Enrollment 100 Women 74% Men 26% Part-time 7%
Nursing Student Activities Sigma Theta Tau, nursing club.
Nursing Student Resources Academic advising; academic or career counseling; assistance for students with disabilities; bookstore; campus computer network; career placement assistance; computer lab; computer-assisted instruction; e-mail services; employment services for current students; externships; housing assistance; interactive nursing skills videos; Internet; learning resource lab; library services; nursing audiovisuals; paid internships; placement services for program completers; remedial services; resume preparation assistance; skills, simulation, or other laboratory; tutoring; unpaid internships.
Library Facilities 450 volumes in health, 400 volumes in nursing; 100 periodical subscriptions health-care related.

BACCALAUREATE PROGRAMS

Degree BSN
Available Programs ADN to Baccalaureate; Generic Baccalaureate; LPN to Baccalaureate.
Study Options Full-time and part-time.
Program Entrance Requirements Minimum overall college GPA of 2.75, transcript of college record, CPR certification, written essay, health exam, health insurance, high school transcript, immunizations, interview, 2 letters of recommendation, professional liability insurance/malpractice insurance, prerequisite course work. Transfer students are accepted. *Application deadline:* 2/1 (fall), 9/1 (spring). *Application fee:* $250.
Advanced Placement Credit given for nursing courses completed elsewhere dependent upon specific evaluations.
Expenses (2015–16) *Tuition:* full-time $20,928; part-time $872 per credit hour. *International tuition:* $20,928 full-time. *Room and board:* $6600; room only: $3800 per academic year. *Required fees:* full-time $2442; part-time $1221 per term.
Financial Aid *Gift aid (need-based):* Federal Pell, FSEOG, state, private, college/university gift aid from institutional funds, United Negro College Fund. *Loans:* Federal Nursing Student Loans, Federal Direct (Subsidized and Unsubsidized Stafford PLUS), Perkins, college/university. *Work-study:* Federal Work-Study. *Financial aid application deadline:* Continuous.
Contact Mrs. Missy Sorter, Program Development and Enrollment Counselor, Division of Nursing, Union College, 3800 South 48th Street, Lincoln, NE 68506. *Telephone:* 402-486-2674. *Fax:* 402-486-2582. *E-mail:* misorter@ucollege.edu.

University of Nebraska Medical Center
College of Nursing
Omaha, Nebraska

http://www.unmc.edu/nursing/
Founded in 1869
DEGREES • BSN • MSN • PHD
Baccalaureate Enrollment 706 Women 88% Men 12%
Graduate Enrollment 349 Women 93% Men 7%
Distance Learning Courses Available.
Nursing Student Activities Nursing Honor Society, Sigma Theta Tau, Student Nurses' Association, nursing club.
Nursing Student Resources Academic advising; academic or career counseling; assistance for students with disabilities; bookstore; campus computer network; career placement assistance; computer lab; computer-assisted instruction; daycare for children of students; e-mail services; employment services for current students; externships; housing assistance; interactive nursing skills videos; Internet; learning resource lab; library services; nursing audiovisuals; other; paid internships; placement services for program completers; remedial services; resume preparation assistance; skills, simulation, or other laboratory; tutoring.

BACCALAUREATE PROGRAMS

Degree BSN
Available Programs Accelerated Baccalaureate; Accelerated RN Baccalaureate; Baccalaureate for Second Degree; Generic Baccalaureate; RN Baccalaureate.
Site Options Lincoln, NE; Kearney, NE; Scottsbluff, NE.
Study Options Full-time.
Program Entrance Requirements Transcript of college record, CPR certification, health insurance, high school transcript, immunizations, prerequisite course work. Transfer students are accepted.
Advanced Placement Credit by examination available. Credit given for nursing courses completed elsewhere dependent upon specific evaluations.
Expenses (2015–16) *Tuition, state resident:* full-time $8626. *Tuition, nonresident:* full-time $26,792. *International tuition:* $26,792 full-time.
Contact Ms. Molly Belieu, Student Services Coordinator, College of Nursing, University of Nebraska Medical Center, 985330 Nebraska Medical Center, Omaha, NE 68198-5330. *Telephone:* 402-559-5102. *E-mail:* molly.handke@unmc.edu.

GRADUATE PROGRAMS

Contact Ms. Rolee Kelly, College of Nursing, University of Nebraska Medical Center, 985330 Nebraska Medical Center, Omaha, NE 68198-5330.

MASTER'S DEGREE PROGRAM
Degree MSN
Available Programs Master's.
Concentrations Available Nursing administration; nursing education. *Clinical nurse specialist programs in:* adult-gerontology acute care. *Nurse practitioner programs in:* adult-gerontology acute care, family health, pediatric, psychiatric/mental health, women's health.
Study Options Full-time and part-time.
Online Degree Options Yes.
Program Entrance Requirements Computer literacy, transcript of college record, CPR certification, immunizations, interview, letters of recommendation, nursing research course, statistics course.

POST-MASTER'S PROGRAM
Areas of Study Nursing administration; nursing education. *Clinical nurse specialist programs in:* adult-gerontology acute care. *Nurse practitioner programs in:* adult-gerontology acute care, family health, pediatric, psychiatric/mental health, women's health.

DOCTORAL DEGREE PROGRAM
Degree PhD
Available Programs Doctorate; Post-Baccalaureate Doctorate.
Areas of Study Faculty preparation, nursing research.
Online Degree Options Yes.
Program Entrance Requirements interview by faculty committee, interview, letters of recommendation, statistics course, vita.
Degree Requirements Dissertation, oral exam, written exam.

POSTDOCTORAL PROGRAM

Postdoctoral Program Contact Dr. Margaret Wilson, Associate Dean for Graduate Programs, College of Nursing, University of Nebraska Medical Center, 985330 Nebraska Medical Center, Omaha, NE 68198-5330. *Telephone:* 402-559-7457. *Fax:* 410-706-0945. *E-mail:* mwilson@unmc.edu.

CONTINUING EDUCATION PROGRAM

Contact Dr. Catherine Bevil, Director, College of Nursing, University of Nebraska Medical Center, 985330 Nebraska Medical Center, Omaha, NE 68198-5330. *Telephone:* 402-559-7487. *E-mail:* cbevil@unmc.edu.

NEVADA

Great Basin College

BSN Program
Elko, Nevada

http://www.gbcnv.edu/programs/show.cgi?BS-NUR
Founded in 1967

DEGREE • BSN
Nursing Program Faculty 7 (29% with doctorates).
Baccalaureate Enrollment 59 **Women** 89% **Men** 11%
Distance Learning Courses Available.
Nursing Student Activities Sigma Theta Tau.
Nursing Student Resources Academic advising; academic or career counseling; assistance for students with disabilities; bookstore; campus computer network; computer lab; computer-assisted instruction; daycare for children of students; e-mail services; Internet; library services; nursing audiovisuals; tutoring.

BACCALAUREATE PROGRAMS

Degree BSN
Available Programs ADN to Baccalaureate; RN Baccalaureate.
Study Options Full-time and part-time.
Online Degree Options Yes (online only).
Program Entrance Requirements Minimum overall college GPA of 3.0, transcript of college record, written essay, 2 letters of recommendation, minimum GPA in nursing prerequisites of 3.0, prerequisite course work, RN licensure. *Application deadline:* 7/1 (fall). *Application fee:* $10.
Expenses (2015–16) *Tuition, state resident:* full-time $2875; part-time $144 per credit. *Tuition, nonresident:* full-time $6040; part-time $302 per credit. *Required fees:* full-time $200; part-time $100 per term.
Financial Aid 5% of baccalaureate students in nursing programs received some form of financial aid in 2014–15. *Gift aid (need-based):* Federal Pell, FSEOG, state, private, college/university gift aid from institutional funds. *Loans:* college/university. *Work-study:* Federal Work-Study, part-time campus jobs. *Financial aid application deadline (priority):* 5/13.
Contact Mrs. Gaye Terras, Admin Assistant, Program Information, BSN Program, Great Basin College, 1500 College Parkway, Elko, NV 89801. *Telephone:* 775-753-2301. *Fax:* 775-753-2151. *E-mail:* gaye.terras@gbcnv.edu.

Nevada State College at Henderson

Nursing Program
Henderson, Nevada

http://www.nsc.nevada.edu/83.asp
Founded in 2002

DEGREE • BSN
Nursing Program Faculty 31 (16% with doctorates).
Baccalaureate Enrollment 312 **Women** 86% **Men** 14% **Part-time** 66%
Distance Learning Courses Available.
Nursing Student Activities Sigma Theta Tau, Student Nurses' Association.

Nursing Student Resources Academic advising; academic or career counseling; assistance for students with disabilities; bookstore; campus computer network; computer lab; computer-assisted instruction; e-mail services; interactive nursing skills videos; Internet; learning resource lab; library services; nursing audiovisuals; skills, simulation, or other laboratory; tutoring.
Library Facilities 1,075 volumes in health, 647 volumes in nursing; 4,981 periodical subscriptions health-care related.

BACCALAUREATE PROGRAMS

Degree BSN
Available Programs Accelerated Baccalaureate for Second Degree; Generic Baccalaureate; RN Baccalaureate.
Study Options Full-time and part-time.
Online Degree Options Yes.
Program Entrance Requirements Minimum overall college GPA of 2.5, transcript of college record, CPR certification, health exam, health insurance, high school transcript, immunizations, minimum GPA in nursing prerequisites of 3.25, prerequisite course work. Transfer students are accepted. *Application deadline:* 3/15 (fall), 9/15 (spring).
Advanced Placement Credit given for nursing courses completed elsewhere dependent upon specific evaluations.
Contact *Telephone:* 702-992-2638. *Fax:* 702-992-2058.

Roseman University of Health Sciences

College of Nursing
Henderson, Nevada

http://www.roseman.edu/
Founded in 2000

DEGREE • BSN
Nursing Program Faculty 77 (16% with doctorates).
Baccalaureate Enrollment 336 **Women** 79% **Men** 21%
Distance Learning Courses Available.
Nursing Student Activities Nursing Honor Society, Student Nurses' Association.
Nursing Student Resources Academic advising; academic or career counseling; assistance for students with disabilities; campus computer network; career placement assistance; computer lab; computer-assisted instruction; e-mail services; interactive nursing skills videos; Internet; learning resource lab; library services; nursing audiovisuals; remedial services; resume preparation assistance; skills, simulation, or other laboratory; unpaid internships.

BACCALAUREATE PROGRAMS

Degree BSN
Available Programs Accelerated Baccalaureate; Accelerated Baccalaureate for Second Degree; Generic Baccalaureate; RN Baccalaureate.
Site Options South Jordan, UT; Las Vegas, NV.
Study Options Full-time.
Online Degree Options Yes (online only).
Program Entrance Requirements Transcript of college record, written essay, health exam, health insurance, immunizations, interview, minimum GPA in nursing prerequisites of 2.75, prerequisite course work. Transfer students are accepted. *Application deadline:* 5/1 (fall), 8/1 (winter), 10/1 (spring), 5/1 (summer). Applications may be processed on a rolling basis for some programs. *Application fee:* $85.
Advanced Placement Credit by examination available. Credit given for nursing courses completed elsewhere dependent upon specific evaluations.
Contact Mr. Erik D. Dillon, Director of Admissions and Enrollment, College of Nursing, Roseman University of Health Sciences, 11 Sunset Way, Henderson, NV 89014. *Telephone:* 702-968-2075. *Fax:* 702-968-2097. *E-mail:* edillon@roseman.edu.

Touro University

School of Nursing
Henderson, Nevada

http://www.touro.edu/
DEGREES • BSN • DNP • MSN
Nursing Program Faculty 10 (60% with doctorates).

Baccalaureate Enrollment 31 **Women** 77.5% **Men** 22.5%
Graduate Enrollment 6 **Women** 83% **Men** 17% **Part-time** 100%
Distance Learning Courses Available.
Nursing Student Activities Sigma Theta Tau, Student Nurses' Association.
Nursing Student Resources Academic advising; assistance for students with disabilities; bookstore; campus computer network; computer lab; computer-assisted instruction; e-mail services; interactive nursing skills videos; Internet; learning resource lab; library services; nursing audiovisuals; remedial services; skills, simulation, or other laboratory; tutoring.
Library Facilities 86 volumes in health; 6,002 periodical subscriptions health-care related.

BACCALAUREATE PROGRAMS

Degree BSN
Available Programs ADN to Baccalaureate; Generic Baccalaureate; RN Baccalaureate.
Study Options Full-time.
Online Degree Options Yes.
Program Entrance Requirements Minimum overall college GPA of 3.0, transcript of college record, CPR certification, health exam, health insurance, immunizations, minimum GPA in nursing prerequisites of 3.0, prerequisite course work, RN licensure. Transfer students are accepted. *Application deadline:* 7/30 (fall), 12/31 (spring). Applications may be processed on a rolling basis for some programs. *Application fee:* $50.
Advanced Placement Credit given for nursing courses completed elsewhere dependent upon specific evaluations.
Contact *Telephone:* 702-777-1751. *Fax:* 702-777-1752.

GRADUATE PROGRAMS

Contact *Telephone:* 702-777-3997. *Fax:* 702-777-1752.

MASTER'S DEGREE PROGRAM
Degree MSN
Available Programs Master's.
Concentrations Available Nursing education.
Study Options Full-time and part-time.
Online Degree Options Yes (online only).
Program Entrance Requirements Clinical experience, computer literacy, minimum overall college GPA of 3.0, transcript of college record, CPR certification, 2 letters of recommendation, statistics course. *Application deadline:* Applications may be processed on a rolling basis for some programs. *Application fee:* $50.
Advanced Placement Credit given for nursing courses completed elsewhere dependent upon specific evaluations.
Degree Requirements 36 total credit hours, thesis or project, comprehensive exam.

DOCTORAL DEGREE PROGRAM
Degree DNP
Available Programs Doctorate.
Areas of Study Individualized study.
Online Degree Options Yes (online only).
Program Entrance Requirements Clinical experience, minimum overall college GPA of 3.0, 3 letters of recommendation, MSN or equivalent, statistics course, vita, writing sample. Application deadline: Applications may be processed on a rolling basis for some programs. Application fee: $50.
Degree Requirements 39 total credit hours, oral exam, residency.

University of Nevada, Las Vegas
School of Nursing
Las Vegas, Nevada

http://www.unlv.edu/nursing
Founded in 1957

DEGREES • BSN • DNP • MSN • PHD
Nursing Program Faculty 37 (68% with doctorates).
Baccalaureate Enrollment 181 **Women** 77% **Men** 23%
Graduate Enrollment 109 **Women** 89% **Men** 11% **Part-time** 60%
Distance Learning Courses Available.
Nursing Student Activities Nursing Honor Society, Sigma Theta Tau, Student Nurses' Association.
Nursing Student Resources Academic advising; academic or career counseling; assistance for students with disabilities; bookstore; campus computer network; career placement assistance; computer lab; computer-

assisted instruction; e-mail services; employment services for current students; interactive nursing skills videos; Internet; learning resource lab; library services; nursing audiovisuals; remedial services; resume preparation assistance; skills, simulation, or other laboratory; tutoring.
Library Facilities 35,800 volumes in health, 12,000 volumes in nursing; 305 periodical subscriptions health-care related.

BACCALAUREATE PROGRAMS

Degree BSN
Available Programs Accelerated Baccalaureate.
Study Options Full-time.
Program Entrance Requirements Minimum overall college GPA of 3.0, transcript of college record, CPR certification, health exam, health insurance, high school transcript, immunizations, minimum GPA in nursing prerequisites of 3.0, prerequisite course work. Transfer students are accepted. *Application deadline:* Applications may be processed on a rolling basis for some programs.
Advanced Placement Credit given for nursing courses completed elsewhere dependent upon specific evaluations.
Expenses (2015–16) *Tuition, state resident:* full-time $16,031; part-time $391 per contact hour. *Tuition, nonresident:* full-time $36,896; part-time $602 per contact hour. *International tuition:* $39,863 full-time. *Room and board:* $12,374; room only: $6934 per academic year. *Required fees:* full-time $1018.
Financial Aid 45% of baccalaureate students in nursing programs received some form of financial aid in 2014–15. *Gift aid (need-based):* Federal Pell, FSEOG, state, private, college/university gift aid from institutional funds. *Loans:* Federal Nursing Student Loans, Federal Direct (Subsidized and Unsubsidized Stafford PLUS), Perkins, state, college/university. *Work-study:* Federal Work-Study, part-time campus jobs. *Financial aid application deadline (priority):* 2/1.
Contact Dr. Marianne Tejada, Undergraduate Coordinator, School of Nursing, University of Nevada, Las Vegas, 4505 Maryland Parkway, Las Vegas, NV 89154-3018. *Telephone:* 702-895-2545. *Fax:* 702-895-4807. *E-mail:* Marianne.Tejadal@unlv.edu.

GRADUATE PROGRAMS

Expenses (2015–16) *Tuition, state resident:* full-time $13,594; part-time $3021 per trimester. *Tuition, nonresident:* full-time $17,158; part-time $3813 per trimester. *International tuition:* $20,125 full-time. *Room and board:* $12,374; room only: $6934 per academic year. *Required fees:* full-time $1581; part-time $542 per term.
Financial Aid 35% of graduate students in nursing programs received some form of financial aid in 2014–15. 4 teaching assistantships with partial tuition reimbursements available (averaging $11,500 per year) were awarded; institutionally sponsored loans, scholarships, and unspecified assistantships also available. *Financial aid application deadline:* 3/1.
Contact Dr. Susan VanBeuge, Coordinator, MSN Program, School of Nursing, University of Nevada, Las Vegas, 4505 Maryland Parkway, Box 453018, Las Vegas, NV 89154-3018. *Telephone:* 702-895-3719. *Fax:* 702-895-4807. *E-mail:* susan.vanbeuge@unlv.edu.

MASTER'S DEGREE PROGRAM
Degree MSN
Available Programs Master's.
Concentrations Available Nursing education. *Nurse practitioner programs in:* family health, pediatric primary care.
Study Options Full-time and part-time.
Online Degree Options Yes (online only).
Program Entrance Requirements Clinical experience, minimum overall college GPA of 3.0, transcript of college record, CPR certification, written essay, immunizations, interview, 2 letters of recommendation, nursing research course, physical assessment course, professional liability insurance/malpractice insurance, prerequisite course work, resume, statistics course. *Application deadline:* 2/1 (fall). *Application fee:* $60.
Advanced Placement Credit given for nursing courses completed elsewhere dependent upon specific evaluations.
Degree Requirements 46 total credit hours, thesis or project.

POST-MASTER'S PROGRAM
Areas of Study Nursing education. *Nurse practitioner programs in:* family health, pediatric primary care.

DOCTORAL DEGREE PROGRAM
Degree DNP
Available Programs Doctorate.
Areas of Study Advanced practice nursing, nursing administration.

Online Degree Options Yes (online only).
Program Entrance Requirements Minimum overall college GPA of 3.5, clinical experience, interview by faculty committee, 3 letters of recommendation, MSN or equivalent, vita. Application deadline: Applications are processed on a rolling basis. Application fee: $60.
Degree Requirements 39 total credit hours, DNP scholarly project, residency.

Degree PhD
Available Programs Doctorate.
Areas of Study Nursing education, nursing research.
Online Degree Options Yes (online only).
Program Entrance Requirements Clinical experience, minimum overall college GPA of 3.5, interview by faculty committee, interview, 3 letters of recommendation, MSN or equivalent, scholarly papers, statistics course, vita, writing sample, GRE General Test. Application deadline: 2/1 (fall). Application fee: $60.
Degree Requirements 62 total credit hours, dissertation, oral exam, written exam.

CONTINUING EDUCATION PROGRAM

Contact Ms. Jill Racicot, Special Projects Coordinator, School of Nursing, University of Nevada, Las Vegas, 4505 Maryland Parkway, Las Vegas, NV 89154-3018. *Telephone:* 702-895-5920. *Fax:* 702-895-4807. *E-mail:* Jill.Racicot@unlv.edu.

University of Nevada, Reno
Orvis School of Nursing
Reno, Nevada

http://www.unr.edu/nursing
Founded in 1874
DEGREES • BSN • DNP • MSN • MSN/MPH
Nursing Program Faculty 34 (47% with doctorates).
Baccalaureate Enrollment 192 **Women** 80% **Men** 20%
Graduate Enrollment 123 **Women** 90% **Men** 10% **Part-time** 60%
Distance Learning Courses Available.
Nursing Student Activities Nursing Honor Society, Sigma Theta Tau, Student Nurses' Association.
Nursing Student Resources Academic advising; academic or career counseling; assistance for students with disabilities; bookstore; campus computer network; career placement assistance; computer lab; computer-assisted instruction; e-mail services; housing assistance; Internet; learning resource lab; library services; nursing audiovisuals; resume preparation assistance; skills, simulation, or other laboratory; tutoring.
Library Facilities 120,213 volumes in health, 6,846 volumes in nursing; 172 periodical subscriptions health-care related.

BACCALAUREATE PROGRAMS

Degree BSN
Available Programs ADN to Baccalaureate; Accelerated Baccalaureate; Accelerated Baccalaureate for Second Degree; Baccalaureate for Second Degree; Generic Baccalaureate; RN Baccalaureate.
Site Options Reno , NV.
Study Options Full-time.
Program Entrance Requirements Transcript of college record, CPR certification, health exam, health insurance, immunizations, interview, minimum GPA in nursing prerequisites of 3.0, professional liability insurance/malpractice insurance, prerequisite course work. Transfer students are accepted. *Application deadline:* 2/26 (fall), 9/26 (spring).
Advanced Placement Credit given for nursing courses completed elsewhere dependent upon specific evaluations.
Expenses (2015–16) *Tuition, state resident:* full-time $6000. *Tuition, nonresident:* full-time $15,000. *Required fees:* full-time $4500.
Contact Kimberly Diane Baxter, Associate Director of Undergraduate Programs, Orvis School of Nursing, University of Nevada, Reno, Mail Stop 0134, Reno, NV 89557. *Telephone:* 775-682-7145. *Fax:* 775-784-4262. *E-mail:* kimbaxter@unr.edu.

GRADUATE PROGRAMS

Expenses (2015–16) *Tuition, state resident:* full-time $31,088; part-time $550 per credit. *Tuition, nonresident:* full-time $75,174. *Room and board:* $929 per academic year.
Financial Aid Research assistantships, teaching assistantships, Federal Work-Study, institutionally sponsored loans, scholarships, and unspecified assistantships available.

Contact Dr. Stephanie DeBoor, Coordinator, Graduate Program, Orvis School of Nursing, University of Nevada, Reno, Pennington Health Sciences Building, Reno, NV 89557-0134. *Telephone:* 775-682-7156. *Fax:* 775-784-4262. *E-mail:* deboors2@unr.edu.

MASTER'S DEGREE PROGRAM
Degrees MSN; MSN/MPH
Available Programs Master's.
Concentrations Available Clinical nurse leader; nursing education. *Nurse practitioner programs in:* adult-gerontology acute care, family health, psychiatric/mental health.
Site Options Reno, NV.
Study Options Full-time and part-time.
Program Entrance Requirements Clinical experience, computer literacy, minimum overall college GPA of 3.0, transcript of college record, CPR certification, written essay, immunizations, 3 letters of recommendation, professional liability insurance/malpractice insurance, resume, statistics course. *Application deadline:* 3/1 (fall), 10/1 (spring). *Application fee:* $60.
Advanced Placement Credit given for nursing courses completed elsewhere dependent upon specific evaluations.
Degree Requirements 48 total credit hours, thesis or project, comprehensive exam.

POST-MASTER'S PROGRAM
Areas of Study Clinical nurse leader; nursing education. *Nurse practitioner programs in:* adult-gerontology acute care, family health, psychiatric/mental health.

DOCTORAL DEGREE PROGRAM
Degree DNP
Available Programs Doctorate; Doctorate for Nurses with Non-Nursing Degrees.
Areas of Study Advanced practice nursing, nursing administration.
Site Options Reno, NV.
Online Degree Options Yes (online only).
Program Entrance Requirements Clinical experience, minimum overall college GPA of 3.5, 2 letters of recommendation, MSN or equivalent, vita, writing sample. Application deadline: 3/15 (fall). Application fee: $60.
Degree Requirements 30 total credit hours, residency.

NEW HAMPSHIRE

Colby-Sawyer College
Department of Nursing
New London, New Hampshire

http://www.colby-sawyer.edu/nursing/index.html
Founded in 1837
DEGREE • BSN
Nursing Program Faculty 14 (.14% with doctorates).
Baccalaureate Enrollment 169 **Women** 93% **Men** 7% **Part-time** 1%
Nursing Student Activities Nursing Honor Society, Student Nurses' Association.
Nursing Student Resources Academic advising; academic or career counseling; assistance for students with disabilities; bookstore; campus computer network; career placement assistance; computer lab; computer-assisted instruction; e-mail services; employment services for current students; housing assistance; interactive nursing skills videos; Internet; learning resource lab; library services; nursing audiovisuals; remedial services; resume preparation assistance; skills, simulation, or other laboratory; tutoring; unpaid internships.
Library Facilities 12,050 volumes in health, 760 volumes in nursing; 135 periodical subscriptions health-care related.

BACCALAUREATE PROGRAMS

Degree BSN
Available Programs Generic Baccalaureate.
Study Options Full-time and part-time.
Program Entrance Requirements Minimum overall college GPA of 2.7, transcript of college record, CPR certification, written essay, health exam, health insurance, high school biology, high school chemistry, high

school foreign language, 3 years high school math, 3 years high school science, high school transcript, immunizations, 2 letters of recommendation, minimum high school GPA of 2.75, minimum GPA in nursing prerequisites of 2.7, prerequisite course work. Transfer students are accepted. *Application deadline:* Applications may be processed on a rolling basis for some programs.
Advanced Placement Credit by examination available. Credit given for nursing courses completed elsewhere dependent upon specific evaluations.
Contact *Telephone:* 603-526-3795. *Fax:* 603-526-3159.

Franklin Pierce University
Master of Science in Nursing
Rindge, New Hampshire

http://www.franklinpierce.edu/
Founded in 1962
DEGREES • BS • MSN
Nursing Program Faculty 4 (50% with doctorates).
Baccalaureate Enrollment 110 **Women** 97% **Men** 3% **Part-time** 100%
Graduate Enrollment 24 **Women** 96% **Men** 4% **Part-time** 100%
Distance Learning Courses Available.
Nursing Student Resources Academic advising; assistance for students with disabilities; bookstore; campus computer network; computer lab; library services.
Library Facilities 200 periodical subscriptions health-care related.

BACCALAUREATE PROGRAMS
Degree BS
Available Programs ADN to Baccalaureate; RN Baccalaureate.
Site Options Concord, NH; Lebanon, NH; Portsmouth, NH.
Study Options Part-time.
Program Entrance Requirements RN licensure. Transfer students are accepted. *Application deadline:* Applications may be processed on a rolling basis for some programs.
Advanced Placement Credit by examination available.
Contact *Telephone:* 603-433-2000 Ext. 2000. *Fax:* 603-899-1067 Ext. 1067.

GRADUATE PROGRAMS
Contact *Telephone:* 603-322-2000. *Fax:* 603-899-1067.

MASTER'S DEGREE PROGRAM
Degree MSN
Available Programs Master's; Master's for Nurses with Non-Nursing Degrees; RN to Master's.
Concentrations Available Nursing administration; nursing education.
Site Options Concord, NH; Lebanon, NH; Portsmouth, NH.
Study Options Part-time.
Program Entrance Requirements Computer literacy, minimum overall college GPA of 2.8, transcript of college record, written essay, interview, 3 letters of recommendation, resume, statistics course. *Application deadline:* Applications may be processed on a rolling basis for some programs.
Degree Requirements 34 total credit hours, thesis or project.

Granite State College
Nursing Department
Concord, New Hampshire

http://www.granite.edu/
Founded in 1972
DEGREE • BSN

BACCALAUREATE PROGRAMS
Degree BSN
Available Programs RN Baccalaureate.
Program Entrance Requirements *Application deadline:* Applications may be processed on a rolling basis for some programs.
Contact Concord Campus, Nursing Department, Granite State College, 25 Hall Street, Concord, NH 03301. *Telephone:* 603-513-1398. *Fax:* 603-513-1389.

Keene State College
Nursing Program
Keene, New Hampshire

http://www.keene.edu/academics/programs/nursing/
Founded in 1909
DEGREE • BS

BACCALAUREATE PROGRAMS
Degree BS
Available Programs Generic Baccalaureate; RN Baccalaureate.
Contact Angela Poirier, Administrative Assistant, Nursing Program, Keene State College, 229 Main Street, Keene, NH 03435. *Telephone:* 603-358-2533. *E-mail:* angela.poirier@keene.edu.

Plymouth State University
RN-BS Completion Program
Plymouth, New Hampshire

http://www.plymouth.edu/department/nursing/degrees-options-minors/rn-bs-completion-program/
Founded in 1871
DEGREE • BS

BACCALAUREATE PROGRAMS
Degree BS
Available Programs RN Baccalaureate.
Contact Laurie Reed, Administrative Assistant, RN-BS Completion Program, Plymouth State University, 17 High Street, MSC #57, Plymouth, NH 03264. *Telephone:* 603-535-2703.
E-mail: lreed@plymouth.edu.

Rivier University
Division of Nursing
Nashua, New Hampshire

http://www.rivier.edu/
Founded in 1933
DEGREES • BS • MS
Nursing Program Faculty 28
Baccalaureate Enrollment 710 **Women** 94% **Men** 6% **Part-time** 45%
Graduate Enrollment 136 **Women** 95% **Men** 5% **Part-time** 89%
Distance Learning Courses Available.
Nursing Student Activities Nursing Honor Society, Sigma Theta Tau, Student Nurses' Association.
Nursing Student Resources Academic advising; academic or career counseling; assistance for students with disabilities; bookstore; campus computer network; career placement assistance; computer lab; computer-assisted instruction; e-mail services; employment services for current students; externships; housing assistance; interactive nursing skills videos; Internet; learning resource lab; library services; nursing audiovisuals; other; remedial services; resume preparation assistance; skills, simulation, or other laboratory; tutoring.
Library Facilities 3,777 volumes in health, 1,170 volumes in nursing; 4,000 periodical subscriptions health-care related.

BACCALAUREATE PROGRAMS
Degree BS
Available Programs ADN to Baccalaureate; Generic Baccalaureate; LPN to Baccalaureate; LPN to RN Baccalaureate; RN Baccalaureate.
Site Options Manchester, NH.
Study Options Full-time and part-time.
Online Degree Options Yes.
Program Entrance Requirements Minimum overall college GPA, transcript of college record, written essay, health exam, health insurance, high school biology, high school chemistry, high school foreign language, 3 years high school math, 2 years high school science, high school transcript, immunizations, 2 letters of recommendation, minimum high school GPA, minimum high school rank, prerequisite course work. Transfer students are accepted. *Application deadline:* Applications may be processed on a rolling basis for some programs. *Application fee:* $25.

Advanced Placement Credit by examination available. Credit given for nursing courses completed elsewhere dependent upon specific evaluations.
Contact *Telephone:* 603-897-8515. *Fax:* 603-897-8808.

GRADUATE PROGRAMS

Contact *Telephone:* 603-897-8528. *Fax:* 603-897-8884.

MASTER'S DEGREE PROGRAM

Degree MS
Available Programs Master's; Master's for Nurses with Non-Nursing Degrees; RN to Master's.
Concentrations Available Nursing education. *Nurse practitioner programs in:* family health, psychiatric/mental health.
Study Options Full-time and part-time.
Program Entrance Requirements Clinical experience, minimum overall college GPA of 3.0, transcript of college record, written essay, immunizations, interview, 2 letters of recommendation, resume, statistics course, GRE, MAT. *Application deadline:* Applications may be processed on a rolling basis for some programs. *Application fee:* $25.
Advanced Placement Credit by examination available. Credit given for nursing courses completed elsewhere dependent upon specific evaluations.
Degree Requirements 43 total credit hours, thesis or project.

POST-MASTER'S PROGRAM

Areas of Study Nursing education. *Nurse practitioner programs in:* family health, psychiatric/mental health.

Saint Anselm College
Department of Nursing
Manchester, New Hampshire

http://www.anselm.edu/Academics/Majors-and-Departments/Nursing.htm
Founded in 1889
DEGREE • BSN
Nursing Program Faculty 31 (26% with doctorates).
Baccalaureate Enrollment 320 **Women** 96% **Men** 4%
Distance Learning Courses Available.
Nursing Student Activities Sigma Theta Tau, Student Nurses' Association, nursing club.
Nursing Student Resources Academic advising; academic or career counseling; assistance for students with disabilities; bookstore; campus computer network; career placement assistance; computer lab; computer-assisted instruction; e-mail services; employment services for current students; externships; housing assistance; interactive nursing skills videos; Internet; learning resource lab; library services; nursing audiovisuals; resume preparation assistance; skills, simulation, or other laboratory; tutoring.
Library Facilities 5,884 volumes in health; 104 periodical subscriptions health-care related.

BACCALAUREATE PROGRAMS

Degree BSN
Available Programs RN Baccalaureate.
Study Options Full-time and part-time.
Program Entrance Requirements Transcript of college record, written essay, health exam, health insurance, high school biology, high school chemistry, high school foreign language, 3 years high school math, 3 years high school science, high school transcript, immunizations, 2 letters of recommendation. Transfer students are accepted. *Application deadline:* 11/15 (fall). *Application fee:* $50.
Advanced Placement Credit by examination available. Credit given for nursing courses completed elsewhere dependent upon specific evaluations.
Expenses (2015–16) *Tuition:* full-time $36,724. *International tuition:* $36,724 full-time. *Room and board:* $13,334 per academic year. *Required fees:* full-time $970.
Financial Aid *Gift aid (need-based):* Federal Pell, FSEOG, state, private, college/university gift aid from institutional funds. *Loans:* Federal Direct (Subsidized and Unsubsidized Stafford PLUS), Perkins. *Work-study:* Federal Work-Study, part-time campus jobs. *Financial aid application deadline:* 3/15.
Contact Mr. Eric Nichols, Director of Admission, Department of Nursing, Saint Anselm College, 100 Saint Anselm Drive, Manchester,

NH 03102-1310. *Telephone:* 603-641-7500. *Fax:* 603-641-7550. *E-mail:* enichols@anselm.edu.

CONTINUING EDUCATION PROGRAM

Contact Ms. Amy Guthrie, Director, Continuing Nursing Education, Department of Nursing, Saint Anselm College, 100 Saint Anselm Drive, #1745, Manchester, NH 03102-1310. *Telephone:* 603-641-7083. *Fax:* 603-641-7089. *E-mail:* aguthrie@anselm.edu.

Southern New Hampshire University
Department of Nursing
Manchester, New Hampshire

http://www.snhu.edu/
Founded in 1932
DEGREES • BS • MSN

BACCALAUREATE PROGRAMS

Degree BS
Available Programs Accelerated RN Baccalaureate.
Online Degree Options Yes (online only).
Contact Judith M. Pare, Director, Department of Nursing, Southern New Hampshire University, 2500 North River Road, Manchester, NH 03106-1045. *Telephone:* 603-314-4828. *E-mail:* j.pare@snhu.edu.

GRADUATE PROGRAMS

Contact Judith M. Pare, Director, Department of Nursing, Southern New Hampshire University, 2500 North River Road, Manchester, NH 03106-1045. *Telephone:* 603-314-4828. *E-mail:* j.pare@snhu.edu.

MASTER'S DEGREE PROGRAM

Degree MSN
Available Programs Master's.
Concentrations Available Clinical nurse leader; nursing education.

University of New Hampshire
Department of Nursing
Durham, New Hampshire

http://www.chhs.unh.edu/nursing
Founded in 1866
DEGREES • BS • DNP • MS
Nursing Program Faculty 13 (75% with doctorates).
Baccalaureate Enrollment 296 **Women** 96% **Men** 4% **Part-time** 15%
Graduate Enrollment 125 **Women** 88% **Men** 12% **Part-time** 20%
Distance Learning Courses Available.
Nursing Student Activities Nursing Honor Society, Sigma Theta Tau, Student Nurses' Association, nursing club.
Nursing Student Resources Academic advising; academic or career counseling; assistance for students with disabilities; bookstore; campus computer network; career placement assistance; computer lab; e-mail services; employment services for current students; externships; interactive nursing skills videos; Internet; learning resource lab; library services; nursing audiovisuals; remedial services; resume preparation assistance; skills, simulation, or other laboratory; tutoring; unpaid internships.

BACCALAUREATE PROGRAMS

Degree BS
Available Programs Generic Baccalaureate.
Study Options Full-time.
Program Entrance Requirements Written essay, health exam, health insurance, high school chemistry, high school foreign language, 4 years high school math, 4 years high school science, high school transcript, immunizations, minimum high school rank 15%, prerequisite course work. *Application deadline:* 2/1 (fall).
Contact Dr. Gene Harkless, Associate Professor and Chair, Department of Nursing, University of New Hampshire, Hewitt Hall, 4 Library Way, Durham, NH 03824-3563. *Telephone:* 603-862-2285. *Fax:* 603-862-4771. *E-mail:* geh@unh.edu.

GRADUATE PROGRAMS

Financial Aid 2 teaching assistantships were awarded; fellowships, research assistantships, Federal Work-Study, scholarships, and tuition waivers (full and partial) also available.
Contact Dr. Pamela DiNapoli, Coordinator, Graduate Program in Nursing, Department of Nursing, University of New Hampshire, Hewitt Hall, 4 Library Way, Durham, NH 03824-3563. *Telephone:* 603-862-3976. *Fax:* 603-862-4771. *E-mail:* ppdn@unh.edu.

MASTER'S DEGREE PROGRAM

Degree MS
Available Programs Accelerated Master's; Accelerated Master's for Non-Nursing College Graduates; Master's; Master's for Nurses with Non-Nursing Degrees.
Concentrations Available Clinical nurse leader. *Nurse practitioner programs in:* family health.
Study Options Full-time and part-time.
Program Entrance Requirements Minimum overall college GPA of 3.0, transcript of college record, written essay, 3 letters of recommendation, nursing research course, statistics course, GRE General Test or MAT. *Application deadline:* 4/1 (fall), 11/1 (spring). Applications may be processed on a rolling basis for some programs.
Advanced Placement Credit given for nursing courses completed elsewhere dependent upon specific evaluations.
Degree Requirements 48 total credit hours.

POST-MASTER'S PROGRAM

Areas of Study *Nurse practitioner programs in:* family health.

DOCTORAL DEGREE PROGRAM

Degree DNP
Available Programs Doctorate.
Areas of Study Advanced practice nursing, clinical practice, clinical research, faculty preparation, health policy, health-care systems, individualized study, nursing education, nursing policy, nursing research, nursing science.
Online Degree Options Yes.
Program Entrance Requirements Clinical experience, minimum overall college GPA of 3.25, interview by faculty committee, 3 letters of recommendation, MSN or equivalent, statistics course, vita. Application deadline: 11/1 (fall), 4/1 (spring). Applications may be processed on a rolling basis for some programs.
Degree Requirements 36 total credit hours, dissertation.

NEW JERSEY

Bloomfield College
Division of Nursing
Bloomfield, New Jersey

http://www.bloomfield.edu/
Founded in 1868
DEGREE • BS
Nursing Program Faculty 16 (50% with doctorates).
Baccalaureate Enrollment 155 **Women** 85% **Men** 15% **Part-time** 30%
Distance Learning Courses Available.
Nursing Student Activities Nursing Honor Society, Sigma Theta Tau, Student Nurses' Association.
Nursing Student Resources Academic advising; academic or career counseling; assistance for students with disabilities; bookstore; campus computer network; career placement assistance; computer lab; computer-assisted instruction; e-mail services; employment services for current students; interactive nursing skills videos; Internet; learning resource lab; library services; nursing audiovisuals; other; placement services for program completers; remedial services; resume preparation assistance; skills, simulation, or other laboratory; tutoring.
Library Facilities 2,000 volumes in health, 2,000 volumes in nursing; 44 periodical subscriptions health-care related.

BACCALAUREATE PROGRAMS

Degree BS
Available Programs Generic Baccalaureate; RN Baccalaureate.
Study Options Full-time and part-time.

Program Entrance Requirements Transcript of college record, CPR certification, health exam, immunizations, minimum GPA in nursing prerequisites of 2.5, prerequisite course work. Transfer students are accepted. *Application deadline:* 5/1 (fall). *Application fee:* $40.
Advanced Placement Credit given for nursing courses completed elsewhere dependent upon specific evaluations.
Expenses (2015–16) *Tuition:* full-time $27,800; part-time $3475 per course. *International tuition:* $27,800 full-time. *Room and board:* $11,300; room only: $5650 per academic year. *Required fees:* full-time $15.
Financial Aid 90% of baccalaureate students in nursing programs received some form of financial aid in 2014–15. *Gift aid (need-based):* Federal Pell, FSEOG, state, private, college/university gift aid from institutional funds. *Loans:* Federal Direct (Subsidized and Unsubsidized Stafford PLUS). *Work-study:* Federal Work-Study, part-time campus jobs. *Financial aid application deadline:* 6/1(priority: 3/15).
Contact Dr. Neddie Serra, Chair, Division of Nursing, Bloomfield College, Bloomfield, NJ 07003. *Telephone:* 973-748-9000 Ext. 1120. *Fax:* 973-743-3998. *E-mail:* neddie_serra@bloomfield.edu.

Caldwell University
Nursing Programs
Caldwell, New Jersey

http://www.caldwell.edu/
Founded in 1939
DEGREE • BSN
Nursing Program Faculty 13 (30% with doctorates).
Baccalaureate Enrollment 150
Distance Learning Courses Available.
Nursing Student Activities Nursing Honor Society, Student Nurses' Association.
Nursing Student Resources Academic advising; academic or career counseling; assistance for students with disabilities; bookstore; campus computer network; computer lab; computer-assisted instruction; e-mail services; employment services for current students; housing assistance; interactive nursing skills videos; Internet; learning resource lab; library services; nursing audiovisuals; paid internships; remedial services; resume preparation assistance; skills, simulation, or other laboratory; tutoring.
Library Facilities 4,794 volumes in health, 97 volumes in nursing; 5,215 periodical subscriptions health-care related.

BACCALAUREATE PROGRAMS

Degree BSN
Available Programs ADN to Baccalaureate; Accelerated Baccalaureate; Accelerated RN Baccalaureate; Baccalaureate for Second Degree; Generic Baccalaureate; RN Baccalaureate.
Study Options Full-time and part-time.
Online Degree Options Yes.
Program Entrance Requirements Minimum overall college GPA of 2.75, transcript of college record, CPR certification, written essay, health exam, health insurance, high school biology, high school chemistry, high school foreign language, 4 years high school math, 3 years high school science, high school transcript, immunizations, 2 letters of recommendation, minimum high school GPA of 2.75, minimum GPA in nursing prerequisites of 2.75, professional liability insurance/malpractice insurance, prerequisite course work. Transfer students are accepted. *Application deadline:* Applications may be processed on a rolling basis for some programs. *Application fee:* $40.
Advanced Placement Credit by examination available.
Contact Ms. Jenny Whitmore, Assistant Director, Admissions, Nursing Programs, Caldwell University, 120 Bloomfield Avenue, Caldwell, NJ 07006. *Telephone:* 973-618-3385. *E-mail:* jwhitmore@caldwell.edu.

The College of New Jersey
School of Nursing, Health and Exercise Science
Ewing, New Jersey

http://www.nursing.pages.tcnj.edu/
Founded in 1855
DEGREES • BSN • MSN
Nursing Program Faculty 45 (22% with doctorates).

Baccalaureate Enrollment 390 Women 89.5% Men 10.5%
Part-time 3%
Graduate Enrollment 36 Women 86% Men 14% Part-time 88%
Nursing Student Activities Sigma Theta Tau, Student Nurses' Association.
Nursing Student Resources Academic advising; academic or career counseling; assistance for students with disabilities; bookstore; campus computer network; career placement assistance; computer lab; computer-assisted instruction; daycare for children of students; e-mail services; employment services for current students; externships; housing assistance; interactive nursing skills videos; Internet; learning resource lab; library services; nursing audiovisuals; paid internships; resume preparation assistance; skills, simulation, or other laboratory; tutoring; unpaid internships.
Library Facilities 30,000 volumes in health, 18,800 volumes in nursing; 228 periodical subscriptions health-care related.

BACCALAUREATE PROGRAMS

Degree BSN
Available Programs Generic Baccalaureate; RN Baccalaureate.
Site Options Hunterdon-Flemington, NJ; Princeton, NJ; New Brunswick, NJ.
Study Options Full-time and part-time.
Program Entrance Requirements Written essay, health exam, high school transcript, immunizations. Transfer students are accepted. *Application deadline:* 1/15 (fall), 11/15 (spring). *Application fee:* $75.
Advanced Placement Credit by examination available. Credit given for nursing courses completed elsewhere dependent upon specific evaluations.
Expenses (2015–16) *Tuition, state resident:* full-time $10,880; part-time $1542 per unit. *Tuition, nonresident:* full-time $21,812; part-time $3088 per unit. *Room and board:* $12,500; room only: $8622 per academic year.
Financial Aid *Gift aid (need-based):* Federal Pell, FSEOG, state, private, college/university gift aid from institutional funds, Federal Nursing. *Loans:* Federal Nursing Student Loans, Federal Direct (Subsidized and Unsubsidized Stafford PLUS), Perkins. *Work-study:* Federal Work-Study. *Financial aid application deadline (priority):* 3/1.
Contact Ms. Ada Swain, Program Assistant, School of Nursing, Health and Exercise Science, The College of New Jersey, PO Box 7718, 2000 Pennington Road, Ewing, NJ 08628-0718. *Telephone:* 609-771-2593. *Fax:* 609-637-5159. *E-mail:* ada.swain@tcnj.edu.

GRADUATE PROGRAMS

Expenses (2015–16) *Tuition, state resident:* full-time $12,510; part-time $695 per credit hour. *Tuition, nonresident:* full-time $19,730; part-time $1096 per credit hour.
Financial Aid Tuition waivers (partial) and unspecified assistantships available.
Contact Dr. Connie Kartoz, Graduate Coordinator Assistant Professor, School of Nursing, Health and Exercise Science, The College of New Jersey, PO Box 7718, 2000 Pennington Road, Ewing, NJ 08628-0718. *Telephone:* 609-771-2509. *E-mail:* kartoz@tcnj.edu.

MASTER'S DEGREE PROGRAM

Degree MSN
Available Programs Master's; RN to Master's.
Concentrations Available Clinical nurse leader. *Clinical nurse specialist programs in:* adult health. *Nurse practitioner programs in:* adult health, family health, neonatal health, school health.
Study Options Full-time and part-time.
Program Entrance Requirements Computer literacy, minimum overall college GPA of 3.0, transcript of college record, written essay, immunizations, interview, 3 letters of recommendation, nursing research course, physical assessment course, professional liability insurance/malpractice insurance, statistics course, GRE General Test. *Application deadline:* 2/1 (fall), 10/1 (winter), 12/1 (spring), 2/1 (summer). *Application fee:* $75.
Advanced Placement Credit given for nursing courses completed elsewhere dependent upon specific evaluations.
Degree Requirements 47 total credit hours, thesis or project.

POST-MASTER'S PROGRAM

Areas of Study *Clinical nurse specialist programs in:* adult health. *Nurse practitioner programs in:* adult health, family health, neonatal health.

College of Saint Elizabeth
Department of Nursing
Morristown, New Jersey

http://www.cse.edu
Founded in 1899
DEGREES • BSN • MSN
Nursing Program Faculty 18 (25% with doctorates).
Baccalaureate Enrollment 254 Women 95% Men 5% Part-time 92%
Graduate Enrollment 48 Women 95% Men 5% Part-time 99%
Nursing Student Activities Nursing Honor Society, Sigma Theta Tau, nursing club.
Nursing Student Resources Academic advising; academic or career counseling; assistance for students with disabilities; bookstore; campus computer network; career placement assistance; computer lab; computer-assisted instruction; e-mail services; employment services for current students; interactive nursing skills videos; Internet; learning resource lab; library services; nursing audiovisuals; other; remedial services; resume preparation assistance; skills, simulation, or other laboratory; tutoring.
Library Facilities 4,246 volumes in health, 702 volumes in nursing; 326 periodical subscriptions health-care related.

BACCALAUREATE PROGRAMS

Degree BSN
Available Programs ADN to Baccalaureate; Accelerated RN Baccalaureate; International Nurse to Baccalaureate; RN Baccalaureate.
Site Options Randolph, NJ; Passaic, NJ; Elizabeth , NJ.
Study Options Full-time and part-time.
Program Entrance Requirements Minimum overall college GPA of 2.0, transcript of college record, CPR certification, health exam, immunizations, prerequisite course work, RN licensure. Transfer students are accepted.
Advanced Placement Credit by examination available. Credit given for nursing courses completed elsewhere dependent upon specific evaluations.
Expenses (2014–15) *Tuition:* part-time $950 per credit.
Financial Aid 75% of baccalaureate students in nursing programs received some form of financial aid in 2013–14.
Contact Dr. Ellen G. Ehrlich, Chairperson, Department of Nursing, College of Saint Elizabeth, 2 Convent Road, Morristown, NJ 07960-6989. *Telephone:* 973-290-4056. *Fax:* 973-290-4177. *E-mail:* eehrlich@cse.edu.

GRADUATE PROGRAMS

Expenses (2014–15) *Tuition:* part-time $1088 per credit.
Financial Aid 70% of graduate students in nursing programs received some form of financial aid in 2013–14.
Contact Dr. Dianne DeLong, Chair of Nursing, Department of Nursing, College of Saint Elizabeth, 2 Convent Road, Morristown, NJ 07960. *Telephone:* 973-290-4037. *Fax:* 973-290-4177. *E-mail:* ddelong@cse.edu.

MASTER'S DEGREE PROGRAM

Degree MSN
Available Programs Master's; Master's for Nurses with Non-Nursing Degrees.
Concentrations Available Nursing education.
Site Options Elizabeth , NJ.
Study Options Part-time.
Program Entrance Requirements Computer literacy, minimum overall college GPA of 3.0, transcript of college record, CPR certification, written essay, 2 letters of recommendation, nursing research course, physical assessment course, resume, statistics course. *Application deadline:* Applications may be processed on a rolling basis for some programs.
Advanced Placement Credit given for nursing courses completed elsewhere dependent upon specific evaluations.
Degree Requirements 37 total credit hours, thesis or project.

POST-MASTER'S PROGRAM
Areas of Study Nursing education.

CONTINUING EDUCATION PROGRAM

Contact Dr. Eileen Carrigg Specchio, Professor, Department of Nursing, College of Saint Elizabeth, 2 Convent Road, Morristown, NJ 07960-

6989. *Telephone:* 973-290-4073. *Fax:* 973-290-4177.
E-mail: especchio@cse.edu.

Fairleigh Dickinson University, Metropolitan Campus

Henry P. Becton School of Nursing and Allied Health
Teaneck, New Jersey

http://www.fduinfo.com/depts/ucnah.php
Founded in 1942

DEGREES • BSN • DNP • MSN
Nursing Program Faculty 17 (47% with doctorates).
Baccalaureate Enrollment 220 **Women** 85% **Men** 15% **Part-time** 21%
Graduate Enrollment 141 **Women** 85% **Men** 15% **Part-time** 52%
Distance Learning Courses Available.
Nursing Student Activities Nursing Honor Society, Sigma Theta Tau, Student Nurses' Association.
Nursing Student Resources Academic advising; academic or career counseling; assistance for students with disabilities; bookstore; campus computer network; career placement assistance; computer lab; computer-assisted instruction; e-mail services; employment services for current students; externships; housing assistance; interactive nursing skills videos; Internet; learning resource lab; library services; nursing audiovisuals; other; placement services for program completers; remedial services; resume preparation assistance; skills, simulation, or other laboratory; tutoring; unpaid internships.
Library Facilities 2,336 volumes in health, 2,336 volumes in nursing; 1,526 periodical subscriptions health-care related.

BACCALAUREATE PROGRAMS

Degree BSN
Available Programs Accelerated Baccalaureate for Second Degree; Generic Baccalaureate; RN Baccalaureate.
Site Options Morristown, NJ; Teaneck, NJ; Summit, NJ.
Study Options Full-time and part-time.
Program Entrance Requirements Minimum overall college GPA of 3.0, transcript of college record, CPR certification, health exam, health insurance, high school biology, high school chemistry, 2 years high school math, 2 years high school science, high school transcript, immunizations, 2 letters of recommendation, professional liability insurance/malpractice insurance. Transfer students are accepted. *Application deadline:* Applications may be processed on a rolling basis for some programs.
Expenses (2015–16) *Tuition:* full-time $35,916; part-time $967 per credit. *International tuition:* $35,916 full-time. *Room and board:* $12,756; room only: $8424 per academic year. *Required fees:* full-time $994; part-time $16 per credit; part-time $199 per term.
Contact Ms. Sylvia Cabassa, Associate Director, Undergraduate Nursing, Henry P. Becton School of Nursing and Allied Health, Fairleigh Dickinson University, Metropolitan Campus, 1000 River Road, H-DH4-02, Teaneck, NJ 07666-1914. *Telephone:* 201-692-2880. *Fax:* 201-692-2388. *E-mail:* scabassa@fdu.edu.

GRADUATE PROGRAMS

Expenses (2015–16) *Tuition:* part-time $1220 per credit. *International tuition:* $1220 full-time. *Room and board:* $12,756; room only: $8424 per academic year. *Required fees:* full-time $994; part-time $16 per credit; part-time $199 per term.
Contact Dr. Elizabeth S. Parietti, Associate Director of Graduate Programs, Henry P. Becton School of Nursing and Allied Health, Fairleigh Dickinson University, Metropolitan Campus, 1000 River Road, H-DH4-02, Teaneck, NJ 07666-1914. *Telephone:* 201-692-2881. *Fax:* 201-692-2388. *E-mail:* parietti@fdu.edu.

MASTER'S DEGREE PROGRAM

Degree MSN
Available Programs Accelerated RN to Master's; Master's; RN to Master's.
Concentrations Available Nursing administration; nursing education; nursing informatics. *Nurse practitioner programs in:* adult health, family health, gerontology, psychiatric/mental health.
Site Options Morristown, NJ; Teaneck, NJ; Summit, NJ.
Study Options Full-time and part-time.

Online Degree Options Yes.
Program Entrance Requirements Clinical experience, minimum overall college GPA of 3.0, transcript of college record, CPR certification, immunizations, 2 letters of recommendation, nursing research course, physical assessment course, professional liability insurance/malpractice insurance, resume, statistics course. *Application deadline:* Applications may be processed on a rolling basis for some programs. *Application fee:* $40.
Advanced Placement Credit given for nursing courses completed elsewhere dependent upon specific evaluations.
Degree Requirements 31 total credit hours, thesis or project.

POST-MASTER'S PROGRAM

Areas of Study Nursing administration; nursing education; nursing informatics. *Nurse practitioner programs in:* adult health, family health, gerontology, psychiatric/mental health.

DOCTORAL DEGREE PROGRAM

Degree DNP
Available Programs Doctorate.
Areas of Study Advanced practice nursing, clinical practice, health policy, health-care systems, human health and illness, information systems, nursing administration, nursing policy, nursing research, nursing science.
Program Entrance Requirements Clinical experience, minimum overall college GPA of 3.5, interview by faculty committee, interview, 3 letters of recommendation, MSN or equivalent, vita, writing sample. Application deadline: Applications may be processed on a rolling basis for some programs.
Degree Requirements 36 total credit hours, dissertation, oral exam, residency.

Felician University

Division of Nursing and Health Management
Lodi, New Jersey

http://www.felician.edu/
Founded in 1942

DEGREES • BSN • MA/MSM • MSN
Nursing Program Faculty 25 (32% with doctorates).
Baccalaureate Enrollment 512 **Women** 92% **Men** 8% **Part-time** 20%
Graduate Enrollment 93 **Women** 89% **Men** 11% **Part-time** 88%
Distance Learning Courses Available.
Nursing Student Activities Nursing Honor Society, Sigma Theta Tau, Student Nurses' Association.
Nursing Student Resources Academic advising; academic or career counseling; assistance for students with disabilities; bookstore; campus computer network; career placement assistance; computer lab; computer-assisted instruction; daycare for children of students; e-mail services; interactive nursing skills videos; Internet; learning resource lab; library services; nursing audiovisuals; placement services for program completers; remedial services; resume preparation assistance; skills, simulation, or other laboratory; tutoring.
Library Facilities 12,519 volumes in health, 12,519 volumes in nursing; 21 periodical subscriptions health-care related.

BACCALAUREATE PROGRAMS

Degree BSN
Available Programs Accelerated Baccalaureate for Second Degree; Generic Baccalaureate.
Site Options East Orange, NJ; Long Branch, NJ; Edison, NJ.
Study Options Full-time and part-time.
Program Entrance Requirements Minimum overall college GPA of 3.0, transcript of college record, written essay, health exam, health insurance, high school biology, high school chemistry, 2 years high school math, 2 years high school science, high school transcript, immunizations, minimum high school GPA of 3.0, minimum GPA in nursing prerequisites of 2.8, professional liability insurance/malpractice insurance. Transfer students are accepted. *Application deadline:* 8/15 (fall), 1/10 (spring). Applications may be processed on a rolling basis for some programs. *Application fee:* $30.
Advanced Placement Credit by examination available. Credit given for nursing courses completed elsewhere dependent upon specific evaluations.
Contact *Telephone:* 201-559-6131. *Fax:* 201-559-6138.

GRADUATE PROGRAMS

Contact *Telephone:* 201-559-6077. *Fax:* 201-559-6138.

MASTER'S DEGREE PROGRAM

Degrees MA/MSM; MSN
Available Programs Accelerated RN to Master's; Master's.
Concentrations Available Nursing administration; nursing education. *Nurse practitioner programs in:* adult health, family health.
Study Options Full-time and part-time.
Online Degree Options Yes.
Program Entrance Requirements Clinical experience, computer literacy, minimum overall college GPA of 3.0, transcript of college record, CPR certification, written essay, immunizations, 2 letters of recommendation, nursing research course, physical assessment course, professional liability insurance/malpractice insurance, prerequisite course work, statistics course. *Application deadline:* Applications may be processed on a rolling basis for some programs. *Application fee:* $40.
Advanced Placement Credit given for nursing courses completed elsewhere dependent upon specific evaluations.
Degree Requirements 46 total credit hours, thesis or project.

POST-MASTER'S PROGRAM

Areas of Study Nursing administration; nursing education. *Nurse practitioner programs in:* adult health, family health.

Georgian Court University

The Georgian Court-Meridian Health School of Nursing
Lakewood, New Jersey

Founded in 1908
DEGREE • BSN

BACCALAUREATE PROGRAMS

Degree BSN
Available Programs Generic Baccalaureate.
Contact *Telephone:* 732-987-2760.

Kean University

Department of Nursing
Union, New Jersey

http://www.kean.edu/KU/School-of-Nursing
Founded in 1855
DEGREES • BSN • MSN • MSN/MPA
Nursing Program Faculty 31 (32% with doctorates).
Baccalaureate Enrollment 313 **Women** 93% **Men** 7% **Part-time** 90%
Graduate Enrollment 102 **Women** 93% **Men** 7% **Part-time** 95%
Nursing Student Activities Nursing Honor Society, Sigma Theta Tau, nursing club.
Nursing Student Resources Academic advising; academic or career counseling; assistance for students with disabilities; bookstore; campus computer network; career placement assistance; computer lab; computer-assisted instruction; daycare for children of students; e-mail services; employment services for current students; housing assistance; interactive nursing skills videos; Internet; learning resource lab; library services; nursing audiovisuals; placement services for program completers; remedial services; resume preparation assistance; tutoring.

BACCALAUREATE PROGRAMS

Degree BSN
Available Programs ADN to Baccalaureate; RN Baccalaureate.
Site Options Branchburg, NJ; Toms River, NJ.
Study Options Full-time and part-time.
Program Entrance Requirements Minimum overall college GPA of 2.0, written essay, 2 letters of recommendation, prerequisite course work, RN licensure. Transfer students are accepted. *Application deadline:* Applications may be processed on a rolling basis for some programs.
Advanced Placement Credit by examination available. Credit given for nursing courses completed elsewhere dependent upon specific evaluations.
Contact *Telephone:* 908-737-3390. *Fax:* 908-737-3393.

GRADUATE PROGRAMS

Contact *Telephone:* 908-737-3390. *Fax:* 908-737-3393.

MASTER'S DEGREE PROGRAM

Degrees MSN; MSN/MPA
Available Programs Accelerated Master's for Nurses with Non-Nursing Degrees; Master's; Master's for Nurses with Non-Nursing Degrees.
Concentrations Available Health-care administration; nursing administration. *Clinical nurse specialist programs in:* community health, school health.
Site Options Toms River, NJ.
Study Options Full-time and part-time.
Program Entrance Requirements Clinical experience, computer literacy, minimum overall college GPA of 3.0, transcript of college record, written essay, immunizations, interview, 2 letters of recommendation, nursing research course, physical assessment course, professional liability insurance/malpractice insurance, statistics course.
Advanced Placement Credit given for nursing courses completed elsewhere dependent upon specific evaluations.
Degree Requirements 36 total credit hours, thesis or project.

Monmouth University

Marjorie K. Unterberg School of Nursing
West Long Branch, New Jersey

http://www.monmouth.edu/
Founded in 1933
DEGREES • BSN • MSN
Nursing Program Faculty 17 (67% with doctorates).
Baccalaureate Enrollment 71 **Women** 93% **Men** 7% **Part-time** 98%
Graduate Enrollment 245 **Women** 97% **Men** 3% **Part-time** 92%
Distance Learning Courses Available.
Nursing Student Activities Sigma Theta Tau, Student Nurses' Association.
Nursing Student Resources Academic advising; academic or career counseling; assistance for students with disabilities; bookstore; campus computer network; career placement assistance; computer lab; computer-assisted instruction; e-mail services; employment services for current students; interactive nursing skills videos; Internet; learning resource lab; library services; nursing audiovisuals; paid internships; remedial services; resume preparation assistance; skills, simulation, or other laboratory; tutoring.
Library Facilities 250,000 volumes in health, 25,000 volumes in nursing; 98 periodical subscriptions health-care related.

BACCALAUREATE PROGRAMS

Degree BSN
Available Programs ADN to Baccalaureate; RN Baccalaureate.
Site Options Red Bank, NJ; Freehold, NJ.
Study Options Full-time and part-time.
Program Entrance Requirements Transcript of college record, health exam, immunizations, 2 letters of recommendation, minimum GPA in nursing prerequisites of 2.0, professional liability insurance/malpractice insurance, prerequisite course work, RN licensure. Transfer students are accepted. *Application deadline:* 7/15 (fall), 11/15 (spring), 5/1 (summer). Applications may be processed on a rolling basis for some programs. *Application fee:* $50.
Advanced Placement Credit by examination available. Credit given for nursing courses completed elsewhere dependent upon specific evaluations.
Contact *Telephone:* 732-571-3443. *Fax:* 732-263-5131.

GRADUATE PROGRAMS

Contact *Telephone:* 732-571-3443. *Fax:* 732-263-5131.

MASTER'S DEGREE PROGRAM

Degree MSN
Available Programs Master's; Master's for Nurses with Non-Nursing Degrees; RN to Master's.
Concentrations Available Nursing administration; nursing education. *Clinical nurse specialist programs in:* forensic nursing, school health. *Nurse practitioner programs in:* adult health, family health, psychiatric/mental health.
Site Options Edison, NJ.
Study Options Full-time and part-time.

Program Entrance Requirements Minimum overall college GPA of 2.75, transcript of college record, immunizations, 2 letters of recommendation, professional liability insurance/malpractice insurance. *Application deadline:* 7/15 (fall), 11/15 (spring), 5/1 (summer). Applications may be processed on a rolling basis for some programs. *Application fee:* $50.

Advanced Placement Credit by examination available. Credit given for nursing courses completed elsewhere dependent upon specific evaluations.

Degree Requirements 42 total credit hours.

POST-MASTER'S PROGRAM

Areas of Study Nursing administration; nursing education. *Clinical nurse specialist programs in:* forensic nursing, school health. *Nurse practitioner programs in:* adult health, family health, psychiatric/mental health.

CONTINUING EDUCATION PROGRAM

Contact *Telephone:* 732-571-3694. *Fax:* 732-263-5131.

New Jersey City University
Department of Nursing
Jersey City, New Jersey

https://www.njcu.edu/nursing/
Founded in 1927
DEGREE • BSN

Nursing Program Faculty 10 (70% with doctorates).
Baccalaureate Enrollment 550 **Women** 85% **Men** 15% **Part-time** 40%
Nursing Student Activities Nursing Honor Society, Sigma Theta Tau, Student Nurses' Association.
Nursing Student Resources Academic advising; academic or career counseling; assistance for students with disabilities; bookstore; campus computer network; computer lab; computer-assisted instruction; daycare for children of students; e-mail services; interactive nursing skills videos; Internet; learning resource lab; library services; nursing audiovisuals; remedial services; skills, simulation, or other laboratory.

BACCALAUREATE PROGRAMS

Degree BSN
Available Programs Accelerated Baccalaureate for Second Degree; RN Baccalaureate.
Site Options Wall Township, NJ; East Orange, NJ.
Study Options Full-time and part-time.
Program Entrance Requirements Minimum overall college GPA of 3.0, transcript of college record, CPR certification, written essay, health exam, immunizations, 2 letters of recommendation, professional liability insurance/malpractice insurance, prerequisite course work, RN licensure. Transfer students are accepted. *Application deadline:* 3/15 (fall), 3/15 (summer). *Application fee:* $35.
Advanced Placement Credit by examination available. Credit given for nursing courses completed elsewhere dependent upon specific evaluations.
Contact Dr. Joyce Wright, Associate Professor, Department of Nursing, New Jersey City University, 2039 Kennedy Boulevard, R405, Jersey City, NJ 07305. *Telephone:* 201-200-3157. *E-mail:* jwright@njcu.edu.

Ramapo College of New Jersey
Master of Science in Nursing Program
Mahwah, New Jersey

http://www.ramapo.edu/rn/
Founded in 1969
DEGREES • BSN • MSN

Nursing Program Faculty 29 (20% with doctorates).
Baccalaureate Enrollment 435 **Women** 90% **Men** 10% **Part-time** 15%
Graduate Enrollment 41 **Women** 95% **Men** 5% **Part-time** 90%
Distance Learning Courses Available.

Nursing Student Activities Nursing Honor Society, Student Nurses' Association.
Nursing Student Resources Academic advising; academic or career counseling; assistance for students with disabilities; bookstore; campus computer network; career placement assistance; computer lab; computer-assisted instruction; e-mail services; employment services for current students; externships; housing assistance; interactive nursing skills videos; Internet; learning resource lab; library services; nursing audiovisuals; placement services for program completers; remedial services; resume preparation assistance; skills, simulation, or other laboratory; tutoring; unpaid internships.
Library Facilities 3,500 volumes in nursing; 200 periodical subscriptions health-care related.

BACCALAUREATE PROGRAMS

Degree BSN
Available Programs Generic Baccalaureate; RN Baccalaureate.
Site Options Englewood, NJ.
Study Options Full-time.
Online Degree Options Yes.
Program Entrance Requirements CPR certification, health exam, 3 years high school science, immunizations, minimum high school GPA of 2.5, minimum high school rank 20%, professional liability insurance/malpractice insurance. Transfer students are accepted. *Application deadline:* 3/1 (fall), 3/1 (spring). Applications may be processed on a rolling basis for some programs. *Application fee:* $60.
Advanced Placement Credit given for nursing courses completed elsewhere dependent upon specific evaluations.
Contact *Telephone:* 201-684-7737. *Fax:* 201-684-7934.

GRADUATE PROGRAMS

Contact *Telephone:* 201-684-7737. *Fax:* 201-684-7934.

MASTER'S DEGREE PROGRAM

Degree MSN
Available Programs Master's.
Concentrations Available Nursing education.
Study Options Full-time and part-time.
Online Degree Options Yes (online only).
Program Entrance Requirements Clinical experience, computer literacy, minimum overall college GPA of 3.0, transcript of college record, CPR certification, 2 letters of recommendation, nursing research course, professional liability insurance/malpractice insurance, statistics course. *Application deadline:* Applications may be processed on a rolling basis for some programs. *Application fee:* $60.
Advanced Placement Credit given for nursing courses completed elsewhere dependent upon specific evaluations.
Degree Requirements 32 total credit hours.

POST-MASTER'S PROGRAM
Areas of Study Nursing education.

CONTINUING EDUCATION PROGRAM

Contact *Telephone:* 201-684-7206. *Fax:* 201-684-7954.

Rider University
RN-BSN Program
Lawrenceville, New Jersey

http://www.rider.edu/
Founded in 1865
DEGREE • BSN

BACCALAUREATE PROGRAMS

Degree BSN
Available Programs RN Baccalaureate.
Online Degree Options Yes (online only).
Contact Rosemary Fliszar, Director, RN-BSN Program, Rider University, 2083 Lawrenceville Road, Lawrenceville, NJ 08648. *Telephone:* 609-895-5435. *E-mail:* rfliszar@rider.edu.

Rowan University
RN to BSN Program
Glassboro, New Jersey

http://www.rowan.edu
Founded in 1923
DEGREES • BSN • MSN
Nursing Program Faculty 15 (80% with doctorates).
Baccalaureate Enrollment 122 **Women** 85% **Men** 15% **Part-time** 100%
Graduate Enrollment 165 **Women** 85% **Men** 15% **Part-time** 100%
Distance Learning Courses Available.
Nursing Student Activities Student Nurses' Association.
Nursing Student Resources Academic advising; bookstore; campus computer network; computer-assisted instruction; e-mail services; interactive nursing skills videos; Internet; learning resource lab; library services; skills, simulation, or other laboratory; tutoring.
Library Facilities 10,000 volumes in health, 10,000 volumes in nursing; 1,000 periodical subscriptions health-care related.

BACCALAUREATE PROGRAMS

Degree BSN
Available Programs RN Baccalaureate.
Site Options Camden, NJ; Stratford, NJ; Sewll, NJ.
Study Options Part-time.
Program Entrance Requirements Minimum overall college GPA of 2.75, transcript of college record, prerequisite course work, RN licensure. *Application deadline:* 7/15 (fall), 11/15 (spring), 3/15 (summer). Applications may be processed on a rolling basis for some programs. *Application fee:* $65.
Expenses (2015–16) *Tuition, state resident:* part-time $570 per credit hour. *Tuition, nonresident:* part-time $570 per credit hour.
Contact Admissions, RN to BSN Program, Rowan University, 201 Mullica Hill Road, Glassboro, NJ 08028. *Telephone:* 856-256-5435. *E-mail:* cgceenrollement@rowan.edu.

GRADUATE PROGRAMS

Expenses (2015–16) *Tuition, state resident:* part-time $700 per credit hour. *Tuition, nonresident:* part-time $700 per credit hour.
Contact Patrice Henry-Thatcher, RN, Academic Program Advisor, RN to BSN Program, Rowan University, 1400 Tanyard Road, Sewell, NJ 08080. *Telephone:* 856-256-5142. *E-mail:* henrythatcher@rowan.edu.

MASTER'S DEGREE PROGRAM
Degree MSN
Available Programs Master's.
Concentrations Available Clinical nurse leader. *Nurse practitioner programs in:* adult-gerontology acute care, family health.
Study Options Part-time.
Program Entrance Requirements Computer literacy, minimum overall college GPA of 3.0, transcript of college record, letters of recommendation, resume, statistics course. *Application deadline:* 7/15 (fall), 11/15 (spring), 3/15 (summer). Applications may be processed on a rolling basis for some programs. *Application fee:* $65.
Advanced Placement Credit given for nursing courses completed elsewhere dependent upon specific evaluations.
Degree Requirements 35 total credit hours.

Rutgers, The State University of New Jersey, Camden
Rutgers School of Nursing–Camden
Camden, New Jersey

http://www.nursing.camden.rutgers.edu/
Founded in 1927
DEGREES • BS • DNP • MSN
Nursing Program Faculty 64 (80% with doctorates).
Baccalaureate Enrollment 645 **Women** 81% **Men** 19% **Part-time** 33%
Graduate Enrollment 101 **Women** 90% **Men** 10% **Part-time** 90%
Distance Learning Courses Available.
Nursing Student Activities Sigma Theta Tau, Student Nurses' Association.

Nursing Student Resources Academic advising; academic or career counseling; assistance for students with disabilities; bookstore; campus computer network; career placement assistance; computer lab; computer-assisted instruction; e-mail services; employment services for current students; externships; housing assistance; interactive nursing skills videos; Internet; learning resource lab; library services; nursing audiovisuals; remedial services; resume preparation assistance; skills, simulation, or other laboratory; tutoring.
Library Facilities 161,463 volumes in health, 9,491 volumes in nursing; 1,389 periodical subscriptions health-care related.

BACCALAUREATE PROGRAMS

Degree BS
Available Programs Accelerated Baccalaureate; Accelerated RN Baccalaureate; Generic Baccalaureate; RN Baccalaureate.
Site Options Atlantic City, NJ; Mercer, NJ.
Study Options Full-time.
Program Entrance Requirements Minimum overall college GPA of 3.0, transcript of college record, CPR certification, written essay, health exam, health insurance, high school biology, high school chemistry, 2 years high school math, high school transcript, immunizations, minimum high school GPA of 3.0, minimum GPA in nursing prerequisites of 3.0, prerequisite course work. Transfer students are accepted. *Application deadline:* 3/15 (fall). *Application fee:* $65.
Expenses (2014–15) *Tuition, state resident:* full-time $10,954; part-time $353 per credit. *Tuition, nonresident:* full-time $25,249; part-time $820 per credit. *International tuition:* $25,249 full-time. *Room and board:* $4736; room only: $3969 per academic year. *Required fees:* full-time $2706; part-time $525 per term.
Financial Aid 90% of baccalaureate students in nursing programs received some form of financial aid in 2013–14. *Gift aid (need-based):* Federal Pell, FSEOG, state, private, college/university gift aid from institutional funds, Federal Nursing. *Loans:* Federal Nursing Student Loans, Federal Direct (Subsidized and Unsubsidized Stafford PLUS), Perkins, state, college/university, alternative loans. *Work-study:* Federal Work-Study, part-time campus jobs. *Financial aid application deadline (priority):* 3/15.
Contact Mahirym Holguin, Administrative Assistant, Rutgers School of Nursing–Camden, Rutgers, The State University of New Jersey, Camden, 311 North Fifth Street, Armitage Hall, Room 407, Camden, NJ 08102. *Telephone:* 856-225-6226. *Fax:* 856-225-6250. *E-mail:* nursecam@camden.rutgers.edu.

GRADUATE PROGRAMS

Expenses (2014–15) *Tuition, state resident:* full-time $17,184; part-time $716 per credit. *Tuition, nonresident:* full-time $25,944; part-time $1081 per credit. *International tuition:* $25,944 full-time. *Room and board:* $5194; room only: $4427 per academic year. *Required fees:* full-time $1466; part-time $1064 per term.
Financial Aid 60% of graduate students in nursing programs received some form of financial aid in 2013–14.
Contact Mr. Thomas Porvaznik, Program Support Specialist, Rutgers School of Nursing–Camden, Rutgers, The State University of New Jersey, Camden, 215 North Third Street, Suite 204, Camden, NJ 08102. *Telephone:* 856-225-6226. *Fax:* 856-225-6250. *E-mail:* Thomas.Porvaznik@rutgers.edu.

MASTER'S DEGREE PROGRAM
Degree MSN
Available Programs Master's.
Concentrations Available *Nurse practitioner programs in:* adult health, family health.
Study Options Full-time and part-time.
Degree Requirements 45 total credit hours.

DOCTORAL DEGREE PROGRAM
Degree DNP
Available Programs Doctorate; Post-Baccalaureate Doctorate.
Areas of Study Advanced practice nursing, aging, bio-behavioral research, biology of health and illness, clinical practice, family health, gerontology, health policy, health promotion/disease prevention, health-care systems, illness and transition, information systems, nurse case management, nursing policy, nursing research, nursing science, urban health.
Program Entrance Requirements Clinical experience, minimum overall college GPA of 3.0, interview by faculty committee, interview, 3 letters of recommendation, vita. Application deadline: 3/30 (spring). Application fee: $65.
Degree Requirements 63 total credit hours, residency.

POSTDOCTORAL PROGRAM

Areas of Study Aging, cancer care, chronic illness, community health, family health, gerontology, health promotion/disease prevention, infection prevention/skin care, nursing informatics, nursing interventions, nursing research, nursing science, outcomes, vulnerable population.
Postdoctoral Program Contact Mr. Thomas Porvaznik, Program Support Specialist, Rutgers School of Nursing–Camden, Rutgers, The State University of New Jersey, Camden, 215 North Third Street, Suite 204, Camden, NJ 08102. *Telephone:* 856-225-2318.
E-mail: porvazta@camden.rutgers.edu.

Rutgers, The State University of New Jersey, Newark

Rutgers School of Nursing
Newark, New Jersey

http://sn.rutgers.edu/
Founded in 1892

DEGREES • BSN • DNP • MSN • MSN/MPH

Nursing Program Faculty 234 (30% with doctorates).
Baccalaureate Enrollment 340 **Women** 85% **Men** 15%
Graduate Enrollment 976 **Women** 80% **Men** 20% **Part-time** 80%
Distance Learning Courses Available.
Nursing Student Activities Nursing Honor Society, Sigma Theta Tau, Student Nurses' Association.
Nursing Student Resources Academic advising; academic or career counseling; assistance for students with disabilities; bookstore; campus computer network; computer lab; computer-assisted instruction; daycare for children of students; e-mail services; housing assistance; interactive nursing skills videos; Internet; learning resource lab; library services; nursing audiovisuals; remedial services; resume preparation assistance; skills, simulation, or other laboratory; tutoring.
Library Facilities 92,000 volumes in health, 3,300 volumes in nursing; 4,500 periodical subscriptions health-care related.

BACCALAUREATE PROGRAMS

Degree BSN
Available Programs Accelerated Baccalaureate for Second Degree; RN Baccalaureate.
Site Options Stratford, NJ.
Study Options Full-time.
Program Entrance Requirements Minimum overall college GPA of 3.3, transcript of college record, CPR certification, written essay, health exam, health insurance, immunizations, 2 letters of recommendation, minimum GPA in nursing prerequisites of 2.75, prerequisite course work. *Application deadline:* 3/15 (fall), 7/15 (spring), 3/15 (summer). *Application fee:* $45.
Advanced Placement Credit given for nursing courses completed elsewhere dependent upon specific evaluations.
Contact *Telephone:* 973-972-5336.

GRADUATE PROGRAMS

Contact *Telephone:* 973-972-5336. *Fax:* 973-972-7904.

MASTER'S DEGREE PROGRAM

Degrees MSN; MSN/MPH
Available Programs Master's; Master's for Nurses with Non-Nursing Degrees; RN to Master's.
Concentrations Available Clinical nurse leader; nurse anesthesia; nurse-midwifery; nursing education; nursing informatics. *Nurse practitioner programs in:* acute care, adult health, family health, gerontology, psychiatric/mental health, women's health.
Site Options Somers Point, NJ; Stratford, NJ; Voorhees, NJ.
Study Options Full-time and part-time.
Online Degree Options Yes.
Program Entrance Requirements Clinical experience, minimum overall college GPA of 3.0, transcript of college record, CPR certification, 2 letters of recommendation, physical assessment course, prerequisite course work, resume, statistics course, GRE. *Application deadline:* 3/15 (fall). *Application fee:* $50.
Advanced Placement Credit given for nursing courses completed elsewhere dependent upon specific evaluations.
Degree Requirements 40 total credit hours.

POST-MASTER'S PROGRAM

Areas of Study Clinical nurse leader; nurse-midwifery; nursing informatics. *Nurse practitioner programs in:* acute care, adult health, family health, gerontology, psychiatric/mental health, women's health.

DOCTORAL DEGREE PROGRAM

Degree DNP
Available Programs Doctorate; Doctorate for Nurses with Non-Nursing Degrees; Post-Baccalaureate Doctorate.
Areas of Study Clinical practice, nursing administration.
Site Options Stratford, NJ.
Program Entrance Requirements Clinical experience, minimum overall college GPA of 3.0, interview by faculty committee, interview, 2 letters of recommendation, MSN or equivalent, statistics course, vita, writing sample. Application deadline: 6/1 (fall), 12/9 (spring). Applications may be processed on a rolling basis for some programs. Application fee: $50.
Degree Requirements 32 total credit hours, dissertation.

CONTINUING EDUCATION PROGRAM

Contact *Telephone:* 973-972-9793. *Fax:* 973-972-7904.

Saint Peter's University

Nursing Program
Jersey City, New Jersey

http://www.saintpeters.edu/
Founded in 1872

DEGREES • BSN • MSN

Nursing Program Faculty 15 (73% with doctorates).
Baccalaureate Enrollment 161 **Women** 85% **Men** 15%
Graduate Enrollment 55 **Women** 99% **Men** 1%
Distance Learning Courses Available.
Nursing Student Activities Nursing Honor Society, Sigma Theta Tau, Student Nurses' Association.
Nursing Student Resources Academic advising; academic or career counseling; assistance for students with disabilities; bookstore; campus computer network; career placement assistance; computer lab; computer-assisted instruction; e-mail services; externships; interactive nursing skills videos; Internet; learning resource lab; library services; nursing audiovisuals; remedial services; resume preparation assistance; skills, simulation, or other laboratory; tutoring.
Library Facilities 7,200 volumes in health; 1,586 periodical subscriptions health-care related.

BACCALAUREATE PROGRAMS

Degree BSN
Available Programs ADN to Baccalaureate; Generic Baccalaureate; RN Baccalaureate.
Site Options Englewood Cliffs, NJ.
Study Options Full-time.
Program Entrance Requirements Minimum overall college GPA of 2.7, transcript of college record, written essay, high school biology, high school chemistry, high school foreign language, 3 years high school math, 3 years high school science, high school transcript, immunizations, 2 letters of recommendation, minimum high school GPA of 3.0. Transfer students are accepted. *Application deadline:* Applications may be processed on a rolling basis for some programs.
Contact *Telephone:* 201-761-7113. *Fax:* 201-761-7105.

GRADUATE PROGRAMS

Contact *Telephone:* 201-761-6272. *Fax:* 201-761-6271.

MASTER'S DEGREE PROGRAM

Degree MSN
Available Programs Master's; Master's for Nurses with Non-Nursing Degrees.
Concentrations Available Nurse case management; nursing administration. *Nurse practitioner programs in:* adult health.
Site Options Englewood Cliffs, NJ.
Study Options Part-time.
Program Entrance Requirements Clinical experience, minimum overall college GPA of 3.0, transcript of college record, written essay, immunizations, 3 letters of recommendation, nursing research course, physical assessment course, professional liability insurance/malpractice

insurance, statistics course. *Application deadline:* 8/25 (fall), 10/24 (winter), 12/15 (spring), 5/5 (summer). *Application fee:* $40.
Degree Requirements 39 total credit hours, thesis or project.

POST-MASTER'S PROGRAM
Areas of Study *Nurse practitioner programs in:* adult health.

Seton Hall University
College of Nursing
South Orange, New Jersey

http://www.shu.edu/academics/nursing/
Founded in 1856
DEGREES • BSN • DNP • MSN • MSN/MBA
Nursing Program Faculty 50 (78% with doctorates).
Baccalaureate Enrollment 832 **Women** 88% **Men** 12% **Part-time** 10%
Graduate Enrollment 236 **Women** 89% **Men** 11% **Part-time** 74%
Distance Learning Courses Available.
Nursing Student Activities Nursing Honor Society, Sigma Theta Tau, Student Nurses' Association.
Nursing Student Resources Academic advising; academic or career counseling; assistance for students with disabilities; bookstore; campus computer network; career placement assistance; computer lab; computer-assisted instruction; e-mail services; employment services for current students; externships; housing assistance; interactive nursing skills videos; Internet; learning resource lab; library services; nursing audiovisuals; paid internships; placement services for program completers; remedial services; resume preparation assistance; skills, simulation, or other laboratory; tutoring; unpaid internships.

BACCALAUREATE PROGRAMS

Degree BSN
Available Programs ADN to Baccalaureate; Accelerated Baccalaureate for Second Degree; Accelerated RN Baccalaureate; Baccalaureate for Second Degree; Generic Baccalaureate; International Nurse to Baccalaureate; RN Baccalaureate.
Site Options Brick/Toms River, NJ; Somerset, NJ; Lakewood, NJ.
Study Options Full-time and part-time.
Program Entrance Requirements Minimum overall college GPA of 3.0, transcript of college record, CPR certification, written essay, health exam, high school biology, high school chemistry, high school foreign language, 3 years high school math, 2 years high school science, high school transcript, immunizations, minimum high school GPA of 3.0, professional liability insurance/malpractice insurance. Transfer students are accepted. *Application deadline:* Applications may be processed on a rolling basis for some programs.
Financial Aid 97% of baccalaureate students in nursing programs received some form of financial aid in 2013–14.
Contact Ms. Kristyn Kent-Wuillermin, Director of Strategic Alliances, Marketing, and Enrollment, College of Nursing, Seton Hall University, 400 South Orange Avenue, South Orange, NJ 07079-2697. *Telephone:* 973-761-9291. *Fax:* 973-761-9607. *E-mail:* kristyn.kent@shu.edu.

GRADUATE PROGRAMS

Financial Aid 91% of graduate students in nursing programs received some form of financial aid in 2013–14. Institutionally sponsored loans, scholarships, traineeships, tuition waivers (partial), and unspecified assistantships available. Aid available to part-time students.
Contact Ms. Kristyn Kent-Wuillermin, Director of Strategic Alliances, Marketing, and Enrollment, College of Nursing, Seton Hall University, 400 South Orange Avenue, South Orange, NJ 07079-2697. *Telephone:* 973-761-9291. *Fax:* 973-761-9607. *E-mail:* kristyn.kent@shu.edu.

MASTER'S DEGREE PROGRAM
Degrees MSN; MSN/MBA
Available Programs Accelerated Master's for Non-Nursing College Graduates; Accelerated Master's for Nurses with Non-Nursing Degrees; Accelerated RN to Master's; Master's; Master's for Non-Nursing College Graduates; Master's for Nurses with Non-Nursing Degrees; RN to Master's.
Concentrations Available Clinical nurse leader; health-care administration; nurse case management; nursing administration. *Nurse practitioner programs in:* adult health, adult-gerontology acute care, pediatric, pediatric primary care, primary care, school health.
Study Options Full-time and part-time.

Online Degree Options Yes (online only).
Program Entrance Requirements Clinical experience, computer literacy, minimum overall college GPA of 3.0, transcript of college record, CPR certification, written essay, immunizations, interview, 2 letters of recommendation, nursing research course, physical assessment course, professional liability insurance/malpractice insurance, prerequisite course work, resume, statistics course. *Application deadline:* 4/15 (fall), 11/1 (spring). Applications may be processed on a rolling basis for some programs. *Application fee:* $75.
Degree Requirements 31 total credit hours, thesis or project.

POST-MASTER'S PROGRAM
Areas of Study Health-care administration; nurse case management; nursing administration. *Nurse practitioner programs in:* adult health, adult-gerontology acute care, pediatric, pediatric primary care, primary care, school health.

DOCTORAL DEGREE PROGRAM
Degree DNP
Available Programs Doctorate; Post-Baccalaureate Doctorate.
Areas of Study Advanced practice nursing, aging, clinical practice, clinical research, faculty preparation, gerontology, health policy, health promotion/disease prevention, health-care systems, illness and transition, individualized study, nurse case management, nursing administration, nursing education, nursing policy, nursing research, nursing science.
Online Degree Options Yes.
Program Entrance Requirements Clinical experience, minimum overall college GPA of 3.0, interview by faculty committee, interview, 2 letters of recommendation, MSN or equivalent, scholarly papers, statistics course, vita, writing sample, GRE (waived for students with GPA of 3.5 or higher).
Degree Requirements 31 total credit hours, dissertation, residency.

Stockton University
Program in Nursing
Galloway, New Jersey

http://www.stockton.edu
Founded in 1969
DEGREES • BSN • MSN
Nursing Program Faculty 6 (66% with doctorates).
Baccalaureate Enrollment 69 **Women** 98% **Men** 2% **Part-time** 80%
Graduate Enrollment 20 **Women** 90% **Men** 10% **Part-time** 95%
Nursing Student Activities Sigma Theta Tau.
Nursing Student Resources Academic advising; academic or career counseling; assistance for students with disabilities; bookstore; campus computer network; computer lab; computer-assisted instruction; daycare for children of students; e-mail services; housing assistance; Internet; learning resource lab; library services; nursing audiovisuals; resume preparation assistance; skills, simulation, or other laboratory; tutoring.
Library Facilities 9,761 volumes in health, 1,258 volumes in nursing; 83 periodical subscriptions health-care related.

BACCALAUREATE PROGRAMS

Degree BSN
Available Programs RN Baccalaureate.
Study Options Full-time and part-time.
Program Entrance Requirements Transfer students are accepted.
Advanced Placement Credit given for nursing courses completed elsewhere dependent upon specific evaluations.
Contact *Telephone:* 609-652-4837.

GRADUATE PROGRAMS

Contact *Telephone:* 609-652-4501.

MASTER'S DEGREE PROGRAM
Degree MSN
Concentrations Available *Nurse practitioner programs in:* adult health.
Study Options Full-time and part-time.
Program Entrance Requirements Clinical experience, computer literacy, minimum overall college GPA of 3.0, transcript of college record, CPR certification, written essay, immunizations, 2 letters of recommendation, nursing research course, physical assessment course, professional liability insurance/malpractice insurance, statistics course.

Advanced Placement Credit given for nursing courses completed elsewhere dependent upon specific evaluations.

Degree Requirements 42 total credit hours, thesis or project.

Thomas Edison State University
W. Cary Edwards School of Nursing
Trenton, New Jersey

http://www.tesu.edu/nursing/
Nursing program founded in 1983

DEGREES • ACCELERATED 2ND DEGREE BSN • RN-BSN • RN-BSN-MSN • BSN-MSN * DNP

Nursing Student Resources Students in the W. Cary Edwards School of Nursing have the opportunity to earn degrees through traditional and non-traditional methods, which take into consideration the individual needs and interests of each student. All post-licensure nursing courses are designed and delivered online. Students in these courses communicate with fellow students and mentors, who guide students in the course and grade assignments and exams, in an asynchronous environment, which allows for a flexible learning schedule. Students may earn credit toward a degree by demonstrating college-level knowledge through testing and assessment of prior learning; by transfer credit for courses taken through other regionally accredited institutions; through the University's e-Pack® courses; and for licenses, certificates and courses taken at work or through military training, if approved and recommended for academic credit.

W. Cary Edwards School of Nursing Mentors The School utilizes mentors, who are off-site nurse educators from a variety of nursing education and service settings to facilitate courses. All mentors have a minimum of a master's degree in nursing with approximately 75% prepared at the doctoral level and many tenured at their home institutions. With its courses offered online, the School has the advantage to draw nurse educators from across the country, resulting in a diverse and experienced group of online nurse mentors. The W. Cary Edwards School of Nursing programs are accredited by the Accreditation Commission for Education in Nursing (ACEN), 3343 Peachtree Road, N.E., Suite 850, Atlanta, GA 30326, (404) 975-5000, http://www.acenursing.org; the Commission on Collegiate Nursing Education (CCNE), One Dupont Circle, N.W., Suite 530, Washington, DC 20036-1120, (202) 887-6791, http://www.aacn.nche.edu/accreditation; and the New Jersey Board of Nursing, P.O. Box 45010, Newark, NJ 07101, (973) 504-6430, www.state.nj.us/lps/ca/medical/nursing.htm.

NURSING DEGREE PROGRAMS

DEGREES · Accelerated 2nd Degree BSN · RN-BSN · RN- BSN-MSN · MSN · DNP

MSN degree has three specialties: Nurse Educator, Nursing Informatics and Nursing Administration

DNP in Systems-Level Leadership

ACCELERATED 2ND DEGREE BSN PROGRAM A 12-month campus-based baccalaureate program designed for adults who already possess a bachelor's degree (non-nursing) completed prior to acceptance and who are interested in becoming registered nurses. The program includes 60 credits of professional nursing completed both online and on campus at Thomas Edison State University in Trenton, N.J. The Accelerated 2nd Degree BSN Program prepares graduates for the National Council Licensure Examination for Registered Nurses (NCLEX-RN). Due to the rigorous nature of this full-time program, outside employment is not recommended.

RN-BSN-MSN * MSN DEGREE PROGRAMS The online RN-BSN-MSN degree programs are designed for experienced registered nurses (RNs) who want an alternative to campus-based instruction. Three options are offered: BSN (Bachelor of Science in Nursing), BSN-MSN (Bachelor of Science in Nursing and Master of Science in Nursing) and MSN (Master of Science in Nursing). Three nursing specialties are offered in the MSN degree: Nurse Educator, Nursing Informatics, and Nursing Administration.

Study Options Online nursing courses offered quarterly; multiple options for credit earning; no time limit for RN-BSN degree completion; with maximum flexibility in transfer credit.

CERTIFICATE PROGRAMS Three 15–18 credit graduate nursing certificate programs—Nurse Educator; Nursing Informatics; and Nursing Administration—are available to RNs with a master's degree in another area of nursing specialty.

DNP – SYSTEMS-LEVEL LEADERSHIP An 18-month online Doctor of Nursing Practice degree program that is practice-focused and prepares nurse experts in specialized areas of advanced nursing practice. The Systems-Level Leadership area of specialty focuses on the improvement of evidence-based outcomes using theoretical knowledge and systems-level initiatives to advance nurse leaders to the highest level of nursing practice.

PROGRAM ENTRANCE REQUIREMENTS
Accelerated 2nd Degree BSN Program

For the Accelerated 2nd Degree BSN Program, admission requirements include a bachelor's degree from a regionally accredited college or university completed prior to admission with an earned cumulative GPA of 3.0 or higher, all science prerequisites completed within five years prior to admission, a grade of B or better in all prerequisite science and math courses, completed general education and nursing prerequisites prior to admission and a criminal background check, drug screen, health and immunization verification, malpractice and health insurance, and CPR certification.

RN-BSN * RN-BSN-MSN

For the RN-BSN and RN-BSN-MSN, admission is open and rolling. RNs can apply any day of the year. In addition to the documentation of their current unencumbered RN license valid in the United States, all applicants must submit a completed online application with $75 fee and have official transcripts of all completed course work sent to the Office of the Registrar (undergraduate students) or Office of Admissions for graduate students. Up to 80 credits may be accepted from a community college, and up to 60 credits will be awarded to diploma graduates based on current licensure. There is no age restriction on credits transferred in to meet general education requirements or lower-division nursing requirements. Any upper-division nursing credits accepted for transfer must be from an accredited baccalaureate or higher degree nursing program, and newer than 10 years at the application date. All credits used in the nursing requirement must have a grade equivalent of C or better. For more information on acceptance of foreign credit, students should visit http://www.tesu.edu/nursing/RN-to-BSNMSN-Admissions-Requirements.cfm. Applicants to the BSN-MSN (BSNM) program will be accepted into the MSN degree on certification for graduation from the BSN degree.

MSN

All previously completed graduate credits transferred in to meet MSN degree and graduate certificate requirements must be newer than seven years at the application date, have a grade equivalent of B or better, and be from a regionally accredited college or university or recognized foreign institution. Up to 9 graduate credits required in the BSN degree may be applied to the MSN degree requirements. For more information: http://www.tesu.edu/nursing/MSN-Admission-Requirements.cfm

DNP

All previously completed graduate credits transferred in to meet DNP degree must be newer than five years at the application date, have a grade equivalent of B or better, and be **from a regionally accredited college or university or recognized foreign institution**. Up to 9 graduate credits may be applied to the DNP degree requirements.

Expenses (2015–16) *Accelerated 2nd Degree BSN Program Tuition,* $36,091. *RN-BSN Tuition, state resident:* $425 per credit. *RN-BSN Tuition, nonresident:* $520 per credit; $645 for the *MSN Degree and Graduate Nursing Certificate Programs. DNP Tuition* $740 per credit. **There are tuition discounts for all nursing programs available for partners.**

Financial Aid 9% of the RNs in the undergraduate nursing program and 6% in the graduate nursing program received some form of financial aid in the first half of 2015–16. Nursing scholarships are also available.

Contact Thomas Edison State University, 111 W. State St., Trenton, NJ 08608. *Telephone:* 888-442-8372. *Email:* nursinginfo@tesu.edu.

William Paterson University of New Jersey
Department of Nursing
Wayne, New Jersey

http://www.wpunj.edu/
Founded in 1855
DEGREES • BSN • DNP • MSN
Nursing Program Faculty 55 (33% with doctorates).
Baccalaureate Enrollment 412 **Women** 81% **Men** 19%
Graduate Enrollment 80 **Women** 95% **Men** 5% **Part-time** 70%
Distance Learning Courses Available.
Nursing Student Activities Sigma Theta Tau, Student Nurses' Association.
Nursing Student Resources Academic advising; academic or career counseling; assistance for students with disabilities; bookstore; campus computer network; career placement assistance; computer lab; computer-assisted instruction; daycare for children of students; e-mail services; employment services for current students; housing assistance; interactive nursing skills videos; Internet; learning resource lab; library services; nursing audiovisuals; placement services for program completers; remedial services; resume preparation assistance; skills, simulation, or other laboratory; tutoring.
Library Facilities 15,000 volumes in health, 12,700 volumes in nursing; 150 periodical subscriptions health-care related.

BACCALAUREATE PROGRAMS
Degree BSN
Available Programs ADN to Baccalaureate; Accelerated Baccalaureate for Second Degree; Generic Baccalaureate; LPN to Baccalaureate; RN Baccalaureate.
Study Options Full-time.
Program Entrance Requirements Minimum overall college GPA of 2.5, transcript of college record, CPR certification, health exam, health insurance, high school biology, high school chemistry, 1 year of high school math, 2 years high school science, high school transcript, immunizations, minimum high school GPA of 3.25, professional liability insurance/malpractice insurance, prerequisite course work. Transfer students are accepted. *Application deadline:* 5/1 (fall). Applications may be processed on a rolling basis for some programs. *Application fee:* $50.
Contact *Telephone:* 973-720-2527. *Fax:* 973-720-2668.

GRADUATE PROGRAMS
Contact *Telephone:* 973-720-3511. *Fax:* 973-720-3517.

MASTER'S DEGREE PROGRAM
Degree MSN
Available Programs Master's; Master's for Nurses with Non-Nursing Degrees.
Concentrations Available Nursing administration; nursing education. *Clinical nurse specialist programs in:* community health. *Nurse practitioner programs in:* adult health, family health.
Site Options Paramus, NJ; Englewood, NJ.
Study Options Full-time and part-time.
Program Entrance Requirements Computer literacy, minimum overall college GPA of 3.0, transcript of college record, CPR certification, written essay, 2 letters of recommendation, nursing research course, physical assessment course, professional liability insurance/malpractice insurance, resume, statistics course, GRE General Test. *Application deadline:* Applications may be processed on a rolling basis for some programs. *Application fee:* $50.
Advanced Placement Credit given for nursing courses completed elsewhere dependent upon specific evaluations.
Degree Requirements 42 total credit hours, thesis or project.

POST-MASTER'S PROGRAM
Areas of Study *Clinical nurse specialist programs in:* school health. *Nurse practitioner programs in:* adult health, family health.

DOCTORAL DEGREE PROGRAM
Degree DNP
Available Programs Doctorate.
Areas of Study Advanced practice nursing, clinical practice, health-care systems, individualized study.
Program Entrance Requirements Clinical experience, minimum overall college GPA of 3.3, interview by faculty committee, letters of rec-ommendation, MSN or equivalent, statistics course, vita, writing sample. Application deadline: 4/15 (fall). Application fee: $75.
Degree Requirements 42 total credit hours.

NEW MEXICO

Brookline College
Department of Nursing
Albuquerque, New Mexico

http://brooklinecollege.edu/
DEGREE • BSN

BACCALAUREATE PROGRAMS
Degree BSN
Available Programs Generic Baccalaureate.
Contact BSN Program, Department of Nursing, Brookline College, 4201 Central Avenue NW, Suite J, Albuquerque, NM 87105-1649. *Telephone:* 505-880-2877.

Eastern New Mexico University
Department of Allied Health–Nursing
Portales, New Mexico

https://www.enmu.edu/
Founded in 1934
DEGREES • BSN • MSN
Nursing Program Faculty 7 (1% with doctorates).
Baccalaureate Enrollment 189 **Part-time** 95%
Graduate Enrollment 30
Distance Learning Courses Available.
Nursing Student Activities Nursing Honor Society.
Nursing Student Resources Academic advising; academic or career counseling; assistance for students with disabilities; bookstore; campus computer network; career placement assistance; computer lab; computer-assisted instruction; e-mail services; housing assistance; Internet; library services; other; resume preparation assistance; tutoring.
Library Facilities 100 volumes in health, 50 volumes in nursing; 15 periodical subscriptions health-care related.

BACCALAUREATE PROGRAMS
Degree BSN
Available Programs ADN to Baccalaureate.
Study Options Full-time and part-time.
Online Degree Options Yes (online only).
Program Entrance Requirements Minimum overall college GPA of 2.0, transcript of college record, CPR certification, immunizations, interview, 3 letters of recommendation, minimum GPA in nursing prerequisites of 2.0, professional liability insurance/malpractice insurance, prerequisite course work, RN licensure. Transfer students are accepted. *Application deadline:* 8/20 (fall), 1/20 (spring), 6/1 (summer).
Advanced Placement Credit given for nursing courses completed elsewhere dependent upon specific evaluations.
Expenses (2015–16) *Tuition, state resident:* part-time $136 per credit hour. *Tuition, nonresident:* part-time $136 per credit hour. *Required fees:* part-time $90 per credit.
Financial Aid *Gift aid (need-based):* Federal Pell, FSEOG, state, private, college/university gift aid from institutional funds. *Loans:* Federal Direct (Subsidized and Unsubsidized Stafford PLUS), Perkins, state, college/university. *Work-study:* Federal Work-Study, part-time campus jobs. *Financial aid application deadline:* Continuous.
Contact Mrs. Crystal Jones, Nursing Program Secretary, Department of Allied Health–Nursing, Eastern New Mexico University, 1500 South Avenue K, Station 12, Portales, NM 88130. *Telephone:* 575-562-2403. *E-mail:* crystal.jones@enmu.edu.

GRADUATE PROGRAMS
Expenses (2015–16) *Tuition, state resident:* part-time $245 per credit hour. *Tuition, nonresident:* part-time $245 per credit hour.

Contact Mrs. Crystal Jones, Nursing Program Secretary, Department of Allied Health–Nursing, Eastern New Mexico University, 1500 South Avenue K, Portales, NM 88130. *Telephone:* 575-562-2403. *E-mail:* crystal.jones@enmu.edu.

MASTER'S DEGREE PROGRAM

Degree MSN
Available Programs Master's.
Concentrations Available Nursing education.
Online Degree Options Yes (online only).
Program Entrance Requirements Minimum overall college GPA of 3.0. *Application deadline:* 8/15 (fall), 1/15 (spring), 6/1 (summer).
Degree Requirements 36 total credit hours.

New Mexico Highlands University
Department of Nursing
Las Vegas, New Mexico

http://www.nmhu.edu/nursing
Founded in 1893
Nursing Program Faculty 6 (20% with doctorates).
Distance Learning Courses Available.
Nursing Student Resources Academic advising; academic or career counseling; assistance for students with disabilities; bookstore; campus computer network; career placement assistance; computer-assisted instruction; e-mail services; employment services for current students; housing assistance; Internet; library services; nursing audiovisuals; placement services for program completers; resume preparation assistance; tutoring.
Library Facilities 500 volumes in nursing; 150 periodical subscriptions health-care related.

New Mexico State University
School of Nursing
Las Cruces, New Mexico

http://schoolofnursing.nmsu.edu/
Founded in 1888
DEGREES • BSN • MSN • PHD
Nursing Program Faculty 30 (35% with doctorates).
Baccalaureate Enrollment 280 Women 84% Men 16% Part-time 15%
Graduate Enrollment 120 Women 88% Men 12% Part-time 25%
Distance Learning Courses Available.
Nursing Student Activities Sigma Theta Tau, Student Nurses' Association.
Nursing Student Resources Academic advising; academic or career counseling; assistance for students with disabilities; bookstore; campus computer network; computer lab; computer-assisted instruction; daycare for children of students; e-mail services; housing assistance; interactive nursing skills videos; Internet; learning resource lab; library services; nursing audiovisuals; paid internships; remedial services; skills, simulation, or other laboratory; tutoring.
Library Facilities 33,000 volumes in health, 17,500 volumes in nursing; 620 periodical subscriptions health-care related.

BACCALAUREATE PROGRAMS

Degree BSN
Available Programs Accelerated Baccalaureate; Generic Baccalaureate; RN Baccalaureate.
Site Options Grants, NM; Alamagordo, NM; Santa Fe, NM.
Study Options Full-time.
Online Degree Options Yes.
Program Entrance Requirements Minimum overall college GPA of 2.0, transcript of college record, CPR certification, health insurance, immunizations, minimum GPA in nursing prerequisites of 2.75, prerequisite course work. Transfer students are accepted. *Application deadline:* 2/1 (fall), 9/1 (winter).
Advanced Placement Credit given for nursing courses completed elsewhere dependent upon specific evaluations.
Expenses (2014–15) *Tuition, state resident:* full-time $3287; part-time $248 per credit hour. *Tuition, nonresident:* full-time $10,329; part-time $796 per credit hour. *International tuition:* $10,330 full-time. *Room and board:* $2700 per academic year. *Required fees:* full-time $500.

Financial Aid 82% of baccalaureate students in nursing programs received some form of financial aid in 2013–14.
Contact Alyce Kolenovsky, Advising Coordinator, School of Nursing, New Mexico State University, PO Box 30001, MSC 3185, Las Cruces, NM 88003-8001. *Telephone:* 575-646-2164. *Fax:* 505-646-6166. *E-mail:* aksky@nmsu.edu.

GRADUATE PROGRAMS

Expenses (2014–15) *Tuition, area resident:* full-time $3543; part-time $268 per credit hour. *Tuition, state resident:* full-time $3453; part-time $268 per credit hour. *Tuition, nonresident:* full-time $10,584; part-time $816 per credit hour. *International tuition:* $10,584 full-time. *Required fees:* full-time $1000; part-time $500 per term.
Financial Aid 73% of graduate students in nursing programs received some form of financial aid in 2013–14. 1 teaching assistantship (averaging $8,130 per year) was awarded; career-related internships or fieldwork, Federal Work-Study, scholarships, traineeships, and unspecified assistantships also available. Aid available to part-time students. *Financial aid application deadline:* 3/1.
Contact Dr. Kathleen M. Huttlinger, Interim Associate Director for Graduate Studies, School of Nursing, New Mexico State University, PO Box 30001, MSC 3185, Las Cruces, NM 88003-8001. *Telephone:* 505-646-8170. *Fax:* 505-646-2167. *E-mail:* huttlin@nmsu.edu.

MASTER'S DEGREE PROGRAM

Degree MSN
Available Programs Master's; Master's for Nurses with Non-Nursing Degrees.
Concentrations Available Nursing administration.
Study Options Full-time and part-time.
Online Degree Options Yes (online only).
Program Entrance Requirements Minimum overall college GPA of 3.0, transcript of college record, CPR certification, written essay, immunizations, 3 letters of recommendation, resume, statistics course, NCLEX exam. *Application deadline:* 2/1 (fall).
Advanced Placement Credit given for nursing courses completed elsewhere dependent upon specific evaluations.
Degree Requirements 36 total credit hours, comprehensive exam.

DOCTORAL DEGREE PROGRAM

Degree PhD
Available Programs Doctorate.
Areas of Study Nursing research.
Online Degree Options Yes (online only).
Program Entrance Requirements Minimum overall college GPA of 3.0, interview by faculty committee, 3 letters of recommendation, MSN or equivalent, statistics course, vita, writing sample, NCLEX exam. Application deadline: 2/1 (fall).
Degree Requirements 60 total credit hours, dissertation, oral exam, written exam.

Northern New Mexico College
College of Nursing and Health Sciences
Española, New Mexico

http://nnmc.edu/
Founded in 1909
DEGREE • BSN
Nursing Program Faculty 5 (20% with doctorates).
Baccalaureate Enrollment 19
Nursing Student Activities Student Nurses' Association.
Nursing Student Resources Academic advising; academic or career counseling; assistance for students with disabilities; bookstore; campus computer network; career placement assistance; computer lab; computer-assisted instruction; e-mail services; interactive nursing skills videos; Internet; learning resource lab; nursing audiovisuals; other; remedial services; skills, simulation, or other laboratory; tutoring.

BACCALAUREATE PROGRAMS

Degree BSN
Available Programs RN Baccalaureate.
Program Entrance Requirements RN licensure.
Contact Director, RN to BSN Program, College of Nursing and Health Sciences, Northern New Mexico College, 921 North Paseo de Onate,

Española, NM 87532. *Telephone:* 505-747-2278.
E-mail: nklebanoff@nnmc.edu.

University of New Mexico
Program in Nursing
Albuquerque, New Mexico

http://nursing.unm.edu/
Founded in 1889
DEGREES • BSN • DNP • MSN • PHD
Nursing Program Faculty 67 (60% with doctorates).
Baccalaureate Enrollment 366 **Women** 83% **Men** 17% **Part-time** 22%
Graduate Enrollment 157 **Women** 87% **Men** 13% **Part-time** 46%
Distance Learning Courses Available.
Nursing Student Activities Sigma Theta Tau, Student Nurses' Association.
Nursing Student Resources Academic advising; academic or career counseling; assistance for students with disabilities; bookstore; campus computer network; career placement assistance; computer lab; computer-assisted instruction; daycare for children of students; e-mail services; housing assistance; interactive nursing skills videos; Internet; learning resource lab; library services; nursing audiovisuals; remedial services; skills, simulation, or other laboratory.
Library Facilities 92,207 volumes in health, 158 volumes in nursing; 2,344 periodical subscriptions health-care related.

BACCALAUREATE PROGRAMS

Degree BSN
Available Programs Generic Baccalaureate; RN Baccalaureate.
Site Options Farmington, NM; Hobbs, NM; Santa Fe, NM.
Study Options Full-time and part-time.
Program Entrance Requirements Minimum overall college GPA of 2.75, transcript of college record, written essay, 2 letters of recommendation, minimum GPA in nursing prerequisites of 2.75, prerequisite course work. Transfer students are accepted. *Application deadline:* 2/15 (fall), 9/15 (spring). *Application fee:* $45.
Advanced Placement Credit given for nursing courses completed elsewhere dependent upon specific evaluations.
Expenses (2015–16) *Tuition, state resident:* part-time $480 per credit hour. *Tuition, nonresident:* part-time $1073 per credit hour. *Required fees:* part-time $400 per term.
Financial Aid 68% of baccalaureate students in nursing programs received some form of financial aid in 2014–15. *Gift aid (need-based):* Federal Pell, FSEOG, state, private, college/university gift aid from institutional funds, United Negro College Fund, Federal Nursing. *Loans:* Federal Nursing Student Loans, Federal Direct (Subsidized and Unsubsidized Stafford PLUS), Perkins, state, college/university. *Work-study:* Federal Work-Study, part-time campus jobs. *Financial aid application deadline (priority):* 3/1.
Contact Ms. Ann Marie Oechsler, Academic Advisement Specialist, Program in Nursing, University of New Mexico, 1 University of New Mexico, MSC09 5350, Albuquerque, NM 87131-0001. *Telephone:* 505-272-4223. *Fax:* 505-272-3970. *E-mail:* aoechsler@salud.unm.edu.

GRADUATE PROGRAMS

Expenses (2015–16) *Tuition, state resident:* part-time $561 per credit hour. *Tuition, nonresident:* part-time $1165 per credit hour. *Required fees:* part-time $600 per term.
Financial Aid 45% of graduate students in nursing programs received some form of financial aid in 2014–15. 11 fellowships (averaging $24,000 per year), 4 research assistantships with partial tuition reimbursements available (averaging $4,054 per year), 13 teaching assistantships with partial tuition reimbursements available (averaging $4,787 per year) were awarded; institutionally sponsored loans, scholarships, and unspecified assistantships also available. Aid available to part-time students. *Financial aid application deadline:* 3/1.
Contact Ms. Jeri Belsher, Student Advisement Coordinator, Program in Nursing, University of New Mexico, College of Nursing, MSC09 5350, 1 University of New Mexico, Albuquerque, NM 87131-0001. *Telephone:* 505-272-4223. *Fax:* 505-272-3970. *E-mail:* jbelsher@salud.unm.edu.

MASTER'S DEGREE PROGRAM

Degree MSN
Available Programs Master's.

Concentrations Available Nurse-midwifery; nursing education. *Nurse practitioner programs in:* acute care, adult-gerontology acute care, family health, pediatric.
Study Options Full-time and part-time.
Online Degree Options Yes (online only).
Program Entrance Requirements Clinical experience, minimum overall college GPA of 3.0, transcript of college record, interview, 3 letters of recommendation, resume. *Application deadline:* 2/15 (fall), 10/15 (spring). *Application fee:* $45.
Advanced Placement Credit given for nursing courses completed elsewhere dependent upon specific evaluations.
Degree Requirements 32 total credit hours, thesis or project, comprehensive exam.

POST-MASTER'S PROGRAM

Areas of Study Nurse-midwifery; nursing education. *Nurse practitioner programs in:* acute care, adult-gerontology acute care, family health, pediatric.

DOCTORAL DEGREE PROGRAM

Degree DNP
Available Programs Doctorate.
Areas of Study Nursing administration.
Online Degree Options Yes.
Program Entrance Requirements Minimum overall college GPA of 3.0, clinical experience, interview by faculty committee, 3 letters of recommendation, MSN or equivalent, scholarly papers, vita, writing sample. Application deadline: 12/1 (summer). Application fee: $60.
Degree Requirements 69 total credit hours, written exam.

Degree PhD
Available Programs Doctorate.
Areas of Study Health policy, nursing research.
Online Degree Options Yes.
Program Entrance Requirements Clinical experience, minimum overall college GPA of 3.0, interview by faculty committee, 3 letters of recommendation, MSN or equivalent, vita, writing sample. Application deadline: 2/15 (summer). Application fee: $45.
Degree Requirements 69 total credit hours, dissertation.

University of Phoenix–New Mexico Campus
College of Nursing
Albuquerque, New Mexico

DEGREES • BSN • MSN • MSN/ED D
Nursing Program Faculty 18 (13% with doctorates).
Baccalaureate Enrollment 24 **Women** 100%
Graduate Enrollment 14 **Women** 100%
Nursing Student Activities Sigma Theta Tau.
Nursing Student Resources Academic advising; academic or career counseling; assistance for students with disabilities; bookstore; campus computer network; computer lab; computer-assisted instruction; e-mail services; interactive nursing skills videos; Internet; learning resource lab; library services; nursing audiovisuals; remedial services; skills, simulation, or other laboratory; tutoring.
Library Facilities 1,300 periodical subscriptions health-care related.

BACCALAUREATE PROGRAMS

Degree BSN
Available Programs Accelerated Baccalaureate.
Site Options Santa Fe, NM; Santa Teresa, NM.
Study Options Full-time.
Program Entrance Requirements Transcript of college record, CPR certification, immunizations, 1 letter of recommendation, RN licensure. Transfer students are accepted.
Advanced Placement Credit by examination available. Credit given for nursing courses completed elsewhere dependent upon specific evaluations.
Contact *Telephone:* 505-821-4800.

GRADUATE PROGRAMS

Contact *Telephone:* 505-821-4800.

MASTER'S DEGREE PROGRAM

Degrees MSN; MSN/Ed D

Available Programs Master's.

Concentrations Available Nursing administration; nursing education.

Site Options Santa Fe, NM; Santa Teresa, NM.

Study Options Full-time.

Online Degree Options Yes.

Program Entrance Requirements Clinical experience, computer literacy, minimum overall college GPA of 2.5, transcript of college record. *Application deadline:* Applications may be processed on a rolling basis for some programs. *Application fee:* $45.

Advanced Placement Credit given for nursing courses completed elsewhere dependent upon specific evaluations.

Degree Requirements 39 total credit hours, thesis or project.

Western New Mexico University

Nursing Department
Silver City, New Mexico

http://nursing.wnmu.edu/

Founded in 1893

DEGREE • BSN

Nursing Program Faculty 16 (30% with doctorates).

Baccalaureate Enrollment 130 **Women** 95% **Men** 5% **Part-time** 88%

Distance Learning Courses Available.

Nursing Student Activities Nursing Honor Society, Student Nurses' Association.

Nursing Student Resources Academic advising; academic or career counseling; assistance for students with disabilities; bookstore; campus computer network; career placement assistance; computer lab; computer-assisted instruction; daycare for children of students; e-mail services; housing assistance; interactive nursing skills videos; Internet; learning resource lab; library services; nursing audiovisuals; placement services for program completers; remedial services; resume preparation assistance; skills, simulation, or other laboratory; tutoring.

Library Facilities 4,980 volumes in health, 4,900 volumes in nursing; 14 periodical subscriptions health-care related.

BACCALAUREATE PROGRAMS

Degree BSN

Available Programs ADN to Baccalaureate; Generic Baccalaureate.

Site Options Deming , NM.

Study Options Full-time and part-time.

Online Degree Options Yes.

Program Entrance Requirements Minimum overall college GPA of 2.5, transcript of college record, CPR certification, immunizations, minimum GPA in nursing prerequisites, prerequisite course work, RN licensure. Transfer students are accepted. *Application deadline:* 7/15 (fall), 7/15 (winter), 11/15 (spring), 4/15 (summer). Applications may be processed on a rolling basis for some programs. *Application fee:* $30.

Advanced Placement Credit given for nursing courses completed elsewhere dependent upon specific evaluations.

Financial Aid 40% of baccalaureate students in nursing programs received some form of financial aid in 2013–14. *Gift aid (need-based):* Federal Pell, FSEOG, state, private, college/university gift aid from institutional funds. *Loans:* Federal Direct (Subsidized and Unsubsidized Stafford PLUS), Perkins, state, college/university. *Work-study:* Federal Work-Study, part-time campus jobs. *Financial aid application deadline (priority):* 3/1.

Contact Ms. Socorro Rico, Executive Assistant, Nursing Department, Western New Mexico University, PO Box 680, Silver City, NM 88062. *Telephone:* 575-538-6972. *Fax:* 575-538-6961. *E-mail:* ricos@wnmu.edu.

NEW YORK

Adelphi University

College of Nursing and Public Health
Garden City, New York

http://www.adelphi.edu/

Founded in 1896

DEGREES • BS • MS • PHD

Nursing Program Faculty 253 (17% with doctorates).

Baccalaureate Enrollment 1,297 **Women** 87.3% **Men** 12.7% **Part-time** 12.1%

Graduate Enrollment 151 **Women** 91.4% **Men** 8.6% **Part-time** 100%

Distance Learning Courses Available.

Nursing Student Activities Nursing Honor Society, Sigma Theta Tau, Student Nurses' Association, nursing club.

Nursing Student Resources Academic advising; academic or career counseling; assistance for students with disabilities; bookstore; campus computer network; career placement assistance; computer lab; computer-assisted instruction; daycare for children of students; e-mail services; employment services for current students; externships; housing assistance; interactive nursing skills videos; Internet; learning resource lab; library services; nursing audiovisuals; paid internships; placement services for program completers; remedial services; resume preparation assistance; skills, simulation, or other laboratory; tutoring; unpaid internships.

Library Facilities 29,918 volumes in health, 2,666 volumes in nursing; 364 periodical subscriptions health-care related.

BACCALAUREATE PROGRAMS

Degree BS

Available Programs Accelerated Baccalaureate for Second Degree; Generic Baccalaureate; RN Baccalaureate.

Site Options Sayville, NY; Manhattan, NY; Poughkeepsie, NY.

Study Options Full-time.

Program Entrance Requirements Minimum overall college GPA of 3.0, transcript of college record, written essay, health exam, high school foreign language, 3 years high school math, 3 years high school science, high school transcript, immunizations, interview, 2 letters of recommendation, minimum high school GPA of 3.0, minimum GPA in nursing prerequisites of 2.7. Transfer students are accepted. *Application deadline:* Applications may be processed on a rolling basis for some programs. *Application fee:* $50.

Advanced Placement Credit given for nursing courses completed elsewhere dependent upon specific evaluations.

Expenses (2015–16) *Tuition:* full-time $32,586; part-time $1015 per credit. *International tuition:* $32,586 full-time. *Room and board:* $13,460; room only: $9570 per academic year. *Required fees:* full-time $3658; part-time $2340 per term.

Financial Aid *Gift aid (need-based):* Federal Pell, FSEOG, state, private, college/university gift aid from institutional funds, United Negro College Fund, endowed and restricted scholarships and grants. *Loans:* Federal Nursing Student Loans, Federal Direct (Subsidized and Unsubsidized Stafford PLUS), Perkins. *Work-study:* Federal Work-Study, part-time campus jobs. *Financial aid application deadline (priority):* 3/1.

Contact Mrs. Christine Murphy, Director of Admissions, College of Nursing and Public Health, Adelphi University, One South Avenue, Levermore Hall, Garden City, NY 11530. *Telephone:* 516-877-3050. *E-mail:* murphy2@adelphi.edu.

GRADUATE PROGRAMS

Expenses (2015–16) *Tuition:* full-time $14,760; part-time $1230 per credit. *International tuition:* $14,760 full-time. *Room and board:* $13,460; room only: $9570 per academic year. *Required fees:* full-time $740; part-time $370 per term.

Financial Aid Research assistantships, career-related internships or fieldwork, tuition waivers (partial), unspecified assistantships, and achievement awards available.

Contact Mrs. Christine Murphy, Director of Admissions, College of Nursing and Public Health, Adelphi University, One South Avenue, Levermore Hall, Garden City, NY 11530. *Telephone:* 516-877-3050. *Fax:* 516-877-3039. *E-mail:* murphy2@adelphi.edu.

MASTER'S DEGREE PROGRAM

Degree MS

Available Programs Master's.

Concentrations Available Health-care administration; nursing administration; nursing education; nursing informatics. *Clinical nurse specialist programs in:* public health. *Nurse practitioner programs in:* adult health.
Study Options Full-time and part-time.
Program Entrance Requirements Clinical experience, computer literacy, minimum overall college GPA of 3.0, transcript of college record, CPR certification, written essay, immunizations, interview, 2 letters of recommendation, nursing research course, professional liability insurance/malpractice insurance, resume, statistics course. *Application deadline:* 3/1 (fall). Applications may be processed on a rolling basis for some programs. *Application fee:* $50.
Advanced Placement Credit given for nursing courses completed elsewhere dependent upon specific evaluations.
Degree Requirements 42 total credit hours, thesis or project, comprehensive exam.

POST-MASTER'S PROGRAM
Areas of Study Health-care administration; nursing administration; nursing education; nursing informatics. *Clinical nurse specialist programs in:* public health. *Nurse practitioner programs in:* adult health.

DOCTORAL DEGREE PROGRAM
Degree PhD
Available Programs Doctorate.
Areas of Study Faculty preparation, health-care systems, nursing administration, nursing education, nursing policy, nursing research, nursing science.
Program Entrance Requirements Minimum overall college GPA of 3.5, interview by faculty committee, interview, 3 letters of recommendation, MSN or equivalent, statistics course, vita, writing sample, GRE. Application deadline: 2/15 (fall). Application fee: $50.
Degree Requirements 54 total credit hours, dissertation, oral exam, written exam.

Binghamton University, State University of New York
Decker School of Nursing
Vestal, New York

http://www.binghamton.edu/dson/
Founded in 1946
DEGREES • BS • DNP • MS • PHD
Nursing Program Faculty 58 (40% with doctorates).
Baccalaureate Enrollment 354
Graduate Enrollment 191
Distance Learning Courses Available.
Nursing Student Activities Sigma Theta Tau, Student Nurses' Association.
Nursing Student Resources Academic advising; assistance for students with disabilities; campus computer network; computer lab; e-mail services; Internet; learning resource lab; library services; skills, simulation, or other laboratory.
Library Facilities 7,000 volumes in health; 9,300 periodical subscriptions health-care related.

BACCALAUREATE PROGRAMS
Degree BS
Available Programs Accelerated RN Baccalaureate; Generic Baccalaureate.
Study Options Full-time and part-time.
Program Entrance Requirements Minimum overall college GPA of 2.7, transcript of college record, CPR certification, written essay, health exam, high school biology, high school chemistry, high school foreign language, 3 years high school math, 2 years high school science, high school transcript, 2 letters of recommendation, minimum high school GPA of 3.0, prerequisite course work. Transfer students are accepted. *Application deadline:* Applications may be processed on a rolling basis for some programs. *Application fee:* $50.
Advanced Placement Credit by examination available. Credit given for nursing courses completed elsewhere dependent upon specific evaluations.
Contact *Telephone:* 607-777-4954. *Fax:* 607-777-4440.

GRADUATE PROGRAMS
Contact *Telephone:* 607-777-4614. *Fax:* 607-777-4440.

MASTER'S DEGREE PROGRAM
Degree MS
Available Programs Master's.
Concentrations Available Nursing administration; nursing education. *Clinical nurse specialist programs in:* community health, family health, gerontology, psychiatric/mental health. *Nurse practitioner programs in:* community health, family health, gerontology, psychiatric/mental health.
Study Options Full-time and part-time.
Program Entrance Requirements Computer literacy, minimum overall college GPA of 3.0, transcript of college record, written essay, 2 letters of recommendation, resume, statistics course, GRE General Test. *Application deadline:* 6/15 (fall), 11/15 (spring). Applications may be processed on a rolling basis for some programs. *Application fee:* $60.
Advanced Placement Credit given for nursing courses completed elsewhere dependent upon specific evaluations.
Degree Requirements 48 total credit hours, thesis or project, comprehensive exam.

POST-MASTER'S PROGRAM
Areas of Study *Nurse practitioner programs in:* community health, family health, gerontology, psychiatric/mental health.

DOCTORAL DEGREE PROGRAM
Degree DNP
Available Programs Doctorate, Post-Baccalaureate Doctorate.
Areas of Study Community health, family health, gerontology, psychiatric/mental health.
Online Degree Options Yes (Post-MS to DNP is online).
Program Entrance Requirements Minimum overall college GPA of 3.0. Application requirements differ between programs; please contact school for complete requirements. Application deadline: 6/1 (fall). Applications may be processed on a rolling basis for some programs. Application fee: $60.
Degree Requirements 77 credits for Post-BS to DNP, 38 credits for Post-MS to DNP, dissertation, oral exam, residency, written exam.

Degree PhD
Available Programs Doctorate; Post-Baccalaureate Doctorate.
Areas of Study Nursing research.
Online Degree Options Yes.
Program Entrance Requirements Clinical experience, minimum overall college GPA of 3.0, interview by faculty committee, interview, 3 letters of recommendation, MSN or equivalent, scholarly papers, statistics course, vita, writing sample, GRE General Test. Application deadline: 6/15 (fall), 11/15 (spring). Applications may be processed on a rolling basis for some programs. Application fee: $60.
Degree Requirements 55 total credit hours, dissertation, written exam.

CONTINUING EDUCATION PROGRAM
Contact *Telephone:* 607-777-4954. *Fax:* 607-777-4440.

The College at Brockport, State University of New York
Department of Nursing
Brockport, New York

http://www.brockport.edu/
Founded in 1867
DEGREE • BSN
Nursing Program Faculty 24 (50% with doctorates).
Baccalaureate Enrollment 200 **Women** 93% **Men** 7% **Part-time** 9%
Distance Learning Courses Available.
Nursing Student Activities Nursing Honor Society, Sigma Theta Tau, Student Nurses' Association.
Nursing Student Resources Academic advising; academic or career counseling; assistance for students with disabilities; bookstore; campus computer network; career placement assistance; computer lab; computer-assisted instruction; daycare for children of students; e-mail services; interactive nursing skills videos; Internet; learning resource lab; library services; nursing audiovisuals; remedial services; resume preparation assistance; skills, simulation, or other laboratory; tutoring.
Library Facilities 18,952 volumes in health, 1,065 volumes in nursing; 257 periodical subscriptions health-care related.

BACCALAUREATE PROGRAMS

Degree BSN
Available Programs ADN to Baccalaureate; Generic Baccalaureate.
Site Options Rochester, NY.
Study Options Full-time and part-time.
Program Entrance Requirements Minimum overall college GPA of 2.75, transcript of college record, CPR certification, health exam, health insurance, high school transcript, immunizations, minimum GPA in nursing prerequisites of 2.0, prerequisite course work. Transfer students are accepted. *Application deadline:* 1/20 (fall).
Advanced Placement Credit given for nursing courses completed elsewhere dependent upon specific evaluations.
Contact *Telephone:* 585-395-2355. *Fax:* 585-395-5312.

College of Mount Saint Vincent
Department of Nursing
Riverdale, New York

http://www.mountsaintvincent.edu/408.htm
Founded in 1911

DEGREES • BS • MSN

Nursing Program Faculty 30 (90% with doctorates).
Baccalaureate Enrollment 520 **Women** 80% **Men** 20% **Part-time** 10%
Graduate Enrollment 100 **Women** 90% **Men** 10% **Part-time** 100%
Nursing Student Activities Sigma Theta Tau, Student Nurses' Association.
Nursing Student Resources Academic advising; academic or career counseling; bookstore; campus computer network; computer lab; computer-assisted instruction; e-mail services; employment services for current students; housing assistance; interactive nursing skills videos; Internet; learning resource lab; library services; nursing audiovisuals; paid internships; remedial services; resume preparation assistance; skills, simulation, or other laboratory; tutoring.
Library Facilities 5,304 volumes in nursing.

BACCALAUREATE PROGRAMS

Degree BS
Available Programs Baccalaureate for Second Degree; Generic Baccalaureate; International Nurse to Baccalaureate; LPN to Baccalaureate; LPN to RN Baccalaureate.
Site Options Manhattan, NY.
Study Options Full-time and part-time.
Program Entrance Requirements Minimum overall college GPA of 2.7, transcript of college record, CPR certification, written essay, health exam, health insurance, high school biology, high school chemistry, high school foreign language, 3 years high school math, 3 years high school science, high school transcript, immunizations, 1 letter of recommendation, minimum high school GPA of 2.7, minimum GPA in nursing prerequisites of 3.0, prerequisite course work. Transfer students are accepted. *Application deadline:* 8/1 (fall), 1/5 (spring). Applications may be processed on a rolling basis for some programs. *Application fee:* $35.
Contact *Telephone:* 718-405-3365. *Fax:* 718-405-3286.

GRADUATE PROGRAMS

Contact *Telephone:* 718-405-3351. *Fax:* 718-405-3286.

MASTER'S DEGREE PROGRAM
Degree MSN
Available Programs Master's.

The College of New Rochelle
School of Nursing
New Rochelle, New York

Founded in 1904

DEGREES • BSN • MS

Nursing Program Faculty 15 (75% with doctorates).
Baccalaureate Enrollment 521 **Women** 90% **Men** 10% **Part-time** 50%
Graduate Enrollment 121 **Women** 90% **Men** 10% **Part-time** 100%
Nursing Student Activities Nursing Honor Society, Sigma Theta Tau, Student Nurses' Association, nursing club.
Nursing Student Resources Academic advising; academic or career counseling; assistance for students with disabilities; bookstore; campus computer network; career placement assistance; computer lab; computer-assisted instruction; e-mail services; housing assistance; interactive nursing skills videos; Internet; learning resource lab; library services; nursing audiovisuals; other; remedial services; resume preparation assistance; skills, simulation, or other laboratory; tutoring.
Library Facilities 8,700 volumes in health, 8,700 volumes in nursing; 165 periodical subscriptions health-care related.

BACCALAUREATE PROGRAMS

Degree BSN
Available Programs Accelerated Baccalaureate for Second Degree; Accelerated RN Baccalaureate; Baccalaureate for Second Degree; Generic Baccalaureate; RN Baccalaureate.
Site Options Bronx, NY.
Study Options Full-time and part-time.
Program Entrance Requirements Transcript of college record, CPR certification, written essay, health exam, health insurance, high school biology, high school chemistry, high school transcript, immunizations. Transfer students are accepted. *Application deadline:* 3/1 (fall), 10/1 (spring). *Application fee:* $35.
Advanced Placement Credit by examination available. Credit given for nursing courses completed elsewhere dependent upon specific evaluations.
Contact *Telephone:* 914-654-5803. *Fax:* 914-654-5994.

GRADUATE PROGRAMS

Contact *Telephone:* 914-654-5803. *Fax:* 914-654-5994.

MASTER'S DEGREE PROGRAM
Degree MS
Available Programs Master's; RN to Master's.
Concentrations Available Health-care administration; nursing administration; nursing education. *Nurse practitioner programs in:* family health.
Site Options New Rochelle, NY.
Study Options Full-time and part-time.
Program Entrance Requirements Clinical experience, minimum overall college GPA of 3.0, transcript of college record, written essay, immunizations, interview, 2 letters of recommendation, physical assessment course, professional liability insurance/malpractice insurance, resume, statistics course.*Application fee:* $35.
Advanced Placement Credit given for nursing courses completed elsewhere dependent upon specific evaluations.
Degree Requirements 40 total credit hours, thesis or project.

POST-MASTER'S PROGRAM
Areas of Study Health-care administration; nursing administration; nursing education. *Clinical nurse specialist programs in:* palliative care. *Nurse practitioner programs in:* family health.

College of Staten Island of the City University of New York
Department of Nursing
Staten Island, New York

http://www.csi.cuny.edu/nursing
Founded in 1955

DEGREES • BS • MS

Nursing Program Faculty 61 (23% with doctorates).
Baccalaureate Enrollment 182 **Women** 87% **Men** 13% **Part-time** 74%
Graduate Enrollment 52 **Women** 99% **Men** 1% **Part-time** 93%
Nursing Student Activities Nursing Honor Society, Sigma Theta Tau.
Nursing Student Resources Academic advising; academic or career counseling; assistance for students with disabilities; bookstore; campus computer network; career placement assistance; computer lab; computer-assisted instruction; daycare for children of students; e-mail services; externships; Internet; learning resource lab; library services; nursing audiovisuals; remedial services; resume preparation assistance; skills, simulation, or other laboratory; tutoring.
Library Facilities 3,700 volumes in health, 1,500 volumes in nursing; 4,900 periodical subscriptions health-care related.

BACCALAUREATE PROGRAMS

Degree BS
Available Programs RN Baccalaureate.
Site Options Brooklyn, NY.

Study Options Full-time and part-time.
Program Entrance Requirements Minimum overall college GPA of 2.5, transcript of college record, CPR certification, health exam, health insurance, high school transcript, immunizations, minimum GPA in nursing prerequisites, professional liability insurance/malpractice insurance, prerequisite course work, RN licensure. Transfer students are accepted. *Application fee:* $65.
Advanced Placement Credit given for nursing courses completed elsewhere dependent upon specific evaluations.
Contact *Telephone:* 718-982-3810. *Fax:* 718-982-3813.

GRADUATE PROGRAMS

Contact *Telephone:* 718-982-3845. *Fax:* 718-982-3813.

MASTER'S DEGREE PROGRAM
Degree MS
Available Programs Master's.
Concentrations Available *Clinical nurse specialist programs in:* adult health, gerontology. *Nurse practitioner programs in:* adult health, gerontology.
Site Options Brooklyn, NY.
Study Options Full-time and part-time.
Program Entrance Requirements Clinical experience, minimum overall college GPA of 3.0, transcript of college record, written essay, immunizations, interview, 2 letters of recommendation, nursing research course, physical assessment course, professional liability insurance/malpractice insurance, prerequisite course work, statistics course. *Application deadline:* Applications may be processed on a rolling basis for some programs. *Application fee:* $65.
Advanced Placement Credit given for nursing courses completed elsewhere dependent upon specific evaluations.
Degree Requirements 48 total credit hours, thesis or project.

POST-MASTER'S PROGRAM
Areas of Study *Nurse practitioner programs in:* adult health, gerontology.

Columbia University
School of Nursing
New York, New York

http://www.nursing.columbia.edu/
Founded in 1754
DEGREES • BS • MS • MSN/MBA • MSN/MPH • PHD
Nursing Program Faculty 77 (92% with doctorates).
Baccalaureate Enrollment 171 **Women** 90% **Men** 10%
Graduate Enrollment 401 **Women** 92% **Men** 8% **Part-time** 62%
Nursing Student Activities Sigma Theta Tau, Student Nurses' Association, nursing club.
Nursing Student Resources Academic advising; academic or career counseling; assistance for students with disabilities; bookstore; campus computer network; computer lab; computer-assisted instruction; daycare for children of students; e-mail services; employment services for current students; housing assistance; interactive nursing skills videos; Internet; learning resource lab; library services; resume preparation assistance; skills, simulation, or other laboratory.
Library Facilities 469,000 volumes in health, 8,220 volumes in nursing.

BACCALAUREATE PROGRAMS

Degree BS
Available Programs Accelerated Baccalaureate; Accelerated Baccalaureate for Second Degree; Accelerated RN Baccalaureate; Baccalaureate for Second Degree.
Study Options Full-time.
Program Entrance Requirements Transcript of college record, written essay, 3 letters of recommendation, prerequisite course work. *Application deadline:* 11/15 (summer). *Application fee:* $65.
Advanced Placement Credit by examination available. Credit given for nursing courses completed elsewhere dependent upon specific evaluations.
Contact *Telephone:* 212-305-5756. *Fax:* 212-305-3680.

GRADUATE PROGRAMS

Contact *Telephone:* 212-305-5756. *Fax:* 212-305-3680.

MASTER'S DEGREE PROGRAM
Degrees MS; MSN/MBA; MSN/MPH
Available Programs Accelerated Master's for Non-Nursing College Graduates; Accelerated Master's for Nurses with Non-Nursing Degrees; Master's; Master's for Non-Nursing College Graduates; Master's for Nurses with Non-Nursing Degrees.
Concentrations Available Nurse anesthesia; nurse-midwifery. *Nurse practitioner programs in:* acute care, adult health, family health, pediatric, psychiatric/mental health.
Study Options Full-time and part-time.
Program Entrance Requirements Clinical experience, minimum overall college GPA of 3.0, transcript of college record, written essay, interview, 3 letters of recommendation, physical assessment course, prerequisite course work, resume, statistics course, GRE General Test. *Application deadline:* 4/15 (fall), 1/15 (summer). *Application fee:* $65.
Advanced Placement Credit by examination available. Credit given for nursing courses completed elsewhere dependent upon specific evaluations.
Degree Requirements 45 total credit hours, thesis or project, comprehensive exam.

POST-MASTER'S PROGRAM
Areas of Study Nurse anesthesia. *Nurse practitioner programs in:* acute care, adult health, family health, pediatric, psychiatric/mental health.

DOCTORAL DEGREE PROGRAM
Degree PhD
Available Programs Doctorate; Doctorate for Nurses with Non-Nursing Degrees; Post-Baccalaureate Doctorate.
Areas of Study Addiction/substance abuse, advanced practice nursing, clinical practice, clinical research, community health, family health, health policy, health promotion/disease prevention, information systems, maternity-newborn, nursing education, nursing policy, nursing research, nursing science, urban health, women's health.
Program Entrance Requirements Minimum overall college GPA of 3.0, interview by faculty committee, interview, 3 letters of recommendation, statistics course, vita, writing sample, GRE General Test. Application deadline: 1/2 (fall). Application fee: $75.
Degree Requirements 60 total credit hours, dissertation, written exam.

POSTDOCTORAL PROGRAM
Areas of Study Nursing informatics, nursing research.
Postdoctoral Program Contact *Telephone:* 212-305-5495.

CONTINUING EDUCATION PROGRAM

Contact *Telephone:* 212-305-1175.

Concordia College–New York
Nursing Program
Bronxville, New York

http://www.concordia-ny.edu/
Founded in 1881
DEGREE • BS
Nursing Program Faculty 6 (50% with doctorates).
Baccalaureate Enrollment 40 **Women** 80% **Men** 20%
Nursing Student Activities Student Nurses' Association.
Nursing Student Resources Academic advising; academic or career counseling; assistance for students with disabilities; bookstore; campus computer network; career placement assistance; computer lab; computer-assisted instruction; e-mail services; housing assistance; interactive nursing skills videos; Internet; learning resource lab; library services; nursing audiovisuals; resume preparation assistance; skills, simulation, or other laboratory; tutoring.

BACCALAUREATE PROGRAMS

Degree BS
Available Programs Accelerated Baccalaureate for Second Degree; Generic Baccalaureate.
Study Options Full-time.
Program Entrance Requirements Minimum overall college GPA of 3.2, transcript of college record, written essay, health exam, health insurance, high school biology, high school chemistry, 3 years high school science, high school transcript, immunizations, interview, 2 letters of recommendation, minimum high school GPA, minimum GPA in nursing prerequisites of 3.0, professional liability insurance/malpractice

insurance, prerequisite course work. Transfer students are accepted. *Application deadline:* 4/1 (winter). *Application fee:* $50.

Advanced Placement Credit given for nursing courses completed elsewhere dependent upon specific evaluations.

Contact *Telephone:* 914-337-9300.

Daemen College
Department of Nursing
Amherst, New York

http://www.daemen.edu/
Founded in 1947

DEGREES • BS • DNP • MS

Nursing Program Faculty 28 (50% with doctorates).
Baccalaureate Enrollment 400 **Women** 88% **Men** 12% **Part-time** 72%
Graduate Enrollment 140 **Women** 88% **Men** 12% **Part-time** 83%
Distance Learning Courses Available.
Nursing Student Activities Sigma Theta Tau, nursing club.
Nursing Student Resources Academic advising; academic or career counseling; assistance for students with disabilities; bookstore; campus computer network; career placement assistance; computer lab; computer-assisted instruction; e-mail services; Internet; learning resource lab; library services; nursing audiovisuals; placement services for program completers; remedial services; resume preparation assistance; skills, simulation, or other laboratory; tutoring.
Library Facilities 10,000 volumes in health, 4,000 volumes in nursing; 250 periodical subscriptions health-care related.

BACCALAUREATE PROGRAMS

Degree BS
Available Programs ADN to Baccalaureate; Accelerated RN Baccalaureate; International Nurse to Baccalaureate; RN Baccalaureate.
Site Options Jamestown, NY; Olean, NY.
Study Options Full-time and part-time.
Program Entrance Requirements Minimum overall college GPA of 2.0, transcript of college record, 2 years high school math, 2 years high school science, high school transcript, immunizations, minimum high school GPA of 3.0. Transfer students are accepted. *Application deadline:* Applications may be processed on a rolling basis for some programs.
Advanced Placement Credit given for nursing courses completed elsewhere dependent upon specific evaluations.
Expenses (2015–16) *Tuition:* full-time $13,000; part-time $425 per credit hour. *International tuition:* $13,000 full-time. *Room and board:* $11,580 per academic year.
Financial Aid 85% of baccalaureate students in nursing programs received some form of financial aid in 2014–15.
Contact Dr. Mary Lou Rusin, Professor and Chair, Department of Nursing, Daemen College, 4380 Main Street, Amherst, NY 14226. *Telephone:* 716-839-8387. *Fax:* 716-839-8403.
E-mail: mrusin@daemen.edu.

GRADUATE PROGRAMS

Expenses (2015–16) *Tuition:* part-time $967 per credit hour. *International tuition:* $967 full-time. *Required fees:* part-time $100 per term.
Financial Aid 85% of graduate students in nursing programs received some form of financial aid in 2014–15. Institutionally sponsored loans and scholarships available. *Financial aid application deadline:* 2/15.
Contact Dr. Mary Lou Rusin, Professor and Chair, Department of Nursing, Daemen College, 4380 Main Street, Amherst, NY 14226. *Telephone:* 716-839-8387. *Fax:* 716-839-8403.
E-mail: mrusin@daemen.edu.

MASTER'S DEGREE PROGRAM

Degree MS
Available Programs Accelerated AD/RN to Master's; Accelerated RN to Master's; Master's; RN to Master's.
Concentrations Available Health-care administration; nursing education. *Nurse practitioner programs in:* adult-gerontology acute care.
Study Options Full-time and part-time.
Program Entrance Requirements Clinical experience, minimum overall college GPA of 3.25, transcript of college record, written essay, immunizations, interview, 3 letters of recommendation, statistics course.

Application deadline: Applications may be processed on a rolling basis for some programs. *Application fee:* $35.
Advanced Placement Credit given for nursing courses completed elsewhere dependent upon specific evaluations.
Degree Requirements 30 total credit hours, thesis or project.

POST-MASTER'S PROGRAM

Areas of Study Health-care administration; nursing education. *Nurse practitioner programs in:* adult-gerontology acute care.

DOCTORAL DEGREE PROGRAM

Degree DNP
Available Programs Doctorate; Post-Baccalaureate Doctorate.
Areas of Study Advanced practice nursing.
Program Entrance Requirements Minimum overall college GPA of 3.25, interview, 3 letters of recommendation, statistics course, vita, writing sample. Application deadline: Applications may be processed on a rolling basis for some programs. Application fee: $35.
Degree Requirements 36 total credit hours.

Dominican College
Department of Nursing
Orangeburg, New York

Founded in 1952

DEGREES • BSN • M SC N

Nursing Program Faculty 14 (21% with doctorates).
Baccalaureate Enrollment 182 **Women** 87% **Men** 13% **Part-time** 43%
Graduate Enrollment 37 **Women** 100% **Part-time** 100%
Nursing Student Activities Nursing Honor Society, Sigma Theta Tau, Student Nurses' Association.
Nursing Student Resources Academic advising; academic or career counseling; assistance for students with disabilities; bookstore; campus computer network; career placement assistance; computer lab; computer-assisted instruction; e-mail services; externships; Internet; learning resource lab; library services; nursing audiovisuals; paid internships; remedial services; resume preparation assistance; skills, simulation, or other laboratory; tutoring.
Library Facilities 5,650 volumes in health; 235 periodical subscriptions health-care related.

BACCALAUREATE PROGRAMS

Degree BSN
Available Programs Accelerated Baccalaureate for Second Degree; Accelerated LPN to Baccalaureate; Accelerated RN Baccalaureate; Generic Baccalaureate; LPN to Baccalaureate; RN Baccalaureate.
Study Options Full-time and part-time.
Program Entrance Requirements Minimum overall college GPA of 2.7, transcript of college record, CPR certification, health exam, health insurance, high school transcript, immunizations, minimum GPA in nursing prerequisites of 2.0, professional liability insurance/malpractice insurance, prerequisite course work. Transfer students are accepted.
Advanced Placement Credit by examination available. Credit given for nursing courses completed elsewhere dependent upon specific evaluations.
Contact *Telephone:* 845-848-6051. *Fax:* 845-398-4891.

GRADUATE PROGRAMS

Contact *Telephone:* 845-848-6026. *Fax:* 845-398-4891.

MASTER'S DEGREE PROGRAM

Degree M Sc N
Available Programs Master's.
Concentrations Available *Nurse practitioner programs in:* family health.
Study Options Full-time and part-time.
Program Entrance Requirements Clinical experience, minimum overall college GPA of 3.0, transcript of college record, written essay, immunizations, 3 letters of recommendation, nursing research course, physical assessment course, professional liability insurance/malpractice insurance, prerequisite course work, statistics course.
Degree Requirements 42 total credit hours, thesis or project.

D'Youville College
School of Nursing
Buffalo, New York

http://www.dyc.edu/academics/nursing/
Founded in 1908

DEGREES • BSN • DNP • MS

Nursing Program Faculty 41 (20% with doctorates).
Baccalaureate Enrollment 654 **Women** 86% **Men** 14% **Part-time** 34%
Graduate Enrollment 155 **Women** 86% **Men** 14% **Part-time** 81%
Distance Learning Courses Available.
Nursing Student Activities Sigma Theta Tau, Student Nurses' Association.
Nursing Student Resources Academic advising; academic or career counseling; assistance for students with disabilities; bookstore; campus computer network; career placement assistance; computer lab; computer-assisted instruction; e-mail services; externships; interactive nursing skills videos; Internet; learning resource lab; library services; nursing audiovisuals; paid internships; placement services for program completers; remedial services; resume preparation assistance; skills, simulation, or other laboratory; tutoring.
Library Facilities 9,714 volumes in health, 930 volumes in nursing; 171 periodical subscriptions health-care related.

BACCALAUREATE PROGRAMS

Degree BSN
Available Programs Generic Baccalaureate; RN Baccalaureate.
Study Options Full-time and part-time.
Program Entrance Requirements Minimum overall college GPA of 2.5, transcript of college record, health exam, health insurance, high school biology, high school chemistry, 1 year of high school math, 1 year of high school science, high school transcript, immunizations, minimum high school GPA of 2.0, minimum high school rank 50%, minimum GPA in nursing prerequisites of 2.0, professional liability insurance/malpractice insurance, prerequisite course work. Transfer students are accepted.
Advanced Placement Credit given for nursing courses completed elsewhere dependent upon specific evaluations.
Expenses (2014–15) *Tuition:* full-time $23,092; part-time $720 per credit hour. *International tuition:* $23,092 full-time. *Room and board:* $10,800 per academic year. *Required fees:* full-time $490.
Financial Aid 90% of baccalaureate students in nursing programs received some form of financial aid in 2013–14. *Gift aid (need-based):* Federal Pell, FSEOG, state, private, college/university gift aid from institutional funds. *Loans:* Federal Nursing Student Loans, Federal Direct (Subsidized and Unsubsidized Stafford PLUS), Perkins. *Work-study:* Federal Work-Study, part-time campus jobs. *Financial aid application deadline (priority):* 2/15.
Contact Dr. Steven Smith, Director of Undergraduate Admissions, School of Nursing, D'Youville College, 320 Porter Avenue, Buffalo, NY 14201. *Telephone:* 716-881-7600. *Fax:* 716-829-7900. *E-mail:* admissions@dyc.edu.

GRADUATE PROGRAMS

Expenses (2014–15) *Tuition:* full-time $25,560; part-time $852 per credit hour. *International tuition:* $25,560 full-time. *Room and board:* $10,520; room only: $8832 per academic year. *Required fees:* full-time $490.
Financial Aid Federal Work-Study, scholarships, traineeships, and unspecified assistantships available.
Contact Mr. Mark Pavone, Director of Graduate Admissions, School of Nursing, D'Youville College, 320 Porter Avenue, Buffalo, NY 14201. *Telephone:* 716-881-8400. *Fax:* 716-829-8408. *E-mail:* pavonem@dyc.edu.

MASTER'S DEGREE PROGRAM

Degree MS
Available Programs Master's.
Concentrations Available Nursing education. *Clinical nurse specialist programs in:* community health, palliative care. *Nurse practitioner programs in:* family health.
Study Options Full-time and part-time.
Program Entrance Requirements Clinical experience, computer literacy, minimum overall college GPA of 3.0, transcript of college record, CPR certification, written essay, immunizations, interview, 2 letters of recommendation, nursing research course, physical assessment course, professional liability insurance/malpractice insurance, prerequisite course work, resume, statistics course.
Advanced Placement Credit given for nursing courses completed elsewhere dependent upon specific evaluations.
Degree Requirements 41 total credit hours, thesis or project.

POST-MASTER'S PROGRAM

Areas of Study *Nurse practitioner programs in:* family health.

DOCTORAL DEGREE PROGRAM

Degree DNP
Available Programs Post-Baccalaureate Doctorate.
Areas of Study Nursing administration.

See display on next page and full description on page 490.

Elmira College
Program in Nursing Education
Elmira, New York

http://www.elmira.edu/
Founded in 1855

DEGREE • BS

Nursing Program Faculty 28 (3% with doctorates).
Baccalaureate Enrollment 279 **Women** 90% **Men** 10% **Part-time** 18%
Nursing Student Activities Nursing Honor Society, Sigma Theta Tau, Student Nurses' Association, nursing club.
Nursing Student Resources Academic advising; academic or career counseling; assistance for students with disabilities; bookstore; campus computer network; career placement assistance; computer lab; computer-assisted instruction; e-mail services; employment services for current students; housing assistance; interactive nursing skills videos; Internet; learning resource lab; library services; nursing audiovisuals; placement services for program completers; resume preparation assistance; skills, simulation, or other laboratory; tutoring; unpaid internships.
Library Facilities 7,461 volumes in health, 5,200 volumes in nursing; 72 periodical subscriptions health-care related.

BACCALAUREATE PROGRAMS

Degree BS
Available Programs Generic Baccalaureate; RN Baccalaureate.
Study Options Full-time and part-time.
Program Entrance Requirements Minimum overall college GPA of 2.7, transcript of college record, written essay, health exam, health insurance, high school biology, high school chemistry, 3 years high school math, 3 years high school science, high school transcript, immunizations, 2 letters of recommendation, minimum high school GPA of 2.5. Transfer students are accepted. *Application deadline:* 8/24 (fall), 11/30 (winter), 3/28 (spring), 6/13 (summer). Applications may be processed on a rolling basis for some programs. *Application fee:* $100.
Advanced Placement Credit by examination available. Credit given for nursing courses completed elsewhere dependent upon specific evaluations.
Expenses (2015–16) *Tuition:* full-time $38,300; part-time $375 per contact hour. *International tuition:* $38,300 full-time. *Room and board:* $12,000; room only: $6400 per academic year. *Required fees:* full-time $1650; part-time $55 per term.
Financial Aid *Gift aid (need-based):* Federal Pell, FSEOG, state, private, college/university gift aid from institutional funds. *Loans:* Federal Direct (Subsidized and Unsubsidized Stafford PLUS), Perkins. *Work-study:* Federal Work-Study, part-time campus jobs. *Financial aid application deadline (priority):* 2/1.
Contact Mr. Christopher Coons, Vice President of Enrollment Management, Program in Nursing Education, Elmira College, One Park Place, Elmira, NY 14901. *Telephone:* 607-735-1806. *Fax:* 607-735-1873. *E-mail:* admissions@elmira.edu.

CONTINUING EDUCATION PROGRAM

Contact Dr. Kathleen J. Lucke, Dean of Health Sciences and Professor of Nurse Education, Program in Nursing Education, Elmira College, One Park Place, Elmira, NY 14901. *Telephone:* 607-735-1890. *Fax:* 607-735-1159. *E-mail:* klucke@elmira.edu.

Excelsior College
School of Nursing
Albany, New York

Founded in 1970

DEGREES • BS • MS

Distance Learning Courses Available.

Nursing Student Activities Sigma Theta Tau.

Nursing Student Resources Academic advising; academic or career counseling; assistance for students with disabilities; bookstore; computer-assisted instruction; e-mail services; Internet; learning resource lab; library services; nursing audiovisuals; other; resume preparation assistance; skills, simulation, or other laboratory; tutoring.

BACCALAUREATE PROGRAMS

Degree BS

Available Programs RN Baccalaureate.

Study Options Part-time.

Program Entrance Requirements Transcript of college record, high school transcript, RN licensure. Transfer students are accepted. *Application deadline:* Applications may be processed on a rolling basis for some programs.

Advanced Placement Credit by examination available. Credit given for nursing courses completed elsewhere dependent upon specific evaluations.

Contact *Telephone:* 518-464-8500. *Fax:* 518-464-8777.

GRADUATE PROGRAMS

Contact *Telephone:* 518-464-8500. *Fax:* 518-464-8777.

MASTER'S DEGREE PROGRAM

Degree MS

Available Programs Master's; RN to Master's.

Concentrations Available Nursing administration; nursing education; nursing informatics.

Study Options Full-time and part-time.

Online Degree Options Yes (online only).

Program Entrance Requirements Computer literacy, minimum overall college GPA of 3, transcript of college record, written essay, resume. *Application deadline:* Applications may be processed on a rolling basis for some programs.

Advanced Placement Credit given for nursing courses completed elsewhere dependent upon specific evaluations.

Degree Requirements 39 total credit hours, thesis or project.

POST-MASTER'S PROGRAM

Areas of Study Nursing education.

Farmingdale State College
Nursing Department
Farmingdale, New York

http://www.farmingdale.edu

Founded in 1912

DEGREE • BS

BACCALAUREATE PROGRAMS

Degree BS

Available Programs Generic Baccalaureate; RN Baccalaureate.

Contact *Telephone:* 631-420-2229. *Fax:* 631-420-2269.

Hartwick College
Department of Nursing
Oneonta, New York

http://www.hartwick.edu/

Founded in 1797

DEGREE • BS

Nursing Program Faculty 11 (18% with doctorates).

Baccalaureate Enrollment 220 **Women** 90% **Men** 10% **Part-time** 6%

Nursing Student Activities Sigma Theta Tau, Student Nurses' Association.

Nursing Student Resources Academic advising; academic or career counseling; assistance for students with disabilities; bookstore; campus computer network; career placement assistance; computer lab; computer-

www.dyc.edu   800.777.3921   716.829.7600

A RECOGNIZED INTERNATIONAL LEADER IN NURSING EDUCATION FOR OVER 70 YEARS

Undergraduate Programs:
Nursing (2-yr. RN to BSN online
- 50% off net tuition)
Nursing (4-yr. BSN)

Masters Program:
Family Nurse Practitioner

Doctoral Program:
Doctor of Nursing Practice

D'Youville
COLLEGE
Educating for life
320 Porter Avenue • Buffalo NY 14201

assisted instruction; e-mail services; employment services for current students; externships; housing assistance; interactive nursing skills videos; Internet; learning resource lab; library services; nursing audiovisuals; placement services for program completers; remedial services; resume preparation assistance; skills, simulation, or other laboratory; tutoring; unpaid internships.

Library Facilities 5,697 volumes in health, 1,199 volumes in nursing; 30 periodical subscriptions health-care related.

BACCALAUREATE PROGRAMS

Degree BS

Available Programs Accelerated Baccalaureate; Accelerated Baccalaureate for Second Degree; Generic Baccalaureate; RN Baccalaureate.

Site Options Albany, NY; Cooperstown, NY.

Study Options Full-time and part-time.

Program Entrance Requirements Minimum overall college GPA of 2.5, transcript of college record, CPR certification, written essay, health exam, high school biology, high school chemistry, high school foreign language, 3 years high school math, 2 years high school science, high school transcript, immunizations, 2 letters of recommendation, minimum high school GPA, minimum GPA in nursing prerequisites of 2.5, professional liability insurance/malpractice insurance. Transfer students are accepted. *Application deadline:* Applications may be processed on a rolling basis for some programs.

Advanced Placement Credit given for nursing courses completed elsewhere dependent upon specific evaluations.

Expenses (2015–16) *Tuition:* full-time $40,630; part-time $1305 per credit hour. *Room and board:* $11,120; room only: $5850 per academic year. *Required fees:* full-time $1300.

Financial Aid *Gift aid (need-based):* Federal Pell, FSEOG, state, private, college/university gift aid from institutional funds. *Loans:* Federal Nursing Student Loans, Federal Direct (Subsidized and Unsubsidized Stafford PLUS), Perkins, college/university, alternative loans. *Work-study:* Federal Work-Study. *Financial aid application deadline:* Continuous.

Contact Dr. Jeanne-Marie E. Havener, Chair and Associate Professor of Nursing, Department of Nursing, Hartwick College, Johnstone Science Center, One Hartwick Drive, Oneonta, NY 13820. *Telephone:* 607-431-4780. *Fax:* 607-431-4850. *E-mail:* havenerj@hartwick.edu.

Helene Fuld College of Nursing

RN to BSN Program
New York, New York

https://www.helenefuld.edu
Founded in 1945

DEGREE • BS

Nursing Program Faculty 12 (7% with doctorates).

Baccalaureate Enrollment 48 **Women** 90% **Men** 10% **Part-time** 15%

Nursing Student Resources Academic advising; academic or career counseling; computer lab; computer-assisted instruction; e-mail services; Internet; library services; skills, simulation, or other laboratory; tutoring.

Library Facilities 1,000 volumes in health, 1,000 volumes in nursing; 2,000 periodical subscriptions health-care related.

BACCALAUREATE PROGRAMS

Degree BS

Available Programs RN Baccalaureate.

Study Options Full-time and part-time.

Program Entrance Requirements Transcript of college record, written essay, immunizations, 2 letters of recommendation, minimum GPA in nursing prerequisites of 2.5, professional liability insurance/malpractice insurance, RN licensure. *Application deadline:* 9/1 (fall). Applications may be processed on a rolling basis for some programs. *Application fee:* $50.

Expenses (2015–16) *Tuition:* full-time $21,780; part-time $575 per credit. *Required fees:* full-time $610; part-time $65 per term.

Financial Aid 83% of baccalaureate students in nursing programs received some form of financial aid in 2014–15. *Gift aid (need-based):* Federal Pell, FSEOG, private. *Financial aid application deadline:* Continuous.

Contact College of Nursing, RN to BSN Program, Helene Fuld College of Nursing, 24 East 120th Street, New York, NY 10035. *Telephone:* 212-616-7200.

Hunter College of the City University of New York

Hunter-Bellevue School of Nursing
New York, New York

http://www.hunter.cuny.edu/schoolhp/nursing
Founded in 1870

DEGREES • BS • DNP • MS • MSN/MPA • MSN/MPH

Nursing Program Faculty 132 (32% with doctorates).

Baccalaureate Enrollment 505 **Women** 84% **Men** 16% **Part-time** 26%

Graduate Enrollment 473 **Women** 88% **Men** 12% **Part-time** 90%

Nursing Student Activities Sigma Theta Tau, Student Nurses' Association.

Nursing Student Resources Academic advising; academic or career counseling; assistance for students with disabilities; bookstore; campus computer network; computer lab; computer-assisted instruction; e-mail services; interactive nursing skills videos; Internet; learning resource lab; library services; nursing audiovisuals; skills, simulation, or other laboratory.

Library Facilities 39,245 volumes in health, 4,295 volumes in nursing; 375 periodical subscriptions health-care related.

BACCALAUREATE PROGRAMS

Degree BS

Available Programs Accelerated Baccalaureate for Second Degree; Generic Baccalaureate; RN Baccalaureate.

Study Options Full-time and part-time.

Program Entrance Requirements Minimum overall college GPA of 3.25, transcript of college record, CPR certification, health exam, immunizations, minimum GPA in nursing prerequisites of 3.0, professional liability insurance/malpractice insurance, prerequisite course work. Transfer students are accepted. *Application deadline:* 2/1 (fall). *Application fee:* $75.

Advanced Placement Credit given for nursing courses completed elsewhere dependent upon specific evaluations.

Expenses (2015–16) *Tuition, state resident:* full-time $6330; part-time $275 per credit. *Tuition, nonresident:* full-time $13,440; part-time $560 per credit. *International tuition:* $13,440 full-time. *Room and board:* room only: $1952 per academic year. *Required fees:* full-time $450; part-time $132 per credit.

Financial Aid 70% of baccalaureate students in nursing programs received some form of financial aid in 2014–15.

Contact Ms. Maria Mendoza, Pre-Nursing Adviser, Hunter-Bellevue School of Nursing, Hunter College of the City University of New York, 425 East 25th Street, New York, NY 10010. *Telephone:* 212-481-4473. *Fax:* 212-481-8237. *E-mail:* prenursingadvising@hunter.cuny.edu.

GRADUATE PROGRAMS

Expenses (2015–16) *Tuition, state resident:* full-time $10,130; part-time $425 per credit. *Tuition, nonresident:* full-time $18,720; part-time $780 per credit. *International tuition:* $18,720 full-time. *Required fees:* full-time $753; part-time $203 per credit.

Financial Aid 50% of graduate students in nursing programs received some form of financial aid in 2014–15. Federal Work-Study, scholarships, traineeships, and tuition waivers (partial) available. Aid available to part-time students. *Financial aid application deadline:* 5/1.

Contact Dr. Lynda Olender, Director of Graduate Program, Hunter-Bellevue School of Nursing, Hunter College of the City University of New York, 425 East 25th Street, New York, NY 10010. *Telephone:* 212-481-3478. *Fax:* 212-481-4427. *E-mail:* lo208@hunter.cuny.edu.

MASTER'S DEGREE PROGRAM

Degrees MS; MSN/MPA; MSN/MPH

Available Programs Master's.

Concentrations Available Nursing administration. *Clinical nurse specialist programs in:* adult health, community health, critical care, psychiatric/mental health, public health, public/community health. *Nurse practitioner programs in:* community health, gerontology, psychiatric/mental health.

Study Options Full-time and part-time.

Program Entrance Requirements Clinical experience, minimum overall college GPA of 3.0, transcript of college record, written essay, immunizations, 2 letters of recommendation, resume, statistics course. *Application deadline:* 4/1 (fall), 11/1 (spring). Applications may be processed on a rolling basis for some programs. *Application fee:* $125.

Advanced Placement Credit given for nursing courses completed elsewhere dependent upon specific evaluations.

Degree Requirements 42 total credit hours, thesis or project.

POST-MASTER'S PROGRAM

Areas of Study *Clinical nurse specialist programs in:* adult health, community health, psychiatric/mental health, public health, public/community health. *Nurse practitioner programs in:* psychiatric/mental health.

DOCTORAL DEGREE PROGRAM

Degree DNP

Available Programs Doctorate; Post-Baccalaureate Doctorate.

Areas of Study Community health, gerontology, neuro-behavior.

Program Entrance Requirements Clinical experience, minimum overall college GPA of 3.5, interview, 2 letters of recommendation, statistics course, vita. Application deadline: 4/1 (fall), 11/1 (spring). Applications may be processed on a rolling basis for some programs. Application fee: $125.

Degree Requirements 90 total credit hours.

CONTINUING EDUCATION PROGRAM

Contact Continuing Education, Hunter-Bellevue School of Nursing, Hunter College of the City University of New York, 695 Park Avenue, East Building, 10th Floor, New York, NY 10021. *Telephone:* 212-650-3850. *Fax:* 212-772-3402. *E-mail:* ce@hunter.cuny.edu.

Keuka College

Division of Nursing
Keuka Park, New York

http://asap.keuka.edu/programs/bs-nursing/
Founded in 1890

DEGREES • BS • MS

Nursing Program Faculty 10 (80% with doctorates).

Baccalaureate Enrollment 178 **Women** 90% **Men** 10%

Graduate Enrollment 45 **Women** 91% **Men** 9%

Distance Learning Courses Available.

Nursing Student Activities Sigma Theta Tau, Student Nurses' Association.

Nursing Student Resources Academic advising; academic or career counseling; assistance for students with disabilities; bookstore; campus computer network; computer lab; computer-assisted instruction; e-mail services; employment services for current students; interactive nursing skills videos; Internet; learning resource lab; library services; nursing audiovisuals; resume preparation assistance; skills, simulation, or other laboratory; tutoring; unpaid internships.

Library Facilities 986 volumes in health, 532 volumes in nursing; 48 periodical subscriptions health-care related.

BACCALAUREATE PROGRAMS

Degree BS

Available Programs Accelerated RN Baccalaureate.

Site Options Rochester, NY; Elmira, NY; Syracuse, NY.

Study Options Full-time.

Program Entrance Requirements Minimum overall college GPA of 2.5, transcript of college record, CPR certification, written essay, health exam, immunizations, 2 letters of recommendation, minimum GPA in nursing prerequisites of 2.5, prerequisite course work, RN licensure. Transfer students are accepted. *Application deadline:* Applications may be processed on a rolling basis for some programs. *Application fee:* $50.

Advanced Placement Credit by examination available. Credit given for nursing courses completed elsewhere dependent upon specific evaluations.

Expenses (2015–16) *Tuition:* full-time $19,210.

Contact Dr. Debra J. Gates, Nursing Division Associate Professor and Chairperson, Division of Nursing, Keuka College, One Keuka Business Park, Penn Yan, NY 14527. *Telephone:* 315-279-5115. *Fax:* 315-279-5105. *E-mail:* dgates@keuka.edu.

GRADUATE PROGRAMS

Expenses (2015–16) *Tuition:* full-time $30,210.

Contact Dr. Debra J. Gates, Nursing Division Associate Professor and Chairperson, Division of Nursing, Keuka College, One Keuka Business Park, Penn Yan, NY 14527. *Telephone:* 315-279-5115. *Fax:* 315-279-5105. *E-mail:* dgates@keuka.edu.

MASTER'S DEGREE PROGRAM

Degree MS

Available Programs Accelerated Master's.

Concentrations Available Nursing education. *Nurse practitioner programs in:* adult-gerontology acute care.

Site Options Rochester, NY; Elmira, NY; Syracuse, NY.

Study Options Full-time.

Program Entrance Requirements Minimum overall college GPA of 3.0, transcript of college record, CPR certification, written essay, immunizations, interview, 3 letters of recommendation, resume. *Application deadline:* Applications may be processed on a rolling basis for some programs. *Application fee:* $50.

Advanced Placement Credit given for nursing courses completed elsewhere dependent upon specific evaluations.

Degree Requirements 38 total credit hours, thesis or project.

POST-MASTER'S PROGRAM

Areas of Study *Nurse practitioner programs in:* adult-gerontology acute care.

Lehman College of the City University of New York

Department of Nursing
Bronx, New York

http://lehman.edu
Founded in 1931

DEGREES • BS • DNS • MS

Nursing Program Faculty 43 (35% with doctorates).

Baccalaureate Enrollment 300 **Women** 80% **Men** 20% **Part-time** 50%

Graduate Enrollment 200 **Women** 90% **Men** 10% **Part-time** 75%

Distance Learning Courses Available.

Nursing Student Activities Nursing Honor Society, Sigma Theta Tau, Student Nurses' Association, nursing club.

Nursing Student Resources Academic advising; academic or career counseling; assistance for students with disabilities; bookstore; campus computer network; career placement assistance; computer lab; computer-assisted instruction; daycare for children of students; e-mail services; employment services for current students; externships; interactive nursing skills videos; Internet; learning resource lab; library services; nursing audiovisuals; paid internships; placement services for program completers; resume preparation assistance; skills, simulation, or other laboratory; tutoring; unpaid internships.

Library Facilities 1,000 volumes in health, 500 volumes in nursing; 200 periodical subscriptions health-care related.

BACCALAUREATE PROGRAMS

Degree BS

Available Programs ADN to Baccalaureate; Accelerated Baccalaureate for Second Degree; Accelerated RN Baccalaureate; Baccalaureate for Second Degree; Generic Baccalaureate; International Nurse to Baccalaureate; RN Baccalaureate.

Site Options New York, NY; Queens, NY.

Study Options Full-time.

Online Degree Options Yes.

Program Entrance Requirements Minimum overall college GPA of 2.0, transcript of college record, health exam, high school transcript, immunizations, minimum GPA in nursing prerequisites of 2.75, professional liability insurance/malpractice insurance, prerequisite course work. Transfer students are accepted. *Application deadline:* 3/15 (fall).

Advanced Placement Credit given for nursing courses completed elsewhere dependent upon specific evaluations.

Contact *Telephone:* 718-960-8214. *Fax:* 718-960-8488.

GRADUATE PROGRAMS

Contact *Telephone:* 718-960-8213. *Fax:* 718-960-8488.

MASTER'S DEGREE PROGRAM

Degree MS

Available Programs Master's; Master's for Nurses with Non-Nursing Degrees.

Concentrations Available Nursing administration; nursing education. *Clinical nurse specialist programs in:* adult health, gerontology, parent-child. *Nurse practitioner programs in:* family health, pediatric.

Site Options New York, NY.

Study Options Full-time and part-time.
Program Entrance Requirements Clinical experience, minimum overall college GPA of 3.0, transcript of college record, written essay, immunizations, interview, 2 letters of recommendation, professional liability insurance/malpractice insurance, prerequisite course work. *Application deadline:* 4/1 (fall), 11/1 (spring). Applications may be processed on a rolling basis for some programs. *Application fee:* $125.
Degree Requirements 43 total credit hours.

POST-MASTER'S PROGRAM

Areas of Study *Nurse practitioner programs in:* family health, pediatric.

DOCTORAL DEGREE PROGRAM

Degree DNS
Available Programs Doctorate.
Areas of Study Urban health.
Site Options New York, NY.
Program Entrance Requirements Clinical experience, minimum overall college GPA of 3.5, interview by faculty committee, interview, letters of recommendation, MSN or equivalent, statistics course, vita, writing sample. Application deadline: 4/1 (fall).
Degree Requirements 51 total credit hours, dissertation, oral exam, written exam, residency.

CONTINUING EDUCATION PROGRAM

Contact *Telephone:* 718-960-8799.

Le Moyne College
Nursing Programs
Syracuse, New York

http://www.lemoyne.edu/nursing
Founded in 1946
DEGREES • BS • MS
Nursing Program Faculty 16 (50% with doctorates).
Baccalaureate Enrollment 316 **Women** 91% **Men** 9% **Part-time** 65%
Graduate Enrollment 40 **Women** 82% **Men** 18% **Part-time** 100%
Distance Learning Courses Available.
Nursing Student Activities Nursing Honor Society, Sigma Theta Tau, Student Nurses' Association, nursing club.
Nursing Student Resources Academic advising; academic or career counseling; assistance for students with disabilities; bookstore; campus computer network; career placement assistance; computer lab; computer-assisted instruction; e-mail services; employment services for current students; housing assistance; interactive nursing skills videos; Internet; learning resource lab; library services; nursing audiovisuals; other; placement services for program completers; remedial services; resume preparation assistance; skills, simulation, or other laboratory; tutoring.
Library Facilities 4,225 volumes in health, 998 volumes in nursing; 8,224 periodical subscriptions health-care related.

BACCALAUREATE PROGRAMS

Degree BS
Available Programs Accelerated Baccalaureate for Second Degree; Baccalaureate for Second Degree; Generic Baccalaureate; RN Baccalaureate.
Site Options Syracuse, NY.
Study Options Full-time and part-time.
Program Entrance Requirements Minimum overall college GPA of 2.6, transcript of college record, written essay, health exam, health insurance, high school biology, high school chemistry, high school foreign language, 3 years high school math, 3 years high school science, high school transcript, immunizations, 3 letters of recommendation, minimum high school GPA of 3.0, minimum high school rank 85%, minimum GPA in nursing prerequisites of 2.5, RN licensure. Transfer students are accepted. *Application deadline:* 2/1 (fall). Applications may be processed on a rolling basis for some programs. *Application fee:* $35.
Advanced Placement Credit given for nursing courses completed elsewhere dependent upon specific evaluations.
Expenses (2015–16) *Tuition:* full-time $31,260. *International tuition:* $31,260 full-time. *Room and board:* $12,540; room only: $7880 per academic year. *Required fees:* full-time $990.
Financial Aid 50% of baccalaureate students in nursing programs received some form of financial aid in 2014–15.
Contact Mr. Grant L. Thatcher, Senior Assistant Director of Admission, Nursing Programs, Le Moyne College, 1419 Salt Springs Road, Syracuse, NY 13214-1301. *Telephone:* 315-445-4300. *Fax:* 315-445-4711. *E-mail:* thatcgr@lemoyne.edu.

GRADUATE PROGRAMS

Expenses (2015–16) *Tuition:* part-time $683 per credit.
Financial Aid 40% of graduate students in nursing programs received some form of financial aid in 2014–15.
Contact Ms. Kristen P. Trapasso, Senior Director of Enrollment Management, Nursing Programs, Le Moyne College, 1419 Salt Springs Road, Syracuse, NY 13214-1301. *Telephone:* 315-445-5444. *Fax:* 315-445-6092. *E-mail:* trapaskp@lemoyne.edu.

MASTER'S DEGREE PROGRAM

Degree MS
Available Programs Master's.
Concentrations Available Nursing administration; nursing education; nursing informatics. *Nurse practitioner programs in:* family health.
Study Options Full-time and part-time.
Program Entrance Requirements Clinical experience, computer literacy, minimum overall college GPA of 3.0, transcript of college record, written essay, immunizations, interview, 2 letters of recommendation, resume. *Application deadline:* 5/1 (fall), 12/15 (spring), 5/1 (summer). *Application fee:* $50.
Advanced Placement Credit given for nursing courses completed elsewhere dependent upon specific evaluations.
Degree Requirements 39 total credit hours, thesis or project.

POST-MASTER'S PROGRAM

Areas of Study Nursing administration; nursing education; nursing informatics. *Nurse practitioner programs in:* family health.

CONTINUING EDUCATION PROGRAM

Contact Ms. Patricia J. Bliss, Director, Center for Continuing Education, Nursing Programs, Le Moyne College, 1419 Salt Springs Road, Syracuse, NY 13214-1301. *Telephone:* 315-445-4141. *Fax:* 315-445-6027. *E-mail:* ceinfo@lemoyne.edu.

Long Island University–LIU Brooklyn
School of Nursing
Brooklyn, New York

http://www.liu.edu
Founded in 1926
DEGREES • BS • MS
Nursing Program Faculty 85 (30% with doctorates).
Baccalaureate Enrollment 789 **Women** 85% **Men** 15% **Part-time** 35%
Graduate Enrollment 240 **Women** 90% **Men** 10% **Part-time** 83%
Nursing Student Activities Nursing Honor Society, Student Nurses' Association, nursing club.
Nursing Student Resources Academic advising; academic or career counseling; assistance for students with disabilities; bookstore; campus computer network; career placement assistance; computer lab; computer-assisted instruction; daycare for children of students; e-mail services; employment services for current students; externships; interactive nursing skills videos; Internet; learning resource lab; library services; nursing audiovisuals; paid internships; remedial services; resume preparation assistance; skills, simulation, or other laboratory; tutoring; unpaid internships.

BACCALAUREATE PROGRAMS

Degree BS
Available Programs ADN to Baccalaureate; Accelerated Baccalaureate for Second Degree; Generic Baccalaureate.
Study Options Full-time and part-time.
Program Entrance Requirements Minimum overall college GPA of 3.0, transcript of college record, CPR certification, health exam, health insurance, high school biology, high school chemistry, 2 years high school math, 2 years high school science, high school transcript, immunizations, interview, minimum high school GPA of 3.0, minimum GPA in nursing prerequisites of 3.0, professional liability insurance/malpractice insurance, prerequisite course work. Transfer students are accepted. *Application deadline:* Applications may be processed on a rolling basis for some programs. *Application fee:* $50.

Advanced Placement Credit given for nursing courses completed elsewhere dependent upon specific evaluations.

Expenses (2015–16) *Tuition:* part-time $1051 per credit. *International tuition:* $1051 full-time. *Required fees:* part-time $442 per term.

Contact Ms. Letitia Galdamez, Director of Advisement, School of Nursing, School of Nursing, Long Island University–LIU Brooklyn, 1 University Plaza, Brooklyn, NY 11201. *Telephone:* 718-488-1059. *Fax:* 718-780-4019. *E-mail:* galdamez@liu.edu.

GRADUATE PROGRAMS

Expenses (2015–16) *Tuition:* part-time $1155 per credit. *Room and board:* $20,238; room only: $15,100 per academic year. *Required fees:* part-time $442 per term.

Financial Aid Scholarships and unspecified assistantships available.

Contact Dr. Anna Acee, Director, School of Nursing, Long Island University–LIU Brooklyn, 1 University Plaza, Brooklyn, NY 11201. *Telephone:* 718-488-1059. *Fax:* 718-780-4019. *E-mail:* anna.acee@liu.edu.

MASTER'S DEGREE PROGRAM

Degree MS

Available Programs Master's; RN to Master's.

Concentrations Available Health-care administration; nursing administration; nursing education. *Nurse practitioner programs in:* adult health, family health.

Site Options Brooklyn, NY.

Study Options Part-time.

Program Entrance Requirements Clinical experience, computer literacy, minimum overall college GPA of 3.0, transcript of college record, CPR certification, immunizations, interview, 3 letters of recommendation, nursing research course, physical assessment course, professional liability insurance/malpractice insurance, prerequisite course work, resume, statistics course. *Application deadline:* 6/30 (fall). *Application fee:* $50.

Advanced Placement Credit given for nursing courses completed elsewhere dependent upon specific evaluations.

Degree Requirements 45 total credit hours, thesis or project.

POST-MASTER'S PROGRAM

Areas of Study Nursing education. *Nurse practitioner programs in:* adult health, family health.

Long Island University–LIU Post
Department of Nursing
Brookville, New York

http://www.liu.edu/post/nursing
Founded in 1954
DEGREES • BS • MS
Nursing Program Faculty 22 (50% with doctorates).
Baccalaureate Enrollment 81 **Women** 93% **Men** 7% **Part-time** 95%
Graduate Enrollment 131 **Women** 92% **Men** 8% **Part-time** 74%
Nursing Student Activities Student Nurses' Association.
Nursing Student Resources Academic advising; academic or career counseling; assistance for students with disabilities; bookstore; campus computer network; career placement assistance; computer lab; computer-assisted instruction; e-mail services; employment services for current students; housing assistance; interactive nursing skills videos; Internet; learning resource lab; library services; nursing audiovisuals; placement services for program completers; remedial services; resume preparation assistance; skills, simulation, or other laboratory; tutoring.
Library Facilities 29,872 volumes in health, 1,683 volumes in nursing; 25,618 periodical subscriptions health-care related.

BACCALAUREATE PROGRAMS

Degree BS

Available Programs Generic Baccalaureate; RN Baccalaureate.

Site Options Brentwood, NY; Manhasset, NY.

Study Options Full-time and part-time.

Program Entrance Requirements Minimum overall college GPA of 3.0, transcript of college record, health exam, health insurance, immunizations, minimum GPA in nursing prerequisites of 3.0, professional liability insurance/malpractice insurance, prerequisite course work, RN licensure. Transfer students are accepted. *Application deadline:* Applications may be processed on a rolling basis for some programs. *Application fee:* $50.

Advanced Placement Credit by examination available. Credit given for nursing courses completed elsewhere dependent upon specific evaluations.

Expenses (2015–16) *Tuition:* full-time $33,678; part-time $1051 per credit. *Room and board:* $12,718; room only: $8200 per academic year. *Required fees:* full-time $1768; part-time $442 per term.

Financial Aid 92% of baccalaureate students in nursing programs received some form of financial aid in 2014–15.

Contact Dr. Mary Infantino, Chairperson and Associate Professor, Department of Nursing, Long Island University–LIU Post, Life Science, Room 270, 720 Northern Boulevard, Brookville, NY 11548-1300. *Telephone:* 516-299-2320. *Fax:* 516-299-2352. *E-mail:* mary.infantino@liu.edu.

GRADUATE PROGRAMS

Expenses (2015–16) *Tuition:* part-time $1155 per credit. *Room and board:* $12,718; room only: $8200 per academic year. *Required fees:* part-time $442 per term.

Financial Aid 72% of graduate students in nursing programs received some form of financial aid in 2014–15. Federal Work-Study and unspecified assistantships available. Aid available to part-time students. *Financial aid application deadline:* 5/15.

Contact Dr. Mary Infantino, Chairperson and Associate Professor, Department of Nursing, Long Island University–LIU Post, Life Science, Room 270, 720 Northern Boulevard, Brookville, NY 11548-1300. *Telephone:* 516-299-2320. *Fax:* 516-299-2352. *E-mail:* mary.infantino@liu.edu.

MASTER'S DEGREE PROGRAM

Degree MS

Available Programs Master's.

Concentrations Available Nursing education. *Nurse practitioner programs in:* family health.

Site Options Brentwood, NY; Manhasset, NY.

Study Options Part-time.

Program Entrance Requirements Clinical experience, computer literacy, minimum overall college GPA of 3.0, transcript of college record, written essay, immunizations, interview, 2 letters of recommendation, nursing research course, physical assessment course, professional liability insurance/malpractice insurance, prerequisite course work, resume, statistics course. *Application deadline:* Applications may be processed on a rolling basis for some programs. *Application fee:* $50.

Advanced Placement Credit given for nursing courses completed elsewhere dependent upon specific evaluations.

Degree Requirements 46 total credit hours.

POST-MASTER'S PROGRAM

Areas of Study Nursing education. *Nurse practitioner programs in:* family health.

Maria College
RN Baccalaureate Completion Program
Albany, New York

Founded in 1958
DEGREE • BSN

BACCALAUREATE PROGRAMS

Degree BSN

Available Programs RN Baccalaureate.

Contact *Telephone:* 518-438-3111 Ext. 2548.

Medgar Evers College of the City University of New York
Department of Nursing
Brooklyn, New York

http://www.mec.cuny.edu/
Founded in 1969
DEGREE • BSN
Nursing Program Faculty 7 (85% with doctorates).
Baccalaureate Enrollment 60 **Women** 98% **Men** 2% **Part-time** 90%
Nursing Student Activities Student Nurses' Association, nursing club.

Nursing Student Resources Academic advising; academic or career counseling; assistance for students with disabilities; bookstore; campus computer network; computer lab; computer-assisted instruction; daycare for children of students; e-mail services; interactive nursing skills videos; Internet; learning resource lab; library services; nursing audiovisuals; remedial services; resume preparation assistance; skills, simulation, or other laboratory; tutoring; unpaid internships.

BACCALAUREATE PROGRAMS

Degree BSN
Available Programs ADN to Baccalaureate; Accelerated RN Baccalaureate.
Study Options Full-time and part-time.
Program Entrance Requirements Minimum overall college GPA of 2.5, transcript of college record, CPR certification, health exam, health insurance, immunizations, professional liability insurance/malpractice insurance, prerequisite course work, RN licensure. Transfer students are accepted.
Advanced Placement Credit given for nursing courses completed elsewhere dependent upon specific evaluations.
Contact *Telephone:* 718-270-6230. *Fax:* 718-270-6235.

Mercy College
Programs in Nursing
Dobbs Ferry, New York

Founded in 1951
DEGREES • BS • MS
Nursing Program Faculty 5 (2% with doctorates).
Baccalaureate Enrollment 333 **Women** 96% **Men** 4% **Part-time** 88%
Graduate Enrollment 100 **Women** 99% **Men** 1% **Part-time** 75%
Distance Learning Courses Available.
Nursing Student Activities Sigma Theta Tau, Student Nurses' Association.
Nursing Student Resources Academic advising; academic or career counseling; assistance for students with disabilities; bookstore; campus computer network; career placement assistance; computer lab; computer-assisted instruction; e-mail services; employment services for current students; Internet; learning resource lab; library services; nursing audiovisuals; remedial services; resume preparation assistance; skills, simulation, or other laboratory; tutoring.
Library Facilities 10,000 volumes in health, 550 volumes in nursing; 180 periodical subscriptions health-care related.

BACCALAUREATE PROGRAMS

Degree BS
Available Programs Accelerated RN Baccalaureate; RN Baccalaureate.
Site Options Dobbs Ferry, NY.
Study Options Full-time and part-time.
Online Degree Options Yes.
Program Entrance Requirements Minimum overall college GPA, transcript of college record, written essay, immunizations, interview, minimum GPA in nursing prerequisites, prerequisite course work, RN licensure. Transfer students are accepted. *Application deadline:* Applications may be processed on a rolling basis for some programs.
Advanced Placement Credit given for nursing courses completed elsewhere dependent upon specific evaluations.
Contact *Telephone:* 914-674-7865. *Fax:* 914-674-7623.

GRADUATE PROGRAMS

Contact *Telephone:* 914-674-7867. *Fax:* 914-674-7623.

MASTER'S DEGREE PROGRAM
Degree MS
Available Programs Accelerated Master's for Non-Nursing College Graduates; Accelerated Master's for Nurses with Non-Nursing Degrees; Accelerated RN to Master's; Master's; Master's for Non-Nursing College Graduates; Master's for Nurses with Non-Nursing Degrees.
Concentrations Available Health-care administration; nursing administration; nursing education.
Site Options Dobbs Ferry, NY.
Study Options Full-time and part-time.
Online Degree Options Yes.
Program Entrance Requirements Clinical experience, minimum overall college GPA of 3.0, transcript of college record, written essay, immunizations, interview, 2 letters of recommendation, professional lia-

bility insurance/malpractice insurance, resume. *Application deadline:* Applications may be processed on a rolling basis for some programs.
Advanced Placement Credit given for nursing courses completed elsewhere dependent upon specific evaluations.
Degree Requirements 36 total credit hours, thesis or project.

POST-MASTER'S PROGRAM
Areas of Study Nursing administration; nursing education.

Molloy College
Division of Nursing
Rockville Centre, New York

http://www.molloy.edu
Founded in 1955
DEGREES • BS • DNP • MS • MS/MBA • PHD
Nursing Program Faculty 216 (20% with doctorates).
Baccalaureate Enrollment 1,480 **Women** 88% **Men** 12% **Part-time** 30%
Graduate Enrollment 502 **Women** 94% **Men** 6% **Part-time** 97%
Nursing Student Activities Sigma Theta Tau, Student Nurses' Association.
Nursing Student Resources Academic advising; academic or career counseling; assistance for students with disabilities; bookstore; campus computer network; career placement assistance; computer lab; computer-assisted instruction; e-mail services; externships; interactive nursing skills videos; Internet; learning resource lab; library services; nursing audiovisuals; remedial services; resume preparation assistance; skills, simulation, or other laboratory; tutoring.
Library Facilities 1,772 volumes in health, 569 volumes in nursing; 58 periodical subscriptions health-care related.

BACCALAUREATE PROGRAMS

Degree BS
Available Programs ADN to Baccalaureate; Accelerated Baccalaureate for Second Degree; Accelerated RN Baccalaureate; Baccalaureate for Second Degree; Generic Baccalaureate; LPN to Baccalaureate; LPN to RN Baccalaureate; RN Baccalaureate.
Site Options Farmingdale, NY; New Hyde Park, NY.
Study Options Full-time and part-time.
Program Entrance Requirements Minimum overall college GPA of 3.0, transcript of college record, written essay, health exam, high school biology, high school chemistry, high school foreign language, 3 years high school math, high school transcript, immunizations, minimum high school GPA of 3.0. Transfer students are accepted. *Application deadline:* Applications may be processed on a rolling basis for some programs. *Application fee:* $30.
Advanced Placement Credit given for nursing courses completed elsewhere dependent upon specific evaluations.
Expenses (2015–16) *Tuition:* full-time $13,490; part-time $890 per credit. *Required fees:* full-time $330; part-time $330 per term.
Financial Aid 87% of baccalaureate students in nursing programs received some form of financial aid in 2014–15. *Gift aid (need-based):* Federal Pell, FSEOG, state, private, college/university gift aid from institutional funds, Federal Nursing, TEACH Grants, TRiO Grants. *Loans:* Federal Nursing Student Loans, Federal Direct (Subsidized and Unsubsidized Stafford PLUS), Perkins, private loans. *Work-study:* Federal Work-Study. *Financial aid application deadline:* 5/1(priority: 4/15).
Contact Marguerite Lane, Dean of Admissions, Division of Nursing, Molloy College, 1000 Hempstead Avenue, PO Box 5002, Rockville Centre, NY 11571-5002. *Telephone:* 516-323-4014.
E-mail: mlane@molloy.edu.

GRADUATE PROGRAMS

Expenses (2015–16) *Tuition:* full-time $8820; part-time $980 per credit. *Required fees:* full-time $615; part-time $430 per term.
Financial Aid 37% of graduate students in nursing programs received some form of financial aid in 2014–15. Research assistantships with partial tuition reimbursements available, teaching assistantships with partial tuition reimbursements available, institutionally sponsored loans, scholarships, and unspecified assistantships available. Aid available to part-time students. *Financial aid application deadline:* 4/1.
Contact Ms. Joanna Forgione, Associate Director of Admissions, Division of Nursing, Molloy College, 1000 Hempstead Avenue, PO Box 5002, Rockville Centre, NY 11571-5002. *Telephone:* 516-323-4013.
E-mail: jforgione@molloy.edu.

MASTER'S DEGREE PROGRAM

Degrees MS; MS/MBA
Available Programs Master's.
Concentrations Available Nursing administration; nursing education; nursing informatics. *Clinical nurse specialist programs in:* adult health. *Nurse practitioner programs in:* adult health, family health, pediatric, pediatric primary care, psychiatric/mental health.
Site Options Farmingdale, NY; New Hyde Park, NY.
Study Options Full-time and part-time.
Program Entrance Requirements Clinical experience, minimum overall college GPA of 3.0, transcript of college record, CPR certification, written essay, immunizations, interview, 3 letters of recommendation, nursing research course, professional liability insurance/malpractice insurance, prerequisite course work, statistics course. *Application deadline:* Applications may be processed on a rolling basis for some programs. *Application fee:* $60.
Advanced Placement Credit given for nursing courses completed elsewhere dependent upon specific evaluations.
Degree Requirements 48 total credit hours, thesis or project.

POST-MASTER'S PROGRAM

Areas of Study Nursing administration; nursing education; nursing informatics. *Clinical nurse specialist programs in:* adult health. *Nurse practitioner programs in:* adult health, family health, pediatric, pediatric primary care, psychiatric/mental health.

DOCTORAL DEGREE PROGRAM

Degree DNP
Available Programs Doctorate.
Areas of Study Advanced practice nursing, clinical practice, clinical research, health policy, health-care systems.
Program Entrance Requirements Minimum overall college GPA of 3.5, clinical experience, interview, interview by faculty committee, 3 letters of recommendation, MSN or equivalent, scholarly papers, statistics course, vita, writing sample. Application deadline: 2/1 (fall). Application fee: $75.
Degree Requirements 37 total credit hours, dissertation, residency.

Degree PhD
Available Programs Doctorate.
Areas of Study Health policy, nursing education, nursing research.
Program Entrance Requirements Clinical experience, minimum overall college GPA of 3.5, interview by faculty committee, interview, 3 letters of recommendation, MSN or equivalent, scholarly papers, statistics course, vita, writing sample. Application deadline: 2/1 (fall). Application fee: $75.
Degree Requirements 45 total credit hours, dissertation.

CONTINUING EDUCATION PROGRAM

Contact Kathleen Lapkowski, Associate Director, Nursing Continuing Education, Division of Nursing, Molloy College, 1000 Hempstead Avenue, PO Box 5002, Rockville Centre, NY 11571-5002. *Telephone:* 516-323-3555. *E-mail:* klapkowski@molloy.edu.

See display on next page and full description on page 502.

Mount Saint Mary College

School of Nursing
Newburgh, New York

http://www.msmc.edu/
Founded in 1960
DEGREES • BSN • MS
Nursing Program Faculty 36 (50% with doctorates).
Nursing Student Activities Sigma Theta Tau, Student Nurses' Association, nursing club.
Nursing Student Resources Academic advising; academic or career counseling; assistance for students with disabilities; bookstore; campus computer network; career placement assistance; computer lab; computer-assisted instruction; e-mail services; employment services for current students; externships; housing assistance; interactive nursing skills videos; Internet; learning resource lab; library services; nursing audiovisuals; paid internships; remedial services; resume preparation assistance; skills, simulation, or other laboratory; tutoring.
Library Facilities 2,443 volumes in health, 1,723 volumes in nursing; 114 periodical subscriptions health-care related.

BACCALAUREATE PROGRAMS

Degree BSN
Available Programs Accelerated Baccalaureate; Accelerated RN Baccalaureate; Generic Baccalaureate; RN Baccalaureate.
Study Options Full-time and part-time.
Program Entrance Requirements Minimum overall college GPA of 2.75, transcript of college record, CPR certification, health exam, high school biology, high school chemistry, 3 years high school math, high school transcript, immunizations, interview. Transfer students are accepted.
Advanced Placement Credit by examination available. Credit given for nursing courses completed elsewhere dependent upon specific evaluations.
Contact *Telephone:* 845-569-3248.

GRADUATE PROGRAMS

Contact *Telephone:* 845-569-3248.

MASTER'S DEGREE PROGRAM

Degree MS
Available Programs Master's.
Concentrations Available *Clinical nurse specialist programs in:* adult health. *Nurse practitioner programs in:* adult health.
Study Options Full-time and part-time.
Program Entrance Requirements Clinical experience, computer literacy, minimum overall college GPA of 3.0, transcript of college record, written essay, immunizations, interview, 3 letters of recommendation, nursing research course, physical assessment course, professional liability insurance/malpractice insurance, resume, statistics course.
Degree Requirements 42 total credit hours, thesis or project.

POST-MASTER'S PROGRAM

Areas of Study Nursing administration; nursing education.

Nazareth College of Rochester

Department of Nursing
Rochester, New York

http://www.naz.edu/
Founded in 1924
DEGREE • BS
Nursing Program Faculty 26 (25% with doctorates).
Baccalaureate Enrollment 195 **Women** 90% **Men** 10% **Part-time** 9%
Distance Learning Courses Available.
Nursing Student Activities Sigma Theta Tau, Student Nurses' Association, nursing club.
Nursing Student Resources Academic advising; academic or career counseling; assistance for students with disabilities; bookstore; campus computer network; career placement assistance; computer lab; computer-assisted instruction; daycare for children of students; e-mail services; employment services for current students; externships; housing assistance; interactive nursing skills videos; Internet; learning resource lab; library services; nursing audiovisuals; resume preparation assistance; skills, simulation, or other laboratory; tutoring.
Library Facilities 267,000 volumes in health, 66,000 volumes in nursing; 44,000 periodical subscriptions health-care related.

BACCALAUREATE PROGRAMS

Degree BS
Available Programs Generic Baccalaureate; LPN to Baccalaureate; RN Baccalaureate.
Study Options Full-time and part-time.
Program Entrance Requirements Minimum overall college GPA of 2.75, transcript of college record, CPR certification, written essay, health exam, high school chemistry, high school transcript, immunizations, minimum high school GPA of 2.75, minimum GPA in nursing prerequisites of 2.5, prerequisite course work. Transfer students are accepted.
Advanced Placement Credit by examination available. Credit given for nursing courses completed elsewhere dependent upon specific evaluations.
Expenses (2015–16) *Tuition:* full-time $30,120; part-time $718 per credit hour. *Room and board:* $12,918 per academic year. *Required fees:* full-time $1400.
Financial Aid 95% of baccalaureate students in nursing programs received some form of financial aid in 2014–15. *Gift aid (need-based):* Federal Pell, FSEOG, state, private, college/university gift aid from insti-

I want to |

Redefine what it means to be a nurse

Help patients beat the odds

Go to one of the top nursing schools in the nation

What are you searching for?

Find it at Molloy College. From our state-of-the-art learning laboratory to innovative clinical practice opportunities, we offer the resources you need to become an effective, humanistic healthcare provider. Whether you're just beginning your education or looking to advance your career, you'll learn from expert faculty in small classes and gain practical experience – all in a nursing program that's one of the most-respected in the nation.

Go ahead. Start something.

Molloy College

molloy.edu | #MolloyLife | 1-888-4-MOLLOY

tutional funds, Federal Nursing. *Loans:* Federal Nursing Student Loans, Federal Direct (Subsidized and Unsubsidized Stafford PLUS), Perkins. *Work-study:* Federal Work-Study. *Financial aid application deadline (priority):* 2/15.

Contact Admissions Office, Department of Nursing, Nazareth College of Rochester, 4245 East Avenue, Rochester, NY 14618-3790. *Telephone:* 585-389-2865. *E-mail:* admissions@naz.edu.

New York City College of Technology of the City University of New York

Department of Nursing
Brooklyn, New York

http://www.citytech.cuny.edu/
Founded in 1946

DEGREE • BS
Nursing Program Faculty 22

BACCALAUREATE PROGRAMS

Degree BS
Available Programs RN Baccalaureate.
Program Entrance Requirements Minimum overall college GPA of 2.5, immunizations, professional liability insurance/malpractice insurance, RN licensure. Transfer students are accepted.
Contact *Telephone:* 718-260-5660. *Fax:* 718-260-5662.

New York Institute of Technology

Department of Nursing
Old Westbury, New York

http://www.nyit.edu/degrees/nursing/
FOUNDED IN 1955
DEGREE • BSN

BACCALAUREATE PROGRAMS

Degree BSN
Available Programs Generic Baccalaureate.
Contact *Telephone:* 516-686-7516.

New York University

College of Nursing
New York, New York

http://www.nyu.edu/nursing/index.html
Founded in 1831

DEGREES • BS • DNP • MS • MS/MPH • PHD
Nursing Program Faculty 285 (25% with doctorates).
Baccalaureate Enrollment 843 **Women** 85.88% **Men** 14.12% **Part-time** 3.8%
Graduate Enrollment 703 **Women** 89% **Men** 11% **Part-time** 92%
Nursing Student Activities Nursing Honor Society, Sigma Theta Tau, Student Nurses' Association, nursing club.
Nursing Student Resources Academic advising; academic or career counseling; assistance for students with disabilities; bookstore; campus computer network; career placement assistance; computer lab; computer-assisted instruction; e-mail services; employment services for current students; externships; housing assistance; Internet; learning resource lab; library services; nursing audiovisuals; remedial services; resume preparation assistance; skills, simulation, or other laboratory; tutoring.
Library Facilities 158,255 volumes in health, 63,258 volumes in nursing; 45,022 periodical subscriptions health-care related.

BACCALAUREATE PROGRAMS

Degree BS
Available Programs Accelerated Baccalaureate for Second Degree; Generic Baccalaureate; RN Baccalaureate.

Study Options Full-time.
Program Entrance Requirements Minimum overall college GPA of 3.0, transcript of college record, CPR certification, written essay, health exam, health insurance, high school foreign language, 3 years high school math, 3 years high school science, high school transcript, immunizations, 1 letter of recommendation, minimum GPA in nursing prerequisites of 2.0. Transfer students are accepted. *Application deadline:* 1/1 (fall), 11/1 (spring). *Application fee:* $70.
Advanced Placement Credit given for nursing courses completed elsewhere dependent upon specific evaluations.
Expenses (2015–16) *Tuition:* full-time $45,278; part-time $2668 per credit. *International tuition:* $45,278 full-time. *Room and board:* $17,580; room only: $13,048 per academic year. *Required fees:* full-time $2472; part-time $470 per term.
Contact Ms. Titilayo Kuti, Assistant Director for Undergraduate Admissions, College of Nursing, New York University, 433 First Avenue, Floor LL1, New York, NY 10010. *Telephone:* 212-998-5336. *Fax:* 212-995-4302. *E-mail:* tok207@nyu.edu.

GRADUATE PROGRAMS

Expenses (2015–16) *Tuition:* full-time $51,744; part-time $1568 per credit. *International tuition:* $51,744 full-time. *Required fees:* full-time $3390.
Financial Aid 7 research assistantships (averaging $25,688 per year) were awarded; scholarships also available.
Contact Ms. Samantha Jaser, Assistant Director of Graduate Student Affairs and Admissions, College of Nursing, New York University, 433 First Avenue, Floor LL1, New York, NY 10010. *Telephone:* 212-992-7653. *Fax:* 212-995-4302. *E-mail:* saj283@nyu.edu.

MASTER'S DEGREE PROGRAM

Degrees MS; MS/MPH
Available Programs Master's.
Concentrations Available Nurse-midwifery; nursing administration; nursing education; nursing informatics. *Nurse practitioner programs in:* adult-gerontology acute care, family health, pediatric, primary care, psychiatric/mental health.
Study Options Full-time and part-time.
Program Entrance Requirements Clinical experience, minimum overall college GPA of 3.0, transcript of college record, CPR certification, written essay, immunizations, 2 letters of recommendation, nursing research course, resume, statistics course. *Application deadline:* 6/15 (fall), 12/1 (spring), 3/1 (summer). Applications may be processed on a rolling basis for some programs. *Application fee:* $80.
Advanced Placement Credit given for nursing courses completed elsewhere dependent upon specific evaluations.
Degree Requirements 48 total credit hours, thesis or project.

POST-MASTER'S PROGRAM

Areas of Study Nurse-midwifery; nursing administration; nursing education; nursing informatics. *Nurse practitioner programs in:* adult-gerontology acute care, family health, gerontology, pediatric, primary care, psychiatric/mental health.

DOCTORAL DEGREE PROGRAM

Degree DNP
Available Programs Doctorate.
Areas of Study Acute care, adult health, gerontology, nurse-midwifery, palliative care, pediatric, psychiatric/mental health.
Program Entrance Requirements Minimum overall college GPA of 3.5, clinical experience, graduate level research course (taken no more than 5 years ago), 2 letters of recommendation, Miller Analogies Test (MAT), MSN or equivalent, RN license, nationally board certified as an NP or certified nurse-midwife. Application deadline: 3/1 (spring). Applications may be processed on a rolling basis for some programs. Application fee: $75.
Degree Requirements 77-89 total credit hours.

Degree PhD
Available Programs Doctorate; Post-Baccalaureate Doctorate.
Areas of Study Nursing research.
Program Entrance Requirements Clinical experience, minimum overall college GPA of 3.0, interview, 3 letters of recommendation, MSN or equivalent, vita, writing sample. Application deadline: 1/15 (fall). Applications may be processed on a rolling basis for some programs. Application fee: $70.
Degree Requirements 45 total credit hours, dissertation, residency.

POSTDOCTORAL PROGRAM

Areas of Study Adolescent health, aging, chronic illness, family health, gerontology, health promotion/disease prevention, nursing interventions, nursing science, outcomes, self-care, vulnerable population.

Postdoctoral Program Contact Dr. Gail D'Eramo Melkus, EdD,C-NP,FAAN, Associate Dean for Research, College of Nursing, New York University, College of Nursing, 433 First Avenue, New York, NY 10010. *Telephone:* 212-998-5356. *Fax:* 212-998-5332. *E-mail:* gail.melkus@nyu.edu.

CONTINUING EDUCATION PROGRAM

Contact Dr. Mattia Gilmartin, Continuing Education Director, College of Nursing, New York University, 433 First Avenue, New York, NY 10010. *Telephone:* 212-992-7128. *Fax:* 212-995-3143. *E-mail:* mjg14@nyu.edu.

Niagara University
Department of Nursing
Niagara Falls, Niagara University, New York

http://www.niagara.edu/nursing
Founded in 1856
DEGREE • BS
Nursing Program Faculty 22 (45% with doctorates).
Baccalaureate Enrollment 208 **Women** 94% **Men** 6%
Distance Learning Courses Available.
Nursing Student Activities Nursing Honor Society, Sigma Theta Tau, Student Nurses' Association.
Nursing Student Resources Academic advising; academic or career counseling; assistance for students with disabilities; bookstore; campus computer network; career placement assistance; computer lab; computer-assisted instruction; e-mail services; employment services for current students; externships; housing assistance; interactive nursing skills videos; Internet; learning resource lab; library services; nursing audiovisuals; paid internships; resume preparation assistance; skills, simulation, or other laboratory; tutoring; unpaid internships.

BACCALAUREATE PROGRAMS

Degree BS
Available Programs Accelerated Baccalaureate for Second Degree; Generic Baccalaureate; RN Baccalaureate.
Site Options Buffalo, NY.
Study Options Full-time.
Program Entrance Requirements Transcript of college record, written essay, health exam, health insurance, high school biology, high school chemistry, 3 years high school science, high school transcript, immunizations, minimum high school GPA of 2.5. Transfer students are accepted. *Application deadline:* 12/20 (fall). Applications may be processed on a rolling basis for some programs. *Application fee:* $35.
Expenses (2015–16) *Tuition:* full-time $28,500; part-time $2700 per course. *Room and board:* $13,000 per academic year. *Required fees:* full-time $650; part-time $70 per term.
Financial Aid 98% of baccalaureate students in nursing programs received some form of financial aid in 2014–15.
Contact Dr. Frances Crosby, RN, Director, Department of Nursing, Niagara University, PO Box 2203, Seton Hall, School of Nursing, Niagara University, NY 14109. *Telephone:* 716-286-8155. *Fax:* 716-286-8763. *E-mail:* fcrosby@niagara.edu.

Nyack College
School of Nursing
Nyack, New York

http://www.nyack.edu/
Founded in 1882
DEGREE • BS
Nursing Program Faculty 5 (60% with doctorates).
Baccalaureate Enrollment 73 **Women** 76% **Men** 24%
Nursing Student Activities Nursing Honor Society, Sigma Theta Tau, Student Nurses' Association.
Nursing Student Resources Academic advising; academic or career counseling; assistance for students with disabilities; bookstore; campus computer network; career placement assistance; computer lab; computer-assisted instruction; e-mail services; employment services for current students; externships; housing assistance; interactive nursing skills videos; Internet; learning resource lab; library services; nursing audiovisuals; remedial services; resume preparation assistance; skills, simulation, or other laboratory; tutoring; unpaid internships.
Library Facilities 179 volumes in health, 90 volumes in nursing; 151 periodical subscriptions health-care related.

BACCALAUREATE PROGRAMS

Degree BS
Available Programs Generic Baccalaureate; LPN to RN Baccalaureate; RN Baccalaureate.
Study Options Full-time.
Online Degree Options Yes.
Program Entrance Requirements Minimum overall college GPA of 2.7, transcript of college record, CPR certification, written essay, health exam, health insurance, high school biology, high school chemistry, high school foreign language, high school math, high school science, high school transcript, immunizations, minimum high school GPA of 2.5, minimum GPA in nursing prerequisites of 2.7, professional liability insurance/malpractice insurance, prerequisite course work. Transfer students are accepted. *Application deadline:* Applications may be processed on a rolling basis for some programs.
Advanced Placement Credit by examination available.
Expenses (2015–16) *Tuition:* full-time $25,000. *Room and board:* $9200 per academic year. *Required fees:* full-time $975.
Financial Aid *Gift aid (need-based):* Federal Pell, FSEOG, state, private, college/university gift aid from institutional funds. *Loans:* Federal Direct (Subsidized and Unsubsidized Stafford PLUS), Perkins. *Work-study:* Federal Work-Study, part-time campus jobs. *Financial aid application deadline (priority):* 3/1.
Contact Ms. Yee Yang, Nursing Admission Counselor. *Telephone:* 845-675-4406. *E-mail:* yee.yang@nyack.edu.

Pace University
Lienhard School of Nursing
New York, New York

http://www.pace.edu/.lienhard
Founded in 1906
DEGREES • BS • DNP • MS
Nursing Program Faculty 176 (27% with doctorates).
Baccalaureate Enrollment 512 **Women** 89% **Men** 11% **Part-time** 23%
Graduate Enrollment 418 **Women** 93% **Men** 7% **Part-time** 99%
Distance Learning Courses Available.
Nursing Student Activities Nursing Honor Society, Sigma Theta Tau, Student Nurses' Association.
Nursing Student Resources Academic advising; academic or career counseling; assistance for students with disabilities; bookstore; campus computer network; career placement assistance; computer lab; computer-assisted instruction; e-mail services; employment services for current students; housing assistance; interactive nursing skills videos; Internet; learning resource lab; library services; nursing audiovisuals; placement services for program completers; resume preparation assistance; skills, simulation, or other laboratory.
Library Facilities 17,370 volumes in health, 2,216 volumes in nursing; 8,261 periodical subscriptions health-care related.

BACCALAUREATE PROGRAMS

Degree BS
Available Programs Accelerated Baccalaureate for Second Degree; Generic Baccalaureate; RN Baccalaureate.
Site Options New York, NY; Pleasantville, NY.
Study Options Full-time and part-time.
Program Entrance Requirements Transcript of college record, CPR certification, written essay, health exam, health insurance, high school biology, high school chemistry, high school foreign language, 4 years high school math, 2 years high school science, high school transcript, immunizations, 2 letters of recommendation, minimum GPA in nursing prerequisites of 2.75. Transfer students are accepted. *Application deadline:* 2/15 (fall). *Application fee:* $50.
Advanced Placement Credit by examination available. Credit given for nursing courses completed elsewhere dependent upon specific evaluations.
Expenses (2015–16) *Tuition:* full-time $39,728; part-time $1140 per credit. *International tuition:* $39,728 full-time. *Room and board:* $15,010 per academic year. *Required fees:* full-time $1553.

Financial Aid *Gift aid (need-based):* Federal Pell, FSEOG, state, private, college/university gift aid from institutional funds. *Loans:* Federal Nursing Student Loans, Federal Direct (Subsidized and Unsubsidized Stafford PLUS), Perkins. *Work-study:* Federal Work-Study. *Financial aid application deadline (priority):* 2/15.
Contact Dr. Martha Greenberg, Associate Professor and Chairperson, Undergraduate Department, Lienhard School of Nursing, Pace University, 861 Bedford Road, Pleasantville, NY 10570. *Telephone:* 914-773-3325. *Fax:* 914-773-3345. *E-mail:* mgreenberg@pace.edu.

GRADUATE PROGRAMS

Expenses (2015–16) *Tuition:* part-time $1150 per credit.
Financial Aid Research assistantships, career-related internships or fieldwork, Federal Work-Study, and tuition waivers (partial) available.
Contact Dr. Joanne K. Singleton, Chair of the Department of Graduate Studies/Director, Doctor of Nursing Program, Lienhard School of Nursing, Pace University, 163 William Street, New York, NY 10038. *Telephone:* 212-618-6010. *E-mail:* jsingleton@pace.edu.

MASTER'S DEGREE PROGRAM

Degree MS
Available Programs Master's; Master's for Nurses with Non-Nursing Degrees.
Concentrations Available Clinical nurse leader; nursing education. *Nurse practitioner programs in:* family health.
Site Options New York, NY; Pleasantville, NY.
Study Options Full-time and part-time.
Online Degree Options Yes.
Program Entrance Requirements Computer literacy, minimum overall college GPA of 3.0, transcript of college record, CPR certification, immunizations, 2 letters of recommendation, nursing research course, professional liability insurance/malpractice insurance, prerequisite course work, resume, statistics course. *Application deadline:* 3/1 (fall). *Application fee:* $70.
Advanced Placement Credit by examination available. Credit given for nursing courses completed elsewhere dependent upon specific evaluations.
Degree Requirements 42 total credit hours, comprehensive exam.

POST-MASTER'S PROGRAM

Areas of Study Clinical nurse leader; nursing education. *Nurse practitioner programs in:* acute care, adult-gerontology acute care, family health.

DOCTORAL DEGREE PROGRAM

Degree DNP
Available Programs Doctorate.
Areas of Study Advanced practice nursing, family health.
Site Options New York, NY.
Program Entrance Requirements Clinical experience, minimum overall college GPA of 3.3, 2 letters of recommendation, MSN or equivalent, vita, writing sample. Application deadline: 3/1 (fall). Application fee: $70.
Degree Requirements 37 total credit hours, residency.

Roberts Wesleyan College

School of Nursing
Rochester, New York

http://www.roberts.edu/Nursing/
Founded in 1866

DEGREES • BSCN • M SC N
Nursing Program Faculty 18 (33% with doctorates).
Baccalaureate Enrollment 367 **Women** 90% **Men** 10% **Part-time** 2%
Graduate Enrollment 54 **Women** 96% **Men** 4%
Distance Learning Courses Available.
Nursing Student Activities Sigma Theta Tau, nursing club.
Nursing Student Resources Academic advising; academic or career counseling; assistance for students with disabilities; bookstore; campus computer network; career placement assistance; computer lab; computer-assisted instruction; e-mail services; employment services for current students; externships; housing assistance; interactive nursing skills videos; Internet; learning resource lab; library services; nursing audiovisuals; placement services for program completers; remedial services; resume preparation assistance; skills, simulation, or other laboratory; tutoring; unpaid internships.

Library Facilities 6,459 volumes in health, 1,219 volumes in nursing; 3,891 periodical subscriptions health-care related.

BACCALAUREATE PROGRAMS

Degree BScN
Available Programs Generic Baccalaureate; RN Baccalaureate.
Site Options Dansville, NY; Buffalo, NY; Rochester, NY; Weedsport, NY.
Study Options Full-time and part-time.
Online Degree Options Yes.
Program Entrance Requirements Minimum overall college GPA of 2.5, transcript of college record, CPR certification, written essay, health exam, health insurance, high school biology, high school chemistry, 3 years high school math, 3 years high school science, high school transcript, immunizations, 3 letters of recommendation, minimum high school GPA, minimum GPA in nursing prerequisites of 2.5, prerequisite course work. Transfer students are accepted. *Application deadline:* 2/1 (fall). Applications may be processed on a rolling basis for some programs.
Expenses (2015–16) *Tuition:* full-time $27,576. *Room and board:* $10,038; room only: $6416 per academic year. *Required fees:* full-time $1460.
Financial Aid 98% of baccalaureate students in nursing programs received some form of financial aid in 2014–15.
Contact Mr. JP Anderson, Associate Vice President for Undergraduate and Seminary Admissions, School of Nursing, Roberts Wesleyan College, 2301 Westside Drive, Rochester, NY 14624. *Telephone:* 585-594-6400. *Fax:* 585-549-6371. *E-mail:* admissions@roberts.edu.

GRADUATE PROGRAMS

Expenses (2015–16) *Tuition:* full-time $16,212. *International tuition:* $16,212 full-time. *Required fees:* full-time $300.
Financial Aid 96% of graduate students in nursing programs received some form of financial aid in 2014–15.
Contact Mrs. Brenda Mutton, Graduate Admissions Coordinator, School of Nursing, Roberts Wesleyan College, 2301 Westside Drive, Rochester, NY 14624-1997. *Telephone:* 585-594-6686. *Fax:* 585-594-6593. *E-mail:* mutton_brenda@roberts.edu.

MASTER'S DEGREE PROGRAM

Degree M Sc N
Available Programs Master's.
Concentrations Available Nursing administration; nursing education.
Study Options Full-time.
Online Degree Options Yes.
Program Entrance Requirements Clinical experience, computer literacy, minimum overall college GPA of 3.0, transcript of college record, written essay, immunizations, interview, 2 letters of recommendation, nursing research course, physical assessment course, prerequisite course work, resume, statistics course. *Application deadline:* Applications may be processed on a rolling basis for some programs.
Degree Requirements 39 total credit hours, thesis or project.

POST-MASTER'S PROGRAM

Areas of Study Nursing administration; nursing education.

The Sage Colleges

Department of Nursing
Troy, New York

http://www.sage.edu/rsc/academics/programs/nursing/

DEGREES • BS • DNS • MS • MS/MBA
Nursing Program Faculty 22 (50% with doctorates).
Baccalaureate Enrollment 358 **Women** 96% **Men** 4% **Part-time** 19%
Graduate Enrollment 230 **Women** 92% **Men** 8% **Part-time** 80%
Nursing Student Activities Nursing Honor Society, Sigma Theta Tau, nursing club.
Nursing Student Resources Academic advising; academic or career counseling; assistance for students with disabilities; bookstore; campus computer network; career placement assistance; computer lab; computer-assisted instruction; e-mail services; employment services for current students; externships; interactive nursing skills videos; Internet; learning resource lab; library services; remedial services; resume preparation assistance; skills, simulation, or other laboratory; tutoring.

BACCALAUREATE PROGRAMS

Degree BS
Available Programs ADN to Baccalaureate; Accelerated Baccalaureate; Accelerated Baccalaureate for Second Degree; Baccalaureate for Second Degree; Generic Baccalaureate; International Nurse to Baccalaureate; LPN to Baccalaureate; RN Baccalaureate.
Site Options Glens Falls, NY; Albany, NY.
Study Options Full-time and part-time.
Program Entrance Requirements Minimum overall college GPA of 3.0, transcript of college record, written essay, health exam, health insurance, high school biology, high school chemistry, 3 years high school math, 3 years high school science, high school transcript, immunizations, interview, 2 letters of recommendation, minimum high school GPA of 3.0, professional liability insurance/malpractice insurance. Transfer students are accepted. *Application deadline:* Applications may be processed on a rolling basis for some programs. *Application fee:* $30.
Advanced Placement Credit by examination available. Credit given for nursing courses completed elsewhere dependent upon specific evaluations.
Expenses (2015–16) *Tuition:* full-time $27,000; part-time $900 per credit hour. *International tuition:* $27,000 full-time. *Room and board:* $12,220; room only: $6330 per academic year.
Financial Aid *Gift aid (need-based):* Federal Pell, FSEOG, state, private, college/university gift aid from institutional funds, Federal Nursing. *Loans:* Federal Direct (Subsidized and Unsubsidized Stafford PLUS), Perkins. *Work-study:* Federal Work-Study, part-time campus jobs. *Financial aid application deadline (priority):* 3/1.
Contact Toni Sposito, Undergraduate Program Secretary, Department of Nursing, The Sage Colleges, 65 1st Street, Ackerman Hall, Room 120, Troy, NY 12180-4115. *Telephone:* 518-244-2231. *Fax:* 518-244-2009. *E-mail:* sposia@sage.edu.

GRADUATE PROGRAMS

Expenses (2015–16) *Tuition:* full-time $12,240; part-time $680 per credit hour. *International tuition:* $12,240 full-time. *Room and board:* $12,220; room only: $6330 per academic year.
Financial Aid Fellowships, research assistantships, Federal Work-Study, scholarships, and unspecified assistantships available.
Contact Dr. Madeline Cafiero, MS Program, Department of Nursing, The Sage Colleges, Troy, NY 12180-4115. *Telephone:* 518-244-4574. *Fax:* 518-244-2009. *E-mail:* nursing@sage.edu.

MASTER'S DEGREE PROGRAM

Degrees MS; MS/MBA
Available Programs Accelerated Master's; Accelerated RN to Master's; Master's.
Concentrations Available Health-care administration; nursing administration; nursing education. *Clinical nurse specialist programs in:* acute care, adult health, gerontology, medical-surgical, psychiatric/mental health. *Nurse practitioner programs in:* acute care, adult health, adult-gerontology acute care, community health, family health, psychiatric/mental health.
Study Options Full-time and part-time.
Program Entrance Requirements Minimum overall college GPA of 3.0, transcript of college record, CPR certification, written essay, 2 letters of recommendation, physical assessment course, professional liability insurance/malpractice insurance, resume.
Advanced Placement Credit given for nursing courses completed elsewhere dependent upon specific evaluations.
Degree Requirements 42 total credit hours, thesis or project.

POST-MASTER'S PROGRAM

Areas of Study Health-care administration; nursing administration; nursing education. *Clinical nurse specialist programs in:* acute care, adult health, gerontology, medical-surgical, psychiatric/mental health. *Nurse practitioner programs in:* acute care, adult health, adult-gerontology acute care, community health, family health, psychiatric/mental health.

DOCTORAL DEGREE PROGRAM

Degree DNS
Available Programs Doctorate.
Areas of Study Faculty preparation, health-care systems, nursing administration, nursing education, nursing policy, nursing research, nursing science.
Program Entrance Requirements Minimum overall college GPA of 3.5, interview by faculty committee, 3 letters of recommendation, MSN or equivalent, statistics course, vita, writing sample.
Degree Requirements 42 total credit hours, dissertation.

CONTINUING EDUCATION PROGRAM

Contact Graduate and Adult Admission, Department of Nursing, The Sage Colleges, 140 New Scotland Avenue, Albany, NY 12208. *Telephone:* 518-292-1774. *E-mail:* spceadm@sage.edu.

St. Francis College
Department of Nursing
Brooklyn Heights, New York

http://www.sfc.edu/page.cfm?p=486
Founded in 1884
DEGREE • BS
Nursing Program Faculty 12 (25% with doctorates).
Baccalaureate Enrollment 798 **Women** 90% **Men** 10% **Part-time** 50%
Distance Learning Courses Available.
Nursing Student Activities Nursing club.
Nursing Student Resources Academic advising; academic or career counseling; assistance for students with disabilities; bookstore; campus computer network; career placement assistance; computer lab; computer-assisted instruction; e-mail services; employment services for current students; externships; housing assistance; interactive nursing skills videos; Internet; learning resource lab; library services; nursing audiovisuals; remedial services; resume preparation assistance; skills, simulation, or other laboratory; tutoring; unpaid internships.

BACCALAUREATE PROGRAMS

Degree BS
Available Programs Generic Baccalaureate; International Nurse to Baccalaureate; RN Baccalaureate; RPN to Baccalaureate.
Study Options Full-time and part-time.
Program Entrance Requirements Minimum overall college GPA of 3.0, transcript of college record, CPR certification, written essay, health exam, health insurance, high school transcript, immunizations, interview, 33 letters of recommendation, minimum high school GPA of 3.0, minimum GPA in nursing prerequisites of 3, professional liability insurance/malpractice insurance, prerequisite course work. Transfer students are accepted.
Advanced Placement Credit by examination available.
Financial Aid *Gift aid (need-based):* Federal Pell, FSEOG, state, private, college/university gift aid from institutional funds. *Loans:* Federal Direct (Subsidized and Unsubsidized Stafford PLUS), Perkins. *Work-study:* Federal Work-Study. *Financial aid application deadline (priority):* 2/15.
Contact Dr. Eleanor Kehoe, Associate Professor, Department of Nursing, St. Francis College, 180 Remsen Street, Brooklyn Heights, NY 11201. *Telephone:* 718-489-5497. *Fax:* 718-489-5408. *E-mail:* ekehoe@sfc.edu.

See display on next page and full description on page 508.

St. John Fisher College
Wegmans School of Nursing
Rochester, New York

http://www.sjfc.edu/academics/nursing/about/index.dot
Founded in 1948
DEGREES • BS • DNP • MS
Nursing Program Faculty 95 (30% with doctorates).
Baccalaureate Enrollment 609 **Women** 88% **Men** 12% **Part-time** 2%
Graduate Enrollment 158 **Women** 96% **Men** 4% **Part-time** 86%
Distance Learning Courses Available.
Nursing Student Activities Sigma Theta Tau, Student Nurses' Association.
Nursing Student Resources Academic advising; academic or career counseling; assistance for students with disabilities; bookstore; campus computer network; career placement assistance; computer lab; computer-assisted instruction; daycare for children of students; e-mail services; employment services for current students; interactive nursing skills videos; Internet; learning resource lab; library services; nursing audiovisuals; resume preparation assistance; skills, simulation, or other laboratory; tutoring.
Library Facilities 30,000 volumes in health, 5,000 volumes in nursing; 200 periodical subscriptions health-care related.

BACCALAUREATE PROGRAMS

Degree BS

Available Programs ADN to Baccalaureate; Accelerated RN Baccalaureate; Baccalaureate for Second Degree; Generic Baccalaureate; RN Baccalaureate.

Study Options Full-time and part-time.

Program Entrance Requirements Minimum overall college GPA of 2.75, transcript of college record, CPR certification, written essay, health exam, health insurance, high school transcript, immunizations, 2 letters of recommendation, minimum high school GPA of 2.0, minimum GPA in nursing prerequisites of 2.40, prerequisite course work. Transfer students are accepted. *Application deadline:* 3/1 (fall), 10/1 (spring). Applications may be processed on a rolling basis for some programs. *Application fee:* $30.

Advanced Placement Credit given for nursing courses completed elsewhere dependent upon specific evaluations.

Expenses (2015–16) *Tuition:* full-time $30,110; part-time $820 per credit hour. *Room and board:* $11,460; room only: $7370 per academic year. *Required fees:* full-time $580.

Financial Aid 95% of baccalaureate students in nursing programs received some form of financial aid in 2014–15. *Gift aid (need-based):* Federal Pell, FSEOG, state, private, college/university gift aid from institutional funds, Federal Nursing. *Loans:* Federal Direct (Subsidized and Unsubsidized Stafford PLUS), Perkins. *Work-study:* Federal Work-Study. *Financial aid application deadline (priority):* 2/15.

Contact Dr. Marilyn Dollinger, Chairperson, Wegmans School of Nursing, St. John Fisher College, 3690 East Avenue, Rochester, NY 14618. *Telephone:* 585-385-8476. *Fax:* 585-385-8466. *E-mail:* mdollinger@sjfc.edu.

GRADUATE PROGRAMS

Expenses (2015–16) *Tuition:* part-time $10,320 per semester. *Required fees:* part-time $120 per term.

Financial Aid 20% of graduate students in nursing programs received some form of financial aid in 2014–15. Scholarships available.

Contact Dr. Colleen Donegan, Graduate Program Director, Wegmans School of Nursing, St. John Fisher College, 3690 East Avenue, Rochester, NY 14618. *Telephone:* 585-899-3788. *Fax:* 585-385-8466. *E-mail:* cdonegan@sjfc.edu.

MASTER'S DEGREE PROGRAM

Degree MS

Available Programs Master's; RN to Master's.

Concentrations Available *Clinical nurse specialist programs in:* adult health. *Nurse practitioner programs in:* adult health, adult-gerontology acute care, psychiatric/mental health.

Study Options Full-time and part-time.

Program Entrance Requirements Computer literacy, minimum overall college GPA of 3.0, transcript of college record, CPR certification, written essay, immunizations, 2 letters of recommendation, nursing research course, physical assessment course, resume, statistics course. *Application deadline:* Applications may be processed on a rolling basis for some programs. *Application fee:* $30.

Advanced Placement Credit given for nursing courses completed elsewhere dependent upon specific evaluations.

Degree Requirements 46 total credit hours, thesis or project, comprehensive exam.

POST-MASTER'S PROGRAM

Areas of Study *Clinical nurse specialist programs in:* adult health. *Nurse practitioner programs in:* adult health, adult-gerontology acute care, psychiatric/mental health.

DOCTORAL DEGREE PROGRAM

Degree DNP

Available Programs Doctorate; Post-Baccalaureate Doctorate.

Areas of Study Advanced practice nursing.

Program Entrance Requirements Clinical experience, minimum overall college GPA of 3.0, interview by faculty committee, letters of recommendation, scholarly papers, vita, writing sample. Application deadline: Applications may be processed on a rolling basis for some programs. Application fee: $30.

Degree Requirements 48 total credit hours, residency.

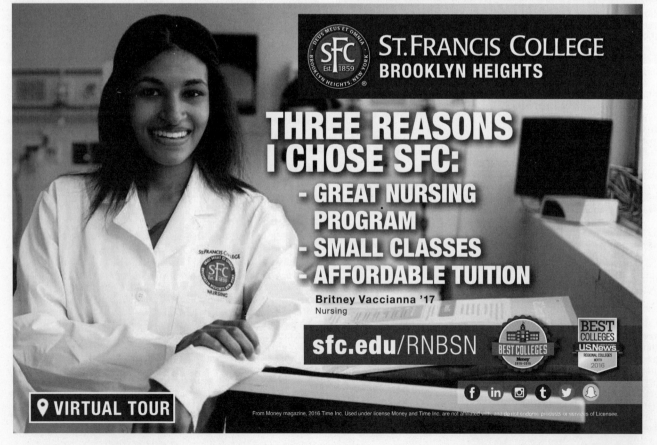

ST. FRANCIS COLLEGE
BROOKLYN HEIGHTS

THREE REASONS I CHOSE SFC:
- GREAT NURSING PROGRAM
- SMALL CLASSES
- AFFORDABLE TUITION

Britney Vaccianna '17
Nursing

sfc.edu/RNBSN

VIRTUAL TOUR

From Money magazine, 2016 Time Inc. Used under license Money and Time Inc. are not affiliated with and do not endorse products or services of Licensee.

St. Joseph's College, New York
Department of Nursing
Brooklyn, New York

http://www.sjcny.edu/
Founded in 1916
DEGREES • BSN • MS
Nursing Program Faculty 22 (41% with doctorates).
Baccalaureate Enrollment 173 **Women** 90% **Men** 10% **Part-time** 95%
Graduate Enrollment 51 **Women** 92% **Men** 8% **Part-time** 100%
Nursing Student Activities Nursing Honor Society, nursing club.
Nursing Student Resources Academic advising; academic or career counseling; assistance for students with disabilities; bookstore; campus computer network; career placement assistance; computer lab; computer-assisted instruction; e-mail services; interactive nursing skills videos; Internet; learning resource lab; library services; nursing audiovisuals; remedial services; resume preparation assistance; skills, simulation, or other laboratory; tutoring.
Library Facilities 15,500 volumes in health, 1,600 volumes in nursing; 18,300 periodical subscriptions health-care related.

BACCALAUREATE PROGRAMS

Degree BSN
Available Programs RN Baccalaureate.
Site Options Patchogue, NY.
Study Options Full-time and part-time.
Program Entrance Requirements Minimum overall college GPA of 2.5, transcript of college record, CPR certification, written essay, health exam, health insurance, immunizations, 2 letters of recommendation, minimum GPA in nursing prerequisites of 2.5, professional liability insurance/malpractice insurance, prerequisite course work, RN licensure. Transfer students are accepted. *Application deadline:* 8/31 (fall), 1/15 (spring). Applications may be processed on a rolling basis for some programs. *Application fee:* $25.
Advanced Placement Credit by examination available. Credit given for nursing courses completed elsewhere dependent upon specific evaluations.
Expenses (2015–16) *Tuition:* part-time $760 per credit. *Required fees:* part-time $13 per credit; part-time $87 per term.
Financial Aid 62% of baccalaureate students in nursing programs received some form of financial aid in 2014–15.
Contact Dr. Florence L. Jerdan, Director, Department of Nursing, St. Joseph's College, New York, 245 Clinton Avenue, Brooklyn, NY 11205-3688. *Telephone:* 718-940-5892. *Fax:* 718-638-8839. *E-mail:* fjerdan@sjcny.edu.

GRADUATE PROGRAMS

Expenses (2015–16) *Tuition:* part-time $780 per credit. *Required fees:* part-time $13 per credit; part-time $171 per term.
Financial Aid 80% of graduate students in nursing programs received some form of financial aid in 2014–15.
Contact Dr. Florence L. Jerdan, Director, Department of Nursing, St. Joseph's College, New York, 245 Clinton Avenue, Brooklyn, NY 11205-3688. *Telephone:* 718-940-5892. *Fax:* 718-638-8839. *E-mail:* fjerdan@sjcny.edu.

MASTER'S DEGREE PROGRAM

Degree MS
Available Programs Master's.
Concentrations Available Nursing education. *Clinical nurse specialist programs in:* adult-gerontology acute care.
Site Options Patchogue, NY.
Study Options Part-time.
Program Entrance Requirements Clinical experience, minimum overall college GPA of 3.0, transcript of college record, CPR certification, written essay, immunizations, interview, 2 letters of recommendation, nursing research course, physical assessment course, professional liability insurance/malpractice insurance, prerequisite course work, resume, statistics course. *Application deadline:* 5/15 (fall). Applications may be processed on a rolling basis for some programs. *Application fee:* $25.

Advanced Placement Credit given for nursing courses completed elsewhere dependent upon specific evaluations.
Degree Requirements 38 total credit hours, thesis or project.

State University of New York at Plattsburgh
Department of Nursing
Plattsburgh, New York

http://www.plattsburgh.edu/nursing
Founded in 1889
DEGREE • BS
Nursing Program Faculty 26 (22% with doctorates).
Baccalaureate Enrollment 411 **Women** 85% **Men** 15% **Part-time** 25%
Distance Learning Courses Available.
Nursing Student Activities Nursing Honor Society, Sigma Theta Tau, Student Nurses' Association, nursing club.
Nursing Student Resources Academic advising; academic or career counseling; assistance for students with disabilities; bookstore; campus computer network; career placement assistance; computer lab; computer-assisted instruction; e-mail services; employment services for current students; externships; interactive nursing skills videos; Internet; learning resource lab; library services; nursing audiovisuals; remedial services; resume preparation assistance; skills, simulation, or other laboratory; tutoring.
Library Facilities 19,450 volumes in health, 200 volumes in nursing; 174 periodical subscriptions health-care related.

BACCALAUREATE PROGRAMS

Degree BS
Available Programs ADN to Baccalaureate; Generic Baccalaureate; RN Baccalaureate.
Site Options Queensbury, NY.
Study Options Full-time and part-time.
Online Degree Options Yes.
Program Entrance Requirements Minimum overall college GPA of 2.5, transcript of college record, high school biology, high school chemistry, 3 years high school math, 3 years high school science, high school transcript, 1 letter of recommendation, minimum GPA in nursing prerequisites of 2.5. *Application deadline:* 12/1 (fall), 11/1 (spring). Applications may be processed on a rolling basis for some programs. *Application fee:* $50.
Expenses (2015–16) *Tuition, state resident:* full-time $6470; part-time $270 per credit hour. *Tuition, nonresident:* full-time $16,320; part-time $680 per credit hour. *International tuition:* $16,500 full-time. *Room and board:* $11,370; room only: $3500 per academic year. *Required fees:* full-time $1484.
Financial Aid 71% of baccalaureate students in nursing programs received some form of financial aid in 2014–15.
Contact Ms. Noreen M. Houck, Chairperson, Department of Nursing, State University of New York at Plattsburgh, 101 Broad Street, Plattsburgh, NY 12901. *Telephone:* 518-564-3124. *Fax:* 518-564-3100. *E-mail:* noreen.houck@plattsburgh.edu.

State University of New York College of Technology at Alfred
Nursing Program
Alfred, New York

Founded in 1908
DEGREE • BSN

BACCALAUREATE PROGRAMS

Degree BSN
Available Programs Generic Baccalaureate.
Online Degree Options Yes.
Contact *Telephone:* 607-587-3680. *Fax:* 315-792-7555.

State University of New York College of Technology at Canton
Nursing Program
Canton, New York

http://www.canton.edu/
Founded in 1906
DEGREE • BS
Nursing Program Faculty 17 (23% with doctorates).
Baccalaureate Enrollment 114 **Women** 88% **Men** 12% **Part-time** 81%
Distance Learning Courses Available.
Nursing Student Activities Nursing Honor Society, Student Nurses' Association.
Nursing Student Resources Academic advising; academic or career counseling; assistance for students with disabilities; bookstore; campus computer network; career placement assistance; computer lab; computer-assisted instruction; e-mail services; employment services for current students; housing assistance; interactive nursing skills videos; Internet; learning resource lab; library services; nursing audiovisuals; remedial services; resume preparation assistance; skills, simulation, or other laboratory; tutoring.

BACCALAUREATE PROGRAMS
Degree BS
Available Programs RN Baccalaureate.
Financial Aid *Gift aid (need-based):* Federal Pell, FSEOG, state, private, college/university gift aid from institutional funds, Bureau of Indian Affairs Grants. *Loans:* Federal Direct (Subsidized and Unsubsidized Stafford PLUS), Perkins, alternative loans. *Work-study:* Federal Work-Study, part-time campus jobs. *Financial aid application deadline (priority):* 3/1.
Contact Peggy LaFrance, RN-BS Curriculum Coordinator, Nursing Program, State University of New York College of Technology at Canton, 34 Cornell Drive, Canton, NY 13617. *E-mail:* lafrancep@canton.edu.

State University of New York College of Technology at Delhi
Bachelor of Science in Nursing Program
Delhi, New York

Founded in 1913
DEGREE • BSN

BACCALAUREATE PROGRAMS
Degree BSN
Available Programs RN Baccalaureate.
Study Options Full-time and part-time.
Online Degree Options Yes (online only).
Program Entrance Requirements RN licensure.
Contact *Telephone:* 607-746-4519.

State University of New York Downstate Medical Center
College of Nursing
Brooklyn, New York

http://www.downstate.edu/nursing/
Founded in 1858
DEGREES • BS • MS • MS/MPH
Nursing Program Faculty 19 (79% with doctorates).
Baccalaureate Enrollment 133 **Women** 93% **Men** 7% **Part-time** 77%
Graduate Enrollment 387 **Women** 90% **Men** 10% **Part-time** 40%
Distance Learning Courses Available.
Nursing Student Activities Student Nurses' Association, nursing club.

Nursing Student Resources Academic advising; academic or career counseling; assistance for students with disabilities; bookstore; campus computer network; computer lab; computer-assisted instruction; e-mail services; housing assistance; interactive nursing skills videos; Internet; learning resource lab; library services; nursing audiovisuals; paid internships; skills, simulation, or other laboratory; unpaid internships.
Library Facilities 357,209 volumes in health, 2,679 volumes in nursing; 619 periodical subscriptions health-care related.

BACCALAUREATE PROGRAMS
Degree BS
Available Programs Accelerated Baccalaureate for Second Degree; RN Baccalaureate.
Study Options Full-time.
Program Entrance Requirements Minimum overall college GPA of 3.0, transcript of college record, written essay, health exam, 2 letters of recommendation, professional liability insurance/malpractice insurance, prerequisite course work. Transfer students are accepted. *Application deadline:* 1/15 (fall), 1/15 (summer). Applications may be processed on a rolling basis for some programs. *Application fee:* $40.
Advanced Placement Credit by examination available.
Expenses (2015–16) *Tuition, state resident:* full-time $3235; part-time $270 per credit. *Tuition, nonresident:* full-time $8160; part-time $680 per credit. *International tuition:* $8160 full-time. *Room and board:* room only: $500 per academic year. *Required fees:* full-time $220; part-time $1 per credit; part-time $13 per term.
Financial Aid 45% of baccalaureate students in nursing programs received some form of financial aid in 2014–15.
Contact Dr. Nellie Bailey, Associate Dean, College of Nursing, State University of New York Downstate Medical Center, 450 Clarkson Avenue, Box 22, Brooklyn, NY 11203. *Telephone:* 718-270-7617. *Fax:* 718-270-7641. *E-mail:* nellie.bailey@downstate.edu.

GRADUATE PROGRAMS
Expenses (2015–16) *Tuition, state resident:* full-time $5435; part-time $453 per credit. *Tuition, nonresident:* full-time $11,105; part-time $841 per credit. *International tuition:* $11,105 full-time. *Required fees:* full-time $219; part-time $1 per credit; part-time $13 per term.
Financial Aid Traineeships and health workforce retraining available.
Contact Dr. Laila N. Sedhom, Associate Dean, College of Nursing, State University of New York Downstate Medical Center, 450 Clarkson Avenue, Box 22, Brooklyn, NY 11203-2098. *Telephone:* 718-270-7605. *Fax:* 718-270-7636. *E-mail:* laila.sedhom@downstate.edu.

MASTER'S DEGREE PROGRAM
Degrees MS; MS/MPH
Available Programs Master's.
Concentrations Available Nurse anesthesia; nurse-midwifery. *Clinical nurse specialist programs in:* adult health, maternity-newborn. *Nurse practitioner programs in:* family health, women's health.
Site Options Brooklyn, NY.
Study Options Full-time and part-time.
Program Entrance Requirements Clinical experience, minimum overall college GPA of 3.0, transcript of college record, CPR certification, written essay, immunizations, interview, 2 letters of recommendation, nursing research course, physical assessment course, professional liability insurance/malpractice insurance, prerequisite course work, resume, statistics course, GRE. *Application deadline:* 1/15 (fall). Applications may be processed on a rolling basis for some programs. *Application fee:* $80.
Advanced Placement Credit given for nursing courses completed elsewhere dependent upon specific evaluations.
Degree Requirements 44 total credit hours, thesis or project.

POST-MASTER'S PROGRAM
Areas of Study *Nurse practitioner programs in:* family health, women's health.

CONTINUING EDUCATION PROGRAM
Contact Ms. Veronica Arikian, PhD, Director of Continuing Education, College of Nursing, State University of New York Downstate Medical Center, 450 Clarkson Avenue, Box 22, Brooklyn, NY 11203. *Telephone:* 718-270-7488. *Fax:* 718-270-7628. *E-mail:* veronica.arikian@downstate.edu.

State University of New York Empire State College
Bachelor of Science in Nursing Program
Saratoga Springs, New York

http://www.esc.edu/nursing
Founded in 1971
DEGREES • BS • MS
Nursing Program Faculty 9 (33% with doctorates).
Baccalaureate Enrollment 1,200 **Women** 92.4% **Men** 7.6% **Part-time** 85.9%
Graduate Enrollment 75
Distance Learning Courses Available.
Nursing Student Activities Sigma Theta Tau.
Nursing Student Resources Academic advising; academic or career counseling; assistance for students with disabilities; bookstore; computer-assisted instruction; e-mail services; Internet; library services; nursing audiovisuals; resume preparation assistance; tutoring.

BACCALAUREATE PROGRAMS

Degree BS
Available Programs RN Baccalaureate.
Online Degree Options Yes (online only).
Program Entrance Requirements Minimum overall college GPA of 2.0, transcript of college record, written essay, RN licensure. Transfer students are accepted. *Application deadline:* 6/1 (fall), 10/1 (spring). *Application fee:* $50.
Advanced Placement Credit by examination available. Credit given for nursing courses completed elsewhere dependent upon specific evaluations.
Expenses (2014–15) *Tuition, area resident:* part-time $245 per credit.
Financial Aid 27% of baccalaureate students in nursing programs received some form of financial aid in 2013–14.
Contact Ms. Erin White, Coordinator of Student Services, Bachelor of Science in Nursing Program, State University of New York Empire State College, 113 West Avenue, Saratoga Springs, NY 12866. *Telephone:* 518-587-2100 Ext. 2812. *Fax:* 518-587-5126. *E-mail:* erin.white@esc.edu.

GRADUATE PROGRAMS

Expenses (2014–15) *Tuition, area resident:* part-time $432 per credit.
Contact Erin White, Coordinator of Student Services, Bachelor of Science in Nursing Program, State University of New York Empire State College, 113 West Avenue, Saratoga Springs, NY 12866. *Telephone:* 518-587-2100 Ext. 3020. *Fax:* 518-587-5126. *E-mail:* erin.white@esc.edu.

MASTER'S DEGREE PROGRAM
Degree MS
Available Programs Master's.
Concentrations Available Nursing education.
Study Options Part-time.
Online Degree Options Yes (online only).
Program Entrance Requirements Clinical experience, minimum overall college GPA of 3.0, transcript of college record, written essay, resume. *Application deadline:* 6/1 (fall), 10/1 (spring). *Application fee:* $50.
Advanced Placement Credit given for nursing courses completed elsewhere dependent upon specific evaluations.
Degree Requirements 42 total credit hours, thesis or project.

State University of New York Polytechnic Institute
School of Nursing and Health Systems
Utica, New York

http://www.sunyit.edu/
Founded in 1966
DEGREES • BS • MS
Nursing Program Faculty 30 (30% with doctorates).
Baccalaureate Enrollment 200 **Women** 96% **Men** 4% **Part-time** 70%
Graduate Enrollment 210 **Women** 90% **Men** 10% **Part-time** 60%

Distance Learning Courses Available.
Nursing Student Activities Nursing Honor Society, Sigma Theta Tau, Student Nurses' Association, nursing club.
Nursing Student Resources Academic advising; academic or career counseling; assistance for students with disabilities; bookstore; campus computer network; career placement assistance; computer lab; computer-assisted instruction; e-mail services; employment services for current students; externships; housing assistance; interactive nursing skills videos; Internet; learning resource lab; library services; nursing audiovisuals; other; placement services for program completers; remedial services; resume preparation assistance; skills, simulation, or other laboratory; tutoring; unpaid internships.
Library Facilities 14,000 volumes in health, 8,500 volumes in nursing; 335 periodical subscriptions health-care related.

BACCALAUREATE PROGRAMS

Degree BS
Available Programs ADN to Baccalaureate; Accelerated Baccalaureate; Accelerated RN Baccalaureate; RN Baccalaureate.
Study Options Full-time and part-time.
Online Degree Options Yes.
Program Entrance Requirements Minimum overall college GPA of 2.75, transcript of college record, health exam, health insurance, high school biology, high school chemistry, 3 years high school math, 3 years high school science, high school transcript, immunizations, minimum high school GPA, minimum high school rank 85%, prerequisite course work. Transfer students are accepted. *Application deadline:* 3/15 (fall). *Application fee:* $50.
Advanced Placement Credit by examination available. Credit given for nursing courses completed elsewhere dependent upon specific evaluations.
Expenses (2015–16) *Tuition, state resident:* full-time $6470; part-time $270 per credit. *Tuition, nonresident:* full-time $16,320; part-time $680 per credit. *International tuition:* $16,320 full-time. *Room and board:* $11,714; room only: $7388 per academic year. *Required fees:* full-time $1270; part-time $53 per credit.
Financial Aid 40% of baccalaureate students in nursing programs received some form of financial aid in 2014–15. *Gift aid (need-based):* Federal Pell, FSEOG, state, private, college/university gift aid from institutional funds. *Loans:* Federal Nursing Student Loans, Federal Direct (Subsidized and Unsubsidized Stafford PLUS), Perkins. *Work-study:* Federal Work-Study, part-time campus jobs. *Financial aid application deadline (priority):* 3/1.
Contact Ms. Gina Liscio, Director of Admissions, School of Nursing and Health Systems, State University of New York Polytechnic Institute, 100 Seymour Road, Utica, NY 13502. *Telephone:* 315-792-7208. *Fax:* 315-792-7837. *E-mail:* admissions@sunyit.edu.

GRADUATE PROGRAMS

Expenses (2015–16) *Tuition, state resident:* full-time $10,870; part-time $453 per credit. *Tuition, nonresident:* full-time $22,210; part-time $925 per credit. *International tuition:* $22,210 full-time. *Room and board:* $12,778; room only: $8452 per academic year. *Required fees:* full-time $1270; part-time $106 per credit.
Financial Aid Federal Work-Study, scholarships, traineeships, and unspecified assistantships available.
Contact Ms. Maryrose Raab, Coordinator of Graduate Center, School of Nursing and Health Systems, State University of New York Polytechnic Institute, 100 Seymour Road, Utica, NY 13502. *Telephone:* 315-792-7297. *Fax:* 315-792-7221. *E-mail:* mb_raab@sunyit.edu.

MASTER'S DEGREE PROGRAM
Degree MS
Available Programs Accelerated AD/RN to Master's; Accelerated RN to Master's; Master's; RN to Master's.
Concentrations Available Nursing administration; nursing education. *Nurse practitioner programs in:* adult health, family health, gerontology.
Study Options Full-time and part-time.
Online Degree Options Yes.
Program Entrance Requirements Clinical experience, computer literacy, minimum overall college GPA of 3.0, transcript of college record, written essay, immunizations, interview, 2 letters of recommendation, nursing research course, physical assessment course, prerequisite course work, resume, statistics course, GRE General Test (if undergraduate GPA less than 3.3). *Application deadline:* 3/1 (fall), 11/1 (spring). *Application fee:* $50.
Advanced Placement Credit given for nursing courses completed elsewhere dependent upon specific evaluations.
Degree Requirements 45 total credit hours, comprehensive exam.

POST-MASTER'S PROGRAM

Areas of Study Nursing administration; nursing education. *Nurse practitioner programs in:* adult health, family health, gerontology.

CONTINUING EDUCATION PROGRAM

Contact Ms. Kathleen Alcott, Continuing Professional Education Program Coordinator, School of Nursing and Health Systems, State University of New York Polytechnic Institute, 100 Seymour Road, Utica, NY 13502. *Telephone:* 315-792-7549. *Fax:* 315-792-7278. *E-mail:* alcottk@sunyit.edu.

State University of New York Upstate Medical University

College of Nursing
Syracuse, New York

http://www.upstate.edu/con
Founded in 1950
DEGREES • BS • MS
Nursing Program Faculty 21 (40% with doctorates).
Baccalaureate Enrollment 136 **Women** 90% **Men** 10% **Part-time** 88%
Graduate Enrollment 277 **Women** 90% **Men** 10% **Part-time** 85%
Distance Learning Courses Available.
Nursing Student Activities Sigma Theta Tau, Student Nurses' Association.
Nursing Student Resources Academic advising; academic or career counseling; assistance for students with disabilities; bookstore; campus computer network; career placement assistance; computer lab; computer-assisted instruction; daycare for children of students; e-mail services; Internet; learning resource lab; library services; skills, simulation, or other laboratory; tutoring.
Library Facilities 220,382 volumes in health, 1,241 volumes in nursing; 4,928 periodical subscriptions health-care related.

BACCALAUREATE PROGRAMS

Degree BS
Available Programs ADN to Baccalaureate.
Site Options Ithaca, NY.
Study Options Full-time and part-time.
Program Entrance Requirements Transcript of college record, CPR certification, written essay, health exam, immunizations, 2 letters of recommendation, prerequisite course work, RN licensure. *Application deadline:* 3/15 (fall), 9/15 (spring). *Application fee:* $50.
Advanced Placement Credit by examination available. Credit given for nursing courses completed elsewhere dependent upon specific evaluations.
Contact *Telephone:* 315-464-4276. *Fax:* 315-464-5168.

GRADUATE PROGRAMS

Contact *Telephone:* 315-464-4276. *Fax:* 315-464-5168.

MASTER'S DEGREE PROGRAM
Degree MS
Available Programs Accelerated RN to Master's; Master's; Master's for Nurses with Non-Nursing Degrees; RN to Master's.
Concentrations Available *Clinical nurse specialist programs in:* medical-surgical. *Nurse practitioner programs in:* adult health, family health, pediatric, psychiatric/mental health.
Site Options Watertown, NY.
Study Options Full-time and part-time.
Program Entrance Requirements Clinical experience, minimum overall college GPA of 3.0, transcript of college record, CPR certification, written essay, immunizations, 3 letters of recommendation, nursing research course, physical assessment course, statistics course. *Application deadline:* 3/15 (fall), 9/15 (spring). *Application fee:* $50.
Advanced Placement Credit by examination available. Credit given for nursing courses completed elsewhere dependent upon specific evaluations.
Degree Requirements 47 total credit hours, thesis or project.

POST-MASTER'S PROGRAM
Areas of Study *Clinical nurse specialist programs in:* medical-surgical. *Nurse practitioner programs in:* adult health, family health, pediatric, psychiatric/mental health.

CONTINUING EDUCATION PROGRAM

Contact *Telephone:* 315-464-4276. *Fax:* 315-464-5168.

Stony Brook University, State University of New York

School of Nursing
Stony Brook, New York

http://www.stonybrook.edu/
Founded in 1957
DEGREES • BS • DNP • MS
Nursing Program Faculty 64 (68% with doctorates).
Baccalaureate Enrollment 382 **Women** 81% **Men** 19% **Part-time** 39%
Graduate Enrollment 864 **Women** 90% **Men** 10% **Part-time** 95%
Distance Learning Courses Available.
Nursing Student Activities Nursing Honor Society, Sigma Theta Tau, Student Nurses' Association, nursing club.
Nursing Student Resources Academic advising; academic or career counseling; assistance for students with disabilities; bookstore; campus computer network; career placement assistance; computer lab; computer-assisted instruction; daycare for children of students; e-mail services; employment services for current students; housing assistance; interactive nursing skills videos; Internet; learning resource lab; library services; nursing audiovisuals; remedial services; resume preparation assistance; skills, simulation, or other laboratory.
Library Facilities 11,022 volumes in health, 5,075 volumes in nursing; 280,000 periodical subscriptions health-care related.

BACCALAUREATE PROGRAMS

Degree BS
Available Programs Accelerated Baccalaureate; Generic Baccalaureate; RN Baccalaureate.
Study Options Full-time and part-time.
Program Entrance Requirements Transcript of college record, CPR certification, written essay, health exam, health insurance, immunizations, interview, 3 letters of recommendation, minimum GPA in nursing prerequisites of 2.8, professional liability insurance/malpractice insurance, prerequisite course work. *Application deadline:* 1/7 (fall), 11/22 (spring), 1/1 (summer). *Application fee:* $50.
Advanced Placement Credit by examination available. Credit given for nursing courses completed elsewhere dependent upon specific evaluations.
Expenses (2015–16) *Tuition, state resident:* full-time $6470; part-time $270 per credit hour. *Tuition, nonresident:* full-time $21,550; part-time $898 per credit hour. *International tuition:* $21,550 full-time. *Room and board:* $12,398; room only: $8460 per academic year. *Required fees:* full-time $2384; part-time $118 per credit; part-time $1189 per term.
Financial Aid 53% of baccalaureate students in nursing programs received some form of financial aid in 2014–15. *Gift aid (need-based):* Federal Pell, FSEOG, state, private, college/university gift aid from institutional funds. *Loans:* Federal Direct (Subsidized and Unsubsidized Stafford PLUS), Perkins. *Work-study:* Federal Work-Study, part-time campus jobs. *Financial aid application deadline (priority):* 3/1.
Contact Mrs. Karen Allard, Senior Staff Assistant, School of Nursing, Stony Brook University, State University of New York, Health Sciences Center, Level 2, Stony Brook, NY 11974-8240. *Telephone:* 631-444-3554. *Fax:* 631-444-3781. *E-mail:* Karen.Allard@stonybrook.edu.

GRADUATE PROGRAMS

Expenses (2015–16) *Tuition, state resident:* full-time $21,740; part-time $453 per credit hour. *Tuition, nonresident:* full-time $44,420; part-time $925 per credit hour. *International tuition:* $44,420 full-time. *Room and board:* $12,398; room only: $8460 per academic year. *Required fees:* full-time $2337; part-time $89 per credit; part-time $752 per term.
Financial Aid 32% of graduate students in nursing programs received some form of financial aid in 2014–15. Fellowships, research assistantships, teaching assistantships, career-related internships or fieldwork, Federal Work-Study, institutionally sponsored loans, and traineeships available. *Financial aid application deadline:* 3/15.
Contact Dolores Bilges, Senior Staff Assistant, School of Nursing, Stony Brook University, State University of New York, Health Sciences Center, Level 2, Stony Brook, NY 11794-8240. *Telephone:* 631-444-2644. *Fax:* 631-444-3136. *E-mail:* dolores.bilges@stonybrook.edu.

MASTER'S DEGREE PROGRAM
Degree MS

Available Programs Master's; RN to Master's.
Concentrations Available Nurse-midwifery; nursing administration; nursing education. *Clinical nurse specialist programs in:* adult health, community health, critical care, family health, parent-child, pediatric, perinatal, psychiatric/mental health, women's health. *Nurse practitioner programs in:* adult health, family health, neonatal health, pediatric, psychiatric/mental health, women's health.
Study Options Part-time.
Online Degree Options Yes.
Program Entrance Requirements Clinical experience, computer literacy, minimum overall college GPA of 3.0, transcript of college record, CPR certification, written essay, immunizations, interview, 3 letters of recommendation, physical assessment course, professional liability insurance/malpractice insurance, prerequisite course work, resume, statistics course. *Application deadline:* 11/19 (summer). *Application fee:* $100.
Advanced Placement Credit by examination available. Credit given for nursing courses completed elsewhere dependent upon specific evaluations.
Degree Requirements 45 total credit hours.

POST-MASTER'S PROGRAM

Areas of Study Nurse-midwifery; nursing administration; nursing education. *Clinical nurse specialist programs in:* adult health, community health, critical care, family health, parent-child, pediatric, perinatal, psychiatric/mental health, women's health. *Nurse practitioner programs in:* adult health, family health, neonatal health, pediatric, psychiatric/mental health, women's health.

DOCTORAL DEGREE PROGRAM

Degree DNP
Available Programs Doctorate.
Areas of Study Advanced practice nursing, biology of health and illness, clinical practice, ethics, health policy, health promotion/disease prevention, health-care systems, individualized study, nursing policy, nursing research.
Program Entrance Requirements Clinical experience, minimum overall college GPA of 3.0, interview by faculty committee, interview, 3 letters of recommendation, MSN or equivalent, vita, writing sample. Application deadline: 12/3 (summer). Application fee: $100.
Degree Requirements 42 total credit hours.

CONTINUING EDUCATION PROGRAM

Contact Mrs. Debra Grimm, RN, Assistant Dean for Business Affairs, Director, Continuing Education, School of Nursing, Stony Brook University, State University of New York, Health Sciences Center, Level 2, Room 226, Stony Brook, NY 11794-8240. *Telephone:* 631-444-3259. *Fax:* 631-444-3136. *E-mail:* Debra.Grimm@stonybrook.edu.

Touro College
School of Nursing
New York, New York

https://www.touro.edu/
Founded in 1971
DEGREE • BS

BACCALAUREATE PROGRAMS

Degree BS
Available Programs Generic Baccalaureate.
Contact Sandra Russo, Chairperson and Director, School of Nursing, Touro College, 902 Quentin Road, New York, NY 10010. *Telephone:* 718-236-2661 Ext. 36308. *E-mail:* sandra.russo@touro.edu.

Trocaire College
Nursing Program
Buffalo, New York

Founded in 1958
DEGREE • BS

BACCALAUREATE PROGRAMS

Degree BS

Available Programs Generic Baccalaureate.
Online Degree Options Yes (online only).
Contact *Telephone:* 716-827-2407.

University at Buffalo, the State University of New York
School of Nursing
Buffalo, New York

http://www.nursing.buffalo.edu/
Founded in 1846
DEGREES • BS • DNP • MS • PHD
Nursing Program Faculty 43 (95% with doctorates).
Baccalaureate Enrollment 250 **Women** 88% **Men** 12% **Part-time** 20%
Graduate Enrollment 198 **Women** 76% **Men** 24% **Part-time** 69%
Distance Learning Courses Available.
Nursing Student Activities Nursing Honor Society, Sigma Theta Tau, Student Nurses' Association.
Nursing Student Resources Academic advising; academic or career counseling; assistance for students with disabilities; bookstore; campus computer network; career placement assistance; computer lab; computer-assisted instruction; daycare for children of students; e-mail services; employment services for current students; externships; housing assistance; interactive nursing skills videos; Internet; learning resource lab; library services; nursing audiovisuals; placement services for program completers; remedial services; resume preparation assistance; skills, simulation, or other laboratory; unpaid internships.
Library Facilities 250,000 volumes in health, 25,000 volumes in nursing; 2,500 periodical subscriptions health-care related.

BACCALAUREATE PROGRAMS

Degree BS
Available Programs Accelerated Baccalaureate for Second Degree; Generic Baccalaureate; RN Baccalaureate.
Study Options Full-time.
Online Degree Options Yes.
Program Entrance Requirements Minimum overall college GPA of 3.0, transcript of college record, CPR certification, written essay, health exam, health insurance, immunizations, minimum GPA in nursing prerequisites of 3.0, prerequisite course work. Transfer students are accepted. *Application deadline:* 2/15 (fall).
Advanced Placement Credit given for nursing courses completed elsewhere dependent upon specific evaluations.
Expenses (2015–16) *Tuition, state resident:* full-time $6470; part-time $270 per credit hour. *Tuition, nonresident:* full-time $21,510; part-time $898 per credit hour. *International tuition:* $21,510 full-time. *Room and board:* $12,761; room only: $7571 per academic year. *Required fees:* full-time $3300; part-time $121 per credit; part-time $450 per term.
Contact Ms. Julie Kim-Proehl, Admissions Coordinator, School of Nursing, University at Buffalo, the State University of New York, Beck Hall, 3435 Main Street, Buffalo, NY 14214. *Telephone:* 716-829-2537. *Fax:* 716-829-2067. *E-mail:* nursing@buffalo.edu.

GRADUATE PROGRAMS

Expenses (2015–16) *Tuition, state resident:* full-time $10,870; part-time $453 per credit hour. *Tuition, nonresident:* full-time $22,210; part-time $925 per credit hour. *International tuition:* $22,210 full-time. *Room and board:* $11,162; room only: $8712 per academic year. *Required fees:* full-time $2800; part-time $180 per credit; part-time $315 per term.
Financial Aid 80% of graduate students in nursing programs received some form of financial aid in 2014–15. 2 fellowships with full and partial tuition reimbursements available (averaging $17,000 per year), 4 research assistantships with full and partial tuition reimbursements available (averaging $10,600 per year), 7 teaching assistantships with full and partial tuition reimbursements available (averaging $10,600 per year) were awarded; scholarships, traineeships, and unspecified assistantships also available. *Financial aid application deadline:* 3/15.
Contact Ms. Ann Taylor, Graduate Program Secretary, School of Nursing, University at Buffalo, the State University of New York, Beck Hall, 3435 Main Street, Buffalo, NY 14214. *Telephone:* 716-829-2537. *Fax:* 716-829-2067. *E-mail:* nursing@buffalo.edu.

MASTER'S DEGREE PROGRAM
Degree MS
Available Programs Master's.

Concentrations Available Nursing administration.
Study Options Full-time and part-time.
Program Entrance Requirements Computer literacy, minimum overall college GPA of 3.0, transcript of college record, CPR certification, written essay, immunizations, interview, 3 letters of recommendation, resume, statistics course, GRE or MAT. *Application deadline:* 7/1 (fall), 12/1 (spring), 4/1 (summer). Applications may be processed on a rolling basis for some programs. *Application fee:* $75.
Advanced Placement Credit given for nursing courses completed elsewhere dependent upon specific evaluations.
Degree Requirements 41 total credit hours, thesis or project.

DOCTORAL DEGREE PROGRAM
Degree DNP
Available Programs Doctorate, Post-Baccalaureate Doctorate.
Areas of Study Addiction/substance abuse, advanced practice nursing, aging, biology of health and illness, clinical nurse leader, clinical practice, community health, critical care, ethics, faculty preparation, family health, gerontology, health policy, health promotion/disease prevention, health-care systems, human health and illness, individualized study, information systems, maternity-newborn, nurse case management, nursing administration, nursing education, nursing policy, nursing research, nursing science, oncology, palliative care, urban health, women's health.
Online Degree Options Yes.
Program Entrance Requirements Minimum overall college GPA of 3.25, clinical experience, interview, interview by faculty committee, 3 letters of recommendation, statistics course, vita, writing sample. Application deadline: 7/1 (fall), 12/1/ (spring), 4/1 (summer). Applications may be processed on a rolling basis. Application fee: $75.
Degree Requirements 93 total credit hours, dissertation.

Degree PhD
Available Programs Doctorate; Post-Baccalaureate Doctorate.
Areas of Study Addiction/substance abuse, advanced practice nursing, aging, biology of health and illness, clinical nurse leader, clinical practice, community health, critical care, ethics, faculty preparation, family health, gerontology, health policy, health promotion/disease prevention, health-care systems, human health and illness, individualized study, information systems, maternity-newborn, nurse case management, nurse executive, nursing administration, nursing education, nursing policy, nursing research, nursing science, oncology, palliative care, urban health, women's health.
Program Entrance Requirements Clinical experience, minimum overall college GPA of 3.25, interview by faculty committee, interview, 3 letters of recommendation, scholarly papers, statistics course, vita, GRE or MAT. Application deadline: 1/15 (fall). Applications may be processed on a rolling basis for some programs. Application fee: $75.
Degree Requirements 79 total credit hours, dissertation.

University of Rochester
School of Nursing
Rochester, New York

http://www.son.rochester.edu/
Founded in 1850
DEGREES • BS • DNP • MS • MSN/PHD • PHD
Contact Ms. Elaine M. Andolina, Director of Admissions, School of Nursing, University of Rochester, Box SON, 601 Elmwood Avenue, Rochester NY 14642. *Telephone:* 585-275-2375. *Fax:* 585-756-8299. *E-mail:* son_admissions@urmc.rochester.edu.

Utica College
Department of Nursing
Utica, New York

http://www.utica.edu/
Founded in 1946
DEGREE • BS
Nursing Program Faculty 83 (6% with doctorates).
Baccalaureate Enrollment 668 **Women** 89% **Men** 11% **Part-time** 60%
Distance Learning Courses Available.
Nursing Student Activities Sigma Theta Tau, Student Nurses' Association.

Nursing Student Resources Academic advising; academic or career counseling; assistance for students with disabilities; bookstore; campus computer network; career placement assistance; computer lab; computer-assisted instruction; e-mail services; employment services for current students; externships; housing assistance; interactive nursing skills videos; Internet; learning resource lab; library services; nursing audiovisuals; paid internships; placement services for program completers; remedial services; resume preparation assistance; skills, simulation, or other laboratory; tutoring; unpaid internships.
Library Facilities 2,652 volumes in health, 1,122 volumes in nursing; 118 periodical subscriptions health-care related.

BACCALAUREATE PROGRAMS
Degree BS
Available Programs Accelerated Baccalaureate for Second Degree; Generic Baccalaureate; RN Baccalaureate.
Site Options Syracuse, NY.
Study Options Full-time and part-time.
Online Degree Options Yes.
Program Entrance Requirements Minimum overall college GPA of 2.8, transcript of college record, written essay, health exam, health insurance, high school biology, high school chemistry, 3 years high school math, 3 years high school science, high school transcript, immunizations, 3 letters of recommendation, minimum high school GPA of 3.0, minimum high school rank 25%, minimum GPA in nursing prerequisites of 2.8. Transfer students are accepted. *Application deadline:* 3/15 (fall), 11/15 (spring). Applications may be processed on a rolling basis for some programs. *Application fee:* $40.
Advanced Placement Credit by examination available. Credit given for nursing courses completed elsewhere dependent upon specific evaluations.
Contact *Telephone:* 315-792-3006. *Fax:* 315-792-3003.

Wagner College
Department of Nursing
Staten Island, New York

http://www.wagner.edu/departments/nursing/
Founded in 1883
DEGREES • BS • MSN
Nursing Program Faculty 17 (90% with doctorates).
Baccalaureate Enrollment 60 **Women** 82% **Men** 18% **Part-time** 5%
Graduate Enrollment 63 **Women** 90% **Men** 10% **Part-time** 95%
Nursing Student Activities Nursing Honor Society, Sigma Theta Tau, Student Nurses' Association.
Nursing Student Resources Academic advising; academic or career counseling; assistance for students with disabilities; bookstore; campus computer network; career placement assistance; computer lab; computer-assisted instruction; e-mail services; externships; housing assistance; interactive nursing skills videos; Internet; learning resource lab; library services; nursing audiovisuals; remedial services; skills, simulation, or other laboratory; tutoring; unpaid internships.
Library Facilities 4,505 volumes in health, 859 volumes in nursing; 87 periodical subscriptions health-care related.

BACCALAUREATE PROGRAMS
Degree BS
Available Programs Baccalaureate for Second Degree; Generic Baccalaureate.
Study Options Full-time.
Program Entrance Requirements Minimum overall college GPA of 3.0, written essay, health exam, health insurance, high school chemistry, high school transcript, immunizations, letters of recommendation, minimum high school GPA of 2.7, minimum GPA in nursing prerequisites of 3.0, prerequisite course work. Transfer students are accepted.
Advanced Placement Credit by examination available. Credit given for nursing courses completed elsewhere dependent upon specific evaluations.
Contact *Telephone:* 718-390-3452. *Fax:* 718-420-4009.

GRADUATE PROGRAMS
Contact *Telephone:* 718-390-3444. *Fax:* 718-420-4009.

MASTER'S DEGREE PROGRAM
Degree MSN

Concentrations Available Nursing education. *Nurse practitioner programs in:* family health.
Study Options Full-time and part-time.
Program Entrance Requirements Clinical experience, minimum overall college GPA of 2.7, transcript of college record, CPR certification, immunizations, interview, 2 letters of recommendation, nursing research course, professional liability insurance/malpractice insurance, resume.
Degree Requirements 44 total credit hours.

POST-MASTER'S PROGRAM

Areas of Study *Nurse practitioner programs in:* family health.

York College of the City University of New York
Program in Nursing
Jamaica, New York

http://www.york.cuny.edu/academics/departments/nursing/nursing-1
Founded in 1967
DEGREE • BS
Nursing Program Faculty 9 (20% with doctorates).
Baccalaureate Enrollment 80 Women 85% Men 15% Part-time 50%
Nursing Student Activities Nursing club.
Nursing Student Resources Academic advising; academic or career counseling; assistance for students with disabilities; bookstore; campus computer network; career placement assistance; computer lab; computer-assisted instruction; daycare for children of students; e-mail services; employment services for current students; Internet; library services; resume preparation assistance; skills, simulation, or other laboratory; tutoring.
Library Facilities 8,714 volumes in health, 567 volumes in nursing.

BACCALAUREATE PROGRAMS

Degree BS
Available Programs ADN to Baccalaureate; RN Baccalaureate.
Program Entrance Requirements Minimum overall college GPA of 3.0, transcript of college record, CPR certification, health exam, immunizations, minimum GPA in nursing prerequisites of 3.0, professional liability insurance/malpractice insurance, prerequisite course work, RN licensure. TransfeSSSSSSSFFCr students are accepted.
Advanced Placement Credit by examination available. Credit given for nursing courses completed elsewhere dependent upon specific evaluations. Contact *Telephone:* 718-262-2165.

NORTH CAROLINA

Appalachian State University
Department of Nursing
Boone, North Carolina

http://www.nursing.appstate.edu/
Founded in 1899
DEGREE • BSN
Nursing Program Faculty 15 (50% with doctorates).
Baccalaureate Enrollment 146 Women 90% Men 10%
Distance Learning Courses Available.
Nursing Student Activities Nursing Honor Society, Sigma Theta Tau, Student Nurses' Association, nursing club.
Nursing Student Resources Academic advising; academic or career counseling; assistance for students with disabilities; bookstore; campus computer network; career placement assistance; computer lab; computer-assisted instruction; e-mail services; interactive nursing skills videos; Internet; learning resource lab; library services; nursing audiovisuals; remedial services; skills, simulation, or other laboratory; tutoring.
Library Facilities 3.2 million volumes in health, 541,000 volumes in nursing; 6,764 periodical subscriptions health-care related.

BACCALAUREATE PROGRAMS

Degree BSN
Available Programs Generic Baccalaureate; RN Baccalaureate.
Study Options Full-time.
Online Degree Options Yes.
Program Entrance Requirements Minimum overall college GPA of 3.0, transcript of college record, CPR certification, health exam, immunizations, minimum GPA in nursing prerequisites of 2.5, professional liability insurance/malpractice insurance, prerequisite course work. Transfer students are accepted. *Application deadline:* 1/15 (fall). *Application fee:* $50.
Contact *Telephone:* 828-262-8039. *Fax:* 828-262-8066.

Barton College
School of Nursing
Wilson, North Carolina

http://www.barton.edu
Founded in 1902
DEGREES • BSN • MSN
Nursing Program Faculty 16 (60% with doctorates).
Baccalaureate Enrollment 120 Women 94.8% Men 5.2%
Graduate Enrollment 24
Nursing Student Activities Nursing Honor Society, Sigma Theta Tau, Student Nurses' Association, nursing club.
Nursing Student Resources Academic advising; academic or career counseling; assistance for students with disabilities; bookstore; campus computer network; career placement assistance; computer lab; computer-assisted instruction; e-mail services; employment services for current students; externships; housing assistance; interactive nursing skills videos; Internet; learning resource lab; library services; nursing audiovisuals; paid internships; placement services for program completers; remedial services; resume preparation assistance; skills, simulation, or other laboratory; tutoring; unpaid internships.
Library Facilities 3,500 volumes in health, 2,250 volumes in nursing; 10,000 periodical subscriptions health-care related.

BACCALAUREATE PROGRAMS

Degree BSN
Available Programs ADN to Baccalaureate; Generic Baccalaureate; RN Baccalaureate.
Study Options Full-time and part-time.
Program Entrance Requirements Minimum overall college GPA of 2.7, transcript of college record, CPR certification, health exam, health insurance, high school biology, high school chemistry, high school transcript, immunizations, minimum GPA in nursing prerequisites of 2.7, professional liability insurance/malpractice insurance, prerequisite course work. Transfer students are accepted. *Application deadline:* 11/1 (fall).
Advanced Placement Credit given for nursing courses completed elsewhere dependent upon specific evaluations.
Expenses (2015–16) *Tuition:* full-time $22,000; part-time $1100 per credit. *Room and board:* $12,000 per academic year. *Required fees:* full-time $2500.
Financial Aid 98% of baccalaureate students in nursing programs received some form of financial aid in 2014–15.
Contact Mrs. Joan Taylor, Department Administrator, School of Nursing, Barton College, PO Box 5000, Wilson, NC 27893-7000. *Telephone:* 252-399-6400. *Fax:* 252-399-6416. *E-mail:* jtaylor@barton.edu.

GRADUATE PROGRAMS

Expenses (2015–16) *Tuition:* full-time $11,000. *Required fees:* full-time $1200.
Contact Dr. Sharon Isenhour Sarvey, Professor and Dean, School of Nursing, Barton College, PO Box 5000, Wilson, NC 27893. *Telephone:* 252-399-6401. *Fax:* 252-399-6416. *E-mail:* sisarvey@barton.edu.

MASTER'S DEGREE PROGRAM
Degree MSN
Available Programs Master's.
Concentrations Available Nursing administration; nursing education.
Study Options Full-time.
Program Entrance Requirements Clinical experience, minimum overall college GPA of 3.0, transcript of college record, CPR certification, immunizations, professional liability insurance/malpractice insurance, statistics course. *Application deadline:* 8/5 (fall), 8/15

(summer). Applications may be processed on a rolling basis for some programs.

Advanced Placement Credit given for nursing courses completed elsewhere dependent upon specific evaluations.

Degree Requirements 39 total credit hours, thesis or project.

Cabarrus College of Health Sciences

Louise Harkey School of Nursing
Concord, North Carolina

http://www.cabarruscollege.edu/
Founded in 1942

DEGREE • BSN

Nursing Program Faculty 3 (25% with doctorates).
Baccalaureate Enrollment 35 **Women** 90% **Men** 10% **Part-time** 50%
Distance Learning Courses Available.
Nursing Student Activities Sigma Theta Tau, Student Nurses' Association, nursing club.
Nursing Student Resources Academic advising; academic or career counseling; assistance for students with disabilities; bookstore; campus computer network; career placement assistance; computer lab; computer-assisted instruction; e-mail services; interactive nursing skills videos; Internet; library services; resume preparation assistance; skills, simulation, or other laboratory.
Library Facilities 500 volumes in health, 300 volumes in nursing; 300 periodical subscriptions health-care related.

BACCALAUREATE PROGRAMS

Degree BSN
Available Programs RN Baccalaureate.
Study Options Full-time and part-time.
Program Entrance Requirements Minimum overall college GPA of 2.5, transcript of college record, CPR certification, written essay, health exam, health insurance, 4 years high school math, immunizations, 2 letters of recommendation, RN licensure. Transfer students are accepted. *Application deadline:* 5/1 (fall), 10/1 (spring). Applications may be processed on a rolling basis for some programs. *Application fee:* $35.
Advanced Placement Credit by examination available.
Contact *Telephone:* 704-403-1756. *Fax:* 704-403-2077.

Duke University

School of Nursing
Durham, North Carolina

https://nursing.duke.edu/
Founded in 1838

DEGREES • BSN • DNP • MSN • PHD

Nursing Program Faculty 88 (95% with doctorates).
Baccalaureate Enrollment 211 **Women** 87% **Men** 13% **Part-time** 1%
Graduate Enrollment 700 **Women** 87% **Men** 13% **Part-time** 70%
Distance Learning Courses Available.
Nursing Student Activities Sigma Theta Tau, Student Nurses' Association.
Nursing Student Resources Academic advising; academic or career counseling; assistance for students with disabilities; bookstore; campus computer network; career placement assistance; computer lab; computer-assisted instruction; e-mail services; Internet; library services; nursing audiovisuals; resume preparation assistance; skills, simulation, or other laboratory.
Library Facilities 114,895 volumes in health, 4,439 volumes in nursing; 13,141 periodical subscriptions health-care related.

BACCALAUREATE PROGRAMS

Degree BSN
Available Programs Accelerated Baccalaureate for Second Degree.
Site Options Durham, NC.
Study Options Full-time.
Program Entrance Requirements Minimum overall college GPA of 3.0, transcript of college record, CPR certification, written essay, health exam, health insurance, immunizations, interview, 3 letters of recommen-

dation, prerequisite course work. *Application deadline:* 12/1 (fall), 5/1 (spring). *Application fee:* $50.
Financial Aid *Gift aid (need-based):* Federal Pell, FSEOG, state, private, college/university gift aid from institutional funds. *Loans:* Federal Direct (Subsidized and Unsubsidized Stafford PLUS), Perkins, college/university, alternative loans. *Work-study:* Federal Work-Study, part-time campus jobs. *Financial aid application deadline:* 3/15.
Contact Mr. Nora Harrington, Admissions Officer, School of Nursing, Duke University, 307 Trent Drive, Box 102400, Durham, NC 27710. *Telephone:* 919-684-4248. *Fax:* 919-668-4693.
E-mail: SONAdmissions@dm.duke.edu.

GRADUATE PROGRAMS

Financial Aid Career-related internships or fieldwork, institutionally sponsored loans, scholarships, traineeships, and tuition waivers (partial) available.
Contact Ms. Nicole Fleming, Admissions Officer, School of Nursing, Duke University, 307 Trent Drive, Box 102400, Durham, NC 27710. *Telephone:* 919-684-4248. *Fax:* 919-668-4693.
E-mail: SONAdmissions@dm.duke.edu.

MASTER'S DEGREE PROGRAM

Degree MSN
Available Programs Master's; RN to Master's.
Concentrations Available Health-care administration; nursing administration; nursing education; nursing informatics. *Nurse practitioner programs in:* acute care, adult health, adult-gerontology acute care, family health, neonatal health, oncology, pediatric, pediatric primary care, primary care, women's health.
Site Options Durham, NC.
Study Options Full-time and part-time.
Online Degree Options Yes.
Program Entrance Requirements Clinical experience, computer literacy, minimum overall college GPA of 3.0, transcript of college record, CPR certification, written essay, immunizations, interview, 3 letters of recommendation, prerequisite course work, resume, statistics course, GRE General Test (waived if undergraduate GPA of 3.4 or higher). *Application deadline:* 12/1 (fall), 5/1 (spring). *Application fee:* $50.
Advanced Placement Credit given for nursing courses completed elsewhere dependent upon specific evaluations.
Degree Requirements 39 total credit hours.

POST-MASTER'S PROGRAM

Areas of Study Health-care administration; nursing administration; nursing education; nursing informatics. *Nurse practitioner programs in:* acute care, adult health, adult-gerontology acute care, family health, neonatal health, oncology, pediatric, pediatric primary care, primary care, women's health.

DOCTORAL DEGREE PROGRAM

Degree DNP
Available Programs Doctorate; Post-Baccalaureate Doctorate.
Areas of Study Advanced practice nursing, aging, critical care, family health, gerontology, health-care systems, illness and transition, information systems, nursing administration, nursing education, nursing policy, nursing research, nursing science, oncology, women's health.
Site Options Durham, NC.
Online Degree Options Yes (online only).
Program Entrance Requirements Clinical experience, minimum overall college GPA of 3.0, interview by faculty committee, interview, 3 letters of recommendation, MSN or equivalent, statistics course, vita, GRE General Test (waived if undergraduate GPA of 3.4 or higher). Application deadline: 2/1 (fall), 5/1 (spring). Application fee: $50.
Degree Requirements 35 total credit hours.

Degree PhD
Available Programs Doctorate, Post-Baccalaureate Doctorate.
Areas of Study Aging, gerontology, health-care systems, illness and transition, information systems, nursing education, nursing policy, nursing research, nursing science, women's health.
Program Entrance Requirements Minimum overall college GPA of 3.5, interview, interview by faculty committee, 3 letters of recommendation, MSN or equivalent, statistics course, vita. Application deadline: 12/1 (fall). Application fee: $80.
Degree Requirements 54 total credit hours, dissertation, written exam.

POSTDOCTORAL PROGRAM

Areas of Study Aging, cancer care, chronic illness, gerontology, health promotion/disease prevention, information systems, neonatal health, nursing informatics, nursing interventions, nursing research, nursing science, vulnerable population, women's health.

Postdoctoral Program Contact Dr. Debra H. Brandon, Director of PhD and Post-Doctoral Fellowship Program, School of Nursing, Duke University, 307 Trent Drive, Box 3322 DUMC, Durham, NC 27710. *Telephone:* 919-684-5376. *Fax:* 919-661-8899. *E-mail:* leslie.barnhouse@duke.edu.

East Carolina University

College of Nursing
Greenville, North Carolina

http://www.nursing.ecu.edu/
Founded in 1907
DEGREES · BSN · DNP · MSN · PHD
Nursing Program Faculty 121 (36% with doctorates).
Baccalaureate Enrollment 666 **Women** 90% **Men** 10% **Part-time** 25%
Graduate Enrollment 517 **Women** 91% **Men** 9% **Part-time** 73%
Distance Learning Courses Available.
Nursing Student Activities Nursing Honor Society, Sigma Theta Tau, Student Nurses' Association.
Nursing Student Resources Academic advising; academic or career counseling; assistance for students with disabilities; bookstore; campus computer network; career placement assistance; computer lab; computer-assisted instruction; e-mail services; employment services for current students; externships; housing assistance; interactive nursing skills videos; Internet; learning resource lab; library services; nursing audiovisuals; remedial services; resume preparation assistance; skills, simulation, or other laboratory; tutoring; unpaid internships.
Library Facilities 36,183 volumes in health, 2,869 volumes in nursing; 1,049 periodical subscriptions health-care related.

BACCALAUREATE PROGRAMS

Degree BSN
Available Programs ADN to Baccalaureate; Accelerated Baccalaureate for Second Degree; Generic Baccalaureate.
Study Options Full-time.
Online Degree Options Yes.
Program Entrance Requirements Minimum overall college GPA of 2.5, transcript of college record, CPR certification, health exam, health insurance, immunizations, professional liability insurance/malpractice insurance, prerequisite course work. Transfer students are accepted. *Application deadline:* 2/1 (fall), 9/1 (spring).
Advanced Placement Credit given for nursing courses completed elsewhere dependent upon specific evaluations.
Expenses (2015–16) *Tuition, state resident:* full-time $4157; part-time $140 per credit hour. *Tuition, nonresident:* full-time $19,731; part-time $667 per credit hour. *International tuition:* $19,731 full-time. *Room and board:* $9319; room only: $5060 per academic year. *Required fees:* full-time $2423; part-time $16 per credit.
Financial Aid *Gift aid (need-based):* Federal Pell, FSEOG, state, private, college/university gift aid from institutional funds, Federal Nursing. *Loans:* Federal Nursing Student Loans, Federal Direct (Subsidized and Unsubsidized Stafford PLUS), Perkins, state. *Work-study:* Federal Work-Study, part-time campus jobs. *Financial aid application deadline (priority):* 3/1.
Contact Ms. Erin Rogers, Executive Director of Student Services, College of Nursing, East Carolina University, Health Sciences Building, Suite 2150, Greenville, NC 27858-4353. *Telephone:* 252-744-6477. *Fax:* 252-744-6391. *E-mail:* ecunursestudentsvc@ecu.edu.

GRADUATE PROGRAMS

Expenses (2015–16) *Tuition, state resident:* full-time $4434; part-time $277 per credit hour. *Tuition, nonresident:* full-time $17,036; part-time $1065 per credit hour. *International tuition:* $17,036 full-time. *Room and board:* $12,640; room only: $5060 per academic year. *Required fees:* full-time $2423; part-time $16 per credit.
Financial Aid Research assistantships, teaching assistantships, Federal Work-Study available.
Contact Dr. Sonya Renae Hardin, Interim Associate Dean of Graduate Programs, College of Nursing, East Carolina University, Health Sciences

Building, Room 3166A, Greenville, NC 27858-4353. *Telephone:* 252-744-6473. *Fax:* 252-744-6391. *E-mail:* hardins@ecu.edu.

MASTER'S DEGREE PROGRAM
Degree MSN
Available Programs Accelerated Master's for Non-Nursing College Graduates; Accelerated Master's for Nurses with Non-Nursing Degrees; Master's; RN to Master's.
Concentrations Available Nurse anesthesia; nurse-midwifery; nursing administration; nursing education. *Nurse practitioner programs in:* neonatal health.
Study Options Full-time and part-time.
Online Degree Options Yes.
Program Entrance Requirements Clinical experience, computer literacy, minimum overall college GPA of 3.0, transcript of college record, CPR certification, written essay, immunizations, interview, 3 letters of recommendation, nursing research course, professional liability insurance/malpractice insurance, prerequisite course work, statistics course, GRE General Test or MAT. *Application deadline:* 3/15 (fall), 10/15 (spring). Applications may be processed on a rolling basis for some programs. *Application fee:* $70.
Advanced Placement Credit given for nursing courses completed elsewhere dependent upon specific evaluations.
Degree Requirements 46 total credit hours, comprehensive exam.

POST-MASTER'S PROGRAM
Areas of Study Nurse anesthesia; nurse-midwifery; nursing administration; nursing education. *Nurse practitioner programs in:* neonatal health.

DOCTORAL DEGREE PROGRAM
Degree DNP
Available Programs Doctorate; Post-Baccalaureate Doctorate.
Areas of Study Advanced practice nursing, family health, nursing administration.
Online Degree Options Yes.
Program Entrance Requirements Clinical experience, minimum overall college GPA of 3.2, interview by faculty committee, interview, 3 letters of recommendation, MSN or equivalent, scholarly papers, statistics course, vita, writing sample. Application deadline: 1/10 (fall). Application fee: $70.
Degree Requirements 36 total credit hours, oral exam, written exam.

Degree PhD
Available Programs Doctorate, Post-Baccalaureate Doctorate.
Areas of Study Nursing science.
Program Entrance Requirements Minimum overall college GPA of 3.2, interview, interview by faculty committee, 3 letters of recommendation, MSN or equivalent, scholarly papers, statistics course, vita, writing sample. Application deadline: 3/15 (fall). Application fee: $70.
Degree Requirements 54 total credit hours, dissertation, oral exam, written exam.

Fayetteville State University
Program in Nursing
Fayetteville, North Carolina

http://www.uncfsu.edu/nursing/
Founded in 1867
DEGREE · BSN

BACCALAUREATE PROGRAMS

Degree BSN
Available Programs Generic Baccalaureate; RN Baccalaureate.
Program Entrance Requirements Minimum overall college GPA of 2.0, transcript of college record, CPR certification, health exam, health insurance, high school biology, 2.0 years high school math, high school transcript, immunizations, minimum high school GPA of 2.0, minimum GPA in nursing prerequisites of 2.0, professional liability insurance/malpractice insurance, prerequisite course work, RN licensure. Transfer students are accepted.
Contact *Telephone:* 910-672-1925.

Gardner-Webb University
School of Nursing
Boiling Springs, North Carolina

http://www.gardner-webb.edu/
Founded in 1905

DEGREES • BSN • DNP • MSN • MSN/MBA
Nursing Program Faculty 52 (40% with doctorates).
Baccalaureate Enrollment 381 **Women** 92% **Men** 8% **Part-time** 37%
Graduate Enrollment 306 **Women** 94% **Men** 6% **Part-time** 17%
Distance Learning Courses Available.
Nursing Student Activities Sigma Theta Tau, Student Nurses' Association.
Nursing Student Resources Academic advising; academic or career counseling; assistance for students with disabilities; bookstore; campus computer network; computer lab; computer-assisted instruction; e-mail services; housing assistance; interactive nursing skills videos; Internet; learning resource lab; library services; nursing audiovisuals; other; paid internships; remedial services; resume preparation assistance; skills, simulation, or other laboratory; tutoring.
Library Facilities 6,002 volumes in health, 2,146 volumes in nursing; 7,808 periodical subscriptions health-care related.

BACCALAUREATE PROGRAMS

Degree BSN
Available Programs ADN to Baccalaureate; Generic Baccalaureate.
Study Options Full-time and part-time.
Online Degree Options Yes.
Program Entrance Requirements Minimum overall college GPA of 3.0, transcript of college record, CPR certification, written essay, high school biology, high school chemistry, high school transcript, immunizations, minimum high school GPA of 3.0, minimum GPA in nursing prerequisites of 3.00, professional liability insurance/malpractice insurance, prerequisite course work. Transfer students are accepted. *Application deadline:* 2/15 (fall). *Application fee:* $40.
Expenses (2015–16) *Tuition:* full-time $13,945; part-time $447 per credit hour. *Room and board:* $9280; room only: $4700 per academic year. *Required fees:* full-time $1870.
Financial Aid 90% of baccalaureate students in nursing programs received some form of financial aid in 2014–15. *Gift aid (need-based):* Federal Pell, FSEOG, state, private, college/university gift aid from institutional funds. *Loans:* Federal Direct (Subsidized and Unsubsidized Stafford PLUS), Perkins, state, alternative loans. *Work-study:* Federal Work-Study, part-time campus jobs. *Financial aid application deadline (priority):* 3/15.
Contact Dr. Candice Rome, Chair, School of Nursing, Gardner-Webb University, PO Box 7309, Boiling Springs, NC 28017. *Telephone:* 704-406-4365. *Fax:* 704-406-3919. *E-mail:* crome@gardner-webb.edu.

GRADUATE PROGRAMS

Expenses (2015–16) *Tuition:* full-time $6888; part-time $574 per credit hour. *Required fees:* full-time $400.
Financial Aid 90% of graduate students in nursing programs received some form of financial aid in 2014–15.
Contact Dr. Cindy Miller, Director of MSN Program, School of Nursing, Gardner-Webb University, PO Box 7309, Boiling Springs, NC 28017. *Telephone:* 704-406-4364. *Fax:* 704-406-3919. *E-mail:* mlmiller@gardner-webb.edu.

MASTER'S DEGREE PROGRAM

Degrees MSN; MSN/MBA
Available Programs Master's; Master's for Non-Nursing College Graduates; RN to Master's.
Concentrations Available Nursing administration; nursing education. *Nurse practitioner programs in:* family health.
Study Options Full-time and part-time.
Online Degree Options Yes.
Program Entrance Requirements Clinical experience, minimum overall college GPA of 3.0, transcript of college record, immunizations, 3 letters of recommendation, statistics course. *Application deadline:* Applications may be processed on a rolling basis for some programs. *Application fee:* $40.
Advanced Placement Credit given for nursing courses completed elsewhere dependent upon specific evaluations.
Degree Requirements 36 total credit hours, thesis or project.

POST-MASTER'S PROGRAM

Areas of Study Nursing administration; nursing education. *Nurse practitioner programs in:* family health.

DOCTORAL DEGREE PROGRAM

Degree DNP
Available Programs Doctorate.
Areas of Study Ethics, faculty preparation, gerontology, health policy, health promotion/disease prevention, health-care systems, human health and illness, information systems, nurse case management, nurse executive, nursing administration, nursing education, nursing policy, nursing research, nursing science.
Program Entrance Requirements Clinical experience, minimum overall college GPA of 3.2, interview by faculty committee, 3 letters of recommendation, MSN or equivalent, vita, writing sample. Application deadline: 10/15 (summer). Application fee: $40.
Degree Requirements 36 total credit hours.

Lees-McRae College
Nursing Program
Banner Elk, North Carolina

http://www.lmc.edu/academics/programs_of_study/nursing-health-sciences/nursing/index.htm
Founded in 1900

DEGREE • BSN
Nursing Program Faculty 6
Baccalaureate Enrollment 51 **Women** 88% **Men** 12%
Distance Learning Courses Available.
Nursing Student Resources Academic advising; academic or career counseling; bookstore; computer lab; computer-assisted instruction; e-mail services; Internet; learning resource lab; library services; nursing audiovisuals; skills, simulation, or other laboratory.

BACCALAUREATE PROGRAMS

Degree BSN
Available Programs ADN to Baccalaureate.
Site Options Spruce Pine, NC.
Study Options Full-time.
Online Degree Options Yes.
Program Entrance Requirements Transcript of college record, CPR certification, immunizations, 2 letters of recommendation, professional liability insurance/malpractice insurance, RN licensure. Transfer students are accepted. *Application deadline:* 8/1 (fall). Applications may be processed on a rolling basis for some programs.
Contact *Telephone:* 828-898-2428. *Fax:* 828-898-2598.

Lenoir-Rhyne University
Program in Nursing
Hickory, North Carolina

http://nur.lr.edu/
Founded in 1891

DEGREES • BS • MSN
Nursing Program Faculty 30 (4% with doctorates).
Baccalaureate Enrollment 300 **Women** 90% **Men** 10% **Part-time** 2%
Graduate Enrollment 45 **Women** 98% **Men** 2% **Part-time** 50%
Distance Learning Courses Available.
Nursing Student Activities Sigma Theta Tau, Student Nurses' Association.
Nursing Student Resources Academic advising; academic or career counseling; assistance for students with disabilities; bookstore; campus computer network; career placement assistance; computer lab; computer-assisted instruction; e-mail services; employment services for current students; externships; housing assistance; interactive nursing skills videos; Internet; learning resource lab; library services; nursing audiovisuals; placement services for program completers; remedial services; resume preparation assistance; skills, simulation, or other laboratory; tutoring; unpaid internships.
Library Facilities 5,000 volumes in health, 4,200 volumes in nursing; 220 periodical subscriptions health-care related.

BACCALAUREATE PROGRAMS

Degree BS
Available Programs ADN to Baccalaureate; Generic Baccalaureate.
Study Options Full-time and part-time.
Program Entrance Requirements Minimum overall college GPA of 3.0, transcript of college record, CPR certification, written essay, health exam, high school chemistry, high school foreign language, 3 years high school math, high school transcript, immunizations, minimum high school GPA of 3.0, minimum GPA in nursing prerequisites of 2.9, prerequisite course work. Transfer students are accepted. *Application deadline:* 3/1 (fall), 4/1 (summer). Applications may be processed on a rolling basis for some programs. *Application fee:* $35.
Advanced Placement Credit by examination available. Credit given for nursing courses completed elsewhere dependent upon specific evaluations.
Financial Aid 100% of baccalaureate students in nursing programs received some form of financial aid in 2013–14.
Contact Dr. Kerry C. Thompson, Chair, School of Nursing, Program in Nursing, Lenoir-Rhyne University, PO Box 7292, Hickory, NC 28603. *Telephone:* 828-328-7282. *Fax:* 828-328-7284.
E-mail: thompsonk@lr.edu.

GRADUATE PROGRAMS

Expenses (2014–15) *Tuition:* part-time $500 per credit hour.
Contact Dr. Kerry C. Thompson, Chair, School of Nursing, Program in Nursing, Lenoir-Rhyne University, Box 7292, Hickory, NC 28601. *Telephone:* 828-328-7282. *E-mail:* thompsonk@lr.edu.

MASTER'S DEGREE PROGRAM

Degree MSN
Available Programs Master's; RN to Master's.
Concentrations Available Health-care administration; nursing education.
Site Options Asheville, NC.
Study Options Full-time and part-time.
Program Entrance Requirements Computer literacy, minimum overall college GPA of 3.0, transcript of college record, CPR certification, immunizations, interview, 2 letters of recommendation, nursing research course, resume, statistics course. *Application deadline:* Applications may be processed on a rolling basis for some programs. *Application fee:* $35.
Advanced Placement Credit given for nursing courses completed elsewhere dependent upon specific evaluations.
Degree Requirements 36 total credit hours, thesis or project.

Methodist University
Department of Nursing
Fayetteville, North Carolina

http://www.methodist.edu/nursing
Founded in 1956
DEGREE • BSN
Nursing Program Faculty 14 (21% with doctorates).
Baccalaureate Enrollment 49
Nursing Student Activities Student Nurses' Association, nursing club.
Nursing Student Resources Academic advising; academic or career counseling; assistance for students with disabilities; bookstore; campus computer network; career placement assistance; computer lab; computer-assisted instruction; e-mail services; employment services for current students; externships; housing assistance; interactive nursing skills videos; Internet; learning resource lab; library services; nursing audiovisuals; other; paid internships; placement services for program completers; remedial services; resume preparation assistance; skills, simulation, or other laboratory; tutoring; unpaid internships.
Library Facilities 1,000 volumes in health, 200 volumes in nursing; 55 periodical subscriptions health-care related.

BACCALAUREATE PROGRAMS

Degree BSN
Available Programs Generic Baccalaureate; RN Baccalaureate.
Study Options Full-time.
Program Entrance Requirements Transcript of college record, CPR certification, health insurance, high school chemistry, high school foreign language, 2 years high school math, immunizations, minimum high school GPA of 2.6, prerequisite course work. Transfer students are accepted. *Application deadline:* 2/15 (fall).

Expenses (2015–16) *Tuition:* full-time $27,830; part-time $928 per credit hour. *Room and board:* $10,804 per academic year. *Required fees:* full-time $1250.
Financial Aid 98% of baccalaureate students in nursing programs received some form of financial aid in 2014–15.
Contact Ms. Jennifer Caviness, Coordinator of Admissions, Department of Nursing, Methodist University, 5400 Ramsey Street, Fayetteville, NC 28314. *Telephone:* 910-630-7578. *Fax:* 910-630-7006.
E-mail: jcaviness@methodist.edu.

North Carolina Agricultural and Technical State University
School of Nursing
Greensboro, North Carolina

http://www.ncat.edu/academics/schools-colleges1/son/index.html
Founded in 1891
DEGREE • BSN
Nursing Program Faculty 29 (15% with doctorates).
Baccalaureate Enrollment 110 **Women** 91% **Men** 9%
Nursing Student Activities Sigma Theta Tau, Student Nurses' Association, nursing club.
Nursing Student Resources Academic advising; academic or career counseling; assistance for students with disabilities; bookstore; campus computer network; career placement assistance; computer lab; computer-assisted instruction; e-mail services; housing assistance; interactive nursing skills videos; Internet; learning resource lab; library services; nursing audiovisuals; remedial services; resume preparation assistance; skills, simulation, or other laboratory; tutoring.

BACCALAUREATE PROGRAMS

Degree BSN
Available Programs Accelerated Baccalaureate for Second Degree; Generic Baccalaureate; RN Baccalaureate.
Site Options Greensboro, NC.
Study Options Full-time.
Program Entrance Requirements Minimum overall college GPA of 2.8, transcript of college record, CPR certification, written essay, health exam, health insurance, high school biology, high school foreign language, 3 years high school math, 3 years high school science, high school transcript, immunizations, minimum high school GPA of 3.0, minimum GPA in nursing prerequisites of 2.8, professional liability insurance/malpractice insurance, prerequisite course work. Transfer students are accepted. *Application deadline:* 2/15 (spring). *Application fee:* $45.
Contact *Telephone:* 336-334-7750. *Fax:* 336-334-7637.

North Carolina Central University
Department of Nursing
Durham, North Carolina

http://www.nccu.edu/
Founded in 1910
DEGREE • BSN
Nursing Program Faculty 30 (4% with doctorates).
Nursing Student Activities Sigma Theta Tau.
Nursing Student Resources Academic advising; academic or career counseling; assistance for students with disabilities; bookstore; campus computer network; career placement assistance; computer lab; computer-assisted instruction; e-mail services; employment services for current students; externships; housing assistance; interactive nursing skills videos; Internet; learning resource lab; library services; nursing audiovisuals; paid internships; placement services for program completers; resume preparation assistance; skills, simulation, or other laboratory; tutoring.

BACCALAUREATE PROGRAMS

Degree BSN
Available Programs Generic Baccalaureate.
Study Options Full-time.

Program Entrance Requirements Minimum overall college GPA of 2.0, transcript of college record, health exam, immunizations, minimum GPA in nursing prerequisites of 2.5, professional liability insurance/malpractice insurance, prerequisite course work. Transfer students are accepted.
Advanced Placement Credit given for nursing courses completed elsewhere dependent upon specific evaluations.
Contact *Telephone:* 919-530-5336. *Fax:* 919-530-5343.

Pfeiffer University
Department of Nursing
Misenheimer, North Carolina

http://misenheimer.pfeiffer.edu/misenheimer/academics/divisions/division-of-applied-health-sciences/nursing-department
Founded in 1885
DEGREE • BS
Nursing Program Faculty 5 (5% with doctorates).
Baccalaureate Enrollment 37
Nursing Student Activities Student Nurses' Association, nursing club.
Nursing Student Resources Academic advising; academic or career counseling; assistance for students with disabilities; bookstore; career placement assistance; computer lab; computer-assisted instruction; e-mail services; externships; Internet; learning resource lab; library services; nursing audiovisuals; remedial services; resume preparation assistance; skills, simulation, or other laboratory; tutoring.

BACCALAUREATE PROGRAMS

Degree BS
Available Programs RN Baccalaureate.
Contact Nursing Department, Department of Nursing, Pfeiffer University, 48380 US Highway 52, Misenheimer, NC 28109. *Telephone:* 800-338-2060. *E-mail:* nursing@pfeiffer.edu.

Queens University of Charlotte
Presbyterian School of Nursing
Charlotte, North Carolina

http://www.queens.edu/nursing/
Founded in 1857
DEGREES • BSN • MSN • MSN/MBA
Nursing Program Faculty 60 (20% with doctorates).
Baccalaureate Enrollment 260 **Women** 95% **Men** 5% **Part-time** 10%
Graduate Enrollment 55 **Women** 95% **Men** 5% **Part-time** 50%
Distance Learning Courses Available.
Nursing Student Activities Nursing Honor Society, Sigma Theta Tau, Student Nurses' Association.
Nursing Student Resources Academic advising; academic or career counseling; assistance for students with disabilities; bookstore; campus computer network; career placement assistance; computer lab; computer-assisted instruction; e-mail services; employment services for current students; externships; housing assistance; interactive nursing skills videos; Internet; learning resource lab; library services; nursing audiovisuals; placement services for program completers; remedial services; resume preparation assistance; skills, simulation, or other laboratory; tutoring; unpaid internships.
Library Facilities 1,703 volumes in health, 713 volumes in nursing; 516 periodical subscriptions health-care related.

BACCALAUREATE PROGRAMS

Degree BSN
Available Programs ADN to Baccalaureate; Accelerated Baccalaureate; Accelerated Baccalaureate for Second Degree; Baccalaureate for Second Degree; Generic Baccalaureate; RN Baccalaureate.
Site Options Charlotte, NC.
Study Options Full-time.
Online Degree Options Yes.
Program Entrance Requirements Minimum overall college GPA of 3.0, transcript of college record, CPR certification, written essay, health exam, health insurance, high school biology, high school chemistry, 2 years high school math, 1 year of high school science, high school transcript, immunizations, minimum high school GPA of 3.0, minimum GPA in nursing prerequisites of 3.0, prerequisite course work. Transfer stu-

dents are accepted. *Application deadline:* 3/15 (fall), 9/21 (spring). *Application fee:* $40.
Advanced Placement Credit given for nursing courses completed elsewhere dependent upon specific evaluations.
Contact *Telephone:* 704-337-2314. *Fax:* 704-337-2415.

GRADUATE PROGRAMS

Contact *Telephone:* 704-337-2314. *Fax:* 704-337-2415.

MASTER'S DEGREE PROGRAM
Degrees MSN; MSN/MBA
Available Programs Master's; RN to Master's.
Concentrations Available Clinical nurse leader; nursing administration; nursing education.
Site Options Charlotte, NC.
Study Options Full-time and part-time.
Online Degree Options Yes (online only).
Program Entrance Requirements Minimum overall college GPA of 3.0, transcript of college record, written essay, professional liability insurance/malpractice insurance, resume. *Application deadline:* Applications may be processed on a rolling basis for some programs. *Application fee:* $40.
Advanced Placement Credit given for nursing courses completed elsewhere dependent upon specific evaluations.
Degree Requirements 36 total credit hours, thesis or project.

CONTINUING EDUCATION PROGRAM

Contact *Telephone:* 704-688-2838.

University of Mount Olive
Department of Nursing
Mount Olive, North Carolina

https://www.umo.edu/
Founded in 1951
DEGREE • BSN

BACCALAUREATE PROGRAMS

Degree BSN
Available Programs RN Baccalaureate.
Online Degree Options Yes (online only).
Contact Joy A. Kieffer, Chair, Department of Nursing, University of Mount Olive, 634 Henderson Street, Mount Olive, NC 28365. *Telephone:* 919-299-4930. *E-mail:* jkieffer@umo.edu.

The University of North Carolina at Chapel Hill
School of Nursing
Chapel Hill, North Carolina

http://nursing.unc.edu/
Founded in 1789
DEGREES • BSN • DNP • MSN • PHD
Nursing Program Faculty 141 (70% with doctorates).
Baccalaureate Enrollment 334 **Women** 84.7% **Men** 15.3%
Graduate Enrollment 324 **Women** 89.2% **Men** 10.8% **Part-time** 39.2%
Distance Learning Courses Available.
Nursing Student Activities Sigma Theta Tau, Student Nurses' Association, nursing club.
Nursing Student Resources Academic advising; academic or career counseling; assistance for students with disabilities; bookstore; campus computer network; career placement assistance; computer lab; computer-assisted instruction; daycare for children of students; e-mail services; employment services for current students; housing assistance; interactive nursing skills videos; Internet; learning resource lab; library services; nursing audiovisuals; other; remedial services; resume preparation assistance; skills, simulation, or other laboratory; tutoring.
Library Facilities 347,000 volumes in health, 9,200 volumes in nursing; 200,000 periodical subscriptions health-care related.

BACCALAUREATE PROGRAMS

Degree BSN
Available Programs Accelerated Baccalaureate; Accelerated Baccalaureate for Second Degree; Baccalaureate for Second Degree; Generic Baccalaureate.
Study Options Full-time.
Program Entrance Requirements Minimum overall college GPA of 2.8, transcript of college record, CPR certification, written essay, health exam, health insurance, high school transcript, immunizations, minimum GPA in nursing prerequisites, professional liability insurance/malpractice insurance, prerequisite course work. Transfer students are accepted. *Application deadline:* 8/10 (spring), 12/22 (summer). *Application fee:* $80.
Advanced Placement Credit given for nursing courses completed elsewhere dependent upon specific evaluations.
Financial Aid 95% of baccalaureate students in nursing programs received some form of financial aid in 2014–15. *Gift aid (need-based):* Federal Pell, FSEOG, state, private, college/university gift aid from institutional funds. *Loans:* Federal Direct (Subsidized and Unsubsidized Stafford PLUS), Perkins, state, college/university, alternative loans. *Work-study:* Federal Work-Study. *Financial aid application deadline (priority):* 3/1.
Contact Ms. Carlee Meritt, Assistant Director for Undergraduate Admissions, School of Nursing, The University of North Carolina at Chapel Hill, CB #7460, Chapel Hill, NC 27599-7460. *Telephone:* 919-966-4260. *Fax:* 919-966-3540. *E-mail:* carlee_meritt@unc.edu.

GRADUATE PROGRAMS

Financial Aid 8 fellowships, 6 research assistantships (averaging $8,000 per year), 10 teaching assistantships (averaging $8,000 per year) were awarded; scholarships, traineeships, and unspecified assistantships also available.
Contact Ms. Emily Sayed, Assistant Director, Graduate Admissions, School of Nursing, The University of North Carolina at Chapel Hill, Carrington Hall, CB #7460, Chapel Hill, NC 27599-7460. *Telephone:* 919-966-4260. *Fax:* 919-966-3540. *E-mail:* sayed@unc.edu.

MASTER'S DEGREE PROGRAM

Degree MSN
Available Programs Master's; RN to Master's.
Concentrations Available Clinical nurse leader; health-care administration; nursing education; nursing informatics. *Nurse practitioner programs in:* adult health, family health, gerontology, pediatric primary care, psychiatric/mental health.
Study Options Full-time and part-time.
Program Entrance Requirements Clinical experience, minimum overall college GPA of 3.0, transcript of college record, CPR certification, written essay, immunizations, 3 letters of recommendation, professional liability insurance/malpractice insurance, resume, statistics course. *Application deadline:* 12/16 (fall). *Application fee:* $85.
Advanced Placement Credit given for nursing courses completed elsewhere dependent upon specific evaluations.
Degree Requirements 42 total credit hours, thesis or project, comprehensive exam.

POST-MASTER'S PROGRAM

Areas of Study Clinical nurse leader; nursing informatics. *Nurse practitioner programs in:* psychiatric/mental health.

DOCTORAL DEGREE PROGRAM

Degree DNP
Available Programs Doctorate.
Areas of Study Advanced practice nursing, family health, gerontology, health policy, health-care systems, information systems, nursing administration, nursing science, oncology.
Program Entrance Requirements Minimum overall college GPA of 3.0, clinical experience, 3 letters of recommendation, statistics course, vita, writing sample. Application deadline: 12/16 (fall). Applications may be processed on a rolling basis for some programs. Application fee: $85.
Degree Requirements 66 total credit hours, Capstone project.

Degree PhD
Available Programs Doctorate; Post-Baccalaureate Doctorate.
Areas of Study Addiction/substance abuse, advanced practice nursing, aging, bio-behavioral research, biology of health and illness, clinical nurse leader, clinical practice, clinical research, ethics, family health, gerontology, health policy, health promotion/disease prevention, health-care systems, human health and illness, illness and transition, individualized study, information systems, legal nurse consultant, maternity-newborn, neuro-behavior, nursing administration, nursing research, nursing science, oncology.
Program Entrance Requirements Clinical experience, minimum overall college GPA of 3.0, 3 letters of recommendation, statistics course, vita, writing sample. Application deadline: 12/16 (fall). Applications may be processed on a rolling basis for some programs. Application fee: $85.
Degree Requirements 54 total credit hours.

POSTDOCTORAL PROGRAM

Areas of Study Addiction/substance abuse, adolescent health, aging, cancer care, chronic illness, community health, family health, gerontology, health promotion/disease prevention, individualized study, infection prevention/skin care, information systems, neuro-behavior, nursing informatics, nursing interventions, nursing research, nursing science, outcomes, self-care, vulnerable population, women's health.
Postdoctoral Program Contact Dr. Barbara Mark, Director, PhD and Post-Doctoral Programs, School of Nursing, The University of North Carolina at Chapel Hill, Carrington Hall, CB #7460, Chapel Hill, NC 27599-7460. *Telephone:* 919-843-6209. *E-mail:* bmark@email.unc.edu.

CONTINUING EDUCATION PROGRAM

Contact Dr. Sonda Oppewal, Director, Center for Lifelong Learning, School of Nursing, The University of North Carolina at Chapel Hill, L400 Carrington Hall, CB #7460, Chapel Hill, NC 27599-7460. *Telephone:* 919-966-3638. *Fax:* 919-966-7298. *E-mail:* oppewal@email.unc.edu.

The University of North Carolina at Charlotte
School of Nursing
Charlotte, North Carolina

http://www.nursing.uncc.edu/
Founded in 1946
DEGREES • BSN • MSN
Nursing Program Faculty 51 (50% with doctorates).
Baccalaureate Enrollment 330 **Women** 92% **Men** 8% **Part-time** 5%
Graduate Enrollment 200 **Women** 80% **Men** 20% **Part-time** 65%
Distance Learning Courses Available.
Nursing Student Activities Sigma Theta Tau, Student Nurses' Association.
Nursing Student Resources Academic advising; academic or career counseling; assistance for students with disabilities; bookstore; campus computer network; career placement assistance; computer lab; computer-assisted instruction; e-mail services; externships; interactive nursing skills videos; Internet; learning resource lab; library services; nursing audiovisuals; resume preparation assistance; skills, simulation, or other laboratory; tutoring.
Library Facilities 39,000 volumes in health, 2,400 volumes in nursing; 160 periodical subscriptions health-care related.

BACCALAUREATE PROGRAMS

Degree BSN
Available Programs ADN to Baccalaureate; Generic Baccalaureate; RN Baccalaureate.
Study Options Full-time.
Program Entrance Requirements Minimum overall college GPA of 2.5, transcript of college record, CPR certification, written essay, health exam, health insurance, high school biology, high school chemistry, high school foreign language, 3 years high school math, 3 years high school science, high school transcript, immunizations, 3 letters of recommendation, minimum GPA in nursing prerequisites of 2.5, prerequisite course work. Transfer students are accepted. *Application deadline:* 1/31 (fall), 8/31 (winter).
Contact *Telephone:* 704-687-4676. *Fax:* 704-687-3180.

GRADUATE PROGRAMS

Contact *Telephone:* 704-687-7992. *Fax:* 704-687-6017.

MASTER'S DEGREE PROGRAM

Degree MSN
Available Programs Master's; RN to Master's.

Concentrations Available Nurse anesthesia; nursing administration; nursing education. *Clinical nurse specialist programs in:* community health. *Nurse practitioner programs in:* adult health, family health.
Study Options Full-time and part-time.
Online Degree Options Yes.
Program Entrance Requirements Clinical experience, computer literacy, minimum overall college GPA of 3.0, transcript of college record, CPR certification, written essay, immunizations, interview, 3 letters of recommendation, nursing research course, professional liability insurance/malpractice insurance, resume, statistics course.

POST-MASTER'S PROGRAM

Areas of Study Nurse anesthesia; nursing administration; nursing education. *Nurse practitioner programs in:* family health.

The University of North Carolina at Greensboro

School of Nursing
Greensboro, North Carolina

http://nursing.uncg.edu
Founded in 1891

DEGREES • BSN • DNP • MSN • MSN/MBA • PHD

Nursing Program Faculty 65 (51% with doctorates).
Baccalaureate Enrollment 399 **Women** 86% **Men** 14%
Graduate Enrollment 205
Distance Learning Courses Available.
Nursing Student Activities Nursing Honor Society, Sigma Theta Tau, Student Nurses' Association, nursing club.
Nursing Student Resources Academic advising; academic or career counseling; assistance for students with disabilities; bookstore; campus computer network; career placement assistance; computer lab; computer-assisted instruction; e-mail services; externships; interactive nursing skills videos; Internet; learning resource lab; library services; nursing audiovisuals; paid internships; placement services for program completers; remedial services; resume preparation assistance; skills, simulation, or other laboratory; tutoring; unpaid internships.
Library Facilities 79 periodical subscriptions health-care related.

BACCALAUREATE PROGRAMS

Degree BSN
Available Programs ADN to Baccalaureate; Baccalaureate for Second Degree; Generic Baccalaureate; RN Baccalaureate.
Site Options Lexington, NC; Greensboro, NC.
Study Options Full-time.
Program Entrance Requirements Minimum overall college GPA of 3.0, transcript of college record, CPR certification, health exam, minimum GPA in nursing prerequisites of 3.0, prerequisite course work. Transfer students are accepted. *Application deadline:* 2/1 (fall). *Application fee:* $55.
Advanced Placement Credit given for nursing courses completed elsewhere dependent upon specific evaluations.
Expenses (2015–16) *Tuition, state resident:* full-time $4129; part-time $516 per credit. *Tuition, nonresident:* full-time $8258; part-time $1032 per credit. *International tuition:* $8258 full-time. *Room and board:* $9743; room only: $6281 per academic year. *Required fees:* full-time $1938; part-time $1938 per term.
Financial Aid 69% of baccalaureate students in nursing programs received some form of financial aid in 2014–15. *Gift aid (need-based):* Federal Pell, FSEOG, state, private, college/university gift aid from institutional funds. *Loans:* Federal Direct (Subsidized and Unsubsidized Stafford PLUS), Perkins, state, college/university. *Work-study:* Federal Work-Study. *Financial aid application deadline (priority):* 3/1.
Contact Dr. Susan A. Letvak, Director, Undergraduate Programs, School of Nursing, The University of North Carolina at Greensboro, PO Box 26170, Greensboro, NC 27402-6170. *Telephone:* 336-256-1024. *Fax:* 336-334-3628. *E-mail:* saletvak@uncg.edu.

GRADUATE PROGRAMS

Expenses (2015–16) *Tuition, state resident:* full-time $4873; part-time $609 per credit. *Tuition, nonresident:* full-time $9746; part-time $1218 per credit. *International tuition:* $9746 full-time. *Room and board:* $9743; room only: $6281 per academic year. *Required fees:* full-time $2572; part-time $103 per credit; part-time $700 per term.

Financial Aid 75% of graduate students in nursing programs received some form of financial aid in 2014–15. Research assistantships with full tuition reimbursements available, career-related internships or fieldwork, Federal Work-Study, scholarships, and traineeships available. Aid available to part-time students.
Contact Dr. Heidi V. Krowchuk, Associate Dean for Academic Programs, School of Nursing, The University of North Carolina at Greensboro, PO Box 26170, Greensboro, NC 27402-6170. *Telephone:* 336-334-4899. *Fax:* 336-334-3628. *E-mail:* hvkrowch@uncg.edu.

MASTER'S DEGREE PROGRAM

Degrees MSN; MSN/MBA
Available Programs Master's.
Concentrations Available Nursing administration; nursing education. *Nurse practitioner programs in:* adult health.
Site Options Raleigh, NC.
Study Options Full-time and part-time.
Online Degree Options Yes (online only).
Program Entrance Requirements Clinical experience, minimum overall college GPA of 3.2, transcript of college record, written essay, 3 letters of recommendation, physical assessment course, statistics course, GRE General Test or MAT. *Application deadline:* Applications may be processed on a rolling basis for some programs. *Application fee:* $65.
Advanced Placement Credit given for nursing courses completed elsewhere dependent upon specific evaluations.
Degree Requirements 38 total credit hours.

POST-MASTER'S PROGRAM

Areas of Study *Nurse practitioner programs in:* adult health.

DOCTORAL DEGREE PROGRAM

Degree DNP
Available Programs Doctorate; Post-Baccalaureate Doctorate.
Areas of Study Advanced practice nursing, gerontology, health-care systems, nursing administration.
Program Entrance Requirements Clinical experience, minimum overall college GPA of 3.2, interview by faculty committee, interview, 3 letters of recommendation, statistics course, vita, writing sample. *Application deadline:* 11/1 (fall). *Application fee:* $60.
Degree Requirements 73 total credit hours, written exam, residency.

Degree PhD
Available Programs Doctorate.
Areas of Study Clinical research, nursing research, nursing science.
Program Entrance Requirements Minimum overall college GPA of 3.0, clinical experience, interview, interview with faculty committee, 3 letters of recommendation, statistics course, vita, writing sample. *Application deadline:* Applications are processed on a rolling basis. *Application fee:* $60.
Degree Requirements 57 total credit hours, dissertation, oral exam, residency, written exam.

The University of North Carolina at Pembroke

Nursing Program
Pembroke, North Carolina

http://www.uncp.edu/nursing/
Founded in 1887

DEGREE • BSN

Nursing Program Faculty 20 (5% with doctorates).
Baccalaureate Enrollment 139
Distance Learning Courses Available.
Nursing Student Activities Student Nurses' Association.
Nursing Student Resources Academic advising; academic or career counseling; assistance for students with disabilities; bookstore; campus computer network; computer lab; computer-assisted instruction; e-mail services; housing assistance; interactive nursing skills videos; Internet; learning resource lab; library services; nursing audiovisuals; remedial services; resume preparation assistance; skills, simulation, or other laboratory; tutoring.

BACCALAUREATE PROGRAMS

Degree BSN
Available Programs Generic Baccalaureate; RN Baccalaureate.
Site Options Southern Pines, NC; Fayetteville, NC; Hamlet, NC.

Study Options Full-time.
Program Entrance Requirements Minimum overall college GPA, health exam, minimum GPA in nursing prerequisites, prerequisite course work, RN licensure. Transfer students are accepted. *Application deadline:* 1/15 (spring).
Advanced Placement Credit given for nursing courses completed elsewhere dependent upon specific evaluations.
Contact *Telephone:* 910-521-6522. *Fax:* 910-521-6178.

The University of North Carolina Wilmington
School of Nursing
Wilmington, North Carolina

http://www.uncw.edu/son
Founded in 1947
DEGREES • BS • MSN
Nursing Program Faculty 58 (50% with doctorates).
Baccalaureate Enrollment 1,021 **Women** 90% **Men** 10% **Part-time** 63%
Graduate Enrollment 85 **Women** 85% **Men** 15% **Part-time** 52%
Distance Learning Courses Available.
Nursing Student Activities Sigma Theta Tau, Student Nurses' Association.
Nursing Student Resources Academic advising; academic or career counseling; assistance for students with disabilities; bookstore; campus computer network; career placement assistance; computer lab; computer-assisted instruction; e-mail services; employment services for current students; externships; housing assistance; interactive nursing skills videos; Internet; learning resource lab; library services; nursing audiovisuals; remedial services; resume preparation assistance; skills, simulation, or other laboratory; tutoring; unpaid internships.
Library Facilities 13,420 volumes in health, 2,869 volumes in nursing; 494 periodical subscriptions health-care related.

BACCALAUREATE PROGRAMS

Degree BS
Available Programs Generic Baccalaureate; RN Baccalaureate.
Study Options Full-time.
Online Degree Options Yes.
Program Entrance Requirements Minimum overall college GPA of 2.7, transcript of college record, CPR certification, health exam, health insurance, immunizations, minimum GPA in nursing prerequisites of 2.7, professional liability insurance/malpractice insurance, prerequisite course work. Transfer students are accepted. *Application deadline:* 12/15 (fall), 7/1 (spring).
Advanced Placement Credit given for nursing courses completed elsewhere dependent upon specific evaluations.
Expenses (2015–16) *Tuition, state resident:* full-time $4188; part-time $141 per credit hour. *Tuition, nonresident:* full-time $18,054; part-time $610 per credit hour. *Room and board:* $9466; room only: $5706 per academic year. *Required fees:* full-time $2503; part-time $16 per credit.
Financial Aid 37% of baccalaureate students in nursing programs received some form of financial aid in 2014–15.
Contact Ms. Jennine Strange, Counselor, School of Nursing, The University of North Carolina Wilmington, 601 South College Road, Wilmington, NC 28403-5995. *Telephone:* 910-962-3208. *Fax:* 910-962-7656. *E-mail:* werbeachm@uncw.edu.

GRADUATE PROGRAMS

Expenses (2015–16) *Tuition, state resident:* full-time $4329. *Tuition, nonresident:* full-time $16,420. *Room and board:* $11,051; room only: $8246 per academic year. *Required fees:* full-time $2459.
Contact Ms. Jennine Strange, CHHS Office of Student Success, School of Nursing, The University of North Carolina Wilmington, 601 South College Road, Wilmington, NC 28403-5995. *Telephone:* 910-962-3208. *Fax:* 910-962-4921. *E-mail:* chhs@uncw.edu.

MASTER'S DEGREE PROGRAM
Degree MSN
Available Programs Master's.
Concentrations Available *Nurse practitioner programs in:* family health.
Study Options Full-time and part-time.

Program Entrance Requirements Clinical experience, computer literacy, minimum overall college GPA of 3.0, transcript of college record, CPR certification, written essay, immunizations, 3 letters of recommendation, physical assessment course, professional liability insurance/malpractice insurance, prerequisite course work, resume, statistics course, GRE General Test. *Application deadline:* 3/1 (fall). *Application fee:* $60.
Advanced Placement Credit given for nursing courses completed elsewhere dependent upon specific evaluations.
Degree Requirements 47 total credit hours, comprehensive exam.

POST-MASTER'S PROGRAM
Areas of Study *Nurse practitioner programs in:* family health.

Western Carolina University
School of Nursing
Cullowhee, North Carolina

http://www.wcu.edu/
Founded in 1889
DEGREES • BSN • MS
Nursing Program Faculty 31 (50% with doctorates).
Baccalaureate Enrollment 200 **Women** 94% **Men** 6%
Graduate Enrollment 122 **Women** 90% **Men** 10%
Distance Learning Courses Available.
Nursing Student Activities Sigma Theta Tau, Student Nurses' Association.
Nursing Student Resources Academic advising; academic or career counseling; assistance for students with disabilities; bookstore; campus computer network; career placement assistance; computer lab; computer-assisted instruction; daycare for children of students; e-mail services; externships; housing assistance; interactive nursing skills videos; Internet; learning resource lab; library services; nursing audiovisuals; resume preparation assistance; skills, simulation, or other laboratory; tutoring.
Library Facilities 10,000 volumes in health, 900 volumes in nursing; 70 periodical subscriptions health-care related.

BACCALAUREATE PROGRAMS

Degree BSN
Available Programs Accelerated Baccalaureate; Generic Baccalaureate; RN Baccalaureate.
Site Options Enka, NC.
Study Options Full-time.
Online Degree Options Yes.
Program Entrance Requirements Minimum overall college GPA of 3.0, transcript of college record, CPR certification, health exam, high school transcript, immunizations, minimum GPA in nursing prerequisites of 2.0, professional liability insurance/malpractice insurance, prerequisite course work. Transfer students are accepted. *Application deadline:* 2/1 (fall), 7/1 (spring). *Application fee:* $45.
Contact *Telephone:* 828-227-7467. *Fax:* 828-227-7052.

GRADUATE PROGRAMS

Contact *Telephone:* 828-670-8810 Ext. 247.

MASTER'S DEGREE PROGRAM
Degree MS
Available Programs Master's.
Concentrations Available Nurse anesthesia; nursing administration; nursing education. *Nurse practitioner programs in:* family health.
Site Options Enka, NC.
Study Options Full-time and part-time.
Online Degree Options Yes.
Program Entrance Requirements Clinical experience, minimum overall college GPA of 3.0, transcript of college record, CPR certification, written essay, immunizations, interview, 3 letters of recommendation, nursing research course, physical assessment course, professional liability insurance/malpractice insurance, resume, statistics course. *Application deadline:* 4/15 (fall), 10/15 (winter). *Application fee:* $45.
Advanced Placement Credit given for nursing courses completed elsewhere dependent upon specific evaluations.
Degree Requirements Thesis or project, comprehensive exam.

POST-MASTER'S PROGRAM
Areas of Study Nursing administration; nursing education. *Nurse practitioner programs in:* family health.

POSTDOCTORAL PROGRAM
Postdoctoral Program Contact *Telephone:* 828-227-7467. *Fax:* 828-227-7071.

Wingate University
Department of Nursing
Wingate, North Carolina

https://www.wingate.edu/
Founded in 1896
DEGREE • BSN

BACCALAUREATE PROGRAMS

Degree BSN
Available Programs RN Baccalaureate.
Contact Dr. Kristen G. Barbee, Director, Department of Nursing, Department of Nursing, Wingate University, 211-A East Wilson Street, Wingate, NC 28174. *Telephone:* 704-233-8653.
E-mail: nursing@wingate.edu.

Winston-Salem State University
Department of Nursing
Winston-Salem, North Carolina

http://www.wssu.edu/
Founded in 1892
DEGREES • BSN • MSN
Nursing Program Faculty 34 (13% with doctorates).
Baccalaureate Enrollment 252 **Women** 77% **Men** 23%
Graduate Enrollment 15
Nursing Student Activities Nursing Honor Society, Sigma Theta Tau, Student Nurses' Association.
Nursing Student Resources Academic advising; academic or career counseling; assistance for students with disabilities; bookstore; campus computer network; computer lab; interactive nursing skills videos; learning resource lab; nursing audiovisuals; skills, simulation, or other laboratory.
Library Facilities 4,381 volumes in health, 2,691 volumes in nursing; 2,205 periodical subscriptions health-care related.

BACCALAUREATE PROGRAMS

Degree BSN
Available Programs ADN to Baccalaureate; Accelerated RN Baccalaureate; Baccalaureate for Second Degree; Generic Baccalaureate; LPN to Baccalaureate; RN Baccalaureate.
Site Options Wilkesboro, NC; Salisbury, NC; Boone, NC.
Study Options Full-time.
Program Entrance Requirements Minimum overall college GPA of 2.6, transcript of college record, CPR certification, health exam, immunizations, professional liability insurance/malpractice insurance, prerequisite course work. Transfer students are accepted.
Advanced Placement Credit by examination available. Credit given for nursing courses completed elsewhere dependent upon specific evaluations.
Contact *Telephone:* 336-750-2560. *Fax:* 336-750-2599.

GRADUATE PROGRAMS

Contact *Telephone:* 336-750-2275. *Fax:* 336-750-2007.

MASTER'S DEGREE PROGRAM
Degree MSN
Available Programs Master's.
Concentrations Available Nursing education. *Nurse practitioner programs in:* family health, psychiatric/mental health.
Study Options Full-time and part-time.
Program Entrance Requirements Clinical experience, transcript of college record, CPR certification, immunizations, interview, 3 letters of recommendation, nursing research course, physical assessment course, professional liability insurance/malpractice insurance, resume, statistics course.
Advanced Placement Credit given for nursing courses completed elsewhere dependent upon specific evaluations.
Degree Requirements 50 total credit hours, thesis or project.

CONTINUING EDUCATION PROGRAM
Contact *Telephone:* 336-750-2665. *Fax:* 336-750-2599.

NORTH DAKOTA

Dickinson State University
Department of Nursing
Dickinson, North Dakota

http://www.dickinsonstate.edu/
Founded in 1918
DEGREE • BSN
Nursing Program Faculty 5 (20% with doctorates).
Baccalaureate Enrollment 33 **Women** 94% **Men** 6% **Part-time** 33%
Nursing Student Activities Student Nurses' Association.
Nursing Student Resources Academic advising; academic or career counseling; assistance for students with disabilities; bookstore; campus computer network; career placement assistance; computer lab; computer-assisted instruction; e-mail services; employment services for current students; externships; housing assistance; interactive nursing skills videos; Internet; learning resource lab; library services; nursing audiovisuals; other; placement services for program completers; remedial services; resume preparation assistance; skills, simulation, or other laboratory; tutoring; unpaid internships.
Library Facilities 1,211 volumes in health, 821 volumes in nursing; 51 periodical subscriptions health-care related.

BACCALAUREATE PROGRAMS

Degree BSN
Available Programs ADN to Baccalaureate; LPN to Baccalaureate; LPN to RN Baccalaureate; RN Baccalaureate.
Study Options Full-time and part-time.
Program Entrance Requirements Minimum overall college GPA of 2.5, transcript of college record, CPR certification, health exam, health insurance, high school chemistry, immunizations, minimum GPA in nursing prerequisites of 2.5, prerequisite course work. Transfer students are accepted. *Application deadline:* 2/1 (fall). Applications may be processed on a rolling basis for some programs.
Advanced Placement Credit given for nursing courses completed elsewhere dependent upon specific evaluations.
Expenses (2015–16) *Tuition, state resident:* full-time $5013; part-time $209 per credit. *Tuition, nonresident:* full-time $7520; part-time $313 per credit. *International tuition:* $7520 full-time. *Room and board:* $6480; room only: $2520 per academic year. *Required fees:* full-time $1759; part-time $48 per credit; part-time $300 per term.
Financial Aid 74% of baccalaureate students in nursing programs received some form of financial aid in 2014–15. *Gift aid (need-based):* Federal Pell, FSEOG, state, private. *Loans:* Federal Nursing Student Loans, Federal Direct (Subsidized and Unsubsidized Stafford PLUS), Perkins, private loans, Alaska Loans. *Work-study:* Federal Work-Study, part-time campus jobs. *Financial aid application deadline (priority):* 4/15.
Contact Dr. Mary Anne Marsh, Chair, Department of Nursing, Dickinson State University, 291 Campus Drive, Dickinson, ND 58601-4896. *Telephone:* 701-483-2133. *Fax:* 701-483-2524.
E-mail: maryanne.marsh@dickinsonstate.edu.

Minot State University
Department of Nursing
Minot, North Dakota

http://www.minotstateu.edu/nursing/
Founded in 1913
DEGREE • BSN
Nursing Program Faculty 22 (27% with doctorates).
Baccalaureate Enrollment 179 **Women** 92% **Men** 8% **Part-time** 20%
Distance Learning Courses Available.
Nursing Student Activities Sigma Theta Tau, Student Nurses' Association.

Nursing Student Resources Academic advising; academic or career counseling; assistance for students with disabilities; bookstore; campus computer network; career placement assistance; computer lab; computer-assisted instruction; e-mail services; housing assistance; interactive nursing skills videos; Internet; learning resource lab; library services; nursing audiovisuals; paid internships; remedial services; resume preparation assistance; skills, simulation, or other laboratory; tutoring; unpaid internships.
Library Facilities 8,500 volumes in health, 1,750 volumes in nursing; 37 periodical subscriptions health-care related.

BACCALAUREATE PROGRAMS

Degree BSN
Available Programs Generic Baccalaureate; RN Baccalaureate.
Study Options Full-time.
Online Degree Options Yes.
Program Entrance Requirements Minimum overall college GPA of 2.75, transcript of college record, CPR certification, written essay, immunizations, 2 letters of recommendation, minimum GPA in nursing prerequisites of 2.8, prerequisite course work. Transfer students are accepted. *Application deadline:* 9/15 (fall), 2/1 (spring). *Application fee:* $25.
Advanced Placement Credit given for nursing courses completed elsewhere dependent upon specific evaluations.
Contact *Telephone:* 701-858-3526. *Fax:* 701-858-4309.

North Dakota State University
Department of Nursing
Fargo, North Dakota

http://www.ndsu.edu/ndsu/nursing/
Founded in 1890
DEGREES • BSN • DNP
Nursing Program Faculty 37
Baccalaureate Enrollment 424 **Women** 89% **Men** 11% **Part-time** 10%
Graduate Enrollment 39 **Women** 87% **Men** 13% **Part-time** 15%
Distance Learning Courses Available.
Nursing Student Activities Sigma Theta Tau, Student Nurses' Association.
Nursing Student Resources Academic advising; academic or career counseling; assistance for students with disabilities; bookstore; campus computer network; career placement assistance; computer lab; computer-assisted instruction; daycare for children of students; e-mail services; employment services for current students; interactive nursing skills videos; Internet; learning resource lab; library services; nursing audiovisuals; paid internships; placement services for program completers; remedial services; resume preparation assistance; skills, simulation, or other laboratory; tutoring.
Library Facilities 8,631 volumes in health, 1,841 volumes in nursing; 121 periodical subscriptions health-care related.

BACCALAUREATE PROGRAMS

Degree BSN
Available Programs Generic Baccalaureate; LPN to Baccalaureate.
Site Options Bismarck, ND.
Study Options Full-time.
Program Entrance Requirements Minimum overall college GPA of 2.75, transcript of college record, CPR certification, written essay, health exam, health insurance, immunizations, 2 letters of recommendation, minimum GPA in nursing prerequisites of 2.75, prerequisite course work. Transfer students are accepted. *Application deadline:* 4/20 (fall), 9/20 (spring). *Application fee:* $50.
Advanced Placement Credit by examination available. Credit given for nursing courses completed elsewhere dependent upon specific evaluations.
Expenses (2014–15) *Tuition, state resident:* full-time $4431; part-time $405 per credit. *Tuition, nonresident:* full-time $6342; part-time $582 per credit.
Financial Aid 85% of baccalaureate students in nursing programs received some form of financial aid in 2013–14.
Contact Ms. Jane Hagen, Academic Assistant, Department of Nursing, North Dakota State University, NDSU Department 2670, PO Box 6050, Fargo, ND 58108-6050. *Telephone:* 701-231-7395. *Fax:* 701-231-6257. *E-mail:* Jane.Hagen@ndsu.edu.

GRADUATE PROGRAMS

Expenses (2014–15) *Tuition, area resident:* full-time $4671; part-time $409 per credit. *Tuition, state resident:* full-time $4671; part-time $506 per credit. *Tuition, nonresident:* full-time $6702; part-time $589 per credit.
Financial Aid 35% of graduate students in nursing programs received some form of financial aid in 2013–14.
Contact Dr. Dean A. Gross, Assistant Professor of Practice and DNP Program Director, Department of Nursing, North Dakota State University, NDSU Department 2670, PO Box 6050, Fargo, ND 58108-6050. *Telephone:* 701-231-8355. *Fax:* 701-231-6257. *E-mail:* dean.gross@ndsu.edu.

DOCTORAL DEGREE PROGRAM
Degree DNP
Available Programs Post-Baccalaureate Doctorate.
Areas of Study Advanced practice nursing, family health.
Site Options Bismarck, ND.
Online Degree Options Yes.
Program Entrance Requirements Clinical experience, minimum overall college GPA of 3.0, interview by faculty committee, 2 letters of recommendation, statistics course, vita, writing sample. Application deadline: 2/28 (fall). Application fee: $50.
Degree Requirements 86 total credit hours, dissertation, oral exam.

University of Jamestown
Department of Nursing
Jamestown, North Dakota

Founded in 1883
DEGREE • BSN
Nursing Program Faculty 11 (9% with doctorates).
Baccalaureate Enrollment 80
Nursing Student Activities Sigma Theta Tau, Student Nurses' Association.
Nursing Student Resources Academic advising; academic or career counseling; bookstore; campus computer network; computer lab; computer-assisted instruction; e-mail services; externships; interactive nursing skills videos; Internet; learning resource lab; library services; nursing audiovisuals; resume preparation assistance; skills, simulation, or other laboratory; tutoring.
Library Facilities 990 volumes in health, 983 volumes in nursing; 163 periodical subscriptions health-care related.

BACCALAUREATE PROGRAMS

Degree BSN
Study Options Full-time and part-time.
Program Entrance Requirements Minimum overall college GPA of 3.0, transcript of college record, written essay, high school transcript, immunizations, prerequisite course work. Transfer students are accepted.
Advanced Placement Credit given for nursing courses completed elsewhere dependent upon specific evaluations.
Contact *Telephone:* 701-252-3467 Ext. 2562. *Fax:* 701-253-4318.

University of Mary
Division of Nursing
Bismarck, North Dakota

http://www.umary.edu/templates/template_degrees.php?degree=Nursing
Founded in 1959
DEGREES • BSN • DNP • MSN • MSN/MBA
Nursing Program Faculty 24 (46% with doctorates).
Baccalaureate Enrollment 132 **Women** 89% **Men** 11%
Graduate Enrollment 158 **Women** 89% **Men** 11% **Part-time** 23%
Distance Learning Courses Available.
Nursing Student Activities Sigma Theta Tau, Student Nurses' Association.
Nursing Student Resources Academic advising; academic or career counseling; assistance for students with disabilities; bookstore; campus computer network; career placement assistance; computer lab; computer-assisted instruction; e-mail services; employment services for current students; externships; housing assistance; interactive nursing skills videos; Internet; library services; nursing audiovisuals; placement services for program completers; resume preparation assistance; skills, simulation, or other laboratory; tutoring; unpaid internships.
Library Facilities 2,825 volumes in health, 720 volumes in nursing; 4,840 periodical subscriptions health-care related.

BACCALAUREATE PROGRAMS

Degree BSN

Available Programs ADN to Baccalaureate; Generic Baccalaureate; LPN to Baccalaureate.

Study Options Full-time and part-time.

Online Degree Options Yes.

Program Entrance Requirements Minimum overall college GPA of 3.0, transcript of college record, CPR certification, written essay, health exam, high school transcript, immunizations, 2 letters of recommendation, minimum GPA in nursing prerequisites of 2.0, prerequisite course work. Transfer students are accepted. *Application deadline:* 11/26 (fall), 3/26 (spring).

Advanced Placement Credit by examination available. Credit given for nursing courses completed elsewhere dependent upon specific evaluations.

Expenses (2015–16) *Tuition:* part-time $515 per credit. *Room and board:* $6136; room only: $2840 per academic year.

Financial Aid 95% of baccalaureate students in nursing programs received some form of financial aid in 2014–15. *Gift aid (need-based):* Federal Pell, FSEOG, state, private, college/university gift aid from institutional funds, TEACH Grants. *Loans:* Federal Nursing Student Loans, Federal Direct (Subsidized and Unsubsidized Stafford PLUS), Perkins, private loans. *Work-study:* Federal Work-Study, part-time campus jobs. *Financial aid application deadline:* Continuous.

Contact Admissions Office, Division of Nursing, University of Mary, 7500 University Drive, Bismarck, ND 58504. *Telephone:* 701-355-8030.

GRADUATE PROGRAMS

Expenses (2015–16) *Tuition:* full-time $12,100; part-time $550 per credit. *Required fees:* full-time $1115.

Financial Aid Fellowships, teaching assistantships available.

Contact Dr. Billie Madler, Graduate Program Director, Division of Nursing, University of Mary, 7500 University Drive, Bismarck, ND 58504. *Telephone:* 701-355-8266. *Fax:* 701-255-7687. *E-mail:* bmadler@umary.edu.

MASTER'S DEGREE PROGRAM

Degrees MSN; MSN/MBA

Available Programs Master's; RN to Master's.

Concentrations Available Nursing administration; nursing education.

Study Options Full-time and part-time.

Online Degree Options Yes (online only).

Program Entrance Requirements Clinical experience, minimum overall college GPA of 2.75, transcript of college record, CPR certification, written essay, immunizations, 2 letters of recommendation, prerequisite course work, resume, statistics course. *Application deadline:* Applications may be processed on a rolling basis for some programs. *Application fee:* $40.

Advanced Placement Credit given for nursing courses completed elsewhere dependent upon specific evaluations.

Degree Requirements 39 total credit hours, thesis or project.

DOCTORAL DEGREE PROGRAM

Degree DNP

Available Programs Post-Baccalaureate Doctorate.

Areas of Study Family health.

Program Entrance Requirements Clinical experience, minimum overall college GPA of 2.75, interview by faculty committee, 2 letters of recommendation, statistics course, writing sample. Application deadline: 2/1 (fall). Application fee: $40.

Degree Requirements 86 total credit hours, written exam.

University of North Dakota

College of Nursing

Grand Forks, North Dakota

http://www.nursing.und.edu/
Founded in 1883

DEGREES • BSN • MS • PHD

Nursing Program Faculty 75 (30% with doctorates).

Baccalaureate Enrollment 304 **Women** 84% **Men** 16% **Part-time** 9%

Graduate Enrollment 264 **Women** 88.1% **Men** 11.9% **Part-time** 52.3%

Distance Learning Courses Available.

Nursing Student Activities Nursing Honor Society, Sigma Theta Tau, Student Nurses' Association.

Nursing Student Resources Academic advising; academic or career counseling; assistance for students with disabilities; bookstore; career placement assistance; computer lab; computer-assisted instruction; daycare for children of students; e-mail services; employment services for current students; externships; housing assistance; interactive nursing skills videos; Internet; learning resource lab; library services; nursing audiovisuals; paid internships; placement services for program completers; remedial services; resume preparation assistance; skills, simulation, or other laboratory; tutoring.

Library Facilities 81,000 volumes in health, 10,200 volumes in nursing; 30,000 periodical subscriptions health-care related.

BACCALAUREATE PROGRAMS

Degree BSN

Available Programs ADN to Baccalaureate; Accelerated Baccalaureate for Second Degree; Baccalaureate for Second Degree; Generic Baccalaureate; LPN to Baccalaureate.

Study Options Full-time and part-time.

Program Entrance Requirements Minimum overall college GPA of 2.5, transcript of college record, CPR certification, written essay, health insurance, immunizations, minimum GPA in nursing prerequisites of 2.5, prerequisite course work. Transfer students are accepted. *Application deadline:* 2/1 (fall), 7/1 (spring).

Advanced Placement Credit by examination available. Credit given for nursing courses completed elsewhere dependent upon specific evaluations.

Contact *Telephone:* 701-777-4534. *Fax:* 701-777-4096.

GRADUATE PROGRAMS

Contact *Telephone:* 701-777-4543. *Fax:* 701-777-4096.

MASTER'S DEGREE PROGRAM

Degree MS

Available Programs Master's.

Concentrations Available Nurse anesthesia; nursing education. *Clinical nurse specialist programs in:* gerontology, psychiatric/mental health, public health. *Nurse practitioner programs in:* family health, gerontology, primary care, psychiatric/mental health.

Study Options Full-time and part-time.

Online Degree Options Yes.

Program Entrance Requirements Clinical experience, minimum overall college GPA of 3.0, transcript of college record, CPR certification, written essay, immunizations, interview, 3 letters of recommendation, prerequisite course work, resume, statistics course. *Application deadline:* 1/15 (fall). *Application fee:* $35.

Advanced Placement Credit given for nursing courses completed elsewhere dependent upon specific evaluations.

Degree Requirements 57 total credit hours, thesis or project.

POST-MASTER'S PROGRAM

Areas of Study Nurse anesthesia; nursing education. *Clinical nurse specialist programs in:* gerontology, psychiatric/mental health. *Nurse practitioner programs in:* family health, gerontology, primary care, psychiatric/mental health.

DOCTORAL DEGREE PROGRAM

Degree PhD

Available Programs Doctorate.

Areas of Study Bio-behavioral research, nursing research.

Online Degree Options Yes (online only).

Program Entrance Requirements Minimum overall college GPA of 3.5, interview by faculty committee, 3 letters of recommendation, MSN or equivalent, statistics course, vita, GRE or MAT. Application deadline: 2/1 (fall). Application fee: $35.

Degree Requirements 90 total credit hours, dissertation, oral exam, written exam.

OHIO

Ashland University

Dwight Schar College of Nursing and Health Sciences
Ashland, Ohio

http://www.ashland.edu/nursing
Founded in 1878
DEGREES • BSN • DNP
Nursing Program Faculty 33 (27% with doctorates).
Baccalaureate Enrollment 424 Women 88% Men 12% Part-time 1%
Graduate Enrollment 21 Women 86% Men 14% Part-time 3%
Distance Learning Courses Available.
Nursing Student Activities Nursing Honor Society, Sigma Theta Tau, Student Nurses' Association, nursing club.
Nursing Student Resources Academic advising; academic or career counseling; assistance for students with disabilities; bookstore; campus computer network; career placement assistance; computer lab; computer-assisted instruction; e-mail services; employment services for current students; housing assistance; interactive nursing skills videos; Internet; learning resource lab; library services; nursing audiovisuals; remedial services; resume preparation assistance; skills, simulation, or other laboratory; tutoring; unpaid internships.

BACCALAUREATE PROGRAMS

Degree BSN
Available Programs ADN to Baccalaureate; Accelerated Baccalaureate; Accelerated Baccalaureate for Second Degree; Baccalaureate for Second Degree; Generic Baccalaureate; RN Baccalaureate.
Study Options Full-time and part-time.
Online Degree Options Yes.
Program Entrance Requirements Minimum overall college GPA of 3.0, transcript of college record, CPR certification, health exam, health insurance, high school transcript, immunizations, minimum high school GPA of 3.0. Transfer students are accepted. *Application deadline:* Applications may be processed on a rolling basis for some programs.
Advanced Placement Credit given for nursing courses completed elsewhere dependent upon specific evaluations.
Financial Aid *Gift aid (need-based):* Federal Pell, FSEOG, state, private, college/university gift aid from institutional funds. *Loans:* Federal Direct (Subsidized and Unsubsidized Stafford PLUS), Perkins, college/university. *Work-study:* Federal Work-Study, part-time campus jobs. *Financial aid application deadline (priority):* 3/15.
Contact Mr. WC Vance, Director of Undergraduate Admissions, Dwight Schar College of Nursing and Health Sciences, Ashland University, 401 College Avenue, Ashland, OH 44805. *Telephone:* 419-289-5052. *E-mail:* wvance@ashland.edu.

GRADUATE PROGRAMS

Expenses (2015–16) *Tuition:* part-time $650 per credit.
Contact Mr. Brock Kertoy, Senior Graduate Admissions Representative, Dwight Schar College of Nursing and Health Sciences, Ashland University, 401 College Avenue, Ashland, OH 44805. *Telephone:* 419-289-4738. *Fax:* 419-289-5999. *E-mail:* bkertoy@ashland.edu.

DOCTORAL DEGREE PROGRAM

Degree DNP
Available Programs Doctorate; Post-Baccalaureate Doctorate.
Areas of Study Clinical practice, family health.
Online Degree Options Yes (online only).
Program Entrance Requirements Clinical experience, minimum overall college GPA of 3.0, interview, letters of recommendation, statistics course, vita, writing sample. Application deadline: Applications may be processed on a rolling basis for some programs. Application fee: $300.
Degree Requirements Dissertation, oral exam, written exam, residency.

Baldwin Wallace University

Accelerated Bachelor of Science in Nursing
Berea, Ohio

http://www.bw.edu/academics/nursing
Founded in 1845
DEGREE • BSN
Nursing Program Faculty 10
Baccalaureate Enrollment 31 Women 81% Men 19%
Nursing Student Resources Academic advising; academic or career counseling; assistance for students with disabilities; bookstore; campus computer network; career placement assistance; computer lab; computer-assisted instruction; e-mail services; employment services for current students; interactive nursing skills videos; Internet; learning resource lab; library services; nursing audiovisuals; placement services for program completers; resume preparation assistance; skills, simulation, or other laboratory; tutoring; unpaid internships.

BACCALAUREATE PROGRAMS

Degree BSN
Available Programs Accelerated Baccalaureate.
Study Options Full-time.
Program Entrance Requirements Minimum overall college GPA of 3.0, transcript of college record, CPR certification, written essay, health exam, immunizations, interview, 2 letters of recommendation, minimum GPA in nursing prerequisites of 3.0, prerequisite course work. *Application deadline:* Applications may be processed on a rolling basis for some programs.
Expenses (2015–16) *Tuition:* full-time $33,215.
Financial Aid *Gift aid (need-based):* Federal Pell, FSEOG, state, private, college/university gift aid from institutional funds. *Loans:* Federal Direct (Subsidized and Unsubsidized Stafford PLUS), Perkins. *Work-study:* Federal Work-Study, part-time campus jobs. *Financial aid application deadline (priority):* 8/15.
Contact Ms. Lydia Avery, Associate Director, Admissions, Accelerated Bachelor of Science in Nursing, Baldwin Wallace University, Admissions Office, 275 Eastland Road, Berea, OH 44017. *Telephone:* 440-826-8016. *E-mail:* lavery@bw.edu.

Capital University

School of Nursing
Columbus, Ohio

http://www.capital.edu/
Founded in 1830
DEGREES • BSN • MN/MBA • MSN • MSN/JD • MSN/MDIV
Nursing Program Faculty 45 (30% with doctorates).
Baccalaureate Enrollment 464 Women 82% Men 18% Part-time 19%
Graduate Enrollment 45 Women 87% Men 13% Part-time 98%
Nursing Student Activities Sigma Theta Tau, Student Nurses' Association.
Nursing Student Resources Academic advising; academic or career counseling; assistance for students with disabilities; bookstore; campus computer network; computer lab; computer-assisted instruction; e-mail services; interactive nursing skills videos; Internet; learning resource lab; library services; nursing audiovisuals; remedial services; resume preparation assistance; skills, simulation, or other laboratory; tutoring; unpaid internships.
Library Facilities 6,209 volumes in health; 82 periodical subscriptions health-care related.

BACCALAUREATE PROGRAMS

Degree BSN
Available Programs ADN to Baccalaureate; Accelerated Baccalaureate for Second Degree; Generic Baccalaureate; RN Baccalaureate.
Study Options Full-time and part-time.
Program Entrance Requirements Minimum overall college GPA of 3.0, transcript of college record, health exam, health insurance, high school biology, high school chemistry, high school foreign language, 3 years high school math, 3 years high school science, high school transcript, immunizations, minimum high school GPA of 3.0. Transfer students are accepted. *Application deadline:* 5/1 (fall), 5/1 (spring). Applications may be processed on a rolling basis for some programs. *Application fee:* $25.

Advanced Placement Credit by examination available. Credit given for nursing courses completed elsewhere dependent upon specific evaluations.

Expenses (2014–15) *Tuition:* full-time $31,990; part-time $1066 per credit. *International tuition:* $31,990 full-time. *Room and board:* $9060; room only: $4020 per academic year. *Required fees:* full-time $1200.

Financial Aid 95% of baccalaureate students in nursing programs received some form of financial aid in 2013–14.

Contact Dr. Renee Dunnington, Vice Chair, Pre-Licensure Programs, School of Nursing, Capital University, 1 College and Main, Columbus, OH 43209-2394. *Telephone:* 614-236-7221. *Fax:* 614-236-6157. *E-mail:* rdunning@capital.edu.

GRADUATE PROGRAMS

Expenses (2014–15) *Tuition:* full-time $5220; part-time $435 per credit. *International tuition:* $5220 full-time. *Required fees:* full-time $25.

Financial Aid 50% of graduate students in nursing programs received some form of financial aid in 2013–14. Career-related internships or fieldwork and traineeships available.

Contact Dr. Heather Janiszewski Goodin, Vice Chair, Post-Licensure Programs, School of Nursing, Capital University, 1 College and Main, Columbus, OH 43209-2394. *Telephone:* 614-236-6380. *Fax:* 614-236-6703. *E-mail:* hjanisze@capital.edu.

MASTER'S DEGREE PROGRAM

Degrees MN/MBA; MSN; MSN/JD; MSN/MDIV
Available Programs Master's; RN to Master's.
Concentrations Available Legal nurse consultant; nursing administration; nursing education. *Clinical nurse specialist programs in:* adult health, gerontology.
Study Options Full-time and part-time.
Program Entrance Requirements Computer literacy, minimum overall college GPA of 3.0, transcript of college record, CPR certification, written essay, immunizations, 3 letters of recommendation, nursing research course, physical assessment course, professional liability insurance/malpractice insurance, resume, statistics course. *Application deadline:* 8/1 (fall), 12/1 (winter), 12/1 (spring), 5/1 (summer). Applications may be processed on a rolling basis for some programs. *Application fee:* $25.
Advanced Placement Credit given for nursing courses completed elsewhere dependent upon specific evaluations.
Degree Requirements 36 total credit hours, comprehensive exam.

POST-MASTER'S PROGRAM

Areas of Study Legal nurse consultant; nursing education. *Clinical nurse specialist programs in:* adult health, gerontology.

Case Western Reserve University
Frances Payne Bolton School of Nursing
Cleveland, Ohio

http://fpb.case.edu/
Founded in 1826
DEGREES • BSN • MSN • MSN/MA • MSN/MPH • PHD
Nursing Program Faculty 99 (65% with doctorates).
Baccalaureate Enrollment 351 **Women** 92% **Men** 8% **Part-time** .85%
Graduate Enrollment 510 **Women** 86% **Men** 14% **Part-time** 34%
Distance Learning Courses Available.
Nursing Student Activities Nursing Honor Society, Sigma Theta Tau, Student Nurses' Association, nursing club.
Nursing Student Resources Academic advising; academic or career counseling; assistance for students with disabilities; bookstore; campus computer network; career placement assistance; computer lab; computer-assisted instruction; e-mail services; employment services for current students; housing assistance; interactive nursing skills videos; Internet; learning resource lab; library services; nursing audiovisuals; other; paid internships; placement services for program completers; remedial services; resume preparation assistance; skills, simulation, or other laboratory; tutoring.
Library Facilities 475,000 volumes in health; 2,500 periodical subscriptions health-care related.

BACCALAUREATE PROGRAMS

Degree BSN
Available Programs Generic Baccalaureate.
Study Options Full-time.

Program Entrance Requirements CPR certification, written essay, health insurance, high school biology, high school chemistry, 2 years high school science, high school transcript, immunizations, 2 letters of recommendation, minimum high school GPA of 3.0. Transfer students are accepted. *Application deadline:* 1/15 (fall).
Advanced Placement Credit given for nursing courses completed elsewhere dependent upon specific evaluations.
Expenses (2014–15) *Tuition:* full-time $42,766; part-time $1782 per credit hour. *International tuition:* $42,766 full-time. *Room and board:* $12,898; room only: $7508 per academic year. *Required fees:* full-time $915.
Financial Aid 100% of baccalaureate students in nursing programs received some form of financial aid in 2013–14. *Gift aid (need-based):* Federal Pell, FSEOG, state, private, college/university gift aid from institutional funds. *Loans:* Federal Nursing Student Loans, Federal Direct (Subsidized and Unsubsidized Stafford PLUS), Perkins, college/university, alternative loans. *Work-study:* Federal Work-Study. *Financial aid application deadline (priority):* 2/15.
Contact Office of Student Services, Frances Payne Bolton School of Nursing, Case Western Reserve University, 10900 Euclid Avenue, Cleveland, OH 44106-4904. *Telephone:* 216-368-2529. *Fax:* 216-368-0124. *E-mail:* admissions@fpb.case.edu.

GRADUATE PROGRAMS

Expenses (2014–15) *Tuition:* full-time $32,724; part-time $1818 per credit hour. *International tuition:* $32,724 full-time. *Required fees:* full-time $490.
Financial Aid 90% of graduate students in nursing programs received some form of financial aid in 2013–14. 12 fellowships with full tuition reimbursements available (averaging $29,145 per year), 12 research assistantships with partial tuition reimbursements available (averaging $15,741 per year), 29 teaching assistantships with partial tuition reimbursements available (averaging $15,741 per year) were awarded; Federal Work-Study, institutionally sponsored loans, scholarships, and tuition waivers (partial) also available. Aid available to part-time students. *Financial aid application deadline:* 5/15.
Contact Office of Student Services, Frances Payne Bolton School of Nursing, Case Western Reserve University, 10900 Euclid Avenue, Cleveland, OH 44106-4904. *Telephone:* 216-368-2529. *Fax:* 216-368-0124. *E-mail:* admissionsfpb@case.edu.

MASTER'S DEGREE PROGRAM

Degrees MSN; MSN/MA; MSN/MPH
Available Programs Accelerated AD/RN to Master's; Master's; Master's for Non-Nursing College Graduates; RN to Master's.
Concentrations Available Nurse anesthesia; nurse-midwifery; nursing education. *Clinical nurse specialist programs in:* oncology, palliative care, psychiatric/mental health. *Nurse practitioner programs in:* acute care, adult health, adult-gerontology acute care, family health, gerontology, neonatal health, oncology, pediatric, pediatric primary care, primary care, psychiatric/mental health, women's health.
Study Options Full-time and part-time.
Program Entrance Requirements Minimum overall college GPA of 3.0, transcript of college record, written essay, immunizations, 3 letters of recommendation, professional liability insurance/malpractice insurance, resume, statistics course, MAT or GRE General Test. *Application deadline:* 6/1 (fall), 10/1 (spring), 3/1 (summer). Applications may be processed on a rolling basis for some programs. *Application fee:* $75.
Advanced Placement Credit given for nursing courses completed elsewhere dependent upon specific evaluations.
Degree Requirements 40 total credit hours.

POST-MASTER'S PROGRAM

Areas of Study Nurse anesthesia; nurse-midwifery; nursing education. *Clinical nurse specialist programs in:* oncology, palliative care, psychiatric/mental health. *Nurse practitioner programs in:* acute care, adult health, adult-gerontology acute care, family health, gerontology, neonatal health, oncology, pediatric, pediatric primary care, primary care, psychiatric/mental health, women's health.

DOCTORAL DEGREE PROGRAM

Degree PhD
Available Programs Doctorate; Doctorate for Nurses with Non-Nursing Degrees; Post-Baccalaureate Doctorate.
Areas of Study Aging, bio-behavioral research, biology of health and illness, clinical research, community health, critical care, ethics, family health, gerontology, health policy, health promotion/disease prevention, health-care systems, human health and illness, illness and transition, information systems, maternity-newborn, neuro-behavior, nursing

administration, nursing policy, nursing research, nursing science, oncology, palliative care, urban health, women's health.
Program Entrance Requirements Minimum overall college GPA of 3.0, interview by faculty committee, 3 letters of recommendation, statistics course, vita, writing sample, GRE General Test, MAT (for DNP). Application deadline: 4/1 (fall), 10/1 (spring). Applications may be processed on a rolling basis for some programs. Application fee: $50.
Degree Requirements 57 total credit hours, dissertation, oral exam, residency.

POSTDOCTORAL PROGRAM
Areas of Study Adolescent health, aging, cancer care, chronic illness, community health, family health, gerontology, health promotion/disease prevention, infection prevention/skin care, information systems, neurobehavior, nursing informatics, nursing interventions, nursing research, nursing science, outcomes, self-care, vulnerable population, women's health.
Postdoctoral Program Contact Dr. Shirley M. Moore, Professor and Associate Dean for Research, Frances Payne Bolton School of Nursing, Case Western Reserve University, 10900 Euclid Avenue, Cleveland, OH 44106-4904. *Telephone:* 216-368-5978. *Fax:* 216-368-3542. *E-mail:* shirley.moore@case.edu.

CONTINUING EDUCATION PROGRAM
Contact Dr. Irena Kenneley, Associate Professor, Frances Payne Bolton School of Nursing, Case Western Reserve University, 10900 Euclid Avenue, Cleveland, OH 44106-4904. *Telephone:* 216-368-4841. *Fax:* 216-368-5303. *E-mail:* ilz@case.edu.

Cedarville University
School of Nursing
Cedarville, Ohio

http://www.cedarville.edu/academics/nursing
Founded in 1887
DEGREES • BSN • MSN
Nursing Program Faculty 18 (44% with doctorates).
Baccalaureate Enrollment 383 **Women** 87.7% **Men** 12.3% **Part-time** 2%
Graduate Enrollment 53 **Women** 92.5% **Men** 7.5% **Part-time** 66%
Distance Learning Courses Available.
Nursing Student Activities Nursing Honor Society, Student Nurses' Association.
Nursing Student Resources Academic advising; academic or career counseling; assistance for students with disabilities; bookstore; campus computer network; career placement assistance; computer lab; computer-assisted instruction; e-mail services; employment services for current students; housing assistance; interactive nursing skills videos; Internet; library services; nursing audiovisuals; paid internships; resume preparation assistance; skills, simulation, or other laboratory; tutoring.
Library Facilities 7,326 volumes in health, 1,366 volumes in nursing; 896 periodical subscriptions health-care related.

BACCALAUREATE PROGRAMS
Degree BSN
Available Programs RN Baccalaureate.
Study Options Full-time and part-time.
Program Entrance Requirements Minimum overall college GPA of 3.0, transcript of college record, CPR certification, written essay, health exam, health insurance, high school biology, high school chemistry, high school foreign language, 4 years high school math, 4 years high school science, high school transcript, immunizations, 1 letter of recommendation, minimum high school GPA of 3.0, minimum GPA in nursing prerequisites of 3.0, professional liability insurance/malpractice insurance, prerequisite course work. Transfer students are accepted. *Application deadline:* Applications may be processed on a rolling basis for some programs. *Application fee:* $30.
Advanced Placement Credit given for nursing courses completed elsewhere dependent upon specific evaluations.
Expenses (2015–16) *Tuition:* part-time $1022 per credit. *Room and board:* $6542; room only: $3708 per academic year.
Financial Aid 97% of baccalaureate students in nursing programs received some form of financial aid in 2014–15. *Gift aid (need-based):* Federal Pell, FSEOG, state, private, college/university gift aid from institutional funds, Federal Nursing. *Loans:* Federal Nursing Student Loans, Federal Direct (Subsidized and Unsubsidized Stafford PLUS), Perkins,

college/university. *Work-study:* Federal Work-Study, part-time campus jobs. *Financial aid application deadline (priority):* 3/1.
Contact Roscoe Smith, Associate Vice President for University Admissions, School of Nursing, Cedarville University, 251 North Main Street, Cedarville, OH 45314-0601. *Telephone:* 800-233-2784. *Fax:* 937-766-2760. *E-mail:* admiss@cedarville.edu.

GRADUATE PROGRAMS
Expenses (2015–16) *Tuition:* part-time $536 per credit. *International tuition:* $536 full-time. *Room and board:* $6542; room only: $3708 per academic year. *Required fees:* full-time $1375; part-time $460 per term.
Financial Aid 72% of graduate students in nursing programs received some form of financial aid in 2014–15.
Contact Jeff Evans, MSN Representative, School of Nursing, Cedarville University, 251 North Main Street, Cedarville, OH 45314. *Telephone:* 888-233-2784. *Fax:* 937-766-3711. *E-mail:* gradadmissions@cedarville.edu.

MASTER'S DEGREE PROGRAM
Degree MSN
Available Programs Master's.
Concentrations Available *Clinical nurse specialist programs in:* family health, public/community health. *Nurse practitioner programs in:* family health.
Study Options Full-time and part-time.
Online Degree Options Yes.
Program Entrance Requirements Clinical experience, computer literacy, minimum overall college GPA of 3.0, transcript of college record, written essay, interview, 3 letters of recommendation, prerequisite course work, resume. *Application deadline:* Applications may be processed on a rolling basis for some programs. *Application fee:* $30.
Degree Requirements 43 total credit hours, thesis or project.

Chamberlain College of Nursing
Chamberlain College of Nursing
Columbus, Ohio

DEGREES • BSN • MSN
Distance Learning Courses Available.

BACCALAUREATE PROGRAMS
Degree BSN
Available Programs Accelerated Baccalaureate; Accelerated Baccalaureate for Second Degree; RN Baccalaureate.
Contact *Telephone:* 888-556-8226.

GRADUATE PROGRAMS
Contact *Telephone:* 888-556-8226.

MASTER'S DEGREE PROGRAM
Degree MSN
Available Programs Master's.

The Christ College of Nursing and Health Sciences
Department of Nursing
Cincinnati, Ohio

http://www.thechristcollege.edu/
DEGREE • BSN
Nursing Program Faculty 32 (1% with doctorates).
Baccalaureate Enrollment 83
Nursing Student Activities Student Nurses' Association, nursing club.
Nursing Student Resources Academic advising; academic or career counseling; assistance for students with disabilities; bookstore; campus computer network; computer lab; e-mail services; interactive nursing skills videos; Internet; learning resource lab; library services; resume preparation assistance; skills, simulation, or other laboratory; tutoring.

BACCALAUREATE PROGRAMS
Degree BSN
Available Programs Generic Baccalaureate; RN Baccalaureate.

Study Options Full-time.

Program Entrance Requirements Minimum overall college GPA of 2.75, transcript of college record, health exam, health insurance, high school biology, 2 years high school math, high school transcript, immunizations, minimum high school GPA of 2.75. Transfer students are accepted.

Contact Dallas McCray-Smith. *Telephone:* 513-585-2401.

Cleveland State University
School of Nursing
Cleveland, Ohio

http://www.csuohio.edu/nursing
Founded in 1964

DEGREES • BSN • MSN • MSN/MBA • PHD
Nursing Program Faculty 33 (33% with doctorates).
Baccalaureate Enrollment 307 **Women** 83% **Men** 17%
Graduate Enrollment 72 **Women** 94% **Men** 6% **Part-time** 100%
Distance Learning Courses Available.
Nursing Student Activities Sigma Theta Tau, Student Nurses' Association.
Nursing Student Resources Academic advising; academic or career counseling; assistance for students with disabilities; bookstore; campus computer network; computer lab; computer-assisted instruction; daycare for children of students; e-mail services; employment services for current students; interactive nursing skills videos; Internet; learning resource lab; library services; nursing audiovisuals; remedial services; resume preparation assistance; skills, simulation, or other laboratory; tutoring.
Library Facilities 6,000 volumes in health, 300 volumes in nursing; 70 periodical subscriptions health-care related.

BACCALAUREATE PROGRAMS
Degree BSN
Available Programs Accelerated Baccalaureate for Second Degree; Generic Baccalaureate; RN Baccalaureate.
Study Options Full-time.
Online Degree Options Yes.
Program Entrance Requirements Minimum overall college GPA of 2.75, transcript of college record, CPR certification, written essay, health exam, health insurance, immunizations, interview, 2 letters of recommendation, minimum GPA in nursing prerequisites of 3.0, prerequisite course work. Transfer students are accepted. *Application deadline:* 3/1 (fall). *Application fee:* $25.
Advanced Placement Credit given for nursing courses completed elsewhere dependent upon specific evaluations.
Expenses (2014–15) *Tuition, state resident:* full-time $9636; part-time $402 per credit. *Tuition, nonresident:* full-time $12,878; part-time $537 per credit. *International tuition:* $12,878 full-time. *Required fees:* full-time $280.
Financial Aid 80% of baccalaureate students in nursing programs received some form of financial aid in 2013–14. *Gift aid (need-based):* Federal Pell, FSEOG, state, private, college/university gift aid from institutional funds. *Loans:* Federal Direct (Subsidized and Unsubsidized Stafford PLUS), Perkins, state, alternative loans. *Work-study:* Federal Work-Study, part-time campus jobs. *Financial aid application deadline (priority):* 2/15.
Contact Mrs. Mary Leanza Manzuk, Recruiter/Advisor, School of Nursing, Cleveland State University, 2121 Euclid Avenue, JH 238, Cleveland, OH 44115-2214. *Telephone:* 216-687-3810. *Fax:* 216-687-3556. *E-mail:* sonadvising@csuohio.edu.

GRADUATE PROGRAMS
Expenses (2014–15) *Tuition, state resident:* part-time $531 per credit. *Tuition, nonresident:* part-time $541 per credit. *Required fees:* part-time $25 per credit.
Financial Aid 50% of graduate students in nursing programs received some form of financial aid in 2013–14.
Contact Ms. Mary Leanza Manzuk, Recruiter/Advisor, School of Nursing, Cleveland State University, 2121 Euclid Avenue, JH 238, Cleveland, OH 44115-2214. *Telephone:* 216-687-3598. *Fax:* 216-687-3556. *E-mail:* sonadvising@csuohio.edu.

MASTER'S DEGREE PROGRAM
Degrees MSN; MSN/MBA
Available Programs Master's.

Concentrations Available Clinical nurse leader; nursing education. *Clinical nurse specialist programs in:* community health, forensic nursing.
Study Options Part-time.
Online Degree Options Yes (online only).
Program Entrance Requirements Computer literacy, minimum overall college GPA of 3.0, transcript of college record, CPR certification, written essay, immunizations, 2 letters of recommendation, professional liability insurance/malpractice insurance, resume, statistics course. *Application deadline:* 4/1 (fall). *Application fee:* $55.
Advanced Placement Credit given for nursing courses completed elsewhere dependent upon specific evaluations.
Degree Requirements 31 total credit hours.

POST-MASTER'S PROGRAM
Areas of Study Nursing education.

DOCTORAL DEGREE PROGRAM
Degree PhD
Available Programs Doctorate.
Areas of Study Nursing education.
Program Entrance Requirements Clinical experience, minimum overall college GPA of 3.25, interview by faculty committee, 2 letters of recommendation, MSN or equivalent, statistics course, vita, writing sample. Application deadline: 2/1 (fall). Application fee: $30.
Degree Requirements 67 total credit hours, dissertation, written exam, residency.

CONTINUING EDUCATION PROGRAM
Contact Noelle Muscatello, Program Coordinator, Continuing Education Programs for Health Care Professionals, School of Nursing, Cleveland State University, 2121 Euclid Avenue, Julka Hall, Room 238, Cleveland, OH 44115. *Telephone:* 216-687-3867. *Fax:* 216-687-3556. *E-mail:* j.n.muscatello@csuohio.edu.

Defiance College
Bachelor's Degree in Nursing
Defiance, Ohio

http://www.defiance.edu/academics/sm/nursing/
Founded in 1850
DEGREE • BSN
Nursing Program Faculty 5
Baccalaureate Enrollment 41 **Women** 63.6% **Men** 36.4% **Part-time** 51.5%
Distance Learning Courses Available.
Nursing Student Resources Academic advising; academic or career counseling; assistance for students with disabilities; bookstore; campus computer network; career placement assistance; computer lab; e-mail services; employment services for current students; housing assistance; Internet; library services; remedial services; resume preparation assistance; tutoring.
Library Facilities 300,083 volumes in health, 67,075 volumes in nursing; 7,416 periodical subscriptions health-care related.

BACCALAUREATE PROGRAMS
Degree BSN
Available Programs ADN to Baccalaureate; Accelerated RN Baccalaureate; RN Baccalaureate.
Study Options Full-time and part-time.
Program Entrance Requirements Minimum overall college GPA of 2.5, transcript of college record, CPR certification, health insurance, high school biology, high school chemistry, 3 years high school math, 3 years high school science, high school transcript, immunizations, interview, minimum high school GPA of 2.25, minimum GPA in nursing prerequisites of 2.75, professional liability insurance/malpractice insurance, prerequisite course work, RN licensure. Transfer students are accepted. *Application deadline:* Applications may be processed on a rolling basis for some programs.
Advanced Placement Credit given for nursing courses completed elsewhere dependent upon specific evaluations.
Expenses (2015–16) *Tuition:* full-time $30,400; part-time $485 per credit hour. *Room and board:* $9850 per academic year. *Required fees:* full-time $742; part-time $100 per term.
Contact Cheryl Hinojosa, RN, Assistant Professor of Practice of Nursing/Director of Nursing, Bachelor's Degree in Nursing, Defiance

College, 701 North Clinton Street, Tenzer 101, Defiance, OH 43512. *Telephone:* 419-783-2448. *Fax:* 419-785-2831. *E-mail:* chinojosa@ defiance.edu.

Fortis College
School of Nursing
Centerville, Ohio

https://www.fortis.edu/
Founded in 1953
DEGREE • BSN

BACCALAUREATE PROGRAMS

Degree BSN
Available Programs RN Baccalaureate.
Contact Admissions, School of Nursing, Fortis College, 555 East Alex Bell Road, Centerville, OH 45459. *Telephone:* 937-433-3410.

Franciscan University of Steubenville
Department of Nursing
Steubenville, Ohio

http://www.franciscan.edu/
Founded in 1946
DEGREES • BSN • MSN
Nursing Program Faculty 15 (20% with doctorates).
Baccalaureate Enrollment 177 **Women** 91% **Men** 9% **Part-time** 5%
Graduate Enrollment 23 **Women** 78% **Men** 22% **Part-time** 83%
Nursing Student Activities Student Nurses' Association.
Nursing Student Resources Academic advising; academic or career counseling; assistance for students with disabilities; bookstore; campus computer network; computer lab; e-mail services; Internet; learning resource lab; library services; resume preparation assistance; tutoring.
Library Facilities 29,761 volumes in health, 8,946 volumes in nursing; 178 periodical subscriptions health-care related.

BACCALAUREATE PROGRAMS

Degree BSN
Available Programs Generic Baccalaureate; RN Baccalaureate; RPN to Baccalaureate.
Study Options Full-time and part-time.
Program Entrance Requirements Minimum overall college GPA of 2.5, transcript of college record, health exam, health insurance, high school biology, high school chemistry, 2 years high school science, high school transcript, immunizations, 2 letters of recommendation, minimum high school GPA of 2.4, minimum GPA in nursing prerequisites of 2.5, professional liability insurance/malpractice insurance, prerequisite course work. Transfer students are accepted.
Advanced Placement Credit by examination available. Credit given for nursing courses completed elsewhere dependent upon specific evaluations.
Contact *Telephone:* 740-283-6324. *Fax:* 740-283-6449.

GRADUATE PROGRAMS

Contact *Telephone:* 740-284-7245. *Fax:* 740-283-6449.

MASTER'S DEGREE PROGRAM
Degree MSN
Available Programs Master's; RN to Master's.
Concentrations Available Nursing education. *Nurse practitioner programs in:* family health.
Study Options Full-time and part-time.
Program Entrance Requirements Clinical experience, minimum overall college GPA of 3.0, transcript of college record, interview, 2 letters of recommendation, nursing research course, physical assessment course, professional liability insurance/malpractice insurance, prerequisite course work, statistics course.

Advanced Placement Credit given for nursing courses completed elsewhere dependent upon specific evaluations.
Degree Requirements 48 total credit hours, thesis or project.

Franklin University
Nursing Program
Columbus, Ohio

Founded in 1902
DEGREE • BSN

BACCALAUREATE PROGRAMS

Degree BSN
Available Programs Accelerated Baccalaureate; Generic Baccalaureate.
Contact *Telephone:* 614-947-6209. *Fax:* 614-255-9678.

Good Samaritan College of Nursing and Health Science
Nursing Program
Cincinnati, Ohio

http://www.gscollege.edu/
DEGREE • BSN

BACCALAUREATE PROGRAMS

Degree BSN
Available Programs RN Baccalaureate.
Program Entrance Requirements *Application deadline:* Applications may be processed on a rolling basis for some programs.
Contact Admissions, Nursing Program, Good Samaritan College of Nursing and Health Science, 375 Dixmyth Avenue, Cincinnati, OH 45220. *Telephone:* 513-862-2743. *Fax:* 513-862-3572.

Hiram College
Nursing Department
Hiram, Ohio

http://www.hiram.edu/nursing
Founded in 1850
DEGREE • BSN
Nursing Program Faculty 18 (20% with doctorates).
Baccalaureate Enrollment 83 **Women** 88% **Men** 12% **Part-time** 1%
Nursing Student Activities Sigma Theta Tau, Student Nurses' Association.
Nursing Student Resources Academic advising; academic or career counseling; assistance for students with disabilities; bookstore; campus computer network; career placement assistance; computer lab; computer-assisted instruction; e-mail services; employment services for current students; externships; interactive nursing skills videos; Internet; learning resource lab; library services; nursing audiovisuals; remedial services; resume preparation assistance; skills, simulation, or other laboratory; tutoring.
Library Facilities 3,846 volumes in health, 869 volumes in nursing; 555 periodical subscriptions health-care related.

BACCALAUREATE PROGRAMS

Degree BSN
Available Programs Generic Baccalaureate.
Study Options Full-time.
Program Entrance Requirements Transcript of college record, written essay, health exam, high school biology, high school chemistry, high school foreign language, high school transcript, immunizations, minimum high school GPA of 2.75. Transfer students are accepted. *Application deadline:* Applications may be processed on a rolling basis for some programs.
Advanced Placement Credit given for nursing courses completed elsewhere dependent upon specific evaluations.
Contact *Telephone:* 330-569-6104. *Fax:* 330-569-6136.

Hondros College
Nursing Programs
Westerville, Ohio

Founded in 1981
DEGREE • BSN

BACCALAUREATE PROGRAMS

Degree BSN
Available Programs Generic Baccalaureate.
Study Options Full-time and part-time.
Online Degree Options Yes (online only).
Program Entrance Requirements Transfer students are accepted.
Contact *Telephone:* 614-508-7277.

Kent State University
College of Nursing
Kent, Ohio

http://www.kent.edu/nursing
Founded in 1910

DEGREES • BSN • DNP • MSN • MSN/MBA • MSN/MPA • PHD

Nursing Program Faculty 140 (20% with doctorates).
Baccalaureate Enrollment 1,223 **Women** 85% **Men** 15% **Part-time** 19%
Graduate Enrollment 523 **Women** 88% **Men** 12% **Part-time** 91%
Distance Learning Courses Available.
Nursing Student Activities Nursing Honor Society, Sigma Theta Tau, Student Nurses' Association.
Nursing Student Resources Academic advising; academic or career counseling; assistance for students with disabilities; bookstore; campus computer network; career placement assistance; computer lab; computer-assisted instruction; e-mail services; employment services for current students; externships; housing assistance; interactive nursing skills videos; Internet; learning resource lab; library services; nursing audiovisuals; other; paid internships; remedial services; resume preparation assistance; skills, simulation, or other laboratory; tutoring; unpaid internships.
Library Facilities 300 periodical subscriptions health-care related.

BACCALAUREATE PROGRAMS

Degree BSN
Available Programs ADN to Baccalaureate; Accelerated Baccalaureate; Accelerated Baccalaureate for Second Degree; Baccalaureate for Second Degree; Generic Baccalaureate; RN Baccalaureate.
Site Options Salem, OH; Burton, OH, OH; Warren, OH; Canton, OH.
Study Options Full-time and part-time.
Program Entrance Requirements Minimum overall college GPA of 2.75, transcript of college record, CPR certification, health exam, high school biology, high school transcript, immunizations, 2 letters of recommendation, minimum high school GPA of 2.75, minimum GPA in nursing prerequisites of 2.75, prerequisite course work. Transfer students are accepted. *Application deadline:* 4/30 (fall), 12/15 (spring).
Advanced Placement Credit given for nursing courses completed elsewhere dependent upon specific evaluations.
Expenses (2014–15) *Tuition, state resident:* full-time $10,012; part-time $456 per credit hour. *Tuition, nonresident:* full-time $17,972; part-time $818 per credit hour. *International tuition:* $17,972 full-time. *Room and board:* $9908; room only: $3500 per academic year. *Required fees:* full-time $150; part-time $75 per term.
Financial Aid 95% of baccalaureate students in nursing programs received some form of financial aid in 2013–14. *Gift aid (need-based):* Federal Pell, FSEOG, state, private, college/university gift aid from institutional funds. *Loans:* Federal Nursing Student Loans, Federal Direct (Subsidized and Unsubsidized Stafford PLUS), Perkins, state, college/university, alternative loans. *Work-study:* Federal Work-Study. *Financial aid application deadline (priority):* 3/1.
Contact Mr. Curtis Good, Director of Student Services, College of Nursing, Kent State University, Henderson Hall, Kent, OH 44242-0001. *Telephone:* 330-672-9972. *Fax:* 330-672-7911. *E-mail:* cjgood@kent.edu.

GRADUATE PROGRAMS

Expenses (2014–15) *Tuition, area resident:* full-time $8730. *Tuition, state resident:* full-time $18,638. *Tuition, nonresident:* full-time $24,794; part-time $827 per credit hour. *International tuition:* $27,658 full-time. *Room and board:* $9908 per academic year. *Required fees:* full-time $60; part-time $10 per credit.
Financial Aid 85% of graduate students in nursing programs received some form of financial aid in 2013–14. Research assistantships with full tuition reimbursements available, teaching assistantships with full tuition reimbursements available, career-related internships or fieldwork, Federal Work-Study, traineeships, and unspecified assistantships available. *Financial aid application deadline:* 2/1.
Contact Dr. Curtis Good, Assistant Dean, Operations and Student Services, College of Nursing, Kent State University, 216 Henderson Hall, PO Box 5190, Kent, OH 44242-0001. *Telephone:* 330-672-7911. *Fax:* 330-672-2061. *E-mail:* cjgood@kent.edu.

MASTER'S DEGREE PROGRAM

Degrees MSN; MSN/MBA; MSN/MPA
Available Programs Accelerated RN to Master's; Master's.
Concentrations Available Health-care administration; nursing education. *Clinical nurse specialist programs in:* adult health, pediatric. *Nurse practitioner programs in:* adult health, adult-gerontology acute care, family health, pediatric primary care, primary care, psychiatric/mental health, women's health.
Study Options Full-time and part-time.
Online Degree Options Yes.
Program Entrance Requirements Clinical experience, computer literacy, minimum overall college GPA of 3.0, transcript of college record, CPR certification, written essay, immunizations, interview, 3 letters of recommendation, professional liability insurance/malpractice insurance, resume, statistics course. *Application deadline:* 2/1 (fall), 11/1 (spring). Applications may be processed on a rolling basis for some programs. *Application fee:* $30.
Advanced Placement Credit given for nursing courses completed elsewhere dependent upon specific evaluations.
Degree Requirements 35 total credit hours.

POST-MASTER'S PROGRAM

Areas of Study Health-care administration; nursing education. *Clinical nurse specialist programs in:* adult health, pediatric. *Nurse practitioner programs in:* adult health, adult-gerontology acute care, family health, pediatric primary care, primary care, psychiatric/mental health, women's health.

DOCTORAL DEGREE PROGRAM

Degree DNP
Available Programs Doctorate.
Areas of Study Aging, clinical practice, family health, gerontology, health policy, health promotion/disease prevention, human health and illness, maternity-newborn, nurse case management, nursing administration, nursing education, nursing research, nursing science, palliative care, women's health.
Online Degree Options Yes.
Program Entrance Requirements Minimum overall college GPA of 3.0, clinical experience, interview, interview by faculty committee, 2 letters of recommendation, BSN or equivalent, MSN or equivalent, scholarly papers, statistics course, vita, writing sample. Application deadline: 7/15 (fall). Applications may be processed on a rolling basis for some programs. Application fee: $30.
Degree Requirements 73-85 total credit hours (post-baccalaureate) or 37 total credit hours (post-master's), oral exam, scholarly project.

Degree PhD
Available Programs Doctorate.
Areas of Study Aging, clinical practice, ethics, family health, gerontology, health policy, health promotion/disease prevention, human health and illness, maternity-newborn, nurse case management, nursing administration, nursing education, nursing research, nursing science, palliative care, women's health.
Program Entrance Requirements Clinical experience, minimum overall college GPA of 3.0, interview by faculty committee, interview, 2 letters of recommendation, MSN or equivalent, scholarly papers, statistics course, vita, writing sample, GRE (for PhD). Application deadline: 7/15 (fall). Applications may be processed on a rolling basis for some programs. Application fee: $30.
Degree Requirements 72 total credit hours, dissertation, oral exam, written exam.

CONTINUING EDUCATION PROGRAM

Contact Shirley Hemminger, Coordinator of Continuing Nursing Education, College of Nursing, Kent State University, PO Box 5190, Kent, OH 44242-0001. *Telephone:* 330-672-8812. *Fax:* 330-672-2433. *E-mail:* shemming@kent.edu.

Kettering College
Division of Nursing
Kettering, Ohio

http://www.kc.edu/nursing
Founded in 1967

DEGREE • BSN
Nursing Program Faculty 15 (15% with doctorates).
Baccalaureate Enrollment 206 **Women** 86% **Men** 14% **Part-time** 52%
Distance Learning Courses Available.
Nursing Student Activities Student Nurses' Association.
Nursing Student Resources Academic advising; academic or career counseling; assistance for students with disabilities; bookstore; campus computer network; computer lab; computer-assisted instruction; e-mail services; externships; interactive nursing skills videos; Internet; learning resource lab; library services; nursing audiovisuals; remedial services; resume preparation assistance; skills, simulation, or other laboratory; tutoring.
Library Facilities 3,403 volumes in health, 1,500 volumes in nursing; 216 periodical subscriptions health-care related.

BACCALAUREATE PROGRAMS

Degree BSN
Available Programs Generic Baccalaureate; LPN to Baccalaureate; RN Baccalaureate.
Study Options Full-time.
Online Degree Options Yes (online only).
Program Entrance Requirements Minimum overall college GPA of 2.5, transcript of college record, CPR certification, health insurance, immunizations, minimum GPA in nursing prerequisites of 2.5, prerequisite course work. Transfer students are accepted. *Application deadline:* 5/20 (fall), 5/25 (spring).
Advanced Placement Credit given for nursing courses completed elsewhere dependent upon specific evaluations.
Expenses (2015–16) *Tuition:* part-time $456 per credit hour. *Room and board:* $11,250 per academic year.
Financial Aid 64% of baccalaureate students in nursing programs received some form of financial aid in 2014–15. *Gift aid (need-based):* Federal Pell, state, private, college/university gift aid from institutional funds. *Loans:* Federal Nursing Student Loans, Federal Direct (Subsidized and Unsubsidized Stafford PLUS), Perkins, college/university. *Work-study:* Federal Work-Study, part-time campus jobs. *Financial aid application deadline (priority):* 3/31.
Contact Dr. Deleise S. Wilson, Director, Division of Nursing, Division of Nursing, Kettering College, 3737 Southern Boulevard, Kettering, OH 45429. *Telephone:* 937-395-5619. *Fax:* 937-395-8810. *E-mail:* deleise.wilson@kc.edu.

Lourdes University
School of Nursing
Sylvania, Ohio

http://www.lourdes.edu/
Founded in 1958

DEGREES • BSN • MSN
Nursing Program Faculty 20 (40% with doctorates).
Baccalaureate Enrollment 235 **Women** 86% **Men** 14% **Part-time** 18%
Graduate Enrollment 107 **Women** 88% **Men** 12% **Part-time** 37%
Nursing Student Activities Nursing Honor Society, Sigma Theta Tau, Student Nurses' Association.
Nursing Student Resources Academic advising; academic or career counseling; assistance for students with disabilities; bookstore; campus computer network; career placement assistance; computer lab; computer-assisted instruction; e-mail services; employment services for current students; housing assistance; interactive nursing skills videos; Internet; learning resource lab; library services; nursing audiovisuals; placement services for program completers; remedial services; resume preparation assistance; skills, simulation, or other laboratory; tutoring.
Library Facilities 1,200 volumes in health, 700 volumes in nursing; 101 periodical subscriptions health-care related.

BACCALAUREATE PROGRAMS

Degree BSN
Available Programs ADN to Baccalaureate; Generic Baccalaureate; LPN to Baccalaureate; LPN to RN Baccalaureate; RN Baccalaureate.
Study Options Full-time.
Program Entrance Requirements Minimum overall college GPA of 2.5, transcript of college record, CPR certification, health exam, high school chemistry, 4 years high school math, 3 years high school science, high school transcript, immunizations, minimum high school GPA of 2.0, minimum GPA in nursing prerequisites of 2.5, professional liability insurance/malpractice insurance, prerequisite course work, RN licensure. Transfer students are accepted. *Application deadline:* 1/2 (fall), 8/1 (winter).
Advanced Placement Credit by examination available. Credit given for nursing courses completed elsewhere dependent upon specific evaluations.
Expenses (2015–16) *Tuition:* full-time $18,970; part-time $633 per credit hour. *Room and board:* $4900 per academic year. *Required fees:* full-time $1000; part-time $50 per credit; part-time $500 per term.
Contact Ms. Pat Yancy, Nursing Advisor/Recruiter, School of Nursing, Lourdes University, 6832 Convent Boulevard, Sylvania, OH 43560. *Telephone:* 419-824-8919. *Fax:* 419-824-3985. *E-mail:* pyancy@lourdes.edu.

GRADUATE PROGRAMS

Expenses (2015–16) *Tuition:* part-time $650 per credit hour. *Room and board:* $4900 per academic year.
Contact Ms. Rebecca Zechman, MSN Coordinator, School of Nursing, Lourdes University, 6832 Convent Boulevard, Sylvania, OH 43560. *Telephone:* 419-824-3972. *Fax:* 419-824-3985. *E-mail:* rzechman@lourdes.edu.

MASTER'S DEGREE PROGRAM
Degree MSN
Available Programs Master's; RN to Master's.
Concentrations Available Nurse anesthesia; nursing administration; nursing education.
Study Options Full-time and part-time.
Program Entrance Requirements Minimum overall college GPA of 3.0, transcript of college record, written essay, interview, letters of recommendation, nursing research course. *Application deadline:* 8/1 (fall), 1/2 (winter). Applications may be processed on a rolling basis for some programs. *Application fee:* $25.
Advanced Placement Credit given for nursing courses completed elsewhere dependent upon specific evaluations.
Degree Requirements 33 total credit hours, thesis or project.

Malone University
School of Nursing
Canton, Ohio

http://www.malone.edu/
Founded in 1892

DEGREES • BSN • MSN
Nursing Program Faculty 35 (23% with doctorates).
Baccalaureate Enrollment 170 **Women** 83.5% **Men** 16.5%
Graduate Enrollment 49 **Women** 80% **Men** 20%
Distance Learning Courses Available.
Nursing Student Activities Sigma Theta Tau, Student Nurses' Association.
Nursing Student Resources Academic advising; academic or career counseling; assistance for students with disabilities; bookstore; campus computer network; career placement assistance; computer lab; computer-assisted instruction; e-mail services; employment services for current students; interactive nursing skills videos; Internet; learning resource lab; library services; nursing audiovisuals; remedial services; resume preparation assistance; skills, simulation, or other laboratory; tutoring; unpaid internships.
Library Facilities 1,509 volumes in health, 1,316 volumes in nursing; 6,246 periodical subscriptions health-care related.

BACCALAUREATE PROGRAMS

Degree BSN

Available Programs ADN to Baccalaureate; Generic Baccalaureate; RN Baccalaureate.

Study Options Full-time and part-time.

Program Entrance Requirements Minimum overall college GPA of 2.5, transcript of college record, CPR certification, health exam, health insurance, high school biology, high school chemistry, 2 years high school math, 3 years high school science, high school transcript, immunizations, 2 letters of recommendation, minimum high school GPA of 3.0, minimum GPA in nursing prerequisites of 2.5, professional liability insurance/malpractice insurance, prerequisite course work. Transfer students are accepted. *Application deadline:* Applications may be processed on a rolling basis for some programs. *Application fee:* $20.

Advanced Placement Credit given for nursing courses completed elsewhere dependent upon specific evaluations.

Financial Aid *Gift aid (need-based):* Federal Pell, FSEOG, state, private, college/university gift aid from institutional funds. *Loans:* Federal Direct (Subsidized and Unsubsidized Stafford PLUS), Perkins, state, college/university, alternative loans. *Work-study:* Federal Work-Study. *Financial aid application deadline:* 7/31(priority: 3/1).

Contact Linda Hoffman, Director of Admissions, School of Nursing, Malone University, 2600 Cleveland Avenue NW, Canton, OH 44709. *Telephone:* 330-471-8145. *Fax:* 330-471-8149. *E-mail:* admissions@malone.edu.

GRADUATE PROGRAMS

Contact Ms. Beth Weingart, Administrative Assistant, School of Nursing, Malone University, 2600 Cleveland Avenue NW, Cant on, OH 44709. *Telephone:* 330-471-8166. *Fax:* 330-471-8607. *E-mail:* eweingart@malone.edu.

MASTER'S DEGREE PROGRAM

Degree MSN

Available Programs Master's.

Concentrations Available *Nurse practitioner programs in:* adult-gerontology acute care, family health.

Study Options Full-time.

Program Entrance Requirements Clinical experience, computer literacy, minimum overall college GPA of 3.0, transcript of college record, CPR certification, written essay, immunizations, interview, 2 letters of recommendation, nursing research course, physical assessment course, professional liability insurance/malpractice insurance, resume, statistics course. *Application deadline:* Applications may be processed on a rolling basis for some programs. *Application fee:* $150.

Advanced Placement Credit given for nursing courses completed elsewhere dependent upon specific evaluations.

Degree Requirements 56 total credit hours, thesis or project.

Mercy College of Ohio
Division of Nursing
Toledo, Ohio

http://www.mercycollege.edu/
Founded in 1993

DEGREE • BSN

Nursing Program Faculty 63 (9.5% with doctorates).

Baccalaureate Enrollment 252 **Women** 88% **Men** 12% **Part-time** 29%

Distance Learning Courses Available.

Nursing Student Activities Sigma Theta Tau, Student Nurses' Association.

Nursing Student Resources Academic advising; academic or career counseling; assistance for students with disabilities; campus computer network; career placement assistance; computer lab; computer-assisted instruction; e-mail services; employment services for current students; housing assistance; interactive nursing skills videos; Internet; learning resource lab; library services; nursing audiovisuals; remedial services; resume preparation assistance; skills, simulation, or other laboratory; tutoring.

Library Facilities 3,580 volumes in health, 800 volumes in nursing; 325 periodical subscriptions health-care related.

BACCALAUREATE PROGRAMS

Degree BSN

Available Programs Generic Baccalaureate; RN Baccalaureate.

Study Options Full-time and part-time.

Online Degree Options Yes.

Program Entrance Requirements Minimum overall college GPA of 2.7, transcript of college record, CPR certification, health exam, health insurance, high school biology, high school chemistry, 2 years high school math, high school transcript, immunizations, minimum high school GPA of 2.7, RN licensure. Transfer students are accepted. *Application deadline:* 8/1 (fall). *Application fee:* $25.

Advanced Placement Credit by examination available.

Expenses (2015–16) *Tuition:* full-time $11,430; part-time $420 per credit hour. *Required fees:* full-time $1100; part-time $35 per credit.

Contact Ms. Lori Edgeworth, Vice President of Enrollment Services, Division of Nursing, Mercy College of Ohio, 2221 Madison Avenue, Toledo, OH 43604. *Telephone:* 888-806-3729. *Fax:* 419-251-1462. *E-mail:* lori.edgeworth@mercycollege.edu.

Miami University
Department of Nursing
Hamilton, Ohio

http://www.regionals.miamioh.edu/nsg/
Founded in 1809

DEGREE • BSN

Nursing Program Faculty 13 (23% with doctorates).

Baccalaureate Enrollment 106 **Women** 98% **Men** 2% **Part-time** 56%

Distance Learning Courses Available.

Nursing Student Activities Sigma Theta Tau, Student Nurses' Association.

Nursing Student Resources Academic advising; academic or career counseling; assistance for students with disabilities; bookstore; campus computer network; computer lab; daycare for children of students; e-mail services; interactive nursing skills videos; Internet; learning resource lab; library services; nursing audiovisuals; resume preparation assistance; tutoring.

Library Facilities 29,000 volumes in nursing; 852 periodical subscriptions health-care related.

BACCALAUREATE PROGRAMS

Degree BSN

Available Programs ADN to Baccalaureate; Generic Baccalaureate; RN Baccalaureate.

Site Options Hamilton, OH; Middletown, OH.

Study Options Full-time and part-time.

Program Entrance Requirements Minimum overall college GPA of 2.5, transcript of college record, health exam, health insurance, high school chemistry, 2 years high school math, 1 year of high school science, high school transcript, immunizations, minimum high school GPA of 3.0, minimum GPA in nursing prerequisites of 2.5, professional liability insurance/malpractice insurance. Transfer students are accepted.

Advanced Placement Credit given for nursing courses completed elsewhere dependent upon specific evaluations.

Contact *Telephone:* 513-785-7751. *Fax:* 513-785-7767.

Miami University Hamilton
Bachelor of Science in Nursing Program
Hamilton, Ohio

Founded in 1968

DEGREE • BSN

Nursing Program Faculty 27 (15% with doctorates).

Baccalaureate Enrollment 116

Distance Learning Courses Available.

Nursing Student Activities Sigma Theta Tau, Student Nurses' Association.

Nursing Student Resources Academic advising; academic or career counseling; assistance for students with disabilities; bookstore; campus computer network; career placement assistance; computer lab; computer-assisted instruction; daycare for children of students; e-mail services; employment services for current students; interactive nursing skills videos; Internet; learning resource lab; library services; nursing audiovisuals; placement services for program completers; remedial services; resume preparation assistance; skills, simulation, or other laboratory; tutoring.

BACCALAUREATE PROGRAMS

Degree BSN
Available Programs Generic Baccalaureate; RN Baccalaureate.
Site Options West Chester, OH; Middletown, OH.
Contact *Telephone:* 513-785-7772. *Fax:* 513-785-7767.

Mount Carmel College of Nursing
Nursing Programs
Columbus, Ohio

http://www.mccn.edu/
Founded in 1903
DEGREES • BSN • DNP • MS
Nursing Program Faculty 94 (17% with doctorates).
Baccalaureate Enrollment 898 **Women** 90% **Men** 10% **Part-time** 30%
Graduate Enrollment 165 **Women** 90% **Men** 10% **Part-time** 56%
Distance Learning Courses Available.
Nursing Student Activities Sigma Theta Tau, Student Nurses' Association.
Nursing Student Resources Academic advising; academic or career counseling; assistance for students with disabilities; bookstore; campus computer network; computer lab; computer-assisted instruction; e-mail services; housing assistance; interactive nursing skills videos; Internet; learning resource lab; library services; nursing audiovisuals; resume preparation assistance; skills, simulation, or other laboratory; tutoring.
Library Facilities 2,265 volumes in health, 2,045 volumes in nursing; 8,665 periodical subscriptions health-care related.

BACCALAUREATE PROGRAMS

Degree BSN
Available Programs Accelerated Baccalaureate for Second Degree; Generic Baccalaureate; RN Baccalaureate.
Site Options Lancaster, OH.
Study Options Full-time.
Online Degree Options Yes.
Program Entrance Requirements Minimum overall college GPA of 2.8, transcript of college record, written essay, health exam, high school biology, high school chemistry, high school foreign language, 3 years high school math, 3 years high school science, high school transcript, immunizations, minimum high school GPA of 3.0. Transfer students are accepted. *Application deadline:* 4/1 (fall), 1/15 (summer). Applications may be processed on a rolling basis for some programs. *Application fee:* $30.
Advanced Placement Credit given for nursing courses completed elsewhere dependent upon specific evaluations.
Contact Kim M. Campbell, Director, Admissions and Recruitment, Nursing Programs, Mount Carmel College of Nursing, 127 South Davis Avenue, Columbus, OH 43222-1504. *Telephone:* 614-234-5144. *Fax:* 614-234-2875. *E-mail:* kcampbell@mccn.edu.

GRADUATE PROGRAMS

Contact Anne Hinze, Graduate Advisor, Nursing Programs, Mount Carmel College of Nursing, 127 South Davis Avenue, Columbus, OH 43222-1504. *Telephone:* 614-234-1135. *Fax:* 614-234-2298. *E-mail:* ahinze@mccn.edu.

MASTER'S DEGREE PROGRAM

Degree MS
Available Programs Master's.
Concentrations Available Nursing administration; nursing education. *Nurse practitioner programs in:* adult-gerontology acute care, family health.
Study Options Full-time and part-time.
Online Degree Options Yes.
Program Entrance Requirements Minimum overall college GPA of 3.0, transcript of college record, CPR certification, written essay, interview, 2 letters of recommendation, nursing research course, resume, statistics course. *Application deadline:* 2/1 (fall), 10/1 (spring). Applications may be processed on a rolling basis for some programs. *Application fee:* $30.
Advanced Placement Credit given for nursing courses completed elsewhere dependent upon specific evaluations.
Degree Requirements 34 total credit hours, thesis or project, comprehensive exam.

POST-MASTER'S PROGRAM

Areas of Study Nursing administration; nursing education. *Nurse practitioner programs in:* adult-gerontology acute care, family health.

DOCTORAL DEGREE PROGRAM

Degree DNP
Available Programs Doctorate.
Online Degree Options Yes (online only).
Program Entrance Requirements Clinical experience, minimum overall college GPA of 3.25, interview, 2 letters of recommendation, MSN or equivalent, statistics course, vita, writing sample. Application deadline: 3/1 (fall). Application fee: $30.
Degree Requirements 35 total credit hours.

Mount St. Joseph University
Department of Nursing
Cincinnati, Ohio

http://www.msj.edu/
Founded in 1920
DEGREES • BSN • MN
Nursing Program Faculty 32 (4% with doctorates).
Baccalaureate Enrollment 287 **Women** 97% **Men** 3% **Part-time** 60%
Graduate Enrollment 21 **Women** 90% **Men** 10%
Nursing Student Activities Nursing Honor Society, Sigma Theta Tau, Student Nurses' Association.
Nursing Student Resources Academic advising; academic or career counseling; assistance for students with disabilities; bookstore; campus computer network; career placement assistance; computer lab; computer-assisted instruction; daycare for children of students; e-mail services; employment services for current students; externships; housing assistance; interactive nursing skills videos; Internet; learning resource lab; library services; nursing audiovisuals; placement services for program completers; remedial services; resume preparation assistance; skills, simulation, or other laboratory; tutoring.
Library Facilities 1,800 volumes in health, 1,200 volumes in nursing; 300 periodical subscriptions health-care related.

BACCALAUREATE PROGRAMS

Degree BSN
Available Programs Accelerated RN Baccalaureate; Generic Baccalaureate.
Site Options Cincinnati, OH; Covington, KY.
Study Options Full-time and part-time.
Program Entrance Requirements Minimum overall college GPA of 2.75, transcript of college record, CPR certification, health exam, health insurance, high school chemistry, 2 years high school math, 2 years high school science, high school transcript, immunizations, interview, minimum high school GPA of 2.75, minimum high school rank 60%, minimum GPA in nursing prerequisites of 2.75, professional liability insurance/malpractice insurance, prerequisite course work. Transfer students are accepted. *Application deadline:* Applications may be processed on a rolling basis for some programs. *Application fee:* $25.
Advanced Placement Credit by examination available. Credit given for nursing courses completed elsewhere dependent upon specific evaluations.
Contact *Telephone:* 513-244-4511. *Fax:* 513-451-2547.

GRADUATE PROGRAMS

Contact *Telephone:* 513-244-4503. *Fax:* 513-451-2547.

MASTER'S DEGREE PROGRAM

Degree MN
Available Programs Accelerated Master's for Non-Nursing College Graduates.
Study Options Full-time.
Program Entrance Requirements Minimum overall college GPA of 3.0, transcript of college record, CPR certification, written essay, immunizations, interview, professional liability insurance/malpractice insurance, prerequisite course work, statistics course. *Application deadline:* Applications may be processed on a rolling basis for some programs. *Application fee:* $50.

Advanced Placement Credit by examination available. Credit given for nursing courses completed elsewhere dependent upon specific evaluations.

Degree Requirements 64 total credit hours, thesis or project.

Mount Vernon Nazarene University
School of Nursing and Health Sciences
Mount Vernon, Ohio

http://www.mvnu.edu/
Founded in 1964
DEGREE • BS
Nursing Program Faculty 10 (10% with doctorates).
Baccalaureate Enrollment 109
Nursing Student Activities Sigma Theta Tau, nursing club.
Nursing Student Resources Academic advising; academic or career counseling; assistance for students with disabilities; bookstore; campus computer network; computer lab; computer-assisted instruction; e-mail services; employment services for current students; interactive nursing skills videos; Internet; learning resource lab; library services; nursing audiovisuals; remedial services; resume preparation assistance; skills, simulation, or other laboratory; tutoring.

BACCALAUREATE PROGRAMS

Degree BS
Available Programs ADN to Baccalaureate; Generic Baccalaureate.
Study Options Full-time and part-time.
Program Entrance Requirements Minimum overall college GPA of 2.75, transcript of college record, CPR certification, health exam, health insurance, immunizations, minimum GPA in nursing prerequisites of 2.0, professional liability insurance/malpractice insurance, prerequisite course work. Transfer students are accepted. *Application deadline:* Applications may be processed on a rolling basis for some programs.
Contact Nursing Program, School of Nursing and Health Sciences, Mount Vernon Nazarene University, 800 Martinsburg Road, Mount Vernon, OH 43050. *Telephone:* 740-392-6868.

Muskingum University
Department of Nursing
New Concord, Ohio

Founded in 1837
DEGREE • BSN

BACCALAUREATE PROGRAMS

Degree BSN
Available Programs Generic Baccalaureate.
Contact *Telephone:* 740-826-6151.

Notre Dame College
Nursing Department
South Euclid, Ohio

http://notredamecollege.edu/academics/academic-divisions/nursing
Founded in 1922
DEGREES • BSN • MSN
Nursing Program Faculty 6 (50% with doctorates).
Baccalaureate Enrollment 325 Women 85% Men 15% Part-time 10%
Graduate Enrollment 7 Women 100%
Distance Learning Courses Available.
Nursing Student Activities Nursing Honor Society, Sigma Theta Tau, Student Nurses' Association, nursing club.
Nursing Student Resources Academic advising; academic or career counseling; assistance for students with disabilities; bookstore; campus computer network; career placement assistance; computer lab; computer-assisted instruction; e-mail services; employment services for current students; housing assistance; interactive nursing skills videos; Internet; learning resource lab; library services; nursing audiovisuals; remedial

services; resume preparation assistance; skills, simulation, or other laboratory; tutoring.
Library Facilities 100 volumes in health, 40 volumes in nursing; 5,000 periodical subscriptions health-care related.

BACCALAUREATE PROGRAMS

Degree BSN
Available Programs Generic Baccalaureate; RN Baccalaureate.
Study Options Full-time.
Online Degree Options Yes.
Program Entrance Requirements Minimum overall college GPA of 2.75, transcript of college record, CPR certification, written essay, health exam, health insurance, high school chemistry, 3 years high school math, 3 years high school science, high school transcript, immunizations, minimum GPA in nursing prerequisites of 2.75, professional liability insurance/malpractice insurance, prerequisite course work. Transfer students are accepted. *Application deadline:* 2/1 (winter), 4/1 (spring). *Application fee:* $30.
Advanced Placement Credit given for nursing courses completed elsewhere dependent upon specific evaluations.
Expenses (2015–16) *Tuition:* full-time $13,410. *Room and board:* $4590; room only: $2275 per academic year. *Required fees:* full-time $350.
Financial Aid 85% of baccalaureate students in nursing programs received some form of financial aid in 2014–15. *Gift aid (need-based):* Federal Pell, FSEOG, state, private, college/university gift aid from institutional funds, Academic Competitiveness Grants, National SMART Grants. *Loans:* Perkins. *Work-study:* Federal Work-Study. *Financial aid application deadline (priority):* 2/15.
Contact *Telephone:* 216-373-5183.

GRADUATE PROGRAMS

Contact Dr. Colleen Sweeney, Director, Graduate Nursing Programs, Nursing Department, Notre Dame College, 4545 College Road, South Euclid, OH 44121. *Telephone:* 216-373-6373. *Fax:* 216-373-5186. *E-mail:* csweeney@ndc.edu.

MASTER'S DEGREE PROGRAM
Degree MSN
Available Programs Master's.
Concentrations Available Nursing education.
Study Options Part-time.
Online Degree Options Yes (online only).
Program Entrance Requirements Clinical experience, minimum overall college GPA of 3.0, transcript of college record, written essay, interview, 3 letters of recommendation, resume. *Application deadline:* 8/14 (fall), 1/9 (spring).
Advanced Placement Credit given for nursing courses completed elsewhere dependent upon specific evaluations.
Degree Requirements 36 total credit hours, thesis or project.

Ohio Northern University
Nursing Program
Ada, Ohio

https://www.onu.edu/academics/college_of_arts_sciences/academic_departments/nursing
Founded in 1871
DEGREE • BSN
Nursing Program Faculty 16 (31% with doctorates).
Distance Learning Courses Available.
Nursing Student Activities Nursing Honor Society, Student Nurses' Association.
Nursing Student Resources Academic advising; academic or career counseling; assistance for students with disabilities; bookstore; campus computer network; career placement assistance; computer lab; computer-assisted instruction; e-mail services; employment services for current students; housing assistance; interactive nursing skills videos; Internet; learning resource lab; library services; nursing audiovisuals; placement services for program completers; remedial services; resume preparation assistance; skills, simulation, or other laboratory; tutoring.

BACCALAUREATE PROGRAMS

Degree BSN
Available Programs Accelerated RN Baccalaureate; Generic Baccalaureate; RN Baccalaureate.

Site Options Findlay, OH; Lima, OH.
Study Options Full-time.
Program Entrance Requirements High school chemistry, 2 years high school math, 2 years high school science, high school transcript, minimum high school GPA of 3.3. Transfer students are accepted. *Application deadline:* Applications may be processed on a rolling basis for some programs.
Advanced Placement Credit given for nursing courses completed elsewhere dependent upon specific evaluations.
Expenses (2014–15) *Tuition:* full-time $28,050; part-time $1145 per credit. *Room and board:* $10,780 per academic year.
Contact Admissions Office, Nursing Program, Ohio Northern University, 525 North Main Street, Ada, OH 45810. *Telephone:* 888-408-4668. *Fax:* 419-772-2821. *E-mail:* admissions-ug@onu.edu.

The Ohio State University
College of Nursing
Columbus, Ohio

http://www.nursing.osu.edu/
Founded in 1870
DEGREES • BSN • DNP • MS • MS/MPH • PHD
Nursing Program Faculty 153 (47% with doctorates).
Baccalaureate Enrollment 688 **Women** 87% **Men** 13% **Part-time** 33%
Graduate Enrollment 629 **Women** 85% **Men** 15% **Part-time** 29%
Distance Learning Courses Available.
Nursing Student Activities Nursing Honor Society, Sigma Theta Tau, Student Nurses' Association, nursing club.
Nursing Student Resources Academic advising; academic or career counseling; assistance for students with disabilities; bookstore; campus computer network; career placement assistance; computer lab; computer-assisted instruction; daycare for children of students; e-mail services; employment services for current students; externships; housing assistance; interactive nursing skills videos; Internet; learning resource lab; library services; nursing audiovisuals; other; paid internships; placement services for program completers; remedial services; resume preparation assistance; skills, simulation, or other laboratory; tutoring; unpaid internships.
Library Facilities 112,764 volumes in health, 12,534 volumes in nursing; 6,297 periodical subscriptions health-care related.

BACCALAUREATE PROGRAMS

Degree BSN
Available Programs Generic Baccalaureate; RN Baccalaureate.
Study Options Full-time.
Online Degree Options Yes.
Program Entrance Requirements Minimum overall college GPA of 3.2, transcript of college record, written essay, minimum GPA in nursing prerequisites of 3.2, prerequisite course work. *Application deadline:* 1/15 (fall), 8/1 (spring). *Application fee:* $60.
Advanced Placement Credit by examination available. Credit given for nursing courses completed elsewhere dependent upon specific evaluations.
Expenses (2015–16) *Tuition, state resident:* full-time $9200; part-time $382 per credit. *Tuition, nonresident:* full-time $30,000; part-time $1245 per credit. *International tuition:* $30,000 full-time. *Room and board:* $10,700; room only: $7000 per academic year. *Required fees:* full-time $2300.
Financial Aid 67% of baccalaureate students in nursing programs received some form of financial aid in 2014–15. *Gift aid (need-based):* Federal Pell, FSEOG, state, private, college/university gift aid from institutional funds. *Loans:* Federal Nursing Student Loans, Federal Direct (Subsidized and Unsubsidized Stafford PLUS), Perkins, college/university. *Work-study:* Federal Work-Study, part-time campus jobs. *Financial aid application deadline (priority):* 2/15.
Contact Ms. Jennifer Marinello, Associate Director, College of Nursing, The Ohio State University, Graduate and Professional Admissions, Student Academic Services Building, Columbus, OH 43210. *Telephone:* 614-292-9444. *Fax:* 614-292-3895. *E-mail:* gpadmissions@osu.edu.

GRADUATE PROGRAMS

Expenses (2015–16) *Tuition, state resident:* full-time $18,000; part-time $723 per credit. *Tuition, nonresident:* full-time $47,000; part-time $1940 per credit. *International tuition:* $47,000 full-time. *Required fees:* full-time $5500; part-time $53 per term.

Financial Aid 67% of graduate students in nursing programs received some form of financial aid in 2014–15. Fellowships, research assistantships, teaching assistantships, Federal Work-Study, institutionally sponsored loans, and unspecified assistantships available. Aid available to part-time students.
Contact Ms. Megan Alexander, Graduate Admissions Counselor, College of Nursing, The Ohio State University, 1585 Neil Avenue, Newton Hall, Columbus, OH 43210-1289. *Telephone:* 614-292-4041. *Fax:* 614-292-9399. *E-mail:* nursing@osu.edu.

MASTER'S DEGREE PROGRAM
Degrees MS; MS/MPH
Available Programs Master's; Master's for Non-Nursing College Graduates; Master's for Nurses with Non-Nursing Degrees; RN to Master's.
Concentrations Available Clinical nurse leader; health-care administration; nurse-midwifery; nursing administration. *Clinical nurse specialist programs in:* adult health. *Nurse practitioner programs in:* acute care, adult health, adult-gerontology acute care, community health, family health, gerontology, neonatal health, pediatric, pediatric primary care, primary care, psychiatric/mental health, women's health.
Study Options Full-time and part-time.
Online Degree Options Yes.
Program Entrance Requirements Minimum overall college GPA of 3.5, transcript of college record, written essay, interview, 3 letters of recommendation, prerequisite course work, resume. *Application deadline:* 1/15 (fall), 10/12 (summer). *Application fee:* $60.
Advanced Placement Credit given for nursing courses completed elsewhere dependent upon specific evaluations.
Degree Requirements 30 total credit hours, thesis or project, comprehensive exam.

POST-MASTER'S PROGRAM
Areas of Study Clinical nurse leader; health-care administration; nurse-midwifery; nursing administration. *Clinical nurse specialist programs in:* adult health. *Nurse practitioner programs in:* acute care, adult health, adult-gerontology acute care, community health, family health, gerontology, neonatal health, pediatric, pediatric primary care, primary care, psychiatric/mental health, women's health.

DOCTORAL DEGREE PROGRAM
Degree DNP
Available Programs Doctorate, Post-Baccalaureate Doctorate.
Areas of Study Addiction/substance abuse, advanced practice nursing, aging, bio-behavioral research, biology of health and illness, clinical nurse leader, clinical practice, clinical research, community health, critical care, ethics, faculty preparation, family health, forensic nursing, gerontology, health policy, health promotion/disease prevention, health-care systems, human health and illness, illness and transition, individualized study, information systems, maternity-newborn, neuro-behavior, nurse case management, nursing administration, nursing education, nursing policy, nursing research, nursing science, oncology, palliative care, urban health, women's health.
Online Degree Options Yes (online only).
Program Entrance Requirements Minimum overall college GPA of 3.5, clinical experience, interview by faculty committee, 3 letters of recommendation, vita, writing sample. Application deadline: 1/15 (fall). Application fee: $60.
Degree Requirements 50 total credit hours, Capstone project, oral exam, residency, written exam.

Degree PhD
Available Programs Doctorate; Post-Baccalaureate Doctorate.
Areas of Study Addiction/substance abuse, advanced practice nursing, aging, bio-behavioral research, biology of health and illness, clinical nurse leader, clinical practice, clinical research, community health, critical care, ethics, faculty preparation, family health, forensic nursing, gerontology, health policy, health promotion/disease prevention, health-care systems, human health and illness, illness and transition, individualized study, information systems, maternity-newborn, neuro-behavior, nurse case management, nursing administration, nursing education, nursing policy, nursing research, nursing science, oncology, palliative care, urban health, women's health.
Program Entrance Requirements Clinical experience, minimum overall college GPA of 3.5, 3 letters of recommendation, vita, writing sample, GRE (for PhD). Application deadline: 12/1 (fall). Application fee: $60.
Degree Requirements 50 total credit hours, dissertation, oral exam, written exam, residency.

CONTINUING EDUCATION PROGRAM

Contact Mr. Tim Raderstorf, Director of the Transformational Learning Academy in Nursing and Health (TLA), College of Nursing, The Ohio State University, 1585 Neil Avenue, Newton Hall, Columbus, OH 43210-1289. *Telephone:* 614-292-2155. *Fax:* 614-292-7976. *E-mail:* Raderstorf.3@osu.edu.

Ohio University

School of Nursing
Athens, Ohio

http://www.ohio.edu/chsp/nrse/
Founded in 1804
DEGREES • BSN • MSN
Nursing Program Faculty 9 (89% with doctorates).
Nursing Student Activities Nursing Honor Society, Sigma Theta Tau.
Nursing Student Resources Academic or career counseling; career placement assistance; computer lab; e-mail services; Internet; library services.

BACCALAUREATE PROGRAMS

Degree BSN
Available Programs Generic Baccalaureate; RN Baccalaureate.
Online Degree Options Yes.
Program Entrance Requirements Transfer students are accepted.
Contact *Telephone:* 740-593-4494. *Fax:* 740-593-0286.

GRADUATE PROGRAMS

Contact *Telephone:* 740-593-4494. *Fax:* 740-593-0144.

MASTER'S DEGREE PROGRAM

Degree MSN
Available Programs Master's.
Concentrations Available Nursing administration; nursing education. *Nurse practitioner programs in:* family health.
Study Options Full-time and part-time.
Program Entrance Requirements Minimum overall college GPA of 3.0, transcript of college record, written essay, 3 letters of recommendation, resume, statistics course.
Advanced Placement Credit given for nursing courses completed elsewhere dependent upon specific evaluations.
Degree Requirements 55 total credit hours.

Otterbein University

Department of Nursing
Westerville, Ohio

http://www.otterbein.edu/
Founded in 1847
DEGREES • BSN • MSN
Nursing Student Activities Nursing Honor Society, Sigma Theta Tau.

BACCALAUREATE PROGRAMS

Degree BSN
Available Programs Accelerated RN Baccalaureate; Generic Baccalaureate; LPN to Baccalaureate; RN Baccalaureate.
Program Entrance Requirements Transfer students are accepted.
Advanced Placement Credit by examination available. Credit given for nursing courses completed elsewhere dependent upon specific evaluations.
Contact *Telephone:* 614-823-1614. *Fax:* 614-823-3131.

GRADUATE PROGRAMS

Contact *Telephone:* 614-823-1614.

MASTER'S DEGREE PROGRAM

Degree MSN
Available Programs Master's.
Concentrations Available Nursing administration; nursing education. *Clinical nurse specialist programs in:* adult health. *Nurse practitioner programs in:* adult health, family health.
Study Options Part-time.

POST-MASTER'S PROGRAM
Areas of Study Nursing education. *Nurse practitioner programs in:* adult health, family health.

CONTINUING EDUCATION PROGRAM

Contact *Telephone:* 614-823-1614.

Shawnee State University

Department of Nursing
Portsmouth, Ohio

http://www.shawnee.edu/
Founded in 1986
DEGREE • BSN
Nursing Program Faculty 9
Nursing Student Activities Student Nurses' Association.
Nursing Student Resources Academic advising; academic or career counseling; assistance for students with disabilities; bookstore; campus computer network; career placement assistance; computer lab; computer-assisted instruction; daycare for children of students; e-mail services; employment services for current students; housing assistance; interactive nursing skills videos; Internet; learning resource lab; library services; nursing audiovisuals; other; placement services for program completers; remedial services; resume preparation assistance; skills, simulation, or other laboratory; tutoring.
Library Facilities 8,273 volumes in health, 870 volumes in nursing; 1,798 periodical subscriptions health-care related.

BACCALAUREATE PROGRAMS

Degree BSN
Available Programs ADN to Baccalaureate; RN Baccalaureate.
Study Options Full-time and part-time.
Program Entrance Requirements Minimum overall college GPA of 2.5, transcript of college record, CPR certification, health exam, health insurance, high school transcript, immunizations, professional liability insurance/malpractice insurance, prerequisite course work, RN licensure. Transfer students are accepted.
Advanced Placement Credit given for nursing courses completed elsewhere dependent upon specific evaluations.
Contact *Telephone:* 740-351-3378. *Fax:* 740-351-3354.

CONTINUING EDUCATION PROGRAM

Contact *Telephone:* 740-351-3281.

The University of Akron

School of Nursing
Akron, Ohio

http://www.uakron.edu/nursing/
Founded in 1870
DEGREES • BSN • MSN • PHD
Nursing Program Faculty 98 (25% with doctorates).
Baccalaureate Enrollment 551 **Women** 78% **Men** 22% **Part-time** 1%
Graduate Enrollment 329 **Women** 87% **Men** 13% **Part-time** 74%
Distance Learning Courses Available.
Nursing Student Activities Nursing Honor Society, Sigma Theta Tau, Student Nurses' Association, nursing club.
Nursing Student Resources Academic advising; academic or career counseling; assistance for students with disabilities; bookstore; campus computer network; career placement assistance; computer lab; computer-assisted instruction; daycare for children of students; e-mail services; employment services for current students; interactive nursing skills videos; Internet; learning resource lab; library services; nursing audiovisuals; remedial services; resume preparation assistance; skills, simulation, or other laboratory; tutoring.
Library Facilities 36,800 volumes in health, 10,258 volumes in nursing; 7,804 periodical subscriptions health-care related.

BACCALAUREATE PROGRAMS

Degree BSN
Available Programs ADN to Baccalaureate; Accelerated Baccalaureate for Second Degree; Accelerated RN Baccalaureate; Generic Baccalaureate; LPN to Baccalaureate.

Site Options Lorain, OH; Orville, OH; Kirtland (Lakeland Community College), OH; Medina, OH; Lakewood (UA Lakewood), OH.
Study Options Full-time and part-time.
Online Degree Options Yes.
Program Entrance Requirements Transcript of college record, CPR certification, health exam, immunizations, minimum GPA in nursing prerequisites of 2.75, prerequisite course work. Transfer students are accepted. *Application deadline:* Applications may be processed on a rolling basis for some programs. *Application fee:* $40.
Advanced Placement Credit given for nursing courses completed elsewhere dependent upon specific evaluations.
Expenses (2014–15) *Tuition, state resident:* full-time $8618; part-time $413 per credit hour. *Tuition, nonresident:* full-time $17,150; part-time $768 per credit hour. *Room and board:* $11,000 per academic year. *Required fees:* full-time $1294; part-time $53 per credit.
Financial Aid 80% of baccalaureate students in nursing programs received some form of financial aid in 2013–14.
Contact School of Nursing, School of Nursing, The University of Akron, Mary Gladwin Hall, 209 Carroll Street, Akron, OH 44325-3701. *Telephone:* 330-972-6674. *Fax:* 330-972-5737.

GRADUATE PROGRAMS

Expenses (2014–15) *Tuition, state resident:* full-time $6316; part-time $421 per credit. *Tuition, nonresident:* full-time $11,229; part-time $721 per credit. *International tuition:* $11,229 full-time. *Required fees:* full-time $416; part-time $35 per credit; part-time $108 per term.
Financial Aid 80% of graduate students in nursing programs received some form of financial aid in 2013–14. 11 teaching assistantships with full tuition reimbursements available were awarded; unspecified assistantships also available.
Contact Ms. Susan Bradford, Student Services Counselor, School of Nursing, The University of Akron, 302 Buchtel Common, Mary Gladwin Hall, Akron, OH 44325-3701. *Telephone:* 330-972-7555. *Fax:* 330-972-5737. *E-mail:* sb14@uakron.edu.

MASTER'S DEGREE PROGRAM

Degree MSN
Available Programs Master's; RN to Master's.
Concentrations Available Nurse anesthesia; nursing administration. *Clinical nurse specialist programs in:* adult health, gerontology. *Nurse practitioner programs in:* adult health, gerontology, pediatric, pediatric primary care, primary care, psychiatric/mental health.
Site Options Lorain, OH; Orville, OH.
Study Options Full-time and part-time.
Program Entrance Requirements Clinical experience, computer literacy, minimum overall college GPA of 3.0, transcript of college record, CPR certification, written essay, immunizations, interview, 3 letters of recommendation, physical assessment course, professional liability insurance/malpractice insurance, prerequisite course work, resume, statistics course. *Application deadline:* Applications may be processed on a rolling basis for some programs. *Application fee:* $45.
Advanced Placement Credit given for nursing courses completed elsewhere dependent upon specific evaluations.
Degree Requirements 53 total credit hours.

POST-MASTER'S PROGRAM

Areas of Study Nurse anesthesia. *Clinical nurse specialist programs in:* adult health, gerontology. *Nurse practitioner programs in:* adult health, family health, gerontology, pediatric, pediatric primary care, primary care, psychiatric/mental health.

DOCTORAL DEGREE PROGRAM

Degree PhD
Available Programs Doctorate.
Areas of Study Advanced practice nursing, aging, clinical practice, community health, critical care, ethics, family health, gerontology, health policy, health promotion/disease prevention, health-care systems, human health and illness, illness and transition, individualized study, maternity-newborn, nursing administration, nursing policy, nursing research, nursing science, women's health.
Program Entrance Requirements Minimum overall college GPA of 3.0, interview by faculty committee, interview, 3 letters of recommendation, MSN or equivalent, vita, writing sample, GRE. Application deadline: Applications may be processed on a rolling basis for some programs. Application fee: $40.
Degree Requirements 72 total credit hours, dissertation, oral exam, written exam, residency.

CONTINUING EDUCATION PROGRAM

Contact Ms. Lisa A. Hart, Associate Instructor, School of Nursing, The University of Akron, 209 Carroll Street, Akron, OH 44325-3701. *Telephone:* 330-972-5924. *Fax:* 330-972-5737. *E-mail:* lahart@uakron.edu.

University of Cincinnati
College of Nursing
Cincinnati, Ohio

http://www.nursing.uc.edu/
Founded in 1819
DEGREES • BSN • MSN • PHD
Nursing Program Faculty 79 (54% with doctorates).
Baccalaureate Enrollment 1,325 **Women** 81% **Men** 19% **Part-time** 29%
Graduate Enrollment 1,720 **Women** 88% **Men** 12% **Part-time** 50%
Distance Learning Courses Available.
Nursing Student Activities Nursing Honor Society, Sigma Theta Tau, Student Nurses' Association, nursing club.
Nursing Student Resources Academic advising; academic or career counseling; assistance for students with disabilities; bookstore; campus computer network; career placement assistance; computer lab; computer-assisted instruction; daycare for children of students; e-mail services; employment services for current students; externships; housing assistance; interactive nursing skills videos; Internet; learning resource lab; library services; nursing audiovisuals; paid internships; remedial services; resume preparation assistance; skills, simulation, or other laboratory; tutoring; unpaid internships.
Library Facilities 225,000 volumes in health, 65,000 volumes in nursing; 110,000 periodical subscriptions health-care related.

BACCALAUREATE PROGRAMS

Degree BSN
Available Programs ADN to Baccalaureate; Accelerated Baccalaureate for Second Degree; Generic Baccalaureate; RN Baccalaureate.
Site Options Batavia, OH.
Study Options Full-time.
Program Entrance Requirements Written essay, health insurance, high school biology, high school chemistry, 4 years high school math, 3 years high school science, high school transcript, minimum high school GPA of 3.0. Transfer students are accepted. *Application deadline:* 3/1 (fall). Applications may be processed on a rolling basis for some programs. *Application fee:* $50.
Advanced Placement Credit by examination available. Credit given for nursing courses completed elsewhere dependent upon specific evaluations.
Expenses (2014–15) *Tuition, state resident:* full-time $9322; part-time $389 per credit hour. *Tuition, nonresident:* full-time $24,656; part-time $1028 per credit hour. *International tuition:* $24,656 full-time. *Room and board:* $10,496; room only: $6274 per academic year. *Required fees:* full-time $2481; part-time $226 per credit; part-time $1358 per term.
Financial Aid 75% of baccalaureate students in nursing programs received some form of financial aid in 2013–14.
Contact Ms. Deborah Gray, Assistant Director, Undergraduate Programs, College of Nursing, University of Cincinnati, PO Box 210038, Office of Student Affairs, Cincinnati, OH 45221-0038. *Telephone:* 513-558-5355. *Fax:* 513-558-7523. *E-mail:* deborah.gray@uc.edu.

GRADUATE PROGRAMS

Expenses (2014–15) *Tuition, state resident:* full-time $12,790; part-time $640 per credit hour. *Tuition, nonresident:* full-time $24,532; part-time $1227 per credit hour. *International tuition:* $24,532 full-time. *Required fees:* full-time $2428; part-time $775 per term.
Financial Aid 75% of graduate students in nursing programs received some form of financial aid in 2013–14. 7 fellowships with full tuition reimbursements available (averaging $13,571 per year), research assistantships with full tuition reimbursements available (averaging $12,000 per year), 8 teaching assistantships with full tuition reimbursements available (averaging $12,000 per year) were awarded; career-related internships or fieldwork, scholarships, traineeships, tuition waivers (partial), and unspecified assistantships also available. Aid available to part-time students. *Financial aid application deadline:* 5/1.
Contact Dr. Jamie Reynolds, Assistant Director, Graduate Programs, College of Nursing, University of Cincinnati, PO Box 210038,

Cincinnati, OH 45221-0038. *Telephone:* 513-558-4394. *Fax:* 513-558-7523. *E-mail:* jamie.reynolds@uc.edu.

MASTER'S DEGREE PROGRAM
Degree MSN
Available Programs Accelerated Master's for Non-Nursing College Graduates; Master's.
Concentrations Available Nurse anesthesia; nurse-midwifery; nursing administration. *Nurse practitioner programs in:* adult-gerontology acute care, family health, neonatal health, occupational health, pediatric, pediatric primary care, women's health.
Study Options Full-time and part-time.
Online Degree Options Yes.
Program Entrance Requirements Clinical experience, minimum overall college GPA of 3.0, transcript of college record, CPR certification, written essay, interview, 3 letters of recommendation, professional liability insurance/malpractice insurance, resume, statistics course, GRE General Test. *Application deadline:* 4/15 (fall), 10/1 (spring), 2/1 (summer). Applications may be processed on a rolling basis for some programs. *Application fee:* $65.
Advanced Placement Credit given for nursing courses completed elsewhere dependent upon specific evaluations.
Degree Requirements 40 total credit hours, thesis or project.

POST-MASTER'S PROGRAM
Areas of Study Nursing education. *Nurse practitioner programs in:* adult-gerontology acute care, family health, neonatal health, pediatric, pediatric primary care, psychiatric/mental health, women's health.

DOCTORAL DEGREE PROGRAM
Degree PhD
Available Programs Doctorate; Post-Baccalaureate Doctorate.
Areas of Study Gerontology, health promotion/disease prevention, health-care systems, individualized study, nursing education, nursing research, nursing science.
Program Entrance Requirements Clinical experience, minimum overall college GPA of 3.25, interview by faculty committee, 3 letters of recommendation, statistics course, vita, writing sample, GRE General Test. Application deadline: 2/16 (fall). Applications may be processed on a rolling basis for some programs. Application fee: $65.
Degree Requirements 90 total credit hours, dissertation, oral exam, written exam, residency.

CONTINUING EDUCATION PROGRAM
Contact Ms. Elizabeth Karle, Program Coordinator, Continuing Education, College of Nursing, University of Cincinnati, PO Box 210038, Cincinnati, OH 45221-0038. *Telephone:* 513-558-5311. *Fax:* 513-558-5054. *E-mail:* elizabeth.karle@uc.edu.

University of Phoenix–Cleveland Campus
College of Nursing
Beachwood, Ohio

Founded in 2000
DEGREES • BSN • MSN
Nursing Program Faculty 10 (20% with doctorates).
Baccalaureate Enrollment 17 **Women** 82.4% **Men** 17.6%
Graduate Enrollment 4 **Women** 100%
Nursing Student Activities Sigma Theta Tau.
Nursing Student Resources Academic advising; academic or career counseling; assistance for students with disabilities; bookstore; campus computer network; computer lab; computer-assisted instruction; e-mail services; interactive nursing skills videos; Internet; learning resource lab; library services; nursing audiovisuals; remedial services; skills, simulation, or other laboratory; tutoring.
Library Facilities 1,300 periodical subscriptions health-care related.

BACCALAUREATE PROGRAMS
Degree BSN
Available Programs Accelerated Baccalaureate.
Site Options Beachwood, OH.
Study Options Full-time.
Program Entrance Requirements Transcript of college record, CPR certification, immunizations, 1 letter of recommendation, RN licensure.

Transfer students are accepted. *Application deadline:* Applications may be processed on a rolling basis for some programs.
Advanced Placement Credit by examination available. Credit given for nursing courses completed elsewhere dependent upon specific evaluations.
Contact *Telephone:* 216-447-8807.

GRADUATE PROGRAMS
Contact *Telephone:* 216-447-8807.

MASTER'S DEGREE PROGRAM
Degree MSN
Available Programs Master's.
Concentrations Available Nursing administration.
Site Options Beachwood, OH.
Study Options Full-time.
Program Entrance Requirements Clinical experience, computer literacy, minimum overall college GPA of 2.5, transcript of college record. *Application deadline:* Applications may be processed on a rolling basis for some programs. *Application fee:* $45.
Advanced Placement Credit given for nursing courses completed elsewhere dependent upon specific evaluations.
Degree Requirements 39 total credit hours, thesis or project.

University of Rio Grande
Holzer School of Nursing
Rio Grande, Ohio

Founded in 1876
DEGREE • BSN
Nursing Program Faculty 9

BACCALAUREATE PROGRAMS
Degree BSN
Available Programs RN Baccalaureate.
Study Options Full-time and part-time.
Contact *Telephone:* 800-282-7201 Ext. 7308. *Fax:* 740-245-7177.

The University of Toledo
College of Nursing
Toledo, Ohio

http://www.utoledo.edu/nursing
Founded in 1872
DEGREES • BSN • DNP • MSN
Nursing Program Faculty 46 (58% with doctorates).
Baccalaureate Enrollment 494 **Women** 79% **Men** 21% **Part-time** 25%
Graduate Enrollment 239 **Women** 87.5% **Men** 12.5% **Part-time** 67.8%
Distance Learning Courses Available.
Nursing Student Activities Sigma Theta Tau, Student Nurses' Association.
Nursing Student Resources Academic advising; academic or career counseling; assistance for students with disabilities; bookstore; campus computer network; computer lab; computer-assisted instruction; e-mail services; employment services for current students; housing assistance; interactive nursing skills videos; Internet; learning resource lab; library services; nursing audiovisuals; remedial services; resume preparation assistance; skills, simulation, or other laboratory; tutoring.
Library Facilities 25,000 volumes in health, 2,000 volumes in nursing; 15,000 periodical subscriptions health-care related.

BACCALAUREATE PROGRAMS
Degree BSN
Available Programs ADN to Baccalaureate; Generic Baccalaureate; RN Baccalaureate.
Site Options Toledo, OH.
Study Options Full-time.
Online Degree Options Yes.
Program Entrance Requirements Minimum overall college GPA of 3.0, transcript of college record, CPR certification, health exam, health insurance, high school biology, high school chemistry, high school foreign language, 3 years high school math, 3 years high school science,

high school transcript, immunizations, minimum high school GPA of 2.75, minimum GPA in nursing prerequisites of 2.0, professional liability insurance/malpractice insurance, prerequisite course work. Transfer students are accepted. *Application deadline:* 5/1 (fall), 9/1 (spring), 1/15 (summer).

Advanced Placement Credit given for nursing courses completed elsewhere dependent upon specific evaluations.

Expenses (2015–16) *Tuition, state resident:* full-time $8052; part-time $335 per credit hour. *Tuition, nonresident:* full-time $17,390; part-time $725 per credit hour. *International tuition:* $17,390 full-time. *Room and board:* $13,116; room only: $9254 per academic year. *Required fees:* full-time $3641.

Financial Aid 96% of baccalaureate students in nursing programs received some form of financial aid in 2014–15. *Gift aid (need-based):* Federal Pell, FSEOG, state, private, college/university gift aid from institutional funds, Federal Nursing, Academic Competitiveness Grants, National SMART Grants, TEACH Grants. *Loans:* Federal Nursing Student Loans, Federal Direct (Subsidized and Unsubsidized Stafford PLUS), Perkins, college/university, alternative loans. *Work-study:* Federal Work-Study. *Financial aid application deadline (priority):* 3/1.

Contact Ms. Kathleen Mitchell, Assistant Dean for Student Services, College of Nursing, The University of Toledo, Mail Stop #1026, 3000 Arlington Avenue, Toledo, OH 43614-2598. *Telephone:* 419-383-5839. *Fax:* 419-383-5894. *E-mail:* kathleen.mitchell@utoledo.edu.

GRADUATE PROGRAMS

Expenses (2015–16) *Tuition, state resident:* full-time $13,165; part-time $549 per credit hour. *Tuition, nonresident:* full-time $23,502; part-time $979 per credit hour. *International tuition:* $23,502 full-time. *Room and board:* $13,116; room only: $9254 per academic year. *Required fees:* full-time $3704.

Financial Aid 93% of graduate students in nursing programs received some form of financial aid in 2014–15. Research assistantships with full and partial tuition reimbursements available, Federal Work-Study, institutionally sponsored loans, scholarships, traineeships, and tuition waivers (full and partial) available.

Contact Mr. David Lymanstall, Graduate Advisor, College of Nursing, The University of Toledo, Mail Stop #1026, 3000 Arlington Avenue, Toledo, OH 43614-2598. *Telephone:* 419-383-5841. *Fax:* 419-383-5894. *E-mail:* david.lymanstall@utoledo.edu.

MASTER'S DEGREE PROGRAM

Degree MSN

Available Programs Master's; Master's for Non-Nursing College Graduates; Master's for Nurses with Non-Nursing Degrees.

Concentrations Available Clinical nurse leader; nursing education. *Nurse practitioner programs in:* family health, gerontology, pediatric primary care, psychiatric/mental health.

Site Options Toledo, OH.

Study Options Full-time and part-time.

Program Entrance Requirements Computer literacy, minimum overall college GPA of 3.0, transcript of college record, CPR certification, written essay, immunizations, 3 letters of recommendation, resume, GRE. *Application deadline:* 12/15 (fall), 9/1 (spring). *Application fee:* $110.

Advanced Placement Credit given for nursing courses completed elsewhere dependent upon specific evaluations.

Degree Requirements 55 total credit hours, thesis or project, comprehensive exam.

POST-MASTER'S PROGRAM

Areas of Study Nursing education. *Nurse practitioner programs in:* family health, pediatric primary care.

DOCTORAL DEGREE PROGRAM

Degree DNP

Available Programs Doctorate; Post-Baccalaureate Doctorate.

Areas of Study Advanced practice nursing, nursing administration.

Site Options Toledo, OH.

Online Degree Options Yes.

Program Entrance Requirements Clinical experience, minimum overall college GPA of 3.0, interview by faculty committee, interview, 3 letters of recommendation, MSN or equivalent, statistics course, vita, writing sample. Application deadline: 12/15 (fall). Application fee: $110.

Degree Requirements 89 total credit hours.

CONTINUING EDUCATION PROGRAM

Contact Dr. Deborah Mattin, Director, Continuing Nursing Education, College of Nursing, The University of Toledo, Mail Stop #1026, 3000 Arlington Avenue, Toledo, OH 43614-2598. *Telephone:* 419-383-5812. *Fax:* 419-383-5894. *E-mail:* deborah.mattin@utoledo.edu.

See display below and full description on page 510.

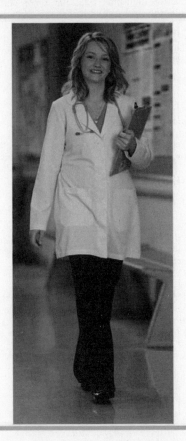

FOCUS YOUR PASSION IN NURSING, BUILD YOUR CAREER!

Enhance your expertise and leadership skills with an advanced degree in nursing from The University of Toledo

POST-BACCALAUREATE DOCTOR OF NURSING PRACTICE (BSN-DNP)

We are committed to:

- Evidence-based practice
- Theoretical and clinical education
- Delivery of high quality care
- Hybrid model of delivery with online & campus course work

To learn more about our Programs visit
www.utoledo.edu/nursing or
call 419.383.5810

COLLEGE of NURSING
THE UNIVERSITY OF TOLEDO

Urbana University
College of Nursing and Allied Health
Urbana, Ohio

http://www.urbana.edu/academics/college-of-nursing-and-allied-health/
Founded in 1850
DEGREES • BSN • MSN
Nursing Program Faculty 2 (100% with doctorates).
Baccalaureate Enrollment 30 **Women** 98% **Men** 2% **Part-time** 100%
Graduate Enrollment 60 **Women** 99% **Men** 1% **Part-time** 100%
Distance Learning Courses Available.
Nursing Student Activities Nursing Honor Society.
Nursing Student Resources Academic advising; academic or career counseling; assistance for students with disabilities; bookstore; campus computer network; career placement assistance; computer lab; computer-assisted instruction; e-mail services; Internet; learning resource lab; library services; nursing audiovisuals; placement services for program completers; remedial services; resume preparation assistance; tutoring.
Library Facilities 320 volumes in health, 250 volumes in nursing; 1,000 periodical subscriptions health-care related.

BACCALAUREATE PROGRAMS

Degree BSN
Available Programs ADN to Baccalaureate.
Site Options Springfield, OH; Dayton, OH.
Study Options Full-time and part-time.
Online Degree Options Yes.
Program Entrance Requirements Minimum overall college GPA of 2.0, transcript of college record, CPR certification, health exam, health insurance, immunizations, 3 letters of recommendation, minimum GPA in nursing prerequisites of 3.0, professional liability insurance/malpractice insurance, RN licensure. Transfer students are accepted. *Application deadline:* Applications may be processed on a rolling basis for some programs.
Expenses (2015–16) *Tuition:* part-time $450 per credit.
Contact Dr. Sue Z. Green, BSN Program Chair, College of Nursing and Allied Health, Urbana University, 579 College Way, Urbana, OH 43078. *Telephone:* 937-772-9258. *E-mail:* sue.green@urbana.edu.

GRADUATE PROGRAMS

Expenses (2015–16) *Tuition:* part-time $515 per credit hour.
Contact Dr. Barbara Miville, MSN Program Chair, College of Nursing and Allied Health, Urbana University, 579 College Way, Urbana, OH 43078. *Telephone:* 937-772-9259. *E-mail:* barb.miville@urbana.edu.

MASTER'S DEGREE PROGRAM
Degree MSN
Available Programs Master's; Master's for Nurses with Non-Nursing Degrees; RN to Master's.
Concentrations Available Nursing administration; nursing education.
Site Options Springfield, OH; Dayton, OH.
Study Options Full-time and part-time.
Online Degree Options Yes.
Program Entrance Requirements Computer literacy, minimum overall college GPA of 2.7, transcript of college record, CPR certification, written essay, immunizations, 3 letters of recommendation, professional liability insurance/malpractice insurance, resume. *Application deadline:* 8/1 (fall), 12/1 (spring), 5/1 (summer). Applications may be processed on a rolling basis for some programs.
Advanced Placement Credit given for nursing courses completed elsewhere dependent upon specific evaluations.
Degree Requirements 36 total credit hours, thesis or project.

CONTINUING EDUCATION PROGRAM

Contact Ms. Renee Crabill, Administrative Assistant, College of Nursing and Allied Health, Urbana University, 579 College Way, Urbana, OH 43078. *Telephone:* 937-772-9254. *E-mail:* renee.crabill@urbana.edu.

Ursuline College
The Breen School of Nursing
Pepper Pike, Ohio

http://www.ursuline.edu/Academics/Nursing/
Founded in 1871
DEGREES • BSN • DNP • MSN • MSN/MBA
Nursing Program Faculty 25 (50% with doctorates).
Baccalaureate Enrollment 265 **Women** 92% **Men** 8%
Graduate Enrollment 280 **Women** 90% **Men** 10% **Part-time** 75%
Distance Learning Courses Available.
Nursing Student Activities Nursing Honor Society, Sigma Theta Tau, Student Nurses' Association.
Nursing Student Resources Academic advising; academic or career counseling; assistance for students with disabilities; bookstore; campus computer network; career placement assistance; computer lab; computer-assisted instruction; e-mail services; employment services for current students; externships; interactive nursing skills videos; Internet; learning resource lab; library services; nursing audiovisuals; placement services for program completers; remedial services; resume preparation assistance; skills, simulation, or other laboratory; tutoring; unpaid internships.

BACCALAUREATE PROGRAMS

Degree BSN
Available Programs ADN to Baccalaureate; Accelerated Baccalaureate; Accelerated Baccalaureate for Second Degree; Accelerated RN Baccalaureate; Baccalaureate for Second Degree; Generic Baccalaureate; RN Baccalaureate.
Study Options Full-time.
Program Entrance Requirements Minimum overall college GPA of 2.5, transcript of college record, CPR certification, written essay, health exam, health insurance, high school biology, high school chemistry, 2 years high school math, 2 years high school science, high school transcript, immunizations, 1 letter of recommendation, minimum high school GPA of 2.75, minimum GPA in nursing prerequisites of 2.75. Transfer students are accepted. *Application deadline:* Applications may be processed on a rolling basis for some programs. *Application fee:* $25.
Advanced Placement Credit given for nursing courses completed elsewhere dependent upon specific evaluations.
Expenses (2015–16) *Tuition:* full-time $28,230. *Room and board:* $9490; room only: $4848 per academic year. *Required fees:* full-time $2600.
Financial Aid 90% of baccalaureate students in nursing programs received some form of financial aid in 2014–15.
Contact Leah Grill, Coordinator, BSN Enrollment, The Breen School of Nursing, Ursuline College, 2550 Lander Road, Pepper Pike, OH 44124-4398. *Telephone:* 440-449-4200. *Fax:* 440-449-4267.

GRADUATE PROGRAMS

Expenses (2015–16) *Tuition:* part-time $1002 per credit. *Required fees:* part-time $230 per credit.
Contact Dr. Janet R. Baker, Associate Dean, Graduate Program, The Breen School of Nursing, Ursuline College, 2550 Lander Road, Pepper Pike, OH 44124-4398. *Telephone:* 440-449-4200 Ext. 8172. *Fax:* 440-684-6053. *E-mail:* jbaker@ursuline.edu.

MASTER'S DEGREE PROGRAM
Degrees MSN; MSN/MBA
Available Programs Master's.
Concentrations Available *Clinical nurse specialist programs in:* adult-gerontology acute care, family health. *Nurse practitioner programs in:* adult-gerontology acute care, family health.
Site Options Kirtland, OH.
Study Options Full-time and part-time.
Program Entrance Requirements Clinical experience, minimum overall college GPA of 3.0, transcript of college record, written essay, 3 letters of recommendation, resume. *Application deadline:* 5/15 (fall), 12/1 (spring). Applications may be processed on a rolling basis for some programs.
Advanced Placement Credit given for nursing courses completed elsewhere dependent upon specific evaluations.
Degree Requirements 39 total credit hours.

POST-MASTER'S PROGRAM
Areas of Study Nurse case management; nursing education. *Clinical nurse specialist programs in:* adult-gerontology acute care, family health,

palliative care. *Nurse practitioner programs in:* adult-gerontology acute care, family health.

DOCTORAL DEGREE PROGRAM
Degree DNP
Available Programs Doctorate; Post-Baccalaureate Doctorate.
Program Entrance Requirements Clinical experience, minimum overall college GPA of 3.0, 2 letters of recommendation, MSN or equivalent. Application deadline: 5/15 (fall), 12/1 (winter). Applications may be processed on a rolling basis for some programs. Application fee: $25.
Degree Requirements 38 total credit hours.

Walsh University
Department of Nursing
North Canton, Ohio

http://www.walsh.edu/
Founded in 1958
DEGREES • BSN • DNP • MSN
Nursing Program Faculty 18 (40% with doctorates).
Baccalaureate Enrollment 245 **Women** 77% **Men** 23% **Part-time** 10%
Graduate Enrollment 32 **Women** 95% **Men** 5% **Part-time** 75%
Distance Learning Courses Available.
Nursing Student Activities Sigma Theta Tau, Student Nurses' Association.
Nursing Student Resources Academic advising; academic or career counseling; assistance for students with disabilities; bookstore; campus computer network; career placement assistance; computer lab; computer-assisted instruction; e-mail services; employment services for current students; housing assistance; interactive nursing skills videos; Internet; learning resource lab; library services; nursing audiovisuals; placement services for program completers; remedial services; resume preparation assistance; skills, simulation, or other laboratory; tutoring.
Library Facilities 4,000 volumes in health, 2,000 volumes in nursing; 114 periodical subscriptions health-care related.

BACCALAUREATE PROGRAMS

Degree BSN
Available Programs Accelerated Baccalaureate for Second Degree; Baccalaureate for Second Degree; Generic Baccalaureate; RN Baccalaureate.
Site Options Medina, OH; Akron, OH; Canton, OH.
Study Options Full-time and part-time.
Program Entrance Requirements Transcript of college record, CPR certification, health exam, health insurance, high school chemistry, high school foreign language, 3 years high school math, 3 years high school science, high school transcript, immunizations, minimum high school GPA of 2.3, minimum GPA in nursing prerequisites of 2.75, professional liability insurance/malpractice insurance, prerequisite course work. Transfer students are accepted. *Application deadline:* 8/15 (fall), 12/31 (spring), 4/15 (summer). Applications may be processed on a rolling basis for some programs. *Application fee:* $25.
Advanced Placement Credit by examination available. Credit given for nursing courses completed elsewhere dependent upon specific evaluations.
Expenses (2015–16) *Tuition:* full-time $26,300; part-time $875 per credit hour. *International tuition:* $26,300 full-time. *Room and board:* $9920; room only: $5260 per academic year. *Required fees:* full-time $1128; part-time $47 per credit.
Financial Aid 95% of baccalaureate students in nursing programs received some form of financial aid in 2014–15.
Contact Dr. Linda G. Linc, Professor and Chair, Department of Nursing, Walsh University, 2020 East Maple Street, North Canton, OH 44720-3336. *Telephone:* 330-490-7251. *Fax:* 330-490-7206. *E-mail:* llinc@walsh.edu.

GRADUATE PROGRAMS

Expenses (2015–16) *Tuition:* full-time $11,610; part-time $645 per credit hour. *International tuition:* $11,610 full-time. *Room and board:* $9920; room only: $2630 per academic year.
Financial Aid 80% of graduate students in nursing programs received some form of financial aid in 2014–15.
Contact Dr. Maria Pappas-Rogich, Director, Graduate Programs, Department of Nursing, Walsh University, 2020 East Maple Street, North Canton, OH 44720. *Telephone:* 330-490-7251. *Fax:* 330-490-7206. *E-mail:* mpappas@walsh.edu.

MASTER'S DEGREE PROGRAM
Degree MSN
Available Programs Accelerated AD/RN to Master's; Accelerated RN to Master's; Master's.
Concentrations Available Nursing education. *Nurse practitioner programs in:* family health.
Study Options Full-time and part-time.
Online Degree Options Yes (online only).
Program Entrance Requirements Minimum overall college GPA of 3.0, transcript of college record, written essay, interview, statistics course. *Application deadline:* Applications may be processed on a rolling basis for some programs. *Application fee:* $25.
Advanced Placement Credit given for nursing courses completed elsewhere dependent upon specific evaluations.
Degree Requirements 36 total credit hours.

POST-MASTER'S PROGRAM
Areas of Study Nursing education. *Nurse practitioner programs in:* family health.

DOCTORAL DEGREE PROGRAM
Degree DNP
Available Programs Post-Baccalaureate Doctorate.
Areas of Study Ethics, health policy, health promotion/disease prevention, health-care systems, information systems, nurse case management, nursing administration, nursing policy, nursing research, nursing science.
Online Degree Options Yes (online only).
Program Entrance Requirements Minimum overall college GPA of 3.0, interview by faculty committee, interview, 2 letters of recommendation, MSN or equivalent, statistics course, writing sample. Application deadline: Applications may be processed on a rolling basis for some programs. Application fee: $25.
Degree Requirements 38 total credit hours, residency.

Wright State University
College of Nursing and Health
Dayton, Ohio

http://nursing.wright.edu/
Founded in 1964
DEGREES • BSN • DNP • MS • MS/MBA
Nursing Program Faculty 68 (33% with doctorates).
Baccalaureate Enrollment 787 **Women** 84% **Men** 16% **Part-time** 35%
Graduate Enrollment 257 **Women** 94% **Men** 6% **Part-time** 86%
Nursing Student Activities Nursing Honor Society, Sigma Theta Tau, Student Nurses' Association, nursing club.
Nursing Student Resources Academic advising; academic or career counseling; assistance for students with disabilities; bookstore; campus computer network; career placement assistance; computer lab; computer-assisted instruction; daycare for children of students; e-mail services; employment services for current students; externships; housing assistance; interactive nursing skills videos; Internet; learning resource lab; library services; nursing audiovisuals; remedial services; resume preparation assistance; skills, simulation, or other laboratory; tutoring.
Library Facilities 111,826 volumes in health, 7,646 volumes in nursing; 1,279 periodical subscriptions health-care related.

BACCALAUREATE PROGRAMS

Degree BSN
Available Programs Baccalaureate for Second Degree; Generic Baccalaureate; RN Baccalaureate.
Study Options Full-time and part-time.
Program Entrance Requirements Minimum overall college GPA of 2.75, transcript of college record, high school transcript, interview, minimum GPA in nursing prerequisites of 2.75, prerequisite course work. Transfer students are accepted. *Application deadline:* 5/15 (fall), 9/15 (spring).
Advanced Placement Credit given for nursing courses completed elsewhere dependent upon specific evaluations.
Expenses (2014–15) *Tuition, state resident:* full-time $8730; part-time $394 per credit hour. *Tuition, nonresident:* full-time $16,910; part-time $770 per credit hour. *International tuition:* $17,008 full-time. *Room and board:* $9108 per academic year. *Required fees:* full-time $800; part-time $400 per term.

Financial Aid 67% of baccalaureate students in nursing programs received some form of financial aid in 2013–14. *Gift aid (need-based):* Federal Pell, FSEOG, state, private, college/university gift aid from institutional funds, United Negro College Fund, Federal Nursing, Choose Ohio First scholarships. *Loans:* Federal Nursing Student Loans, Federal Direct (Subsidized and Unsubsidized Stafford PLUS), Perkins, state, college/university, private loans. *Work-study:* Federal Work-Study. *Financial aid application deadline (priority):* 3/1.

Contact Dr. Sherrill Smith, Assistant Dean, Undergraduate Education, College of Nursing and Health, Wright State University, 3640 Colonel Glenn Highway, Dayton, OH 45435. *Telephone:* 937-775-3132. *Fax:* 937-775-4571. *E-mail:* sherrill.smith@wright.edu.

GRADUATE PROGRAMS

Expenses (2014–15) *Tuition, state resident:* full-time $12,788; part-time $590 per credit hour. *Tuition, nonresident:* full-time $21,724; part-time $1005 per credit hour. *International tuition:* $21,822 full-time.

Financial Aid 43% of graduate students in nursing programs received some form of financial aid in 2013–14. 15 fellowships with full tuition reimbursements available were awarded; research assistantships, teaching assistantships, Federal Work-Study, institutionally sponsored loans, and unspecified assistantships also available. Aid available to part-time students. *Financial aid application deadline:* 6/1.

Contact Dr. Deborah Ulrich, Associate Dean, College of Nursing and Health, Wright State University, 3640 Colonel Glenn Highway, Dayton, OH 45435. *Telephone:* 937-775-3132. *Fax:* 937-775-4571. *E-mail:* deborah.ulrich@wright.edu.

MASTER'S DEGREE PROGRAM

Degrees MS; MS/MBA

Available Programs Master's.

Concentrations Available Health-care administration; nursing administration; nursing education. *Clinical nurse specialist programs in:* adult health, adult-gerontology acute care, community health, pediatric, public health, school health. *Nurse practitioner programs in:* adult-gerontology acute care, family health, neonatal health, pediatric, pediatric primary care, psychiatric/mental health.

Study Options Full-time and part-time.

Online Degree Options Yes.

Program Entrance Requirements Clinical experience, computer literacy, minimum overall college GPA of 3.0, transcript of college record, written essay, interview, 2 letters of recommendation, physical assessment course, resume, statistics course, GRE General Test. *Application deadline:* Applications may be processed on a rolling basis for some programs. *Application fee:* $40.

Advanced Placement Credit given for nursing courses completed elsewhere dependent upon specific evaluations.

Degree Requirements Thesis or project.

POST-MASTER'S PROGRAM

Areas of Study *Clinical nurse specialist programs in:* adult-gerontology acute care. *Nurse practitioner programs in:* family health, pediatric, pediatric primary care.

DOCTORAL DEGREE PROGRAM

Degree DNP

Available Programs Doctorate.

Areas of Study Advanced practice nursing, biology of health and illness, clinical practice, community health, family health, health policy, health promotion/disease prevention, health-care systems, information systems, nursing administration, nursing policy, nursing science.

Online Degree Options Yes (online only).

Program Entrance Requirements Clinical experience, minimum overall college GPA of 3.3, interview by faculty committee, 3 letters of recommendation, MSN or equivalent, statistics course, vita, writing sample. Application deadline: 4/1 (fall). Application fee: $40.

Degree Requirements 36 total credit hours, residency.

CONTINUING EDUCATION PROGRAM

Contact Ms. Harriet Knowles, College of Nursing and Health, Wright State University, 3640 Colonel Glenn Highway, Dayton, OH 45435. *Telephone:* 937-775-3132. *Fax:* 937-775-4571. *E-mail:* harriet.knowles@wright.edu.

Xavier University
School of Nursing
Cincinnati, Ohio

http://www.xavier.edu/msn/About-the-School-of-Nursing.cfm
Founded in 1831

DEGREES • BSN • DNP • MSN • MSN/ED D • MSN/MBA
Nursing Program Faculty 80 (14% with doctorates).
Baccalaureate Enrollment 432 **Women** 90% **Men** 10% **Part-time** 2%
Graduate Enrollment 223 **Women** 90% **Men** 10% **Part-time** 98%
Nursing Student Activities Sigma Theta Tau, nursing club.
Nursing Student Resources Academic advising; academic or career counseling; assistance for students with disabilities; bookstore; campus computer network; career placement assistance; computer lab; computer-assisted instruction; e-mail services; employment services for current students; externships; housing assistance; interactive nursing skills videos; Internet; learning resource lab; library services; nursing audiovisuals; remedial services; resume preparation assistance; skills, simulation, or other laboratory; tutoring.
Library Facilities 8,900 volumes in health, 1,160 volumes in nursing; 200 periodical subscriptions health-care related.

BACCALAUREATE PROGRAMS

Degree BSN

Available Programs Generic Baccalaureate.

Study Options Full-time and part-time.

Program Entrance Requirements Minimum overall college GPA of 2.7, transcript of college record, written essay, high school chemistry, high school foreign language, 3 years high school math, 2 years high school science, high school transcript, minimum high school GPA of 3.0. *Application deadline:* 1/15 (fall). Applications may be processed on a rolling basis for some programs.

Advanced Placement Credit given for nursing courses completed elsewhere dependent upon specific evaluations.

Expenses (2015–16) *Tuition:* part-time $654 per credit. *Room and board:* $11,380; room only: $6300 per academic year.

Financial Aid 85% of baccalaureate students in nursing programs received some form of financial aid in 2014–15.

Contact Mrs. Marilyn Volk Gomez, Academic Program Director, School of Nursing, Xavier University, 3800 Victory Parkway, Cincinnati, OH 45207-7351. *Telephone:* 513-745-4392. *Fax:* 513-745-1087. *E-mail:* gomez@xavier.edu.

GRADUATE PROGRAMS

Expenses (2015–16) *Tuition:* part-time $606 per credit.
Contact Mrs. Marilyn Volk Gomez, Academic Program Director, School of Nursing, Xavier University, 3800 Victory Parkway, Cincinnati, OH 45207-7351. *Telephone:* 513-745-4392. *Fax:* 513-745-1087. *E-mail:* gomez@xavier.edu.

MASTER'S DEGREE PROGRAM

Degrees MSN; MSN/Ed D; MSN/MBA

Available Programs Accelerated Master's for Non-Nursing College Graduates; Master's; Master's for Nurses with Non-Nursing Degrees; RN to Master's.

Concentrations Available Clinical nurse leader; nursing administration; nursing education; nursing informatics. *Nurse practitioner programs in:* family health.

Study Options Full-time and part-time.

Program Entrance Requirements Minimum overall college GPA of 2.8, transcript of college record, written essay, 3 letters of recommendation, resume, statistics course, GRE. *Application deadline:* Applications may be processed on a rolling basis for some programs.

Advanced Placement Credit given for nursing courses completed elsewhere dependent upon specific evaluations.

Degree Requirements 36 total credit hours, thesis or project.

POST-MASTER'S PROGRAM

Areas of Study *Nurse practitioner programs in:* family health.

DOCTORAL DEGREE PROGRAM

Degree DNP

Available Programs Doctorate.

Areas of Study Nursing science.

Program Entrance Requirements Minimum overall college GPA of 3.3, 3 letters of recommendation, MSN or equivalent, scholarly papers,

statistics course, vita, writing sample. Application deadline: Applications may be processed on a rolling basis for some programs.
Degree Requirements 40 total credit hours.

Youngstown State University
Department of Nursing
Youngstown, Ohio

http://web.ysu.edu/bchhs/nursing
Founded in 1908
DEGREES • BSN • MSN
Nursing Program Faculty 46 (33% with doctorates).
Baccalaureate Enrollment 300
Graduate Enrollment 86 **Women** 74% **Men** 26% **Part-time** 57%
Distance Learning Courses Available.
Nursing Student Activities Nursing Honor Society, Sigma Theta Tau, Student Nurses' Association.
Nursing Student Resources Academic advising; academic or career counseling; assistance for students with disabilities; bookstore; campus computer network; career placement assistance; computer lab; computer-assisted instruction; e-mail services; employment services for current students; housing assistance; interactive nursing skills videos; Internet; learning resource lab; library services; nursing audiovisuals; other; placement services for program completers; remedial services; resume preparation assistance; skills, simulation, or other laboratory; tutoring.
Library Facilities 23,808 volumes in health, 1,265 volumes in nursing; 9,877 periodical subscriptions health-care related.

BACCALAUREATE PROGRAMS

Degree BSN
Available Programs ADN to Baccalaureate; Generic Baccalaureate; RN Baccalaureate.
Site Options Cleveland, OH; Boardman, OH; Akron, OH.
Study Options Full-time.
Program Entrance Requirements Minimum overall college GPA of 2.5, transcript of college record, CPR certification, health exam, health insurance, high school biology, high school chemistry, 3 years high school math, 3 years high school science, high school transcript, immunizations, minimum high school GPA, minimum high school rank, minimum GPA in nursing prerequisites of 3.0, prerequisite course work. Transfer students are accepted.
Advanced Placement Credit by examination available. Credit given for nursing courses completed elsewhere dependent upon specific evaluations.
Contact Ms. Susanne Miller, Nursing Advisor, Department of Nursing, Youngstown State University, One University Plaza, Youngstown, OH 44555. *Telephone:* 330-941-1820. *E-mail:* smmiller04@ysu.edu.

GRADUATE PROGRAMS

Expenses (2014–15) *Tuition, area resident:* full-time $10,881; part-time $906 per credit hour. *Tuition, state resident:* full-time $11,121; part-time $926 per credit hour. *Tuition, nonresident:* full-time $14,091; part-time $1174 per credit hour. *Room and board:* $8645 per academic year. *Required fees:* full-time $230.
Financial Aid Federal Work-Study, institutionally sponsored loans, and scholarships available.
Contact Dr. Valerie O'Dell, MSN Director, Department of Nursing, Youngstown State University, One University Plaza, Youngstown, OH 44555. *Telephone:* 330-941-2177. *Fax:* 330-941-2025. *E-mail:* vmodell@ysu.edu.

MASTER'S DEGREE PROGRAM
Degree MSN
Available Programs Master's.
Concentrations Available Nurse anesthesia; nursing education. *Clinical nurse specialist programs in:* adult-gerontology acute care, school health. *Nurse practitioner programs in:* family health.
Site Options Cleveland, OH; Boardman, OH; Akron, OH.
Study Options Full-time and part-time.
Program Entrance Requirements Clinical experience, computer literacy, transcript of college record, CPR certification, written essay, immunizations, nursing research course, physical assessment course, prerequisite course work, resume, GRE General Test.
Advanced Placement Credit given for nursing courses completed elsewhere dependent upon specific evaluations.

Degree Requirements Thesis or project.

POST-MASTER'S PROGRAM
Areas of Study Nursing education. *Nurse practitioner programs in:* family health.

OKLAHOMA

Bacone College
Department of Nursing
Muskogee, Oklahoma

Founded in 1880
DEGREE • BSN
Nursing Program Faculty 8
Baccalaureate Enrollment 16 **Women** 100%
Nursing Student Activities Student Nurses' Association, nursing club.
Nursing Student Resources Academic advising; bookstore; campus computer network; computer lab; computer-assisted instruction; interactive nursing skills videos; Internet; learning resource lab; library services; nursing audiovisuals; remedial services; skills, simulation, or other laboratory.

BACCALAUREATE PROGRAMS

Degree BSN
Available Programs Accelerated RN Baccalaureate.
Program Entrance Requirements Transcript of college record, CPR certification, health exam, health insurance, immunizations, 2 letters of recommendation, minimum GPA in nursing prerequisites of 2.5, prerequisite course work, RN licensure.
Contact *Telephone:* 888-682-5514.

East Central University
Department of Nursing
Ada, Oklahoma

http://www.ecok.edu
Founded in 1909
DEGREE • BS
Nursing Program Faculty 17 (31% with doctorates).
Baccalaureate Enrollment 495 **Women** 86% **Men** 14% **Part-time** 14%
Distance Learning Courses Available.
Nursing Student Activities Student Nurses' Association.
Nursing Student Resources Academic advising; academic or career counseling; assistance for students with disabilities; bookstore; campus computer network; career placement assistance; computer lab; computer-assisted instruction; daycare for children of students; e-mail services; employment services for current students; externships; housing assistance; interactive nursing skills videos; Internet; learning resource lab; library services; nursing audiovisuals; other; placement services for program completers; resume preparation assistance; skills, simulation, or other laboratory; tutoring.
Library Facilities 2,236 volumes in health, 893 volumes in nursing; 266 periodical subscriptions health-care related.

BACCALAUREATE PROGRAMS

Degree BS
Available Programs ADN to Baccalaureate; Generic Baccalaureate.
Site Options Ardmore, OK; McAlester, OK; Durant, OK.
Study Options Full-time and part-time.
Program Entrance Requirements Minimum overall college GPA of 2.5, transcript of college record, CPR certification, health exam, immunizations, minimum GPA in nursing prerequisites of 2.5, professional liability insurance/malpractice insurance, prerequisite course work. Transfer students are accepted. *Application deadline:* 9/17 (spring).
Advanced Placement Credit given for nursing courses completed elsewhere dependent upon specific evaluations.
Contact *Telephone:* 580-310-5434. *Fax:* 580-310-5785.

Langston University
School of Nursing and Health Professions
Langston, Oklahoma

http://www.langston.edu/academics/colleges/nursing-health-professions/nursing-health-professions
Founded in 1897

DEGREE • BSN
Nursing Program Faculty 16 (13% with doctorates).
Nursing Student Activities Student Nurses' Association, nursing club.
Nursing Student Resources Academic advising; academic or career counseling; assistance for students with disabilities; bookstore; campus computer network; career placement assistance; computer lab; computer-assisted instruction; daycare for children of students; e-mail services; housing assistance; interactive nursing skills videos; Internet; learning resource lab; library services; nursing audiovisuals; remedial services; resume preparation assistance; skills, simulation, or other laboratory; tutoring.
Library Facilities 35,397 volumes in health, 2,664 volumes in nursing; 978 periodical subscriptions health-care related.

BACCALAUREATE PROGRAMS

Degree BSN
Available Programs Generic Baccalaureate; LPN to Baccalaureate; RN Baccalaureate.
Site Options Tulsa, OK.
Study Options Full-time and part-time.
Program Entrance Requirements Minimum overall college GPA of 2.5, transcript of college record, written essay, health exam, immunizations, minimum GPA in nursing prerequisites of 2.5, professional liability insurance/malpractice insurance, prerequisite course work. Transfer students are accepted.
Advanced Placement Credit by examination available. Credit given for nursing courses completed elsewhere dependent upon specific evaluations.
Contact *Telephone:* 405-466-3411. *Fax:* 405-466-2195.

Northeastern State University
Department of Nursing
Tahlequah, Oklahoma

http://academics.nsuok.edu/healthprofessions/HealthProHome.aspx
Founded in 1846

DEGREES • BSN • MSN
Nursing Program Faculty 3 (75% with doctorates).
Baccalaureate Enrollment 125 **Women** 92% **Men** 8% **Part-time** 95%
Graduate Enrollment 25 **Women** 95% **Men** 5% **Part-time** 100%
Distance Learning Courses Available.
Nursing Student Activities Sigma Theta Tau, Student Nurses' Association.
Nursing Student Resources Academic advising; academic or career counseling; assistance for students with disabilities; bookstore; campus computer network; career placement assistance; computer lab; computer-assisted instruction; e-mail services; employment services for current students; housing assistance; interactive nursing skills videos; Internet; library services; nursing audiovisuals; placement services for program completers; remedial services; resume preparation assistance; tutoring.
Library Facilities 21,000 volumes in health, 15,500 volumes in nursing; 1,000 periodical subscriptions health-care related.

BACCALAUREATE PROGRAMS

Degree BSN
Available Programs Accelerated RN Baccalaureate; RN Baccalaureate.
Study Options Full-time and part-time.
Online Degree Options Yes (online only).
Program Entrance Requirements Minimum overall college GPA of 2.0, transcript of college record, CPR certification, health exam, immunizations, 3 letters of recommendation, minimum GPA in nursing prerequisites of 2.0, professional liability insurance/malpractice insurance, prerequisite course work, RN licensure. Transfer students are accepted. *Application deadline:* 8/1 (fall), 1/1 (spring), 6/1 (summer).
Advanced Placement Credit given for nursing courses completed elsewhere dependent upon specific evaluations.

Expenses (2015–16) *Tuition, state resident:* full-time $148. *Tuition, nonresident:* full-time $393. *Room and board:* room only: $3181 per academic year.
Financial Aid 94% of baccalaureate students in nursing programs received some form of financial aid in 2014–15.
Contact Dr. Diana Mashburn, Chair, RN-BSN Program, Department of Nursing, Northeastern State University, PO Box 549, Muskogee, OK 74402-0549. *Telephone:* 918-781-5410. *Fax:* 918-781-5411. *E-mail:* downindd@nsuok.edu.

GRADUATE PROGRAMS
Expenses (2015–16) *Tuition, state resident:* full-time $190. *Tuition, nonresident:* full-time $463.
Financial Aid 80% of graduate students in nursing programs received some form of financial aid in 2014–15.
Contact Dr. Heather Fenton, EdD, Chair, MSN-Education Program, Department of Nursing, Northeastern State University, PO Box 549, Muskogee, OK 74402-0549. *Telephone:* 918-781-5410. *Fax:* 918-781-5411. *E-mail:* fentonh@nsuok.edu.

MASTER'S DEGREE PROGRAM
Degree MSN
Available Programs Master's.
Concentrations Available Nursing education.
Study Options Full-time and part-time.
Online Degree Options Yes (online only).
Program Entrance Requirements Minimum overall college GPA of 3.0, transcript of college record, CPR certification, immunizations, 3 letters of recommendation, nursing research course, professional liability insurance/malpractice insurance, statistics course. *Application deadline:* 8/1 (fall), 1/1 (spring), 6/1 (summer).
Advanced Placement Credit given for nursing courses completed elsewhere dependent upon specific evaluations.
Degree Requirements 32 total credit hours, thesis or project.

Northwestern Oklahoma State University
Division of Nursing
Alva, Oklahoma

http://www.nwosu.edu/nursing
Founded in 1897

DEGREE • BSN
Nursing Program Faculty 11 (60% with doctorates).
Baccalaureate Enrollment 85 **Women** 94% **Men** 6% **Part-time** 1%
Distance Learning Courses Available.
Nursing Student Activities Nursing Honor Society, Student Nurses' Association.
Nursing Student Resources Academic advising; academic or career counseling; assistance for students with disabilities; bookstore; campus computer network; career placement assistance; computer lab; computer-assisted instruction; e-mail services; housing assistance; interactive nursing skills videos; Internet; learning resource lab; library services; nursing audiovisuals; remedial services; skills, simulation, or other laboratory; tutoring.
Library Facilities 59 periodical subscriptions health-care related.

BACCALAUREATE PROGRAMS

Degree BSN
Available Programs ADN to Baccalaureate; Accelerated Baccalaureate; Baccalaureate for Second Degree; Generic Baccalaureate; LPN to Baccalaureate; LPN to RN Baccalaureate; RN Baccalaureate.
Site Options Enid, OK; Woodward, OK; Alva, OK.
Study Options Full-time and part-time.
Online Degree Options Yes.
Program Entrance Requirements Minimum overall college GPA of 2.5, transcript of college record, CPR certification, health exam, health insurance, immunizations, 2 letters of recommendation, minimum high school GPA of 2.5, minimum GPA in nursing prerequisites of 2.5, professional liability insurance/malpractice insurance, prerequisite course work. Transfer students are accepted. *Application deadline:* 1/20 (fall), 2/2 (spring). *Application fee:* $15.
Advanced Placement Credit by examination available. Credit given for nursing courses completed elsewhere dependent upon specific evaluations.

Financial Aid 85% of baccalaureate students in nursing programs received some form of financial aid in 2014–15. *Gift aid (need-based):* Federal Pell, FSEOG, state, private, college/university gift aid from institutional funds. *Loans:* Federal Direct (Subsidized and Unsubsidized Stafford PLUS). *Work-study:* Federal Work-Study, part-time campus jobs. *Financial aid application deadline:* Continuous.
Contact Dr. Shelly Wells, Division Chair and Associate Professor, Division of Nursing, Northwestern Oklahoma State University, 709 Oklahoma Boulevard, Alva, OK 73717-2799. *Telephone:* 580-327-8489. *Fax:* 580-327-8434. *E-mail:* scwells@nwosu.edu.

Oklahoma Baptist University
School of Nursing
Shawnee, Oklahoma

http://www.okbu.edu/
Founded in 1910
DEGREES • BSN • MSN
Nursing Program Faculty 12 (50% with doctorates).
Baccalaureate Enrollment 235 **Women** 95% **Men** 5% **Part-time** 4%
Graduate Enrollment 12 **Women** 100% **Part-time** 50%
Distance Learning Courses Available.
Nursing Student Activities Sigma Theta Tau, Student Nurses' Association.
Nursing Student Resources Academic advising; academic or career counseling; assistance for students with disabilities; bookstore; campus computer network; career placement assistance; computer lab; computer-assisted instruction; e-mail services; externships; interactive nursing skills videos; Internet; learning resource lab; library services; nursing audiovisuals; remedial services; resume preparation assistance; skills, simulation, or other laboratory; tutoring; unpaid internships.
Library Facilities 10,000 volumes in health, 5,500 volumes in nursing; 65 periodical subscriptions health-care related.

BACCALAUREATE PROGRAMS
Degree BSN
Available Programs ADN to Baccalaureate; Baccalaureate for Second Degree; Generic Baccalaureate; LPN to Baccalaureate; LPN to RN Baccalaureate; RN Baccalaureate.
Study Options Full-time and part-time.
Online Degree Options Yes (online only).
Program Entrance Requirements Minimum overall college GPA of 2.8, transcript of college record, CPR certification, health exam, health insurance, high school chemistry, high school transcript, immunizations, minimum GPA in nursing prerequisites of 2.8, professional liability insurance/malpractice insurance, prerequisite course work. Transfer students are accepted. *Application deadline:* 5/1 (fall), 10/1 (winter), 10/1 (spring), 5/1 (summer). *Application fee:* $50.
Advanced Placement Credit given for nursing courses completed elsewhere dependent upon specific evaluations.
Expenses (2015–16) *Tuition:* full-time $22,710; part-time $650 per credit hour. *International tuition:* $22,710 full-time. *Room and board:* $7010; room only: $3250 per academic year. *Required fees:* full-time $525.
Contact Dr. Lepaine Sharp-McHenry, Dean, School of Nursing, Oklahoma Baptist University, 500 West University, Box 61805, Shawnee, OK 74804. *Telephone:* 405-585-4450. *Fax:* 405-585-4474. *E-mail:* Lepaine.McHenry@okbu.edu.

GRADUATE PROGRAMS
Contact Dr. Rhonda Richards, Dean, College of Graduate and Professional Studies, School of Nursing, Oklahoma Baptist University, 3800 North May Avenue, Oklahoma City, OK 73112. *Telephone:* 405-585-4601. *Fax:* 405-585-4646. *E-mail:* Rhonda.Richards@okbu.edu.

MASTER'S DEGREE PROGRAM
Degree MSN
Available Programs Master's; RN to Master's.
Concentrations Available Nursing education.
Study Options Full-time and part-time.
Online Degree Options Yes (online only).
Program Entrance Requirements Clinical experience, minimum overall college GPA of 3.0, transcript of college record, CPR certification, written essay, 1 letter of recommendation, nursing research course, professional liability insurance/malpractice insurance, resume, statistics course. *Application deadline:* 7/30 (fall), 12/20 (winter), 7/30

(spring), 7/30 (summer). Applications may be processed on a rolling basis for some programs. *Application fee:* $50.
Degree Requirements 35 total credit hours, thesis or project.

Oklahoma Christian University
Nursing Program
Oklahoma City, Oklahoma

Founded in 1950
DEGREE • BSN

BACCALAUREATE PROGRAMS
Degree BSN
Available Programs Generic Baccalaureate.
Program Entrance Requirements Minimum overall college GPA of 2.75, 3 letters of recommendation.
Contact *Telephone:* 405-425-1921.

Oklahoma City University
Kramer School of Nursing
Oklahoma City, Oklahoma

http://www.okcu.edu/nursing
Founded in 1904
DEGREES • BSN • DNP • MSN • PHD
Nursing Program Faculty 49 (31% with doctorates).
Baccalaureate Enrollment 290 **Women** 86% **Men** 14% **Part-time** 10%
Graduate Enrollment 151 **Women** 87% **Men** 13% **Part-time** 65%
Distance Learning Courses Available.
Nursing Student Activities Sigma Theta Tau, Student Nurses' Association.
Nursing Student Resources Academic advising; academic or career counseling; assistance for students with disabilities; bookstore; campus computer network; career placement assistance; computer lab; computer-assisted instruction; e-mail services; employment services for current students; housing assistance; interactive nursing skills videos; Internet; learning resource lab; library services; nursing audiovisuals; placement services for program completers; remedial services; resume preparation assistance; skills, simulation, or other laboratory; tutoring.
Library Facilities 2,714 volumes in health, 590 volumes in nursing; 234 periodical subscriptions health-care related.

BACCALAUREATE PROGRAMS
Degree BSN
Available Programs ADN to Baccalaureate; Accelerated Baccalaureate; Accelerated Baccalaureate for Second Degree; Baccalaureate for Second Degree; Generic Baccalaureate; International Nurse to Baccalaureate; RN Baccalaureate.
Site Options Lawton, OK; Ardmore , OK.
Study Options Full-time and part-time.
Program Entrance Requirements Minimum overall college GPA of 3.0, transcript of college record, CPR certification, health insurance, high school transcript, immunizations, minimum GPA in nursing prerequisites of 3.0, prerequisite course work. Transfer students are accepted. *Application deadline:* 8/1 (fall), 12/1 (spring), 4/1 (summer). Applications may be processed on a rolling basis for some programs. *Application fee:* $50.
Advanced Placement Credit by examination available. Credit given for nursing courses completed elsewhere dependent upon specific evaluations.
Expenses (2014–15) *Tuition:* full-time $24,740; part-time $840 per credit hour. *International tuition:* $24,740 full-time. *Room and board:* $9210 per academic year. *Required fees:* full-time $6720; part-time $210 per credit.
Financial Aid 85% of baccalaureate students in nursing programs received some form of financial aid in 2013–14.
Contact Ms. Debbie Taber, Intake Specialist, Kramer School of Nursing, Oklahoma City University, 2501 North Blackwelder Avenue, Oklahoma City, OK 73106-1493. *Telephone:* 405-208-5924. *Fax:* 405-208-5914. *E-mail:* djtaber@okcu.edu.

GRADUATE PROGRAMS
Expenses (2014–15) *Tuition:* full-time $11,232; part-time $936 per credit hour. *International tuition:* $11,232 full-time. *Room and board:* $9210

per academic year. *Required fees:* full-time $2520; part-time $210 per credit.

Financial Aid 92% of graduate students in nursing programs received some form of financial aid in 2013–14.

Contact Mrs. Shelley Cassada, Graduate Specialist, Kramer School of Nursing, Oklahoma City University, 2501 North Blackwelder Avenue, Oklahoma City, OK 73106-1493. *Telephone:* 405-208-5960. *Fax:* 405-208-5914. *E-mail:* neallisoncatalfu@okcu.edu.

MASTER'S DEGREE PROGRAM

Degree MSN

Available Programs Accelerated AD/RN to Master's; Accelerated Master's; Accelerated Master's for Nurses with Non-Nursing Degrees; Accelerated RN to Master's; Master's; Master's for Nurses with Non-Nursing Degrees; RN to Master's.

Concentrations Available Nursing administration; nursing education.

Study Options Full-time and part-time.

Program Entrance Requirements Minimum overall college GPA of 3.0, transcript of college record, written essay, nursing research course, physical assessment course, statistics course. *Application deadline:* 8/1 (fall), 12/1 (spring), 4/1 (summer). Applications may be processed on a rolling basis for some programs. *Application fee:* $50.

Advanced Placement Credit given for nursing courses completed elsewhere dependent upon specific evaluations.

Degree Requirements 33 total credit hours, thesis or project.

DOCTORAL DEGREE PROGRAM

Degree DNP

Available Programs Doctorate, Doctorate for Nurses with Non-Nursing Degrees, Post-Baccalaureate Doctorate.

Areas of Study Clinical practice, nursing administration, nursing education.

Program Entrance Requirements Minimum overall college GPA of 3.5, clinical experience, interview by faculty committee, MSN or equivalent, statistics course, vita, writing sample. Application deadline: 4/1 (fall). Application fee: $50.

Degree Requirements 90 total credit hours, dissertation, oral exam, residency, written exam.

Degree PhD

Available Programs Doctorate; Doctorate for Nurses with Non-Nursing Degrees; Post-Baccalaureate Doctorate.

Areas of Study Nursing administration, nursing education.

Program Entrance Requirements Clinical experience, minimum overall college GPA of 3.5, interview by faculty committee, 3 letters of recommendation, MSN or equivalent, statistics course, vita, writing sample. Application deadline: 4/1 (fall). Application fee: $50.

Degree Requirements 90 total credit hours, dissertation, oral exam, written exam, residency.

CONTINUING EDUCATION PROGRAM

Contact Mr. Christopher Black, Director of Communications and Outreach, Kramer School of Nursing, Oklahoma City University, 2501 North Blackwelder Avenue, Oklahoma City, OK 73106-1493. *Telephone:* 405-208-5832. *Fax:* 405-208-5914. *E-mail:* cblack@okcu.edu.

Oklahoma Panhandle State University

Bachelor of Science in Nursing Program
Goodwell, Oklahoma

http://www.opsu.edu/
Founded in 1909

DEGREE • BSN

Nursing Program Faculty 4

Baccalaureate Enrollment 57 **Women** 90% **Men** 10% **Part-time** 73%

Distance Learning Courses Available.

Nursing Student Activities Student Nurses' Association.

Nursing Student Resources Academic advising; academic or career counseling; assistance for students with disabilities; bookstore; campus computer network; computer-assisted instruction; e-mail services; Internet; library services.

Library Facilities 1,019 volumes in health, 380 volumes in nursing; 2,032 periodical subscriptions health-care related.

BACCALAUREATE PROGRAMS

Degree BSN

Available Programs ADN to Baccalaureate.

Study Options Full-time and part-time.

Online Degree Options Yes (online only).

Program Entrance Requirements Minimum overall college GPA of 2.0, transcript of college record, CPR certification, immunizations, minimum GPA in nursing prerequisites of 2.0, RN licensure. Transfer students are accepted. *Application deadline:* 8/1 (fall), 1/10 (spring), 5/20 (summer).

Advanced Placement Credit given for nursing courses completed elsewhere dependent upon specific evaluations.

Contact *Telephone:* 580-349-1520. *Fax:* 580-349-1529.

Oklahoma Wesleyan University

School of Nursing
Bartlesville, Oklahoma

http://www.okwu.edu/
Founded in 1909

DEGREE • BSN

Nursing Program Faculty 56 (58% with doctorates).

Baccalaureate Enrollment 140 **Women** 96% **Men** 4%

Distance Learning Courses Available.

Nursing Student Resources Academic advising; academic or career counseling; assistance for students with disabilities; bookstore; campus computer network; computer lab; computer-assisted instruction; interactive nursing skills videos; Internet; learning resource lab; library services; nursing audiovisuals; skills, simulation, or other laboratory.

Library Facilities 946 volumes in health, 483 volumes in nursing; 40 periodical subscriptions health-care related.

BACCALAUREATE PROGRAMS

Degree BSN

Available Programs ADN to Baccalaureate; Accelerated RN Baccalaureate; Baccalaureate for Second Degree; Generic Baccalaureate; International Nurse to Baccalaureate; LPN to Baccalaureate; RN Baccalaureate.

Site Options McAlester, OK; Oklahoma City, OK; Tulsa, OK.

Study Options Full-time.

Program Entrance Requirements Minimum overall college GPA of 2.3, transcript of college record, CPR certification, health exam, health insurance, immunizations, 2 letters of recommendation, minimum GPA in nursing prerequisites of 2.75, professional liability insurance/malpractice insurance, prerequisite course work, RN licensure. Transfer students are accepted. *Application deadline:* 6/1 (fall). Applications may be processed on a rolling basis for some programs.

Advanced Placement Credit by examination available. Credit given for nursing courses completed elsewhere dependent upon specific evaluations.

Expenses (2015–16) *Tuition:* full-time $21,930; part-time $900 per hour. *Room and board:* $7082; room only: $3858 per academic year.

Financial Aid *Gift aid (need-based):* Federal Pell, FSEOG, state, private, college/university gift aid from institutional funds. *Loans:* Federal Direct (Subsidized and Unsubsidized Stafford PLUS), Perkins, college/university. *Work-study:* Federal Work-Study, part-time campus jobs. *Financial aid application deadline (priority):* 3/1.

Contact Mrs. Jessica L. Johnson, Interim Dean, School of Nursing, Oklahoma Wesleyan University, 2201 Silver Lake Road, Bartlesville, OK 74006. *Telephone:* 918-335-6854. *E-mail:* jljohnson@okwu.edu.

Oral Roberts University

Anna Vaughn School of Nursing
Tulsa, Oklahoma

http://www.oru.edu/
Founded in 1963

DEGREE • BSN

Nursing Program Faculty 29 (10% with doctorates).

Baccalaureate Enrollment 174 **Women** 85% **Men** 15% **Part-time** 2%

Distance Learning Courses Available.

Nursing Student Activities Sigma Theta Tau, Student Nurses' Association.

Nursing Student Resources Academic advising; academic or career counseling; assistance for students with disabilities; bookstore; campus computer network; computer lab; computer-assisted instruction; e-mail services; employment services for current students; housing assistance; interactive nursing skills videos; Internet; learning resource lab; library services; nursing audiovisuals; remedial services; resume preparation assistance; skills, simulation, or other laboratory; tutoring.
Library Facilities 97,285 volumes in health, 37,104 volumes in nursing; 525 periodical subscriptions health-care related.

BACCALAUREATE PROGRAMS

Degree BSN
Available Programs ADN to Baccalaureate; Generic Baccalaureate; RN Baccalaureate.
Study Options Full-time and part-time.
Program Entrance Requirements Minimum overall college GPA of 3.0, transcript of college record, CPR certification, health exam, health insurance, high school biology, high school chemistry, 2 years high school math, 2 years high school science, high school transcript, immunizations, minimum high school GPA of 2.5, minimum GPA in nursing prerequisites of 2.5. Transfer students are accepted. *Application deadline:* 7/31 (fall), 12/10 (spring). *Application fee:* $35.
Advanced Placement Credit given for nursing courses completed elsewhere dependent upon specific evaluations.
Expenses (2015–16) *Tuition:* full-time $23,896; part-time $998 per credit hour. *International tuition:* $23,896 full-time. *Room and board:* room only: $6400 per academic year. *Required fees:* full-time $1596.
Financial Aid 98% of baccalaureate students in nursing programs received some form of financial aid in 2014–15. *Gift aid (need-based):* Federal Pell, FSEOG, state, private, college/university gift aid from institutional funds. *Loans:* Federal Direct (Subsidized and Unsubsidized Stafford PLUS), Perkins. *Work-study:* Federal Work-Study, part-time campus jobs. *Financial aid application deadline (priority):* 3/1.
Contact Dr. Kenda Jezek, Dean, Anna Vaughn School of Nursing, Oral Roberts University, 7777 South Lewis Avenue, Tulsa, OK 74171. *Telephone:* 918-495-6198. *Fax:* 918-495-6020. *E-mail:* kjezek@oru.edu.

Rogers State University
Nursing Program
Claremore, Oklahoma

Founded in 1909
DEGREE • BSN
Baccalaureate Enrollment 18 **Women** 94% **Men** 6%
Distance Learning Courses Available.
Nursing Student Activities Student Nurses' Association.
Nursing Student Resources Academic advising; academic or career counseling; assistance for students with disabilities; bookstore; campus computer network; career placement assistance; computer lab; computer-assisted instruction; daycare for children of students; e-mail services; housing assistance; interactive nursing skills videos; Internet; learning resource lab; library services; nursing audiovisuals; placement services for program completers; remedial services; resume preparation assistance; skills, simulation, or other laboratory.

BACCALAUREATE PROGRAMS

Degree BSN
Available Programs ADN to Baccalaureate.
Site Options Bartlesville, OK.
Program Entrance Requirements Minimum overall college GPA, CPR certification, health exam, health insurance, immunizations, minimum GPA in nursing prerequisites, RN licensure. Transfer students are accepted.
Contact *Telephone:* 918-343-7885. *Fax:* 918-343-7628.

Southern Nazarene University
School of Nursing
Bethany, Oklahoma

http://www.snu.edu/
Founded in 1899
DEGREES • BS • MS
Nursing Program Faculty 35 (40% with doctorates).

Baccalaureate Enrollment 101 **Women** 90% **Men** 10% **Part-time** 10%
Graduate Enrollment 34 **Women** 90% **Men** 10%
Distance Learning Courses Available.
Nursing Student Activities Sigma Theta Tau, Student Nurses' Association.
Nursing Student Resources Academic advising; academic or career counseling; assistance for students with disabilities; bookstore; campus computer network; career placement assistance; computer lab; computer-assisted instruction; e-mail services; employment services for current students; externships; housing assistance; interactive nursing skills videos; Internet; learning resource lab; library services; nursing audiovisuals; paid internships; remedial services; skills, simulation, or other laboratory; tutoring.

BACCALAUREATE PROGRAMS

Degree BS
Available Programs ADN to Baccalaureate; Baccalaureate for Second Degree; Generic Baccalaureate; LPN to Baccalaureate.
Study Options Full-time.
Program Entrance Requirements Minimum overall college GPA of 2.75, transcript of college record, CPR certification, health exam, health insurance, immunizations, minimum GPA in nursing prerequisites of 2.75, professional liability insurance/malpractice insurance, prerequisite course work. Transfer students are accepted. *Application deadline:* 12/5 (fall). Applications may be processed on a rolling basis for some programs.
Advanced Placement Credit by examination available. Credit given for nursing courses completed elsewhere dependent upon specific evaluations.
Contact *Telephone:* 405-717-6217. *Fax:* 405-717-6264.

GRADUATE PROGRAMS

Contact *Telephone:* 405-717-6217. *Fax:* 405-717-6264.

MASTER'S DEGREE PROGRAM
Degree MS
Available Programs Accelerated Master's; Accelerated Master's for Nurses with Non-Nursing Degrees.
Concentrations Available Nursing administration; nursing education.
Site Options Tulsa, OK.
Study Options Full-time.
Program Entrance Requirements Clinical experience, computer literacy, minimum overall college GPA of 3.0, transcript of college record, immunizations, interview, 3 letters of recommendation, nursing research course, physical assessment course, resume, statistics course. *Application deadline:* Applications may be processed on a rolling basis for some programs.
Advanced Placement Credit given for nursing courses completed elsewhere dependent upon specific evaluations.
Degree Requirements 39 total credit hours, thesis or project.

Southwestern Oklahoma State University
School of Nursing
Weatherford, Oklahoma

http://www.swosu.edu/academics/nursing/index.asp
Founded in 1901
DEGREE • BSN
Nursing Program Faculty 12 (17% with doctorates).
Baccalaureate Enrollment 77 **Women** 88% **Men** 12%
Distance Learning Courses Available.
Nursing Student Activities Sigma Theta Tau, Student Nurses' Association, nursing club.
Nursing Student Resources Academic advising; academic or career counseling; assistance for students with disabilities; bookstore; campus computer network; computer lab; computer-assisted instruction; e-mail services; externships; housing assistance; interactive nursing skills videos; Internet; learning resource lab; library services; nursing audiovisuals; remedial services; skills, simulation, or other laboratory; tutoring.
Library Facilities 284 periodical subscriptions health-care related.

BACCALAUREATE PROGRAMS

Degree BSN

Available Programs ADN to Baccalaureate; Generic Baccalaureate; RN Baccalaureate.
Site Options Weatherford, OK; Oklahoma City, OK; Elk City, OK.
Study Options Full-time.
Online Degree Options Yes.
Program Entrance Requirements Minimum overall college GPA of 2.5, transcript of college record, CPR certification, immunizations, letters of recommendation, minimum GPA in nursing prerequisites of 2.0, professional liability insurance/malpractice insurance, prerequisite course work. Transfer students are accepted. *Application deadline:* 2/1 (fall).
Advanced Placement Credit given for nursing courses completed elsewhere dependent upon specific evaluations.
Expenses (2014–15) *Tuition, state resident:* full-time $5850. *Tuition, nonresident:* full-time $12,000. *International tuition:* $12,000 full-time. *Room and board:* $2060 per academic year. *Required fees:* full-time $1650.
Financial Aid 70% of baccalaureate students in nursing programs received some form of financial aid in 2013–14. *Gift aid (need-based):* Federal Pell, FSEOG, state, private, college/university gift aid from institutional funds. *Loans:* Federal Direct (Subsidized and Unsubsidized Stafford PLUS). *Work-study:* Federal Work-Study. *Financial aid application deadline:* 3/1.
Contact Ms. Pam Colvard, Administrative Assistant, School of Nursing, Southwestern Oklahoma State University, 100 Campus Drive, Weatherford, OK 73096-3098. *Telephone:* 580-774-3261. *Fax:* 580-774-7075. *E-mail:* pam.colvard@swosu.edu.

University of Central Oklahoma
Department of Nursing
Edmond, Oklahoma

http://www.uco.edu/cms/nursing
Founded in 1890
DEGREES • BSN • MS
Nursing Program Faculty 43 (2% with doctorates).
Baccalaureate Enrollment 301 **Women** 90% **Men** 10% **Part-time** 1%
Graduate Enrollment 48 **Women** 99% **Men** 1% **Part-time** 2%
Nursing Student Activities Nursing Honor Society, Sigma Theta Tau, Student Nurses' Association.
Nursing Student Resources Academic advising; academic or career counseling; assistance for students with disabilities; bookstore; campus computer network; career placement assistance; computer lab; computer-assisted instruction; e-mail services; externships; housing assistance; interactive nursing skills videos; Internet; learning resource lab; library services; nursing audiovisuals; paid internships; placement services for program completers; remedial services; resume preparation assistance; skills, simulation, or other laboratory; tutoring.
Library Facilities 5,685 volumes in health, 737 volumes in nursing.

BACCALAUREATE PROGRAMS

Degree BSN
Available Programs Generic Baccalaureate; LPN to Baccalaureate; RN Baccalaureate.
Study Options Full-time and part-time.
Program Entrance Requirements Minimum overall college GPA of 2.5, transcript of college record, CPR certification, immunizations, professional liability insurance/malpractice insurance, prerequisite course work. Transfer students are accepted. *Application deadline:* 9/11 (fall), 1/29 (spring). *Application fee:* $25.
Advanced Placement Credit given for nursing courses completed elsewhere dependent upon specific evaluations.
Expenses (2015–16) *Tuition, state resident:* full-time $7736; part-time $276 per credit hour. *International tuition:* $16,020 full-time. *Room and board:* $7470; room only: $3620 per academic year. *Required fees:* full-time $2047.
Financial Aid 35% of baccalaureate students in nursing programs received some form of financial aid in 2014–15. *Gift aid (need-based):* Federal Pell, FSEOG, state, private, college/university gift aid from institutional funds. *Loans:* Federal Direct (Subsidized and Unsubsidized Stafford PLUS). *Work-study:* Federal Work-Study, part-time campus jobs. *Financial aid application deadline:* Continuous.
Contact Vicki Addison, Administrative Assistant, Department of Nursing, University of Central Oklahoma, 100 North University Drive, Edmond, OK 73034-5209. *Telephone:* 405-974-5000.
E-mail: vaddison@uco.edu.

GRADUATE PROGRAMS

Expenses (2015–16) *Tuition, area resident:* full-time $5952; part-time $2976 per credit hour. *International tuition:* $12,061 full-time. *Room and board:* $7470; room only: $3620 per academic year. *Required fees:* full-time $1316; part-time $73 per credit.
Financial Aid 30% of graduate students in nursing programs received some form of financial aid in 2014–15.
Contact Dr. Nancy Dentlinger, Master's Coordinator, Department of Nursing, University of Central Oklahoma, 100 North University Drive, Edmond, OK 73034. *Telephone:* 405-974-5379. *Fax:* 405-974-3848. *E-mail:* ndentlinger@uco.edu.

MASTER'S DEGREE PROGRAM
Degree MS
Available Programs Master's.
Concentrations Available Nursing education.
Study Options Full-time and part-time.
Program Entrance Requirements Minimum overall college GPA of 3.0, transcript of college record, CPR certification, immunizations, 3 letters of recommendation, professional liability insurance/malpractice insurance, prerequisite course work, statistics course. *Application deadline:* 4/1 (fall), 11/1 (spring). *Application fee:* $50.
Advanced Placement Credit given for nursing courses completed elsewhere dependent upon specific evaluations.
Degree Requirements 34 total credit hours, thesis or project, comprehensive exam.

University of Oklahoma Health Sciences Center
College of Nursing
Oklahoma City, Oklahoma

http://nursing.ouhsc.edu/
Founded in 1890
DEGREES • BSN • MS • PHD
Nursing Program Faculty 185 (16% with doctorates).
Baccalaureate Enrollment 892 **Women** 85% **Men** 15% **Part-time** 4%
Graduate Enrollment 256 **Women** 93% **Men** 7% **Part-time** 71%
Distance Learning Courses Available.
Nursing Student Activities Sigma Theta Tau, Student Nurses' Association.
Nursing Student Resources Academic advising; academic or career counseling; assistance for students with disabilities; bookstore; campus computer network; computer lab; computer-assisted instruction; e-mail services; employment services for current students; housing assistance; Internet; learning resource lab; library services; nursing audiovisuals; skills, simulation, or other laboratory; tutoring.

BACCALAUREATE PROGRAMS

Degree BSN
Available Programs ADN to Baccalaureate; Accelerated Baccalaureate for Second Degree; Generic Baccalaureate; LPN to RN Baccalaureate.
Site Options Lawton, OK; Tulsa, OK.
Study Options Full-time.
Program Entrance Requirements Minimum overall college GPA of 2.5, transcript of college record, high school transcript, minimum GPA in nursing prerequisites of 2.5, prerequisite course work. Transfer students are accepted. *Application deadline:* 1/15 (fall). *Application fee:* $65.
Advanced Placement Credit by examination available. Credit given for nursing courses completed elsewhere dependent upon specific evaluations.
Contact *Telephone:* 405-271-2128. *Fax:* 405-271-7341.

GRADUATE PROGRAMS

Contact *Telephone:* 405-271-2128. *Fax:* 405-271-7341.

MASTER'S DEGREE PROGRAM
Degree MS
Available Programs Master's; Master's for Non-Nursing College Graduates.
Concentrations Available Clinical nurse leader; health-care administration; nursing education. *Clinical nurse specialist programs in:* acute care. *Nurse practitioner programs in:* adult health, family health, neonatal health, pediatric.
Site Options Lawton, OK; Tulsa, OK.

Study Options Full-time and part-time.

Online Degree Options Yes.

Program Entrance Requirements Computer literacy, minimum overall college GPA of 3.0, transcript of college record, 3 letters of recommendation, nursing research course, professional liability insurance/malpractice insurance, prerequisite course work, statistics course. *Application deadline:* 3/1 (fall), 8/1 (spring), 1/15 (summer). *Application fee:* $65.

Advanced Placement Credit given for nursing courses completed elsewhere dependent upon specific evaluations.

Degree Requirements 38 total credit hours, thesis or project, comprehensive exam.

POST-MASTER'S PROGRAM

Areas of Study Clinical nurse leader; health-care administration; nursing education. *Nurse practitioner programs in:* adult health, family health, neonatal health, pediatric.

DOCTORAL DEGREE PROGRAM

Degree PhD

Available Programs Doctorate.

Areas of Study Nursing education.

Program Entrance Requirements Minimum overall college GPA of 3.5, interview by faculty committee, 3 letters of recommendation, scholarly papers, statistics course, vita, writing sample. Application deadline: 4/14 (fall). Application fee: $65.

Degree Requirements 90 total credit hours, dissertation, oral exam, written exam.

CONTINUING EDUCATION PROGRAM

Contact *Telephone:* 405-271-2428. *Fax:* 405-271-7341.

University of Phoenix–Oklahoma City Campus

College of Health and Human Services
Oklahoma City, Oklahoma

Founded in 1976

Nursing Program Faculty 1

Nursing Student Activities Sigma Theta Tau.

Nursing Student Resources Academic advising; academic or career counseling; assistance for students with disabilities; bookstore; campus computer network; computer lab; computer-assisted instruction; e-mail services; interactive nursing skills videos; Internet; learning resource lab; library services; nursing audiovisuals; skills, simulation, or other laboratory; tutoring.

Library Facilities 1,300 periodical subscriptions health-care related.

University of Phoenix–Tulsa Learning Center

College of Health and Human Services
Tulsa, Oklahoma

Founded in 1998

Nursing Student Activities Sigma Theta Tau.

Nursing Student Resources Academic advising; academic or career counseling; assistance for students with disabilities; bookstore; campus computer network; computer lab; computer-assisted instruction; e-mail services; interactive nursing skills videos; Internet; learning resource lab; library services; nursing audiovisuals; remedial services; skills, simulation, or other laboratory; tutoring.

Library Facilities 1,300 periodical subscriptions health-care related.

The University of Tulsa

School of Nursing
Tulsa, Oklahoma

http://www.utulsa.edu/nursing
Founded in 1894

DEGREE • BSN

Nursing Program Faculty 17 (35% with doctorates).

Baccalaureate Enrollment 80 **Women** 88% **Men** 12% **Part-time** 2%

Nursing Student Activities Sigma Theta Tau, Student Nurses' Association.

Nursing Student Resources Academic advising; academic or career counseling; assistance for students with disabilities; bookstore; campus computer network; career placement assistance; computer lab; computer-assisted instruction; daycare for children of students; e-mail services; employment services for current students; externships; housing assistance; interactive nursing skills videos; Internet; learning resource lab; library services; nursing audiovisuals; placement services for program completers; remedial services; resume preparation assistance; skills, simulation, or other laboratory; tutoring.

Library Facilities 4,300 volumes in nursing; 8,168 periodical subscriptions health-care related.

BACCALAUREATE PROGRAMS

Degree BSN

Available Programs Generic Baccalaureate; LPN to RN Baccalaureate; RN Baccalaureate.

Site Options Tulsa, OK.

Study Options Full-time.

Program Entrance Requirements Minimum overall college GPA of 2.5, transcript of college record, CPR certification, written essay, health exam, immunizations, minimum GPA in nursing prerequisites. Transfer students are accepted. *Application deadline:* 2/1 (fall). Applications may be processed on a rolling basis for some programs.

Advanced Placement Credit by examination available. Credit given for nursing courses completed elsewhere dependent upon specific evaluations.

Expenses (2015–16) *Tuition:* full-time $40,484. *Room and board:* room only: $6394 per academic year. *Required fees:* full-time $1025.

Financial Aid *Gift aid (need-based):* Federal Pell, FSEOG, state, private, college/university gift aid from institutional funds. *Loans:* Federal Direct (Subsidized and Unsubsidized Stafford PLUS), Perkins. *Work-study:* Federal Work-Study, part-time campus jobs. *Financial aid application deadline (priority):* 3/1.

Contact Dr. Deborah L. Greubel, Director, School of Nursing, The University of Tulsa, 800 South Tucker Drive, Tulsa, OK 74104-9700. *Telephone:* 918-631-2920. *Fax:* 918-631-2068. *E-mail:* deb-greubel@utulsa.edu.

OREGON

Concordia University

Nursing Program
Portland, Oregon

http://www.cu-portland.edu/
Founded in 1905

DEGREE • BSN

BACCALAUREATE PROGRAMS

Degree BSN

Available Programs Generic Baccalaureate.

Study Options Full-time.

Program Entrance Requirements Transfer students are accepted.

Contact Donna Bachand, Interim Director of Nursing Program, Nursing Program, Concordia University, 2811 NE Holman Street, Portland, OR 97211. *Telephone:* 503-280-8538. *E-mail:* dbachand@cu-portland.edu.

George Fox University
Nursing Department
Newberg, Oregon

*http://www.georgefox.edu/academics/undergrad/departments
/nursing/index.html*
Founded in 1891

DEGREE • BSN
Nursing Program Faculty 15 (20% with doctorates).
Baccalaureate Enrollment 110 **Women** 91% **Men** 9%
Nursing Student Activities Nursing club.
Nursing Student Resources Academic advising; academic or career counseling; assistance for students with disabilities; bookstore; campus computer network; career placement assistance; computer lab; computer-assisted instruction; e-mail services; employment services for current students; housing assistance; interactive nursing skills videos; Internet; learning resource lab; library services; nursing audiovisuals; remedial services; resume preparation assistance; skills, simulation, or other laboratory; tutoring.
Library Facilities 490 volumes in health, 100 volumes in nursing; 5,600 periodical subscriptions health-care related.

BACCALAUREATE PROGRAMS
Degree BSN
Available Programs Generic Baccalaureate.
Study Options Full-time.
Program Entrance Requirements Minimum overall college GPA of 2.8, transcript of college record, CPR certification, written essay, immunizations, 2 letters of recommendation, minimum GPA in nursing prerequisites of 2.8, prerequisite course work. Transfer students are accepted. *Application deadline:* 10/2 (fall). *Application fee:* $50.
Contact *Telephone:* 503-554-2950. *Fax:* 503-554-3900.

Linfield College
School of Nursing
McMinnville, Oregon

http://www.linfield.edu/portland
Founded in 1849

DEGREE • BSN
Nursing Program Faculty 65 (26% with doctorates).
Baccalaureate Enrollment 347 **Women** 83% **Men** 17% **Part-time** 2%
Distance Learning Courses Available.
Nursing Student Activities Nursing Honor Society, Sigma Theta Tau, Student Nurses' Association, nursing club.
Nursing Student Resources Academic advising; academic or career counseling; assistance for students with disabilities; bookstore; campus computer network; computer lab; computer-assisted instruction; e-mail services; employment services for current students; housing assistance; Internet; learning resource lab; library services; nursing audiovisuals; resume preparation assistance; skills, simulation, or other laboratory.
Library Facilities 7,201 volumes in health, 1,482 volumes in nursing; 249 periodical subscriptions health-care related.

BACCALAUREATE PROGRAMS
Degree BSN
Available Programs ADN to Baccalaureate; Accelerated Baccalaureate for Second Degree; Baccalaureate for Second Degree; Generic Baccalaureate; RN Baccalaureate.
Site Options Portland, OR.
Study Options Full-time.
Online Degree Options Yes.
Program Entrance Requirements Minimum overall college GPA of 2.9, transcript of college record, CPR certification, written essay, health exam, health insurance, immunizations, 1 letter of recommendation, minimum GPA in nursing prerequisites of 3.0, professional liability insurance/malpractice insurance, prerequisite course work. Transfer students are accepted. *Application deadline:* 2/1 (fall), 8/1 (spring), 2/1 (summer). *Application fee:* $65.
Advanced Placement Credit given for nursing courses completed elsewhere dependent upon specific evaluations.
Expenses (2015–16) *Tuition:* full-time $38,300; part-time $1192 per credit hour. *International tuition:* $38,300 full-time. *Room and board:*

$7480; room only: $4280 per academic year. *Required fees:* full-time $1467.
Financial Aid *Gift aid (need-based):* Federal Pell, FSEOG, state, private, college/university gift aid from institutional funds. *Loans:* Federal Direct (Subsidized and Unsubsidized Stafford PLUS), Perkins, private loans. *Work-study:* Federal Work-Study, part-time campus jobs. *Financial aid application deadline (priority):* 2/1.
Contact Mr. Todd McCollum, Director, Enrollment Services, School of Nursing, Linfield College, 2255 NW Northrup Street, Portland, OR 97210. *Telephone:* 503-413-7830. *Fax:* 503-413-6283.
E-mail: tmccoll@linfield.edu.

CONTINUING EDUCATION PROGRAM
Contact Ms. Jessica Cunningham, Assistant Director of Admissions, School of Nursing, Linfield College, 416 Linfield Avenue, McMinnville, OR, OR 97128. *Telephone:* 503-883-2478.
E-mail: jcunning@linfield.edu.

Oregon Health & Science University
School of Nursing
Portland, Oregon

http://www.ohsu.edu/xd/education/schools/school-of-nursing/
Founded in 1974

DEGREES • BS • MN • PHD
Nursing Program Faculty 199 (41% with doctorates).
Baccalaureate Enrollment 848 **Women** 84% **Men** 16% **Part-time** 73%
Graduate Enrollment 259 **Women** 81% **Men** 19% **Part-time** 11.6%
Distance Learning Courses Available.
Nursing Student Activities Nursing Honor Society, Sigma Theta Tau, Student Nurses' Association, nursing club.
Nursing Student Resources Academic advising; academic or career counseling; assistance for students with disabilities; bookstore; campus computer network; career placement assistance; computer lab; computer-assisted instruction; e-mail services; externships; interactive nursing skills videos; Internet; learning resource lab; library services; nursing audiovisuals; other; resume preparation assistance; skills, simulation, or other laboratory; tutoring.
Library Facilities 260,674 volumes in health, 8,678 volumes in nursing; 40,816 periodical subscriptions health-care related.

BACCALAUREATE PROGRAMS
Degree BS
Available Programs Accelerated Baccalaureate; Generic Baccalaureate; RN Baccalaureate.
Site Options Klamath Falls, Ashland, Monmouth, and LaGrande, OR.
Study Options Full-time.
Program Entrance Requirements Minimum overall college GPA of 3.0, transcript of college record, minimum GPA in nursing prerequisites of 3.0, prerequisite course work. Transfer students are accepted. *Application deadline:* 2/15 (fall). *Application fee:* $45.
Advanced Placement Credit given for nursing courses completed elsewhere dependent upon specific evaluations.
Expenses (2015–16) *Tuition, state resident:* full-time $10,620; part-time $354 per credit. *Tuition, nonresident:* full-time $19,400; part-time $649 per credit. *International tuition:* $19,400 full-time. *Required fees:* full-time $5415; part-time $1579 per term.
Financial Aid *Gift aid (need-based):* Federal Pell, FSEOG, state, private, college/university gift aid from institutional funds. *Loans:* Federal Nursing Student Loans, Federal Direct (Subsidized and Unsubsidized Stafford PLUS), Perkins, college/university, alternative loans. *Work-study:* Federal Work-Study.
Contact Admissions Counselor, School of Nursing, Oregon Health & Science University, Office of Admissions SN-ADM, 3455 SW U.S. Veterans Hospital Road, Portland, OR 97239-2491. *Telephone:* 503-494-7725. *Fax:* 503-494-6433. *E-mail:* proginfo@ohsu.edu.

GRADUATE PROGRAMS
Expenses (2015–16) *Tuition, state resident:* full-time $19,740; part-time $564 per credit. *Tuition, nonresident:* full-time $25,515; part-time $729 per credit. *International tuition:* $25,515 full-time. *Required fees:* full-time $7220; part-time $1565 per term.

Financial Aid Fellowships, research assistantships, teaching assistantships, career-related internships or fieldwork, Federal Work-Study, institutionally sponsored loans, scholarships, and traineeships available.
Contact Admissions Counselor, School of Nursing, Oregon Health & Science University, Office of Admissions SN-ADM, 3455 SW U.S. Veterans Hospital Road, Portland, OR 97239-2491. *Telephone:* 503-494-7725. *Fax:* 503-494-4350. *E-mail:* proginfo@ohsu.edu.

MASTER'S DEGREE PROGRAM
Degree MN
Available Programs Accelerated Master's for Non-Nursing College Graduates; Master's.
Concentrations Available Health-care administration; nurse anesthesia; nurse-midwifery; nursing education. *Nurse practitioner programs in:* adult-gerontology acute care, family health, pediatric, pediatric primary care, psychiatric/mental health.
Study Options Full-time and part-time.
Program Entrance Requirements Clinical experience, computer literacy, minimum overall college GPA of 3.0, transcript of college record, CPR certification, written essay, immunizations, interview, 3 letters of recommendation, resume, statistics course, GRE General Test. *Application deadline:* 1/4 (fall). Applications may be processed on a rolling basis for some programs. *Application fee:* $65.
Advanced Placement Credit given for nursing courses completed elsewhere dependent upon specific evaluations.
Degree Requirements 70 total credit hours.

POST-MASTER'S PROGRAM
Areas of Study Health-care administration; nurse-midwifery; nursing education. *Nurse practitioner programs in:* adult-gerontology acute care, family health, pediatric, pediatric primary care, psychiatric/mental health.

DOCTORAL DEGREE PROGRAM
Degree PhD
Available Programs Doctorate; Post-Baccalaureate Doctorate.
Areas of Study Advanced practice nursing, aging, clinical practice, ethics, faculty preparation, family health, gerontology, health policy, health promotion/disease prevention, health-care systems, human health and illness, illness and transition, maternity-newborn, nursing policy, nursing research, nursing science, women's health.
Program Entrance Requirements Clinical experience, minimum overall college GPA of 3.0, interview by faculty committee, interview, 3 letters of recommendation, MSN or equivalent, scholarly papers, statistics course, vita, writing sample, GRE General Test. Application deadline: 1/15 (fall). Applications may be processed on a rolling basis for some programs. Application fee: $65.
Degree Requirements 90 total credit hours, dissertation, oral exam, written exam, residency.

POSTDOCTORAL PROGRAM
Areas of Study Adolescent health, aging, chronic illness, family health, gerontology, health promotion/disease prevention, nursing interventions, nursing research, nursing science, outcomes, self-care, vulnerable population, women's health.
Postdoctoral Program Contact Academic Programs Counselor, School of Nursing, Oregon Health & Science University, Office of Admissions SN-ADM, 3455 SW U.S. Veterans Hospital Road, Portland, OR 97239-2491. *Telephone:* 503-494-7725. *Fax:* 503-494-4350. *E-mail:* proginfo@ohsu.edu.

CONTINUING EDUCATION PROGRAM
Contact Paula McNeil, Director of Continuing Education, School of Nursing, Oregon Health & Science University, Office of Continuing Education, SN-4N, 3455 SW U.S. Veterans Hospital Road, Portland, OR 97239-2491. *Telephone:* 503-494-6772. *Fax:* 503-494-4350. *E-mail:* snconted@ohsu.edu.

University of Portland
School of Nursing
Portland, Oregon

http://www.nursing.up.edu/
Founded in 1901
DEGREES • BSN • DNP • MS
Nursing Program Faculty 60 (33% with doctorates).
Baccalaureate Enrollment 687 **Women** 90% **Men** 10%

Graduate Enrollment 42 **Women** 93% **Men** 7%
Distance Learning Courses Available.
Nursing Student Activities Sigma Theta Tau, Student Nurses' Association, nursing club.
Nursing Student Resources Academic advising; academic or career counseling; assistance for students with disabilities; bookstore; campus computer network; career placement assistance; computer lab; computer-assisted instruction; daycare for children of students; e-mail services; employment services for current students; housing assistance; interactive nursing skills videos; Internet; learning resource lab; library services; nursing audiovisuals; remedial services; resume preparation assistance; skills, simulation, or other laboratory; tutoring.
Library Facilities 3,296 volumes in health, 939 volumes in nursing; 1,859 periodical subscriptions health-care related.

BACCALAUREATE PROGRAMS
Degree BSN
Available Programs Generic Baccalaureate.
Study Options Full-time.
Program Entrance Requirements Minimum overall college GPA of 2.7, transcript of college record, CPR certification, written essay, health exam, health insurance, high school chemistry, high school transcript, immunizations, 1 letter of recommendation, minimum high school GPA of 2.7, minimum GPA in nursing prerequisites of 2.7, prerequisite course work. Transfer students are accepted. *Application deadline:* 1/15 (fall), 2/1 (spring). *Application fee:* $50.
Advanced Placement Credit by examination available. Credit given for nursing courses completed elsewhere dependent upon specific evaluations.
Expenses (2015–16) *Tuition:* full-time $47,370. *Room and board:* $13,558 per academic year. *Required fees:* full-time $2273.
Financial Aid 97% of baccalaureate students in nursing programs received some form of financial aid in 2014–15. *Gift aid (need-based):* Federal Pell, FSEOG, state, private, college/university gift aid from institutional funds, United Negro College Fund, Federal Nursing. *Loans:* Federal Nursing Student Loans, Federal Direct (Subsidized and Unsubsidized Stafford PLUS), Perkins. *Work-study:* Federal Work-Study, part-time campus jobs. *Financial aid application deadline (priority):* 3/1.
Contact Mr. Jason McDonald, Dean of Admissions, School of Nursing, University of Portland, 5000 North Willamette Boulevard, Portland, OR 97203-5798. *Telephone:* 503-943-7147. *E-mail:* mcdonaja@up.edu.

GRADUATE PROGRAMS
Expenses (2015–16) *Tuition:* part-time $1120 per credit. *Room and board:* $14,128 per academic year. *Required fees:* part-time $55 per term.
Financial Aid 76% of graduate students in nursing programs received some form of financial aid in 2014–15. Fellowships, research assistantships, Federal Work-Study and scholarships available. Aid available to part-time students. *Financial aid application deadline:* 3/1.
Contact Ms. Becca Fischer, Graduate Program Coordinator, School of Nursing, University of Portland, 5000 North Willamette Boulevard, MSC-153, Portland, OR 97203-5798. *Telephone:* 503-943-7423. *Fax:* 503-943-7729. *E-mail:* fischer@up.edu.

MASTER'S DEGREE PROGRAM
Degree MS
Available Programs Master's.
Concentrations Available Clinical nurse leader; nursing education.
Study Options Full-time and part-time.
Program Entrance Requirements Computer literacy, minimum overall college GPA of 3.0, transcript of college record, written essay, interview, 2 letters of recommendation, resume, statistics course, GRE General Test or MAT. *Application deadline:* 1/15 (summer). Applications may be processed on a rolling basis for some programs.
Advanced Placement Credit given for nursing courses completed elsewhere dependent upon specific evaluations.
Degree Requirements 42 total credit hours, thesis or project.

DOCTORAL DEGREE PROGRAM
Degree DNP
Available Programs Doctorate; Post-Baccalaureate Doctorate.
Areas of Study Advanced practice nursing.
Program Entrance Requirements Minimum overall college GPA of 3.0, interview by faculty committee, 3 letters of recommendation, statistics course, vita, writing sample, GRE General Test or MAT. Application deadline: 1/15 (summer). Applications may be processed on a rolling basis for some programs.
Degree Requirements Oral exam, residency.

PENNSYLVANIA

Alvernia University

Nursing
Reading, Pennsylvania

http://www.alvernia.edu/
Founded in 1958
DEGREES • BSN • MSN • MSN/ED D
Nursing Program Faculty 13 (7% with doctorates).
Baccalaureate Enrollment 252 **Women** 96% **Men** 4% **Part-time** 10%
Nursing Student Activities Nursing Honor Society, Sigma Theta Tau, Student Nurses' Association.
Nursing Student Resources Academic advising; academic or career counseling; assistance for students with disabilities; bookstore; campus computer network; computer lab; computer-assisted instruction; e-mail services; employment services for current students; externships; interactive nursing skills videos; Internet; learning resource lab; library services; nursing audiovisuals; remedial services; resume preparation assistance; skills, simulation, or other laboratory; tutoring.
Library Facilities 3,015 volumes in health, 995 volumes in nursing; 89 periodical subscriptions health-care related.

BACCALAUREATE PROGRAMS

Degree BSN
Available Programs Generic Baccalaureate; LPN to Baccalaureate; LPN to RN Baccalaureate; RN Baccalaureate.
Site Options Reading, PA.
Study Options Full-time.
Program Entrance Requirements Minimum overall college GPA of 2.7, transcript of college record, CPR certification, written essay, health exam, health insurance, high school biology, high school chemistry, 2 years high school math, 2 years high school science, high school transcript, immunizations, 2 letters of recommendation, minimum high school GPA of 2.7, minimum GPA in nursing prerequisites of 2.7. Transfer students are accepted.
Advanced Placement Credit by examination available. Credit given for nursing courses completed elsewhere dependent upon specific evaluations.
Contact Dr. Deborah Greenawald, Nursing Department Chair, Nursing, Alvernia University, 400 Saint Bernardine Street, Reading, PA 19607. *Telephone:* 610-796-8217. *Fax:* 610-796-8464. *E-mail:* Deborah.Greenawald@alvernia.edu.

GRADUATE PROGRAMS

Contact Dr. Vera Brancato, RN to BSN and MSN Coordinator, Nursing, Alvernia University, 400 Saint Bernardine Street, Reading, PA 19607. *Telephone:* 610-790-1958. *Fax:* 610-796-8464. *E-mail:* Vera.Brancato@alvernia.edu.

MASTER'S DEGREE PROGRAM

Degrees MSN; MSN/Ed D
Available Programs Master's; RN to Master's.
Concentrations Available *Clinical nurse specialist programs in:* acute care, adult health, adult-gerontology acute care, cardiovascular, critical care, family health, forensic nursing, gerontology, home health care, medical-surgical, oncology.
Site Options Schuylkill Haven, PA; Reading, PA.
Study Options Part-time.
Program Entrance Requirements Clinical experience, computer literacy, minimum overall college GPA of 3.0, transcript of college record, CPR certification, immunizations, interview, physical assessment course, professional liability insurance/malpractice insurance, resume, statistics course.
Advanced Placement Credit given for nursing courses completed elsewhere dependent upon specific evaluations.
Degree Requirements 36 total credit hours.

CONTINUING EDUCATION PROGRAM

Contact Ms. Mary Arbogast, Nursing Outreach Coordinator, Nursing, Alvernia University, 400 Saint Bernardine Street, Reading, PA 19607. *Telephone:* 610-796-8429. *Fax:* 610-796-8367. *E-mail:* mary.arbogast@alvernia.edu.

Bloomsburg University of Pennsylvania

Department of Nursing
Bloomsburg, Pennsylvania

http://www.bloomu.edu/nursing
Founded in 1839
DEGREES • BSN • MSN • MSN/MBA
Nursing Program Faculty 42 (40% with doctorates).
Baccalaureate Enrollment 423 **Women** 86.9% **Men** 13.1% **Part-time** 9.8%
Graduate Enrollment 109 **Women** 74.3% **Men** 25.7% **Part-time** 67.9%
Distance Learning Courses Available.
Nursing Student Activities Sigma Theta Tau, Student Nurses' Association.
Nursing Student Resources Academic advising; academic or career counseling; assistance for students with disabilities; bookstore; campus computer network; career placement assistance; computer lab; computer-assisted instruction; daycare for children of students; e-mail services; employment services for current students; externships; housing assistance; interactive nursing skills videos; Internet; learning resource lab; library services; nursing audiovisuals; paid internships; placement services for program completers; remedial services; resume preparation assistance; skills, simulation, or other laboratory; tutoring; unpaid internships.
Library Facilities 3,350 volumes in health, 1,732 volumes in nursing; 5,457 periodical subscriptions health-care related.

BACCALAUREATE PROGRAMS

Degree BSN
Available Programs Accelerated Baccalaureate for Second Degree; Baccalaureate for Second Degree; Generic Baccalaureate; LPN to RN Baccalaureate.
Site Options Danville, PA.
Study Options Full-time.
Program Entrance Requirements Transcript of college record, high school biology, high school chemistry, 2 years high school math, 3 years high school science, high school transcript, minimum high school GPA of 3.0, minimum high school rank 80%. Transfer students are accepted. *Application deadline:* 11/15 (fall). *Application fee:* $35.
Advanced Placement Credit by examination available.
Expenses (2015–16) *Tuition, state resident:* full-time $7060; part-time $294 per credit. *Tuition, nonresident:* full-time $17,650; part-time $735 per credit. *Room and board:* $8480; room only: $8360 per academic year. *Required fees:* full-time $2266.
Financial Aid *Gift aid (need-based):* Federal Pell, FSEOG, state, private, college/university gift aid from institutional funds. *Loans:* Federal Direct (Subsidized and Unsubsidized Stafford PLUS), Perkins, state, alternative loans. *Work-study:* Federal Work-Study, part-time campus jobs. *Financial aid application deadline (priority):* 3/15.
Contact Dr. Michelle Ficca, Department Chairperson, Department of Nursing, Bloomsburg University of Pennsylvania, 400 East 2nd Street, Room 3109, MCHS, Bloomsburg, PA 17815. *Telephone:* 570-389-4423. *Fax:* 570-389-5008. *E-mail:* mficca@bloomu.edu.

GRADUATE PROGRAMS

Expenses (2015–16) *Tuition, state resident:* part-time $470 per credit. *Tuition, nonresident:* part-time $705 per credit. *Required fees:* part-time $75 per term.
Financial Aid 66% of graduate students in nursing programs received some form of financial aid in 2014–15. Unspecified assistantships available.
Contact Dr. Noreen Chikotas, Coordinator of Graduate Program, Department of Nursing, Bloomsburg University of Pennsylvania, 400 East Second Street, Room 3211, MCHS, Bloomsburg, PA 17815. *Telephone:* 570-389-4609. *Fax:* 570-389-5008. *E-mail:* nchikota@bloomu.edu.

MASTER'S DEGREE PROGRAM

Degrees MSN; MSN/MBA
Available Programs Master's; RN to Master's.
Concentrations Available Nurse anesthesia; nursing administration. *Nurse practitioner programs in:* family health, gerontology.
Study Options Full-time and part-time.

Program Entrance Requirements Clinical experience, computer literacy, minimum overall college GPA of 3.0, transcript of college record, CPR certification, written essay, immunizations, interview, 3 letters of recommendation, nursing research course, physical assessment course, professional liability insurance/malpractice insurance, resume, statistics course. *Application deadline:* 7/1 (fall), 8/1 (spring). *Application fee:* $35.

Degree Requirements 39 total credit hours, comprehensive exam.

California University of Pennsylvania
Department of Nursing
California, Pennsylvania

http://www.calu.edu/academics/colleges/eberly/nursing/index.htm
Founded in 1852

DEGREE • BSN
Nursing Program Faculty 5 (60% with doctorates).
Baccalaureate Enrollment 145 **Women** 83% **Men** 17% **Part-time** 92%
Nursing Student Activities Sigma Theta Tau.
Nursing Student Resources Academic advising; academic or career counseling; assistance for students with disabilities; bookstore; campus computer network; career placement assistance; computer lab; computer-assisted instruction; daycare for children of students; e-mail services; employment services for current students; Internet; library services; nursing audiovisuals; placement services for program completers; remedial services; resume preparation assistance; tutoring.
Library Facilities 3,840 volumes in health, 2,010 volumes in nursing; 80 periodical subscriptions health-care related.

BACCALAUREATE PROGRAMS
Degree BSN
Available Programs RN Baccalaureate.
Site Options West Mifflin, PA.
Study Options Full-time and part-time.
Program Entrance Requirements Minimum overall college GPA of 2.0, transcript of college record, CPR certification, health exam, health insurance, immunizations, 2 letters of recommendation, professional liability insurance/malpractice insurance, prerequisite course work, RN licensure. Transfer students are accepted.
Advanced Placement Credit by examination available. Credit given for nursing courses completed elsewhere dependent upon specific evaluations.
Contact *Telephone:* 724-938-5739. *Fax:* 724-938-1612.

Carlow University
College of Health and Wellness
Pittsburgh, Pennsylvania

http://www.carlow.edu/Nursing.aspx
Founded in 1929

DEGREES • BSN • DNP • MSN • MSN/MBA
Nursing Program Faculty 25 (15% with doctorates).
Baccalaureate Enrollment 334 **Women** 95% **Men** 5% **Part-time** 27%
Graduate Enrollment 352 **Women** 91% **Men** 9% **Part-time** 20%
Distance Learning Courses Available.
Nursing Student Activities Nursing Honor Society, Sigma Theta Tau, Student Nurses' Association.
Nursing Student Resources Academic advising; academic or career counseling; assistance for students with disabilities; bookstore; campus computer network; career placement assistance; computer lab; computer-assisted instruction; e-mail services; employment services for current students; externships; Internet; learning resource lab; library services; nursing audiovisuals; other; placement services for program completers; remedial services; resume preparation assistance; skills, simulation, or other laboratory; tutoring; unpaid internships.
Library Facilities 2,293 volumes in health, 998 volumes in nursing; 2,810 periodical subscriptions health-care related.

BACCALAUREATE PROGRAMS
Degree BSN

Available Programs Accelerated RN Baccalaureate; Generic Baccalaureate; RN Baccalaureate.
Site Options Cranberry Township, PA; Greensburg, PA.
Study Options Full-time and part-time.
Online Degree Options Yes.
Program Entrance Requirements Transcript of college record, health insurance, high school biology, high school chemistry, 2 years high school math, 3 years high school science, high school transcript, minimum high school GPA of 3.0, minimum GPA in nursing prerequisites of 3.0, prerequisite course work. Transfer students are accepted. *Application deadline:* Applications may be processed on a rolling basis for some programs.
Advanced Placement Credit by examination available. Credit given for nursing courses completed elsewhere dependent upon specific evaluations.
Expenses (2015–16) *Tuition:* full-time $26,604; part-time $846 per credit. *International tuition:* $26,604 full-time. *Room and board:* $10,572; room only: $5406 per academic year. *Required fees:* full-time $228.
Contact Ms. Wivinia Chmura, Director, Admissions, College of Health and Wellness, Carlow University, 3333 Fifth Avenue, Admissions Office, Pittsburgh, PA 15213. *Telephone:* 412-578-6059.
E-mail: admissions@carlow.edu.

GRADUATE PROGRAMS
Expenses (2015–16) *Tuition:* full-time $10,768; part-time $923 per credit. *International tuition:* $10,768 full-time.
Contact Ms. Kimberly Lipniskis, Associate Director, Graduate Admissions, College of Health and Wellness, Carlow University, 3333 Fifth Avenue, Pittsburgh, PA 15213. *Telephone:* 412-578-6059. *Fax:* 412-578-6321. *E-mail:* admissions@carlow.edu.

MASTER'S DEGREE PROGRAM
Degrees MSN; MSN/MBA
Available Programs Master's.
Concentrations Available Nurse case management; nursing administration; nursing education. *Nurse practitioner programs in:* family health.
Site Options Cranberry Township, PA; Greensburg, PA.
Study Options Full-time and part-time.
Program Entrance Requirements Clinical experience, computer literacy, minimum overall college GPA of 3.0, transcript of college record, CPR certification, written essay, interview, professional liability insurance/malpractice insurance, resume, statistics course. *Application deadline:* Applications may be processed on a rolling basis for some programs.
Advanced Placement Credit by examination available. Credit given for nursing courses completed elsewhere dependent upon specific evaluations.
Degree Requirements 50 total credit hours.

POST-MASTER'S PROGRAM
Areas of Study *Nurse practitioner programs in:* family health.

DOCTORAL DEGREE PROGRAM
Degree DNP
Available Programs Doctorate.
Areas of Study Advanced practice nursing, clinical practice, clinical research, faculty preparation, individualized study, nurse executive, nursing administration, nursing education, nursing research.
Program Entrance Requirements Minimum overall college GPA of 3.0, interview by faculty committee, interview, 2 letters of recommendation, MSN or equivalent, writing sample. Application deadline: Applications may be processed on a rolling basis for some programs.
Degree Requirements 30 total credit hours.

Cedar Crest College
Department of Nursing
Allentown, Pennsylvania

http://www.cedarcrest.edu/
Founded in 1867

DEGREES • BS • MSN
Nursing Program Faculty 33 (21% with doctorates).
Baccalaureate Enrollment 271 **Women** 91% **Men** 9% **Part-time** 73%
Graduate Enrollment 12 **Women** 100% **Part-time** 100%
Distance Learning Courses Available.

Nursing Student Activities Nursing Honor Society, Sigma Theta Tau, Student Nurses' Association.

Nursing Student Resources Academic advising; academic or career counseling; assistance for students with disabilities; bookstore; campus computer network; career placement assistance; computer lab; computer-assisted instruction; e-mail services; interactive nursing skills videos; Internet; learning resource lab; library services; nursing audiovisuals; remedial services; skills, simulation, or other laboratory; tutoring.

BACCALAUREATE PROGRAMS

Degree BS
Available Programs Baccalaureate for Second Degree; Generic Baccalaureate; LPN to Baccalaureate; RN Baccalaureate.
Site Options Reading, PA.
Study Options Full-time and part-time.
Online Degree Options Yes.
Program Entrance Requirements Minimum overall college GPA of 2.5, CPR certification, written essay, health exam, health insurance, high school biology, high school chemistry, 3 years high school math, 2 years high school science, high school transcript, immunizations, minimum GPA in nursing prerequisites of 2.7, prerequisite course work. Transfer students are accepted. *Application deadline:* Applications may be processed on a rolling basis for some programs.
Advanced Placement Credit given for nursing courses completed elsewhere dependent upon specific evaluations.
Expenses (2015–16) *Tuition:* full-time $35,000; part-time $881 per credit. *Room and board:* $10,765 per academic year.
Financial Aid *Gift aid (need-based):* Federal Pell, FSEOG, state, private, college/university gift aid from institutional funds, Federal Nursing. *Loans:* Federal Nursing Student Loans, Federal Direct (Subsidized and Unsubsidized Stafford PLUS), Perkins. *Work-study:* Federal Work-Study, part-time campus jobs. *Financial aid application deadline (priority):* 5/1.
Contact Office of Admissions, Department of Nursing, Cedar Crest College, 100 College Drive, Allentown, PA 18104. *Telephone:* 610-740-3780. *Fax:* 610-606-4647. *E-mail:* cccadmis@cedarcrest.edu.

GRADUATE PROGRAMS

Expenses (2015–16) *Tuition:* part-time $772 per credit.
Contact Dr. Wendy Robb, Graduate Program Director, Department of Nursing, Cedar Crest College, 100 College Drive, Allentown, PA 18104. *Telephone:* 610-606-4666 Ext. 3480. *E-mail:* wjrobb@cedarcrest.edu.

MASTER'S DEGREE PROGRAM

Degree MSN
Available Programs Master's.
Site Options Reading, PA.
Study Options Part-time.
Online Degree Options Yes.
Program Entrance Requirements Clinical experience, minimum overall college GPA of 3.0, transcript of college record, CPR certification, immunizations, interview, 3 letters of recommendation, nursing research course, physical assessment course, resume, statistics course. *Application deadline:* Applications may be processed on a rolling basis for some programs. *Application fee:* $30.
Advanced Placement Credit given for nursing courses completed elsewhere dependent upon specific evaluations.
Degree Requirements 38 total credit hours, thesis or project.

Chatham University
Nursing Programs
Pittsburgh, Pennsylvania

http://www.chatham.edu/
Founded in 1869

DEGREES • BSN • DNP • MSN
Nursing Program Faculty 27 (80% with doctorates).
Baccalaureate Enrollment 100 **Women** 84% **Men** 16% **Part-time** 80%
Graduate Enrollment 150 **Women** 88% **Men** 12% **Part-time** 53%
Distance Learning Courses Available.
Nursing Student Activities Nursing Honor Society, Sigma Theta Tau.
Nursing Student Resources Academic advising; academic or career counseling; assistance for students with disabilities; bookstore; campus computer network; career placement assistance; computer lab; e-mail services; employment services for current students; housing assistance; Internet; library services; other; placement services for program completers; remedial services; resume preparation assistance; tutoring.

Library Facilities 1,747 volumes in health, 1,732 volumes in nursing; 967 periodical subscriptions health-care related.

BACCALAUREATE PROGRAMS

Degree BSN
Available Programs RN Baccalaureate; RPN to Baccalaureate.
Study Options Full-time and part-time.
Program Entrance Requirements Written essay, health insurance, high school transcript, immunizations, 2 letters of recommendation. Transfer students are accepted. *Application deadline:* 4/15 (fall), 11/1 (spring). Applications may be processed on a rolling basis for some programs.
Advanced Placement Credit by examination available. Credit given for nursing courses completed elsewhere dependent upon specific evaluations.
Financial Aid *Gift aid (need-based):* Federal Pell, FSEOG, state, private, college/university gift aid from institutional funds. *Loans:* Federal Direct (Subsidized and Unsubsidized Stafford PLUS), Perkins. *Work-study:* Federal Work-Study, part-time campus jobs. *Financial aid application deadline:* Continuous.
Contact Ms. Elana DiPietro, Admission Counselor, Nursing Programs, Chatham University, Berry Hall, Woodland Road, Pittsburgh, PA 15232. *Telephone:* 412-365-1298. *Fax:* 412-365-1609.
E-mail: edipietro@chatham.edu.

GRADUATE PROGRAMS

Expenses (2014–15) *Tuition:* part-time $782 per credit. *Required fees:* part-time $22 per credit.
Financial Aid 75% of graduate students in nursing programs received some form of financial aid in 2013–14.
Contact Mr. David A. Vey, Assistant Director of Online Admission, Nursing Programs, Chatham University, Admission Office, Woodland Road, Pittsburgh, PA 15232. *Telephone:* 412-365-1498. *Fax:* 412-365-1609. *E-mail:* dvey@chatham.edu.

MASTER'S DEGREE PROGRAM

Degree MSN
Available Programs Master's.
Concentrations Available Nursing administration; nursing education; nursing informatics.
Study Options Full-time and part-time.
Online Degree Options Yes.
Program Entrance Requirements Minimum overall college GPA of 3.0, transcript of college record, written essay, resume. *Application deadline:* 8/15 (fall). Applications may be processed on a rolling basis for some programs.
Advanced Placement Credit given for nursing courses completed elsewhere dependent upon specific evaluations.
Degree Requirements 36 total credit hours, thesis or project.

DOCTORAL DEGREE PROGRAM

Degree DNP
Available Programs Doctorate.
Online Degree Options Yes (online only).
Program Entrance Requirements Clinical experience, minimum overall college GPA of 3.0, 2 letters of recommendation, MSN or equivalent, vita, writing sample. Application deadline: 5/1 (fall), 11/1 (spring). Applications may be processed on a rolling basis for some programs.
Degree Requirements 27 total credit hours, residency.

Clarion University of Pennsylvania
School of Nursing
Oil City, Pennsylvania

http://www.clarion.edu/
Founded in 1867

DEGREES • BSN • DNP • MSN
Nursing Program Faculty 25 (25% with doctorates).
Baccalaureate Enrollment 217 **Women** 85.3% **Men** 14.7% **Part-time** 93.4%
Graduate Enrollment 94 **Women** 97.9% **Men** 2.1% **Part-time** 100%
Distance Learning Courses Available.
Nursing Student Activities Nursing Honor Society, Sigma Theta Tau, Student Nurses' Association, nursing club.

Nursing Student Resources Academic advising; academic or career counseling; assistance for students with disabilities; bookstore; campus computer network; career placement assistance; computer lab; computer-assisted instruction; daycare for children of students; e-mail services; employment services for current students; externships; housing assistance; interactive nursing skills videos; Internet; learning resource lab; library services; nursing audiovisuals; placement services for program completers; remedial services; resume preparation assistance; skills, simulation, or other laboratory; tutoring.
Library Facilities 12,000 volumes in health, 7,000 volumes in nursing; 300 periodical subscriptions health-care related.

BACCALAUREATE PROGRAMS

Degree BSN
Available Programs ADN to Baccalaureate; RN Baccalaureate.
Site Options Oil City, PA.
Study Options Full-time and part-time.
Online Degree Options Yes (online only).
Program Entrance Requirements Minimum overall college GPA of 2.5, transcript of college record, CPR certification, health exam, health insurance, high school transcript, immunizations, minimum GPA in nursing prerequisites of 2.0, professional liability insurance/malpractice insurance, RN licensure. Transfer students are accepted. *Application deadline:* 8/1 (fall), 12/1 (winter). Applications may be processed on a rolling basis for some programs. *Application fee:* $35.
Expenses (2015–16) *Tuition, state resident:* full-time $7060; part-time $294 per credit hour. *Tuition, nonresident:* full-time $7624; part-time $318 per credit hour. *International tuition:* $7624 full-time. *Required fees:* full-time $1896; part-time $948 per term.
Financial Aid 50% of baccalaureate students in nursing programs received some form of financial aid in 2014–15.
Contact Ms. Deb Kelly, PhD, Chairperson, Nursing Department, School of Nursing, Clarion University of Pennsylvania, 1801 West First Street, Oil City, PA 16301. *Telephone:* 814-393-1261. *Fax:* 814-676-0251. *E-mail:* dkelly@clarion.edu.

GRADUATE PROGRAMS

Expenses (2015–16) *Tuition, state resident:* full-time $9306; part-time $517 per credit hour. *Tuition, nonresident:* full-time $10,044; part-time $558 per credit hour. *International tuition:* $10,044 full-time. *Required fees:* full-time $2844.
Financial Aid 75% of graduate students in nursing programs received some form of financial aid in 2014–15. 2 research assistantships with full tuition reimbursements available (averaging $4,660 per year) were awarded. *Financial aid application deadline:* 3/1.
Contact Dr. Deborah Ciesielka, Coordinator, MSN Family Nurse Practitioner Program, School of Nursing, Clarion University of Pennsylvania, 4900 Friendship Avenue, Pittsburgh, PA 15224. *Telephone:* 412-578-7277. *E-mail:* dciesielka@clarion.edu.

MASTER'S DEGREE PROGRAM

Degree MSN
Available Programs Master's.
Concentrations Available *Nurse practitioner programs in:* family health.
Site Options Edinboro, PA; Pittsburgh, PA.
Study Options Full-time and part-time.
Program Entrance Requirements Clinical experience, computer literacy, minimum overall college GPA of 3.0, transcript of college record, written essay, interview, 2 letters of recommendation, resume, statistics course. *Application deadline:* 4/1 (fall), 11/1 (winter), 11/1 (spring), 4/1 (summer). *Application fee:* $40.
Advanced Placement Credit given for nursing courses completed elsewhere dependent upon specific evaluations.
Degree Requirements 45 total credit hours, thesis or project, comprehensive exam.

POST-MASTER'S PROGRAM

Areas of Study *Nurse practitioner programs in:* family health.

DOCTORAL DEGREE PROGRAM

Degree DNP
Available Programs Doctorate.
Areas of Study Advanced practice nursing.
Site Options Oil City, PA.
Online Degree Options Yes (online only).
Program Entrance Requirements Clinical experience, minimum overall college GPA of 3.25, interview by faculty committee, 2 letters of recommendation, MSN or equivalent, vita, writing sample. Application

deadline: Applications may be processed on a rolling basis for some programs. Application fee: $40.
Degree Requirements 34 total credit hours, dissertation.

DeSales University
Department of Nursing and Health
Center Valley, Pennsylvania

http://www.desales.edu/
Founded in 1964
DEGREES • BSN • DNP • MSN • MSN/MBA
Nursing Program Faculty 74 (23% with doctorates).
Baccalaureate Enrollment 313 **Women** 85% **Men** 15% **Part-time** 37%
Graduate Enrollment 103 **Women** 96% **Men** 4% **Part-time** 51%
Nursing Student Activities Nursing Honor Society, Sigma Theta Tau, Student Nurses' Association.
Nursing Student Resources Academic advising; academic or career counseling; assistance for students with disabilities; bookstore; campus computer network; career placement assistance; computer lab; computer-assisted instruction; e-mail services; employment services for current students; externships; housing assistance; interactive nursing skills videos; Internet; learning resource lab; library services; nursing audiovisuals; paid internships; placement services for program completers; remedial services; resume preparation assistance; skills, simulation, or other laboratory; tutoring; unpaid internships.
Library Facilities 3,171 volumes in health, 1,107 volumes in nursing; 2,151 periodical subscriptions health-care related.

BACCALAUREATE PROGRAMS

Degree BSN
Available Programs ADN to Baccalaureate; Accelerated Baccalaureate; Accelerated RN Baccalaureate; Baccalaureate for Second Degree; Generic Baccalaureate; RN Baccalaureate.
Study Options Full-time and part-time.
Program Entrance Requirements Minimum overall college GPA of 2.5, transcript of college record, written essay, high school biology, high school chemistry, high school foreign language, 2 years high school math, 3 years high school science, high school transcript, 2 letters of recommendation, minimum high school GPA of 2.5, minimum high school rank 33%, minimum GPA in nursing prerequisites of 2.0. Transfer students are accepted. *Application deadline:* Applications may be processed on a rolling basis for some programs. *Application fee:* $30.
Advanced Placement Credit by examination available. Credit given for nursing courses completed elsewhere dependent upon specific evaluations.
Expenses (2014–15) *Tuition:* full-time $31,000; part-time $1290 per credit. *International tuition:* $31,000 full-time. *Room and board:* $11,620 per academic year.
Financial Aid 86% of baccalaureate students in nursing programs received some form of financial aid in 2013–14. *Gift aid (need-based):* Federal Pell, FSEOG, state, private, college/university gift aid from institutional funds. *Loans:* Federal Nursing Student Loans, Federal Direct (Subsidized and Unsubsidized Stafford PLUS), Perkins. *Work-study:* Federal Work-Study, part-time campus jobs. *Financial aid application deadline:* 5/1(priority: 2/15).
Contact Dr. Mary Elizabeth Doyle-Tadduni, Chair, Nursing and Health Department, Department of Nursing and Health, DeSales University, 2755 Station Avenue, Center Valley, PA 18034-9568. *Telephone:* 610-282-1100 Ext. 1285. *Fax:* 610-282-2091.
E-mail: maryelizabeth.doyletadduni@desales.edu.

GRADUATE PROGRAMS

Expenses (2014–15) *Tuition:* part-time $1090 per credit. *Room and board:* $11,620 per academic year.
Financial Aid 18% of graduate students in nursing programs received some form of financial aid in 2013–14.
Contact Dr. Carol G. Mest, Director of Graduate Program in Nursing, Department of Nursing and Health, DeSales University, 2755 Station Avenue, Center Valley, PA 18034-9568. *Telephone:* 610-282-1100 Ext. 1664. *Fax:* 610-282-2091. *E-mail:* carol.mest@desales.edu.

MASTER'S DEGREE PROGRAM

Degrees MSN; MSN/MBA
Available Programs Accelerated AD/RN to Master's; Accelerated RN to Master's; Master's; RN to Master's.

Concentrations Available Clinical nurse leader; health-care administration; nursing administration; nursing education. *Clinical nurse specialist programs in:* adult health, gerontology. *Nurse practitioner programs in:* family health, gerontology.
Study Options Full-time and part-time.
Program Entrance Requirements Clinical experience, minimum overall college GPA of 3.3, transcript of college record, CPR certification, written essay, interview, 3 letters of recommendation, physical assessment course, professional liability insurance/malpractice insurance, prerequisite course work, statistics course. *Application deadline:* Applications may be processed on a rolling basis for some programs. *Application fee:* $35.
Advanced Placement Credit given for nursing courses completed elsewhere dependent upon specific evaluations.
Degree Requirements 47 total credit hours.

POST-MASTER'S PROGRAM

Areas of Study Nursing education. *Clinical nurse specialist programs in:* adult health, gerontology. *Nurse practitioner programs in:* family health, gerontology.

DOCTORAL DEGREE PROGRAM

Degree DNP
Available Programs Doctorate.
Areas of Study Clinical nurse leader, clinical practice, nursing administration.
Program Entrance Requirements Clinical experience, minimum overall college GPA of 3.3, 3 letters of recommendation, MSN or equivalent, vita, writing sample. Application deadline: 4/15 (fall). Application fee: $50.
Degree Requirements 45 total credit hours.

CONTINUING EDUCATION PROGRAM

Contact Dr. Mary Elizabeth Doyle-Tadduni, Chair, Nursing and Health Department, Department of Nursing and Health, DeSales University, 2755 Station Avenue, Center Valley, PA 18034-9568. *Telephone:* 610-282-1100 Ext. 1285. *Fax:* 610-282-2091.
E-mail: maryelizabeth.doyletadduni@desales.edu.

Drexel University
College of Nursing and Health Professions
Philadelphia, Pennsylvania

http://www.drexel.edu/cnhp
Founded in 1891
DEGREES • BSN • DR NP • MSN
Nursing Program Faculty 73 (52% with doctorates).
Baccalaureate Enrollment 1,696 **Women** 87% **Men** 13% **Part-time** 46%
Graduate Enrollment 1,010 **Women** 89% **Men** 11% **Part-time** 96%
Distance Learning Courses Available.
Nursing Student Activities Nursing Honor Society, Sigma Theta Tau, Student Nurses' Association, nursing club.
Nursing Student Resources Academic advising; academic or career counseling; assistance for students with disabilities; bookstore; campus computer network; career placement assistance; computer lab; computer-assisted instruction; e-mail services; housing assistance; interactive nursing skills videos; Internet; learning resource lab; library services; nursing audiovisuals; paid internships; placement services for program completers; remedial services; resume preparation assistance; skills, simulation, or other laboratory; tutoring.
Library Facilities 51,000 volumes in health, 5,015 volumes in nursing; 63,000 periodical subscriptions health-care related.

BACCALAUREATE PROGRAMS

Degree BSN
Available Programs Accelerated Baccalaureate; Accelerated Baccalaureate for Second Degree; Generic Baccalaureate; RN Baccalaureate.
Site Options Philadelphia, PA.
Study Options Full-time.
Program Entrance Requirements CPR certification, written essay, health insurance, high school biology, high school chemistry, 3 years high school math, 2 years high school science, high school transcript, immunizations, 2 letters of recommendation. Transfer students are accepted. *Application deadline:* 1/15 (fall). *Application fee:* $75.
Contact *Telephone:* 215-895-6732. *Fax:* 215-895-5939.

GRADUATE PROGRAMS

Contact *Telephone:* 215-762-3999. *Fax:* 215-762-1259.

MASTER'S DEGREE PROGRAM

Degree MSN
Available Programs Master's; RN to Master's.
Concentrations Available Clinical nurse leader; nurse anesthesia; nursing administration; nursing education. *Clinical nurse specialist programs in:* women's health. *Nurse practitioner programs in:* acute care, adult health, family health, pediatric, psychiatric/mental health, women's health.
Site Options Philadelphia, PA.
Study Options Full-time and part-time.
Online Degree Options Yes.
Program Entrance Requirements Clinical experience, computer literacy, minimum overall college GPA of 3.0, transcript of college record, CPR certification, written essay, immunizations, 2 letters of recommendation, resume. *Application deadline:* 1/1 (fall). Applications may be processed on a rolling basis for some programs. *Application fee:* $75.
Advanced Placement Credit given for nursing courses completed elsewhere dependent upon specific evaluations.
Degree Requirements 55 total credit hours, thesis or project, comprehensive exam.

POST-MASTER'S PROGRAM

Areas of Study Nursing administration; nursing education. *Nurse practitioner programs in:* family health, pediatric.

DOCTORAL DEGREE PROGRAM

Degree Dr NP
Available Programs Doctorate.
Areas of Study Clinical practice, faculty preparation, nursing administration, nursing education, nursing research, nursing science.
Site Options Philadelphia, PA.
Online Degree Options Yes (online only).
Program Entrance Requirements Clinical experience, minimum overall college GPA of 3.25, interview by faculty committee, interview, 2 letters of recommendation, vita, writing sample, GRE General Test. Application deadline: 6/1 (fall).
Degree Requirements 48 total credit hours, dissertation, oral exam, written exam, residency.

CONTINUING EDUCATION PROGRAM

Contact *Telephone:* 215-762-8521. *Fax:* 215-762-7778.

Duquesne University
School of Nursing
Pittsburgh, Pennsylvania

http://www.duq.edu/nursing
Founded in 1878
DEGREES • BSN • MSN • PHD
Nursing Program Faculty 128 (36% with doctorates).
Baccalaureate Enrollment 739 **Women** 88% **Men** 12% **Part-time** 7%
Graduate Enrollment 262 **Women** 90% **Men** 10% **Part-time** 44%
Distance Learning Courses Available.
Nursing Student Activities Nursing Honor Society, Sigma Theta Tau, Student Nurses' Association, nursing club.
Nursing Student Resources Academic advising; academic or career counseling; assistance for students with disabilities; bookstore; campus computer network; career placement assistance; computer lab; computer-assisted instruction; daycare for children of students; e-mail services; employment services for current students; externships; housing assistance; interactive nursing skills videos; Internet; learning resource lab; library services; nursing audiovisuals; paid internships; placement services for program completers; remedial services; resume preparation assistance; skills, simulation, or other laboratory; tutoring; unpaid internships.
Library Facilities 31,885 volumes in health, 1,371 volumes in nursing; 9,679 periodical subscriptions health-care related.

BACCALAUREATE PROGRAMS

Degree BSN
Available Programs ADN to Baccalaureate; Accelerated Baccalaureate for Second Degree; Generic Baccalaureate.
Study Options Full-time and part-time.

Program Entrance Requirements Minimum overall college GPA of 3.0, transcript of college record, written essay, high school biology, high school chemistry, high school foreign language, 2 years high school math, 3 years high school science, high school transcript, 1 letter of recommendation, minimum high school GPA of 3.0, minimum high school rank 40%. Transfer students are accepted. *Application deadline:* 5/1 (fall), 10/1 (spring). Applications may be processed on a rolling basis for some programs. *Application fee:* $50.

Advanced Placement Credit by examination available.

Expenses (2015–16) *Tuition:* full-time $33,778; part-time $1119 per credit. *International tuition:* $33,778 full-time.

Financial Aid 99% of baccalaureate students in nursing programs received some form of financial aid in 2014–15.

Contact Ms. Gina Plocki, Nursing Recruiter, School of Nursing, Duquesne University, 600 Forbes Avenue, Pittsburgh, PA 15282-1760. *Telephone:* 412-396-6534. *Fax:* 412-396-6346. *E-mail:* plockir@duq.edu.

GRADUATE PROGRAMS

Expenses (2015–16) *Tuition:* part-time $1218 per credit.

Financial Aid 76% of graduate students in nursing programs received some form of financial aid in 2014–15. 5 research assistantships with partial tuition reimbursements available (averaging $1,800 per year), 7 teaching assistantships with partial tuition reimbursements available (averaging $1,957 per year) were awarded; institutionally sponsored loans, scholarships, traineeships, tuition waivers (partial), and unspecified assistantships also available. Aid available to part-time students. *Financial aid application deadline:* 7/1.

Contact Ms. Susan Hardner, Nursing Recruiter, School of Nursing, Duquesne University, 600 Forbes Avenue, Pittsburgh, PA 15282-1760. *Telephone:* 412-396-4945. *Fax:* 412-396-6346. *E-mail:* hardnersue@duq.edu.

MASTER'S DEGREE PROGRAM

Degree MSN
Available Programs Master's.

Concentrations Available Nursing education. *Clinical nurse specialist programs in:* forensic nursing. *Nurse practitioner programs in:* family health.

Study Options Full-time and part-time.

Online Degree Options Yes (online only).

Program Entrance Requirements Clinical experience, computer literacy, minimum overall college GPA of 3.0, transcript of college record, written essay, 2 letters of recommendation, nursing research course, physical assessment course, prerequisite course work, resume, statistics course. *Application deadline:* 3/1 (summer). Applications may be processed on a rolling basis for some programs.

Advanced Placement Credit given for nursing courses completed elsewhere dependent upon specific evaluations.

Degree Requirements 45 total credit hours, comprehensive exam.

POST-MASTER'S PROGRAM

Areas of Study Nursing education. *Clinical nurse specialist programs in:* forensic nursing. *Nurse practitioner programs in:* family health.

DOCTORAL DEGREE PROGRAM

Degree PhD
Available Programs Doctorate.
Areas of Study Ethics, forensic nursing, nursing research.
Online Degree Options Yes (online only).

Program Entrance Requirements Minimum overall college GPA of 3.5, interview by faculty committee, 3 letters of recommendation, MSN or equivalent, scholarly papers, statistics course, vita, writing sample. Application deadline: 2/1 (summer).

Degree Requirements 56 total credit hours, dissertation, oral exam, written exam, residency.

CONTINUING EDUCATION PROGRAM

Contact Mr. Sean Flaherty, Outcomes Coordinator, School of Nursing, Duquesne University, 600 Forbes Avenue, Pittsburgh, PA 15282-1760. *Telephone:* 412-396-2067. *Fax:* 412-396-6346. *E-mail:* flahert2@duq.edu.

See display below and full description on page 488.

Become the nurse you were meant to be.

Earn a degree that prepares you for a lifetime of caring. You'll change lives—both yours, and your patients'.

Undergraduate Programs
- BSN
- RN-BSN (100% online)
- Second Degree BSN
- Biomedical Engineering (BME)-BSN

Online Graduate Programs
- MSN
- Post-Master's Certificates
- PhD in Nursing
- DNP

DUQUESNE UNIVERSITY
School of Nursing

Pittsburgh, Pa.

duq.edu/nursing
nursing@duq.edu

Eastern University
Program in Nursing
St. Davids, Pennsylvania

http://www.eastern.edu/academics/programs/nursing-department-undergraduate
Founded in 1952

DEGREE • BSN
Nursing Program Faculty 8 (50% with doctorates).
Baccalaureate Enrollment 95 **Women** 92% **Men** 8%
Distance Learning Courses Available.
Nursing Student Activities Sigma Theta Tau, Student Nurses' Association.
Nursing Student Resources Academic advising; academic or career counseling; assistance for students with disabilities; bookstore; campus computer network; career placement assistance; computer lab; computer-assisted instruction; e-mail services; employment services for current students; externships; Internet; learning resource lab; library services; nursing audiovisuals; placement services for program completers; remedial services; resume preparation assistance; skills, simulation, or other laboratory; tutoring; unpaid internships.
Library Facilities 5,858 volumes in health, 3,000 volumes in nursing; 821 periodical subscriptions health-care related.

BACCALAUREATE PROGRAMS
Degree BSN
Available Programs Accelerated RN Baccalaureate; Baccalaureate for Second Degree; Generic Baccalaureate.
Site Options Harrisburg, PA.
Study Options Full-time.
Program Entrance Requirements Minimum overall college GPA of 3.0, transcript of college record, CPR certification, written essay, health exam, health insurance, high school chemistry, high school transcript, immunizations, interview, 2 letters of recommendation, minimum GPA in nursing prerequisites of 3.0, professional liability insurance/malpractice insurance, prerequisite course work, RN licensure. *Application deadline:* Applications may be processed on a rolling basis for some programs. *Application fee:* $40.
Expenses (2015–16) *Tuition:* full-time $30,250; part-time $595 per credit hour. *Room and board:* $10,500; room only: $5500 per academic year. *Required fees:* full-time $600; part-time $33 per credit.
Contact Ms. Christina Theodos, RN-BSN/BSN TWO Program Advisor, Program in Nursing, Eastern University, 1300 Eagle Road, St. Davids, PA 19087. *Telephone:* 800-732-7669. *Fax:* 610-341-1474. *E-mail:* ctheodus@eastern.edu.

East Stroudsburg University of Pennsylvania
Department of Nursing
East Stroudsburg, Pennsylvania

http://www4.esu.edu/
Founded in 1893

DEGREE • BS
Nursing Program Faculty 14 (77% with doctorates).
Baccalaureate Enrollment 166 **Women** 75% **Men** 25%
Nursing Student Activities Nursing Honor Society, Sigma Theta Tau, Student Nurses' Association, nursing club.
Nursing Student Resources Academic advising; academic or career counseling; assistance for students with disabilities; bookstore; campus computer network; career placement assistance; computer lab; computer-assisted instruction; daycare for children of students; e-mail services; employment services for current students; externships; housing assistance; interactive nursing skills videos; Internet; learning resource lab; library services; nursing audiovisuals; other; placement services for program completers; remedial services; resume preparation assistance; skills, simulation, or other laboratory; tutoring; unpaid internships.
Library Facilities 16,810 volumes in health, 2,035 volumes in nursing; 495 periodical subscriptions health-care related.

BACCALAUREATE PROGRAMS
Degree BS
Available Programs Generic Baccalaureate; RN Baccalaureate.

Study Options Full-time.
Program Entrance Requirements Minimum overall college GPA of 2.75, transcript of college record, health exam, 2 years high school math, 2 years high school science, high school transcript, immunizations, minimum high school GPA of 3.0, minimum high school rank 75%, minimum GPA in nursing prerequisites of 2.75. Transfer students are accepted. *Application deadline:* 5/1 (fall), 1/1 (winter), 1/1 (spring). Applications may be processed on a rolling basis for some programs. *Application fee:* $100.
Advanced Placement Credit by examination available. Credit given for nursing courses completed elsewhere dependent upon specific evaluations.
Contact *Telephone:* 570-422-3569. *Fax:* 570-422-3848.

Edinboro University of Pennsylvania
Department of Nursing
Edinboro, Pennsylvania

http://www.edinboro.edu/
Founded in 1857

DEGREE • BSN
Nursing Program Faculty 21 (62% with doctorates).
Baccalaureate Enrollment 274 **Women** 91% **Men** 9% **Part-time** .02%
Distance Learning Courses Available.
Nursing Student Activities Sigma Theta Tau, Student Nurses' Association, nursing club.
Nursing Student Resources Academic advising; academic or career counseling; assistance for students with disabilities; bookstore; campus computer network; career placement assistance; computer lab; computer-assisted instruction; daycare for children of students; e-mail services; employment services for current students; housing assistance; interactive nursing skills videos; Internet; learning resource lab; library services; nursing audiovisuals; remedial services; resume preparation assistance; skills, simulation, or other laboratory; tutoring.
Library Facilities 500 volumes in health, 100 volumes in nursing; 105 periodical subscriptions health-care related.

BACCALAUREATE PROGRAMS
Degree BSN
Available Programs Accelerated Baccalaureate; Accelerated Baccalaureate for Second Degree; Generic Baccalaureate.
Site Options Erie, PA.
Study Options Full-time and part-time.
Program Entrance Requirements Minimum overall college GPA of 3.0, CPR certification, health exam, high school biology, high school chemistry, 2 years high school math, 2 years high school science, high school transcript, immunizations, minimum high school rank 40%, minimum GPA in nursing prerequisites of 3.00, professional liability insurance/malpractice insurance. *Application deadline:* 8/15 (fall), 1/15 (spring). Applications may be processed on a rolling basis for some programs. *Application fee:* $30.
Expenses (2015–16) *Tuition, state resident:* full-time $11,361; part-time $294 per credit. *Tuition, nonresident:* full-time $12,029; part-time $309 per credit. *Room and board:* $9500; room only: $8000 per academic year. *Required fees:* full-time $2476.
Contact Dr. Thomas R. White, Chairperson, Department of Nursing, Department of Nursing, Edinboro University of Pennsylvania, Human Services Building, #125, 215 Scotland Road, Edinboro, PA 16444. *Telephone:* 814-732-2900. *Fax:* 814-732-2536. *E-mail:* twhite@edinboro.edu.

Gannon University
Villa Maria School of Nursing
Erie, Pennsylvania

http://www.gannon.edu/Academic-Offerings/Health-Professions-and-Sciences/Villa-Maria-School-of-Nursing/
Founded in 1925

DEGREES • BSN • DNP • MSN
Nursing Program Faculty 16 (20% with doctorates).
Baccalaureate Enrollment 350 **Women** 88% **Men** 12% **Part-time** 5%
Graduate Enrollment 97 **Women** 68% **Men** 32% **Part-time** 38%

Distance Learning Courses Available.
Nursing Student Activities Nursing Honor Society, Sigma Theta Tau.
Nursing Student Resources Academic advising; academic or career counseling; assistance for students with disabilities; bookstore; campus computer network; career placement assistance; computer lab; computer-assisted instruction; e-mail services; employment services for current students; externships; housing assistance; interactive nursing skills videos; Internet; learning resource lab; library services; nursing audiovisuals; other; paid internships; placement services for program completers; remedial services; resume preparation assistance; skills, simulation, or other laboratory; tutoring; unpaid internships.
Library Facilities 140,000 volumes in health, 20,000 volumes in nursing; 3,000 periodical subscriptions health-care related.

BACCALAUREATE PROGRAMS

Degree BSN
Available Programs ADN to Baccalaureate; Baccalaureate for Second Degree; Generic Baccalaureate; International Nurse to Baccalaureate; RN Baccalaureate.
Study Options Full-time and part-time.
Online Degree Options Yes.
Program Entrance Requirements Minimum overall college GPA of 2.7, transcript of college record, CPR certification, written essay, health exam, health insurance, high school biology, high school chemistry, 4 years high school math, 2 years high school science, high school transcript, immunizations, 1 letter of recommendation, minimum high school GPA of 2.5, minimum high school rank 40%, minimum GPA in nursing prerequisites of 2.7. Transfer students are accepted. *Application deadline:* Applications may be processed on a rolling basis for some programs. *Application fee:* $25.
Contact *Telephone:* 814-871-5470. *Fax:* 814-871-5662.

GRADUATE PROGRAMS

Contact *Telephone:* 814-871-5547. *Fax:* 814-871-5662.

MASTER'S DEGREE PROGRAM
Degree MSN
Available Programs Accelerated AD/RN to Master's; Accelerated RN to Master's; Master's; RN to Master's.
Concentrations Available Nurse anesthesia; nursing administration. *Nurse practitioner programs in:* family health.
Study Options Full-time and part-time.
Program Entrance Requirements Clinical experience, computer literacy, minimum overall college GPA of 3.0, transcript of college record, CPR certification, written essay, immunizations, interview, 3 letters of recommendation, nursing research course, professional liability insurance/malpractice insurance, prerequisite course work, statistics course, GRE General Test. *Application deadline:* Applications may be processed on a rolling basis for some programs. *Application fee:* $50.
Advanced Placement Credit given for nursing courses completed elsewhere dependent upon specific evaluations.
Degree Requirements 46 total credit hours, thesis or project.

POST-MASTER'S PROGRAM
Areas of Study Nurse anesthesia; nursing administration. *Nurse practitioner programs in:* family health.

DOCTORAL DEGREE PROGRAM
Degree DNP
Available Programs Doctorate.
Areas of Study Clinical practice, family health.
Program Entrance Requirements Clinical experience, minimum overall college GPA of 3.0, interview by faculty committee, 3 letters of recommendation, MSN or equivalent, statistics course, vita, writing sample. Application deadline: Applications may be processed on a rolling basis for some programs. Application fee: $50.
Degree Requirements 42 total credit hours, dissertation, residency.

Gwynedd Mercy University
Frances M. Maguire School of Nursing and Health Professions
Gwynedd Valley, Pennsylvania

Founded in 1948
DEGREES • BSN • MSN
Nursing Program Faculty 21 (43% with doctorates).

Baccalaureate Enrollment 85 **Women** 95% **Men** 5% **Part-time** 28%
Graduate Enrollment 40 **Women** 85% **Men** 15% **Part-time** 80%
Nursing Student Activities Sigma Theta Tau, Student Nurses' Association.
Nursing Student Resources Academic advising; bookstore; campus computer network; computer lab; computer-assisted instruction; daycare for children of students; e-mail services; interactive nursing skills videos; learning resource lab; library services; nursing audiovisuals; resume preparation assistance; skills, simulation, or other laboratory; tutoring.

BACCALAUREATE PROGRAMS

Degree BSN
Available Programs ADN to Baccalaureate; Accelerated RN Baccalaureate; RN Baccalaureate.
Site Options Fort Washington, PA.
Study Options Full-time and part-time.
Program Entrance Requirements Minimum overall college GPA of 2.8, transcript of college record, CPR certification, health exam, health insurance, high school biology, high school chemistry, 2 years high school math, high school transcript, immunizations, letters of recommendation, minimum high school rank 33%, minimum GPA in nursing prerequisites, professional liability insurance/malpractice insurance, RN licensure. Transfer students are accepted.
Advanced Placement Credit by examination available. Credit given for nursing courses completed elsewhere dependent upon specific evaluations.
Contact *Telephone:* 215-646-7300 Ext. 425. *Fax:* 215-641-5556 Ext. 528.

GRADUATE PROGRAMS

Contact *Telephone:* 215-646-7300 Ext. 407. *Fax:* 215-542-5789.

MASTER'S DEGREE PROGRAM
Degree MSN
Available Programs Master's; RN to Master's.
Concentrations Available *Clinical nurse specialist programs in:* gerontology, oncology, pediatric. *Nurse practitioner programs in:* adult health, pediatric.
Study Options Full-time and part-time.
Program Entrance Requirements Clinical experience, minimum overall college GPA of 3.0, transcript of college record, written essay, immunizations, interview, 2 letters of recommendation, physical assessment course, professional liability insurance/malpractice insurance, statistics course, GRE General Test or MAT.
Advanced Placement Credit by examination available. Credit given for nursing courses completed elsewhere dependent upon specific evaluations.
Degree Requirements 43 total credit hours.

POST-MASTER'S PROGRAM
Areas of Study *Nurse practitioner programs in:* adult health, pediatric.

Holy Family University
School of Nursing and Allied Health Professions
Philadelphia, Pennsylvania

http://www.holyfamily.edu/choosing-holy-family-u/academics/schools-of-study/philadelphia-school-of-nursing
Founded in 1954
DEGREES • BSN • MSN
Nursing Program Faculty 32 (44% with doctorates).
Baccalaureate Enrollment 658 **Women** 84% **Men** 16% **Part-time** 23%
Graduate Enrollment 68 **Women** 91% **Men** 9% **Part-time** 90%
Distance Learning Courses Available.
Nursing Student Activities Nursing Honor Society, Sigma Theta Tau, Student Nurses' Association, nursing club.
Nursing Student Resources Academic advising; academic or career counseling; assistance for students with disabilities; bookstore; campus computer network; career placement assistance; computer lab; computer-assisted instruction; e-mail services; employment services for current students; externships; housing assistance; interactive nursing skills videos; Internet; learning resource lab; library services; nursing audiovisuals; other; remedial services; resume preparation assistance; skills, simulation, or other laboratory; tutoring; unpaid internships.

Library Facilities 8,159 volumes in health, 2,177 volumes in nursing; 279 periodical subscriptions health-care related.

BACCALAUREATE PROGRAMS

Degree BSN

Available Programs Accelerated Baccalaureate; Accelerated Baccalaureate for Second Degree; Baccalaureate for Second Degree; Generic Baccalaureate; International Nurse to Baccalaureate.

Site Options Newtown, PA; Philadelphia, PA; Bensalem, PA.

Study Options Full-time and part-time.

Program Entrance Requirements Minimum overall college GPA of 3.0, transcript of college record, CPR certification, health exam, health insurance, high school biology, high school chemistry, high school foreign language, 3 years high school math, 3 years high school science, high school transcript, immunizations, 2 letters of recommendation, minimum high school GPA of 3.0, minimum high school rank 60%, minimum GPA in nursing prerequisites of 2.75, prerequisite course work. Transfer students are accepted. *Application deadline:* 8/1 (fall), 1/5 (spring), 4/30 (summer). Applications may be processed on a rolling basis for some programs. *Application fee:* $25.

Expenses (2015–16) *Tuition:* full-time $28,198; part-time $603 per credit hour. *International tuition:* $28,198 full-time. *Room and board:* $13,576; room only: $7140 per academic year. *Required fees:* full-time $970; part-time $108 per term.

Financial Aid 77% of baccalaureate students in nursing programs received some form of financial aid in 2014–15. *Gift aid (need-based):* Federal Pell, FSEOG, state, private, college/university gift aid from institutional funds. *Loans:* Federal Nursing Student Loans, Federal Direct (Subsidized and Unsubsidized Stafford PLUS), Perkins. *Work-study:* Federal Work-Study. *Financial aid application deadline (priority):* 3/1.

Contact Lauren A. Campbell, Executive Director of Admissions, School of Nursing and Allied Health Professions, Holy Family University, 9801 Frankford Avenue, Philadelphia, PA 19114-2094. *Telephone:* 215-637-3050. *Fax:* 215-281-1022. *E-mail:* admissions@holyfamily.edu.

GRADUATE PROGRAMS

Expenses (2015–16) *Tuition:* part-time $722 per credit hour. *Required fees:* part-time $134 per term.

Financial Aid 33% of graduate students in nursing programs received some form of financial aid in 2014–15.

Contact Jaimie Anderson, Assistant Director of Admissions, School of Nursing and Allied Health Professions, Holy Family University, 9801 Frankford Avenue, Philadelphia, PA 19114-2094. *Telephone:* 267-341-3327. *E-mail:* gradstudy@holyfamily.edu.

MASTER'S DEGREE PROGRAM

Degree MSN

Available Programs Accelerated Master's; Master's; Master's for Nurses with Non-Nursing Degrees.

Concentrations Available Nursing administration; nursing education. *Clinical nurse specialist programs in:* public/community health.

Site Options Philadelphia, PA.

Study Options Full-time and part-time.

Program Entrance Requirements Computer literacy, minimum overall college GPA of 3.0, transcript of college record, CPR certification, written essay, immunizations, interview, 2 letters of recommendation, nursing research course, professional liability insurance/malpractice insurance, prerequisite course work, resume, statistics course. *Application deadline:* 8/1 (fall), 12/20 (spring), 5/10 (summer). Applications may be processed on a rolling basis for some programs. *Application fee:* $25.

Advanced Placement Credit given for nursing courses completed elsewhere dependent upon specific evaluations.

Degree Requirements 30 total credit hours, thesis or project, comprehensive exam.

POST-MASTER'S PROGRAM

Areas of Study Nursing administration; nursing education. *Clinical nurse specialist programs in:* public/community health.

CONTINUING EDUCATION PROGRAM

Contact Dr. Mary Wombwell, Professor, School of Nursing and Allied Health Professions, Holy Family University, 9801 Frankford Avenue, Philadelphia, PA 19114. *Telephone:* 267-341-3374. *Fax:* 215-637-6598. *E-mail:* mwombwell@holyfamily.edu.

Immaculata University
Division of Nursing
Immaculata, Pennsylvania

http://www.immaculata.edu/nursing/
Founded in 1920

DEGREES • BSN • MSN

Nursing Program Faculty 80 (50% with doctorates).

Baccalaureate Enrollment 1,125 **Women** 92% **Men** 8% **Part-time** 90%

Graduate Enrollment 105 **Women** 97% **Men** 3% **Part-time** 100%

Nursing Student Activities Sigma Theta Tau, Student Nurses' Association.

Nursing Student Resources Academic advising; academic or career counseling; assistance for students with disabilities; bookstore; campus computer network; career placement assistance; computer lab; computer-assisted instruction; e-mail services; employment services for current students; externships; interactive nursing skills videos; Internet; learning resource lab; library services; nursing audiovisuals; placement services for program completers; resume preparation assistance; skills, simulation, or other laboratory; tutoring.

Library Facilities 1,500 volumes in health, 1,500 volumes in nursing; 115 periodical subscriptions health-care related.

BACCALAUREATE PROGRAMS

Degree BSN

Available Programs Accelerated RN Baccalaureate; Generic Baccalaureate; RN Baccalaureate.

Site Options Philadelphia, PA; Abington, PA; Christiana, DE.

Study Options Full-time.

Online Degree Options Yes (online only).

Program Entrance Requirements Transcript of college record, CPR certification, written essay, health exam, high school chemistry, high school foreign language, 2 years high school math, 3 years high school science, high school transcript, immunizations, interview, 2 letters of recommendation, minimum high school GPA of 3.0, prerequisite course work. Transfer students are accepted. *Application deadline:* 1/31 (fall). *Application fee:* $35.

Advanced Placement Credit by examination available.

Expenses (2014–15) *Tuition:* full-time $32,000; part-time $510 per credit. *International tuition:* $32,000 full-time. *Room and board:* $12,190; room only: $6890 per academic year. *Required fees:* full-time $1000; part-time $50 per term.

Financial Aid 75% of baccalaureate students in nursing programs received some form of financial aid in 2013–14. *Gift aid (need-based):* Federal Pell, FSEOG, state, private, college/university gift aid from institutional funds. *Loans:* Perkins. *Financial aid application deadline (priority):* 2/15.

Contact Ms. Gwen Dreibelbis, Admissions Counselor, Division of Nursing, Immaculata University, 1145 King Road, Immaculata, PA 19345. *Telephone:* 610-647-4400 Ext. 3013. *Fax:* 610-640-0836. *E-mail:* gdreibelbis@immaculata.edu.

GRADUATE PROGRAMS

Expenses (2014–15) *Tuition:* part-time $660 per credit. *International tuition:* $660 full-time. *Required fees:* full-time $250.

Financial Aid 25% of graduate students in nursing programs received some form of financial aid in 2013–14.

Contact Dr. Jane Tang, Coordinator, MSN Program, Division of Nursing, Immaculata University, 1145 King Road, Immaculata, PA 19345-0691. *Telephone:* 610-647-4400 Ext. 3309. *Fax:* 610-640-0286. *E-mail:* jtang@immaculata.edu.

MASTER'S DEGREE PROGRAM

Degree MSN

Available Programs Master's; Master's for Non-Nursing College Graduates.

Concentrations Available Nursing administration; nursing education.

Site Options Abington, PA; Christiana, DE.

Study Options Part-time.

Program Entrance Requirements Minimum overall college GPA of 3.0, transcript of college record, written essay, interview, 3 letters of recommendation, physical assessment course, statistics course. *Application deadline:* Applications may be processed on a rolling basis for some programs. *Application fee:* $50.

Advanced Placement Credit given for nursing courses completed elsewhere dependent upon specific evaluations.
Degree Requirements 39 total credit hours, thesis or project.

Indiana University of Pennsylvania
Department of Nursing and Allied Health
Indiana, Pennsylvania

http://www.iup.edu/rn-alliedhealth
Founded in 1875
DEGREES • BSN • MS • PHD
Nursing Program Faculty 43 (42% with doctorates).
Baccalaureate Enrollment 652 **Women** 86% **Men** 14% **Part-time** 6%
Graduate Enrollment 58 **Women** 88% **Men** 12% **Part-time** 82%
Distance Learning Courses Available.
Nursing Student Activities Nursing Honor Society, Sigma Theta Tau, Student Nurses' Association, nursing club.
Nursing Student Resources Academic advising; academic or career counseling; assistance for students with disabilities; bookstore; campus computer network; career placement assistance; computer lab; computer-assisted instruction; e-mail services; employment services for current students; housing assistance; interactive nursing skills videos; Internet; learning resource lab; library services; nursing audiovisuals; remedial services; resume preparation assistance; skills, simulation, or other laboratory; tutoring.
Library Facilities 5,758 volumes in health, 3,395 volumes in nursing; 225 periodical subscriptions health-care related.

BACCALAUREATE PROGRAMS

Degree BSN
Available Programs Baccalaureate for Second Degree; Generic Baccalaureate; LPN to Baccalaureate.
Study Options Full-time and part-time.
Program Entrance Requirements Minimum overall college GPA of 3.0, transcript of college record, high school chemistry, 3 years high school math, high school transcript, minimum high school GPA of 3.0, prerequisite course work. Transfer students are accepted. *Application deadline:* Applications may be processed on a rolling basis for some programs. *Application fee:* $50.
Advanced Placement Credit given for nursing courses completed elsewhere dependent upon specific evaluations.
Expenses (2015–16) *Tuition, area resident:* full-time $7060; part-time $294 per credit. *Tuition, state resident:* full-time $12,000; part-time $500 per credit. *Tuition, nonresident:* full-time $17,650; part-time $735 per credit. *Room and board:* $11,312 per academic year. *Required fees:* full-time $2876; part-time $149 per credit.
Financial Aid 88% of baccalaureate students in nursing programs received some form of financial aid in 2014–15.
Contact Mr. Chris Kitas, Associate Director of Institutional Research, Planning and Assessment, Department of Nursing and Allied Health, Indiana University of Pennsylvania, Institutional Research Planning and Assessment, 404 Sutton Hall, Indiana, PA 15705. *Telephone:* 724-357-5562. *Fax:* 724-357-3833. *E-mail:* Chris.Kitas@iup.edu.

GRADUATE PROGRAMS

Expenses (2015–16) *Tuition, state resident:* part-time $520 per credit. *Tuition, nonresident:* part-time $779 per credit.
Financial Aid 7 fellowships (averaging $564 per year), 5 research assistantships (averaging $2,920 per year), 2 teaching assistantships (averaging $23,305 per year) were awarded; career-related internships or fieldwork, Federal Work-Study, scholarships, and unspecified assistantships also available.
Contact Dr. Theresa Marie Gropelli, Chairperson, Department of Nursing and Allied Health, Department of Nursing and Allied Health, Indiana University of Pennsylvania, 1010 Oakland Avenue, Indiana, PA 15705-1087. *Telephone:* 724-357-2557. *Fax:* 724-357-3267. *E-mail:* tgropell@iup.edu.

MASTER'S DEGREE PROGRAM
Degree MS
Available Programs Master's; Master's for Nurses with Non-Nursing Degrees.
Concentrations Available Nursing administration; nursing education.
Site Options Monroeville, PA; Freeport, PA.

Study Options Part-time.
Program Entrance Requirements Clinical experience, minimum overall college GPA of 3.0, transcript of college record, written essay, 2 letters of recommendation, nursing research course, resume, statistics course. *Application deadline:* Applications may be processed on a rolling basis for some programs. *Application fee:* $50.
Advanced Placement Credit given for nursing courses completed elsewhere dependent upon specific evaluations.
Degree Requirements 36 total credit hours, thesis or project.

DOCTORAL DEGREE PROGRAM
Degree PhD
Available Programs Doctorate.
Areas of Study Nursing education.
Program Entrance Requirements Minimum overall college GPA of 3.5, interview by faculty committee, 2 letters of recommendation, MSN or equivalent, statistics course, vita, writing sample, GRE. Application deadline: Applications may be processed on a rolling basis for some programs. Application fee: $50.
Degree Requirements 60 total credit hours, dissertation, oral exam, written exam, residency.

La Roche College
Department of Nursing and Nursing Management
Pittsburgh, Pennsylvania

http://www.laroche.edu/
Founded in 1963
DEGREES • BSN • MSN
Nursing Program Faculty 11 (90% with doctorates).
Baccalaureate Enrollment 84 **Women** 90% **Men** 10% **Part-time** 80%
Graduate Enrollment 25 **Women** 90% **Men** 10% **Part-time** 90%
Distance Learning Courses Available.
Nursing Student Activities Sigma Theta Tau.
Nursing Student Resources Academic advising; academic or career counseling; assistance for students with disabilities; bookstore; campus computer network; computer lab; e-mail services; externships; Internet; library services; resume preparation assistance; tutoring.
Library Facilities 850 periodical subscriptions health-care related.

BACCALAUREATE PROGRAMS

Degree BSN
Available Programs Accelerated RN Baccalaureate; LPN to RN Baccalaureate; RN Baccalaureate.
Study Options Full-time and part-time.
Online Degree Options Yes (online only).
Program Entrance Requirements Minimum overall college GPA of 3.0, transcript of college record, CPR certification, written essay, health exam, health insurance, high school chemistry, high school transcript, immunizations, interview, 2 letters of recommendation, minimum high school GPA of 3.0, professional liability insurance/malpractice insurance, RN licensure. Transfer students are accepted. *Application deadline:* Applications may be processed on a rolling basis for some programs. *Application fee:* $50.
Advanced Placement Credit by examination available. Credit given for nursing courses completed elsewhere dependent upon specific evaluations.
Contact *Telephone:* 412-536-1266. *Fax:* 412-536-1283.

GRADUATE PROGRAMS

Contact *Telephone:* 412-536-1262. *Fax:* 412-536-1283.

MASTER'S DEGREE PROGRAM
Degree MSN
Available Programs Master's; RN to Master's.
Concentrations Available Nurse anesthesia; nursing administration; nursing education.
Study Options Full-time and part-time.
Online Degree Options Yes (online only).
Program Entrance Requirements Clinical experience, minimum overall college GPA of 3.0, transcript of college record, immunizations, interview, 2 letters of recommendation, professional liability insurance/malpractice insurance, resume. *Application deadline:* Applications may be processed on a rolling basis for some programs. *Application fee:* $50.

Advanced Placement Credit given for nursing courses completed else-where dependent upon specific evaluations.
Degree Requirements 36 total credit hours, thesis or project.

CONTINUING EDUCATION PROGRAM

Contact *Telephone:* 412-536-1260. *Fax:* 412-536-1283.

La Salle University
School of Nursing and Health Sciences
Philadelphia, Pennsylvania

http://www.lasalle.edu/schools/snhs/
Founded in 1863
DEGREES • BSN • MSN • MSN/MBA
Nursing Program Faculty 45 (32% with doctorates).
Nursing Student Activities Sigma Theta Tau, Student Nurses' Association, nursing club.
Nursing Student Resources Academic advising; academic or career counseling; assistance for students with disabilities; bookstore; campus computer network; career placement assistance; computer lab; computer-assisted instruction; e-mail services; employment services for current students; externships; housing assistance; interactive nursing skills videos; Internet; learning resource lab; library services; nursing audiovisuals; placement services for program completers; remedial services; resume preparation assistance; skills, simulation, or other laboratory; tutoring.
Library Facilities 8,350 volumes in nursing; 310 periodical subscriptions health-care related.

BACCALAUREATE PROGRAMS

Degree BSN
Available Programs Baccalaureate for Second Degree; Generic Baccalaureate; LPN to Baccalaureate; RN Baccalaureate.
Site Options Newtown, PA.
Study Options Full-time and part-time.
Program Entrance Requirements Minimum overall college GPA of 2.75, transcript of college record, CPR certification, written essay, health exam, health insurance, high school biology, high school chemistry, 3 years high school math, 3 years high school science, high school transcript, immunizations, interview, 2 letters of recommendation, minimum high school GPA of 3.0, minimum high school rank 25%, minimum GPA in nursing prerequisites of 2.75, professional liability insurance/malpractice insurance, prerequisite course work. Transfer students are accepted.
Advanced Placement Credit by examination available. Credit given for nursing courses completed elsewhere dependent upon specific evaluations.
Contact *Telephone:* 215-951-1430. *Fax:* 215-951-1896.

GRADUATE PROGRAMS

Contact *Telephone:* 215-951-1413. *Fax:* 215-951-1896.

MASTER'S DEGREE PROGRAM
Degrees MSN; MSN/MBA
Available Programs Master's; RN to Master's.
Concentrations Available Nurse anesthesia; nursing administration. *Clinical nurse specialist programs in:* adult health, public health. *Nurse practitioner programs in:* adult health, family health.
Site Options Newtown, PA.
Study Options Full-time and part-time.
Program Entrance Requirements Clinical experience, minimum overall college GPA of 3.0, transcript of college record, CPR certification, written essay, immunizations, interview, 2 letters of recommendation, nursing research course, physical assessment course, professional liability insurance/malpractice insurance, resume, statistics course.
Advanced Placement Credit given for nursing courses completed elsewhere dependent upon specific evaluations.
Degree Requirements 41 total credit hours.

POST-MASTER'S PROGRAM
Areas of Study Nurse anesthesia; nursing administration; nursing education. *Clinical nurse specialist programs in:* adult health, public health. *Nurse practitioner programs in:* adult health, family health.

CONTINUING EDUCATION PROGRAM

Contact *Telephone:* 215-951-1432. *Fax:* 215-951-1896.

Lock Haven University of Pennsylvania
Nursing Program
Lock Haven, Pennsylvania

https://www.lhup.edu/
Founded in 1870
DEGREE • BSN

BACCALAUREATE PROGRAMS

Degree BSN
Available Programs Accelerated Baccalaureate; RN Baccalaureate.
Study Options Full-time and part-time.
Program Entrance Requirements RN licensure.
Contact *Telephone:* 814-768-3430.

Mansfield University of Pennsylvania
Department of Health Sciences–Nursing
Mansfield, Pennsylvania

http://www.mansfield.edu/
Founded in 1857
DEGREES • BSN • MSN
Nursing Program Faculty 12 (50% with doctorates).
Baccalaureate Enrollment 186 **Women** 95% **Men** 5% **Part-time** 5%
Graduate Enrollment 52 **Women** 98% **Men** 2% **Part-time** 100%
Distance Learning Courses Available.
Nursing Student Activities Nursing Honor Society, Student Nurses' Association, nursing club.
Nursing Student Resources Academic advising; academic or career counseling; assistance for students with disabilities; bookstore; campus computer network; career placement assistance; computer lab; daycare for children of students; e-mail services; employment services for current students; housing assistance; Internet; learning resource lab; library services; nursing audiovisuals; remedial services; resume preparation assistance; skills, simulation, or other laboratory; tutoring.
Library Facilities 1,300 volumes in health, 500 volumes in nursing; 550 periodical subscriptions health-care related.

BACCALAUREATE PROGRAMS

Degree BSN
Available Programs Generic Baccalaureate; RN Baccalaureate.
Site Options Sayre, PA.
Study Options Full-time and part-time.
Program Entrance Requirements Minimum overall college GPA of 2.7, transcript of college record, CPR certification, health exam, health insurance, high school biology, high school chemistry, 2 years high school math, 2 years high school science, high school transcript, immunizations, minimum high school GPA of 2.7, minimum high school rank 60%, professional liability insurance/malpractice insurance. Transfer students are accepted. *Application deadline:* Applications may be processed on a rolling basis for some programs. *Application fee:* $25.
Advanced Placement Credit by examination available. Credit given for nursing courses completed elsewhere dependent upon specific evaluations.
Contact *Telephone:* 570-662-4243. *Fax:* 570-662-4121.

GRADUATE PROGRAMS

Contact *Telephone:* 570-662-4522. *Fax:* 570-662-4137.

MASTER'S DEGREE PROGRAM
Degree MSN
Available Programs Master's.
Concentrations Available Nursing administration; nursing education.
Study Options Part-time.
Online Degree Options Yes (online only).
Program Entrance Requirements Minimum overall college GPA of 3.0, transcript of college record, 1 letter of recommendation, nursing research course, prerequisite course work. *Application deadline:* Applications may be processed on a rolling basis for some programs. *Application fee:* $25.

Advanced Placement Credit given for nursing courses completed elsewhere dependent upon specific evaluations.
Degree Requirements 33 total credit hours, thesis or project.

Marywood University
Department of Nursing
Scranton, Pennsylvania

http://www.marywood.edu/nursing/index.html
Founded in 1915
DEGREES • BSN • MSN • MSN/MPH
Nursing Program Faculty 16 (50% with doctorates).
Baccalaureate Enrollment 117 **Women** 90% **Men** 10% **Part-time** 5%
Graduate Enrollment 17 **Women** 100% **Part-time** 90%
Distance Learning Courses Available.
Nursing Student Activities Sigma Theta Tau, Student Nurses' Association.
Nursing Student Resources Academic advising; academic or career counseling; assistance for students with disabilities; bookstore; campus computer network; computer lab; daycare for children of students; e-mail services; employment services for current students; interactive nursing skills videos; Internet; learning resource lab; library services; nursing audiovisuals; skills, simulation, or other laboratory; tutoring.
Library Facilities 7,400 volumes in health, 3,006 volumes in nursing; 750 periodical subscriptions health-care related.

BACCALAUREATE PROGRAMS

Degree BSN
Available Programs ADN to Baccalaureate; Generic Baccalaureate; International Nurse to Baccalaureate; LPN to Baccalaureate; RN Baccalaureate.
Study Options Full-time and part-time.
Program Entrance Requirements Transcript of college record, high school biology, high school chemistry, 1 year of high school math, high school transcript, 1 letter of recommendation. Transfer students are accepted.
Advanced Placement Credit given for nursing courses completed elsewhere dependent upon specific evaluations.
Contact *Telephone:* 570-348-6211 Ext. 2374. *Fax:* 570-961-4761.

GRADUATE PROGRAMS

Contact *Telephone:* 570-348-6211 Ext. 2475. *Fax:* 570-961-4761.

MASTER'S DEGREE PROGRAM
Degrees MSN; MSN/MPH
Available Programs Master's.
Concentrations Available Nursing administration.
Study Options Full-time and part-time.
Program Entrance Requirements Clinical experience, minimum overall college GPA of 3.0, transcript of college record, written essay, 2 letters of recommendation, nursing research course, physical assessment course, statistics course.
Degree Requirements 39 total credit hours, thesis or project.

CONTINUING EDUCATION PROGRAM

Contact *Telephone:* 570-340-6060. *Fax:* 570-961-4776.

Messiah College
Department of Nursing
Mechanicsburg, Pennsylvania

http://www.messiah.edu/
Founded in 1909
DEGREES • BSN • MSN
Nursing Program Faculty 33 (18% with doctorates).
Baccalaureate Enrollment 202 **Women** 96% **Men** 4% **Part-time** 5%
Graduate Enrollment 30 **Women** 97% **Men** 3% **Part-time** 57%
Nursing Student Activities Nursing Honor Society, Sigma Theta Tau, Student Nurses' Association, nursing club.
Nursing Student Resources Academic advising; academic or career counseling; assistance for students with disabilities; bookstore; campus computer network; career placement assistance; computer lab; computer-assisted instruction; e-mail services; employment services for current students; interactive nursing skills videos; Internet; learning resource lab; library services; nursing audiovisuals; remedial services; resume preparation assistance; skills, simulation, or other laboratory; tutoring.
Library Facilities 6,669 volumes in health, 671 volumes in nursing; 8,402 periodical subscriptions health-care related.

BACCALAUREATE PROGRAMS

Degree BSN
Available Programs Generic Baccalaureate.
Study Options Full-time and part-time.
Program Entrance Requirements Minimum overall college GPA of 3.0, transcript of college record, CPR certification, written essay, health exam, health insurance, high school foreign language, 2 years high school math, 2 years high school science, high school transcript, immunizations, minimum high school rank 66%, minimum GPA in nursing prerequisites of 2.7, prerequisite course work. Transfer students are accepted. *Application deadline:* 4/15 (fall), 10/15 (spring). Applications may be processed on a rolling basis for some programs. *Application fee:* $20.
Advanced Placement Credit given for nursing courses completed elsewhere dependent upon specific evaluations.
Expenses (2015–16) *Tuition:* full-time $31,410; part-time $1310 per credit hour. *Room and board:* $9630; room only: $5100 per academic year. *Required fees:* full-time $1770; part-time $35 per credit hour.
Financial Aid 99% of baccalaureate students in nursing programs received some form of financial aid in 2014–15.
Contact Dana Britton, Director of Admissions, Department of Nursing, Messiah College, Suite 3005, One College Avenue, Mechanicsburg, PA 17055. *Telephone:* 800-233-4220. *Fax:* 717-796-5374.
E-mail: admiss@messiah.edu.

GRADUATE PROGRAMS

Expenses (2015–16) *Tuition:* full-time $12,810; part-time $610 per credit hour. *Required fees:* full-time $210; part-time $30 per course.
Financial Aid 79% of graduate students in nursing programs received some form of financial aid in 2014–15.
Contact Matthew Reitnour, Director of Graduate and Non-traditional enrollment, Department of Nursing, Messiah College, Graduate Admissions Office, One College Avenue, Suite 3060, Mechanicsburg, PA 17055. *Telephone:* 717-796-5061. *Fax:* 717-691-2307.
E-mail: GradPrograms@messiah.edu.

MASTER'S DEGREE PROGRAM
Degree MSN
Available Programs Master's; RN to Master's.
Concentrations Available Nursing education.
Study Options Full-time and part-time.
Online Degree Options Yes (online only).
Program Entrance Requirements Clinical experience, minimum overall college GPA of 3.0, transcript of college record, written essay, 3 letters of recommendation, nursing research course, physical assessment course, prerequisite course work, resume, statistics course. *Application deadline:* 3/29 (fall), 11/2 (winter), 11/2 (spring), 1/25 (summer). Applications may be processed on a rolling basis for some programs. *Application fee:* $30.
Degree Requirements 39 total credit hours, thesis or project, comprehensive exam.

Millersville University of Pennsylvania
Department of Nursing
Millersville, Pennsylvania

http://www.millersville.edu/nursing/
Founded in 1855
DEGREES • BSN • MSN
Nursing Program Faculty 10 (60% with doctorates).
Baccalaureate Enrollment 101 **Women** 95% **Men** 5% **Part-time** 90%
Graduate Enrollment 110 **Women** 86% **Men** 14% **Part-time** 100%
Nursing Student Activities Sigma Theta Tau.
Nursing Student Resources Academic advising; academic or career counseling; assistance for students with disabilities; bookstore; computer lab; e-mail services; interactive nursing skills videos; Internet; library services; nursing audiovisuals; resume preparation assistance.
Library Facilities 82 periodical subscriptions health-care related.

BACCALAUREATE PROGRAMS

Degree BSN
Available Programs RN Baccalaureate.
Site Options Harrisburg, PA.
Study Options Full-time and part-time.
Program Entrance Requirements Minimum overall college GPA of 2.0, transcript of college record, RN licensure. Transfer students are accepted. *Application deadline:* Applications may be processed on a rolling basis for some programs. *Application fee:* $40.
Contact *Telephone:* 717-872-3376. *Fax:* 717-871-4877.

GRADUATE PROGRAMS

Contact *Telephone:* 717-871-5341. *Fax:* 717-871-4887.

MASTER'S DEGREE PROGRAM

Degree MSN
Available Programs Master's.
Concentrations Available Nursing education. *Nurse practitioner programs in:* family health.
Study Options Part-time.
Program Entrance Requirements Clinical experience, minimum overall college GPA of 3.0, transcript of college record, interview, 3 letters of recommendation, nursing research course, physical assessment course, resume, statistics course. *Application deadline:* 1/15 (spring). *Application fee:* $40.
Degree Requirements Thesis or project.

POST-MASTER'S PROGRAM

Areas of Study Nursing education. *Nurse practitioner programs in:* family health.

Misericordia University
Department of Nursing
Dallas, Pennsylvania

http://www.misericordia.edu/nursing
Founded in 1924

DEGREES • BSN • MSN
Nursing Program Faculty 34 (5% with doctorates).
Baccalaureate Enrollment 243 **Women** 89% **Men** 11% **Part-time** 35%
Graduate Enrollment 45 **Women** 95% **Men** 5% **Part-time** 100%
Distance Learning Courses Available.
Nursing Student Activities Nursing Honor Society, Sigma Theta Tau, Student Nurses' Association, nursing club.
Nursing Student Resources Academic advising; academic or career counseling; assistance for students with disabilities; bookstore; campus computer network; career placement assistance; computer lab; computer-assisted instruction; e-mail services; employment services for current students; externships; housing assistance; interactive nursing skills videos; Internet; learning resource lab; library services; nursing audiovisuals; placement services for program completers; remedial services; resume preparation assistance; skills, simulation, or other laboratory; tutoring.
Library Facilities 6 volumes in health, 5 volumes in nursing; 15 periodical subscriptions health-care related.

BACCALAUREATE PROGRAMS

Degree BSN
Available Programs Accelerated RN Baccalaureate; Baccalaureate for Second Degree; Generic Baccalaureate; RN Baccalaureate.
Study Options Full-time and part-time.
Program Entrance Requirements Minimum overall college GPA of 3.0, transcript of college record, CPR certification, health exam, health insurance, high school biology, high school chemistry, 4 years high school math, high school transcript, immunizations, letters of recommendation, minimum high school GPA of 2.8, minimum high school rank 50%, minimum GPA in nursing prerequisites of 3.0, professional liability insurance/malpractice insurance. Transfer students are accepted. *Application deadline:* 8/1 (fall), 8/1 (winter), 12/1 (spring), 4/1 (summer). Applications may be processed on a rolling basis for some programs. *Application fee:* $35.
Advanced Placement Credit by examination available. Credit given for nursing courses completed elsewhere dependent upon specific evaluations.
Financial Aid *Gift aid (need-based):* Federal Pell, FSEOG, state, private, college/university gift aid from institutional funds, Federal Nursing. *Loans:* Federal Nursing Student Loans, Federal Direct (Subsidized and Unsubsidized Stafford PLUS), Perkins, state. *Work-study:* Federal Work-Study. *Financial aid application deadline (priority):* 3/1.
Contact Mr. Glenn Bozinski, Admissions, Department of Nursing, Misericordia University, 301 Lake Street, Dallas, PA 18612. *Telephone:* 570-674-6434. *E-mail:* gbozinsk@misericordia.edu.

GRADUATE PROGRAMS

Expenses (2015–16) *Tuition:* full-time $12,600; part-time $700 per credit. *International tuition:* $12,600 full-time.
Financial Aid Teaching assistantships, career-related internships or fieldwork, scholarships, traineeships, tuition waivers (partial), and unspecified assistantships available.
Contact Ms. Maureen Sheridan, Adult Education Counselor, Graduate Programs, Department of Nursing, Misericordia University, 301 Lake Street, Dallas, PA 18612. *Telephone:* 570-674-6451. *Fax:* 570-674-8902. *E-mail:* msherida@misericordia.edu.

MASTER'S DEGREE PROGRAM

Degree MSN
Available Programs Master's; RN to Master's.
Concentrations Available Nursing education. *Clinical nurse specialist programs in:* family health. *Nurse practitioner programs in:* family health.
Study Options Part-time.
Program Entrance Requirements Clinical experience, computer literacy, minimum overall college GPA of 3.0, transcript of college record, written essay, 3 letters of recommendation, nursing research course, physical assessment course, professional liability insurance/malpractice insurance, statistics course. *Application deadline:* 7/18 (fall), 7/18 (winter), 12/1 (spring), 4/1 (summer). Applications may be processed on a rolling basis for some programs. *Application fee:* $200.
Advanced Placement Credit given for nursing courses completed elsewhere dependent upon specific evaluations.
Degree Requirements 46 total credit hours, thesis or project.

POST-MASTER'S PROGRAM

Areas of Study Nursing education. *Clinical nurse specialist programs in:* family health. *Nurse practitioner programs in:* family health.

Moravian College
Department of Nursing
Bethlehem, Pennsylvania

http://www.moravian.edu/
Founded in 1742

DEGREES • BSN • MSN
Nursing Program Faculty 61 (23% with doctorates).
Baccalaureate Enrollment 267 **Women** 83% **Men** 17% **Part-time** 33%
Graduate Enrollment 65 **Women** 92% **Men** 8% **Part-time** 100%
Nursing Student Activities Sigma Theta Tau, Student Nurses' Association.
Nursing Student Resources Academic advising; academic or career counseling; assistance for students with disabilities; bookstore; campus computer network; career placement assistance; computer lab; computer-assisted instruction; e-mail services; employment services for current students; externships; housing assistance; interactive nursing skills videos; Internet; learning resource lab; library services; nursing audiovisuals; placement services for program completers; remedial services; resume preparation assistance; skills, simulation, or other laboratory; tutoring.
Library Facilities 4,600 volumes in health, 1,900 volumes in nursing; 275 periodical subscriptions health-care related.

BACCALAUREATE PROGRAMS

Degree BSN
Available Programs Accelerated Baccalaureate; Accelerated Baccalaureate for Second Degree; Baccalaureate for Second Degree; Generic Baccalaureate; RN Baccalaureate.
Study Options Full-time.
Program Entrance Requirements Minimum overall college GPA of 3.0, transcript of college record, CPR certification, written essay, health exam, health insurance, high school biology, high school chemistry, high school foreign language, 3 years high school math, 3 years high school science, high school transcript, immunizations, 1 letter of recommendation, minimum high school GPA of 3.4, minimum GPA in nursing prerequisites of 3.0, prerequisite course work. Transfer students are accepted. *Application deadline:* 3/1 (fall).

Advanced Placement Credit by examination available. Credit given for nursing courses completed elsewhere dependent upon specific evaluations.

Expenses (2015–16) *Tuition:* full-time $37,251; part-time $1670 per course. *International tuition:* $37,251 full-time. *Room and board:* $11,868; room only: $6792 per academic year. *Required fees:* full-time $1021; part-time $15 per credit; part-time $45 per term.

Financial Aid 96% of baccalaureate students in nursing programs received some form of financial aid in 2014–15. *Gift aid (need-based):* Federal Pell, FSEOG, state, private, college/university gift aid from institutional funds. *Loans:* Federal Direct (Subsidized and Unsubsidized Stafford PLUS), Perkins. *Work-study:* Federal Work-Study, part-time campus jobs. *Financial aid application deadline (priority):* 3/1.

Contact Mr. Scott Dams, Executive Director of Admission, Department of Nursing, Moravian College, 1200 Main Street, Bethlehem, PA 18018. *Telephone:* 800-441-3191. *E-mail:* damss@moravian.edu.

GRADUATE PROGRAMS

Expenses (2015–16) *Tuition:* part-time $818 per credit hour. *International tuition:* $818 full-time. *Required fees:* part-time $35 per credit; part-time $45 per term.

Contact Dr. Lori Hoffman, RN, MS Program Coordinator, Department of Nursing, Moravian College, 1200 Main Street, Bethlehem, PA 18018. *Telephone:* 610-625-7769. *Fax:* 610-625-7861. *E-mail:* hoffmanl@moravian.edu.

MASTER'S DEGREE PROGRAM

Degree MSN

Available Programs Master's; Master's for Nurses with Non-Nursing Degrees.

Concentrations Available Clinical nurse leader; nursing administration; nursing education. *Nurse practitioner programs in:* adult health, adult-gerontology acute care, gerontology, primary care.

Study Options Part-time.

Program Entrance Requirements Computer literacy, minimum overall college GPA of 3.0, transcript of college record, written essay, 2 letters of recommendation, prerequisite course work, resume, statistics course. *Application deadline:* 4/1 (fall). Applications may be processed on a rolling basis for some programs. *Application fee:* $40.

Advanced Placement Credit given for nursing courses completed elsewhere dependent upon specific evaluations.

Degree Requirements 43 total credit hours, thesis or project.

Mount Aloysius College
Division of Nursing
Cresson, Pennsylvania

http://www.mtaloy.edu/
Founded in 1939

DEGREE • BSN

Nursing Program Faculty 40 (15% with doctorates).

Baccalaureate Enrollment 194 **Women** 86% **Men** 14% **Part-time** 91%

Distance Learning Courses Available.

Nursing Student Activities Student Nurses' Association.

Nursing Student Resources Academic advising; academic or career counseling; assistance for students with disabilities; bookstore; campus computer network; computer lab; computer-assisted instruction; daycare for children of students; e-mail services; interactive nursing skills videos; Internet; learning resource lab; library services; nursing audiovisuals; remedial services; resume preparation assistance; skills, simulation, or other laboratory; tutoring.

Library Facilities 6,000 volumes in health, 900 volumes in nursing; 525 periodical subscriptions health-care related.

BACCALAUREATE PROGRAMS

Degree BSN

Available Programs ADN to Baccalaureate; Accelerated RN Baccalaureate; LPN to RN Baccalaureate; RN Baccalaureate.

Site Options Johnstown, PA; Altoona, PA.

Study Options Full-time and part-time.

Online Degree Options Yes.

Program Entrance Requirements Transcript of college record, health exam, high school transcript, immunizations, RN licensure. Transfer students are accepted. *Application deadline:* Applications may be processed on a rolling basis for some programs. *Application fee:* $30.

Advanced Placement Credit by examination available. Credit given for nursing courses completed elsewhere dependent upon specific evaluations.

Expenses (2015–16) *Tuition:* full-time $23,380; part-time $775 per credit. *International tuition:* $23,380 full-time. *Room and board:* $9552; room only: $4804 per academic year. *Required fees:* full-time $1060.

Financial Aid *Gift aid (need-based):* Federal Pell, FSEOG, state, private, college/university gift aid from institutional funds. *Loans:* Federal Nursing Student Loans, Federal Direct (Subsidized and Unsubsidized Stafford PLUS), Perkins, alternative loans. *Work-study:* Federal Work-Study. *Financial aid application deadline (priority):* 4/1.

Contact Dr. Cynthia R. King, Dean of Nursing, Division of Nursing, Mount Aloysius College, 7373 Admiral Peary Highway, Cresson, PA 16630. *Telephone:* 814-886-6401. *Fax:* 814-886-6374. *E-mail:* cking@mtaloy.edu.

CONTINUING EDUCATION PROGRAM

Contact Mr. Matthew Bodenschatz, Director of Graduate and Continuing Education, Division of Nursing, Mount Aloysius College, 7373 Admiral Peary Highway, Cresson, PA 16630. *Telephone:* 814-886-6383. *Fax:* 814-886-6441. *E-mail:* rmbodenschatz@mtaloy.edu.

Neumann University
Program in Nursing and Health Sciences
Aston, Pennsylvania

http://www.neumann.edu/
Founded in 1965

DEGREES • BS • MS

Nursing Program Faculty 37 (14% with doctorates).

Baccalaureate Enrollment 585 **Women** 87.9% **Men** 12.1% **Part-time** 40.2%

Graduate Enrollment 34 **Women** 100% **Part-time** 100%

Nursing Student Activities Nursing Honor Society, Sigma Theta Tau, Student Nurses' Association, nursing club.

Nursing Student Resources Academic advising; academic or career counseling; assistance for students with disabilities; bookstore; campus computer network; career placement assistance; computer lab; computer-assisted instruction; e-mail services; employment services for current students; externships; housing assistance; interactive nursing skills videos; Internet; learning resource lab; library services; nursing audiovisuals; paid internships; remedial services; resume preparation assistance; skills, simulation, or other laboratory; tutoring; unpaid internships.

Library Facilities 600 volumes in health, 540 volumes in nursing; 6,500 periodical subscriptions health-care related.

BACCALAUREATE PROGRAMS

Degree BS

Available Programs ADN to Baccalaureate; Accelerated RN Baccalaureate; Baccalaureate for Second Degree; Generic Baccalaureate; International Nurse to Baccalaureate; LPN to Baccalaureate; LPN to RN Baccalaureate.

Study Options Full-time and part-time.

Program Entrance Requirements Minimum overall college GPA of 2.5, transcript of college record, health exam, health insurance, high school biology, high school chemistry, high school foreign language, 2 years high school math, 4 years high school science, high school transcript, immunizations, minimum high school GPA of 2.5, minimum GPA in nursing prerequisites of 2.5, prerequisite course work. Transfer students are accepted. *Application deadline:* Applications may be processed on a rolling basis for some programs.

Advanced Placement Credit by examination available. Credit given for nursing courses completed elsewhere dependent upon specific evaluations.

Expenses (2015–16) *Tuition:* full-time $25,792; part-time $589 per credit. *Room and board:* $3557 per academic year.

Financial Aid 98% of baccalaureate students in nursing programs received some form of financial aid in 2014–15.

Contact Ms. Casey Downie, Admissions Counselor, Program in Nursing and Health Sciences, Neumann University, One Neumann Drive, Aston, PA 19014-1298. *Telephone:* 610-558-5614. *Fax:* 610-361-2548. *E-mail:* downiec@neumann.edu.

GRADUATE PROGRAMS

Contact Ms. Kittie Pain, Associate Director, Admissions, Program in Nursing and Health Sciences, Neumann University, One Neumann Drive,

Aston, PA 19014-1298. *Telephone:* 800-963-8626 Ext. 5613. *Fax:* 610-558-5652. *E-mail:* nursediv@neumann.edu.

MASTER'S DEGREE PROGRAM
Degree MS
Available Programs Master's.
Concentrations Available Nursing education. *Nurse practitioner programs in:* adult health.
Study Options Full-time and part-time.
Program Entrance Requirements Computer literacy, minimum overall college GPA of 3.0, transcript of college record, CPR certification, immunizations, interview, 2 letters of recommendation, nursing research course, physical assessment course, professional liability insurance/malpractice insurance, prerequisite course work, statistics course, GRE or MAT. *Application deadline:* Applications may be processed on a rolling basis for some programs.
Advanced Placement Credit given for nursing courses completed elsewhere dependent upon specific evaluations.
Degree Requirements 43 total credit hours, thesis or project.

POST-MASTER'S PROGRAM
Areas of Study Nursing education. *Nurse practitioner programs in:* adult health.

Penn State University Park
School of Nursing
State College, University Park, Pennsylvania

http://www.nursing.psu.edu/
Founded in 1855
DEGREES • BS • MS • MSN/PHD • PHD
Nursing Program Faculty 110 (20% with doctorates).
Baccalaureate Enrollment 824 **Women** 95% **Men** 5% **Part-time** 43%
Graduate Enrollment 61 **Women** 92% **Men** 8% **Part-time** 59%
Distance Learning Courses Available.
Nursing Student Activities Sigma Theta Tau, Student Nurses' Association.
Nursing Student Resources Academic advising; academic or career counseling; assistance for students with disabilities; bookstore; campus computer network; career placement assistance; computer lab; computer-assisted instruction; daycare for children of students; e-mail services; employment services for current students; externships; housing assistance; interactive nursing skills videos; Internet; learning resource lab; library services; nursing audiovisuals; paid internships; remedial services; resume preparation assistance; skills, simulation, or other laboratory; tutoring.
Library Facilities 244,000 volumes in health; 3,500 periodical subscriptions health-care related.

BACCALAUREATE PROGRAMS
Degree BS
Available Programs ADN to Baccalaureate; Generic Baccalaureate; RN Baccalaureate.
Site Options Uniontown, PA; New Kensington, PA; Harrisburg, PA; Hershey, PA; University Park, PA; Altoona, PA; Mont Alto, PA; Sharon, PA; Scranton, PA.
Study Options Full-time.
Online Degree Options Yes.
Program Entrance Requirements Transcript of college record, 3 years high school math, 3 years high school science, high school transcript. Transfer students are accepted. *Application deadline:* 11/30 (fall). *Application fee:* $50.
Advanced Placement Credit given for nursing courses completed elsewhere dependent upon specific evaluations.
Contact *Telephone:* 814-863-8185. *Fax:* 814-863-2925.

GRADUATE PROGRAMS
Contact *Telephone:* 814-863-2211. *Fax:* 814-865-2925.

MASTER'S DEGREE PROGRAM
Degrees MS; MSN/PhD
Available Programs Master's.
Concentrations Available Nursing administration. *Clinical nurse specialist programs in:* adult health, community health, gerontology. *Nurse practitioner programs in:* adult health, family health.
Site Options Hershey, PA; University Park, PA.

Study Options Full-time and part-time.
Online Degree Options Yes.
Program Entrance Requirements Computer literacy, minimum overall college GPA of 3.0, transcript of college record, CPR certification, written essay, immunizations, 2 letters of recommendation, professional liability insurance/malpractice insurance. *Application deadline:* Applications may be processed on a rolling basis for some programs. *Application fee:* $65.
Advanced Placement Credit given for nursing courses completed elsewhere dependent upon specific evaluations.
Degree Requirements 43 total credit hours, thesis or project.

POST-MASTER'S PROGRAM
Areas of Study *Nurse practitioner programs in:* family health.

DOCTORAL DEGREE PROGRAM
Degree PhD
Available Programs Doctorate.
Areas of Study Bio-behavioral research, faculty preparation, gerontology, human health and illness, illness and transition, individualized study, nursing research, nursing science.
Site Options Hershey, PA; University Park, PA.
Program Entrance Requirements Minimum overall college GPA of 3.5, interview, 3 letters of recommendation, MSN or equivalent, writing sample. Application deadline: Applications may be processed on a rolling basis for some programs. Application fee: $65.
Degree Requirements 58 total credit hours, dissertation, oral exam, written exam, residency.

POSTDOCTORAL PROGRAM
Areas of Study Gerontology.
Postdoctoral Program Contact *Telephone:* 814-865-9337. *Fax:* 814-865-2925.

CONTINUING EDUCATION PROGRAM
Contact *Telephone:* 814-865-8469. *Fax:* 814-865-3779.

Pennsylvania College of Health Sciences
Bachelor of Science in Nursing Program
Lancaster, Pennsylvania

Founded in 1903
DEGREE • BSN

BACCALAUREATE PROGRAMS
Degree BSN
Available Programs RN Baccalaureate.
Program Entrance Requirements Minimum overall college GPA of 2.0, RN licensure.
Contact *Telephone:* 800-622-5443.

Pennsylvania College of Technology
School of Health Sciences
Williamsport, Pennsylvania

https://www.pct.edu/catalog/majors/BGN.shtml
Founded in 1965
DEGREE • BSN
Nursing Program Faculty 35 (33% with doctorates).
Baccalaureate Enrollment 178 **Women** 84% **Men** 16%
Distance Learning Courses Available.
Nursing Student Activities Student Nurses' Association.
Nursing Student Resources Academic advising; academic or career counseling; assistance for students with disabilities; bookstore; campus computer network; career placement assistance; computer lab; computer-assisted instruction; daycare for children of students; e-mail services; employment services for current students; externships; housing assistance; interactive nursing skills videos; Internet; learning resource lab; library services; nursing audiovisuals; placement services for program

completers; remedial services; resume preparation assistance; skills, simulation, or other laboratory; tutoring.
Library Facilities 638 volumes in nursing; 187 periodical subscriptions health-care related.

BACCALAUREATE PROGRAMS

Degree BSN
Available Programs ADN to Baccalaureate; RN Baccalaureate.
Site Options Williamsport, PA.
Study Options Full-time and part-time.
Online Degree Options Yes.
Program Entrance Requirements Minimum overall college GPA of 3.0, transcript of college record, 2 years high school math, high school transcript, minimum GPA in nursing prerequisites of 3.0. Transfer students are accepted. *Application deadline:* 12/1 (fall), 5/1 (spring). *Application fee:* $50.
Advanced Placement Credit by examination available. Credit given for nursing courses completed elsewhere dependent upon specific evaluations.
Expenses (2015–16) *Tuition, state resident:* full-time $27,498; part-time $527 per credit hour. *Tuition, nonresident:* full-time $34,158; part-time $791 per credit hour. *International tuition:* $34,158 full-time. *Room and board:* $5144; room only: $3148 per academic year. *Required fees:* full-time $40.
Financial Aid *Gift aid (need-based):* Federal Pell, FSEOG, state, private, college/university gift aid from institutional funds. *Loans:* Federal Direct (Subsidized and Unsubsidized Stafford PLUS). *Work-study:* Federal Work-Study. *Financial aid application deadline (priority):* 4/15.
Contact Dr. Sandra L. Richmond, Director of Nursing, School of Health Sciences, Pennsylvania College of Technology, One College Avenue, Williamsport, PA 17701. *Telephone:* 570-327-4525. *Fax:* 570-320-5263. *E-mail:* slr8@pct.edu.

Robert Morris University
School of Nursing and Health Sciences
Moon Township, Pennsylvania

http://www.rmu.edu/web/cms/schools/snhs/nursing/Pages/default.aspx
Founded in 1921
DEGREES • BSN • DNP • MSN
Nursing Program Faculty 66 (41% with doctorates).
Baccalaureate Enrollment 459 **Women** 87.3% **Men** 12.7% **Part-time** 31%
Graduate Enrollment 197 **Women** 86.8% **Men** 13.2% **Part-time** 100%
Distance Learning Courses Available.
Nursing Student Activities Nursing Honor Society, Sigma Theta Tau, Student Nurses' Association.
Nursing Student Resources Academic advising; academic or career counseling; assistance for students with disabilities; bookstore; campus computer network; career placement assistance; computer lab; computer-assisted instruction; e-mail services; employment services for current students; externships; housing assistance; interactive nursing skills videos; Internet; learning resource lab; library services; nursing audiovisuals; paid internships; placement services for program completers; remedial services; resume preparation assistance; skills, simulation, or other laboratory; tutoring; unpaid internships.

BACCALAUREATE PROGRAMS

Degree BSN
Available Programs Baccalaureate for Second Degree; Generic Baccalaureate; RN Baccalaureate.
Study Options Full-time and part-time.
Online Degree Options Yes.
Program Entrance Requirements Minimum overall college GPA of 3.0, transcript of college record, written essay, health exam, health insurance, high school biology, high school chemistry, 2 years high school math, 2 years high school science, high school transcript, immunizations, 2 letters of recommendation, minimum high school GPA of 3.0, minimum GPA in nursing prerequisites of 2.0, prerequisite course work. Transfer students are accepted. *Application deadline:* 5/1 (fall), 11/1 (spring). Applications may be processed on a rolling basis for some programs. *Application fee:* $30.
Advanced Placement Credit given for nursing courses completed elsewhere dependent upon specific evaluations.

Expenses (2015–16) *Tuition:* full-time $28,970; part-time $930 per credit hour. *Room and board:* $12,130; room only: $5760 per academic year. *Required fees:* full-time $864.
Financial Aid 84% of baccalaureate students in nursing programs received some form of financial aid in 2014–15.
Contact Enrollment Services, School of Nursing and Health Sciences, Robert Morris University, 6001 University Boulevard, Moon Township, PA 15108-1189. *Telephone:* 412-397-5200. *Fax:* 412-397-2425. *E-mail:* admissionsoffice@rmu.edu.

GRADUATE PROGRAMS

Expenses (2015–16) *Tuition:* part-time $495 per credit hour. *Required fees:* part-time $420 per term.
Financial Aid 26% of graduate students in nursing programs received some form of financial aid in 2014–15. Federal Work-Study, institutionally sponsored loans, and unspecified assistantships available. *Financial aid application deadline:* 5/1.
Contact Office of Graduate Admissions, School of Nursing and Health Sciences, Robert Morris University, 6001 University Boulevard, Moon Township, PA 15108-1189. *Telephone:* 800-762-0097. *Fax:* 412-397-2425. *E-mail:* GraduateAdmissions@rmu.edu.

MASTER'S DEGREE PROGRAM

Degree MSN
Available Programs Master's; RN to Master's.
Concentrations Available Nursing education.
Study Options Part-time.
Online Degree Options Yes.
Program Entrance Requirements Clinical experience, minimum overall college GPA of 3.25, transcript of college record, CPR certification, written essay, interview, 2 letters of recommendation, resume, statistics course. *Application deadline:* 5/1 (fall). Applications may be processed on a rolling basis for some programs. *Application fee:* $35.
Degree Requirements 36 total credit hours, thesis or project.

DOCTORAL DEGREE PROGRAM

Degree DNP
Available Programs Doctorate; Post-Baccalaureate Doctorate.
Areas of Study Advanced practice nursing.
Program Entrance Requirements Clinical experience, minimum overall college GPA of 3.25, interview by faculty committee, 2 letters of recommendation, vita, writing sample. Application deadline: 5/1 (fall). Applications may be processed on a rolling basis for some programs. Application fee: $35.
Degree Requirements 86 total credit hours.

Saint Francis University
Department of Nursing
Loretto, Pennsylvania

http://www.francis.edu/nursing/
Founded in 1847
DEGREE • BSN
Nursing Program Faculty 7 (1% with doctorates).
Baccalaureate Enrollment 85 **Women** 90% **Men** 10%
Nursing Student Activities Student Nurses' Association, nursing club.
Nursing Student Resources Academic advising; academic or career counseling; assistance for students with disabilities; bookstore; campus computer network; career placement assistance; computer lab; computer-assisted instruction; e-mail services; employment services for current students; externships; interactive nursing skills videos; Internet; learning resource lab; library services; nursing audiovisuals; resume preparation assistance; skills, simulation, or other laboratory; tutoring.
Library Facilities 150,000 volumes in health, 120,000 volumes in nursing; 25 periodical subscriptions health-care related.

BACCALAUREATE PROGRAMS

Degree BSN
Available Programs Generic Baccalaureate.
Study Options Full-time and part-time.
Program Entrance Requirements Transcript of college record, high school biology, high school chemistry, 2 years high school math, 2 years high school science, high school transcript, minimum high school GPA of 3.0, minimum high school rank 50%, minimum GPA in nursing prerequisites of 2.7, prerequisite course work. Transfer students are accepted.

Application deadline: Applications may be processed on a rolling basis for some programs. *Application fee:* $30.
Advanced Placement Credit by examination available. Credit given for nursing courses completed elsewhere dependent upon specific evaluations.
Contact *Telephone:* 814-472-3027. *Fax:* 814-472-3849.

Slippery Rock University of Pennsylvania
Department of Nursing
Slippery Rock, Pennsylvania

http://www.sru.edu/academics/colleges/ches/nursing/Pages/Welcome.aspx
Founded in 1889
DEGREE • BSN
Nursing Program Faculty 7 (100% with doctorates).
Baccalaureate Enrollment 230 **Women** 95% **Men** 5% **Part-time** 97%
Distance Learning Courses Available.
Nursing Student Activities Sigma Theta Tau.
Nursing Student Resources Academic advising; academic or career counseling; assistance for students with disabilities; bookstore; campus computer network; career placement assistance; computer lab; computer-assisted instruction; daycare for children of students; e-mail services; employment services for current students; housing assistance; Internet; library services; nursing audiovisuals; placement services for program completers; resume preparation assistance; tutoring.
Library Facilities 7,214 volumes in health, 925 volumes in nursing; 1,299 periodical subscriptions health-care related.

BACCALAUREATE PROGRAMS

Degree BSN
Available Programs ADN to Baccalaureate; RN Baccalaureate.
Study Options Full-time and part-time.
Online Degree Options Yes (online only).
Program Entrance Requirements Minimum overall college GPA of 2.5, transcript of college record, minimum GPA in nursing prerequisites of 2.5, professional liability insurance/malpractice insurance, RN licensure. Transfer students are accepted. *Application deadline:* Applications may be processed on a rolling basis for some programs. *Application fee:* $30.
Advanced Placement Credit by examination available. Credit given for nursing courses completed elsewhere dependent upon specific evaluations.
Contact *Telephone:* 724-738-4921. *Fax:* 724-738-2509.

Temple University
Department of Nursing
Philadelphia, Pennsylvania

http://www.temple.edu/nursing
Founded in 1884
DEGREES • BSN • DNP • MSN
Nursing Program Faculty 37 (50% with doctorates).
Baccalaureate Enrollment 400 **Women** 85% **Men** 15% **Part-time** 62%
Graduate Enrollment 120 **Women** 95% **Men** 5% **Part-time** 100%
Distance Learning Courses Available.
Nursing Student Activities Nursing Honor Society, Sigma Theta Tau, Student Nurses' Association, nursing club.
Nursing Student Resources Academic advising; academic or career counseling; assistance for students with disabilities; bookstore; campus computer network; career placement assistance; computer lab; computer-assisted instruction; e-mail services; externships; housing assistance; interactive nursing skills videos; Internet; learning resource lab; library services; nursing audiovisuals; remedial services; resume preparation assistance; skills, simulation, or other laboratory; tutoring.
Library Facilities 60,374 volumes in health, 1,350 volumes in nursing; 1,350 periodical subscriptions health-care related.

BACCALAUREATE PROGRAMS

Degree BSN
Available Programs Generic Baccalaureate; RN Baccalaureate.

Study Options Full-time.
Program Entrance Requirements Minimum overall college GPA of 3.0, transcript of college record, CPR certification, written essay, health exam, health insurance, high school biology, high school chemistry, high school foreign language, 3 years high school math, 3 years high school science, high school transcript, immunizations, interview, minimum high school GPA of 3.0, minimum GPA in nursing prerequisites of 3.0, prerequisite course work. Transfer students are accepted. *Application deadline:* 2/15 (fall). *Application fee:* $50.
Advanced Placement Credit given for nursing courses completed elsewhere dependent upon specific evaluations.
Contact *Telephone:* 215-707-4618. *Fax:* 215-707-1599.

GRADUATE PROGRAMS

Contact *Telephone:* 215-707-3789. *Fax:* 215-707-1599.

MASTER'S DEGREE PROGRAM
Degree MSN
Available Programs Master's.
Concentrations Available Nursing education. *Clinical nurse specialist programs in:* psychiatric/mental health. *Nurse practitioner programs in:* adult health, family health, pediatric.
Study Options Full-time and part-time.
Program Entrance Requirements Clinical experience, minimum overall college GPA of 3.0, transcript of college record, CPR certification, written essay, immunizations, interview, 2 letters of recommendation, nursing research course, physical assessment course, professional liability insurance/malpractice insurance, statistics course, GRE General Test or MAT.
Advanced Placement Credit given for nursing courses completed elsewhere dependent upon specific evaluations.
Degree Requirements 36 total credit hours.

POST-MASTER'S PROGRAM
Areas of Study Nursing education. *Clinical nurse specialist programs in:* psychiatric/mental health. *Nurse practitioner programs in:* adult health, family health, pediatric.

DOCTORAL DEGREE PROGRAM
Degree DNP
Available Programs Doctorate.
Program Entrance Requirements GRE General Test or MAT.

Thomas Jefferson University
Department of Nursing
Philadelphia, Pennsylvania

http://www.tju.edu/
Founded in 1824
DEGREES • BSN • DNP • MSN
Nursing Program Faculty 38 (42% with doctorates).
Nursing Student Activities Nursing Honor Society, Sigma Theta Tau, Student Nurses' Association.
Nursing Student Resources Academic advising; academic or career counseling; assistance for students with disabilities; bookstore; campus computer network; career placement assistance; computer lab; computer-assisted instruction; e-mail services; interactive nursing skills videos; Internet; learning resource lab; library services; nursing audiovisuals; paid internships; placement services for program completers; remedial services; resume preparation assistance; skills, simulation, or other laboratory; tutoring.
Library Facilities 146,000 volumes in health, 4,700 volumes in nursing; 2,100 periodical subscriptions health-care related.

BACCALAUREATE PROGRAMS

Degree BSN
Available Programs ADN to Baccalaureate; Accelerated Baccalaureate; Accelerated Baccalaureate for Second Degree; Accelerated RN Baccalaureate; Baccalaureate for Second Degree; Generic Baccalaureate; RN Baccalaureate.
Site Options Atlantic City, NJ; Philadelphia, PA.
Study Options Full-time and part-time.
Program Entrance Requirements Minimum overall college GPA of 2.9, transcript of college record, CPR certification, written essay, health exam, health insurance, high school transcript, immunizations, 2 letters

of recommendation, prerequisite course work. Transfer students are accepted.

Advanced Placement Credit by examination available. Credit given for nursing courses completed elsewhere dependent upon specific evaluations.

Contact *Telephone:* 215-503-8104. *Fax:* 215-503-0376.

GRADUATE PROGRAMS

Contact *Telephone:* 215-503-8057. *Fax:* 215-932-1468.

MASTER'S DEGREE PROGRAM

Degree MSN

Available Programs Accelerated Master's; Accelerated RN to Master's; Master's; Master's for Non-Nursing College Graduates; Master's for Nurses with Non-Nursing Degrees; RN to Master's.

Concentrations Available Nurse anesthesia; nursing education; nursing informatics. *Clinical nurse specialist programs in:* acute care, adult health, community health, critical care, home health care, medical-surgical, oncology, pediatric, public health. *Nurse practitioner programs in:* acute care, adult health, family health, neonatal health, oncology, pediatric.

Site Options Philadelphia, PA.

Study Options Full-time and part-time.

Program Entrance Requirements Clinical experience, computer literacy, minimum overall college GPA of 3.0, transcript of college record, CPR certification, written essay, interview, 3 letters of recommendation, nursing research course, physical assessment course, professional liability insurance/malpractice insurance, resume, statistics course.

Advanced Placement Credit given for nursing courses completed elsewhere dependent upon specific evaluations.

Degree Requirements 36 total credit hours.

POST-MASTER'S PROGRAM

Areas of Study Nursing education; nursing informatics. *Nurse practitioner programs in:* acute care, adult health, family health, neonatal health, oncology, pediatric.

DOCTORAL DEGREE PROGRAM

Degree DNP

Available Programs Doctorate.

Areas of Study Advanced practice nursing, clinical practice, individualized study.

Program Entrance Requirements Clinical experience, minimum overall college GPA of 3.2, interview by faculty committee, interview, 3 letters of recommendation, MSN or equivalent, scholarly papers, statistics course, vita, writing sample.

Degree Requirements 36 total credit hours, written exam, residency.

CONTINUING EDUCATION PROGRAM

Contact *Telephone:* 215-503-8057. *Fax:* 215-503-0376.

University of Pennsylvania
School of Nursing
Philadelphia, Pennsylvania

http://www.nursing.upenn.edu
Founded in 1740

DEGREES • BSN • MSN • MSN/MBA • MSN/MPH • MSN/PHD • PHD

Nursing Program Faculty 339 (21% with doctorates).
Baccalaureate Enrollment 587 **Women** 90% **Men** 10% **Part-time** 1%
Graduate Enrollment 584 **Women** 90% **Men** 10% **Part-time** 64%
Nursing Student Activities Nursing Honor Society, Sigma Theta Tau, Student Nurses' Association.
Nursing Student Resources Academic advising; academic or career counseling; assistance for students with disabilities; bookstore; campus computer network; career placement assistance; computer lab; computer-assisted instruction; daycare for children of students; e-mail services; employment services for current students; externships; housing assistance; interactive nursing skills videos; Internet; learning resource lab; library services; nursing audiovisuals; other; paid internships; placement services for program completers; remedial services; resume preparation assistance; skills, simulation, or other laboratory; tutoring; unpaid internships.

BACCALAUREATE PROGRAMS

Degree BSN

Available Programs Accelerated Baccalaureate; Accelerated Baccalaureate for Second Degree; Baccalaureate for Second Degree; Generic Baccalaureate.

Study Options Full-time.

Program Entrance Requirements Minimum overall college GPA of 3.0, transcript of college record, written essay, health exam, health insurance, high school biology, high school chemistry, high school foreign language, 4 years high school math, 4 years high school science, high school transcript, immunizations, interview, 2 letters of recommendation, minimum high school GPA of 3.0, minimum high school rank 10%. Transfer students are accepted. *Application deadline:* 1/1 (fall). *Application fee:* $80.

Advanced Placement Credit given for nursing courses completed elsewhere dependent upon specific evaluations.

Expenses (2015–16) *Tuition:* full-time $43,838; part-time $5596 per course. *International tuition:* $43,838 full-time. *Room and board:* $13,900; room only: $9060 per academic year. *Required fees:* full-time $5689; part-time $604 per credit.

Contact Office of Enrollment Management, School of Nursing, University of Pennsylvania, 418 Curie Boulevard, Philadelphia, PA 19104-4217. *Telephone:* 215-898-4271. *Fax:* 215-573-8439. *E-mail:* admissions@nursing.upenn.edu.

GRADUATE PROGRAMS

Expenses (2015–16) *Tuition:* full-time $38,060; part-time $4784 per course. *International tuition:* $38,060 full-time. *Room and board:* $18,310; room only: $13,065 per academic year. *Required fees:* full-time $3966; part-time $432 per credit.

Financial Aid Fellowships, research assistantships, teaching assistantships, institutionally sponsored loans, scholarships, traineeships, and unspecified assistantships available.

Contact Carol Ladden, Director, Graduate Enrollment, School of Nursing, University of Pennsylvania, 418 Curie Boulevard, Philadelphia, PA 19104-4217. *Telephone:* 215-898-4271. *Fax:* 215-573-8439. *E-mail:* admissions@nursing.upenn.edu.

MASTER'S DEGREE PROGRAM

Degrees MSN; MSN/MBA; MSN/MPH; MSN/PhD

Available Programs Accelerated Master's for Non-Nursing College Graduates; Accelerated Master's for Nurses with Non-Nursing Degrees; Master's.

Concentrations Available Health-care administration; nurse anesthesia; nurse-midwifery; nursing administration. *Clinical nurse specialist programs in:* acute care, adult health, pediatric. *Nurse practitioner programs in:* acute care, adult health, adult-gerontology acute care, family health, gerontology, neonatal health, pediatric, primary care, psychiatric/mental health, women's health.

Study Options Full-time and part-time.

Program Entrance Requirements Clinical experience, computer literacy, minimum overall college GPA of 3.0, transcript of college record, CPR certification, written essay, immunizations, interview, 3 letters of recommendation, prerequisite course work, resume, statistics course, GRE General Test. *Application deadline:* Please refer to website for specific program deadlines. *Application fee:* $80.

Advanced Placement Credit given for nursing courses completed elsewhere dependent upon specific evaluations.

Degree Requirements 36 total credit hours.

POST-MASTER'S PROGRAM

Areas of Study Health-care administration; nurse anesthesia; nurse-midwifery; nursing administration; nursing education. *Clinical nurse specialist programs in:* acute care, adult health, maternity-newborn, medical-surgical, pediatric. *Nurse practitioner programs in:* acute care, adult health, adult-gerontology acute care, family health, gerontology, neonatal health, oncology, pediatric, primary care, psychiatric/mental health, women's health.

DOCTORAL DEGREE PROGRAM

Degree PhD

Available Programs Doctorate; Post-Baccalaureate Doctorate.

Areas of Study Addiction/substance abuse, aging, bio-behavioral research, biology of health and illness, clinical practice, community health, critical care, ethics, faculty preparation, family health, gerontology, health policy, health promotion/disease prevention, health-care systems, human health and illness, illness and transition, individualized study, information systems, maternity-newborn, neuro-behavior, nursing administration, nursing policy, nursing research, nursing science, oncology, palliative care, urban health, women's health.

Program Entrance Requirements Minimum overall college GPA of 3.5, interview by faculty committee, interview, 3 letters of recommendation, MSN or equivalent, statistics course, vita, writing sample, GRE General Test. Application deadline: 12/1 (fall). Application fee: $80.

Degree Requirements 42 total credit hours, dissertation, oral exam, written exam, residency.

POSTDOCTORAL PROGRAM

Areas of Study Adolescent health, aging, chronic illness, community health, family health, gerontology, health promotion/disease prevention, individualized study, nursing interventions, nursing research, nursing science, outcomes, self-care, vulnerable population, women's health.

Postdoctoral Program Contact Dr. Abigail Cohen, Assistant Dean for Nursing Research, School of Nursing, University of Pennsylvania, 418 Curie Boulevard, Claire M. Fagin Hall, 4th Floor, Philadelphia, PA 19104-4271. *Telephone:* 215-898-8523. *Fax:* 215-898-3056. *E-mail:* research@nursing.upenn.edu.

University of Pittsburgh
School of Nursing
Pittsburgh, Pennsylvania

http://www.nursing.pitt.edu/
Founded in 1787

DEGREES • BSN • MSN • PHD

Nursing Program Faculty 120 (78% with doctorates).

Baccalaureate Enrollment 547 **Women** 91% **Men** 9% **Part-time** 1.7%

Graduate Enrollment 382 **Women** 81% **Men** 19% **Part-time** 42%

Distance Learning Courses Available.

Nursing Student Activities Nursing Honor Society, Sigma Theta Tau, Student Nurses' Association.

Nursing Student Resources Academic advising; academic or career counseling; assistance for students with disabilities; bookstore; campus computer network; career placement assistance; computer lab; computer-assisted instruction; daycare for children of students; e-mail services; employment services for current students; externships; housing assistance; interactive nursing skills videos; Internet; learning resource lab; library services; nursing audiovisuals; other; paid internships; placement services for program completers; remedial services; resume preparation assistance; skills, simulation, or other laboratory; tutoring.

Library Facilities 149,631 volumes in health, 7,641 volumes in nursing; 6,138 periodical subscriptions health-care related.

BACCALAUREATE PROGRAMS

Degree BSN

Available Programs Accelerated Baccalaureate for Second Degree; Generic Baccalaureate; RN Baccalaureate.

Site Options Johnstown, PA.

Study Options Full-time.

Program Entrance Requirements Minimum overall college GPA of 3.0, transcript of college record, written essay, health exam, health insurance, high school biology, high school chemistry, 4 years high school math, 3 years high school science, high school transcript, immunizations, 1 letter of recommendation, minimum high school GPA of 3.3, minimum GPA in nursing prerequisites of 3.0. Transfer students are accepted. *Application fee:* $45.

Advanced Placement Credit by examination available.

Expenses (2015–16) *Tuition, state resident:* full-time $21,770; part-time $907 per credit. *Tuition, nonresident:* full-time $35,662; part-time $1485 per credit. *International tuition:* $35,662 full-time. *Required fees:* full-time $924; part-time $294 per term.

Financial Aid 75% of baccalaureate students in nursing programs received some form of financial aid in 2014–15. *Gift aid (need-based):* Federal Pell, FSEOG, state, private, college/university gift aid from institutional funds, Federal Nursing. *Loans:* Federal Nursing Student Loans, Federal Direct (Subsidized and Unsubsidized Stafford PLUS), Perkins, state, college/university. *Work-study:* Federal Work-Study. *Financial aid application deadline (priority):* 3/1.

Contact Mrs. Suzanne Brody, Associate Director of Student Services Recruitment, School of Nursing, University of Pittsburgh, 239 Victoria Building, 3500 Victoria Street, Pittsburgh, PA 15261. *Telephone:* 412-624-1291. *Fax:* 412-624-2409. *E-mail:* brodys@pitt.edu.

GRADUATE PROGRAMS

Expenses (2015–16) *Tuition, state resident:* full-time $37,392; part-time $1016 per credit. *Tuition, nonresident:* full-time $43,290; part-time $1179 per credit. *International tuition:* $43,290 full-time. *Required fees:* full-time $1236; part-time $217 per term.

Financial Aid 83% of graduate students in nursing programs received some form of financial aid in 2014–15. 37 fellowships with full and partial tuition reimbursements available (averaging $15,529 per year), 12 research assistantships with full and partial tuition reimbursements available (averaging $13,346 per year), 14 teaching assistantships with full and partial tuition reimbursements available (averaging $14,707 per year) were awarded; scholarships, traineeships, and unspecified assistantships also available. Aid available to part-time students. *Financial aid application deadline:* 7/1.

Contact Mrs. Suzanne Brody, Associate Director of Student Services Recruitment, School of Nursing, University of Pittsburgh, 239 Victoria Building, 3500 Victoria Street, Pittsburgh, PA 15261. *Telephone:* 412-624-1291. *Fax:* 412-624-2409. *E-mail:* brodys@pitt.edu.

MASTER'S DEGREE PROGRAM

Degree MSN

Available Programs Master's; RN to Master's.

Concentrations Available Clinical nurse leader; nurse anesthesia; nursing administration; nursing informatics. *Nurse practitioner programs in:* neonatal health.

Site Options Johnstown, PA; Greensburg, PA; Bradford, PA.

Study Options Full-time and part-time.

Online Degree Options Yes.

Program Entrance Requirements Clinical experience, minimum overall college GPA of 3.0, transcript of college record, CPR certification, written essay, immunizations, interview, 3 letters of recommendation, professional liability insurance/malpractice insurance, resume, statistics course, GRE or MAT. *Application fee:* $50.

Advanced Placement Credit by examination available. Credit given for nursing courses completed elsewhere dependent upon specific evaluations.

Degree Requirements 42 total credit hours, comprehensive exam.

POST-MASTER'S PROGRAM

Areas of Study Nursing education; nursing informatics. *Nurse practitioner programs in:* adult-gerontology acute care, neonatal health, psychiatric/mental health, school health.

DOCTORAL DEGREE PROGRAM

Degree PhD

Available Programs Doctorate; Post-Baccalaureate Doctorate.

Areas of Study Nursing research, nursing science.

Program Entrance Requirements Minimum overall college GPA of 3.5, interview by faculty committee, interview, 3 letters of recommendation, MSN or equivalent, statistics course, vita, writing sample, GRE. Application fee: $50.

Degree Requirements 64 total credit hours, dissertation.

POSTDOCTORAL PROGRAM

Areas of Study Nursing research, nursing science.

Postdoctoral Program Contact Dr. Catherine Bender, Professor, PhD Program Director, School of Nursing, University of Pittsburgh, 3500 Victoria Street, Pittsburgh, PA 15261. *Telephone:* 412-624-3594. *Fax:* 412-383-7293. *E-mail:* cbe100@pitt.edu.

CONTINUING EDUCATION PROGRAM

Contact Mrs. Mary Rodgers Schubert, Director Continuing Nursing Education, School of Nursing, University of Pittsburgh, 225 Victoria Building, 3500 Victoria Street, Pittsburgh, PA 15261. *Telephone:* 412-624-9079. *Fax:* 412-624-1215. *E-mail:* mschuber@pitt.edu; conted@pitt.edu.

University of Pittsburgh at Bradford

Department of Nursing
Bradford, Pennsylvania

http://www.upb.pitt.edu/
Founded in 1963

DEGREE • BSN

Nursing Program Faculty 10 (30% with doctorates).
Baccalaureate Enrollment 15 **Women** 80% **Men** 20% **Part-time** 13%
Distance Learning Courses Available.
Nursing Student Activities Nursing club.
Nursing Student Resources Academic advising; academic or career counseling; assistance for students with disabilities; bookstore; campus computer network; career placement assistance; computer lab; computer-assisted instruction; e-mail services; employment services for current students; externships; housing assistance; Internet; learning resource lab; library services; nursing audiovisuals; remedial services; resume preparation assistance; skills, simulation, or other laboratory; tutoring; unpaid internships.
Library Facilities 737 volumes in health, 568 volumes in nursing; 13 periodical subscriptions health-care related.

BACCALAUREATE PROGRAMS

Degree BSN
Available Programs Generic Baccalaureate; RN Baccalaureate.
Study Options Full-time and part-time.
Program Entrance Requirements Transcript of college record, CPR certification, health exam, health insurance, high school transcript, immunizations, minimum high school GPA of 2.5, minimum GPA in nursing prerequisites of 2.5, professional liability insurance/malpractice insurance, prerequisite course work, RN licensure. Transfer students are accepted. *Application deadline:* Applications may be processed on a rolling basis for some programs. *Application fee:* $45.
Advanced Placement Credit by examination available. Credit given for nursing courses completed elsewhere dependent upon specific evaluations.
Expenses (2015–16) *Tuition, state resident:* full-time $15,952; part-time $664 per credit. *Tuition, nonresident:* full-time $29,672; part-time $1236 per credit. *International tuition:* $29,672 full-time. *Room and board:* $9380; room only: $5228 per academic year. *Required fees:* full-time $932; part-time $161 per term.
Financial Aid 100% of baccalaureate students in nursing programs received some form of financial aid in 2014–15.
Contact Mr. Alexander Nazemetz, Nursing Admissions, Department of Nursing, University of Pittsburgh at Bradford, 300 Campus Drive, Bradford, PA 16701. *Telephone:* 800-872-1787. *Fax:* 814-362-5150. *E-mail:* nazemetz@pitt.edu.

The University of Scranton

Department of Nursing
Scranton, Pennsylvania

http://www.scranton.edu/academics/pcps/nursing/index.shtml
Founded in 1888

DEGREES • BSN • MSN

Nursing Program Faculty 58 (69% with doctorates).
Baccalaureate Enrollment 310 **Women** 91% **Men** 9% **Part-time** 1%
Graduate Enrollment 79 **Women** 85% **Men** 15% **Part-time** 50%
Nursing Student Activities Nursing Honor Society, Sigma Theta Tau, Student Nurses' Association, nursing club.
Nursing Student Resources Academic advising; academic or career counseling; bookstore; campus computer network; career placement assistance; computer lab; computer-assisted instruction; e-mail services; employment services for current students; interactive nursing skills videos; Internet; learning resource lab; library services; nursing audiovisuals; placement services for program completers; remedial services; resume preparation assistance; skills, simulation, or other laboratory; tutoring.

Library Facilities 28,400 volumes in health, 8,484 volumes in nursing; 106 periodical subscriptions health-care related.

BACCALAUREATE PROGRAMS

Degree BSN
Available Programs Baccalaureate for Second Degree; Generic Baccalaureate; LPN to RN Baccalaureate; RN Baccalaureate.
Study Options Full-time and part-time.
Program Entrance Requirements Minimum overall college GPA of 2.5, transcript of college record, written essay, health exam, health insurance, high school biology, high school chemistry, high school foreign language, 3 years high school math, 3 years high school science, high school transcript, immunizations, minimum high school GPA of 3.2, minimum high school rank 30%, minimum GPA in nursing prerequisites of 2.7. Transfer students are accepted. *Application deadline:* 3/1 (fall). Applications may be processed on a rolling basis for some programs. *Application fee:* $200.
Advanced Placement Credit by examination available. Credit given for nursing courses completed elsewhere dependent upon specific evaluations.
Expenses (2014–15) *Tuition:* full-time $39,556; part-time $1017 per credit. *Room and board:* $14,022; room only: $8410 per academic year. *Required fees:* full-time $1000.
Financial Aid 80% of baccalaureate students in nursing programs received some form of financial aid in 2013–14. *Gift aid (need-based):* Federal Pell, FSEOG, state, private, college/university gift aid from institutional funds. *Loans:* Federal Direct (Subsidized and Unsubsidized Stafford PLUS), Perkins. *Work-study:* Federal Work-Study, part-time campus jobs. *Financial aid application deadline (priority):* 2/15.
Contact Dr. Dona Carpenter, Chairperson, Department of Nursing, The University of Scranton, 800 Linden Street, McGurrin Hall, Scranton, PA 18510-4595. *Telephone:* 570-941-4195. *Fax:* 570-941-7903. *E-mail:* dona.carpenter@scranton.edu.

GRADUATE PROGRAMS

Expenses (2014–15) *Tuition:* part-time $940 per credit hour. *Room and board:* $8926; room only: $7536 per academic year.
Financial Aid 90% of graduate students in nursing programs received some form of financial aid in 2013–14. 6 teaching assistantships with full and partial tuition reimbursements available (averaging $6,600 per year) were awarded; career-related internships or fieldwork, Federal Work-Study, and unspecified assistantships also available. Aid available to part-time students. *Financial aid application deadline:* 3/1.
Contact Dr. Mary Jane Hanson, Director, Graduate Nursing Program, Department of Nursing, The University of Scranton, 800 Linden Street, McGurrin Hall, Scranton, PA 18510-4595. *Telephone:* 570-941-4060. *Fax:* 570-941-7903. *E-mail:* maryjane.hanson@scranton.edu.

MASTER'S DEGREE PROGRAM

Degree MSN
Available Programs Accelerated AD/RN to Master's; Accelerated RN to Master's; Master's; RN to Master's.
Concentrations Available Nurse anesthesia; nursing education. *Clinical nurse specialist programs in:* adult health. *Nurse practitioner programs in:* family health.
Study Options Full-time and part-time.
Program Entrance Requirements Clinical experience, minimum overall college GPA of 3.0, transcript of college record, CPR certification, written essay, immunizations, interview, 3 letters of recommendation, nursing research course, physical assessment course, professional liability insurance/malpractice insurance, prerequisite course work, statistics course. *Application deadline:* 8/1 (fall), 1/1 (spring). Applications may be processed on a rolling basis for some programs. *Application fee:* $50.
Advanced Placement Credit given for nursing courses completed elsewhere dependent upon specific evaluations.
Degree Requirements 46 total credit hours, comprehensive exam.

POST-MASTER'S PROGRAM

Areas of Study Nurse anesthesia; nursing education. *Clinical nurse specialist programs in:* adult health. *Nurse practitioner programs in:* family health.

Villanova University
College of Nursing
Villanova, Pennsylvania

http://www.nursing.villanova.edu/
Founded in 1842

DEGREES • BSN • DNP • MSN • PHD

Nursing Program Faculty 105 (71% with doctorates).
Baccalaureate Enrollment 777 **Women** 91.5% **Men** 8.5% **Part-time** 21%
Graduate Enrollment 324 **Women** 91% **Men** 9% **Part-time** 39%
Distance Learning Courses Available.
Nursing Student Activities Nursing Honor Society, Sigma Theta Tau, Student Nurses' Association, nursing club.
Nursing Student Resources Academic advising; academic or career counseling; assistance for students with disabilities; bookstore; campus computer network; career placement assistance; computer lab; computer-assisted instruction; e-mail services; employment services for current students; housing assistance; interactive nursing skills videos; Internet; learning resource lab; library services; nursing audiovisuals; remedial services; resume preparation assistance; skills, simulation, or other laboratory; tutoring.
Library Facilities 15,235 volumes in health, 1,806 volumes in nursing; 1,586 periodical subscriptions health-care related.

BACCALAUREATE PROGRAMS

Degree BSN

Available Programs ADN to Baccalaureate; Accelerated Baccalaureate for Second Degree; Accelerated RN Baccalaureate; Baccalaureate for Second Degree; Generic Baccalaureate; International Nurse to Baccalaureate; RN Baccalaureate.
Study Options Full-time and part-time.
Program Entrance Requirements Minimum overall college GPA of 3.0, transcript of college record, CPR certification, written essay, health exam, health insurance, high school biology, high school chemistry, high school foreign language, 3 years high school math, 3 years high school science, high school transcript, immunizations, 2 letters of recommendation, minimum high school GPA of 3.0, minimum GPA in nursing prerequisites. Transfer students are accepted. *Application deadline:* 11/1 (fall), 1/15 (winter). *Application fee:* $80.
Advanced Placement Credit given for nursing courses completed elsewhere dependent upon specific evaluations.
Expenses (2015–16) *Tuition:* full-time $46,966; part-time $1960 per credit. *International tuition:* $46,966 full-time. *Room and board:* $12,707; room only: $6737 per academic year. *Required fees:* full-time $650; part-time $150 per credit; part-time $325 per term.
Financial Aid 61% of baccalaureate students in nursing programs received some form of financial aid in 2014–15. *Gift aid (need-based):* Federal Pell, FSEOG, state, private, college/university gift aid from institutional funds, endowed and restricted scholarships and grants. *Loans:* Federal Nursing Student Loans, Federal Direct (Subsidized and Unsubsidized Stafford PLUS), Perkins, alternative loans. *Work-study:* Federal Work-Study, part-time campus jobs. *Financial aid application deadline:* 2/7.
Contact Dr. Angelina A. Arcamone, Assistant Dean and Director, Undergraduate Program, College of Nursing, Villanova University, Driscoll Hall, 800 Lancaster Avenue, Villanova, PA 19085-1690. *Telephone:* 610-519-4926. *Fax:* 610-519-7650. *E-mail:* angelina.arcamone@villanova.edu.

GRADUATE PROGRAMS

Expenses (2015–16) *Tuition:* full-time $15,066; part-time $837 per credit. *International tuition:* $15,066 full-time. *Required fees:* part-time $50 per term.
Financial Aid 49% of graduate students in nursing programs received some form of financial aid in 2014–15. 5 teaching assistantships with full tuition reimbursements available (averaging $15,475 per year) were awarded; institutionally sponsored loans, scholarships, traineeships, tuition waivers (full), and unspecified assistantships also available. *Financial aid application deadline:* 7/1.
Contact Dr. Marguerite K. Schlag, Assistant Dean and Director, Graduate Program, College of Nursing, Villanova University, Driscoll Hall, 800 Lancaster Avenue, Villanova, PA 19085-1690. *Telephone:* 610-519-4934. *Fax:* 610-519-7997. *E-mail:* marguerite.schlag@villanova.edu.

MASTER'S DEGREE PROGRAM
Degree MSN
Available Programs Master's.
Concentrations Available Nurse anesthesia; nursing education. *Nurse practitioner programs in:* adult health, family health, pediatric.
Site Options Philadelphia, PA; Chester, PA.
Study Options Full-time and part-time.
Program Entrance Requirements Clinical experience, computer literacy, minimum overall college GPA of 3.0, transcript of college record, CPR certification, written essay, immunizations, 3 letters of recommendation, nursing research course, physical assessment course, professional liability insurance/malpractice insurance, resume, statistics course, GRE or MAT. *Application deadline:* 7/1 (fall), 11/1 (spring), 4/1 (summer). Applications may be processed on a rolling basis for some programs. *Application fee:* $50.
Advanced Placement Credit given for nursing courses completed elsewhere dependent upon specific evaluations.
Degree Requirements 45 total credit hours, thesis or project.

POST-MASTER'S PROGRAM
Areas of Study Nurse anesthesia; nursing education. *Nurse practitioner programs in:* adult health, family health, pediatric.

DOCTORAL DEGREE PROGRAM
Degree DNP
Available Programs Doctorate.
Areas of Study Advanced practice nursing, health policy, nursing administration.
Program Entrance Requirements Minimum overall college GPA of 3.5, clinical experience, interview, 3 letters of recommendation, MSN or equivalent, statistics course, vita, writing sample. *Application deadline:* Applications are processed on a rolling basis. *Application fee:* $70.
Degree Requirements 35 total credit hours, Capstone project, written exam.

Degree PhD
Available Programs Doctorate.
Areas of Study Faculty preparation, nursing education, nursing research.
Program Entrance Requirements Clinical experience, minimum overall college GPA of 3.5, interview, 3 letters of recommendation, MSN or equivalent, scholarly papers, vita, writing sample, GRE. *Application deadline:* 12/1 (fall), 12/1 (summer). *Application fee:* $70.
Degree Requirements 51 total credit hours, dissertation, oral exam, written exam.

CONTINUING EDUCATION PROGRAM

Contact Dr. Lynore DeSilets, Assistant Dean and Director, Continuing Education, College of Nursing, Villanova University, Driscoll Hall, 800 Lancaster Avenue, Villanova, PA 19085-1690. *Telephone:* 610-519-4931. *Fax:* 610-519-6780. *E-mail:* lyn.desilets@villanova.edu.

Waynesburg University
Department of Nursing
Waynesburg, Pennsylvania

http://www.waynesburg.edu/
Founded in 1849

DEGREES • BSN • DNP • MSN • MSN/MBA

Nursing Program Faculty 48 (39% with doctorates).
Baccalaureate Enrollment 337 **Women** 91% **Men** 9%
Graduate Enrollment 240 **Women** 95% **Men** 5% **Part-time** 95%
Nursing Student Activities Sigma Theta Tau, Student Nurses' Association.
Nursing Student Resources Academic advising; academic or career counseling; assistance for students with disabilities; bookstore; campus computer network; career placement assistance; computer lab; computer-assisted instruction; e-mail services; employment services for current students; externships; Internet; learning resource lab; library services; nursing audiovisuals; paid internships; placement services for program completers; remedial services; resume preparation assistance; skills, simulation, or other laboratory; tutoring.
Library Facilities 4,500 volumes in nursing; 46 periodical subscriptions health-care related.

BACCALAUREATE PROGRAMS

Degree BSN

Available Programs Accelerated Baccalaureate; Accelerated Baccalaureate for Second Degree; Generic Baccalaureate; LPN to Baccalaureate.
Site Options Monroeville, PA; Canonsburg, PA; Wexford, PA.
Study Options Full-time.
Program Entrance Requirements Minimum overall college GPA of 3.0, transcript of college record, CPR certification, health exam, health insurance, high school biology, high school chemistry, 2 years high school math, 2 years high school science, high school transcript, immunizations, minimum high school GPA of 3.0, minimum GPA in nursing prerequisites of 3.0, professional liability insurance/malpractice insurance, prerequisite course work. Transfer students are accepted. *Application deadline:* Applications may be processed on a rolling basis for some programs. *Application fee:* $75.
Advanced Placement Credit by examination available.
Contact *Telephone:* 724-852-3356. *Fax:* 724-852-3220.

GRADUATE PROGRAMS

Contact *Telephone:* 412-824-3700.

MASTER'S DEGREE PROGRAM

Degrees MSN; MSN/MBA
Available Programs Accelerated Master's; Accelerated Master's for Nurses with Non-Nursing Degrees; Accelerated RN to Master's.
Concentrations Available Nursing administration; nursing education; nursing informatics.
Site Options Monroeville, PA; Canonsburg, PA; Wexford, PA.
Study Options Part-time.
Program Entrance Requirements Clinical experience, computer literacy, minimum overall college GPA of 3.0, transcript of college record, written essay, 2 letters of recommendation, resume, statistics course. *Application deadline:* Applications may be processed on a rolling basis for some programs. *Application fee:* $75.
Degree Requirements 36 total credit hours, thesis or project.

DOCTORAL DEGREE PROGRAM

Degree DNP
Available Programs Doctorate; Post-Baccalaureate Doctorate.
Areas of Study Advanced practice nursing, health-care systems, nursing administration.
Site Options Monroeville, PA.
Program Entrance Requirements Minimum overall college GPA of 3.0, interview by faculty committee, interview, letters of recommendation, MSN or equivalent, statistics course, vita, writing sample. Application deadline: Applications may be processed on a rolling basis for some programs.
Degree Requirements 80 total credit hours, oral exam, written exam, residency.

West Chester University of Pennsylvania
Department of Nursing
West Chester, Pennsylvania

http://www.wcupa.edu/_academics/Healthsciences/nursing/
Founded in 1871
DEGREES • BSN • MSN
Nursing Program Faculty 40 (28% with doctorates).
Baccalaureate Enrollment 384 **Women** 88% **Men** 12% **Part-time** 28%
Graduate Enrollment 42 **Women** 93% **Men** 7% **Part-time** 81%
Distance Learning Courses Available.
Nursing Student Activities Nursing Honor Society, Sigma Theta Tau, Student Nurses' Association.
Nursing Student Resources Academic advising; academic or career counseling; assistance for students with disabilities; bookstore; campus computer network; career placement assistance; computer lab; computer-assisted instruction; e-mail services; employment services for current students; externships; housing assistance; interactive nursing skills videos; Internet; learning resource lab; library services; nursing audiovisuals; remedial services; resume preparation assistance; skills, simulation, or other laboratory; tutoring.
Library Facilities 88 volumes in nursing; 173 periodical subscriptions health-care related.

BACCALAUREATE PROGRAMS

Degree BSN

Available Programs Accelerated Baccalaureate for Second Degree; Generic Baccalaureate; RN Baccalaureate.
Study Options Full-time and part-time.
Program Entrance Requirements Written essay, health exam, health insurance, high school biology, high school chemistry, 3 years high school math, 3 years high school science, high school transcript, minimum high school GPA, minimum high school rank. *Application deadline:* Applications may be processed on a rolling basis for some programs. *Application fee:* $45.
Advanced Placement Credit given for nursing courses completed elsewhere dependent upon specific evaluations.
Contact *Telephone:* 610-436-2693. *Fax:* 610-436-3083.

GRADUATE PROGRAMS

Contact *Telephone:* 610-436-2331. *Fax:* 610-436-3083.

MASTER'S DEGREE PROGRAM

Degree MSN
Available Programs Master's.
Concentrations Available Nursing administration; nursing education. *Clinical nurse specialist programs in:* public health.
Study Options Full-time and part-time.
Program Entrance Requirements Clinical experience, minimum overall college GPA of 2.8, transcript of college record, written essay, interview, 2 letters of recommendation, physical assessment course, resume, statistics course. *Application deadline:* Applications may be processed on a rolling basis for some programs. *Application fee:* $45.
Advanced Placement Credit given for nursing courses completed elsewhere dependent upon specific evaluations.
Degree Requirements 39 total credit hours, comprehensive exam.

Widener University
School of Nursing
Chester, Pennsylvania

http://www.widener.edu/
Founded in 1821
DEGREES • BSN • MSN • MSN/PHD • PHD
Nursing Program Faculty 115 (32% with doctorates).
Baccalaureate Enrollment 678 **Women** 90% **Men** 10%
Graduate Enrollment 187 **Women** 93% **Men** 7% **Part-time** 89%
Distance Learning Courses Available.
Nursing Student Activities Nursing Honor Society, Sigma Theta Tau, Student Nurses' Association.
Nursing Student Resources Academic advising; academic or career counseling; assistance for students with disabilities; bookstore; campus computer network; career placement assistance; computer lab; computer-assisted instruction; e-mail services; employment services for current students; housing assistance; interactive nursing skills videos; Internet; learning resource lab; library services; nursing audiovisuals; placement services for program completers; remedial services; resume preparation assistance; skills, simulation, or other laboratory; tutoring.
Library Facilities 15,003 volumes in health, 2,643 volumes in nursing; 717 periodical subscriptions health-care related.

BACCALAUREATE PROGRAMS

Degree BSN
Available Programs ADN to Baccalaureate; Generic Baccalaureate; RN Baccalaureate.
Study Options Full-time.
Program Entrance Requirements Minimum overall college GPA of 3.0, transcript of college record, health exam, health insurance, high school biology, high school chemistry, high school foreign language, 3 years high school math, 3 years high school science, high school transcript, immunizations, minimum high school GPA of 2.85, minimum GPA in nursing prerequisites of 3.0. Transfer students are accepted. *Application deadline:* Applications may be processed on a rolling basis for some programs.
Advanced Placement Credit by examination available. Credit given for nursing courses completed elsewhere dependent upon specific evaluations.
Expenses (2015–16) *Tuition:* full-time $40,418. *International tuition:* $40,418 full-time. *Room and board:* $13,924 per academic year. *Required fees:* full-time $1510.
Financial Aid 98% of baccalaureate students in nursing programs received some form of financial aid in 2014–15.

Contact Dr. Rose Schwartz, RN, Director, Prelicensure BSN, School of Nursing, Widener University, One University Place, Chester, PA 19013-5892. *Telephone:* 610-499-4211. *Fax:* 610-499-4216. *E-mail:* raschwartz@widener.edu.

GRADUATE PROGRAMS

Expenses (2015–16) *Tuition:* part-time $944 per credit hour.
Financial Aid 48% of graduate students in nursing programs received some form of financial aid in 2014–15. Career-related internships or fieldwork, Federal Work-Study, and traineeships available. Aid available to part-time students. *Financial aid application deadline:* 4/1.
Contact Mrs. Betty Boyles, Administrative Assistant for Graduate Programs, School of Nursing, Widener University, One University Place, Chester, PA 19013-5892. *Telephone:* 610-499-4208. *Fax:* 610-499-4216. *E-mail:* eaboyles@widener.edu.

MASTER'S DEGREE PROGRAM

Degrees MSN; MSN/PhD
Available Programs Master's; Master's for Nurses with Non-Nursing Degrees.
Concentrations Available Nursing education. *Clinical nurse specialist programs in:* adult-gerontology acute care. *Nurse practitioner programs in:* family health.
Site Options Harrisburg, PA.
Study Options Full-time and part-time.
Program Entrance Requirements Clinical experience, computer literacy, minimum overall college GPA of 3.0, transcript of college record, immunizations, interview, 2 letters of recommendation, nursing research course, resume, statistics course, GRE General Test. *Application deadline:* 6/1 (fall), 11/1 (spring), 3/1 (summer). Applications may be processed on a rolling basis for some programs.
Advanced Placement Credit given for nursing courses completed elsewhere dependent upon specific evaluations.
Degree Requirements 42 total credit hours.

POST-MASTER'S PROGRAM

Areas of Study Nursing education. *Clinical nurse specialist programs in:* adult-gerontology acute care. *Nurse practitioner programs in:* family health.

DOCTORAL DEGREE PROGRAM

Degree PhD
Available Programs Doctorate.
Areas of Study Faculty preparation, nursing education, nursing research, nursing science.
Program Entrance Requirements Minimum overall college GPA of 3.5, interview, 2 letters of recommendation, MSN or equivalent, statistics course, vita, writing sample, GRE General Test. Application deadline: 7/1 (fall), 11/1 (spring), 3/1 (summer). Applications may be processed on a rolling basis for some programs.
Degree Requirements 63 total credit hours, dissertation, written exam.

CONTINUING EDUCATION PROGRAM

Contact Ms. Tracey Swanson, Administrative Assistant, School of Nursing, Widener University, One University Place, Chester, PA 19013. *Telephone:* 610-499-4213. *Fax:* 610-499-4216. *E-mail:* thswanson@widener.edu.

Wilkes University
Department of Nursing
Wilkes-Barre, Pennsylvania

http://www.wilkes.edu/
Founded in 1933

DEGREES • BS • MS
Nursing Program Faculty 25 (20% with doctorates).
Baccalaureate Enrollment 300 **Women** 90% **Men** 10% **Part-time** 15%
Graduate Enrollment 65 **Women** 85% **Men** 15% **Part-time** 75%
Distance Learning Courses Available.
Nursing Student Activities Sigma Theta Tau, Student Nurses' Association, nursing club.
Nursing Student Resources Academic advising; academic or career counseling; assistance for students with disabilities; bookstore; campus computer network; career placement assistance; computer lab; computer-assisted instruction; daycare for children of students; e-mail services; employment services for current students; externships; housing assis-

tance; interactive nursing skills videos; Internet; learning resource lab; library services; nursing audiovisuals; paid internships; placement services for program completers; remedial services; resume preparation assistance; skills, simulation, or other laboratory; tutoring; unpaid internships.
Library Facilities 13,450 volumes in health, 13,000 volumes in nursing; 70 periodical subscriptions health-care related.

BACCALAUREATE PROGRAMS

Degree BS
Available Programs ADN to Baccalaureate; Accelerated Baccalaureate for Second Degree; Accelerated LPN to Baccalaureate; Accelerated RN Baccalaureate; Generic Baccalaureate; LPN to RN Baccalaureate; RN Baccalaureate.
Study Options Full-time and part-time.
Program Entrance Requirements Minimum overall college GPA of 2.0, transcript of college record, CPR certification, health exam, health insurance, high school biology, high school chemistry, 2 years high school math, 3 years high school science, high school transcript, immunizations, minimum high school GPA, professional liability insurance/malpractice insurance. Transfer students are accepted.
Advanced Placement Credit by examination available. Credit given for nursing courses completed elsewhere dependent upon specific evaluations.
Contact *Telephone:* 570-408-4074. *Fax:* 570-408-7807.

GRADUATE PROGRAMS

Contact *Telephone:* 570-408-4078. *Fax:* 570-408-7807.

MASTER'S DEGREE PROGRAM

Degree MS
Available Programs Accelerated AD/RN to Master's; Accelerated RN to Master's; Master's; Master's for Non-Nursing College Graduates; RN to Master's.
Concentrations Available Nursing administration; nursing education. *Clinical nurse specialist programs in:* gerontology, psychiatric/mental health.
Study Options Full-time and part-time.
Program Entrance Requirements Clinical experience, minimum overall college GPA of 3.0, transcript of college record, CPR certification, immunizations, interview, 3 letters of recommendation, nursing research course, physical assessment course, professional liability insurance/malpractice insurance, statistics course.
Advanced Placement Credit given for nursing courses completed elsewhere dependent upon specific evaluations.
Degree Requirements 37 total credit hours, thesis or project.

POST-MASTER'S PROGRAM

Areas of Study Nursing administration; nursing education. *Clinical nurse specialist programs in:* gerontology, psychiatric/mental health.

CONTINUING EDUCATION PROGRAM
Contact *Telephone:* 570-408-4462.

York College of Pennsylvania
Department of Nursing
York, Pennsylvania

http://www.ycp.edu/academics/academic-departments/nursing/
Founded in 1787

DEGREES • BS • DNP • MS
Nursing Program Faculty 69 (36% with doctorates).
Baccalaureate Enrollment 521 **Women** 90% **Men** 10% **Part-time** 4%
Graduate Enrollment 79 **Women** 80% **Men** 20% **Part-time** 53%
Nursing Student Activities Sigma Theta Tau, Student Nurses' Association, nursing club.
Nursing Student Resources Academic advising; academic or career counseling; assistance for students with disabilities; bookstore; campus computer network; career placement assistance; computer lab; computer-assisted instruction; e-mail services; employment services for current students; externships; housing assistance; interactive nursing skills videos; Internet; learning resource lab; library services; nursing audiovisuals; paid internships; placement services for program completers; remedial services; resume preparation assistance; skills, simulation, or other laboratory; tutoring.

Library Facilities 6,681 volumes in health, 1,226 volumes in nursing; 83 periodical subscriptions health-care related.

BACCALAUREATE PROGRAMS

Degree BS

Available Programs ADN to Baccalaureate; Baccalaureate for Second Degree; Generic Baccalaureate; RN Baccalaureate.

Study Options Full-time and part-time.

Program Entrance Requirements Minimum overall college GPA of 2.8, transcript of college record, CPR certification, health exam, health insurance, high school biology, high school chemistry, high school foreign language, 3 years high school math, 3 years high school science, high school transcript, immunizations, 2 letters of recommendation, minimum high school GPA of 3.4, minimum GPA in nursing prerequisites of 2.8, professional liability insurance/malpractice insurance, prerequisite course work. *Application deadline:* Applications may be processed on a rolling basis for some programs.

Advanced Placement Credit by examination available. Credit given for nursing courses completed elsewhere dependent upon specific evaluations.

Expenses (2015–16) *Tuition:* full-time $16,480; part-time $510 per credit. *Room and board:* $10,160; room only: $5700 per academic year. *Required fees:* full-time $1760; part-time $380 per term.

Financial Aid 99% of baccalaureate students in nursing programs received some form of financial aid in 2014–15.

Contact Karen S. March, Chairperson and Professor, Department of Nursing, York College of Pennsylvania, 441 Country Club Road, York, PA 17403-3651. *Telephone:* 717-815-1243. *Fax:* 717-849-1651. *E-mail:* kmarch@ycp.edu.

GRADUATE PROGRAMS

Expenses (2015–16) *Tuition:* part-time $765 per credit. *Required fees:* part-time $1260 per term.

Contact Dr. Kimberly Fenstermacher, Director, Department of Nursing, York College of Pennsylvania, 441 Country Club Road, York, PA 17403-3651. *Telephone:* 717-815-1383. *Fax:* 717-849-1651. *E-mail:* kfenster@ycp.edu.

MASTER'S DEGREE PROGRAM

Degree MS

Available Programs Master's.

Concentrations Available Nurse anesthesia; nursing education. *Clinical nurse specialist programs in:* adult-gerontology acute care. *Nurse practitioner programs in:* adult-gerontology acute care.

Study Options Part-time.

Program Entrance Requirements Clinical experience, computer literacy, minimum overall college GPA of 3.0, transcript of college record, CPR certification, written essay, immunizations, interview, 2 letters of recommendation, nursing research course, physical assessment course, professional liability insurance/malpractice insurance, resume, statistics course. *Application deadline:* 7/1 (fall), 11/1 (spring), 3/1 (summer). Applications may be processed on a rolling basis for some programs. *Application fee:* $50.

Advanced Placement Credit given for nursing courses completed elsewhere dependent upon specific evaluations.

Degree Requirements 41 total credit hours, thesis or project.

POST-MASTER'S PROGRAM

Areas of Study *Nurse practitioner programs in:* adult-gerontology acute care.

DOCTORAL DEGREE PROGRAM

Degree DNP

Available Programs Doctorate.

Areas of Study Advanced practice nursing, clinical practice, health policy, health-care systems, individualized study, information systems, nursing policy, nursing science.

Program Entrance Requirements Clinical experience, minimum overall college GPA of 3.5, interview by faculty committee, 2 letters of recommendation, MSN or equivalent, statistics course, vita, writing sample. Application deadline: 12/15 (summer). Applications may be processed on a rolling basis for some programs. Application fee: $50.

Degree Requirements 37 total credit hours, residency.

PUERTO RICO

Inter American University of Puerto Rico, Aguadilla Campus
Nursing Program
Aguadilla, Puerto Rico

Founded in 1957

DEGREE • BSN
Nursing Program Faculty 20 (20% with doctorates).
Baccalaureate Enrollment 397 **Women** 69% **Men** 31%
Nursing Student Activities Student Nurses' Association.
Nursing Student Resources Academic advising; assistance for students with disabilities; campus computer network; computer lab; computer-assisted instruction; e-mail services; interactive nursing skills videos; Internet; learning resource lab; library services; nursing audiovisuals; skills, simulation, or other laboratory; tutoring.
Library Facilities 36 periodical subscriptions health-care related.

BACCALAUREATE PROGRAMS

Degree BSN
Available Programs RN Baccalaureate.
Site Options Aguadilla, PR.
Study Options Full-time.
Program Entrance Requirements Minimum overall college GPA of 2.50, transcript of college record, CPR certification, high school transcript, immunizations, minimum high school GPA of 2.50. Transfer students are accepted.
Advanced Placement Credit given for nursing courses completed elsewhere dependent upon specific evaluations.
Contact *Telephone:* 787-891-0925.

Inter American University of Puerto Rico, Arecibo Campus
Nursing Program
Arecibo, Puerto Rico

http://www.arecibo.inter.edu/portal/default.htm
Founded in 1957

DEGREES • BSN • MSN
Nursing Program Faculty 59 (6% with doctorates).
Baccalaureate Enrollment 870
Graduate Enrollment 30
Nursing Student Activities Student Nurses' Association.
Nursing Student Resources Academic advising; academic or career counseling; assistance for students with disabilities; bookstore; campus computer network; computer lab; computer-assisted instruction; e-mail services; employment services for current students; externships; interactive nursing skills videos; Internet; learning resource lab; library services; nursing audiovisuals; remedial services; resume preparation assistance; skills, simulation, or other laboratory; tutoring.
Library Facilities 560 volumes in nursing.

BACCALAUREATE PROGRAMS

Degree BSN
Available Programs Generic Baccalaureate.
Study Options Full-time and part-time.
Program Entrance Requirements Transcript of college record, CPR certification, high school transcript, immunizations, minimum high school GPA of 2.5. Transfer students are accepted. *Application deadline:* Applications may be processed on a rolling basis for some programs.
Contact Undergraduate Program, Nursing Program, Inter American University of Puerto Rico, Arecibo Campus, Arecibo, PR 00614-4050. *Telephone:* 787-878-5475.

GRADUATE PROGRAMS

Contact Dr. Frances Cortés, Department Director, Nursing Program, Inter American University of Puerto Rico, Arecibo Campus, PO Box 4050, Arecibo, PR 00614. *E-mail:* fcortes@arecibo.inter.edu.

MASTER'S DEGREE PROGRAM

Degree MSN

Available Programs Master's.

Concentrations Available *Clinical nurse specialist programs in:* acute care, medical-surgical.

Study Options Full-time and part-time.

Program Entrance Requirements Clinical experience, minimum overall college GPA of 2.5, transcript of college record, CPR certification, immunizations, interview, 2 letters of recommendation, resume.

Degree Requirements 41 total credit hours, thesis or project.

Inter American University of Puerto Rico, Metropolitan Campus

Carmen Torres de Tiburcio School of Nursing
San Juan, Puerto Rico

http://www.metro.inter.edu/index.asp

Founded in 1960

DEGREE • BSN

Nursing Program Faculty 26 (27% with doctorates).

Baccalaureate Enrollment 312 **Women** 57% **Men** 43%

Nursing Student Activities Student Nurses' Association.

Nursing Student Resources Academic advising; academic or career counseling; assistance for students with disabilities; bookstore; campus computer network; career placement assistance; computer lab; computer-assisted instruction; daycare for children of students; e-mail services; employment services for current students; externships; interactive nursing skills videos; Internet; learning resource lab; library services; nursing audiovisuals; paid internships; placement services for program completers; remedial services; skills, simulation, or other laboratory; tutoring.

Library Facilities 36,000 volumes in health, 21,759 volumes in nursing; 2,090 periodical subscriptions health-care related.

BACCALAUREATE PROGRAMS

Degree BSN

Available Programs ADN to Baccalaureate; Accelerated Baccalaureate; Generic Baccalaureate.

Study Options Full-time and part-time.

Program Entrance Requirements Minimum overall college GPA of 2.0, transcript of college record, CPR certification, health exam, health insurance, high school transcript, immunizations, 2 letters of recommendation, minimum high school rank 4%, minimum GPA in nursing prerequisites of 2. Transfer students are accepted.

Advanced Placement Credit by examination available. Credit given for nursing courses completed elsewhere dependent upon specific evaluations.

Contact *Telephone:* 787-763-3066. *Fax:* 787-250-1242 Ext. 2159.

Pontifical Catholic University of Puerto Rico

Department of Nursing
Ponce, Puerto Rico

http://www.pucpr.edu/

Founded in 1948

DEGREE • BSN

Library Facilities 1,499 volumes in nursing.

BACCALAUREATE PROGRAMS

Degree BSN

Available Programs Generic Baccalaureate.

Program Entrance Requirements Minimum overall college GPA of 2.0, CPR certification, health exam, health insurance, immunizations, interview, letters of recommendation, minimum high school GPA of 2.5, prerequisite course work.

Contact *Telephone:* 787-841-2000 Ext. 1604.

Universidad Adventista de las Antillas

Department of Nursing
Mayagüez, Puerto Rico

Founded in 1957

DEGREE • BSN

Nursing Program Faculty 11 (18% with doctorates).

Baccalaureate Enrollment 257 **Women** 69% **Men** 31% **Part-time** 1%

Nursing Student Activities Nursing club.

Nursing Student Resources Academic advising; academic or career counseling; assistance for students with disabilities; campus computer network; computer lab; computer-assisted instruction; e-mail services; employment services for current students; housing assistance; interactive nursing skills videos; Internet; learning resource lab; library services; nursing audiovisuals; remedial services; resume preparation assistance; skills, simulation, or other laboratory; tutoring; unpaid internships.

Library Facilities 2,488 volumes in health, 1,556 volumes in nursing; 29 periodical subscriptions health-care related.

BACCALAUREATE PROGRAMS

Degree BSN

Available Programs Generic Baccalaureate; RN Baccalaureate.

Study Options Full-time.

Program Entrance Requirements Minimum overall college GPA of 2.3, transcript of college record, health exam, health insurance, high school transcript, immunizations, interview, 2 letters of recommendation, minimum high school GPA of 2.5. Transfer students are accepted.

Advanced Placement Credit given for nursing courses completed elsewhere dependent upon specific evaluations.

Contact *Telephone:* 787-834-9595 Ext. 2209. *Fax:* 787-834-9597.

CONTINUING EDUCATION PROGRAM

Contact *Telephone:* 787-834-9595 Ext. 2284. *Fax:* 787-834-9597.

Universidad del Turabo

Nursing Program
Gurabo, Puerto Rico

Founded in 1972

DEGREE • BS

BACCALAUREATE PROGRAMS

Degree BS

Available Programs Generic Baccalaureate.

Contact *Telephone:* 787-743-7979.

Universidad Metropolitana

Department of Nursing
San Juan, Puerto Rico

http://www.suagm.edu/umet/oa_pe_cs_programas.asp?cn_id=686

Founded in 1980

DEGREE • BSN

Library Facilities 5,438 volumes in health; 110 periodical subscriptions health-care related.

BACCALAUREATE PROGRAMS

Degree BSN

Contact *Telephone:* 787-766-1717 Ext. 6422. *Fax:* 787-769-7663.

University of Puerto Rico in Arecibo

Department of Nursing
Arecibo, Puerto Rico

http://www.upra.edu/
Founded in 1967
DEGREE • BSN
Nursing Program Faculty 21

BACCALAUREATE PROGRAMS

Degree BSN
Available Programs Generic Baccalaureate.
Contact *Telephone:* 787-878-2830. *Fax:* 787-880-4972.

University of Puerto Rico in Humacao

Department of Nursing
Humacao, Puerto Rico

http://www1.uprh.edu/enfe/
Founded in 1962
DEGREE • BSN
Nursing Program Faculty 16 (12% with doctorates).
Baccalaureate Enrollment 221 **Women** 77% **Men** 23%
Nursing Student Activities Student Nurses' Association.
Nursing Student Resources Academic advising; academic or career counseling; assistance for students with disabilities; campus computer network; career placement assistance; computer lab; computer-assisted instruction; daycare for children of students; e-mail services; employment services for current students; Internet; learning resource lab; library services; nursing audiovisuals; other; resume preparation assistance; skills, simulation, or other laboratory; tutoring.
Library Facilities 800 volumes in health, 83 volumes in nursing; 8,623 periodical subscriptions health-care related.

BACCALAUREATE PROGRAMS

Degree BSN
Available Programs Generic Baccalaureate.
Study Options Full-time.
Program Entrance Requirements Transcript of college record, health exam, health insurance, high school transcript, immunizations. Transfer students are accepted. *Application deadline:* 1/30 (winter).
Financial Aid 86% of baccalaureate students in nursing programs received some form of financial aid in 2013–14.
Contact Dra. Francisca Rodriguez, Director, Department of Nursing, University of Puerto Rico in Humacao, Humacao, PR 00791. *Telephone:* 787-850-9346. *Fax:* 787-850-9411. *E-mail:* f_rodriguez@webmail.uprh.edu.

University of Puerto Rico, Mayagüez Campus

Department of Nursing
Mayagüez, Puerto Rico

http://www.uprm.edu/enfe/
Founded in 1911
DEGREE • BSN
Nursing Program Faculty 21 (10% with doctorates).
Nursing Student Activities Nursing Honor Society, Sigma Theta Tau, Student Nurses' Association.
Nursing Student Resources Academic advising; academic or career counseling; assistance for students with disabilities; bookstore; campus computer network; career placement assistance; computer lab; computer-assisted instruction; e-mail services; employment services for current students; interactive nursing skills videos; Internet; learning resource lab; library services; nursing audiovisuals; paid internships; placement services for program completers; remedial services; resume preparation assistance; skills, simulation, or other laboratory; tutoring.
Library Facilities 68 periodical subscriptions health-care related.

BACCALAUREATE PROGRAMS

Degree BSN
Available Programs Generic Baccalaureate.
Study Options Full-time.
Program Entrance Requirements High school transcript, immunizations. Transfer students are accepted.
Advanced Placement Credit by examination available.
Contact *Telephone:* 787-263-3482. *Fax:* 787-832-3875.

CONTINUING EDUCATION PROGRAM

Contact *Telephone:* 787-265-3842. *Fax:* 787-832-3875.

University of Puerto Rico, Medical Sciences Campus

School of Nursing
San Juan, Puerto Rico

http://www.md.rcm.upr.edu/
Founded in 1950
DEGREES • BSN • MSN
Nursing Program Faculty 37 (25% with doctorates).
Baccalaureate Enrollment 241 **Women** 85% **Men** 15% **Part-time** 12%
Graduate Enrollment 158 **Women** 79% **Men** 21% **Part-time** 6%
Nursing Student Activities Sigma Theta Tau, Student Nurses' Association.
Nursing Student Resources Academic advising; academic or career counseling; assistance for students with disabilities; computer lab; computer-assisted instruction; e-mail services; employment services for current students; interactive nursing skills videos; Internet; library services; nursing audiovisuals; skills, simulation, or other laboratory; tutoring.
Library Facilities 7,830 volumes in health, 1,143 volumes in nursing; 1,215 periodical subscriptions health-care related.

BACCALAUREATE PROGRAMS

Degree BSN
Available Programs ADN to Baccalaureate; Generic Baccalaureate.
Study Options Full-time and part-time.
Program Entrance Requirements Minimum overall college GPA of 2.0, transcript of college record, health exam, immunizations, interview, minimum high school GPA of 2.0, prerequisite course work. Transfer students are accepted.
Contact *Telephone:* 787-758-2525 Ext. 1984. *Fax:* 787-281-0721.

GRADUATE PROGRAMS

Contact *Telephone:* 787-758-2525 Ext. 3105. *Fax:* 787-281-0721.

MASTER'S DEGREE PROGRAM
Degree MSN
Available Programs Master's.
Concentrations Available Nurse anesthesia; nursing administration; nursing education. *Clinical nurse specialist programs in:* adult health, community health, critical care, gerontology, maternity-newborn, pediatric, psychiatric/mental health.
Site Options Mayaguez, PR.
Study Options Full-time and part-time.
Program Entrance Requirements Clinical experience, minimum overall college GPA of 2.5, transcript of college record, immunizations, interview, resume, statistics course, GRE or EXADEP.
Degree Requirements 48 total credit hours, thesis or project.

CONTINUING EDUCATION PROGRAM

Contact *Telephone:* 787-758-2525 Ext. 2102. *Fax:* 787-281-0721.

RHODE ISLAND

New England Institute of Technology
Nursing Department
East Greenwich, Rhode Island

http://www.neit.edu/
Founded in 1940
DEGREE • BSN

BACCALAUREATE PROGRAMS

Degree BSN
Available Programs RN Baccalaureate.
Contact Dayle EdD, MS, MEd, RN, Assistant Provost and Director of Nursing, Nursing Department, New England Institute of Technology, One New England Tech Boulevard, East Greenwich, RI 02818. *Telephone:* 401-467-7744. *E-mail:* djoseph@neit.edu.

Rhode Island College
Department of Nursing
Providence, Rhode Island

http://www.ric.edu/nursing
Founded in 1854
DEGREES • BSN • MSN
Nursing Program Faculty 49 (39% with doctorates).
Baccalaureate Enrollment 415 **Women** 89% **Men** 11% **Part-time** 38%
Graduate Enrollment 43 **Women** 98% **Men** 2% **Part-time** 98%
Distance Learning Courses Available.
Nursing Student Activities Sigma Theta Tau, Student Nurses' Association, nursing club.
Nursing Student Resources Academic advising; academic or career counseling; assistance for students with disabilities; bookstore; campus computer network; career placement assistance; computer lab; computer-assisted instruction; daycare for children of students; e-mail services; employment services for current students; housing assistance; interactive nursing skills videos; Internet; learning resource lab; library services; nursing audiovisuals; paid internships; placement services for program completers; remedial services; resume preparation assistance; skills, simulation, or other laboratory; tutoring.
Library Facilities 574 volumes in nursing; 63 periodical subscriptions health-care related.

BACCALAUREATE PROGRAMS

Degree BSN
Available Programs Baccalaureate for Second Degree; Generic Baccalaureate; RN Baccalaureate.
Site Options Providence, RI.
Study Options Full-time and part-time.
Program Entrance Requirements Minimum overall college GPA of 2.7, CPR certification, health exam, health insurance, high school biology, high school chemistry, high school foreign language, 4 years high school math, 2 years high school science, high school transcript, immunizations, letters of recommendation, minimum GPA in nursing prerequisites of 3.0, prerequisite course work. Transfer students are accepted. *Application deadline:* 10/15 (fall), 4/15 (spring).
Advanced Placement Credit given for nursing courses completed elsewhere dependent upon specific evaluations.
Contact *Telephone:* 401-456-8014. *Fax:* 401-456-8206.

GRADUATE PROGRAMS

Contact *Telephone:* 401-456-9720. *Fax:* 401-456-8206.

MASTER'S DEGREE PROGRAM
Degree MSN
Available Programs Master's.
Concentrations Available *Clinical nurse specialist programs in:* acute care, adult health, community health. *Nurse practitioner programs in:* acute care, adult health.
Site Options Providence, RI.

Study Options Full-time and part-time.
Program Entrance Requirements Minimum overall college GPA of 3.0, transcript of college record, written essay, letters of recommendation, resume, statistics course. *Application deadline:* 2/15 (fall). *Application fee:* $50.
Advanced Placement Credit given for nursing courses completed elsewhere dependent upon specific evaluations.
Degree Requirements 45 total credit hours, thesis or project.

Salve Regina University
Department of Nursing
Newport, Rhode Island

http://www.salve.edu/academics/departments/nur/
Founded in 1934
DEGREE • BS
Nursing Program Faculty 23 (18% with doctorates).
Baccalaureate Enrollment 314 **Women** 91% **Men** 9% **Part-time** 15%
Nursing Student Activities Sigma Theta Tau, Student Nurses' Association, nursing club.
Nursing Student Resources Academic advising; academic or career counseling; assistance for students with disabilities; bookstore; campus computer network; career placement assistance; computer lab; computer-assisted instruction; e-mail services; housing assistance; interactive nursing skills videos; Internet; learning resource lab; library services; nursing audiovisuals; paid internships; resume preparation assistance; skills, simulation, or other laboratory; tutoring; unpaid internships.
Library Facilities 6,882 volumes in health, 1,081 volumes in nursing; 76 periodical subscriptions health-care related.

BACCALAUREATE PROGRAMS

Degree BS
Available Programs Generic Baccalaureate; RN Baccalaureate.
Site Options Warwick, RI.
Study Options Full-time and part-time.
Program Entrance Requirements Minimum overall college GPA of 2.7, transcript of college record, written essay, high school biology, high school chemistry, high school foreign language, 3 years high school math, 3 years high school science, high school transcript, 2 letters of recommendation, minimum GPA in nursing prerequisites of 2.0, prerequisite course work. Transfer students are accepted. *Application deadline:* 2/1 (fall). Applications may be processed on a rolling basis for some programs. *Application fee:* $50.
Advanced Placement Credit by examination available. Credit given for nursing courses completed elsewhere dependent upon specific evaluations.
Contact *Telephone:* 888-467-2583. *Fax:* 401-848-2823.

CONTINUING EDUCATION PROGRAM

Contact *Telephone:* 800-637-0002. *Fax:* 401-341-2973.

University of Rhode Island
College of Nursing
Kingston, Rhode Island

http://www.uri.edu/nursing
Founded in 1892
DEGREES • BS • MS • PHD
Nursing Program Faculty 30 (50% with doctorates).
Baccalaureate Enrollment 851 **Women** 87% **Men** 13% **Part-time** 10%
Graduate Enrollment 120 **Women** 95% **Men** 5% **Part-time** 70%
Distance Learning Courses Available.
Nursing Student Activities Sigma Theta Tau, Student Nurses' Association, nursing club.
Nursing Student Resources Academic advising; academic or career counseling; assistance for students with disabilities; bookstore; campus computer network; career placement assistance; computer lab; computer-assisted instruction; e-mail services; externships; housing assistance; interactive nursing skills videos; Internet; learning resource lab; library services; nursing audiovisuals; remedial services; resume preparation assistance; skills, simulation, or other laboratory; tutoring; unpaid internships.

BACCALAUREATE PROGRAMS

Degree BS
Available Programs ADN to Baccalaureate; RN Baccalaureate.
Site Options Providence, RI.
Study Options Full-time and part-time.
Online Degree Options Yes.
Program Entrance Requirements Minimum overall college GPA of 2.5, transcript of college record, CPR certification, written essay, health exam, high school biology, high school foreign language, 3 years high school math, 2 years high school science, high school transcript, immunizations, 2 letters of recommendation, minimum high school rank 30%, minimum GPA in nursing prerequisites of 2.5, prerequisite course work. Transfer students are accepted. *Application deadline:* 2/1 (fall), 11/1 (spring).
Advanced Placement Credit given for nursing courses completed elsewhere dependent upon specific evaluations.
Expenses (2015–16) *Tuition, state resident:* full-time $12,862. *Tuition, nonresident:* full-time $28,852. *International tuition:* $28,852 full-time. *Room and board:* $11,956 per academic year. *Required fees:* full-time $750.
Financial Aid *Gift aid (need-based):* Federal Pell, FSEOG, state, private, college/university gift aid from institutional funds. *Loans:* Federal Nursing Student Loans, Federal Direct (Subsidized and Unsubsidized Stafford PLUS), Perkins, college/university. *Work-study:* Federal Work-Study. *Financial aid application deadline (priority):* 3/1.
Contact Undergraduate Admissions Office, College of Nursing, University of Rhode Island, Newman Hall, 14 Upper College Road, Kingston, RI 02881. *Telephone:* 401-874-7100.

GRADUATE PROGRAMS

Expenses (2015–16) *Tuition, area resident:* full-time $11,796; part-time $655 per credit. *Tuition, state resident:* full-time $24,206; part-time $1345 per credit. *Tuition, nonresident:* full-time $17,694; part-time $983 per credit. *Required fees:* full-time $3538; part-time $42 per credit.
Financial Aid 1 research assistantship (averaging $16,300 per year), 7 teaching assistantships (averaging $12,500 per year) were awarded.
Contact Dr. Patricia Burbank, Associate Dean, College of Nursing, University of Rhode Island, White Hall, Kingston, RI 02881. *Telephone:* 401-874-2766. *E-mail:* pburbank@uri.edu.

MASTER'S DEGREE PROGRAM

Degree MS
Available Programs Master's; RN to Master's.
Concentrations Available Nursing education. *Clinical nurse specialist programs in:* gerontology. *Nurse practitioner programs in:* acute care, family health, gerontology.
Site Options Providence, RI.
Study Options Full-time and part-time.
Program Entrance Requirements Clinical experience, minimum overall college GPA of 3.0, transcript of college record, written essay, immunizations, 3 letters of recommendation, nursing research course, professional liability insurance/malpractice insurance, resume, statistics course, GRE or MAT. *Application deadline:* 4/15 (fall), 10/15 (spring). *Application fee:* $65.
Advanced Placement Credit given for nursing courses completed elsewhere dependent upon specific evaluations.
Degree Requirements 41 total credit hours, thesis or project, comprehensive exam.

POST-MASTER'S PROGRAM

Areas of Study Nursing education. *Clinical nurse specialist programs in:* gerontology. *Nurse practitioner programs in:* acute care, family health, gerontology.

DOCTORAL DEGREE PROGRAM

Degree PhD
Available Programs Doctorate.
Areas of Study Nursing research, nursing science.
Site Options Providence, RI.
Program Entrance Requirements Clinical experience, minimum overall college GPA of 3.0, interview, 3 letters of recommendation, MSN or equivalent, scholarly papers, statistics course, vita, writing sample, GRE. Application deadline: 4/15 (fall), 10/15 (spring). Application fee: $65.
Degree Requirements 61 total credit hours, dissertation, oral exam, written exam, residency.

SOUTH CAROLINA

Anderson University
School of Nursing
Anderson, South Carolina

http://www.andersonuniversity.edu/son.aspx
Founded in 1911
DEGREE • BSN
Nursing Program Faculty 22 (27% with doctorates).
Baccalaureate Enrollment 83 **Women** 75% **Men** 25%
Distance Learning Courses Available.
Nursing Student Activities Student Nurses' Association.
Nursing Student Resources Academic advising; academic or career counseling; assistance for students with disabilities; bookstore; campus computer network; career placement assistance; computer lab; e-mail services; interactive nursing skills videos; Internet; learning resource lab; library services; nursing audiovisuals; placement services for program completers; resume preparation assistance; skills, simulation, or other laboratory; unpaid internships.
Library Facilities 1,000 volumes in health, 96 volumes in nursing; 11,000 periodical subscriptions health-care related.

BACCALAUREATE PROGRAMS

Degree BSN
Available Programs ADN to Baccalaureate; Accelerated Baccalaureate; Accelerated Baccalaureate for Second Degree; Generic Baccalaureate.
Study Options Full-time.
Program Entrance Requirements Minimum overall college GPA of 3.0, CPR certification, health exam, health insurance, immunizations, professional liability insurance/malpractice insurance. Transfer students are accepted. *Application deadline:* Applications may be processed on a rolling basis for some programs. *Application fee:* $25.
Expenses (2014–15) *Tuition:* full-time $21,660; part-time $535 per credit. *Room and board:* $5281; room only: $3105 per academic year. *Required fees:* full-time $3000.
Financial Aid 75% of baccalaureate students in nursing programs received some form of financial aid in 2013–14. *Gift aid (need-based):* Federal Pell, FSEOG, state, private, college/university gift aid from institutional funds. *Loans:* Federal Direct (Subsidized and Unsubsidized Stafford PLUS), Perkins, state, private loans. *Work-study:* Federal Work-Study, part-time campus jobs. *Financial aid application deadline:* 7/30(priority: 3/1).
Contact Lydia Price, Admission Counselor, School of Nursing, Anderson University, 316 Boulevard, Anderson, SC 29621. *Telephone:* 864-622-6037. *Fax:* 864-231-2033.
E-mail: lydiaprice@andersonuniversity.edu.

Charleston Southern University
Wingo School of Nursing
Charleston, South Carolina

http://www.csuniv.edu/
Founded in 1964
DEGREES • BSN • MSN
Nursing Program Faculty 20 (25% with doctorates).
Baccalaureate Enrollment 178 **Women** 90% **Men** 10%
Graduate Enrollment 32 **Women** 99% **Men** 1%
Distance Learning Courses Available.
Nursing Student Activities Sigma Theta Tau, Student Nurses' Association.
Nursing Student Resources Academic advising; academic or career counseling; assistance for students with disabilities; bookstore; campus computer network; career placement assistance; computer lab; computer-assisted instruction; e-mail services; externships; interactive nursing skills videos; Internet; learning resource lab; library services; nursing audiovisuals; remedial services; resume preparation assistance; skills, simulation, or other laboratory; tutoring.
Library Facilities 2,400 volumes in health, 250 volumes in nursing; 55 periodical subscriptions health-care related.

BACCALAUREATE PROGRAMS

Degree BSN

Available Programs ADN to Baccalaureate; Generic Baccalaureate; RN Baccalaureate.

Study Options Full-time.

Online Degree Options Yes.

Program Entrance Requirements Minimum overall college GPA of 2.75, transcript of college record, CPR certification, health exam, health insurance, immunizations, minimum GPA in nursing prerequisites of 3.0, professional liability insurance/malpractice insurance, prerequisite course work. Transfer students are accepted. *Application deadline:* 3/15 (fall).

Advanced Placement Credit given for nursing courses completed elsewhere dependent upon specific evaluations.

Financial Aid 90% of baccalaureate students in nursing programs received some form of financial aid in 2013–14.

Contact Dr. Andreea Meier, Dean of Nursing, Wingo School of Nursing, Charleston Southern University, 9200 University Boulevard, PO Box 118087, Charleston, SC 29423-8087. *Telephone:* 843-863-7826. *Fax:* 843-863-7540. *E-mail:* ameier@csuniv.edu.

GRADUATE PROGRAMS

Financial Aid 95% of graduate students in nursing programs received some form of financial aid in 2013–14.

Contact Dr. Andreea Meier, Dean, Wingo School of Nursing, Charleston Southern University, 9200 University Boulevard, PO Box 118087, Charleston, SC 29423. *Telephone:* 843-863-7826. *Fax:* 843-863-7540. *E-mail:* ameier@csuniv.edu.

MASTER'S DEGREE PROGRAM

Degree MSN

Available Programs Master's; RN to Master's.

Concentrations Available Health-care administration; nursing administration; nursing education.

Study Options Full-time.

Online Degree Options Yes (online only).

Program Entrance Requirements Clinical experience, minimum overall college GPA of 3.0, transcript of college record, written essay, 3 letters of recommendation, resume. *Application deadline:* 6/31 (fall). *Application fee:* $20.

Advanced Placement Credit given for nursing courses completed elsewhere dependent upon specific evaluations.

Degree Requirements 39 total credit hours, thesis or project.

Clemson University
School of Nursing
Clemson, South Carolina

http://www.clemson.edu/hehd/departments/nursing/
Founded in 1889

DEGREES • BS • MS

Nursing Program Faculty 22 (71% with doctorates).

Baccalaureate Enrollment 402 **Women** 99% **Men** 1%

Graduate Enrollment 82 **Women** 90% **Men** 10% **Part-time** 54%

Distance Learning Courses Available.

Nursing Student Activities Nursing Honor Society, Sigma Theta Tau, Student Nurses' Association.

Nursing Student Resources Academic advising; academic or career counseling; assistance for students with disabilities; bookstore; campus computer network; career placement assistance; computer lab; computer-assisted instruction; e-mail services; employment services for current students; externships; housing assistance; interactive nursing skills videos; Internet; learning resource lab; library services; nursing audiovisuals; other; remedial services; resume preparation assistance; skills, simulation, or other laboratory; tutoring; unpaid internships.

Library Facilities 29,800 volumes in health, 5,548 volumes in nursing; 877 periodical subscriptions health-care related.

BACCALAUREATE PROGRAMS

Degree BS

Available Programs Accelerated Baccalaureate; Generic Baccalaureate; RN Baccalaureate.

Site Options Greenville, SC.

Study Options Full-time and part-time.

Program Entrance Requirements Minimum overall college GPA of 2.5, transcript of college record, CPR certification, health insurance, high school biology, high school chemistry, 3 years high school math, 3 years high school science, high school transcript, immunizations, minimum

high school GPA of 2.5, professional liability insurance/malpractice insurance, prerequisite course work. Transfer students are accepted.

Advanced Placement Credit by examination available. Credit given for nursing courses completed elsewhere dependent upon specific evaluations.

Contact *Telephone:* 864-656-5463. *Fax:* 864-656-2464.

GRADUATE PROGRAMS

Contact *Telephone:* 864-250-8881. *Fax:* 864-250-6711.

MASTER'S DEGREE PROGRAM

Degree MS

Available Programs Master's.

Concentrations Available Nursing administration; nursing education. *Nurse practitioner programs in:* adult health, family health, gerontology.

Site Options Greenville, SC.

Study Options Full-time and part-time.

Program Entrance Requirements Clinical experience, computer literacy, minimum overall college GPA of 3.0, transcript of college record, CPR certification, written essay, immunizations, 2 letters of recommendation, nursing research course, physical assessment course, professional liability insurance/malpractice insurance, prerequisite course work, resume, statistics course, GRE General Test. *Application deadline:* 4/1 (fall), 10/1 (spring).

Advanced Placement Credit given for nursing courses completed elsewhere dependent upon specific evaluations.

Degree Requirements 45 total credit hours, thesis or project, comprehensive exam.

POST-MASTER'S PROGRAM

Areas of Study Nursing administration; nursing education. *Nurse practitioner programs in:* adult health, family health, gerontology.

DOCTORAL DEGREE PROGRAM

Program Entrance Requirements GRE General Test.

Coastal Carolina University
Nursing Completion Program
Conway, South Carolina

http://www.coastal.edu/nursing
Founded in 1954

DEGREE • BSN

Nursing Program Faculty 6 (83% with doctorates).

Baccalaureate Enrollment 75 **Women** 90% **Men** 10% **Part-time** 10%

Distance Learning Courses Available.

Nursing Student Activities Nursing club.

Nursing Student Resources Academic advising; academic or career counseling; assistance for students with disabilities; bookstore; campus computer network; computer lab; computer-assisted instruction; e-mail services; interactive nursing skills videos; Internet; learning resource lab; library services; nursing audiovisuals; remedial services; resume preparation assistance; skills, simulation, or other laboratory; tutoring.

Library Facilities 1,719 volumes in health, 109 volumes in nursing; 716 periodical subscriptions health-care related.

BACCALAUREATE PROGRAMS

Degree BSN

Available Programs ADN to Baccalaureate; RN Baccalaureate.

Site Options Myrtle Beach, SC.

Study Options Full-time and part-time.

Program Entrance Requirements Minimum overall college GPA of 2.0, CPR certification, health exam, health insurance, immunizations, professional liability insurance/malpractice insurance, prerequisite course work, RN licensure. Transfer students are accepted. *Application deadline:* Applications may be processed on a rolling basis for some programs. *Application fee:* $45.

Expenses (2014–15) *Tuition, state resident:* part-time $429 per credit hour. *Tuition, nonresident:* part-time $979 per credit hour.

Financial Aid *Gift aid (need-based):* Federal Pell, FSEOG, state, private, college/university gift aid from institutional funds. *Loans:* Federal Direct (Subsidized and Unsubsidized Stafford PLUS), Perkins, state. *Work-study:* Federal Work-Study, part-time campus jobs. *Financial aid application deadline (priority):* 3/1.

Contact Dr. Wanda Dooley, Director, RN-to-BSN Completion Program, Nursing Completion Program, Coastal Carolina University, PO Box 261954, Conway, SC 29528-6054. *E-mail:* wdooley@coastal.edu.

Francis Marion University
Department of Nursing
Florence, South Carolina

http://www.fmarion.edu/
Founded in 1970

DEGREE • BSN
Nursing Program Faculty 13 (38% with doctorates).
Baccalaureate Enrollment 213 **Women** 86% **Men** 14%
Distance Learning Courses Available.
Nursing Student Activities Nursing Honor Society, Sigma Theta Tau, Student Nurses' Association.
Nursing Student Resources Academic advising; academic or career counseling; assistance for students with disabilities; bookstore; campus computer network; career placement assistance; computer lab; computer-assisted instruction; daycare for children of students; e-mail services; externships; housing assistance; interactive nursing skills videos; Internet; learning resource lab; library services; nursing audiovisuals; paid internships; placement services for program completers; remedial services; resume preparation assistance; skills, simulation, or other laboratory; tutoring; unpaid internships.

BACCALAUREATE PROGRAMS

Degree BSN
Available Programs ADN to Baccalaureate; Generic Baccalaureate.
Study Options Full-time.
Online Degree Options Yes.
Program Entrance Requirements Transcript of college record, CPR certification, written essay, health insurance, immunizations, 3 letters of recommendation, minimum GPA in nursing prerequisites of 3.0, prerequisite course work. Transfer students are accepted. *Application deadline:* 3/1 (fall), 10/1 (spring). *Application fee:* $78.
Contact *Telephone:* 843-661-1226. *Fax:* 843-661-1696.

Lander University
School of Nursing
Greenwood, South Carolina

http://www.lander.edu/nursing/
Founded in 1872

DEGREE • BSN
Nursing Program Faculty 21 (10% with doctorates).
Baccalaureate Enrollment 273 **Women** 92% **Men** 8% **Part-time** 16%
Distance Learning Courses Available.
Nursing Student Activities Sigma Theta Tau, Student Nurses' Association.
Nursing Student Resources Academic advising; academic or career counseling; assistance for students with disabilities; bookstore; campus computer network; career placement assistance; computer lab; computer-assisted instruction; e-mail services; externships; housing assistance; interactive nursing skills videos; Internet; learning resource lab; library services; nursing audiovisuals; resume preparation assistance; skills, simulation, or other laboratory.
Library Facilities 6,209 volumes in health, 1,145 volumes in nursing; 36 periodical subscriptions health-care related.

BACCALAUREATE PROGRAMS

Degree BSN
Available Programs Accelerated Baccalaureate; Accelerated Baccalaureate for Second Degree; Accelerated RN Baccalaureate; Baccalaureate for Second Degree; Generic Baccalaureate; RN Baccalaureate.
Site Options Greenwood, SC.
Study Options Full-time and part-time.
Online Degree Options Yes.
Program Entrance Requirements Minimum overall college GPA of 2.6, transcript of college record, CPR certification, health exam, health insurance, immunizations, professional liability insurance/malpractice insurance, prerequisite course work. Transfer students are accepted.

Application deadline: Applications may be processed on a rolling basis for some programs. *Application fee:* $35.
Advanced Placement Credit given for nursing courses completed elsewhere dependent upon specific evaluations.
Contact *Telephone:* 864-388-8307. *Fax:* 864-388-8125.

Medical University of South Carolina
College of Nursing
Charleston, South Carolina

http://www.musc.edu/nursing
Founded in 1824

DEGREES • BSN • MSN • PHD
Nursing Program Faculty 42 (88% with doctorates).
Baccalaureate Enrollment 288 **Women** 83% **Men** 17% **Part-time** 1%
Graduate Enrollment 289 **Women** 94% **Men** 6% **Part-time** 35%
Distance Learning Courses Available.
Nursing Student Activities Sigma Theta Tau, Student Nurses' Association.
Nursing Student Resources Academic advising; academic or career counseling; assistance for students with disabilities; bookstore; campus computer network; computer lab; computer-assisted instruction; e-mail services; interactive nursing skills videos; Internet; learning resource lab; library services; nursing audiovisuals; other; resume preparation assistance; skills, simulation, or other laboratory; tutoring.
Library Facilities 35,000 volumes in health, 2,230 volumes in nursing; 25,000 periodical subscriptions health-care related.

BACCALAUREATE PROGRAMS

Degree BSN
Available Programs ADN to Baccalaureate; Accelerated Baccalaureate; Accelerated Baccalaureate for Second Degree.
Site Options Charleston, SC.
Study Options Full-time.
Program Entrance Requirements Minimum overall college GPA of 3.0, transcript of college record, CPR certification, written essay, health exam, health insurance, immunizations, 3 letters of recommendation, minimum GPA in nursing prerequisites of 3.0, prerequisite course work. *Application deadline:* 1/15 (fall), 9/15 (spring). *Application fee:* $95.
Advanced Placement Credit by examination available. Credit given for nursing courses completed elsewhere dependent upon specific evaluations.
Financial Aid 87% of baccalaureate students in nursing programs received some form of financial aid in 2014–15. *Gift aid (need-based):* Federal Pell, FSEOG, state, private, college/university gift aid from institutional funds, Federal Nursing, Scholarships for Disadvantaged Students (SDS). *Loans:* Federal Nursing Student Loans, Federal Direct (Subsidized and Unsubsidized Stafford PLUS), Perkins, state, alternative loans, Health Professions Student Loans (HPSL), Loans for Disadvantaged Students program, Primary Care Loans. *Work-study:* Federal Work-Study.
Contact Mrs. Mardi Long, Program Coordinator, College of Nursing, Medical University of South Carolina, 99 Jonathan Lucas Street, MSC 160, Charleston, SC 29425-1600. *Telephone:* 843-792-6683. *Fax:* 843-792-9258. *E-mail:* longm@musc.edu.

GRADUATE PROGRAMS

Financial Aid 68% of graduate students in nursing programs received some form of financial aid in 2014–15. Federal Work-Study, scholarships, and traineeships available. Aid available to part-time students. *Financial aid application deadline:* 3/10.
Contact Dr. Catherine Durham, Director of Graduate Programs, College of Nursing, Medical University of South Carolina, 99 Jonathan Lucas Street, MSC 160, Charleston, SC 29425-1600. *Telephone:* 843-792-3585. *Fax:* 843-792-5395. *E-mail:* durhamc@musc.edu.

MASTER'S DEGREE PROGRAM
Degree MSN
Available Programs Master's.
Concentrations Available *Nurse practitioner programs in:* adult health, family health, gerontology, pediatric, primary care.
Site Options Charleston, SC.
Study Options Full-time and part-time.
Online Degree Options Yes (online only).

Program Entrance Requirements Minimum overall college GPA of 3.0, transcript of college record, CPR certification, written essay, immunizations, 3 letters of recommendation, prerequisite course work, resume, statistics course. *Application deadline:* 3/15 (fall). *Application fee:* $95.

Advanced Placement Credit given for nursing courses completed elsewhere dependent upon specific evaluations.

Degree Requirements 60 total credit hours, thesis or project, comprehensive exam.

DOCTORAL DEGREE PROGRAM

Degree PhD

Available Programs Doctorate; Doctorate for Nurses with Non-Nursing Degrees; Post-Baccalaureate Doctorate.

Areas of Study Community health, family health, nursing administration, nursing education, nursing policy, nursing research, nursing science.

Site Options Charleston, SC.

Online Degree Options Yes (online only).

Program Entrance Requirements Minimum overall college GPA of 3.5, interview by faculty committee, interview, 3 letters of recommendation, MSN or equivalent, statistics course, vita, writing sample. Application deadline: 3/1 (fall). Applications may be processed on a rolling basis for some programs. Application fee: $95.

Degree Requirements 45 total credit hours, dissertation, oral exam, written exam.

POSTDOCTORAL PROGRAM

Postdoctoral Program Contact Dr. William Basco, Program Director, College of Nursing, Medical University of South Carolina, Rutledge Towers, MSC 106, Charleston, SC 29425. *Telephone:* 843-876-6512. *Fax:* 843-876-8709. *E-mail:* bascob@musc.edu.

Newberry College

Department of Nursing
Newberry, South Carolina

http://www.newberry.edu/academics/areasofstudy/nursing.aspx
Founded in 1856

DEGREE • BSN

Nursing Program Faculty 6 (17% with doctorates).

Baccalaureate Enrollment 44 **Women** 75% **Men** 25% **Part-time** 2.3%

Distance Learning Courses Available.

Nursing Student Activities Student Nurses' Association.

Nursing Student Resources Academic advising; academic or career counseling; assistance for students with disabilities; bookstore; campus computer network; career placement assistance; computer-assisted instruction; e-mail services; Internet; learning resource lab; library services; nursing audiovisuals; resume preparation assistance; skills, simulation, or other laboratory; tutoring.

BACCALAUREATE PROGRAMS

Degree BSN

Available Programs ADN to Baccalaureate; Generic Baccalaureate.

Study Options Full-time.

Program Entrance Requirements Transcript of college record, minimum GPA in nursing prerequisites of 2.75, prerequisite course work. Transfer students are accepted. *Application deadline:* 5/1 (fall).

Advanced Placement Credit given for nursing courses completed elsewhere dependent upon specific evaluations.

Expenses (2015–16) *Tuition:* full-time $22,050; part-time $735 per credit hour. *Room and board:* $12,725; room only: $8000 per academic year. *Required fees:* full-time $3350; part-time $68 per credit.

Contact Dr. Betsy M. McDowell, Department Chair, Department of Nursing, Newberry College, 2100 College Street, Newberry, SC 29108. *Telephone:* 800-845-4955. *E-mail:* mcdowell@newberry.edu.

University of South Carolina

College of Nursing
Columbia, South Carolina

http://www.sc.edu/nursing
Founded in 1801

DEGREES • BSN • DNP • MSN • PHD

Nursing Program Faculty 101 (73% with doctorates).

Baccalaureate Enrollment 1,146 **Women** 92% **Men** 8% **Part-time** 3.2%

Graduate Enrollment 349 **Women** 91% **Men** 9% **Part-time** 66.2%

Distance Learning Courses Available.

Nursing Student Activities Nursing Honor Society, Sigma Theta Tau, Student Nurses' Association, nursing club.

Nursing Student Resources Academic advising; academic or career counseling; assistance for students with disabilities; bookstore; campus computer network; career placement assistance; computer lab; computer-assisted instruction; daycare for children of students; e-mail services; employment services for current students; externships; housing assistance; interactive nursing skills videos; Internet; learning resource lab; library services; nursing audiovisuals; paid internships; placement services for program completers; remedial services; resume preparation assistance; skills, simulation, or other laboratory; tutoring; unpaid internships.

Library Facilities 76,116 volumes in health, 6,931 volumes in nursing; 16,390 periodical subscriptions health-care related.

BACCALAUREATE PROGRAMS

Degree BSN

Available Programs Accelerated RN Baccalaureate; Generic Baccalaureate.

Site Options Lancaster, SC; Walterboro, SC; Allendale, SC.

Study Options Full-time and part-time.

Online Degree Options Yes.

Program Entrance Requirements Minimum overall college GPA of 3.0, transcript of college record, high school biology, high school chemistry, high school foreign language, 4 years high school math, 3 years high school science, high school transcript, immunizations, minimum GPA in nursing prerequisites of 3.0. Transfer students are accepted. *Application deadline:* 12/1 (fall), 11/1 (spring), 12/1 (summer). *Application fee:* $50.

Advanced Placement Credit by examination available. Credit given for nursing courses completed elsewhere dependent upon specific evaluations.

Expenses (2015–16) *Tuition, state resident:* full-time $11,082; part-time $462 per credit hour. *Tuition, nonresident:* full-time $29,898; part-time $1246 per credit hour. *International tuition:* $29,898 full-time. *Room and board:* $10,398; room only: $6832 per academic year. *Required fees:* full-time $4355.

Financial Aid 61% of baccalaureate students in nursing programs received some form of financial aid in 2014–15. *Gift aid (need-based):* Federal Pell, FSEOG, state, private, college/university gift aid from institutional funds, United Negro College Fund, Federal Nursing, USC Opportunity Grants, Gamecock Guarantee. *Loans:* Federal Nursing Student Loans, Federal Direct (Subsidized and Unsubsidized Stafford PLUS), Perkins. *Work-study:* Federal Work-Study, part-time campus jobs. *Financial aid application deadline (priority):* 4/1.

Contact Ms. Heidi Waltz, Student Services Manager, College of Nursing, University of South Carolina, College of Nursing, 1601 Greene Street, Columbia, SC 29208-4001. *Telephone:* 803-777-7412. *Fax:* 803-777-0616. *E-mail:* waltzh@mailbox.sc.edu.

GRADUATE PROGRAMS

Expenses (2015–16) *Tuition, state resident:* full-time $17,136; part-time $714 per credit hour. *Tuition, nonresident:* full-time $31,284; part-time $1304 per credit hour. *International tuition:* $31,284 full-time. *Required fees:* full-time $4280; part-time $174 per term.

Financial Aid 50% of graduate students in nursing programs received some form of financial aid in 2014–15. 1 fellowship (averaging $1,200 per year), 3 research assistantships with partial tuition reimbursements available (averaging $2,790 per year), 11 teaching assistantships (averaging $5,533 per year) were awarded; scholarships, traineeships, and unspecified assistantships also available. *Financial aid application deadline:* 4/1.

Contact Office of Academic Affairs, College of Nursing, University of South Carolina, College of Nursing, 1601 Greene Street, Columbia, SC

29208-4001. *Telephone:* 803-777-7412. *Fax:* 803-777-2305. *E-mail:* nursinq@mailbox.sc.edu.

MASTER'S DEGREE PROGRAM
Degree MSN
Available Programs Accelerated Master's; Master's.
Concentrations Available Nursing administration. *Nurse practitioner programs in:* adult-gerontology acute care, family health, psychiatric/mental health.
Study Options Full-time and part-time.
Online Degree Options Yes (online only).
Program Entrance Requirements Minimum overall college GPA of 3.0, transcript of college record, written essay, immunizations, 3 letters of recommendation, resume, GRE General Test, MAT. *Application deadline:* 4/1 (fall), 10/1 (spring), 3/1 (summer). *Application fee:* $50.
Advanced Placement Credit given for nursing courses completed elsewhere dependent upon specific evaluations.
Degree Requirements 45 total credit hours, comprehensive exam.

POST-MASTER'S PROGRAM
Areas of Study Nursing administration. *Nurse practitioner programs in:* adult-gerontology acute care, family health, psychiatric/mental health.

DOCTORAL DEGREE PROGRAM
Degree DNP
Available Programs Doctorate, Post-Baccalaureate Doctorate.
Areas of Study Adult-gerontology acute care, family health, nurse executive, psychiatric/mental health.
Online Degree Options Yes.
Program Entrance Requirements Minimum overall college GPA of 3.0, interview by faculty committee, 3 letters of recommendation, vita, writing sample. Application deadline: 4/1 (fall), 10/1 (spring), 3/1 (summer). Application fee: $50.
Degree Requirements 33 total credit hours (post-master's) or 60-75 (post-BSN) credit hours, dissertation, residency.

Degree PhD
Available Programs Doctorate; Post-Baccalaureate Doctorate.
Areas of Study Addiction/substance abuse, bio-behavioral research, clinical research, family health, health promotion/disease prevention, health-care systems, individualized study, nursing research, nursing science, palliative care, women's health.
Program Entrance Requirements Minimum overall college GPA of 3.0, interview by faculty committee, 3 letters of recommendation, scholarly papers, statistics course, vita, writing sample, GRE General Test. Application deadline: 2/1 (fall). Application fee: $50.
Degree Requirements 57 total credit hours, dissertation, oral exam, written exam, residency.

POSTDOCTORAL PROGRAM
Areas of Study Addiction/substance abuse, cancer care, community health, health promotion/disease prevention, individualized study, nursing interventions, nursing research, nursing science, vulnerable population.
Postdoctoral Program Contact Dr. Bernardine M. Pinto, Associate Dean for Research and Professor, College of Nursing, University of South Carolina, 1601 Greene Street, Columbia, SC 29208-4001. *Telephone:* 803-777-9272. *Fax:* 803-777-5935. *E-mail:* pintob@mailbox.sc.edu.

CONTINUING EDUCATION PROGRAM
Contact Ms. Ellen C. Synovec, Clinical Associate Professor, College of Nursing, University of South Carolina, 1601 Greene Street, Columbia, SC 29208-4001. *Telephone:* 803-777-4889. *Fax:* 803-777-6800. *E-mail:* synove@mailbox.sc.edu.

University of South Carolina Aiken
School of Nursing
Aiken, South Carolina

http://www.usca.edu/nursing/
Founded in 1961
DEGREE • BSN
Nursing Program Faculty 16 (50% with doctorates).
Baccalaureate Enrollment 230 **Women** 85% **Men** 15% **Part-time** 2%

Distance Learning Courses Available.
Nursing Student Activities Nursing Honor Society, Sigma Theta Tau, Student Nurses' Association.
Nursing Student Resources Academic advising; academic or career counseling; assistance for students with disabilities; bookstore; campus computer network; career placement assistance; computer lab; computer-assisted instruction; daycare for children of students; e-mail services; employment services for current students; externships; housing assistance; interactive nursing skills videos; Internet; learning resource lab; library services; nursing audiovisuals; placement services for program completers; resume preparation assistance; skills, simulation, or other laboratory; tutoring.
Library Facilities 200 volumes in health, 100 volumes in nursing; 100 periodical subscriptions health-care related.

BACCALAUREATE PROGRAMS
Degree BSN
Available Programs ADN to Baccalaureate; Generic Baccalaureate; RN Baccalaureate.
Study Options Full-time.
Online Degree Options Yes.
Program Entrance Requirements Transcript of college record, CPR certification, written essay, health exam, immunizations, 2 letters of recommendation, minimum GPA in nursing prerequisites of 3.00, prerequisite course work. Transfer students are accepted. *Application deadline:* 3/15 (fall), 10/15 (spring).
Advanced Placement Credit given for nursing courses completed elsewhere dependent upon specific evaluations.
Expenses (2015–16) *Tuition, state resident:* full-time $9588; part-time $399 per credit hour. *Tuition, nonresident:* full-time $19,182; part-time $799 per credit hour. *International tuition:* $19,182 full-time. *Room and board:* $7290; room only: $4740 per academic year. *Required fees:* full-time $290; part-time $9 per credit; part-time $25 per term.
Financial Aid 75% of baccalaureate students in nursing programs received some form of financial aid in 2014–15.
Contact Ms. Kathy Simmons, Administrative Assistant, School of Nursing, University of South Carolina Aiken, 471 University Parkway, Aiken, SC 29801. *Telephone:* 803-648-3392. *Fax:* 803-641-3725. *E-mail:* kathers@usca.edu.

University of South Carolina Beaufort
Nursing Program
Bluffton, South Carolina

http://www.uscb.edu/
Founded in 1959
DEGREE • BSN
Nursing Program Faculty 15 (60% with doctorates).
Baccalaureate Enrollment 73 **Women** 88.7% **Men** 11.3% **Part-time** 39%
Distance Learning Courses Available.
Nursing Student Activities Student Nurses' Association.
Nursing Student Resources Academic advising; academic or career counseling; assistance for students with disabilities; bookstore; campus computer network; career placement assistance; computer lab; computer-assisted instruction; e-mail services; employment services for current students; externships; housing assistance; interactive nursing skills videos; Internet; learning resource lab; library services; nursing audiovisuals; paid internships; remedial services; resume preparation assistance; skills, simulation, or other laboratory; tutoring; unpaid internships.
Library Facilities 2,273 volumes in health, 198 volumes in nursing; 120 periodical subscriptions health-care related.

BACCALAUREATE PROGRAMS
Degree BSN
Available Programs Generic Baccalaureate; RN Baccalaureate.
Site Options Beaufort, SC.
Study Options Full-time.
Program Entrance Requirements Minimum overall college GPA of 3.0, transcript of college record, CPR certification, health exam, health insurance, immunizations, 2 letters of recommendation, minimum GPA in nursing prerequisites of 3.0, prerequisite course work. Transfer students are accepted. *Application deadline:* 8/1 (spring). *Application fee:* $65.

Advanced Placement Credit by examination available. Credit given for nursing courses completed elsewhere dependent upon specific evaluations.

Expenses (2015–16) *Tuition, state resident:* full-time $4731; part-time $394 per credit hour. *Tuition, nonresident:* full-time $9798; part-time $817 per credit hour. *International tuition:* $9798 full-time. *Room and board:* room only: $3440 per academic year. *Required fees:* full-time $3576; part-time $1778 per term.

Contact Dr. Rose Kearney-Nunnery, Professor and Chair, Department of Nursing, Nursing Program, University of South Carolina Beaufort, 1 University Boulevard, Bluffton, SC 29909. *Telephone:* 843-208-8124. *E-mail:* nursing@uscb.edu.

University of South Carolina Upstate

Mary Black School of Nursing
Spartanburg, South Carolina

https://www.uscupstate.edu/academics/nursing/default.aspx?id=2287

Founded in 1967

DEGREES • BSN • MSN

Nursing Program Faculty 80 (16% with doctorates).

Baccalaureate Enrollment 543 **Women** 92% **Men** 8% **Part-time** 15%

Graduate Enrollment 9 **Women** 88% **Men** 12% **Part-time** 33%

Distance Learning Courses Available.

Nursing Student Activities Nursing Honor Society, Sigma Theta Tau, Student Nurses' Association.

Nursing Student Resources Academic advising; academic or career counseling; assistance for students with disabilities; bookstore; campus computer network; career placement assistance; computer lab; computer-assisted instruction; daycare for children of students; e-mail services; employment services for current students; externships; housing assistance; interactive nursing skills videos; Internet; learning resource lab; library services; nursing audiovisuals; paid internships; resume preparation assistance; skills, simulation, or other laboratory; tutoring; unpaid internships.

Library Facilities 214,998 volumes in health, 23,359 volumes in nursing; 2,160 periodical subscriptions health-care related.

BACCALAUREATE PROGRAMS

Degree BSN

Available Programs Generic Baccalaureate; RN Baccalaureate.

Site Options Greenville, SC.

Study Options Full-time and part-time.

Online Degree Options Yes.

Program Entrance Requirements Transcript of college record, CPR certification, health exam, health insurance, immunizations, minimum GPA in nursing prerequisites of 2.75, professional liability insurance/malpractice insurance, prerequisite course work. Transfer students are accepted. *Application deadline:* 1/15 (fall), 5/1 (spring).

Advanced Placement Credit by examination available. Credit given for nursing courses completed elsewhere dependent upon specific evaluations.

Expenses (2014–15) *Tuition, state resident:* full-time $10,068; part-time $420 per credit hour. *Tuition, nonresident:* full-time $20,418; part-time $851 per credit hour. *International tuition:* $20,418 full-time. *Room and board:* $4200; room only: $3000 per academic year. *Required fees:* full-time $1100; part-time $54 per credit.

Financial Aid 85% of baccalaureate students in nursing programs received some form of financial aid in 2013–14. *Gift aid (need-based):* Federal Pell, FSEOG, state, private, college/university gift aid from institutional funds. *Loans:* Federal Direct (Subsidized and Unsubsidized Stafford PLUS), Perkins, state, private loans. *Work-study:* Federal Work-Study, part-time campus jobs. *Financial aid application deadline (priority):* 3/1.

Contact Dr. Katharine M. Gibb, Dean, Mary Black School of Nursing, University of South Carolina Upstate, 800 University Way, Spartanburg, SC 29303. *Telephone:* 864-503-5444. *Fax:* 864-503-5405. *E-mail:* kgibb@uscupstate.edu.

GRADUATE PROGRAMS

Expenses (2014–15) *Tuition, state resident:* full-time $12,024; part-time $501 per credit hour. *Tuition, nonresident:* full-time $25,770; part-time $1074 per credit hour. *International tuition:* $25,770 full-time. *Required fees:* full-time $285; part-time $35 per term.

Financial Aid 20% of graduate students in nursing programs received some form of financial aid in 2013–14.

Contact Dr. Katharine M. Gibb, EdD, Dean, Mary Black School of Nursing, University of South Carolina Upstate, 800 University way, Spartanburg, SC 29303. *Telephone:* 864-503-5444. *Fax:* 864-503-5405. *E-mail:* kgibb@uscupstate.edu.

MASTER'S DEGREE PROGRAM

Degree MSN

Available Programs Master's.

Concentrations Available Clinical nurse leader.

Study Options Full-time and part-time.

Online Degree Options Yes.

Program Entrance Requirements Minimum overall college GPA of 3.0, transcript of college record, 3 letters of recommendation, resume. *Application deadline:* 6/30 (fall).

Advanced Placement Credit given for nursing courses completed elsewhere dependent upon specific evaluations.

Degree Requirements 38 total credit hours, thesis or project.

SOUTH DAKOTA

Augustana University

Department of Nursing
Sioux Falls, South Dakota

http://www.augie.edu/nursing

Founded in 1860

DEGREE • BA

Nursing Program Faculty 10 (3% with doctorates).

Baccalaureate Enrollment 117 **Women** 90% **Men** 10% **Part-time** 14%

Nursing Student Activities Sigma Theta Tau, Student Nurses' Association.

Nursing Student Resources Academic advising; academic or career counseling; assistance for students with disabilities; bookstore; campus computer network; career placement assistance; computer lab; computer-assisted instruction; daycare for children of students; e-mail services; employment services for current students; housing assistance; interactive nursing skills videos; Internet; learning resource lab; library services; nursing audiovisuals; remedial services; resume preparation assistance; skills, simulation, or other laboratory; tutoring; unpaid internships.

BACCALAUREATE PROGRAMS

Degree BA

Available Programs Accelerated Baccalaureate; Generic Baccalaureate.

Study Options Full-time and part-time.

Program Entrance Requirements Minimum overall college GPA of 2.7, transcript of college record, CPR certification, written essay, health exam, health insurance, high school transcript, immunizations, 2 letters of recommendation, minimum high school GPA of 3.0, minimum GPA in nursing prerequisites of 2.7, prerequisite course work. Transfer students are accepted. *Application deadline:* 2/15 (fall). Applications may be processed on a rolling basis for some programs.

Advanced Placement Credit given for nursing courses completed elsewhere dependent upon specific evaluations.

Contact Jennie Holland, Health Sciences Program Manager, Department of Nursing, Augustana University, 2001 South Summit Avenue, Nursing, Sioux Falls, SD 57197. *Telephone:* 605-274-4727. *E-mail:* jholland@augie.edu.

Dakota Wesleyan University
The Arlene Gates Department of Nursing
Mitchell, South Dakota

http://www.dwu.edu/nursing/
Founded in 1885
DEGREE • BSN

BACCALAUREATE PROGRAMS

Degree BSN
Available Programs RN Baccalaureate.
Contact Department of Nursing, The Arlene Gates Department of Nursing, Dakota Wesleyan University, 1200 West University Avenue, Mitchell, SD 57301. *Telephone:* 800-333-8506.

Mount Marty College
Nursing Program
Yankton, South Dakota

http://www.mtmc.edu/
Founded in 1936
DEGREES • BSN • MSN
Nursing Program Faculty 14 (14% with doctorates).
Baccalaureate Enrollment 80 **Women** 84% **Men** 16% **Part-time** 9%
Graduate Enrollment 10 **Women** 80% **Men** 20% **Part-time** 90%
Distance Learning Courses Available.
Nursing Student Activities Sigma Theta Tau, Student Nurses' Association, nursing club.
Nursing Student Resources Academic advising; academic or career counseling; assistance for students with disabilities; bookstore; campus computer network; career placement assistance; computer lab; computer-assisted instruction; daycare for children of students; e-mail services; employment services for current students; externships; housing assistance; interactive nursing skills videos; Internet; learning resource lab; library services; nursing audiovisuals; paid internships; placement services for program completers; remedial services; resume preparation assistance; skills, simulation, or other laboratory; tutoring; unpaid internships.
Library Facilities 8,750 volumes in health, 5,350 volumes in nursing; 70 periodical subscriptions health-care related.

BACCALAUREATE PROGRAMS

Degree BSN
Available Programs ADN to Baccalaureate; Accelerated LPN to Baccalaureate; Generic Baccalaureate; International Nurse to Baccalaureate; LPN to Baccalaureate; LPN to RN Baccalaureate; RN Baccalaureate.
Site Options Watertown, SD.
Study Options Full-time and part-time.
Program Entrance Requirements Minimum overall college GPA of 2.8, transcript of college record, CPR certification, health exam, health insurance, high school transcript, immunizations, prerequisite course work. Transfer students are accepted. *Application deadline:* Applications may be processed on a rolling basis for some programs.
Advanced Placement Credit given for nursing courses completed elsewhere dependent upon specific evaluations.
Expenses (2015–16) *Tuition:* full-time $22,336. *International tuition:* $22,336 full-time. *Room and board:* $7326 per academic year. *Required fees:* full-time $2920.
Financial Aid *Gift aid (need-based):* Federal Pell, FSEOG, state, private, college/university gift aid from institutional funds. *Loans:* Federal Nursing Student Loans, Federal Direct (Subsidized and Unsubsidized Stafford PLUS), Perkins, state, college/university. *Work-study:* Federal Work-Study, part-time campus jobs. *Financial aid application deadline (priority):* 3/1.
Contact Dr. Alfred Lupien, Chair and Director, Division of Nursing, Nursing Program, Mount Marty College, 1105 West 8th Street, Yankton, SD 57078-3724. *Telephone:* 605-668-1526. *Fax:* 605-668-1618. *E-mail:* alfred.lupien@mtmc.edu.

GRADUATE PROGRAMS

Expenses (2015–16) *Tuition:* part-time $545 per credit hour.
Contact Josephine Garcia, Interim Family Nurse Practitioner Track Coordinator, Nursing Program, Mount Marty College, 1105 W. 8th Street, Yankton, SD 57078. *Telephone:* 605-668-1435. *Fax:* 605-668-1618. *E-mail:* josephine.garcia@mtmc.edu.

MASTER'S DEGREE PROGRAM
Degree MSN
Available Programs Master's; Master's for Non-Nursing College Graduates; Master's for Nurses with Non-Nursing Degrees; RN to Master's.
Concentrations Available *Nurse practitioner programs in:* family health.
Site Options Sioux Falls, SD.
Study Options Full-time and part-time.
Program Entrance Requirements Clinical experience, computer literacy, minimum overall college GPA of 3.0, transcript of college record, CPR certification, written essay, immunizations, interview, 3 letters of recommendation, nursing research course, physical assessment course, professional liability insurance/malpractice insurance, prerequisite course work, resume, statistics course. *Application deadline:* 3/1 (fall). *Application fee:* $35.
Advanced Placement Credit given for nursing courses completed elsewhere dependent upon specific evaluations.
Degree Requirements 46 total credit hours, thesis or project.

POST-MASTER'S PROGRAM
Areas of Study *Nurse practitioner programs in:* family health.

National American University
School of Nursing
Rapid City, South Dakota

Founded in 1941
DEGREE • BSN

BACCALAUREATE PROGRAMS

Degree BSN
Available Programs Generic Baccalaureate.
Contact *Telephone:* 303-876-7181. *Fax:* 303-876-7105.

Presentation College
Department of Nursing
Aberdeen, South Dakota

http://www.presentation.edu/
Founded in 1951
DEGREE • BSN
Nursing Program Faculty 21 (9% with doctorates).
Baccalaureate Enrollment 185 **Women** 95% **Men** 5% **Part-time** 24%
Distance Learning Courses Available.
Nursing Student Activities Nursing Honor Society, Sigma Theta Tau, Student Nurses' Association, nursing club.
Nursing Student Resources Academic advising; academic or career counseling; assistance for students with disabilities; bookstore; campus computer network; career placement assistance; computer lab; computer-assisted instruction; e-mail services; employment services for current students; externships; interactive nursing skills videos; Internet; learning resource lab; library services; nursing audiovisuals; placement services for program completers; remedial services; resume preparation assistance; skills, simulation, or other laboratory; tutoring; unpaid internships.
Library Facilities 378 volumes in health, 353 volumes in nursing; 2,172 periodical subscriptions health-care related.

BACCALAUREATE PROGRAMS

Degree BSN
Available Programs ADN to Baccalaureate; Baccalaureate for Second Degree; Generic Baccalaureate; LPN to RN Baccalaureate; RN Baccalaureate.
Site Options Fargo , ND; Fairmont, MN.
Study Options Full-time and part-time.
Online Degree Options Yes.
Program Entrance Requirements Minimum overall college GPA of 2.5, transcript of college record, CPR certification, written essay, health exam, high school biology, high school chemistry, 2 years high school math, high school transcript, immunizations, 2 letters of recommendation, minimum high school GPA of 2.7, minimum GPA in nursing pre-

requisites of 2.5, prerequisite course work. Transfer students are accepted. *Application deadline:* 3/1 (fall).

Advanced Placement Credit by examination available. Credit given for nursing courses completed elsewhere dependent upon specific evaluations.

Contact *Telephone:* 605-229-8492. *Fax:* 605-229-8489.

South Dakota State University
College of Nursing
Brookings, South Dakota

http://www.sdstate.edu/nurs/
Founded in 1881

DEGREES • BS • DNP • MS • PHD
Nursing Program Faculty 210 (15% with doctorates).
Baccalaureate Enrollment 753
Graduate Enrollment 193
Distance Learning Courses Available.
Nursing Student Activities Nursing Honor Society, Sigma Theta Tau, Student Nurses' Association, nursing club.
Nursing Student Resources Academic advising; academic or career counseling; assistance for students with disabilities; bookstore; campus computer network; career placement assistance; computer lab; computer-assisted instruction; e-mail services; employment services for current students; externships; housing assistance; interactive nursing skills videos; Internet; learning resource lab; library services; nursing audiovisuals; paid internships; placement services for program completers; remedial services; resume preparation assistance; skills, simulation, or other laboratory; tutoring; unpaid internships.
Library Facilities 31,419 volumes in health, 26,105 volumes in nursing; 5,711 periodical subscriptions health-care related.

BACCALAUREATE PROGRAMS

Degree BS
Available Programs Accelerated RN Baccalaureate; Baccalaureate for Second Degree; RN Baccalaureate.
Site Options Rapid City, SD; Aberdeen, SD; Sioux Falls, SD.
Study Options Full-time.
Online Degree Options Yes.
Program Entrance Requirements Minimum overall college GPA of 2.7, transcript of college record, CPR certification, health exam, health insurance, immunizations, minimum GPA in nursing prerequisites of 2.7, professional liability insurance/malpractice insurance, prerequisite course work. Transfer students are accepted. *Application deadline:* 1/25 (fall), 9/25 (spring).
Advanced Placement Credit given for nursing courses completed elsewhere dependent upon specific evaluations.
Contact Dr. Linda Herrick, Associate Dean for Undergraduate Nursing, College of Nursing, South Dakota State University, 1060 Campanile Avenue, SWG 363, Brookings, SD 57007-0098. *Telephone:* 605-688-6153. *E-mail:* linda.herrick@sdstate.edu.

GRADUATE PROGRAMS

Expenses (2015–16) *Tuition, state resident:* full-time $5922; part-time $219 per credit. *Tuition, nonresident:* full-time $12,534; part-time $464 per credit. *International tuition:* $12,534 full-time.
Financial Aid 2 fellowships, 1 research assistantship, 3 teaching assistantships were awarded; career-related internships or fieldwork, Federal Work-Study, scholarships, and unspecified assistantships also available.
Contact Dr. Mary Minton, Associate Dean for Graduate Nursing, College of Nursing, South Dakota State University, 1060 Campanile Avenue, SWG 217, Brookings, SD 57007-0098. *Telephone:* 605-688-4114. *E-mail:* mary.minton@sdstate.edu.

MASTER'S DEGREE PROGRAM
Degree MS
Available Programs Master's; RN to Master's.
Concentrations Available Clinical nurse leader; nursing administration; nursing education. *Nurse practitioner programs in:* family health.
Site Options Rapid City, SD; Sioux Falls, SD.
Study Options Full-time and part-time.
Online Degree Options Yes.
Program Entrance Requirements Clinical experience, minimum overall college GPA of 3.0, transcript of college record, CPR certifi-

cation, written essay, immunizations, interview, 3 letters of recommendation, professional liability insurance/malpractice insurance, statistics course. *Application deadline:* 3/15 (fall). *Application fee:* $100.
Advanced Placement Credit given for nursing courses completed elsewhere dependent upon specific evaluations.
Degree Requirements 53 total credit hours, comprehensive exam.

POST-MASTER'S PROGRAM
Areas of Study Clinical nurse leader; nursing education. *Nurse practitioner programs in:* family health.

DOCTORAL DEGREE PROGRAM
Degree DNP
Available Programs Doctorate, Post-Baccalaureate Doctorate.
Areas of Study Advanced practice nursing, clinical practice, clinical research, family health.
Program Entrance Requirements Minimum overall college GPA of 3.3, clinical experience, interview, interview by faculty committee, 3 letters of recommendations, MSN or equivalent (for post-Master's), statistics course, vita. Application deadline: 3/15 (fall). Application fee: $100.
Degree Requirements 28-78 total credit depending on program, Capstone project, oral exam, written exam.

Degree PhD
Available Programs Doctorate; Post-Baccalaureate Doctorate.
Areas of Study Nursing research.
Site Options Rapid City, SD; Sioux Falls, SD.
Program Entrance Requirements Clinical experience, minimum overall college GPA of 3.3, interview by faculty committee, interview, 4 letters of recommendation, MSN or equivalent, scholarly papers, statistics course, vita, writing sample. Application deadline: 3/15 (fall). Application fee: $100.
Degree Requirements 60–90 total credit hours, dissertation, oral exam, written exam.

CONTINUING EDUCATION PROGRAM

Contact Ms. Linda Lemme, Program Assistant II, College of Nursing, South Dakota State University, 1060 Campanile Avenue, SWG 255, Brookings, SD 57007-0098. *Telephone:* 605-688-5745. *E-mail:* Linda.Lemme@sdstate.edu.

University of Sioux Falls
School of Nursing
Sioux Falls, South Dakota

http://www.usiouxfalls.edu/nursing
Founded in 1883

DEGREE • BSN
Nursing Program Faculty 5 (20% with doctorates).
Baccalaureate Enrollment 169
Distance Learning Courses Available.
Nursing Student Activities Nursing Honor Society, Sigma Theta Tau, Student Nurses' Association.
Nursing Student Resources Academic advising; academic or career counseling; assistance for students with disabilities; bookstore; campus computer network; career placement assistance; computer lab; computer-assisted instruction; e-mail services; employment services for current students; interactive nursing skills videos; Internet; learning resource lab; library services; nursing audiovisuals; other; placement services for program completers; remedial services; resume preparation assistance; skills, simulation, or other laboratory; tutoring.

BACCALAUREATE PROGRAMS

Degree BSN
Available Programs Accelerated Baccalaureate; Generic Baccalaureate; RN Baccalaureate.
Online Degree Options Yes.
Program Entrance Requirements Minimum overall college GPA of 2.75, written essay, letters of recommendation, minimum high school GPA of 2.75, prerequisite course work, RN licensure.
Contact *Telephone:* 605-331-6697.

The University of South Dakota
Department of Nursing
Vermillion, South Dakota

http://www.usd.edu/health-sciences/nursing/
Founded in 1862
DEGREE • BSN
Nursing Program Faculty 88 (.16% with doctorates).
Baccalaureate Enrollment 437 **Women** 88% **Men** 12% **Part-time** .5%
Distance Learning Courses Available.
Nursing Student Activities Sigma Theta Tau, Student Nurses' Association.
Nursing Student Resources Academic advising; academic or career counseling; assistance for students with disabilities; bookstore; campus computer network; computer lab; e-mail services; interactive nursing skills videos; Internet; learning resource lab; library services; nursing audiovisuals; skills, simulation, or other laboratory; tutoring.

BACCALAUREATE PROGRAMS

Degree BSN
Available Programs Generic Baccalaureate; RN Baccalaureate.
Site Options Sioux Falls, SD; Rapid City, SD.
Study Options Full-time.
Online Degree Options Yes.
Program Entrance Requirements Minimum overall college GPA of 2.7, transcript of college record, health exam, health insurance, immunizations, 3 letters of recommendation, minimum GPA in nursing prerequisites of 2.7, prerequisite course work. Transfer students are accepted. *Application deadline:* 2/1 (fall), 8/1 (spring).
Advanced Placement Credit given for nursing courses completed elsewhere dependent upon specific evaluations.
Expenses (2015–16) *Tuition, state resident:* full-time $4197; part-time $145 per credit hour. *Tuition, nonresident:* full-time $6295; part-time $217 per credit hour. *Room and board:* $7174; room only: $3988 per academic year.
Financial Aid 78% of baccalaureate students in nursing programs received some form of financial aid in 2014–15.
Contact USD Nursing Program Office, Department of Nursing, The University of South Dakota, 414 East Clark Street, Vermillion, SD 57069. *Telephone:* 605-677-5006. *E-mail:* nursing@usd.edu.

TENNESSEE

Aquinas College
School of Nursing
Nashville, Tennessee

http://www.aquinas.edu/nursing/
Founded in 1961
DEGREES • BSN • MSN
Nursing Program Faculty 29 (33% with doctorates).
Baccalaureate Enrollment 65 **Women** 87% **Men** 13% **Part-time** 23%
Nursing Student Activities Nursing Honor Society.
Nursing Student Resources Academic advising; academic or career counseling; assistance for students with disabilities; bookstore; campus computer network; career placement assistance; computer lab; computer-assisted instruction; e-mail services; employment services for current students; interactive nursing skills videos; Internet; learning resource lab; library services; nursing audiovisuals; remedial services; resume preparation assistance; skills, simulation, or other laboratory; tutoring.
Library Facilities 2,290 volumes in health, 1,220 volumes in nursing; 1,300 periodical subscriptions health-care related.

BACCALAUREATE PROGRAMS

Degree BSN
Available Programs ADN to Baccalaureate; Generic Baccalaureate.
Study Options Full-time and part-time.
Program Entrance Requirements Minimum overall college GPA of 2.75, transcript of college record, CPR certification, written essay, health exam, health insurance, high school chemistry, high school transcript, immunizations, 2 letters of recommendation, minimum high school GPA

of 2.75, minimum GPA in nursing prerequisites of 2.75, professional liability insurance/malpractice insurance, prerequisite course work, RN licensure. Transfer students are accepted. *Application deadline:* Applications may be processed on a rolling basis for some programs.
Advanced Placement Credit by examination available. Credit given for nursing courses completed elsewhere dependent upon specific evaluations.
Expenses (2015–16) *Tuition:* full-time $9975; part-time $680 per credit hour. *Room and board:* $4450; room only: $2850 per academic year. *Required fees:* full-time $225.
Contact Dr. Elizabeth Cooper, RN, Dean, School of Nursing, School of Nursing, Aquinas College, 4210 Harding Pike, Nashville, TN 37205. *Telephone:* 615-297-2008. *Fax:* 615-783-0562. *E-mail:* coopere@aquinascollege.edu.

GRADUATE PROGRAMS

Expenses (2015–16) *Tuition:* full-time $12,420; part-time $690 per credit hour. *Required fees:* full-time $95.
Contact Dr. Elizabeth Cooper, RN, Dean, School of Nursing, School of Nursing, Aquinas College, 4210 Harding Pike, Nashville, TN 37205. *Telephone:* 615-297-2008. *Fax:* 615-783-0562. *E-mail:* coopere@aquinascollege.edu.

MASTER'S DEGREE PROGRAM
Degree MSN
Available Programs Master's.
Concentrations Available Nursing education.
Study Options Full-time and part-time.
Program Entrance Requirements Computer literacy, minimum overall college GPA of 3.0, transcript of college record, CPR certification, written essay, immunizations, interview, 2 letters of recommendation, professional liability insurance/malpractice insurance, resume, statistics course. *Application deadline:* Applications may be processed on a rolling basis for some programs.
Advanced Placement Credit by examination available. Credit given for nursing courses completed elsewhere dependent upon specific evaluations.
Degree Requirements 40 total credit hours, thesis or project.

POST-MASTER'S PROGRAM
Areas of Study Nursing education.

Austin Peay State University
School of Nursing
Clarksville, Tennessee

http://www.apsu.edu/nursing01
Founded in 1927
DEGREES • BSN • MSN
Nursing Program Faculty 39 (29% with doctorates).
Baccalaureate Enrollment 295 **Women** 87.11% **Men** 12.89%
Graduate Enrollment 207 **Women** 87.92% **Men** 12.08% **Part-time** 86.47%
Distance Learning Courses Available.
Nursing Student Activities Nursing Honor Society, Sigma Theta Tau, Student Nurses' Association.
Nursing Student Resources Academic advising; academic or career counseling; assistance for students with disabilities; bookstore; campus computer network; computer lab; computer-assisted instruction; daycare for children of students; e-mail services; employment services for current students; interactive nursing skills videos; Internet; library services; nursing audiovisuals; remedial services; resume preparation assistance; skills, simulation, or other laboratory; tutoring.
Library Facilities 4,700 volumes in health, 800 volumes in nursing; 80 periodical subscriptions health-care related.

BACCALAUREATE PROGRAMS

Degree BSN
Available Programs ADN to Baccalaureate; Baccalaureate for Second Degree; Generic Baccalaureate; RN Baccalaureate.
Study Options Full-time.
Program Entrance Requirements Minimum overall college GPA of 3.0, transcript of college record, immunizations, minimum GPA in nursing prerequisites of 3.0, prerequisite course work. Transfer students are accepted. *Application deadline:* 5/1 (fall), 9/1 (spring).

Expenses (2014–15) *Tuition, state resident:* full-time $3780; part-time $309 per credit hour. *Tuition, nonresident:* full-time $11,508; part-time $913 per credit hour. *Room and board:* $8706; room only: $5600 per academic year. *Required fees:* full-time $400; part-time $25 per credit; part-time $200 per term.

Financial Aid 68% of baccalaureate students in nursing programs received some form of financial aid in 2013–14. *Gift aid (need-based):* Federal Pell, FSEOG, state, private, college/university gift aid from institutional funds. *Loans:* Federal Direct (Subsidized and Unsubsidized Stafford PLUS), Perkins. *Work-study:* Federal Work-Study, part-time campus jobs. *Financial aid application deadline:* Continuous.

Contact Ms. Debbie Cochener, Administrative Specialist/Pre-Nursing Advisor, School of Nursing, Austin Peay State University, PO Box 4658, Clarksville, TN 37044. *Telephone:* 931-221-7708. *Fax:* 931-221-7595. *E-mail:* cochenerd@apsu.edu.

GRADUATE PROGRAMS

Expenses (2014–15) *Tuition, state resident:* full-time $4437; part-time $439 per credit hour. *Tuition, nonresident:* full-time $10,422; part-time $1158 per credit hour. *Required fees:* full-time $450; part-time $25 per credit; part-time $225 per term.

Financial Aid 63% of graduate students in nursing programs received some form of financial aid in 2013–14.

Contact Dr. Michele Robertson, Coordinator of the MSN RODP, School of Nursing, Austin Peay State University, PO Box 4658, Clarksville, TN 37044. *Telephone:* 931-221-7489. *Fax:* 931-221-7595. *E-mail:* robertsonm@apsu.edu.

MASTER'S DEGREE PROGRAM

Degree MSN

Available Programs Master's.

Concentrations Available Nursing administration; nursing education; nursing informatics. *Nurse practitioner programs in:* family health.

Study Options Full-time and part-time.

Online Degree Options Yes (online only).

Program Entrance Requirements Minimum overall college GPA of 3.0, transcript of college record, statistics course. *Application deadline:* 6/15 (fall), 10/15 (spring), 2/1 (summer). Applications may be processed on a rolling basis for some programs. *Application fee:* $25.

Advanced Placement Credit given for nursing courses completed elsewhere dependent upon specific evaluations.

Degree Requirements 46 total credit hours.

POST-MASTER'S PROGRAM

Areas of Study Nursing administration; nursing education; nursing informatics. *Nurse practitioner programs in:* family health.

Baptist College of Health Sciences

Nursing Division
Memphis, Tennessee

http://www.bchs.edu/
Founded in 1994

DEGREE • BSN

Nursing Program Faculty 53 (26% with doctorates).
Baccalaureate Enrollment 501 **Women** 88% **Men** 12% **Part-time** 77%
Distance Learning Courses Available.
Nursing Student Activities Sigma Theta Tau, Student Nurses' Association.
Nursing Student Resources Academic advising; academic or career counseling; assistance for students with disabilities; bookstore; campus computer network; career placement assistance; computer lab; computer-assisted instruction; e-mail services; employment services for current students; externships; housing assistance; interactive nursing skills videos; Internet; learning resource lab; library services; nursing audiovisuals; paid internships; placement services for program completers; resume preparation assistance; skills, simulation, or other laboratory; tutoring.
Library Facilities 21 volumes in health, 2 volumes in nursing; 50,340 periodical subscriptions health-care related.

BACCALAUREATE PROGRAMS

Degree BSN

Available Programs Generic Baccalaureate; LPN to Baccalaureate; RN Baccalaureate.

Study Options Full-time.

Program Entrance Requirements Minimum overall college GPA of 2.8, transcript of college record, CPR certification, health exam, health insurance, 2 years high school math, 2 years high school science, high school transcript, immunizations, minimum high school GPA of 2.7, minimum GPA in nursing prerequisites of 2.6, prerequisite course work, RN licensure. Transfer students are accepted. *Application deadline:* 3/15 (fall), 7/15 (spring), 11/15 (summer). Applications may be processed on a rolling basis for some programs. *Application fee:* $25.

Advanced Placement Credit by examination available. Credit given for nursing courses completed elsewhere dependent upon specific evaluations.

Expenses (2015–16) *Tuition:* full-time $13,440. *International tuition:* $13,440 full-time. *Room and board:* $1400; room only: $1100 per academic year. *Required fees:* full-time $2192.

Financial Aid 97% of baccalaureate students in nursing programs received some form of financial aid in 2014–15.

Contact Ms. Lissa Morgan, Director of Admissions, Nursing Division, Baptist College of Health Sciences, 1003 Monroe Avenue, Memphis, TN 38104. *Telephone:* 901-572-2441. *Fax:* 901-572-2461. *E-mail:* lissa.morgan@bchs.edu.

Belmont University

School of Nursing
Nashville, Tennessee

http://www.belmont.edu/nursing
Founded in 1951

DEGREES • BSN • DNP • MSN

Nursing Program Faculty 65 (19% with doctorates).
Baccalaureate Enrollment 458 **Women** 91% **Men** 9% **Part-time** 8%
Graduate Enrollment 67 **Women** 87% **Men** 13% **Part-time** 35%
Nursing Student Activities Nursing Honor Society, Sigma Theta Tau, Student Nurses' Association.
Nursing Student Resources Academic advising; academic or career counseling; assistance for students with disabilities; bookstore; campus computer network; career placement assistance; computer lab; computer-assisted instruction; e-mail services; employment services for current students; externships; housing assistance; interactive nursing skills videos; Internet; learning resource lab; library services; nursing audiovisuals; placement services for program completers; remedial services; resume preparation assistance; skills, simulation, or other laboratory; tutoring.
Library Facilities 6,000 volumes in health, 800 volumes in nursing; 7,500 periodical subscriptions health-care related.

BACCALAUREATE PROGRAMS

Degree BSN

Available Programs ADN to Baccalaureate; Accelerated Baccalaureate; Accelerated Baccalaureate for Second Degree; Baccalaureate for Second Degree; Generic Baccalaureate; LPN to RN Baccalaureate; RN Baccalaureate.

Study Options Full-time and part-time.

Program Entrance Requirements Minimum overall college GPA of 3.0, transcript of college record, CPR certification, written essay, health exam, health insurance, high school biology, high school chemistry, 3 years high school math, 3 years high school science, high school transcript, immunizations, 1 letter of recommendation, minimum high school GPA of 3.0, minimum GPA in nursing prerequisites of 3.0. Transfer students are accepted. *Application deadline:* Applications may be processed on a rolling basis for some programs. *Application fee:* $50.

Advanced Placement Credit by examination available. Credit given for nursing courses completed elsewhere dependent upon specific evaluations.

Financial Aid 85% of baccalaureate students in nursing programs received some form of financial aid in 2013–14. *Gift aid (need-based):* Federal Pell, FSEOG, state, private, college/university gift aid from institutional funds. *Loans:* Federal Direct (Subsidized and Unsubsidized Stafford PLUS), Perkins. *Work-study:* Federal Work-Study. *Financial aid application deadline (priority):* 3/1.

Contact Ms. Madison Rhodes, Admissions Coordinator, School of Nursing, Belmont University, 1900 Belmont Boulevard, Nashville, TN 37212-3757. *Telephone:* 615-460-6120. *Fax:* 615-460-6125. *E-mail:* madison.rhodes@belmont.edu.

GRADUATE PROGRAMS

Financial Aid 95% of graduate students in nursing programs received some form of financial aid in 2013–14. Scholarships and traineeships available. *Financial aid application deadline:* 3/1.
Contact Dr. Leslie Higgins, Director, Graduate Program, School of Nursing, Belmont University, 1900 Belmont Boulevard, Nashville, TN 37212-3757. *Telephone:* 615-460-6027. *Fax:* 615-460-6125. *E-mail:* leslie.higgins@mail.belmont.edu.

MASTER'S DEGREE PROGRAM
Degree MSN
Available Programs Master's.
Concentrations Available Nursing education. *Nurse practitioner programs in:* family health.
Study Options Full-time and part-time.
Program Entrance Requirements Clinical experience, minimum overall college GPA of 3.0, transcript of college record, CPR certification, written essay, immunizations, interview, 2 letters of recommendation, resume, GRE. *Application fee:* $50.
Advanced Placement Credit given for nursing courses completed elsewhere dependent upon specific evaluations.
Degree Requirements 41 total credit hours, comprehensive exam.

POST-MASTER'S PROGRAM
Areas of Study Nursing education. *Nurse practitioner programs in:* family health.

DOCTORAL DEGREE PROGRAM
Degree DNP
Available Programs Doctorate; Post-Baccalaureate Doctorate.
Areas of Study Advanced practice nursing, aging, clinical practice, clinical research, community health, family health, gerontology, health policy, health promotion/disease prevention, health-care systems, human health and illness, illness and transition, individualized study, maternity-newborn, nursing administration, nursing policy, nursing research, palliative care, women's health.
Program Entrance Requirements Clinical experience, minimum overall college GPA of 3.0, interview, 2 letters of recommendation, statistics course, vita, writing sample. Application deadline: Applications may be processed on a rolling basis for some programs.
Degree Requirements 75 total credit hours, oral exam, written exam.

Bethel University
Nursing Program
McKenzie, Tennessee

http://www.bethelu.edu/academics/colleges_and_schools/college_of_health_sciences/don
Founded in 1842
DEGREE • BSN
Nursing Program Faculty 11
Baccalaureate Enrollment 63 **Women** 80% **Men** 20%
Distance Learning Courses Available.
Nursing Student Activities Student Nurses' Association.
Nursing Student Resources Academic advising; academic or career counseling; assistance for students with disabilities; bookstore; campus computer network; career placement assistance; computer lab; computer-assisted instruction; e-mail services; housing assistance; interactive nursing skills videos; Internet; learning resource lab; library services; nursing audiovisuals; remedial services; resume preparation assistance; skills, simulation, or other laboratory; tutoring.
Library Facilities 1,146 volumes in nursing; 99 periodical subscriptions health-care related.

BACCALAUREATE PROGRAMS
Degree BSN
Available Programs ADN to Baccalaureate; Generic Baccalaureate.
Study Options Full-time.
Online Degree Options Yes.
Program Entrance Requirements Minimum overall college GPA of 2.75, transcript of college record, CPR certification, health exam, health insurance, immunizations, minimum GPA in nursing prerequisites of 2.0, professional liability insurance/malpractice insurance, prerequisite course work. Transfer students are accepted. *Application deadline:* 3/1 (spring). *Application fee:* $25.

Advanced Placement Credit given for nursing courses completed elsewhere dependent upon specific evaluations.
Expenses (2015–16) *Tuition:* full-time $15,714; part-time $440 per credit. *Room and board:* $10,000; room only: $6928 per academic year. *Required fees:* full-time $1000.
Financial Aid 73% of baccalaureate students in nursing programs received some form of financial aid in 2014–15.
Contact Ms. Mary Bess Griffith, Director, Nursing Program, Bethel University, 325 Cherry Avenue, McKenzie, TN 38201. *Telephone:* 731-352-6472. *Fax:* 731-352-4589. *E-mail:* griffithmb@bethelu.edu.

Carson-Newman University
Department of Nursing
Jefferson City, Tennessee

http://www.cn.edu/
Founded in 1851
DEGREES • BSN • MSN
Nursing Program Faculty 27 (33% with doctorates).
Baccalaureate Enrollment 116 **Women** 88.8% **Men** 11.2% **Part-time** 2.5%
Graduate Enrollment 49 **Women** 89.8% **Men** 10.2% **Part-time** 85.7%
Distance Learning Courses Available.
Nursing Student Activities Sigma Theta Tau, Student Nurses' Association.
Nursing Student Resources Academic advising; academic or career counseling; assistance for students with disabilities; bookstore; campus computer network; career placement assistance; computer lab; computer-assisted instruction; daycare for children of students; e-mail services; employment services for current students; housing assistance; interactive nursing skills videos; Internet; learning resource lab; library services; nursing audiovisuals; placement services for program completers; remedial services; resume preparation assistance; skills, simulation, or other laboratory; tutoring.
Library Facilities 8,700 volumes in health, 4,396 volumes in nursing; 5,370 periodical subscriptions health-care related.

BACCALAUREATE PROGRAMS
Degree BSN
Available Programs Accelerated Baccalaureate; Generic Baccalaureate; RN Baccalaureate.
Study Options Full-time.
Online Degree Options Yes.
Program Entrance Requirements Minimum overall college GPA of 2.75, transcript of college record, health insurance, high school transcript, immunizations, minimum GPA in nursing prerequisites of 2.75, prerequisite course work. Transfer students are accepted. *Application deadline:* Applications may be processed on a rolling basis for some programs.
Advanced Placement Credit by examination available. Credit given for nursing courses completed elsewhere dependent upon specific evaluations.
Expenses (2015–16) *Tuition:* full-time $24,200; part-time $1010 per credit hour. *International tuition:* $24,200 full-time. *Room and board:* $9630; room only: $5290 per academic year. *Required fees:* full-time $1195; part-time $390 per term.
Contact Dr. Angela F. Wood, RN, Chair, Department of Nursing, Department of Nursing, Carson-Newman University, 1646 Russell Avenue, C-N Box 71883, Jefferson City, TN 37760. *Telephone:* 865-471-3442. *Fax:* 865-471-4574. *E-mail:* awood@cn.edu.

GRADUATE PROGRAMS
Expenses (2015–16) *Tuition:* part-time $575 per credit hour. *Room and board:* $4815; room only: $2645 per academic year. *Required fees:* part-time $140 per term.
Contact Dr. Kimberly S. Bolton, Graduate Program Director, Graduate Studies in Nursing, Department of Nursing, Carson-Newman University, 1646 Russell Avenue, C-N Box 71883, Jefferson City, TN 37760. *Telephone:* 865-471-4056. *Fax:* 865-471-4574. *E-mail:* kbolton@cn.edu.

MASTER'S DEGREE PROGRAM
Degree MSN
Available Programs Master's.
Concentrations Available Nursing education. *Nurse practitioner programs in:* family health.
Study Options Full-time and part-time.

Program Entrance Requirements Minimum overall college GPA of 3.0, transcript of college record, written essay, interview, 3 letters of recommendation, GRE (minimum score of 300 within ten years of application). *Application deadline:* 3/15 (fall), 10/15 (spring).
Advanced Placement Credit given for nursing courses completed elsewhere dependent upon specific evaluations.
Degree Requirements 45 total credit hours, thesis or project, comprehensive exam.

POST-MASTER'S PROGRAM
Areas of Study Nursing education. *Nurse practitioner programs in:* family health.

Christian Brothers University
RN to BSN Program
Memphis, Tennessee

http://www.cbu.edu/nursing
Founded in 1871
DEGREE • BSN
Nursing Program Faculty 4 (75% with doctorates).
Baccalaureate Enrollment 64 **Women** 90% **Men** 10% **Part-time** 16%
Nursing Student Activities Sigma Theta Tau.
Nursing Student Resources Academic advising; academic or career counseling; assistance for students with disabilities; bookstore; campus computer network; career placement assistance; computer lab; computer-assisted instruction; e-mail services; housing assistance; interactive nursing skills videos; Internet; learning resource lab; library services; nursing audiovisuals; remedial services; resume preparation assistance; skills, simulation, or other laboratory; tutoring.

BACCALAUREATE PROGRAMS
Degree BSN
Available Programs RN Baccalaureate.
Study Options Full-time and part-time.
Program Entrance Requirements Minimum overall college GPA, transcript of college record, CPR certification, written essay, immunizations, interview, 2 letters of recommendation, RN licensure. Transfer students are accepted. *Application deadline:* 8/10 (fall), 12/20 (spring). Applications may be processed on a rolling basis for some programs. *Application fee:* $25.
Advanced Placement Credit given for nursing courses completed elsewhere dependent upon specific evaluations.
Expenses (2015–16) *Tuition:* full-time $14,000.
Financial Aid 98% of baccalaureate students in nursing programs received some form of financial aid in 2014–15.
Contact Dr. Peggy Veeser, Director and Professor, RN to BSN Program, Christian Brothers University, 650 East Parkway South, Box 89, Memphis, TN 38104. *Telephone:* 901-321-3339. *Fax:* 901-321-3324. *E-mail:* pveeser@cbu.edu.

Cumberland University
Rudy School of Nursing and Health Professions
Lebanon, Tennessee

http://www.cumberland.edu/Nursing/
Founded in 1842
DEGREE • BSN
Nursing Program Faculty 57 (14% with doctorates).
Baccalaureate Enrollment 343 **Women** 78% **Men** 22% **Part-time** 29%
Distance Learning Courses Available.
Nursing Student Activities Sigma Theta Tau, Student Nurses' Association.
Nursing Student Resources Academic advising; academic or career counseling; assistance for students with disabilities; bookstore; campus computer network; career placement assistance; computer lab; computer-assisted instruction; e-mail services; externships; housing assistance; interactive nursing skills videos; Internet; learning resource lab; library services; nursing audiovisuals; remedial services; resume preparation assistance; skills, simulation, or other laboratory; tutoring.
Library Facilities 125 volumes in health, 66 volumes in nursing; 25 periodical subscriptions health-care related.

BACCALAUREATE PROGRAMS
Degree BSN
Available Programs ADN to Baccalaureate; Accelerated Baccalaureate; Accelerated Baccalaureate for Second Degree; Accelerated RN Baccalaureate; Baccalaureate for Second Degree; Generic Baccalaureate; RN Baccalaureate.
Site Options Mt. Juliet, TN.
Study Options Full-time and part-time.
Online Degree Options Yes.
Program Entrance Requirements Minimum overall college GPA of 3.0, transcript of college record, CPR certification, written essay, health exam, health insurance, high school transcript, immunizations, minimum high school GPA of 2.75, minimum GPA in nursing prerequisites of 3.0, professional liability insurance/malpractice insurance, prerequisite course work. Transfer students are accepted. *Application deadline:* 6/5 (fall), 10/2 (spring), 2/6 (summer). Applications may be processed on a rolling basis for some programs. *Application fee:* $25.
Advanced Placement Credit by examination available. Credit given for nursing courses completed elsewhere dependent upon specific evaluations.
Expenses (2015–16) *Tuition:* full-time $20,160; part-time $840 per credit. *International tuition:* $20,160 full-time. *Room and board:* $8200; room only: $7050 per academic year. *Required fees:* full-time $1050; part-time $315 per credit; part-time $525 per term.
Contact Dr. Carole Ann Bach, Professor and Dean, Rudy School of Nursing and Health Professions, Cumberland University, One Cumberland Square, McFarland Site, Lebanon, TN 37087-3554. *Telephone:* 615-547-1200. *Fax:* 615-449-1368. *E-mail:* cbach@cumberland.edu.

East Tennessee State University
College of Nursing
Johnson City, Tennessee

http://www.etsu.edu/nursing
Founded in 1911
DEGREES • BSN • DNP • MSN • PHD
Nursing Program Faculty 70 (36% with doctorates).
Baccalaureate Enrollment 679 **Women** 80% **Men** 20% **Part-time** 10%
Graduate Enrollment 432 **Women** 90% **Men** 10% **Part-time** 50%
Distance Learning Courses Available.
Nursing Student Activities Nursing Honor Society, Sigma Theta Tau, Student Nurses' Association.
Nursing Student Resources Academic advising; academic or career counseling; assistance for students with disabilities; bookstore; campus computer network; career placement assistance; computer lab; computer-assisted instruction; daycare for children of students; e-mail services; employment services for current students; externships; housing assistance; interactive nursing skills videos; Internet; learning resource lab; library services; nursing audiovisuals; remedial services; resume preparation assistance; skills, simulation, or other laboratory; tutoring.

BACCALAUREATE PROGRAMS
Degree BSN
Available Programs ADN to Baccalaureate; Accelerated Baccalaureate for Second Degree; Accelerated RN Baccalaureate; Baccalaureate for Second Degree; Generic Baccalaureate; LPN to Baccalaureate; RN Baccalaureate.
Site Options Cleveland, TN; Kingsport, TN; Sevierville, TN; Pellissippi, TN.
Study Options Full-time and part-time.
Online Degree Options Yes.
Program Entrance Requirements Minimum overall college GPA of 2.6, transcript of college record, minimum GPA in nursing prerequisites of 2.6, prerequisite course work. Transfer students are accepted. *Application deadline:* 10/1 (fall), 2/1 (spring). *Application fee:* $45.
Advanced Placement Credit given for nursing courses completed elsewhere dependent upon specific evaluations.
Expenses (2015–16) *Tuition, state resident:* full-time $4983; part-time $365 per credit hour. *Tuition, nonresident:* full-time $13,000; part-time $1057 per credit hour. *Room and board:* $3300; room only: $2000 per academic year.
Financial Aid 90% of baccalaureate students in nursing programs received some form of financial aid in 2014–15.
Contact Mr. Scott Vaughn, Director, Student Services, College of Nursing, East Tennessee State University, PO Box 70664, Office of

Student Services, Johnson City, TN 37614. *Telephone:* 423-439-4578. *Fax:* 423-439-4522. *E-mail:* nursing@etsu.edu.

GRADUATE PROGRAMS

Expenses (2015–16) *Tuition, state resident:* full-time $11,000; part-time $519 per credit hour. *Tuition, nonresident:* full-time $13,500; part-time $773 per credit hour. *Room and board:* $3300; room only: $1000 per academic year. *Required fees:* full-time $600; part-time $50 per credit.

Financial Aid 80% of graduate students in nursing programs received some form of financial aid in 2014–15. 9 research assistantships with full and partial tuition reimbursements available (averaging $4,500 per year), 1 teaching assistantship (averaging $6,000 per year) were awarded; career-related internships or fieldwork, institutionally sponsored loans, scholarships, and unspecified assistantships also available. *Financial aid application deadline:* 7/1.

Contact Ms. Amy Bower, Coordinator, College of Nursing, East Tennessee State University, PO Box 70664, Office of Student Services, Johnson City, TN 37614. *Telephone:* 423-439-4578. *Fax:* 423-439-4522. *E-mail:* bowera@etsu.edu.

MASTER'S DEGREE PROGRAM

Degree MSN

Available Programs Master's; RN to Master's.

Concentrations Available Nursing administration; nursing education; nursing informatics. *Nurse practitioner programs in:* family health.

Study Options Full-time and part-time.

Online Degree Options Yes (online only).

Program Entrance Requirements Minimum overall college GPA of 3.0, transcript of college record, written essay, 3 letters of recommendation, resume, statistics course. *Application deadline:* 2/1 (fall), 7/1 (spring), 12/1 (summer). *Application fee:* $35.

Advanced Placement Credit given for nursing courses completed elsewhere dependent upon specific evaluations.

Degree Requirements 46 total credit hours, comprehensive exam.

POST-MASTER'S PROGRAM

Areas of Study Nursing administration; nursing education; nursing informatics. *Nurse practitioner programs in:* family health.

DOCTORAL DEGREE PROGRAM

Degree DNP

Available Programs Doctorate, Doctorate for Nurses with Non-Nursing Degrees, Post-Baccalaureate Doctorate.

Areas of Study Advanced practice nursing, gerontology, nursing administration, psychiatric/mental health.

Online Degree Options Yes.

Program Entrance Requirements Minimum overall college GPA of 3.0, clinical experience, interview by faculty committee, letters of recommendation, BSN or MSN or equivalent, vita, writing sample. Application deadline: 2/1 for BSN to DNP (fall), 10/1 for MSN to DNP (spring). Application fee: $35.

Degree Requirements 79-85 total credit hours, residency.

Degree PhD

Available Programs Doctorate.

Areas of Study Individualized study.

Program Entrance Requirements Clinical experience, minimum overall college GPA of 3.0, interview by faculty committee, 3 letters of recommendation, MSN or equivalent, statistics course, vita, writing sample, GRE General Test. Application deadline: 2/1 (spring). Application fee: $35.

Degree Requirements 62 total credit hours, dissertation, written exam, residency.

CONTINUING EDUCATION PROGRAM

Contact Ms. Patti Harnois-Church, Instructor, College of Nursing, East Tennessee State University, PO Box 70629, 807 University Parkway, Johnson City, TN 37614-1709. *Telephone:* 423-439-4052. *E-mail:* harnoischurc@etsu.edu.

Freed-Hardeman University
Department of Nursing
Henderson, Tennessee

http://www.fhu.edu/nursing
Founded in 1869
DEGREE • BSN
Nursing Program Faculty 7 (38% with doctorates).
Baccalaureate Enrollment 45
Nursing Student Activities Student Nurses' Association.
Nursing Student Resources Academic advising; academic or career counseling; assistance for students with disabilities; bookstore; campus computer network; computer-assisted instruction; e-mail services; employment services for current students; housing assistance; interactive nursing skills videos; Internet; library services; nursing audiovisuals; remedial services; resume preparation assistance; skills, simulation, or other laboratory; tutoring.

BACCALAUREATE PROGRAMS

Degree BSN
Available Programs Generic Baccalaureate.
Site Options Dickson, TN.
Study Options Full-time.
Program Entrance Requirements Minimum overall college GPA of 2.8, transcript of college record, health exam, immunizations, minimum GPA in nursing prerequisites of 2.5, prerequisite course work. Transfer students are accepted. *Application deadline:* 2/1 (fall).
Contact Dr. Christopher J. White, Chair, Department of Nursing, Department of Nursing, Freed-Hardeman University, 158 East Main Street, Henderson, TN 38340. *Telephone:* 731-989-6965. *Fax:* 731-989-6316. *E-mail:* cjwhite@fhu.edu.

King University
School of Nursing
Bristol, Tennessee

http://www.king.edu/
Founded in 1867
DEGREES • BSN • MSN • MSN/MBA
Nursing Program Faculty 31 (26% with doctorates).
Baccalaureate Enrollment 366 **Women** 96% **Men** 4%
Graduate Enrollment 35 **Women** 99% **Men** 1%
Distance Learning Courses Available.
Nursing Student Activities Student Nurses' Association.
Nursing Student Resources Academic advising; academic or career counseling; assistance for students with disabilities; bookstore; campus computer network; career placement assistance; computer lab; computer-assisted instruction; e-mail services; employment services for current students; externships; interactive nursing skills videos; Internet; learning resource lab; library services; nursing audiovisuals; paid internships; remedial services; resume preparation assistance; skills, simulation, or other laboratory; tutoring.
Library Facilities 929 volumes in health, 158 volumes in nursing; 87 periodical subscriptions health-care related.

BACCALAUREATE PROGRAMS

Degree BSN
Available Programs Accelerated RN Baccalaureate; Generic Baccalaureate.
Site Options Kingsport, TN.
Study Options Full-time.
Program Entrance Requirements Minimum overall college GPA of 2.0, transcript of college record, CPR certification, written essay, health exam, health insurance, high school biology, high school chemistry, high school foreign language, 2 years high school math, 2 years high school science, high school transcript, immunizations, minimum high school GPA of 2.6, minimum high school rank 25%, minimum GPA in nursing prerequisites of 2.75. Transfer students are accepted. *Application deadline:* 6/1 (fall). *Application fee:* $100.
Contact *Telephone:* 423-652-4841. *Fax:* 423-652-4833.

GRADUATE PROGRAMS

Contact *Telephone:* 423-652-4841. *Fax:* 423-652-4833.

MASTER'S DEGREE PROGRAM

Degrees MSN; MSN/MBA

Available Programs Accelerated RN to Master's; Master's.

Concentrations Available *Clinical nurse specialist programs in:* acute care, adult health, oncology.

Study Options Full-time.

Program Entrance Requirements Clinical experience, computer literacy, minimum overall college GPA of 3.0, transcript of college record, CPR certification, written essay, immunizations, 2 letters of recommendation, nursing research course, physical assessment course, resume, statistics course. *Application deadline:* 4/15 (fall). *Application fee:* $100.

Degree Requirements 39 total credit hours, thesis or project.

Lincoln Memorial University

Caylor School of Nursing
Harrogate, Tennessee

http://www.lmunet.edu/academics/nursing/index2.shtml
Founded in 1897

DEGREES • BSN • MSN

Nursing Program Faculty 50 (57% with doctorates).

Baccalaureate Enrollment 70 **Women** 80% **Men** 20%

Graduate Enrollment 65

Nursing Student Activities Student Nurses' Association.

Nursing Student Resources Academic advising; academic or career counseling; bookstore; campus computer network; career placement assistance; computer lab; e-mail services; externships; interactive nursing skills videos; Internet; learning resource lab; library services; nursing audiovisuals; other; placement services for program completers; skills, simulation, or other laboratory; tutoring.

Library Facilities 1,230 volumes in health, 630 volumes in nursing; 36 periodical subscriptions health-care related.

BACCALAUREATE PROGRAMS

Degree BSN

Available Programs ADN to Baccalaureate; Accelerated Baccalaureate; Generic Baccalaureate; RN Baccalaureate.

Site Options Knoxville, TN.

Study Options Full-time.

Program Entrance Requirements Minimum overall college GPA of 2.75, transcript of college record, CPR certification, immunizations, professional liability insurance/malpractice insurance, prerequisite course work, RN licensure. Transfer students are accepted. *Application deadline:* Applications may be processed on a rolling basis for some programs.

Contact *Telephone:* 423-869-3611. *Fax:* 423-869-6444.

GRADUATE PROGRAMS

Contact *Telephone:* 423-869-6283. *Fax:* 423-869-6244.

MASTER'S DEGREE PROGRAM

Degree MSN

Available Programs Master's.

Concentrations Available Nurse anesthesia. *Nurse practitioner programs in:* family health, psychiatric/mental health.

Site Options Knoxville, TN.

Study Options Full-time and part-time.

Program Entrance Requirements Clinical experience, computer literacy, transcript of college record, CPR certification, written essay, immunizations, interview, 3 letters of recommendation, professional liability insurance/malpractice insurance, prerequisite course work, statistics course. *Application deadline:* Applications may be processed on a rolling basis for some programs.

POST-MASTER'S PROGRAM

Areas of Study *Nurse practitioner programs in:* family health, psychiatric/mental health.

Lipscomb University

Department of Nursing
Nashville, Tennessee

Founded in 1891

DEGREE • BSN

BACCALAUREATE PROGRAMS

Degree BSN

Available Programs Generic Baccalaureate.

Contact *Telephone:* 615-996-6650.

Martin Methodist College

Division of Nursing
Pulaski, Tennessee

http://www.martinmethodist.edu/
Founded in 1870

DEGREE • BSN

Nursing Program Faculty 7 (43% with doctorates).

Baccalaureate Enrollment 71 **Women** 96% **Men** 4%

Distance Learning Courses Available.

Nursing Student Activities Student Nurses' Association.

Nursing Student Resources Academic advising; academic or career counseling; bookstore; campus computer network; career placement assistance; computer lab; computer-assisted instruction; e-mail services; employment services for current students; housing assistance; interactive nursing skills videos; Internet; learning resource lab; library services; nursing audiovisuals; placement services for program completers; remedial services; resume preparation assistance; skills, simulation, or other laboratory; tutoring; unpaid internships.

Library Facilities 875 volumes in nursing; 400 periodical subscriptions health-care related.

BACCALAUREATE PROGRAMS

Degree BSN

Available Programs Generic Baccalaureate.

Study Options Full-time.

Program Entrance Requirements Transcript of college record, CPR certification, health insurance, immunizations, minimum GPA in nursing prerequisites, prerequisite course work. Transfer students are accepted. *Application deadline:* 2/1 (fall), 2/1 (winter). *Application fee:* $30.

Contact *Telephone:* 931-424-7395. *Fax:* 931-363-9891.

Middle Tennessee State University

School of Nursing
Murfreesboro, Tennessee

http://www.mtsu.edu/
Founded in 1911

DEGREES • BSN • MSN

Nursing Program Faculty 45 (65% with doctorates).

Baccalaureate Enrollment 300 **Women** 85% **Men** 15%

Graduate Enrollment 100 **Women** 80% **Men** 20% **Part-time** 50%

Distance Learning Courses Available.

Nursing Student Activities Sigma Theta Tau, Student Nurses' Association.

Nursing Student Resources Academic advising; academic or career counseling; assistance for students with disabilities; bookstore; campus computer network; career placement assistance; computer lab; computer-assisted instruction; e-mail services; interactive nursing skills videos; Internet; learning resource lab; library services; nursing audiovisuals; remedial services; resume preparation assistance; skills, simulation, or other laboratory; tutoring.

Library Facilities 100 volumes in health, 45 volumes in nursing; 100 periodical subscriptions health-care related.

BACCALAUREATE PROGRAMS

Degree BSN

Available Programs Generic Baccalaureate; LPN to RN Baccalaureate; RN Baccalaureate.
Study Options Full-time.
Online Degree Options Yes.
Program Entrance Requirements Minimum overall college GPA of 2.8, transcript of college record, CPR certification, health exam, health insurance, immunizations, interview, minimum GPA in nursing prerequisites of 2.75, professional liability insurance/malpractice insurance, prerequisite course work. Transfer students are accepted. *Application deadline:* 2/1 (fall), 10/1 (spring).
Advanced Placement Credit by examination available. Credit given for nursing courses completed elsewhere dependent upon specific evaluations.
Contact *Telephone:* 615-898-2437. *Fax:* 615-898-5441.

GRADUATE PROGRAMS

Contact *Telephone:* 615-898-2437. *Fax:* 615-898-5441.

MASTER'S DEGREE PROGRAM
Degree MSN
Available Programs Accelerated AD/RN to Master's; Master's.
Concentrations Available Nursing administration; nursing education; nursing informatics. *Nurse practitioner programs in:* family health.
Site Options multiple cities.
Study Options Full-time and part-time.
Online Degree Options Yes.
Program Entrance Requirements Minimum overall college GPA of 3.0, transcript of college record, 3 letters of recommendation, prerequisite course work, resume. *Application deadline:* Applications may be processed on a rolling basis for some programs.
Degree Requirements 43 total credit hours, thesis or project.

POST-MASTER'S PROGRAM
Areas of Study *Nurse practitioner programs in:* family health.

Milligan College
Department of Nursing
Milligan College, Tennessee

http://www.milligan.edu/BSN/
Founded in 1866
DEGREE • BSN
Nursing Program Faculty 10 (25% with doctorates).
Baccalaureate Enrollment 195 **Women** 90% **Men** 10%
Nursing Student Activities Nursing Honor Society, Student Nurses' Association.
Nursing Student Resources Academic advising; academic or career counseling; assistance for students with disabilities; bookstore; campus computer network; career placement assistance; computer lab; computer-assisted instruction; e-mail services; employment services for current students; externships; interactive nursing skills videos; Internet; learning resource lab; library services; nursing audiovisuals; placement services for program completers; remedial services; resume preparation assistance; skills, simulation, or other laboratory; tutoring; unpaid internships.
Library Facilities 2,430 volumes in health, 184 volumes in nursing; 340 periodical subscriptions health-care related.

BACCALAUREATE PROGRAMS

Degree BSN
Available Programs ADN to Baccalaureate; Baccalaureate for Second Degree; Generic Baccalaureate; LPN to Baccalaureate; LPN to RN Baccalaureate; RN Baccalaureate.
Study Options Full-time and part-time.
Program Entrance Requirements Minimum overall college GPA of 2.5, transcript of college record, CPR certification, written essay, health exam, immunizations, letters of recommendation, minimum GPA in nursing prerequisites of 2.5, professional liability insurance/malpractice insurance, prerequisite course work. Transfer students are accepted. *Application deadline:* Applications may be processed on a rolling basis for some programs. *Application fee:* $30.
Advanced Placement Credit given for nursing courses completed elsewhere dependent upon specific evaluations.
Contact *Telephone:* 423-461-8655. *Fax:* 423-461-8982.

South College
Department of Nursing
Knoxville, Tennessee

Founded in 1882
DEGREE • BSN
Nursing Program Faculty 14 (25% with doctorates).
Baccalaureate Enrollment 75 **Women** 90% **Men** 10%
Nursing Student Activities Student Nurses' Association.
Nursing Student Resources Academic advising; academic or career counseling; assistance for students with disabilities; bookstore; campus computer network; career placement assistance; computer lab; computer-assisted instruction; e-mail services; externships; interactive nursing skills videos; Internet; learning resource lab; library services; nursing audiovisuals; placement services for program completers; resume preparation assistance; skills, simulation, or other laboratory; tutoring.

BACCALAUREATE PROGRAMS

Degree BSN
Available Programs Generic Baccalaureate.
Study Options Full-time.
Program Entrance Requirements CPR certification, written essay, health exam, immunizations, interview, 2 letters of recommendation, minimum GPA in nursing prerequisites of 2.5. Transfer students are accepted. *Application fee:* $25.
Advanced Placement Credit by examination available. Credit given for nursing courses completed elsewhere dependent upon specific evaluations.
Contact *Telephone:* 865-251-1800.

Southern Adventist University
School of Nursing
Collegedale, Tennessee

http://www.southern.edu/nursing
Founded in 1892
DEGREES • BS • DNP • MSN • MSN/MBA
Nursing Program Faculty 28 (32% with doctorates).
Baccalaureate Enrollment 156 **Women** 81% **Men** 19% **Part-time** 63%
Graduate Enrollment 191 **Women** 80% **Men** 20% **Part-time** 48%
Distance Learning Courses Available.
Nursing Student Activities Nursing Honor Society, Sigma Theta Tau, nursing club.
Nursing Student Resources Academic advising; academic or career counseling; assistance for students with disabilities; bookstore; campus computer network; career placement assistance; computer lab; computer-assisted instruction; e-mail services; employment services for current students; housing assistance; interactive nursing skills videos; Internet; learning resource lab; library services; nursing audiovisuals; remedial services; resume preparation assistance; skills, simulation, or other laboratory; tutoring.
Library Facilities 6,835 volumes in health, 2,114 volumes in nursing; 7,831 periodical subscriptions health-care related.

BACCALAUREATE PROGRAMS

Degree BS
Available Programs ADN to Baccalaureate.
Site Options Chattanooga, TN.
Study Options Full-time and part-time.
Online Degree Options Yes.
Program Entrance Requirements Minimum overall college GPA of 2.5, transcript of college record, CPR certification, health exam, health insurance, high school transcript, immunizations, interview, minimum GPA in nursing prerequisites of 2.0, prerequisite course work, RN licensure. Transfer students are accepted. *Application deadline:* 2/1 (fall), 9/1 (winter). Applications may be processed on a rolling basis for some programs. *Application fee:* $40.
Advanced Placement Credit given for nursing courses completed elsewhere dependent upon specific evaluations.
Expenses (2015–16) *Tuition:* full-time $20,240; part-time $820 per credit hour. *International tuition:* $24,500 full-time. *Room and board:* $5850; room only: $3700 per academic year. *Required fees:* full-time $1500; part-time $120 per credit; part-time $850 per term.

Financial Aid 80% of baccalaureate students in nursing programs received some form of financial aid in 2014–15. *Gift aid (need-based):* Federal Pell, FSEOG, state, private, college/university gift aid from institutional funds. *Loans:* Federal Nursing Student Loans, Federal Direct (Subsidized and Unsubsidized Stafford PLUS), Perkins, college/university. *Work-study:* Federal Work-Study, part-time campus jobs. *Financial aid application deadline (priority):* 3/31.

Contact Mrs. Sylvia D. Mayer, RN, Director of Admissions and Progressions, School of Nursing, Southern Adventist University, PO Box 370, Collegedale, TN 37315-0370. *Telephone:* 423-236-2941. *Fax:* 423-236-1940. *E-mail:* smayer@southern.edu.

GRADUATE PROGRAMS

Expenses (2015–16) *Tuition:* full-time $15,390; part-time $600 per credit hour. *International tuition:* $21,390 full-time. *Room and board:* $13,038; room only: $9888 per academic year. *Required fees:* full-time $1500; part-time $120 per credit; part-time $850 per term.

Financial Aid 85% of graduate students in nursing programs received some form of financial aid in 2014–15.

Contact Mrs. Diane Proffitt, Applications Manager, School of Nursing, Southern Adventist University, PO Box 370, Collegedale, TN 37315-0370. *Telephone:* 423-236-2957. *Fax:* 423-236-1940.
E-mail: dproffit@southern.edu.

MASTER'S DEGREE PROGRAM

Degrees MSN; MSN/MBA

Available Programs Accelerated RN to Master's; Master's.

Concentrations Available Health-care administration; nursing education. *Nurse practitioner programs in:* acute care, adult health, family health, primary care, psychiatric/mental health.

Study Options Full-time and part-time.

Online Degree Options Yes (online only).

Program Entrance Requirements Clinical experience, minimum overall college GPA of 3.0, transcript of college record, CPR certification, written essay, immunizations, interview, 2 letters of recommendation, physical assessment course, prerequisite course work, resume, statistics course. *Application deadline:* 5/1 (fall), 10/1 (winter). Applications may be processed on a rolling basis for some programs. *Application fee:* $40.

Advanced Placement Credit given for nursing courses completed elsewhere dependent upon specific evaluations.

Degree Requirements 46 total credit hours, thesis or project.

POST-MASTER'S PROGRAM

Areas of Study Nursing education. *Nurse practitioner programs in:* acute care, adult health, family health, primary care, psychiatric/mental health.

DOCTORAL DEGREE PROGRAM

Degree DNP

Available Programs Doctorate.

Areas of Study Advanced practice nursing, health promotion/disease prevention.

Online Degree Options Yes (online only).

Program Entrance Requirements Clinical experience, minimum overall college GPA of 3.0, interview by faculty committee, interview, 3 letters of recommendation, MSN or equivalent, scholarly papers, statistics course, vita, writing sample. Application deadline: 7/1 (fall), 11/1 (winter), 9/1 (spring), 4/1 (summer). Applications may be processed on a rolling basis for some programs. Application fee: $25.

Degree Requirements 42 total credit hours.

CONTINUING EDUCATION PROGRAM

Contact Mrs. Sylvia Mayer, Director of Admissions and Progressions, School of Nursing, Southern Adventist University, PO Box 370, Collegedale, TN 37315-0370. *Telephone:* 423-236-2941. *Fax:* 423-236-1940. *E-mail:* smayer@southern.edu.

Tennessee State University

Division of Nursing
Nashville, Tennessee

http://www.tnstate.edu/nursing/
Founded in 1912

DEGREES • BSN • MSN
Nursing Program Faculty 54 (41% with doctorates).

Baccalaureate Enrollment 119 **Women** 80% **Men** 20% **Part-time** 21%
Graduate Enrollment 275 **Women** 93% **Men** 7% **Part-time** 80%
Distance Learning Courses Available.
Nursing Student Activities Sigma Theta Tau.
Nursing Student Resources Academic advising; academic or career counseling; assistance for students with disabilities; bookstore; campus computer network; career placement assistance; computer lab; computer-assisted instruction; e-mail services; employment services for current students; interactive nursing skills videos; Internet; learning resource lab; library services; nursing audiovisuals; remedial services; resume preparation assistance; skills, simulation, or other laboratory; tutoring.
Library Facilities 50,000 volumes in health, 25,000 volumes in nursing; 300 periodical subscriptions health-care related.

BACCALAUREATE PROGRAMS

Degree BSN

Available Programs Generic Baccalaureate; RN Baccalaureate.

Site Options Nashville, TN.

Study Options Full-time.

Program Entrance Requirements Minimum overall college GPA of 2.8, transcript of college record, CPR certification, health exam, health insurance, immunizations, minimum high school GPA of 2.8, minimum GPA in nursing prerequisites of 2.8, professional liability insurance/malpractice insurance, prerequisite course work. Transfer students are accepted. *Application deadline:* 3/1 (fall).

Expenses (2015–16) *Tuition, state resident:* full-time $7112; part-time $318 per credit hour. *Tuition, nonresident:* full-time $19,832; part-time $848 per credit hour. *International tuition:* $20,250 full-time. *Room and board:* $10,130; room only: $6780 per academic year. *Required fees:* full-time $750; part-time $25 per credit.

Financial Aid *Gift aid (need-based):* Federal Pell, FSEOG, state, private, college/university gift aid from institutional funds. *Loans:* Federal Direct (Subsidized and Unsubsidized Stafford PLUS), Perkins. *Work-study:* Federal Work-Study, part-time campus jobs. *Financial aid application deadline (priority):* 4/1.

Contact Ms. Kathy Gretton, Interim, BSN Program Director, Division of Nursing, Tennessee State University, 3500 John A. Merritt Boulevard, Box 9590, Nashville, TN 37209-1561. *Telephone:* 615-963-7615. *Fax:* 615-963-5593. *E-mail:* kwilson29@tnstate.edu.

GRADUATE PROGRAMS

Expenses (2015–16) *Tuition, state resident:* full-time $9384; part-time $474 per credit hour. *Tuition, nonresident:* full-time $21,652; part-time $1056 per credit hour. *Required fees:* full-time $513; part-time $64 per credit.

Financial Aid Research assistantships, teaching assistantships available.

Contact Dr. Maria A. Revell, MSN Program Director, Division of Nursing, Tennessee State University, 3500 John A. Merritt Boulevard, Box 9590, Nashville, TN 37209-1561. *Telephone:* 615-963-5255. *Fax:* 615-963-7614. *E-mail:* mrevell1@tnstate.edu.

MASTER'S DEGREE PROGRAM

Degree MSN

Available Programs RN to Master's.

Concentrations Available Nursing administration; nursing education. *Nurse practitioner programs in:* family health.

Site Options Nashville, TN.

Study Options Full-time and part-time.

Online Degree Options Yes.

Program Entrance Requirements Minimum overall college GPA of 3.0, transcript of college record, CPR certification, written essay, immunizations, 3 letters of recommendation, nursing research course, physical assessment course, professional liability insurance/malpractice insurance, resume, GRE General Test or MAT. *Application deadline:* 6/15 (fall), 10/15 (spring), 2/15 (summer). *Application fee:* $35.

Advanced Placement Credit given for nursing courses completed elsewhere dependent upon specific evaluations.

Degree Requirements 49 total credit hours, comprehensive exam.

POST-MASTER'S PROGRAM

Areas of Study Nursing administration; nursing education. *Nurse practitioner programs in:* family health.

Tennessee Technological University
Whitson-Hester School of Nursing
Cookeville, Tennessee

http://www.tntech.edu/nursing
Founded in 1915
DEGREES • BSN • M SC N • MSN
Nursing Program Faculty 20 (35% with doctorates).
Baccalaureate Enrollment 283 **Women** 84% **Men** 16% **Part-time** 1.7%
Graduate Enrollment 116 **Women** 86% **Men** 14% **Part-time** 82%
Distance Learning Courses Available.
Nursing Student Activities Sigma Theta Tau, Student Nurses' Association.
Nursing Student Resources Academic advising; academic or career counseling; assistance for students with disabilities; bookstore; campus computer network; career placement assistance; computer lab; computer-assisted instruction; daycare for children of students; e-mail services; employment services for current students; externships; housing assistance; Internet; learning resource lab; library services; nursing audiovisuals; paid internships; placement services for program completers; remedial services; resume preparation assistance; skills, simulation, or other laboratory; tutoring; unpaid internships.
Library Facilities 312,892 volumes in health, 11,893 volumes in nursing; 96 periodical subscriptions health-care related.

BACCALAUREATE PROGRAMS

Degree BSN
Available Programs ADN to Baccalaureate; Baccalaureate for Second Degree; Generic Baccalaureate; RN Baccalaureate.
Study Options Full-time.
Program Entrance Requirements Minimum overall college GPA of 3.0, transcript of college record, CPR certification, written essay, health exam, high school biology, high school foreign language, 4 years high school math, 2 years high school science, high school transcript, immunizations, minimum high school GPA of 3.0, minimum GPA in nursing prerequisites of 2.0, professional liability insurance/malpractice insurance, prerequisite course work. Transfer students are accepted. *Application deadline:* 2/1 (fall), 6/1 (spring).
Advanced Placement Credit given for nursing courses completed elsewhere dependent upon specific evaluations.
Expenses (2015–16) *Tuition, state resident:* full-time $8011; part-time $358 per credit hour. *Tuition, nonresident:* full-time $15,432; part-time $643 per credit hour. *International tuition:* $15,432 full-time. *Room and board:* $8382; room only: $4590 per academic year. *Required fees:* full-time $1114.
Contact Mr. Ben Clark, Academic Advisor, Whitson-Hester School of Nursing, Tennessee Technological University, Box 5001, Cookeville, TN 38505-0001. *Telephone:* 931-372-3229. *Fax:* 931-372-6244.
E-mail: Bclark@tntech.edu.

GRADUATE PROGRAMS

Expenses (2015–16) *Tuition, state resident:* part-time $561 per credit hour. *Tuition, nonresident:* part-time $1267 per credit hour.
Contact Mr. Ben Clark, Academic Advisor, Whitson-Hester School of Nursing, Tennessee Technological University, Box 5001, Cookeville, TN 38505-0001. *Telephone:* 931-372-3229. *Fax:* 931-372-6244.
E-mail: bclark@tntech.edu.

MASTER'S DEGREE PROGRAM

Degrees M Sc N; MSN
Available Programs Master's.
Concentrations Available Nursing administration; nursing education.
Nurse practitioner programs in: family health.
Study Options Full-time and part-time.
Online Degree Options Yes (online only).
Program Entrance Requirements Computer literacy, minimum overall college GPA of 3.0, transcript of college record, CPR certification, written essay, immunizations, 3 letters of recommendation, nursing research course, professional liability insurance/malpractice insurance, resume, statistics course. *Application deadline:* 8/1 (fall), 12/1 (spring), 5/1 (summer). Applications may be processed on a rolling basis for some programs. *Application fee:* $25.
Advanced Placement Credit given for nursing courses completed elsewhere dependent upon specific evaluations.

Degree Requirements 46 total credit hours, thesis or project.

Tennessee Wesleyan College
Fort Sanders Nursing Department
Knoxville, Tennessee

http://www.twcnet.edu/admissions/nursing-program/
Founded in 1857
DEGREE • BSN
Nursing Program Faculty 18 (6% with doctorates).
Baccalaureate Enrollment 128 **Women** 89% **Men** 11% **Part-time** 3%
Distance Learning Courses Available.
Nursing Student Activities Nursing Honor Society, Sigma Theta Tau, Student Nurses' Association.
Nursing Student Resources Academic advising; assistance for students with disabilities; bookstore; campus computer network; computer lab; e-mail services; Internet; library services; nursing audiovisuals; other; skills, simulation, or other laboratory.
Library Facilities 5,000 volumes in health, 4,000 volumes in nursing; 135 periodical subscriptions health-care related.

BACCALAUREATE PROGRAMS

Degree BSN
Available Programs ADN to Baccalaureate; Generic Baccalaureate; RN Baccalaureate.
Site Options Knoxville, TN.
Study Options Full-time.
Program Entrance Requirements Minimum overall college GPA of 2.7, transcript of college record, CPR certification, written essay, health exam, high school transcript, immunizations, interview, minimum GPA in nursing prerequisites of 2.7, prerequisite course work. Transfer students are accepted. *Application deadline:* 1/15 (fall). *Application fee:* $25.
Advanced Placement Credit given for nursing courses completed elsewhere dependent upon specific evaluations.
Contact *Telephone:* 865-777-5100. *Fax:* 865-777-5114.

Union University
School of Nursing
Jackson, Tennessee

http://www.uu.edu/academics/son/
Founded in 1823
DEGREES • BSN • MSN
Nursing Program Faculty 28 (36% with doctorates).
Baccalaureate Enrollment 285 **Women** 93% **Men** 7% **Part-time** 56%
Graduate Enrollment 55 **Women** 80% **Men** 20% **Part-time** 4%
Nursing Student Activities Nursing Honor Society, Sigma Theta Tau, Student Nurses' Association.
Nursing Student Resources Academic advising; academic or career counseling; assistance for students with disabilities; bookstore; campus computer network; career placement assistance; computer lab; computer-assisted instruction; e-mail services; employment services for current students; housing assistance; Internet; learning resource lab; library services; nursing audiovisuals; resume preparation assistance; skills, simulation, or other laboratory; tutoring.
Library Facilities 6,005 volumes in nursing; 1,284 periodical subscriptions health-care related.

BACCALAUREATE PROGRAMS

Degree BSN
Available Programs Accelerated Baccalaureate for Second Degree; Generic Baccalaureate; LPN to Baccalaureate; RN Baccalaureate.
Site Options Germantown, TN.
Study Options Full-time.
Program Entrance Requirements Minimum overall college GPA of 2.8, transcript of college record, CPR certification, health exam, immunizations, minimum GPA in nursing prerequisites of 2.8, prerequisite course work. Transfer students are accepted.
Advanced Placement Credit by examination available. Credit given for nursing courses completed elsewhere dependent upon specific evaluations.
Contact *Telephone:* 731-661-5538. *Fax:* 731-661-5504.

GRADUATE PROGRAMS

Contact *Telephone:* 731-661-5538. *Fax:* 901-661-5504.

MASTER'S DEGREE PROGRAM
Degree MSN
Available Programs Master's.
Concentrations Available Nurse anesthesia; nursing administration; nursing education. *Clinical nurse specialist programs in:* adult health, pediatric. *Nurse practitioner programs in:* family health.
Site Options Germantown, TN.
Study Options Full-time and part-time.
Program Entrance Requirements Minimum overall college GPA of 3.0, transcript of college record, CPR certification, written essay, immunizations, interview, 3 letters of recommendation, professional liability insurance/malpractice insurance, GRE.
Advanced Placement Credit given for nursing courses completed elsewhere dependent upon specific evaluations.
Degree Requirements 46 total credit hours.

POST-MASTER'S PROGRAM
Areas of Study Nursing administration; nursing education. *Clinical nurse specialist programs in:* adult health, pediatric. *Nurse practitioner programs in:* family health.

CONTINUING EDUCATION PROGRAM

Contact *Telephone:* 731-661-5152. *Fax:* 731-661-5504.

University of Memphis
Loewenberg School of Nursing
Memphis, Tennessee

http://www.nursing.memphis.edu/
Founded in 1912
DEGREES • BSN • MSN
Nursing Program Faculty 65 (22% with doctorates).
Baccalaureate Enrollment 441 **Women** 91% **Men** 9% **Part-time** 15%
Graduate Enrollment 124 **Women** 92% **Men** 8% **Part-time** 75%
Distance Learning Courses Available.
Nursing Student Activities Sigma Theta Tau, Student Nurses' Association.
Nursing Student Resources Academic advising; academic or career counseling; assistance for students with disabilities; bookstore; campus computer network; career placement assistance; computer lab; computer-assisted instruction; daycare for children of students; e-mail services; externships; housing assistance; interactive nursing skills videos; Internet; learning resource lab; library services; nursing audiovisuals; paid internships; remedial services; resume preparation assistance; skills, simulation, or other laboratory; tutoring.
Library Facilities 74,513 volumes in health; 878 periodical subscriptions health-care related.

BACCALAUREATE PROGRAMS

Degree BSN
Available Programs ADN to Baccalaureate; Accelerated Baccalaureate; Accelerated Baccalaureate for Second Degree; Accelerated RN Baccalaureate; Baccalaureate for Second Degree; Generic Baccalaureate; RN Baccalaureate.
Site Options Jackson, TN.
Study Options Full-time.
Program Entrance Requirements Minimum overall college GPA of 2.7, transcript of college record, CPR certification, health exam, high school biology, high school chemistry, high school foreign language, 3 years high school math, 2 years high school science, high school transcript, immunizations, minimum high school GPA of 3.0, minimum GPA in nursing prerequisites of 2.4, prerequisite course work. Transfer students are accepted.
Advanced Placement Credit by examination available. Credit given for nursing courses completed elsewhere dependent upon specific evaluations.
Contact *Telephone:* 901-678-2003. *Fax:* 901-678-4906.

GRADUATE PROGRAMS

Contact *Telephone:* 901-678-2003. *Fax:* 901-678-4906.

MASTER'S DEGREE PROGRAM
Degree MSN
Available Programs Accelerated Master's for Nurses with Non-Nursing Degrees; Master's; Master's for Non-Nursing College Graduates; Master's for Nurses with Non-Nursing Degrees.
Concentrations Available Nursing administration; nursing education. *Nurse practitioner programs in:* family health.
Site Options Jackson, TN.
Study Options Full-time and part-time.
Online Degree Options Yes.
Program Entrance Requirements Minimum overall college GPA of 2.8, CPR certification, immunizations, 3 letters of recommendation, professional liability insurance/malpractice insurance.
Advanced Placement Credit given for nursing courses completed elsewhere dependent upon specific evaluations.
Degree Requirements 45 total credit hours, comprehensive exam.

POST-MASTER'S PROGRAM
Areas of Study *Nurse practitioner programs in:* family health.

The University of Tennessee
College of Nursing
Knoxville, Tennessee

https://nursing.utk.edu/Pages/default.aspx
Founded in 1794
DEGREES • BSN • MSN • MSN/PHD • PHD
Nursing Program Faculty 58 (64% with doctorates).
Baccalaureate Enrollment 523 **Women** 88% **Men** 12% **Part-time** 8%
Graduate Enrollment 160 **Women** 85% **Men** 15% **Part-time** 40.6%
Distance Learning Courses Available.
Nursing Student Activities Sigma Theta Tau, Student Nurses' Association.
Nursing Student Resources Academic advising; academic or career counseling; assistance for students with disabilities; bookstore; campus computer network; computer lab; computer-assisted instruction; e-mail services; employment services for current students; externships; interactive nursing skills videos; Internet; learning resource lab; library services; nursing audiovisuals; remedial services; skills, simulation, or other laboratory; tutoring.
Library Facilities 59,214 volumes in health, 3,711 volumes in nursing; 572 periodical subscriptions health-care related.

BACCALAUREATE PROGRAMS

Degree BSN
Available Programs Accelerated Baccalaureate; Generic Baccalaureate; RN Baccalaureate.
Study Options Full-time and part-time.
Program Entrance Requirements Transcript of college record, CPR certification, written essay, health exam, health insurance, high school biology, high school chemistry, 3 years high school math, 2 years high school science, high school transcript, immunizations, interview, minimum high school GPA of 3.2, minimum GPA in nursing prerequisites of 3.2, professional liability insurance/malpractice insurance, prerequisite course work. Transfer students are accepted. *Application deadline:* 12/1 (fall), 12/1 (summer). *Application fee:* $30.
Advanced Placement Credit given for nursing courses completed elsewhere dependent upon specific evaluations.
Contact *Telephone:* 865-974-7604. *Fax:* 865-974-3569.

GRADUATE PROGRAMS

Contact *Telephone:* 865-974-4151. *Fax:* 865-974-3569.

MASTER'S DEGREE PROGRAM
Degrees MSN; MSN/PhD
Available Programs Master's.
Concentrations Available Nurse anesthesia; nursing administration. *Clinical nurse specialist programs in:* pediatric, psychiatric/mental health. *Nurse practitioner programs in:* family health, pediatric, psychiatric/mental health.
Study Options Full-time and part-time.
Program Entrance Requirements Minimum overall college GPA of 3.0, transcript of college record, CPR certification, written essay, immunizations, 3 letters of recommendation, physical assessment course, professional liability insurance/malpractice insurance, prerequisite course

work, statistics course, GRE General Test. *Application deadline:* 2/1 (fall), 10/1 (spring), 10/1 (summer). *Application fee:* $30.
Advanced Placement Credit given for nursing courses completed elsewhere dependent upon specific evaluations.
Degree Requirements 41 total credit hours, comprehensive exam.

POST-MASTER'S PROGRAM

Areas of Study Nurse anesthesia; nursing administration; nursing education. *Clinical nurse specialist programs in:* pediatric, psychiatric/mental health. *Nurse practitioner programs in:* family health, pediatric, psychiatric/mental health.

DOCTORAL DEGREE PROGRAM

Degree PhD
Available Programs Doctorate; Post-Baccalaureate Doctorate.
Areas of Study Advanced practice nursing, bio-behavioral research, biology of health and illness, faculty preparation, family health, health policy, health promotion/disease prevention, health-care systems, human health and illness, individualized study, neuro-behavior, nursing administration, nursing education, nursing policy, nursing research, nursing science, women's health.
Online Degree Options Yes (online only).
Program Entrance Requirements Minimum overall college GPA of 3.0, interview by faculty committee, interview, 3 letters of recommendation, writing sample, GRE General Test. Application deadline: 2/1 (fall), 10/1 (summer). Application fee: $30.
Degree Requirements 67 total credit hours, dissertation, oral exam, written exam, residency.

CONTINUING EDUCATION PROGRAM

Contact *Telephone:* 865-974-7598. *Fax:* 865-974-3569.

The University of Tennessee at Chattanooga
School of Nursing
Chattanooga, Tennessee

http://www.utc.edu/Academic/Nursing
Founded in 1886
DEGREES • BSN • DNP • MSN
Nursing Program Faculty 31 (63% with doctorates).
Baccalaureate Enrollment 293 **Women** 87% **Men** 13% **Part-time** 36%
Graduate Enrollment 93 **Women** 67% **Men** 33% **Part-time** 55%
Distance Learning Courses Available.
Nursing Student Activities Sigma Theta Tau, Student Nurses' Association.
Nursing Student Resources Academic advising; academic or career counseling; assistance for students with disabilities; bookstore; campus computer network; career placement assistance; computer lab; computer-assisted instruction; daycare for children of students; e-mail services; employment services for current students; interactive nursing skills videos; Internet; learning resource lab; library services; nursing audiovisuals; skills, simulation, or other laboratory; tutoring.
Library Facilities 19,370 volumes in health, 3,100 volumes in nursing; 200 periodical subscriptions health-care related.

BACCALAUREATE PROGRAMS

Degree BSN
Available Programs ADN to Baccalaureate; Baccalaureate for Second Degree; Generic Baccalaureate.
Study Options Full-time.
Online Degree Options Yes (online only).
Program Entrance Requirements Minimum overall college GPA of 3.0, transcript of college record, CPR certification, written essay, health exam, health insurance, high school transcript, immunizations, minimum GPA in nursing prerequisites of 2.50, professional liability insurance/malpractice insurance, prerequisite course work. Transfer students are accepted. *Application deadline:* 4/1 (fall), 10/1 (spring).
Advanced Placement Credit given for nursing courses completed elsewhere dependent upon specific evaluations.
Expenses (2015–16) *Tuition, state resident:* full-time $8356; part-time $4178 per semester. *Tuition, nonresident:* full-time $24,474; part-time $12,237 per semester. *International tuition:* $24,474 full-time. *Room and board:* $3000; room only: $2500 per academic year. *Required fees:* full-time $1378; part-time $53 per credit; part-time $689 per term.

Financial Aid 90% of baccalaureate students in nursing programs received some form of financial aid in 2014–15. *Gift aid (need-based):* Federal Pell, FSEOG, state, private, college/university gift aid from institutional funds. *Loans:* Federal Direct (Subsidized and Unsubsidized Stafford PLUS), Perkins, private loans. *Work-study:* Federal Work-Study, part-time campus jobs. *Financial aid application deadline:* 5/1.
Contact April Michele Anderson, BSN Professional Advisor, School of Nursing, The University of Tennessee at Chattanooga, 615 McCallie Avenue, Department 1051, Chattanooga, TN 37403-2598. *Telephone:* 423-425-4670. *Fax:* 423-425-4668. *E-mail:* april-anderson@utc.edu.

GRADUATE PROGRAMS

Expenses (2015–16) *Tuition, state resident:* full-time $9670; part-time $4835 per semester. *Tuition, nonresident:* full-time $25,788; part-time $12,894 per semester. *International tuition:* $25,788 full-time. *Required fees:* full-time $954; part-time $53 per credit; part-time $477 per term.
Financial Aid 90% of graduate students in nursing programs received some form of financial aid in 2014–15. Career-related internships or fieldwork and scholarships available. Aid available to part-time students.
Contact Sarah Dolores Wright, Coordinator, Nursing Programs and Business Operations, School of Nursing, The University of Tennessee at Chattanooga, 615 McCallie Avenue, Department 1051, Chattanooga, TN 37403-2598. *Telephone:* 423-425-4750. *Fax:* 423-425-4668. *E-mail:* sarah-d-wright@utc.edu.

MASTER'S DEGREE PROGRAM

Degree MSN
Available Programs Master's.
Concentrations Available Nurse anesthesia. *Nurse practitioner programs in:* acute care, family health.
Site Options Tupelo, MS.
Study Options Full-time and part-time.
Program Entrance Requirements Clinical experience, computer literacy, minimum overall college GPA of 3.0, transcript of college record, CPR certification, written essay, immunizations, interview, 3 letters of recommendation, professional liability insurance/malpractice insurance, resume, GRE General Test, MAT. *Application deadline:* 6/1 (spring), 8/1 (summer). *Application fee:* $30.
Advanced Placement Credit given for nursing courses completed elsewhere dependent upon specific evaluations.
Degree Requirements 48 total credit hours, comprehensive exam.

POST-MASTER'S PROGRAM

Areas of Study Nurse anesthesia. *Nurse practitioner programs in:* acute care, family health.

DOCTORAL DEGREE PROGRAM

Degree DNP
Available Programs Doctorate; Post-Baccalaureate Doctorate.
Areas of Study Nursing administration.
Online Degree Options Yes (online only).
Program Entrance Requirements Clinical experience, minimum overall college GPA of 3.0, interview by faculty committee, interview, 3.0 letters of recommendation, MSN or equivalent, vita. Application deadline: 6/1 (spring). Application fee: $30.
Degree Requirements 36 total credit hours, residency.

The University of Tennessee at Martin
Department of Nursing
Martin, Tennessee

http://www.utm.edu/
Founded in 1900
DEGREE • BSN
Nursing Program Faculty 15 (20% with doctorates).
Baccalaureate Enrollment 198 **Women** 88% **Men** 12% **Part-time** 27%
Distance Learning Courses Available.
Nursing Student Activities Nursing Honor Society, Sigma Theta Tau, Student Nurses' Association, nursing club.
Nursing Student Resources Academic advising; academic or career counseling; assistance for students with disabilities; bookstore; campus computer network; career placement assistance; computer lab; computer-assisted instruction; daycare for children of students; e-mail services; employment services for current students; housing assistance; interactive nursing skills videos; Internet; learning resource lab; library services;

nursing audiovisuals; remedial services; resume preparation assistance; skills, simulation, or other laboratory; tutoring.

Library Facilities 1,772 volumes in health, 1,645 volumes in nursing; 10,803 periodical subscriptions health-care related.

BACCALAUREATE PROGRAMS

Degree BSN

Available Programs ADN to Baccalaureate; Generic Baccalaureate; LPN to RN Baccalaureate.

Site Options Ripley, TN; Selmer, TN; Parsons, TN.

Study Options Full-time.

Program Entrance Requirements Minimum overall college GPA of 2.0, transcript of college record, CPR certification, written essay, health exam, health insurance, high school biology, high school chemistry, high school foreign language, 3 years high school math, 2 years high school science, high school transcript, immunizations, interview, minimum high school GPA of 3.0, minimum GPA in nursing prerequisites of 2.0, professional liability insurance/malpractice insurance, prerequisite course work. Transfer students are accepted. *Application deadline:* 2/1 (fall).

Advanced Placement Credit by examination available. Credit given for nursing courses completed elsewhere dependent upon specific evaluations.

Contact *Telephone:* 731-881-7138. *Fax:* 731-881-7939.

The University of Tennessee Health Science Center

College of Nursing
Memphis, Tennessee

http://www.uthsc.edu/nursing
Founded in 1911

DEGREES • BSN • DNP • MSN • PHD

Nursing Program Faculty 46 (76% with doctorates).

Baccalaureate Enrollment 135 **Women** 84% **Men** 16%

Graduate Enrollment 274 **Women** 82% **Men** 18% **Part-time** .09%

Distance Learning Courses Available.

Nursing Student Activities Sigma Theta Tau, Student Nurses' Association, nursing club.

Nursing Student Resources Academic advising; academic or career counseling; assistance for students with disabilities; bookstore; campus computer network; computer lab; computer-assisted instruction; e-mail services; externships; interactive nursing skills videos; Internet; learning resource lab; library services; nursing audiovisuals; other; remedial services; resume preparation assistance; skills, simulation, or other laboratory; tutoring.

Library Facilities 124,967 volumes in health, 9,011 volumes in nursing; 7,727 periodical subscriptions health-care related.

BACCALAUREATE PROGRAMS

Degree BSN

Available Programs ADN to Baccalaureate; Accelerated Baccalaureate; Accelerated Baccalaureate for Second Degree; Accelerated RN Baccalaureate; RN Baccalaureate.

Study Options Full-time and part-time.

Online Degree Options Yes.

Program Entrance Requirements Minimum overall college GPA of 3.0, transcript of college record, CPR certification, written essay, health exam, high school transcript, immunizations, 3 letters of recommendation, prerequisite course work. Transfer students are accepted. *Application deadline:* 1/15 (fall), 9/1 (spring). *Application fee:* $45.

Advanced Placement Credit by examination available.

Expenses (2015–16) *Tuition, area resident:* full-time $10,440; part-time $348 per credit hour. *Tuition, state resident:* full-time $10,680; part-time $356 per credit hour. *Tuition, nonresident:* full-time $33,360; part-time $1112 per credit hour. *International tuition:* $33,360 full-time. *Required fees:* full-time $465; part-time $70 per credit.

Financial Aid 89% of baccalaureate students in nursing programs received some form of financial aid in 2014–15.

Contact Ms. Jamie Overton, Director, Student Affairs, College of Nursing, The University of Tennessee Health Science Center, 920 Madison Avenue, Suite 1021, Memphis, TN 38163. *Telephone:* 901-448-6139. *Fax:* 901-448-4121. *E-mail:* joverton@uthsc.edu.

GRADUATE PROGRAMS

Expenses (2015–16) *Tuition, area resident:* full-time $6105; part-time $679 per credit hour. *Tuition, state resident:* full-time $5309; part-time $591 per credit hour. *Tuition, nonresident:* full-time $15,181; part-time $1707 per credit hour. *International tuition:* $15,181 full-time. *Required fees:* full-time $465; part-time $70 per credit.

Financial Aid 94% of graduate students in nursing programs received some form of financial aid in 2014–15. 3 research assistantships (averaging $75,000 per year) were awarded; Federal Work-Study, institutionally sponsored loans, scholarships, and traineeships also available. *Financial aid application deadline:* 3/15.

Contact Jamie Overton, Director, Student Affairs, College of Nursing, The University of Tennessee Health Science Center, 920 Madison Avenue, Suite 1021, Memphis, TN 38163. *Telephone:* 901-448-6139. *Fax:* 901-448-4121. *E-mail:* joverton@uthsc.edu.

MASTER'S DEGREE PROGRAM

Degree MSN

Available Programs Accelerated Master's; Accelerated Master's for Nurses with Non-Nursing Degrees; Master's; Master's for Nurses with Non-Nursing Degrees.

Concentrations Available Clinical nurse leader.

Study Options Full-time.

Program Entrance Requirements Computer literacy, minimum overall college GPA of 3.0, transcript of college record, CPR certification, written essay, immunizations, interview, 3 letters of recommendation, prerequisite course work, resume, statistics course. *Application deadline:* 1/15 (fall). *Application fee:* $65.

Advanced Placement Credit by examination available.

Degree Requirements 83 total credit hours, thesis or project.

DOCTORAL DEGREE PROGRAM

Degree DNP

Available Programs Doctorate; Post-Baccalaureate Doctorate.

Areas of Study Advanced practice nursing, clinical practice, critical care, family health, gerontology.

Online Degree Options Yes (online only).

Program Entrance Requirements Minimum overall college GPA of 3.0, interview by faculty committee, interview, 3 letters of recommendation, vita, writing sample. Application deadline: 1/15 (fall), 9/1 (summer). Application fee: $65.

Degree Requirements 62 total credit hours.

Degree PhD

Available Programs Doctorate, Post-Baccalaureate Doctorate.

Areas of Study Nursing research.

Program Entrance Requirements Minimum overall college GPA of 3.0, interview, interview by faculty committee, 3 letters of recommendation, vita, writing sample. Application deadline: 2/1 (fall). Application fee: $65.

Degree Requirements 65 total credit hours (for MSN) or 77 total credits (for post-BSN), dissertation.

CONTINUING EDUCATION PROGRAM

Contact Dr. Tommie L. Norris, DNS, Associate Dean for Evaluation and Effectiveness, College of Nursing, The University of Tennessee Health Science Center, 920 Madison Avenue, Suite 1005, Memphis, TN 38163. *Telephone:* 901-448-7377. *Fax:* 901-448-4121. *E-mail:* tnorris4@uthsc.edu.

Vanderbilt University

Vanderbilt University School of Nursing
Nashville, Tennessee

http://www.nursing.vanderbilt.edu/
Founded in 1873

DEGREES • DNP • MSN • MSN/MDIV • MSN/MTS • PHD

Nursing Program Faculty 174 (63% with doctorates).

Graduate Enrollment 876 **Women** 89% **Men** 11% **Part-time** 43%

Distance Learning Courses Available.

Nursing Student Activities Nursing Honor Society, Sigma Theta Tau.

Nursing Student Resources Academic advising; academic or career counseling; assistance for students with disabilities; bookstore; campus computer network; career placement assistance; computer lab; computer-assisted instruction; e-mail services; housing assistance; interactive nursing skills videos; Internet; learning resource lab; library services;

nursing audiovisuals; remedial services; resume preparation assistance; skills, simulation, or other laboratory; tutoring.

Library Facilities 190,156 volumes in health; 3,816 periodical subscriptions health-care related.

GRADUATE PROGRAMS

Expenses (2014–15) *Tuition:* full-time $46,605; part-time $1195 per credit hour. *Required fees:* full-time $3879.

Financial Aid 86% of graduate students in nursing programs received some form of financial aid in 2013–14. Scholarships available. Aid available to part-time students. *Financial aid application deadline:* 3/15.

Contact Patricia Peerman, Assistant Dean of Enrollment Management, Vanderbilt University School of Nursing, Vanderbilt University, 207 Godchaux Hall, Nashville, TN 37240. *Telephone:* 615-322-3800. *Fax:* 615-343-0333. *E-mail:* paddy.peerman@vanderbilt.edu.

MASTER'S DEGREE PROGRAM

Degrees MSN; MSN/MDIV; MSN/MTS

Available Programs Master's; Master's for Non-Nursing College Graduates; RN to Master's.

Concentrations Available Health-care administration; nurse-midwifery; nursing administration; nursing informatics. *Nurse practitioner programs in:* adult health, adult-gerontology acute care, family health, neonatal health, pediatric, pediatric primary care, psychiatric/mental health, women's health.

Study Options Full-time and part-time.

Online Degree Options Yes (online only).

Program Entrance Requirements Computer literacy, minimum overall college GPA of 3.0, transcript of college record, CPR certification, written essay, immunizations, 3 letters of recommendation, prerequisite course work, statistics course, GRE General Test (taken within the past 5 years). *Application deadline:* 11/1 (fall). Applications may be processed on a rolling basis for some programs. *Application fee:* $50.

Advanced Placement Credit by examination available. Credit given for nursing courses completed elsewhere dependent upon specific evaluations.

Degree Requirements 39 total credit hours.

POST-MASTER'S PROGRAM

Areas of Study Health-care administration; nurse-midwifery; nursing administration; nursing informatics. *Nurse practitioner programs in:* adult health, adult-gerontology acute care, family health, neonatal health, pediatric, pediatric primary care, psychiatric/mental health, women's health.

DOCTORAL DEGREE PROGRAM

Degree DNP

Available Programs Doctorate.

Areas of Study Biology of health and illness, clinical practice, community health, critical care, family health, gerontology, health policy, health promotion/disease prevention, health-care systems, human health and illness, information systems, maternity-newborn, nursing administration, nursing policy, palliative care, women's health.

Program Entrance Requirements Minimum overall college GPA of 3.5, interview by faculty committee, 3 letters of recommendation, MSN or equivalent, statistics course, vita, writing sample, GRE General Test. Application deadline: 11/1 (fall). Applications may be processed on a rolling basis for some programs. Application fee: $50.

Degree Requirements 74 total credit hours, oral exam.

Degree PhD

Available Programs Doctorate.

Areas of Study Clinical research, nursing research.

Program Entrance Requirements Minimum overall college GPA of 3.5, interview by faculty committee, 3 letters of recommendation, MSN or equivalent, statistics course, vita, writing sample. Application deadline: 1/15 (fall).

Degree Requirements 72 semester credit hours, dissertation, oral exam.

POSTDOCTORAL PROGRAM

Areas of Study Individualized study.

Postdoctoral Program Contact Dr. Ann Minnick, Director, Vanderbilt University School of Nursing, Vanderbilt University, 415 Godchaux Hall, Nashville, TN 37240. *Telephone:* 615-343-2998. *Fax:* 615-343-5898. *E-mail:* ann.minnick@vanderbilt.edu.

TEXAS

Abilene Christian University
School of Nursing
Abilene, Texas

http://www.acu.edu/
Founded in 1906
DEGREE • BSN

BACCALAUREATE PROGRAMS

Degree BSN

Available Programs Generic Baccalaureate.

Program Entrance Requirements Transcript of college record, high school transcript, immunizations, prerequisite course work. *Application deadline:* 2/1 (fall).

Contact School of Nursing, School of Nursing, Abilene Christian University, ACU Box 28035, Abilene, TX 79699-9103. *Telephone:* 325-674-2081. *Fax:* 325-674-6256.

Angelo State University
Department of Nursing and Rehabilitation Sciences
San Angelo, Texas

http://www.angelo.edu/dept/nursing
Founded in 1928
DEGREES • BSN • MSN

Nursing Program Faculty 29 (41% with doctorates).

Baccalaureate Enrollment 253 **Women** 82% **Men** 18% **Part-time** 35%

Graduate Enrollment 83 **Women** 82% **Men** 18% **Part-time** 65%

Distance Learning Courses Available.

Nursing Student Activities Nursing Honor Society, Sigma Theta Tau, Student Nurses' Association.

Nursing Student Resources Academic advising; academic or career counseling; assistance for students with disabilities; bookstore; campus computer network; computer lab; computer-assisted instruction; e-mail services; housing assistance; interactive nursing skills videos; Internet; learning resource lab; library services; nursing audiovisuals; remedial services; skills, simulation, or other laboratory; tutoring.

Library Facilities 8,958 volumes in health, 5,241 volumes in nursing; 135 periodical subscriptions health-care related.

BACCALAUREATE PROGRAMS

Degree BSN

Available Programs Generic Baccalaureate; RN Baccalaureate.

Study Options Full-time.

Online Degree Options Yes.

Program Entrance Requirements Minimum overall college GPA of 2.5, transcript of college record, CPR certification, health insurance, immunizations, 2 letters of recommendation, prerequisite course work. Transfer students are accepted. *Application deadline:* 2/15 (fall), 9/1 (spring).

Expenses (2014–15) *Tuition, state resident:* full-time $5628; part-time $157 per credit hour. *Tuition, nonresident:* full-time $18,564; part-time $519 per credit hour. *Room and board:* $7602; room only: $4707 per academic year. *Required fees:* full-time $5036; part-time $513 per credit; part-time $1771 per term.

Financial Aid 72% of baccalaureate students in nursing programs received some form of financial aid in 2013–14.

Contact Ms. Crystal M. Nelms, Academic College Advisor, Department of Nursing and Rehabilitation Sciences, Angelo State University, ASU Station #10911, San Angelo, TX 76909. *Telephone:* 325-942-2630. *Fax:* 325-942-2631. *E-mail:* chhs@angelo.edu.

GRADUATE PROGRAMS

Expenses (2014–15) *Tuition, state resident:* full-time $7248; part-time $202 per credit hour. *Tuition, nonresident:* full-time $20,184; part-time $564 per credit hour. *Room and board:* $7602; room only: $4707 per academic year. *Required fees:* full-time $4916; part-time $1731 per term.

Financial Aid 68% of graduate students in nursing programs received some form of financial aid in 2013–14. 1 research assistantship (aver-

aging $7,490 per year) was awarded; career-related internships or fieldwork, Federal Work-Study, and scholarships also available. Aid available to part-time students. *Financial aid application deadline:* 3/1.
Contact Dr. Molly Walker, Graduate Adviser, MSN Program, Department of Nursing and Rehabilitation Sciences, Angelo State University, ASU Station #10902, San Angelo, TX 76909. *Telephone:* 325-942-2224. *Fax:* 325-942-2236. *E-mail:* molly.walker@angelo.edu.

MASTER'S DEGREE PROGRAM
Degree MSN
Available Programs Master's; Master's for Non-Nursing College Graduates; RN to Master's.
Concentrations Available Nursing education. *Clinical nurse specialist programs in:* adult health, medical-surgical. *Nurse practitioner programs in:* family health.
Study Options Full-time and part-time.
Online Degree Options Yes (online only).
Program Entrance Requirements Minimum overall college GPA of 3.0, transcript of college record, CPR certification, written essay, immunizations, 3 letters of recommendation, physical assessment course, prerequisite course work, statistics course. *Application deadline:* 4/1 (fall), 10/1 (spring), 4/1 (summer). *Application fee:* $40.
Advanced Placement Credit given for nursing courses completed elsewhere dependent upon specific evaluations.
Degree Requirements 39 total credit hours, comprehensive exam.

Baptist Health System School of Health Professions
RN-BSN Program
San Antonio, Texas

http://www.bshp.edu/future-students/programs/bachelors
DEGREE • BSN

BACCALAUREATE PROGRAMS
Degree BSN
Available Programs RN Baccalaureate.
Contact Admissions Advisor, RN-BSN Program, Baptist Health System School of Health Professions, 8400 Datapoint Drive, Dallas, TX 78229. *Telephone:* 210-297-9637.

Baylor University
Louise Herrington School of Nursing
Dallas, Texas

http://www.baylor.edu/nursing
Founded in 1845
DEGREES • BSN • DNP • MSN
Nursing Program Faculty 80 (29% with doctorates).
Baccalaureate Enrollment 416 **Women** 94% **Men** 6%
Graduate Enrollment 44 **Women** 89% **Men** 11% **Part-time** 18%
Distance Learning Courses Available.
Nursing Student Activities Sigma Theta Tau, Student Nurses' Association.
Nursing Student Resources Academic advising; academic or career counseling; assistance for students with disabilities; campus computer network; career placement assistance; computer lab; e-mail services; employment services for current students; housing assistance; interactive nursing skills videos; Internet; learning resource lab; library services; nursing audiovisuals; placement services for program completers; resume preparation assistance; skills, simulation, or other laboratory; tutoring.
Library Facilities 4,826 volumes in health, 4,826 volumes in nursing; 74 periodical subscriptions health-care related.

BACCALAUREATE PROGRAMS
Degree BSN
Available Programs Accelerated Baccalaureate for Second Degree; Generic Baccalaureate.
Study Options Full-time.
Program Entrance Requirements Transcript of college record, CPR certification, health exam, health insurance, immunizations, interview, minimum GPA in nursing prerequisites of 3.0, prerequisite course work.

Transfer students are accepted. *Application deadline:* 1/15 (fall), 5/31 (spring), 11/1 (summer). *Application fee:* $45.
Advanced Placement Credit by examination available. Credit given for nursing courses completed elsewhere dependent upon specific evaluations.
Expenses (2015–16) *Tuition:* full-time $36,360; part-time $1515 per credit hour. *International tuition:* $36,360 full-time. *Required fees:* full-time $3838.
Financial Aid 92% of baccalaureate students in nursing programs received some form of financial aid in 2014–15. *Gift aid (need-based):* Federal Pell, FSEOG, state, college/university gift aid from institutional funds. *Loans:* Federal Nursing Student Loans, Federal Direct (Subsidized and Unsubsidized Stafford PLUS), Perkins, state, private loans. *Work-study:* Federal Work-Study, part-time campus jobs. *Financial aid application deadline (priority):* 3/1.
Contact Recruiter, Louise Herrington School of Nursing, Baylor University, 3700 Worth Street, Dallas, TX 75246. *Telephone:* 214-820-3361. *Fax:* 214-820-3835. *E-mail:* BU_Nursing@baylor.edu.

GRADUATE PROGRAMS
Expenses (2015–16) *Tuition:* full-time $27,270; part-time $1515 per credit hour. *International tuition:* $27,270 full-time. *Required fees:* full-time $3838.
Financial Aid 100% of graduate students in nursing programs received some form of financial aid in 2014–15. 1 teaching assistantship (averaging $4,167 per year) was awarded; Federal Work-Study, scholarships, and unspecified assistantships also available. Aid available to part-time students. *Financial aid application deadline:* 6/30.
Contact Dr. Tanya Sudia, Director, Graduate Program (Interim), Louise Herrington School of Nursing, Baylor University, 3700 Worth Street, Dallas, TX 75246. *Telephone:* 214-820-3361. *Fax:* 214-820-4770. *E-mail:* tanya_sudia@baylor.edu.

MASTER'S DEGREE PROGRAM
Degree MSN
Available Programs Master's.
Concentrations Available Health-care administration.
Study Options Full-time.
Online Degree Options Yes (online only).
Program Entrance Requirements Clinical experience, minimum overall college GPA of 3.0, transcript of college record, CPR certification, written essay, immunizations, interview, 3 letters of recommendation, prerequisite course work, statistics course, GRE General Test or MAT. *Application deadline:* 4/1 (fall), 10/1 (spring). Applications may be processed on a rolling basis for some programs. *Application fee:* $65.
Advanced Placement Credit given for nursing courses completed elsewhere dependent upon specific evaluations.
Degree Requirements 36 total credit hours, thesis or project, comprehensive exam.

DOCTORAL DEGREE PROGRAM
Degree DNP
Available Programs Doctorate.
Areas of Study Advanced practice nursing, family health, maternity-newborn.
Program Entrance Requirements Clinical experience, minimum overall college GPA of 3.0, interview by faculty committee, interview, 3 letters of recommendation, MSN or equivalent, statistics course, writing sample, GRE General Test. Application deadline: 2/1 (fall). Application fee: $65.
Degree Requirements 75 total credit hours, residency.

Concordia University Texas
School of Nursing
Austin, Texas

http://www.concordia.edu/page.cfm?page_ID=1187
Founded in 1926
DEGREES • BSN • MSN
Nursing Program Faculty 10
Distance Learning Courses Available.

BACCALAUREATE PROGRAMS
Degree BSN
Available Programs Generic Baccalaureate.
Site Options Austin, TX.

Program Entrance Requirements *Application deadline:* 5/15 (fall), 10/1 (spring).
Contact Kathryn Lauchner, PhD, Director of School of Nursing/Assistant Dean, College of Science, School of Nursing, Concordia University Texas, 11400 Concordia University Drive, Austin, TX 78726. *Telephone:* 512-313-5514.
E-mail: kathy.lauchner@concordia.edu.

GRADUATE PROGRAMS

MASTER'S DEGREE PROGRAM
Degree MSN
Available Programs Accelerated Master's; Master's; RN to Master's.

East Texas Baptist University
Department of Nursing
Marshall, Texas

http://www.etbu.edu/nursing/
Founded in 1912
DEGREE • BSN
Nursing Program Faculty 8 (25% with doctorates).
Baccalaureate Enrollment 43 **Women** 95% **Men** 5%
Nursing Student Activities Student Nurses' Association.
Nursing Student Resources Academic advising; academic or career counseling; assistance for students with disabilities; bookstore; campus computer network; computer lab; computer-assisted instruction; e-mail services; employment services for current students; housing assistance; interactive nursing skills videos; Internet; learning resource lab; library services; nursing audiovisuals; remedial services; resume preparation assistance; skills, simulation, or other laboratory; tutoring.
Library Facilities 568 volumes in health, 291 volumes in nursing; 2,100 periodical subscriptions health-care related.

BACCALAUREATE PROGRAMS
Degree BSN
Available Programs Generic Baccalaureate.
Study Options Full-time.
Program Entrance Requirements Transcript of college record, CPR certification, health insurance, immunizations, 2 letters of recommendation, minimum GPA in nursing prerequisites of 2.8, prerequisite course work. Transfer students are accepted. *Application deadline:* 1/15 (fall).
Advanced Placement Credit given for nursing courses completed elsewhere dependent upon specific evaluations.
Contact *Telephone:* 903-923-2210. *Fax:* 903-938-9225.

Hardin-Simmons University
Patty Hanks Shelton School of Nursing
Abilene, Texas

See description of programs under Patty Hanks Shelton School of Nursing (Abilene, Texas).

Houston Baptist University
School of Nursing and Allied Health
Houston, Texas

http://www.hbu.edu/University-Catalog/Catalog-School-of-Nursing-and-Allied-Health.aspx
Founded in 1960
DEGREE • BSN
Nursing Program Faculty 19 (15% with doctorates).
Baccalaureate Enrollment 190 **Women** 95% **Men** 5% **Part-time** 20%
Nursing Student Activities Nursing Honor Society, Sigma Theta Tau, Student Nurses' Association.
Nursing Student Resources Academic advising; academic or career counseling; assistance for students with disabilities; bookstore; career placement assistance; computer lab; e-mail services; employment services for current students; externships; housing assistance; interactive nursing skills videos; Internet; learning resource lab; library services;

nursing audiovisuals; paid internships; placement services for program completers; remedial services; resume preparation assistance; skills, simulation, or other laboratory; tutoring; unpaid internships.
Library Facilities 4,276 volumes in health, 1,200 volumes in nursing; 117 periodical subscriptions health-care related.

BACCALAUREATE PROGRAMS
Degree BSN
Available Programs Generic Baccalaureate; RN Baccalaureate.
Site Options Houston, TX.
Study Options Full-time.
Program Entrance Requirements Minimum overall college GPA of 3.0, transcript of college record, CPR certification, health exam, health insurance, immunizations, minimum GPA in nursing prerequisites of 3.0, prerequisite course work. Transfer students are accepted. *Application deadline:* 3/1 (fall), 9/1 (spring).
Advanced Placement Credit by examination available.
Financial Aid 80% of baccalaureate students in nursing programs received some form of financial aid in 2013–14. *Gift aid (need-based):* Federal Pell, FSEOG, state, private, college/university gift aid from institutional funds. *Loans:* Federal Direct (Subsidized and Unsubsidized Stafford PLUS). *Work-study:* Federal Work-Study, part-time campus jobs. *Financial aid application deadline:* 4/15(priority: 3/1).
Contact Dr. Renae Schumann, Dean, School of Nursing and Allied Health, School of Nursing and Allied Health, Houston Baptist University, 7502 Fondren Street, Houston, TX 77074. *Telephone:* 281-649-3680. *Fax:* 281-649-3340. *E-mail:* rschumann@hbu.edu.

Lamar University
Department of Nursing
Beaumont, Texas

http://www.lamar.edu/nursing/
Founded in 1923
DEGREES • BSN • MSN • MSN/MBA
Nursing Program Faculty 42 (24% with doctorates).
Baccalaureate Enrollment 530 **Women** 83% **Men** 17% **Part-time** 39%
Graduate Enrollment 52 **Women** 85% **Men** 15% **Part-time** 85%
Distance Learning Courses Available.
Nursing Student Activities Sigma Theta Tau, Student Nurses' Association.
Nursing Student Resources Academic advising; academic or career counseling; assistance for students with disabilities; bookstore; campus computer network; computer lab; computer-assisted instruction; e-mail services; employment services for current students; housing assistance; interactive nursing skills videos; Internet; learning resource lab; library services; nursing audiovisuals; remedial services; resume preparation assistance; skills, simulation, or other laboratory; tutoring.
Library Facilities 7,166 volumes in health, 3,318 volumes in nursing; 1,059 periodical subscriptions health-care related.

BACCALAUREATE PROGRAMS
Degree BSN
Available Programs ADN to Baccalaureate; Generic Baccalaureate; RN Baccalaureate.
Study Options Full-time.
Online Degree Options Yes.
Program Entrance Requirements Minimum overall college GPA of 2.0, transcript of college record, CPR certification, health exam, immunizations, minimum GPA in nursing prerequisites of 2.5, professional liability insurance/malpractice insurance, prerequisite course work. Transfer students are accepted. *Application deadline:* 3/1 (fall), 9/1 (spring). *Application fee:* $25.
Advanced Placement Credit given for nursing courses completed elsewhere dependent upon specific evaluations.
Expenses (2015–16) *Tuition, state resident:* full-time $2760; part-time $230 per credit hour. *Tuition, nonresident:* full-time $7440; part-time $620 per credit hour. *Room and board:* $8302; room only: $5252 per academic year. *Required fees:* part-time $150 per term.
Contact Academic Advisor, Department of Nursing, Lamar University, PO Box 10079, Beaumont, TX 77710. *Telephone:* 409-880-8822. *E-mail:* nursing@lamar.edu.

GRADUATE PROGRAMS
Expenses (2015–16) *Tuition, state resident:* full-time $3950; part-time $496 per credit hour. *Tuition, nonresident:* full-time $7460; part-time

$886 per credit hour. *Room and board:* $8302; room only: $5252 per academic year.

Contact Dr. Ruthie Robinson, Director of Graduate Nursing Studies, Department of Nursing, Lamar University, PO Box 10081, Beaumont, TX 77710. *Telephone:* 409-880-7720. *Fax:* 409-880-8698. *E-mail:* ruthie.robinson@lamar.edu.

MASTER'S DEGREE PROGRAM

Degrees MSN; MSN/MBA
Available Programs Master's; RN to Master's.
Concentrations Available Nursing administration; nursing education.
Study Options Full-time and part-time.
Online Degree Options Yes (online only).
Program Entrance Requirements Computer literacy, minimum overall college GPA of 3.0, transcript of college record, CPR certification, immunizations, professional liability insurance/malpractice insurance, prerequisite course work, statistics course. *Application deadline:* Applications may be processed on a rolling basis for some programs. *Application fee:* $25.
Advanced Placement Credit given for nursing courses completed elsewhere dependent upon specific evaluations.
Degree Requirements 37 total credit hours, thesis or project.

POST-MASTER'S PROGRAM

Areas of Study Nursing administration; nursing education.

CONTINUING EDUCATION PROGRAM

Contact Dr. Cindy Stinson, Coordinator of Continuing Education, Department of Nursing, Lamar University, PO Box 10081, Beaumont, TX 77710. *Telephone:* 409-880-8833. *Fax:* 409-880-1865. *E-mail:* cynthia.stinson@lamar.edu.

Lubbock Christian University
Department of Nursing
Lubbock, Texas

Founded in 1957
DEGREE • BSN
Nursing Program Faculty 5 (40% with doctorates).

BACCALAUREATE PROGRAMS

Degree BSN
Available Programs RN Baccalaureate.
Study Options Part-time.
Program Entrance Requirements Minimum overall college GPA of 2.5, transcript of college record, CPR certification, health exam, immunizations, interview, 2 letters of recommendation, minimum high school GPA, minimum GPA in nursing prerequisites of 2.5, professional liability insurance/malpractice insurance, prerequisite course work, RN licensure. Transfer students are accepted.

McMurry University
Patty Hanks Shelton School of Nursing
Abilene, Texas

See description of programs under Patty Hanks Shelton School of Nursing (Abilene, Texas).

Midwestern State University
Wilson School of Nursing
Wichita Falls, Texas

http://www.mwsu.edu/academics/hs2/nursing/
Founded in 1922
DEGREES • BSN • MSN
Nursing Program Faculty 25 (30% with doctorates).
Baccalaureate Enrollment 482 **Women** 83% **Men** 17% **Part-time** 23%
Graduate Enrollment 122 **Women** 82% **Men** 18% **Part-time** 34%
Distance Learning Courses Available.

Nursing Student Activities Nursing Honor Society, Sigma Theta Tau, Student Nurses' Association.
Nursing Student Resources Academic advising; academic or career counseling; assistance for students with disabilities; bookstore; campus computer network; career placement assistance; computer lab; computer-assisted instruction; e-mail services; employment services for current students; externships; housing assistance; interactive nursing skills videos; Internet; learning resource lab; library services; nursing audiovisuals; other; placement services for program completers; remedial services; resume preparation assistance; skills, simulation, or other laboratory; tutoring.
Library Facilities 10,000 volumes in health, 5,000 volumes in nursing; 6,000 periodical subscriptions health-care related.

BACCALAUREATE PROGRAMS

Degree BSN
Available Programs ADN to Baccalaureate; Accelerated Baccalaureate; Generic Baccalaureate; RN Baccalaureate.
Study Options Full-time and part-time.
Program Entrance Requirements Transcript of college record, CPR certification, health exam, health insurance, immunizations, minimum GPA in nursing prerequisites of 3.0, professional liability insurance/malpractice insurance, prerequisite course work. Transfer students are accepted. *Application deadline:* 3/15 (fall), 9/30 (spring). *Application fee:* $25.
Advanced Placement Credit given for nursing courses completed elsewhere dependent upon specific evaluations.
Financial Aid 80% of baccalaureate students in nursing programs received some form of financial aid in 2013–14. *Gift aid (need-based):* Federal Pell, FSEOG, state, private, college/university gift aid from institutional funds, state nursing scholarships. *Loans:* Federal Direct (Subsidized and Unsubsidized Stafford PLUS), Perkins, state, college/university, private loans. *Work-study:* Federal Work-Study, part-time campus jobs. *Financial aid application deadline (priority):* 3/1.
Contact Mrs. Robin Lockhart, BSN Programs Coordinator, Wilson School of Nursing, Midwestern State University, 3410 Taft Boulevard, Bridwell Hall, Wichita Falls, TX 76308. *Telephone:* 940-397-4614. *Fax:* 940-397-4911. *E-mail:* robin.lockhart@mwsu.edu.

GRADUATE PROGRAMS

Financial Aid 50% of graduate students in nursing programs received some form of financial aid in 2013–14. Teaching assistantships with partial tuition reimbursements available, career-related internships or fieldwork, Federal Work-Study, institutionally sponsored loans, scholarships, tuition waivers (partial), and unspecified assistantships available. Aid available to part-time students. *Financial aid application deadline:* 3/1.
Contact Dr. Debra G. Walker, Graduate Coordinator, Wilson School of Nursing, Midwestern State University, 3410 Taft Boulevard, Bridwell Hall 308C, Wichita Falls, TX 76308. *Telephone:* 940-397-4600. *Fax:* 940-397-4911. *E-mail:* debra.walker@mwsu.edu.

MASTER'S DEGREE PROGRAM

Degree MSN
Available Programs Master's; RN to Master's.
Concentrations Available Nursing education. *Nurse practitioner programs in:* family health, psychiatric/mental health.
Study Options Full-time and part-time.
Online Degree Options Yes.
Program Entrance Requirements Clinical experience, minimum overall college GPA of 3.0, transcript of college record, CPR certification, immunizations, interview, professional liability insurance/malpractice insurance, statistics course, GRE General Test or MAT. *Application deadline:* 7/1 (fall), 11/1 (spring), 4/15 (summer). Applications may be processed on a rolling basis for some programs. *Application fee:* $35.
Advanced Placement Credit by examination available. Credit given for nursing courses completed elsewhere dependent upon specific evaluations.
Degree Requirements 40 total credit hours, thesis or project.

POST-MASTER'S PROGRAM

Areas of Study Nursing education. *Nurse practitioner programs in:* family health, psychiatric/mental health.

CONTINUING EDUCATION PROGRAM

Contact Dr. Betty Bowles, Coordinator, Professional Outreach Center, Wilson School of Nursing, Midwestern State University, 3410 Taft

Boulevard, Wichita Falls, TX 76308. *Telephone:* 940-397-4048. *Fax:* 940-397-4513. *E-mail:* betty.bowles@mwsu.edu.

Patty Hanks Shelton School of Nursing
Abilene, Texas

http://www.phssn.edu/

DEGREES • BSN • MSN

Nursing Program Faculty 17 (30% with doctorates).
Baccalaureate Enrollment 131 **Women** 89% **Men** 11% **Part-time** 9%
Graduate Enrollment 18 **Women** 73% **Men** 27%
Distance Learning Courses Available.
Nursing Student Activities Nursing Honor Society, Sigma Theta Tau, Student Nurses' Association.
Nursing Student Resources Academic advising; academic or career counseling; assistance for students with disabilities; bookstore; campus computer network; career placement assistance; computer lab; computer-assisted instruction; e-mail services; employment services for current students; externships; interactive nursing skills videos; Internet; learning resource lab; library services; nursing audiovisuals; remedial services; resume preparation assistance; skills, simulation, or other laboratory; tutoring.
Library Facilities 9,200 volumes in health, 1,300 volumes in nursing; 140 periodical subscriptions health-care related.

BACCALAUREATE PROGRAMS

Degree BSN
Available Programs Generic Baccalaureate; RN Baccalaureate.
Study Options Full-time.
Program Entrance Requirements Minimum overall college GPA of 3.0, transcript of college record, CPR certification, health exam, health insurance, immunizations, 2 letters of recommendation, minimum GPA in nursing prerequisites of 3.0, professional liability insurance/malpractice insurance, prerequisite course work. Transfer students are accepted. *Application deadline:* 6/13 (fall), 10/13 (spring).
Advanced Placement Credit by examination available. Credit given for nursing courses completed elsewhere dependent upon specific evaluations.
Contact *Telephone:* 325-671-2353. *Fax:* 325-671-2386.

GRADUATE PROGRAMS

Contact *Telephone:* 325-671-2367. *Fax:* 325-671-2386.

MASTER'S DEGREE PROGRAM

Degree MSN
Available Programs Master's.
Concentrations Available Nursing education. *Nurse practitioner programs in:* family health.
Study Options Full-time and part-time.
Program Entrance Requirements Clinical experience, minimum overall college GPA of 3.5, transcript of college record, CPR certification, written essay, immunizations, interview, 3 letters of recommendation, physical assessment course, professional liability insurance/malpractice insurance, resume, statistics course. *Application deadline:* 8/12 (fall).
Advanced Placement Credit given for nursing courses completed elsewhere dependent upon specific evaluations.
Degree Requirements 49 total credit hours.

POST-MASTER'S PROGRAM

Areas of Study *Nurse practitioner programs in:* family health.

CONTINUING EDUCATION PROGRAM

Contact *Telephone:* 325-671-2399. *Fax:* 325-671-2386.

Prairie View A&M University
College of Nursing
Houston, Texas

http://www.pvamu.edu/nursing
Founded in 1878

DEGREES • BSN • MSN

Nursing Program Faculty 66 (26% with doctorates).
Baccalaureate Enrollment 447 **Women** 85% **Men** 15% **Part-time** 19%
Graduate Enrollment 103 **Women** 95% **Men** 5% **Part-time** 78%
Distance Learning Courses Available.
Nursing Student Activities Nursing Honor Society, Sigma Theta Tau, Student Nurses' Association, nursing club.
Nursing Student Resources Academic advising; academic or career counseling; assistance for students with disabilities; bookstore; campus computer network; career placement assistance; computer lab; computer-assisted instruction; e-mail services; employment services for current students; interactive nursing skills videos; Internet; learning resource lab; library services; nursing audiovisuals; placement services for program completers; resume preparation assistance; skills, simulation, or other laboratory; tutoring.
Library Facilities 355,707 volumes in health, 7,899 volumes in nursing; 9,283 periodical subscriptions health-care related.

BACCALAUREATE PROGRAMS

Degree BSN
Available Programs Generic Baccalaureate; LPN to Baccalaureate; RN Baccalaureate.
Site Options Woodlands, TX; College Station, TX.
Study Options Full-time and part-time.
Program Entrance Requirements Minimum overall college GPA of 2.5, transcript of college record, CPR certification, health exam, immunizations, minimum GPA in nursing prerequisites of 2.0, professional liability insurance/malpractice insurance, prerequisite course work. Transfer students are accepted. *Application deadline:* 3/1 (fall), 10/1 (spring). *Application fee:* $25.
Advanced Placement Credit given for nursing courses completed elsewhere dependent upon specific evaluations.
Contact *Telephone:* 713-797-7031. *Fax:* 713-797-7092.

GRADUATE PROGRAMS

Contact *Telephone:* 713-797-7015. *Fax:* 713-797-7011.

MASTER'S DEGREE PROGRAM

Degree MSN
Available Programs Master's.
Concentrations Available Nursing administration; nursing education. *Nurse practitioner programs in:* family health.
Study Options Full-time and part-time.
Program Entrance Requirements Clinical experience, minimum overall college GPA of 2.75, transcript of college record, CPR certification, immunizations, interview, 3 letters of recommendation, physical assessment course, prerequisite course work, resume, statistics course, MAT or GRE. *Application deadline:* 6/1 (fall), 10/1 (spring), 4/1 (summer). *Application fee:* $25.
Advanced Placement Credit by examination available. Credit given for nursing courses completed elsewhere dependent upon specific evaluations.
Degree Requirements 53 total credit hours, thesis or project.

POST-MASTER'S PROGRAM

Areas of Study Nursing administration; nursing education. *Nurse practitioner programs in:* family health.

Sam Houston State University
Nursing Program
Huntsville, Texas

http://www.shsu.edu/nursing
Founded in 1879

DEGREE • BSN

Nursing Program Faculty 26 (25% with doctorates).
Baccalaureate Enrollment 209 **Women** 85% **Men** 15%
Distance Learning Courses Available.

Nursing Student Activities Sigma Theta Tau, Student Nurses' Association, nursing club.

Nursing Student Resources Academic advising; academic or career counseling; assistance for students with disabilities; bookstore; campus computer network; career placement assistance; computer lab; computer-assisted instruction; e-mail services; employment services for current students; externships; housing assistance; interactive nursing skills videos; Internet; learning resource lab; library services; nursing audiovisuals; placement services for program completers; remedial services; resume preparation assistance; skills, simulation, or other laboratory; tutoring.

BACCALAUREATE PROGRAMS

Degree BSN

Available Programs ADN to Baccalaureate; Baccalaureate for Second Degree; Generic Baccalaureate; International Nurse to Baccalaureate; LPN to Baccalaureate; LPN to RN Baccalaureate; RN Baccalaureate.
Site Options The Woodlands, TX.
Study Options Full-time.
Program Entrance Requirements Minimum overall college GPA of 3.0, transcript of college record, CPR certification, health exam, health insurance, immunizations, minimum GPA in nursing prerequisites of 3.0, professional liability insurance/malpractice insurance, prerequisite course work. Transfer students are accepted. *Application deadline:* 6/1 (fall), 10/1 (spring).
Expenses (2015–16) *Tuition, state resident:* full-time $7546. *Tuition, nonresident:* full-time $15,000. *Required fees:* full-time $1500.
Contact Anne S. Stiles, PhD, Professor and Chair, Nursing Program, Sam Houston State University, 1 Financial Plaza, Suite 215, Huntsville, TX 77340. *Telephone:* 936-294-2379. *E-mail:* Astiles@shsu.edu.

Schreiner University
Bachelor of Science in Nursing
Kerrville, Texas

http://www.schreiner.edu/academics/majors-and-programs/bachelor-of-science-in-nursing/index.aspx
Founded in 1923
DEGREE • BSN

BACCALAUREATE PROGRAMS

Degree BSN
Available Programs RN Baccalaureate.
Contact Nursing Programs, Bachelor of Science in Nursing, Schreiner University, 2100 Memorial Boulevard, Kerrville, TX 78028-5697. *Telephone:* 800-343-4919.

Southwestern Adventist University
Department of Nursing
Keene, Texas

http://www.swau.edu/
Founded in 1894
DEGREE • BS
Nursing Program Faculty 10 (38% with doctorates).
Baccalaureate Enrollment 93 **Women** 82% **Men** 18% **Part-time** 28%
Nursing Student Activities Student Nurses' Association.
Nursing Student Resources Academic advising; academic or career counseling; assistance for students with disabilities; bookstore; campus computer network; computer lab; computer-assisted instruction; e-mail services; externships; interactive nursing skills videos; Internet; learning resource lab; library services; nursing audiovisuals; remedial services; resume preparation assistance; skills, simulation, or other laboratory; tutoring.
Library Facilities 1,791 volumes in health, 847 volumes in nursing; 5,168 periodical subscriptions health-care related.

BACCALAUREATE PROGRAMS

Degree BS
Available Programs Generic Baccalaureate; LPN to RN Baccalaureate; RN Baccalaureate.
Study Options Full-time and part-time.

Program Entrance Requirements Transcript of college record, CPR certification, health exam, health insurance, immunizations, 3 letters of recommendation, minimum GPA in nursing prerequisites of 2.75, prerequisite course work. *Application deadline:* 8/15 (spring).
Advanced Placement Credit by examination available.
Contact *Telephone:* 817-202-6670. *Fax:* 817-202-6713.

Stephen F. Austin State University
Richard and Lucille Dewitt School of Nursing
Nacogdoches, Texas

http://www.fp.sfasu.edu/nursing/
Founded in 1923
DEGREE • BSN
Nursing Program Faculty 33 (38% with doctorates).
Baccalaureate Enrollment 285
Distance Learning Courses Available.
Nursing Student Activities Sigma Theta Tau, Student Nurses' Association.
Nursing Student Resources Academic advising; academic or career counseling; assistance for students with disabilities; bookstore; campus computer network; career placement assistance; computer lab; computer-assisted instruction; e-mail services; employment services for current students; housing assistance; interactive nursing skills videos; Internet; learning resource lab; library services; nursing audiovisuals; remedial services; resume preparation assistance; skills, simulation, or other laboratory; tutoring.

BACCALAUREATE PROGRAMS

Degree BSN
Available Programs Generic Baccalaureate; RN Baccalaureate.
Site Options Nacogdoches, TX.
Study Options Full-time.
Program Entrance Requirements Minimum overall college GPA of 2.5, transcript of college record, CPR certification, written essay, health insurance, high school transcript, immunizations, 3 letters of recommendation, minimum GPA in nursing prerequisites of 2.75, professional liability insurance/malpractice insurance, prerequisite course work. Transfer students are accepted. *Application deadline:* 2/1 (fall), 8/15 (spring).
Advanced Placement Credit given for nursing courses completed elsewhere dependent upon specific evaluations.
Contact Dr. Sara E. Bishop, Interim Director, Richard and Lucille Dewitt School of Nursing, Stephen F. Austin State University, SFA Box 6156, Nacogdoches, TX 75962. *Telephone:* 936-468-7704. *Fax:* 936-468-7752.

Tarleton State University
Department of Nursing
Stephenville, Texas

http://www.tarleton.edu/nursing
Founded in 1899
DEGREES • BSN • MSN
Nursing Program Faculty 32 (31% with doctorates).
Baccalaureate Enrollment 353
Graduate Enrollment 19
Distance Learning Courses Available.
Nursing Student Activities Sigma Theta Tau, Student Nurses' Association.
Nursing Student Resources Academic advising; academic or career counseling; assistance for students with disabilities; bookstore; campus computer network; career placement assistance; computer lab; computer-assisted instruction; e-mail services; employment services for current students; Internet; learning resource lab; library services; nursing audiovisuals; remedial services; resume preparation assistance; skills, simulation, or other laboratory; tutoring.

BACCALAUREATE PROGRAMS

Degree BSN
Available Programs ADN to Baccalaureate; Generic Baccalaureate; LPN to Baccalaureate.
Site Options Fort Worth, TX; Waco, TX.

Study Options Full-time and part-time.
Program Entrance Requirements Transcript of college record, CPR certification, written essay, health insurance, immunizations, 3 letters of recommendation, minimum GPA in nursing prerequisites of 3.0, professional liability insurance/malpractice insurance, prerequisite course work. Transfer students are accepted.
Contact Dr. Dok Woods, Director of Undergraduate Nursing Program, Department of Nursing, Tarleton State University, Box T-0500, Stephenville, TX 76402. *Telephone:* 254-968-9139. *Fax:* 254-968-9716. *E-mail:* woods@tarleton.edu.

GRADUATE PROGRAMS

Contact Dr. Jennifer J. Yeager, Director of the Graduate Nursing Program, Department of Nursing, Tarleton State University, Box T-0500, Stephenville, TX 76402. *Telephone:* 254-968-9139. *E-mail:* jyeager@tarleton.edu.

MASTER'S DEGREE PROGRAM
Degree MSN
Available Programs Master's; RN to Master's.
Concentrations Available Nursing administration; nursing education.
Site Options Fort Worth, TX.
Study Options Full-time and part-time.
Program Entrance Requirements Minimum overall college GPA of 3.0, transcript of college record, written essay, 3 letters of recommendation, resume, statistics course.
Degree Requirements Thesis or project, comprehensive exam.

CONTINUING EDUCATION PROGRAM

Contact Ms. Nancy Gaither, Coordinator of Nursing Professional Development, Department of Nursing, Tarleton State University, Box T-0500, Stephenville, TX 76402. *Telephone:* 254-968-0535. *E-mail:* gaither@tarleton.edu.

Texas A&M Health Science Center
College of Nursing
College Station, Texas

http://www.tamhsc.edu
Founded in 1999
DEGREES • BSN • MSN
Nursing Program Faculty 44 (39% with doctorates).
Baccalaureate Enrollment 145 Women 89% Men 11% Part-time 2%
Graduate Enrollment 44 Women 87% Men 13% Part-time 43%
Distance Learning Courses Available.
Nursing Student Activities Sigma Theta Tau, Student Nurses' Association, nursing club.
Nursing Student Resources Academic advising; assistance for students with disabilities; bookstore; campus computer network; career placement assistance; computer lab; computer-assisted instruction; e-mail services; externships; interactive nursing skills videos; Internet; learning resource lab; library services; nursing audiovisuals; remedial services; resume preparation assistance; skills, simulation, or other laboratory; tutoring.
Library Facilities 4 million volumes in health, 1.5 million volumes in nursing; 123,000 periodical subscriptions health-care related.

BACCALAUREATE PROGRAMS

Degree BSN
Available Programs ADN to Baccalaureate; Accelerated Baccalaureate for Second Degree; Generic Baccalaureate; RN Baccalaureate.
Site Options McAllen, TX; Round Rock, TX.
Study Options Full-time.
Online Degree Options Yes.
Program Entrance Requirements Minimum overall college GPA of 3.0, transcript of college record, CPR certification, written essay, health exam, health insurance, high school foreign language, immunizations, 1 letter of recommendation, minimum GPA in nursing prerequisites of 2.75, professional liability insurance/malpractice insurance, prerequisite course work. Transfer students are accepted. *Application deadline:* 8/1 (winter), 2/1 (summer). *Application fee:* $50.
Advanced Placement Credit by examination available. Credit given for nursing courses completed elsewhere dependent upon specific evaluations.

Expenses (2014–15) *Tuition, state resident:* full-time $8563; part-time $279 per credit hour. *Tuition, nonresident:* full-time $19,808; part-time $645 per credit hour. *International tuition:* $19,808 full-time.
Financial Aid 89% of baccalaureate students in nursing programs received some form of financial aid in 2013–14.
Contact Kathryn Willis Cochran, Associate Dean for Student Affairs, College of Nursing, Texas A&M Health Science Center, 8447 State Highway 47, Bryan, TX 77807-3260. *Telephone:* 979-436-0110. *Fax:* 979-436-0098. *E-mail:* cochran@tamhsc.edu.

GRADUATE PROGRAMS

Expenses (2014–15) *Tuition, state resident:* full-time $6923; part-time $410 per credit hour. *Tuition, nonresident:* full-time $13,439; part-time $772 per credit hour. *International tuition:* $13,439 full-time.
Contact Kathryn Cochran, Associate Dean for Student Affairs, College of Nursing, Texas A&M Health Science Center, 8447 State Highway 47, Bryan, TX 77807-3260. *Telephone:* 979-436-0121. *Fax:* 979-436-0098. *E-mail:* cochran@tamhsc.edu.

MASTER'S DEGREE PROGRAM
Degree MSN
Available Programs Accelerated Master's; Master's; RN to Master's.
Concentrations Available Nursing education. *Nurse practitioner programs in:* family health.
Study Options Full-time and part-time.
Online Degree Options Yes (online only).
Program Entrance Requirements Minimum overall college GPA of 3.0, transcript of college record, CPR certification, written essay, immunizations, 3 letters of recommendation, professional liability insurance/malpractice insurance, resume, statistics course. *Application deadline:* 8/1 (spring). *Application fee:* $50.
Advanced Placement Credit given for nursing courses completed elsewhere dependent upon specific evaluations.
Degree Requirements 36 total credit hours.

CONTINUING EDUCATION PROGRAM

Contact Pat Ehlert, Point for CE and Clinical Assistant Professor, College of Nursing, Texas A&M Health Science Center, 8447 State Highway 47, Bryan, TX 77807-3260. *Telephone:* 979-436-0135. *Fax:* 979-436-0098. *E-mail:* ehlert@tamhsc.edu.

Texas A&M International University
Canseco School of Nursing
Laredo, Texas

Founded in 1969
DEGREES • BSN • MSN
Nursing Program Faculty 24 (17% with doctorates).
Baccalaureate Enrollment 117 Women 74.4% Men 25.6% Part-time 1%
Graduate Enrollment 40 Women 82.5% Men 17.5% Part-time 100%
Distance Learning Courses Available.
Nursing Student Activities Nursing Honor Society, Student Nurses' Association.
Nursing Student Resources Academic advising; academic or career counseling; assistance for students with disabilities; bookstore; campus computer network; career placement assistance; computer lab; computer-assisted instruction; daycare for children of students; e-mail services; employment services for current students; externships; housing assistance; interactive nursing skills videos; Internet; learning resource lab; library services; nursing audiovisuals; paid internships; placement services for program completers; remedial services; resume preparation assistance; skills, simulation, or other laboratory; tutoring.
Library Facilities 14,285 volumes in health, 1,804 volumes in nursing; 8,751 periodical subscriptions health-care related.

BACCALAUREATE PROGRAMS

Degree BSN
Available Programs Generic Baccalaureate; RN Baccalaureate.
Study Options Full-time.
Program Entrance Requirements Minimum overall college GPA of 2.5, transcript of college record, CPR certification, written essay, health exam, immunizations, 2 letters of recommendation, minimum high school GPA of 2.5, minimum GPA in nursing prerequisites of 2.5, prereq-

uisite course work. Transfer students are accepted. *Application deadline:* 6/1 (fall). *Application fee:* $25.

Advanced Placement Credit given for nursing courses completed elsewhere dependent upon specific evaluations.

Contact *Telephone:* 956-326-2450. *Fax:* 956-326-2449.

GRADUATE PROGRAMS

Contact *Telephone:* 956-326-2450. *Fax:* 956-326-2449.

MASTER'S DEGREE PROGRAM

Degree MSN

Available Programs Master's.

Concentrations Available Nursing administration. *Nurse practitioner programs in:* family health.

Study Options Full-time and part-time.

Program Entrance Requirements Clinical experience, minimum overall college GPA of 3.0, transcript of college record, CPR certification, written essay, immunizations, interview, 2 letters of recommendation, nursing research course. *Application deadline:* 6/1 (fall). *Application fee:* $25.

Advanced Placement Credit given for nursing courses completed elsewhere dependent upon specific evaluations.

Degree Requirements 45 total credit hours.

Texas A&M University–Commerce

Nursing Department
Commerce, Texas

http://www.tamuc.edu/
Founded in 1889

DEGREE • BSN

Nursing Program Faculty 8 (38% with doctorates).
Baccalaureate Enrollment 83
Nursing Student Activities Sigma Theta Tau, Student Nurses' Association.
Nursing Student Resources Academic advising; academic or career counseling; assistance for students with disabilities; bookstore; campus computer network; career placement assistance; computer lab; computer-assisted instruction; daycare for children of students; e-mail services; employment services for current students; externships; housing assistance; interactive nursing skills videos; Internet; learning resource lab; library services; nursing audiovisuals; resume preparation assistance; skills, simulation, or other laboratory; tutoring.
Library Facilities 6,097 volumes in health, 179 volumes in nursing; 552 periodical subscriptions health-care related.

BACCALAUREATE PROGRAMS

Degree BSN

Available Programs Generic Baccalaureate; RN Baccalaureate.
Study Options Full-time.
Program Entrance Requirements Transcript of college record, written essay, minimum GPA in nursing prerequisites. Transfer students are accepted. *Application deadline:* 5/15 (fall). *Application fee:* $40.
Expenses (2015–16) *Tuition, state resident:* full-time $10,000. *Tuition, nonresident:* full-time $21,000.
Contact Angie Proctor, Mentor Center.
E-mail: Angie.Proctor@tamuc.edu.

Texas A&M University–Corpus Christi

College of Nursing and Health Sciences
Corpus Christi, Texas

http://conhs.tamucc.edu/index.html
Founded in 1947

DEGREES • BSN • MSN

Nursing Program Faculty 109 (45% with doctorates).
Baccalaureate Enrollment 488 **Women** 79% **Men** 21% **Part-time** 13%
Graduate Enrollment 388 **Women** 84% **Men** 16% **Part-time** 99%
Distance Learning Courses Available.

Nursing Student Activities Nursing Honor Society, Sigma Theta Tau, Student Nurses' Association.
Nursing Student Resources Academic advising; academic or career counseling; assistance for students with disabilities; bookstore; campus computer network; career placement assistance; computer lab; computer-assisted instruction; e-mail services; employment services for current students; housing assistance; interactive nursing skills videos; Internet; learning resource lab; library services; nursing audiovisuals; placement services for program completers; remedial services; resume preparation assistance; skills, simulation, or other laboratory; tutoring.
Library Facilities 500 volumes in health, 350 volumes in nursing; 100 periodical subscriptions health-care related.

BACCALAUREATE PROGRAMS

Degree BSN

Available Programs ADN to Baccalaureate; Accelerated Baccalaureate; Accelerated Baccalaureate for Second Degree; Baccalaureate for Second Degree; Generic Baccalaureate; RN Baccalaureate.
Study Options Full-time and part-time.
Online Degree Options Yes.
Program Entrance Requirements Minimum overall college GPA of 3.0, transcript of college record, CPR certification, health insurance, immunizations, professional liability insurance/malpractice insurance, prerequisite course work. Transfer students are accepted. *Application deadline:* 2/15 (fall), 2/15 (winter), 7/31 (spring), 10/31 (summer). *Application fee:* $45.
Advanced Placement Credit by examination available. Credit given for nursing courses completed elsewhere dependent upon specific evaluations.
Expenses (2015–16) *Tuition, state resident:* full-time $7558; part-time $354 per contact hour. *Tuition, nonresident:* full-time $20,406; part-time $706 per contact hour. *International tuition:* $20,406 full-time. *Required fees:* full-time $4944; part-time $380 per credit; part-time $1649 per term.
Financial Aid 80% of baccalaureate students in nursing programs received some form of financial aid in 2014–15. *Gift aid (need-based):* Federal Pell, FSEOG, state, college/university gift aid from institutional funds. *Loans:* Federal Direct (Subsidized and Unsubsidized Stafford PLUS), Perkins, state, college/university. *Work-study:* Federal Work-Study, part-time campus jobs. *Financial aid application deadline (priority):* 3/31.
Contact Dr. Christina Murphey, Undergraduate Chair, College of Nursing and Health Sciences, Texas A&M University–Corpus Christi, 6300 Ocean Drive, Unit 5805, Corpus Christi, TX 78412-5503. *Telephone:* 361-825-2244. *Fax:* 361-825-2484.
E-mail: Christina.murpheyl@tamucc.edu.

GRADUATE PROGRAMS

Expenses (2015–16) *Tuition, state resident:* full-time $5871; part-time $372 per contact hour. *Tuition, nonresident:* full-time $15,648; part-time $734 per contact hour. *International tuition:* $15,648 full-time. *Required fees:* full-time $3714.
Financial Aid 45% of graduate students in nursing programs received some form of financial aid in 2014–15.
Contact Dr. Linda Gibson-Young, Graduate Department Chair, College of Nursing and Health Sciences, Texas A&M University–Corpus Christi, 6300 Ocean Drive, Unit 5805, Corpus Christi, TX 78412. *Telephone:* 361-825-2798. *Fax:* 361-825-2484.
E-mail: linda.gibson-young@tamucc.edu.

MASTER'S DEGREE PROGRAM

Degree MSN

Available Programs Master's; RN to Master's.
Concentrations Available Nursing administration; nursing education. *Nurse practitioner programs in:* family health.
Study Options Part-time.
Online Degree Options Yes (online only).
Program Entrance Requirements Minimum overall college GPA of 3.0, transcript of college record, CPR certification, written essay, immunizations, 3 letters of recommendation, resume, statistics course. *Application deadline:* 4/15 (fall), 11/15 (spring), 4/15 (summer). *Application fee:* $40.
Advanced Placement Credit given for nursing courses completed elsewhere dependent upon specific evaluations.
Degree Requirements 49 total credit hours, thesis or project.

POST-MASTER'S PROGRAM

Areas of Study Nursing administration; nursing education. *Nurse practitioner programs in:* family health.

CONTINUING EDUCATION PROGRAM

Contact Ms. Yvonne Serna, Chair of Continuing Education Committee, College of Nursing and Health Sciences, Texas A&M University–Corpus Christi, 6300 Ocean Drive, Island Hall, Room 342, Corpus Christi, TX 78412-5503. *Telephone:* 361-825-3790. *Fax:* 361-825-2484. *E-mail:* Yvonne.serna@tamucc.edu.

Texas A&M University–Texarkana

Nursing Department
Texarkana, Texas

http://www.tamut.edu/
Founded in 1971

DEGREES • BSN • MSN
Nursing Program Faculty 3 (100% with doctorates).
Baccalaureate Enrollment 50 **Women** 87% **Men** 13% **Part-time** 50%
Graduate Enrollment 12 **Women** 92% **Men** 8% **Part-time** 100%
Distance Learning Courses Available.
Nursing Student Resources Academic advising; academic or career counseling; assistance for students with disabilities; bookstore; campus computer network; career placement assistance; computer lab; computer-assisted instruction; e-mail services; Internet; library services; nursing audiovisuals; remedial services; resume preparation assistance; tutoring; unpaid internships.
Library Facilities 8,743 volumes in health, 2,558 volumes in nursing; 80 periodical subscriptions health-care related.

BACCALAUREATE PROGRAMS

Degree BSN
Available Programs ADN to Baccalaureate.
Study Options Full-time and part-time.
Online Degree Options Yes (online only).
Program Entrance Requirements Minimum overall college GPA of 2.8, transcript of college record, CPR certification, health insurance, immunizations, letters of recommendation, minimum GPA in nursing prerequisites, professional liability insurance/malpractice insurance, pre-requisite course work, RN licensure. Transfer students are accepted. *Application deadline:* 7/15 (fall).
Advanced Placement Credit given for nursing courses completed elsewhere dependent upon specific evaluations.
Expenses (2015–16) *Tuition, area resident:* full-time $7500; part-time $294 per credit hour. *Tuition, state resident:* full-time $7884; part-time $327 per credit hour. *Tuition, nonresident:* full-time $17,000; part-time $719 per credit hour. *International tuition:* $17,000 full-time.
Contact Dr. Kathy Missildine, Associate Dean, STEM/Director of Nursing, Nursing Department, Texas A&M University–Texarkana, 7101 University Boulevard, Texarkana, TX 75503. *Telephone:* 903-2233177. *Fax:* 903-223-3107. *E-mail:* kmissildine@tamut.edu.

GRADUATE PROGRAMS

Expenses (2015–16) *Tuition, area resident:* full-time $7072; part-time $294 per credit hour. *Tuition, state resident:* full-time $7848; part-time $327 per credit hour. *Tuition, nonresident:* full-time $17,000; part-time $719 per credit hour. *International tuition:* $17,000 full-time.
Contact Dr. Kathy Missildine, Associate Dean, STEM/Director of Nursing, Nursing Department, Texas A&M University–Texarkana, 7107 University Boulevard, Texarkana, TX 75503. *Telephone:* 903-223-3177. *E-mail:* kmissildine@tamut.edu.

MASTER'S DEGREE PROGRAM
Degree MSN
Available Programs Master's.
Concentrations Available Nursing administration.
Study Options Full-time and part-time.
Online Degree Options Yes (online only).
Program Entrance Requirements Minimum overall college GPA of 3.0, transcript of college record, CPR certification, written essay, immunizations, 2 letters of recommendation, professional liability insurance/malpractice insurance, resume. *Application deadline:* 7/15 (fall).
Degree Requirements 36 total credit hours, thesis or project.

Texas Christian University

Harris College of Nursing
Fort Worth, Texas

http://www.nursing.tcu.edu/
Founded in 1873

DEGREES • BSN • DNP • MSN
Nursing Program Faculty 60 (62% with doctorates).
Baccalaureate Enrollment 768 **Women** 92% **Men** 8%
Graduate Enrollment 276 **Women** 74% **Men** 26% **Part-time** 6%
Distance Learning Courses Available.
Nursing Student Activities Sigma Theta Tau, Student Nurses' Association.
Nursing Student Resources Academic advising; academic or career counseling; assistance for students with disabilities; bookstore; campus computer network; career placement assistance; computer lab; computer-assisted instruction; e-mail services; employment services for current students; externships; interactive nursing skills videos; Internet; learning resource lab; library services; nursing audiovisuals; other; placement services for program completers; remedial services; resume preparation assistance; skills, simulation, or other laboratory; tutoring; unpaid internships.
Library Facilities 27,670 volumes in health, 2,777 volumes in nursing; 249 periodical subscriptions health-care related.

BACCALAUREATE PROGRAMS

Degree BSN
Available Programs Accelerated Baccalaureate; Accelerated Baccalaureate for Second Degree; Generic Baccalaureate.
Study Options Full-time and part-time.
Program Entrance Requirements Minimum overall college GPA of 2.5, transcript of college record, CPR certification, written essay, health insurance, high school foreign language, 2 years high school math, 4 years high school science, high school transcript, immunizations, minimum high school GPA of 3.0, minimum GPA in nursing prerequisites of 2.5, prerequisite course work. Transfer students are accepted. *Application deadline:* 2/1 (fall), 10/1 (spring). *Application fee:* $40.
Advanced Placement Credit by examination available. Credit given for nursing courses completed elsewhere dependent upon specific evaluations.
Expenses (2015–16) *Tuition:* full-time $40,630; part-time $1715 per contact hour. *Room and board:* $11,800; room only: $7100 per academic year. *Required fees:* full-time $1107.
Financial Aid *Gift aid (need-based):* Federal Pell, FSEOG, state, private, college/university gift aid from institutional funds. *Loans:* Federal Nursing Student Loans, Federal Direct (Subsidized and Unsubsidized Stafford PLUS), Perkins, state. *Work-study:* Federal Work-Study, part-time campus jobs. *Financial aid application deadline:* 5/1.
Contact Mrs. Marinda Allender, Director, Undergraduate Nursing Studies, Harris College of Nursing, Texas Christian University, TCU Box 298620, Fort Worth, TX 76129. *Telephone:* 817-257-6743. *Fax:* 817-257-7944. *E-mail:* s.lockwood@tcu.edu.

GRADUATE PROGRAMS

Expenses (2015–16) *Tuition:* part-time $1415 per credit hour.
Contact Ms. Mary Jane Allred, Administrative Program Specialist, Harris College of Nursing, Texas Christian University, TCU Box 298627, Fort Worth, TX 76129. *Telephone:* 817-257-6726. *Fax:* 817-257-8383. *E-mail:* m.allred@tcu.edu.

MASTER'S DEGREE PROGRAM
Degree MSN
Available Programs Master's.
Concentrations Available Clinical nurse leader; nursing education. *Clinical nurse specialist programs in:* adult health, gerontology, pediatric.
Study Options Full-time and part-time.
Online Degree Options Yes (online only).
Program Entrance Requirements Clinical experience, computer literacy, minimum overall college GPA of 3.0, transcript of college record, CPR certification, written essay, immunizations, 3 letters of recommendation, prerequisite course work, resume. *Application deadline:* 4/1 (fall), 9/1 (spring), 2/1 (summer). Applications may be processed on a rolling basis for some programs. *Application fee:* $60.
Advanced Placement Credit given for nursing courses completed elsewhere dependent upon specific evaluations.
Degree Requirements 40 total credit hours, thesis or project.

POST-MASTER'S PROGRAM

Areas of Study Clinical nurse leader; nursing education. *Clinical nurse specialist programs in:* adult health, gerontology, pediatric.

DOCTORAL DEGREE PROGRAM

Degree DNP
Available Programs Doctorate.
Areas of Study Advanced practice nursing, nursing administration.
Online Degree Options Yes (online only).
Program Entrance Requirements Clinical experience, minimum overall college GPA of 3.0, interview by faculty committee, 3 letters of recommendation, MSN or equivalent, vita, writing sample. Application deadline: 11/15 (summer). Application fee: $60.
Degree Requirements 30 total credit hours, oral exam.

Degree DNP
Available Programs Doctorate.
Areas of Study Advanced practice nursing.
Program Entrance Requirements Minimum overall college GPA of 3.0, clinical experience, interview by faculty committee, 3 letters of recommendation, writing sample, vita. Application deadline: 7/1 (summer). Application fee: $60.
Degree Requirements 80-86 total credit hours, written exam.

CONTINUING EDUCATION PROGRAM

Contact Mrs. Laura Thielke, Primary Nurse Planner, Harris College of Nursing, Texas Christian University, TCU Box 298620, Fort Worth, TX 76129. *Telephone:* 817-257-5457. *Fax:* 817-257-7944. *E-mail:* l.thielke@tcu.edu.

Texas State University

St. David's School of Nursing
San Marcos, Texas

http://www.nursing.txstate.edu
Founded in 1899
DEGREES • BSN • MSN
Nursing Program Faculty 36 (25% with doctorates).
Baccalaureate Enrollment 183 **Women** 87% **Men** 13% **Part-time** .5%
Graduate Enrollment 71 **Women** 89% **Men** 11% **Part-time** 1%
Distance Learning Courses Available.
Nursing Student Activities Nursing Honor Society, Student Nurses' Association, nursing club.
Nursing Student Resources Academic advising; academic or career counseling; assistance for students with disabilities; bookstore; campus computer network; computer lab; computer-assisted instruction; e-mail services; interactive nursing skills videos; Internet; library services; nursing audiovisuals; remedial services; resume preparation assistance; skills, simulation, or other laboratory; tutoring.
Library Facilities 39,615 volumes in health, 917 volumes in nursing; 11,734 periodical subscriptions health-care related.

BACCALAUREATE PROGRAMS

Degree BSN
Available Programs Generic Baccalaureate.
Site Options Round Rock, TX.
Study Options Full-time.
Program Entrance Requirements Minimum overall college GPA of 2.9, transcript of college record, CPR certification, written essay, health exam, health insurance, high school foreign language, immunizations, 2 letters of recommendation, minimum GPA in nursing prerequisites of 3.0, professional liability insurance/malpractice insurance, prerequisite course work. *Application deadline:* 1/15 (fall). *Application fee:* $25.
Expenses (2015–16) *Tuition, state resident:* full-time $12,200. *Tuition, nonresident:* full-time $26,240. *International tuition:* $26,240 full-time. *Required fees:* full-time $2500.
Financial Aid 90% of baccalaureate students in nursing programs received some form of financial aid in 2014–15. *Gift aid (need-based):* Federal Pell, FSEOG, state, private, college/university gift aid from institutional funds. *Loans:* Federal Direct (Subsidized and Unsubsidized Stafford PLUS), Perkins, state, college/university, short-term emergency loans. *Work-study:* Federal Work-Study, part-time campus jobs. *Financial aid application deadline (priority):* 4/1.
Contact Ms. Lynn Heimerl, Admissions and Retention Coordinator, St. David's School of Nursing, Texas State University, 1555 University

Drive, Round Rock, TX 78665. *Telephone:* 512-716-2900. *Fax:* 512-716-2949. *E-mail:* lh46@txstate.edu.

GRADUATE PROGRAMS

Expenses (2015–16) *Tuition, state resident:* full-time $19,068. *Tuition, nonresident:* full-time $29,960. *International tuition:* $29,960 full-time. *Required fees:* full-time $4200.
Financial Aid 50% of graduate students in nursing programs received some form of financial aid in 2014–15.
Contact Dr. Shirley A. Levenson, School of Nursing, St. David's School of Nursing, Texas State University, 1555 University Drive, Round Rock, TX 78665. *Telephone:* 512-716-2900. *Fax:* 512-716-2911. *E-mail:* sal11@txstate.edu.

MASTER'S DEGREE PROGRAM

Degree MSN
Available Programs Master's.
Concentrations Available *Nurse practitioner programs in:* family health.
Site Options Round Rock, TX.
Study Options Full-time.
Online Degree Options Yes (online only).
Program Entrance Requirements Clinical experience, computer literacy, minimum overall college GPA of 3.0, transcript of college record, CPR certification, written essay, immunizations, 3 letters of recommendation, nursing research course, professional liability insurance/malpractice insurance, resume, statistics course. *Application deadline:* 4/1 (fall). *Application fee:* $40.
Advanced Placement Credit given for nursing courses completed elsewhere dependent upon specific evaluations.
Degree Requirements 48 total credit hours, thesis or project.

Texas Tech University Health Sciences Center

School of Nursing
Lubbock, Texas

http://www.ttuhsc.edu/son
Founded in 1969
DEGREES • BSN • DNP • MSN
Nursing Program Faculty 159 (48% with doctorates).
Baccalaureate Enrollment 1,029 **Women** 88% **Men** 12% **Part-time** 13.2%
Graduate Enrollment 600 **Women** 81.5% **Men** 18.5% **Part-time** 89.5%
Distance Learning Courses Available.
Nursing Student Activities Sigma Theta Tau, Student Nurses' Association.
Nursing Student Resources Academic advising; academic or career counseling; assistance for students with disabilities; bookstore; campus computer network; career placement assistance; computer lab; computer-assisted instruction; e-mail services; Internet; learning resource lab; library services; nursing audiovisuals; other; resume preparation assistance; skills, simulation, or other laboratory; tutoring.
Library Facilities 320,818 volumes in health, 6,583 volumes in nursing; 28,960 periodical subscriptions health-care related.

BACCALAUREATE PROGRAMS

Degree BSN
Available Programs ADN to Baccalaureate; Accelerated Baccalaureate for Second Degree; Generic Baccalaureate; RN Baccalaureate.
Site Options Odessa, TX; Abilene, TX.
Study Options Full-time.
Online Degree Options Yes (online only).
Program Entrance Requirements Transcript of college record, CPR certification, immunizations, interview, minimum GPA in nursing prerequisites of 3.0, prerequisite course work. *Application deadline:* 1/15 (fall), 8/31 (spring), 1/15 (summer). *Application fee:* $40.
Advanced Placement Credit given for nursing courses completed elsewhere dependent upon specific evaluations.
Expenses (2015–16) *Tuition, state resident:* full-time $2805; part-time $187 per credit hour. *Tuition, nonresident:* full-time $8655; part-time $577 per credit hour. *Required fees:* full-time $1471; part-time $1471 per term.

Financial Aid 65% of baccalaureate students in nursing programs received some form of financial aid in 2014–15.

Contact Ms. Elizabeth Martinez, Unit Coordinator, School of Nursing, Texas Tech University Health Sciences Center, 3601 4th Street, MS 6264, Lubbock, TX 79430. *Telephone:* 806-743-9234. *Fax:* 806-743-1648. *E-mail:* elizabeth.martinez@ttuhsc.edu.

GRADUATE PROGRAMS

Expenses (2015–16) *Tuition, state resident:* full-time $2133; part-time $237 per credit hour. *Tuition, nonresident:* full-time $5643; part-time $627 per credit hour. *Required fees:* full-time $947; part-time $947 per term.

Financial Aid 51% of graduate students in nursing programs received some form of financial aid in 2014–15. Institutionally sponsored loans, scholarships, and traineeships available. Aid available to part-time students. *Financial aid application deadline:* 12/1.

Contact Ms. Georgina Barrera, MSN Student Affairs Coordinator, School of Nursing, Texas Tech University Health Sciences Center, 3601 4th Street, MS 6264, Lubbock, TX 79430. *Telephone:* 806-743-2762. *Fax:* 806-743-2324. *E-mail:* georgina.barrera@ttuhsc.edu.

MASTER'S DEGREE PROGRAM

Degree MSN

Available Programs Master's.

Concentrations Available Nurse-midwifery; nursing administration; nursing education; nursing informatics. *Nurse practitioner programs in:* acute care, adult-gerontology acute care, family health, pediatric primary care, primary care.

Study Options Part-time.

Online Degree Options Yes (online only).

Program Entrance Requirements Clinical experience, computer literacy, minimum overall college GPA of 3.0, transcript of college record, CPR certification, written essay, immunizations, 3 letters of recommendation, resume. *Application deadline:* 2/15 (fall), 8/1 (spring). *Application fee:* $40.

Advanced Placement Credit given for nursing courses completed elsewhere dependent upon specific evaluations.

Degree Requirements 48 total credit hours.

POST-MASTER'S PROGRAM

Areas of Study Nurse-midwifery; nursing education; nursing informatics. *Nurse practitioner programs in:* acute care, adult-gerontology acute care, family health, pediatric primary care, primary care.

DOCTORAL DEGREE PROGRAM

Degree DNP

Available Programs Doctorate.

Areas of Study Advanced practice nursing, nurse executive.

Program Entrance Requirements Clinical experience, minimum overall college GPA of 3.0, interview by faculty committee, interview, 3 letters of recommendation, MSN or equivalent, statistics course, vita, writing sample. Application deadline: 1/15 (summer). Application fee: $40.

Degree Requirements 45 total credit hours.

Texas Tech University Health Sciences Center El Paso

Texas Tech University Health Sciences Center El Paso
El Paso, Texas

DEGREE • BSN

Nursing Program Faculty 14 (57% with doctorates).

Baccalaureate Enrollment 137 **Women** 82% **Men** 18% **Part-time** 6%

Distance Learning Courses Available.

Nursing Student Activities Student Nurses' Association, nursing club.

Nursing Student Resources Academic advising; academic or career counseling; assistance for students with disabilities; campus computer network; computer lab; computer-assisted instruction; e-mail services; interactive nursing skills videos; Internet; learning resource lab; library services; nursing audiovisuals; remedial services; skills, simulation, or other laboratory; tutoring.

Library Facilities 50,000 volumes in health, 1,000 volumes in nursing; 26,000 periodical subscriptions health-care related.

BACCALAUREATE PROGRAMS

Degree BSN

Available Programs ADN to Baccalaureate; Accelerated Baccalaureate.

Study Options Full-time and part-time.

Online Degree Options Yes.

Program Entrance Requirements Minimum overall college GPA of 2.5, transcript of college record, written essay, interview, minimum GPA in nursing prerequisites of 2.5, prerequisite course work. Transfer students are accepted. *Application deadline:* 2/1 (fall), 8/15 (spring), 4/1 (summer). *Application fee:* $40.

Advanced Placement Credit by examination available.

Expenses (2015–16) *Tuition, state resident:* full-time $9537. *Tuition, nonresident:* full-time $29,427. *Required fees:* full-time $6402.

Financial Aid 98% of baccalaureate students in nursing programs received some form of financial aid in 2014–15.

Contact Jeanne Novotny, PhD, RN, FAAN, Founding Dean and Professor, Texas Tech University Health Sciences Center El Paso, 210 North Concepcion, El Paso, TX 79905. *Telephone:* 915-215-6124. *E-mail:* jeanne.novotny@ttuhsc.edu.

Texas Woman's University
College of Nursing
Denton, Texas

http://www.twu.edu/nursing
Founded in 1901

DEGREES • BS • MS • MS/MHA • PHD

Nursing Program Faculty 238 (37% with doctorates).

Baccalaureate Enrollment 1,013 **Women** 90% **Men** 10%

Graduate Enrollment 918 **Women** 93% **Men** 7%

Distance Learning Courses Available.

Nursing Student Activities Nursing Honor Society, Sigma Theta Tau, Student Nurses' Association, nursing club.

Nursing Student Resources Academic advising; academic or career counseling; assistance for students with disabilities; bookstore; campus computer network; career placement assistance; computer lab; computer-assisted instruction; e-mail services; employment services for current students; interactive nursing skills videos; Internet; learning resource lab; library services; nursing audiovisuals; placement services for program completers; remedial services; resume preparation assistance; skills, simulation, or other laboratory; tutoring; unpaid internships.

Library Facilities 250,000 volumes in health, 26,463 volumes in nursing; 2,644 periodical subscriptions health-care related.

BACCALAUREATE PROGRAMS

Degree BS

Available Programs Baccalaureate for Second Degree; Generic Baccalaureate; RN Baccalaureate.

Site Options Dallas, TX; Houston, TX.

Study Options Full-time and part-time.

Online Degree Options Yes.

Program Entrance Requirements Transcript of college record, CPR certification, high school transcript, immunizations, minimum GPA in nursing prerequisites of 3.0, professional liability insurance/malpractice insurance, prerequisite course work. Transfer students are accepted. *Application deadline:* 2/1 (fall), 9/1 (spring). *Application fee:* $30.

Advanced Placement Credit given for nursing courses completed elsewhere dependent upon specific evaluations.

Contact Heather Close, Nursing Admissions Coordinator, College of Nursing, Texas Woman's University, PO Box 425498, Denton, TX 76204. *Telephone:* 940-898-2401. *Fax:* 940-898-2437. *E-mail:* nursing@twu.edu.

GRADUATE PROGRAMS

Financial Aid 10 research assistantships (averaging $5,600 per year), 1 teaching assistantship (averaging $5,600 per year) were awarded; career-related internships or fieldwork, Federal Work-Study, institutionally sponsored loans, scholarships, traineeships, and unspecified assistantships also available.

Contact Dr. Ruth Johnson, Associate Dean of the Graduate School, College of Nursing, Texas Woman's University, PO Box 425649, Denton, TX 76204. *Telephone:* 940-898-3415. *E-mail:* rjohnson@twu.edu.

MASTER'S DEGREE PROGRAM

Degrees MS; MS/MHA

Available Programs Master's; RN to Master's.

Concentrations Available Clinical nurse leader; health-care administration; nursing administration; nursing education. *Nurse practitioner programs in:* adult health, adult-gerontology acute care, family health, pediatric, women's health.
Site Options Dallas, TX; Houston, TX.
Study Options Full-time and part-time.
Online Degree Options Yes.
Program Entrance Requirements Clinical experience, minimum overall college GPA of 3.0, transcript of college record, CPR certification, immunizations, professional liability insurance/malpractice insurance, statistics course, GRE or MAT. *Application deadline:* 2/1 (fall), 9/1 (spring).
Advanced Placement Credit given for nursing courses completed elsewhere dependent upon specific evaluations.
Degree Requirements 48 total credit hours, thesis or project.

POST-MASTER'S PROGRAM

Areas of Study *Nurse practitioner programs in:* adult health, adult-gerontology acute care, family health, pediatric, women's health.

DOCTORAL DEGREE PROGRAM

Degree PhD
Available Programs Doctorate.
Areas of Study Nursing research, nursing science, women's health.
Site Options Dallas, TX; Houston, TX.
Online Degree Options Yes.
Program Entrance Requirements Minimum overall college GPA of 3.5, 2 letters of recommendation, MSN or equivalent, statistics course, vita, GRE (preferred minimum score 153 [500 old version] Verbal, 144 [500 old version] Quantitative, 4 Analytical).
Degree Requirements 60 total credit hours, dissertation, oral exam, written exam.

University of Houston

School of Nursing
Houston, Texas

http://www.uh.edu/nursing
Founded in 1927
DEGREES • BSN • MSN

BACCALAUREATE PROGRAMS

Degree BSN
Available Programs Accelerated Baccalaureate for Second Degree; RN Baccalaureate.
Contact *Telephone:* 361-570-4848.

GRADUATE PROGRAMS

Contact *Telephone:* 361-570-4848.

MASTER'S DEGREE PROGRAM

Degree MSN
Available Programs Master's; RN to Master's.
Concentrations Available Nursing administration; nursing education.
Program Entrance Requirements GRE or MAT.

University of Mary Hardin-Baylor

College of Nursing
Belton, Texas

http://www.umhb.edu/
Founded in 1845
DEGREES • BSN • MSN
Nursing Program Faculty 66 (19% with doctorates).
Baccalaureate Enrollment 502 **Women** 90% **Men** 10%
Graduate Enrollment 42 **Women** 97% **Men** 3% **Part-time** 4%
Distance Learning Courses Available.
Nursing Student Activities Nursing Honor Society, Sigma Theta Tau, Student Nurses' Association.
Nursing Student Resources Academic advising; academic or career counseling; assistance for students with disabilities; bookstore; campus computer network; career placement assistance; computer lab; e-mail services; employment services for current students; housing assistance;

Internet; learning resource lab; library services; nursing audiovisuals; placement services for program completers; remedial services; resume preparation assistance; skills, simulation, or other laboratory; tutoring.
Library Facilities 8,116 volumes in health, 6,339 volumes in nursing; 145 periodical subscriptions health-care related.

BACCALAUREATE PROGRAMS

Degree BSN
Available Programs ADN to Baccalaureate; Generic Baccalaureate.
Study Options Full-time and part-time.
Program Entrance Requirements Minimum overall college GPA of 3.0, transcript of college record, CPR certification, written essay, health exam, health insurance, high school transcript, immunizations, minimum GPA in nursing prerequisites of 3.0, prerequisite course work. Transfer students are accepted. *Application deadline:* 3/1 (fall), 10/1 (spring). Applications may be processed on a rolling basis for some programs.
Advanced Placement Credit given for nursing courses completed elsewhere dependent upon specific evaluations.
Expenses (2015–16) *Tuition:* full-time $23,850; part-time $795 per credit hour. *International tuition:* $23,850 full-time. *Room and board:* $6920; room only: $5020 per academic year. *Required fees:* full-time $3750.
Financial Aid 95% of baccalaureate students in nursing programs received some form of financial aid in 2014–15. *Gift aid (need-based):* Federal Pell, FSEOG, state, private, college/university gift aid from institutional funds. *Loans:* Federal Direct (Subsidized and Unsubsidized Stafford PLUS), Perkins, state. *Work-study:* Federal Work-Study, part-time campus jobs. *Financial aid application deadline (priority):* 3/1.
Contact Dr. Sharon Souter, Dean and Professor, College of Nursing, University of Mary Hardin-Baylor, Box 8015, 900 College Street, Belton, TX 76513-2599. *Telephone:* 254-295-4665. *Fax:* 254-295-4141. *E-mail:* lpehl@umhb.edu.

GRADUATE PROGRAMS

Expenses (2015–16) *Tuition:* full-time $14,670; part-time $815 per credit hour. *International tuition:* $14,670 full-time. *Required fees:* full-time $2250.
Financial Aid 30% of graduate students in nursing programs received some form of financial aid in 2014–15.
Contact Dr. Carrie Johnson, Director and Associate Professor, College of Nursing, University of Mary Hardin-Baylor, Box 8015, 900 College Street, Belton, TX 76513-2599. *Telephone:* 254-295-4178. *Fax:* 254-295-4141. *E-mail:* cjohnson@umhb.edu.

MASTER'S DEGREE PROGRAM

Degree MSN
Available Programs Master's.
Concentrations Available Clinical nurse leader; nursing education. *Nurse practitioner programs in:* family health.
Study Options Full-time and part-time.
Program Entrance Requirements Clinical experience, computer literacy, minimum overall college GPA of 3.0, transcript of college record, CPR certification, written essay, immunizations, interview, 2 letters of recommendation, nursing research course, physical assessment course, professional liability insurance/malpractice insurance, prerequisite course work, statistics course. *Application deadline:* 4/1 (fall). Applications may be processed on a rolling basis for some programs. *Application fee:* $50.
Advanced Placement Credit given for nursing courses completed elsewhere dependent upon specific evaluations.
Degree Requirements 36 total credit hours, comprehensive exam.

POST-MASTER'S PROGRAM

Areas of Study Clinical nurse leader; nursing education. *Nurse practitioner programs in:* family health.

University of St. Thomas

Carol and Odis Peavy School of Nursing
Houston, Texas

http://www.stthom.edu/Home/Index.aqf
Founded in 1947
DEGREE • BSN

BACCALAUREATE PROGRAMS

Degree BSN
Available Programs RN Baccalaureate.

Contact Poldi Tschirch, Dean and Professor, Carol and Odis Peavy School of Nursing, University of St. Thomas, 3812 Montrose Boulevard, Houston, TX 77006. *Telephone:* 713-525-6991. *E-mail:* tschirp@stthom.edu.

The University of Texas at Arlington
College of Nursing
Arlington, Texas

http://www.uta.edu/nursing
Founded in 1895
DEGREES • BSN • MSN • MSN/MBA • MSN/MHA • MSN/MPH • PHD
Nursing Program Faculty 145 (31% with doctorates).
Baccalaureate Enrollment 12,717 **Women** 82% **Men** 18% **Part-time** 70%
Graduate Enrollment 2,190 **Women** 87% **Men** 13% **Part-time** 93%
Distance Learning Courses Available.
Nursing Student Activities Nursing Honor Society, Sigma Theta Tau, Student Nurses' Association, nursing club.
Nursing Student Resources Academic advising; academic or career counseling; assistance for students with disabilities; bookstore; campus computer network; career placement assistance; computer lab; computer-assisted instruction; e-mail services; interactive nursing skills videos; Internet; learning resource lab; library services; nursing audiovisuals; remedial services; resume preparation assistance; skills, simulation, or other laboratory; tutoring.
Library Facilities 36,000 volumes in health, 23,300 volumes in nursing; 530 periodical subscriptions health-care related.

BACCALAUREATE PROGRAMS

Degree BSN
Available Programs ADN to Baccalaureate; Accelerated Baccalaureate; Accelerated Baccalaureate for Second Degree; Accelerated RN Baccalaureate; Baccalaureate for Second Degree; Generic Baccalaureate; RN Baccalaureate.
Study Options Full-time and part-time.
Online Degree Options Yes.
Program Entrance Requirements Minimum overall college GPA of 2.5, transcript of college record, CPR certification, health insurance, immunizations, minimum high school GPA of 2.5, minimum GPA in nursing prerequisites of 2.5, professional liability insurance/malpractice insurance, prerequisite course work. Transfer students are accepted. *Application deadline:* 1/5 (fall), 6/1 (spring). *Application fee:* $60.
Advanced Placement Credit given for nursing courses completed elsewhere dependent upon specific evaluations.
Expenses (2015–16) *Tuition, state resident:* full-time $8878; part-time $1004 per unit. *Tuition, nonresident:* full-time $18,774; part-time $1455 per unit. *International tuition:* $18,774 full-time. *Room and board:* $8970; room only: $4428 per academic year. *Required fees:* full-time $528; part-time $22 per credit.
Financial Aid 54% of baccalaureate students in nursing programs received some form of financial aid in 2014–15. *Gift aid (need-based):* Federal Pell, FSEOG, state, private, college/university gift aid from institutional funds, United Negro College Fund. *Loans:* Federal Direct (Subsidized and Unsubsidized Stafford PLUS), Perkins, state. *Work-study:* Federal Work-Study, part-time campus jobs. *Financial aid application deadline (priority):* 4/15.
Contact Dr. Ceil Flores, Assistant Dean, Office of Enrollment and Student Services, College of Nursing, The University of Texas at Arlington, 411 South Nedderman Drive, Box 19407, Arlington, TX 76019-0407. *Telephone:* 817-272-2776. *Fax:* 817-272-5006. *E-mail:* nursing@uta.edu.

GRADUATE PROGRAMS

Expenses (2015–16) *Tuition, state resident:* full-time $10,200; part-time $1300 per unit. *Tuition, nonresident:* full-time $15,757; part-time $1809 per unit. *International tuition:* $15,757 full-time. *Room and board:* $8970; room only: $4428 per academic year. *Required fees:* full-time $1728; part-time $96 per credit.
Financial Aid 60% of graduate students in nursing programs received some form of financial aid in 2014–15. 22 fellowships with partial tuition reimbursements available (averaging $4,473 per year), 6 research assistantships (averaging $8,873 per year), 24 teaching assistantships (aver-

aging $6,202 per year) were awarded; career-related internships or fieldwork, scholarships, and traineeships also available. *Financial aid application deadline:* 6/1.
Contact Dr. Judy Leflore, Professor, College of Nursing, The University of Texas at Arlington, 411 South Nedderman Drive, Box 19407, Arlington, TX 76019-0407. *Telephone:* 214-213-6645. *E-mail:* jleflore@uta.edu.

MASTER'S DEGREE PROGRAM
Degrees MSN; MSN/MBA; MSN/MHA; MSN/MPH
Available Programs Master's.
Concentrations Available Health-care administration; nursing administration; nursing education. *Nurse practitioner programs in:* acute care, adult health, family health, gerontology, neonatal health, pediatric, psychiatric/mental health.
Site Options Fort Worth, TX; Dallas, TX.
Study Options Full-time and part-time.
Online Degree Options Yes.
Program Entrance Requirements Clinical experience, minimum overall college GPA of 3.0, transcript of college record, CPR certification, written essay, immunizations, statistics course, GRE General Test if GPA less than 3.0. *Application deadline:* 6/1 (fall), 10/15 (spring). *Application fee:* $70.
Advanced Placement Credit given for nursing courses completed elsewhere dependent upon specific evaluations.
Degree Requirements 48 total credit hours, thesis or project, comprehensive exam.

POST-MASTER'S PROGRAM
Areas of Study *Nurse practitioner programs in:* acute care, adult health, family health, gerontology, neonatal health, pediatric, psychiatric/mental health.

DOCTORAL DEGREE PROGRAM
Degree PhD
Available Programs Doctorate; Post-Baccalaureate Doctorate.
Areas of Study Faculty preparation, nursing education, nursing research.
Program Entrance Requirements Clinical experience, minimum overall college GPA of 3.0, interview by faculty committee, interview, 3 letters of recommendation, statistics course, GRE General Test (waived for MSN-to-PhD applicants). *Application deadline:* 6/15 (fall), 10/15 (spring). *Application fee:* $70.
Degree Requirements 54 total credit hours, dissertation, residency.

The University of Texas at Austin
School of Nursing
Austin, Texas

http://www.utexas.edu/nursing
Founded in 1883
DEGREES • BSN • MSN • PHD
Nursing Program Faculty 82 (54% with doctorates).
Baccalaureate Enrollment 791 **Women** 90.5% **Men** 9.5% **Part-time** 13%
Graduate Enrollment 300 **Women** 88% **Men** 12% **Part-time** 24%
Distance Learning Courses Available.
Nursing Student Activities Nursing Honor Society, Sigma Theta Tau, Student Nurses' Association, nursing club.
Nursing Student Resources Academic advising; academic or career counseling; assistance for students with disabilities; bookstore; campus computer network; career placement assistance; computer lab; computer-assisted instruction; e-mail services; externships; interactive nursing skills videos; Internet; learning resource lab; library services; nursing audiovisuals; other; remedial services; resume preparation assistance; skills, simulation, or other laboratory; tutoring; unpaid internships.
Library Facilities 100,000 volumes in health, 80,000 volumes in nursing; 504 periodical subscriptions health-care related.

BACCALAUREATE PROGRAMS

Degree BSN
Available Programs Generic Baccalaureate; RN Baccalaureate.
Study Options Full-time.
Program Entrance Requirements Minimum overall college GPA of 2.75, transcript of college record, CPR certification, written essay, 3 years high school math, 2 years high school science, high school transcript, 3 letters of recommendation, minimum GPA in nursing prerequisites of

2.75, professional liability insurance/malpractice insurance, prerequisite course work. Transfer students are accepted. *Application deadline:* 8/1 (fall), 2/15 (spring). *Application fee:* $50.

Advanced Placement Credit by examination available. Credit given for nursing courses completed elsewhere dependent upon specific evaluations.

Expenses (2014–15) *Tuition, state resident:* full-time $10,738; part-time $1558 per credit hour. *Tuition, nonresident:* full-time $30,502; part-time $5615 per credit hour. *International tuition:* $30,502 full-time. *Room and board:* $11,456 per academic year. *Required fees:* full-time $2530.

Financial Aid 54% of baccalaureate students in nursing programs received some form of financial aid in 2013–14. *Gift aid (need-based):* Federal Pell, FSEOG, state, private, college/university gift aid from institutional funds. *Loans:* Federal Direct (Subsidized and Unsubsidized Stafford PLUS), Perkins, state. *Work-study:* Federal Work-Study, part-time campus jobs. *Financial aid application deadline (priority):* 3/31.

Contact Christina Jarvis, Student Affairs Office, School of Nursing, The University of Texas at Austin, 1710 Red River Street, Austin, TX 78701-1412. *Telephone:* 512-232-4780. *Fax:* 512-232-4777. *E-mail:* sar@mail.nur.utexas.edu.

GRADUATE PROGRAMS

Expenses (2014–15) *Tuition, state resident:* full-time $9482; part-time $3461 per semester. *Tuition, nonresident:* full-time $17,250; part-time $5733 per semester. *International tuition:* $17,520 full-time.

Financial Aid 76% of graduate students in nursing programs received some form of financial aid in 2013–14. Fellowships, research assistantships, teaching assistantships, scholarships and traineeships available. *Financial aid application deadline:* 2/1.

Contact Ms. Tracy Demchuk, Assistant Director Graduate Academic Services, School of Nursing, The University of Texas at Austin, 1710 Red River Street, Graduate Student Services, Austin, TX 78701-1499. *Telephone:* 512-471-7927. *Fax:* 512-232-4777. *E-mail:* nugrad@uts.cc.utexas.edu.

MASTER'S DEGREE PROGRAM

Degree MSN

Available Programs Accelerated Master's for Non-Nursing College Graduates; Master's; Master's for Nurses with Non-Nursing Degrees.

Concentrations Available Nursing administration. *Clinical nurse specialist programs in:* adult health. *Nurse practitioner programs in:* family health, pediatric, psychiatric/mental health.

Study Options Full-time and part-time.

Program Entrance Requirements Minimum overall college GPA of 3.0, transcript of college record, written essay, interview, 3 letters of recommendation, prerequisite course work, resume, statistics course, GRE General Test. *Application deadline:* 12/1 (fall), 10/1 (summer). *Application fee:* $65.

Advanced Placement Credit given for nursing courses completed elsewhere dependent upon specific evaluations.

Degree Requirements 39 total credit hours.

POST-MASTER'S PROGRAM

Areas of Study *Clinical nurse specialist programs in:* adult health. *Nurse practitioner programs in:* family health, pediatric, psychiatric/mental health.

DOCTORAL DEGREE PROGRAM

Degree PhD

Available Programs Doctorate; Doctorate for Nurses with Non-Nursing Degrees; Post-Baccalaureate Doctorate.

Areas of Study Addiction/substance abuse, aging, bio-behavioral research, clinical practice, community health, ethics, family health, gerontology, health promotion/disease prevention, health-care systems, human health and illness, illness and transition, individualized study, information systems, maternity-newborn, nursing administration, nursing research, nursing science, oncology, women's health.

Program Entrance Requirements Minimum overall college GPA of 3.0, interview, 3 letters of recommendation, MSN or equivalent, statistics course, vita, writing sample, GRE General Test. Application deadline: 12/1 (fall), 10/1 (summer). Application fee: $65.

Degree Requirements 57 total credit hours, dissertation, oral exam.

POSTDOCTORAL PROGRAM

Postdoctoral Program Contact Dr. Lorraine Walker, Professor, School of Nursing, The University of Texas at Austin, 1700 Red River Street, Austin, TX 78701. *Telephone:* 512-232-4751. *Fax:* 512-232-4777. *E-mail:* lwalker@mail.nur.utexas.edu.

The University of Texas at Brownsville
Department of Nursing
Brownsville, Texas

http://www.utb.edu/vpaa/nursing/pages/default.aspx
Founded in 1973

DEGREES • BSN • MSN
Nursing Program Faculty 13 (62% with doctorates).
Baccalaureate Enrollment 91 **Women** 74% **Men** 26% **Part-time** 82%
Graduate Enrollment 53 **Women** 77% **Men** 23% **Part-time** 47%
Distance Learning Courses Available.
Nursing Student Activities Nursing club.
Nursing Student Resources Academic advising; academic or career counseling; assistance for students with disabilities; bookstore; campus computer network; career placement assistance; computer lab; computer-assisted instruction; daycare for children of students; e-mail services; employment services for current students; housing assistance; interactive nursing skills videos; Internet; learning resource lab; library services; nursing audiovisuals; remedial services; resume preparation assistance; skills, simulation, or other laboratory; tutoring.

BACCALAUREATE PROGRAMS

Degree BSN

Available Programs ADN to Baccalaureate.

Study Options Full-time and part-time.

Online Degree Options Yes (online only).

Program Entrance Requirements Minimum overall college GPA of 2.5, transcript of college record, CPR certification, immunizations, minimum GPA in nursing prerequisites of 2.5, professional liability insurance/malpractice insurance, prerequisite course work, RN licensure. Transfer students are accepted. *Application deadline:* 3/1 (fall), 11/1 (spring).

Advanced Placement Credit by examination available.

Contact *Telephone:* 956-882-5071. *Fax:* 956-882-5100.

GRADUATE PROGRAMS

Contact *Telephone:* 956-882-5079. *Fax:* 956-882-5100.

MASTER'S DEGREE PROGRAM

Degree MSN

Available Programs Master's; Master's for Nurses with Non-Nursing Degrees.

Concentrations Available Nursing administration; nursing education. *Clinical nurse specialist programs in:* public health.

Study Options Full-time and part-time.

Online Degree Options Yes (online only).

Program Entrance Requirements Computer literacy, minimum overall college GPA of 3.0, transcript of college record, CPR certification, written essay, immunizations, interview, professional liability insurance/malpractice insurance, resume, statistics course. *Application deadline:* 4/1 (fall), 10/1 (spring). *Application fee:* $25.

Advanced Placement Credit given for nursing courses completed elsewhere dependent upon specific evaluations.

Degree Requirements 37 total credit hours, thesis or project.

CONTINUING EDUCATION PROGRAM

Contact *Telephone:* 956-882-5084. *Fax:* 956-882-5100.

The University of Texas at El Paso
School of Nursing
El Paso, Texas

http://www.utep.edu/
Founded in 1913

DEGREES • BSN • DNP • MSN
Nursing Program Faculty 79 (27% with doctorates).
Baccalaureate Enrollment 505 **Women** 75% **Men** 25% **Part-time** 5%
Graduate Enrollment 314 **Women** 82% **Men** 18% **Part-time** 10%
Distance Learning Courses Available.
Nursing Student Activities Nursing Honor Society, Sigma Theta Tau, Student Nurses' Association.

Nursing Student Resources Academic advising; academic or career counseling; assistance for students with disabilities; bookstore; campus computer network; career placement assistance; computer lab; computer-assisted instruction; e-mail services; employment services for current students; interactive nursing skills videos; Internet; learning resource lab; library services; nursing audiovisuals; paid internships; remedial services; skills, simulation, or other laboratory; tutoring.

Library Facilities 71,389 volumes in health, 13,043 volumes in nursing; 314 periodical subscriptions health-care related.

BACCALAUREATE PROGRAMS

Degree BSN

Available Programs Accelerated Baccalaureate; Generic Baccalaureate; RN Baccalaureate.

Site Options El Paso, TX.

Study Options Full-time and part-time.

Program Entrance Requirements Minimum overall college GPA of 2.0, transcript of college record, CPR certification, health exam, high school biology, high school math, high school science, high school transcript, immunizations, minimum GPA in nursing prerequisites of 2.5, professional liability insurance/malpractice insurance, prerequisite course work. Transfer students are accepted. *Application deadline:* 2/28 (fall), 9/30 (spring), 2/28 (summer).

Advanced Placement Credit by examination available. Credit given for nursing courses completed elsewhere dependent upon specific evaluations.

Financial Aid 67% of baccalaureate students in nursing programs received some form of financial aid in 2013–14.

Contact Dr. Gloria E. McKee, Assistant Dean, Undergraduate Education, School of Nursing, The University of Texas at El Paso, 500 West University Avenue, El Paso, TX 79968. *Telephone:* 915-747-7246. *Fax:* 915-747-8295. *E-mail:* gmckee@utep.edu.

GRADUATE PROGRAMS

Financial Aid Research assistantships (averaging $18,825 per year), teaching assistantships (averaging $18,000 per year) were awarded; fellowships, institutionally sponsored loans, scholarships, tuition waivers (partial), and unspecified assistantships also available.

Contact Dr. Leslie Robbins, Assistant Dean, Graduate Education, School of Nursing, The University of Texas at El Paso, 500 West University Avenue, El Paso, TX 79968. *Telephone:* 915-747-7227. *Fax:* 915-747-8295. *E-mail:* lhrobbins@utep.edu.

MASTER'S DEGREE PROGRAM

Degree MSN

Available Programs Master's.

Concentrations Available Nursing administration; nursing education. *Nurse practitioner programs in:* adult-gerontology acute care, family health, pediatric primary care.

Site Options El Paso, TX.

Study Options Full-time and part-time.

Online Degree Options Yes (online only).

Program Entrance Requirements Clinical experience, computer literacy, minimum overall college GPA of 3.0, transcript of college record, CPR certification, written essay, immunizations, interview, resume. *Application deadline:* Applications may be processed on a rolling basis for some programs. *Application fee:* $45.

Advanced Placement Credit given for nursing courses completed elsewhere dependent upon specific evaluations.

Degree Requirements 49 total credit hours, comprehensive exam.

POST-MASTER'S PROGRAM

Areas of Study Nursing administration; nursing education. *Nurse practitioner programs in:* adult-gerontology acute care, family health, pediatric primary care.

DOCTORAL DEGREE PROGRAM

Degree DNP

Available Programs Doctorate.

Site Options El Paso, TX.

Program Entrance Requirements Clinical experience, minimum overall college GPA of 3.0, interview by faculty committee, 3 letters of recommendation, MSN or equivalent, vita, GRE. Application deadline: 3/15 (fall). Application fee: $45.

Degree Requirements 45 total credit hours.

The University of Texas at Tyler
Program in Nursing
Tyler, Texas

http://www.uttyler.edu/nursing
Founded in 1971

DEGREES • BSN • MSN • MSN/MBA • PHD

Nursing Program Faculty 65 (25% with doctorates).

Baccalaureate Enrollment 650 **Women** 70% **Men** 30% **Part-time** 15%

Graduate Enrollment 175 **Women** 88% **Men** 12% **Part-time** 88%

Distance Learning Courses Available.

Nursing Student Activities Nursing Honor Society, Sigma Theta Tau, Student Nurses' Association, nursing club.

Nursing Student Resources Academic advising; academic or career counseling; assistance for students with disabilities; bookstore; campus computer network; career placement assistance; computer lab; computer-assisted instruction; e-mail services; employment services for current students; externships; interactive nursing skills videos; Internet; learning resource lab; library services; nursing audiovisuals; resume preparation assistance; skills, simulation, or other laboratory; tutoring.

Library Facilities 11,000 volumes in health, 5,500 volumes in nursing; 150 periodical subscriptions health-care related.

BACCALAUREATE PROGRAMS

Degree BSN

Available Programs ADN to Baccalaureate; Accelerated RN Baccalaureate; Generic Baccalaureate; International Nurse to Baccalaureate; LPN to Baccalaureate; LPN to RN Baccalaureate; RN Baccalaureate.

Site Options Longview, TX; Palestine, TX.

Study Options Full-time and part-time.

Online Degree Options Yes (online only).

Program Entrance Requirements Minimum overall college GPA of 2.75, transcript of college record, CPR certification, immunizations, minimum GPA in nursing prerequisites of 2.75, professional liability insurance/malpractice insurance, prerequisite course work. Transfer students are accepted. *Application deadline:* 2/15 (fall), 9/15 (spring).

Advanced Placement Credit given for nursing courses completed elsewhere dependent upon specific evaluations.

Financial Aid 70% of baccalaureate students in nursing programs received some form of financial aid in 2013–14.

Contact Mrs. Tammie Cooper, Nurse Recruiter/Advising, Program in Nursing, The University of Texas at Tyler, 3900 University Boulevard, Tyler, TX 75799. *Telephone:* 903-565-5534. *Fax:* 903-565-5901. *E-mail:* tcooper@uttyler.edu.

GRADUATE PROGRAMS

Financial Aid 60% of graduate students in nursing programs received some form of financial aid in 2013–14. 1 fellowship (averaging $10,000 per year), 3 research assistantships (averaging $2,200 per year) were awarded; institutionally sponsored loans and scholarships also available. *Financial aid application deadline:* 7/1.

Contact Ms. Christina Chatman, Graduate Advisor, Program in Nursing, The University of Texas at Tyler, 3900 University Boulevard, Tyler, TX 75799. *Telephone:* 903-566-7243. *Fax:* 903-565-5534. *E-mail:* cchatman@uttyler.edu.

MASTER'S DEGREE PROGRAM

Degrees MSN; MSN/MBA

Available Programs Accelerated AD/RN to Master's; Accelerated RN to Master's; Master's; RN to Master's.

Concentrations Available Nursing administration; nursing education. *Nurse practitioner programs in:* family health, pediatric.

Study Options Full-time and part-time.

Online Degree Options Yes (online only).

Program Entrance Requirements Computer literacy, minimum overall college GPA of 3.0, transcript of college record, CPR certification, written essay, immunizations, 4 letters of recommendation, nursing research course, prerequisite course work, resume, statistics course, GRE General Test or MAT, GMAT. *Application deadline:* 3/15 (fall), 10/15 (spring).

Advanced Placement Credit given for nursing courses completed elsewhere dependent upon specific evaluations.

Degree Requirements 36 total credit hours, thesis or project, comprehensive exam.

POST-MASTER'S PROGRAM

Areas of Study Nursing administration; nursing education. *Nurse practitioner programs in:* family health, pediatric.

DOCTORAL DEGREE PROGRAM

Degree PhD
Available Programs Doctorate.
Areas of Study Nursing science.
Program Entrance Requirements Minimum overall college GPA of 3.0, interview by faculty committee, 3 letters of recommendation, MSN or equivalent, scholarly papers, statistics course, vita, writing sample.
Degree Requirements 65 total credit hours, dissertation, written exam.

The University of Texas Health Science Center at Houston

School of Nursing
Houston, Texas

https://nursing.uth.edu/
Founded in 1972

DEGREES • BSN • MSN • MSN/MPH • PHD
Nursing Program Faculty 100 (82% with doctorates).
Baccalaureate Enrollment 597 **Women** 84% **Men** 16% **Part-time** 24%
Graduate Enrollment 576 **Women** 83% **Men** 17% **Part-time** 59%
Distance Learning Courses Available.
Nursing Student Activities Sigma Theta Tau, Student Nurses' Association.
Nursing Student Resources Academic advising; academic or career counseling; assistance for students with disabilities; bookstore; campus computer network; computer lab; computer-assisted instruction; daycare for children of students; e-mail services; employment services for current students; housing assistance; interactive nursing skills videos; Internet; learning resource lab; library services; nursing audiovisuals; skills, simulation, or other laboratory; tutoring.

BACCALAUREATE PROGRAMS

Degree BSN
Available Programs ADN to Baccalaureate; Generic Baccalaureate.
Study Options Full-time.
Program Entrance Requirements Transcript of college record, CPR certification, health exam, immunizations, minimum GPA in nursing prerequisites of 2.75, prerequisite course work. Transfer students are accepted. *Application deadline:* 3/15 (fall), 8/15 (spring), 1/15 (summer). *Application fee:* $60.
Advanced Placement Credit given for nursing courses completed elsewhere dependent upon specific evaluations.
Expenses (2015–16) *Tuition, state resident:* full-time $9120; part-time $190 per credit hour. *Tuition, nonresident:* full-time $37,200; part-time $775 per credit hour. *International tuition:* $37,200 full-time. *Required fees:* full-time $2965; part-time $62 per credit; part-time $988 per term.
Financial Aid 64% of baccalaureate students in nursing programs received some form of financial aid in 2014–15. *Gift aid (need-based):* Federal Pell, FSEOG, state, private, college/university gift aid from institutional funds. *Loans:* Federal Nursing Student Loans, Federal Direct (Subsidized and Unsubsidized Stafford PLUS), Perkins, state, college/university, alternative loans.
Contact Linda S. Brannon, M.Ed., Executive Director, Student Affairs and Admissions, School of Nursing, The University of Texas Health Science Center at Houston, 6901 Bertner Avenue, Suite 216, Houston, TX 77030. *Telephone:* 713-500-2101. *Fax:* 713-500-2107.
E-mail: Linda.S.Brannon@uth.tmc.edu.

GRADUATE PROGRAMS

Expenses (2015–16) *Tuition, state resident:* full-time $7808; part-time $244 per credit hour. *Tuition, nonresident:* full-time $30,272; part-time $946 per credit hour. *International tuition:* $30,272 full-time. *Required fees:* full-time $1905; part-time $60 per credit; part-time $635 per term.
Financial Aid 33% of graduate students in nursing programs received some form of financial aid in 2014–15. Research assistantships with tuition reimbursements available, teaching assistantships with tuition reimbursements available, institutionally sponsored loans, scholarships, traineeships, and tuition waivers available. Aid available to part-time students.
Contact Linda S. Brannon, M.Ed., Executive Director, Student Affairs and Admissions, School of Nursing, The University of Texas Health

Science Center at Houston, 6901 Bertner Avenue, Suite 216, Houston, TX 77030. *Telephone:* 713-500-2101. *Fax:* 713-500-2107.
E-mail: Linda.S.Brannon@uth.tmc.edu.

MASTER'S DEGREE PROGRAM

Degrees MSN; MSN/MPH
Available Programs Master's.
Concentrations Available Nurse anesthesia; nursing administration; nursing education. *Nurse practitioner programs in:* acute care, adult health, family health, gerontology, psychiatric/mental health.
Study Options Full-time and part-time.
Program Entrance Requirements Clinical experience, minimum overall college GPA of 3.0, transcript of college record, CPR certification, immunizations, interview, 3 letters of recommendation, prerequisite course work, resume, statistics course, GRE or MAT. *Application deadline:* 1/1 (fall), 10/15 (spring), 1/1 (summer). Applications may be processed on a rolling basis for some programs. *Application fee:* $60.
Advanced Placement Credit given for nursing courses completed elsewhere dependent upon specific evaluations.
Degree Requirements 41 total credit hours.

POST-MASTER'S PROGRAM

Areas of Study Nursing administration; nursing education. *Nurse practitioner programs in:* acute care, adult health, family health, gerontology, psychiatric/mental health.

DOCTORAL DEGREE PROGRAM

Degree PhD
Available Programs Doctorate.
Areas of Study Addiction/substance abuse, advanced practice nursing, aging, bio-behavioral research, biology of health and illness, clinical practice, clinical research, community health, critical care, ethics, faculty preparation, family health, forensic nursing, gerontology, health policy, health promotion/disease prevention, health-care systems, human health and illness, illness and transition, individualized study, information systems, legal nurse consultant, maternity-newborn, neuro-behavior, nurse case management, nurse executive, nursing administration, nursing education, nursing policy, nursing research, nursing science, oncology, palliative care, urban health, women's health.
Program Entrance Requirements Clinical experience, minimum overall college GPA of 3.0, interview by faculty committee, 3 letters of recommendation, MSN or equivalent, vita, writing sample, GRE. *Application deadline:* 4/1 (fall). *Application fee:* $60.
Degree Requirements 66 total credit hours, dissertation.

CONTINUING EDUCATION PROGRAM

Contact Dr. Vaunette P. Fay, Associate Professor of Clinical Nursing, School of Nursing, The University of Texas Health Science Center at Houston, 6901 Bertner Avenue, Suite 846, Houston, TX 77030. *Telephone:* 713-500-2116. *Fax:* 713-500-2026. *E-mail:* vaunette.p.fay@uth.tmc.edu.

The University of Texas Health Science Center at San Antonio

School of Nursing
San Antonio, Texas

http://www.nursing.uthscsa.edu/
Founded in 1976

DEGREES • BSN • MSN • PHD
Nursing Program Faculty 122 (63% with doctorates).
Baccalaureate Enrollment 558 **Women** 84.59% **Men** 15.41% **Part-time** 2.15%
Graduate Enrollment 258 **Women** 16% **Men** 84% **Part-time** 41%
Distance Learning Courses Available.
Nursing Student Activities Nursing Honor Society, Sigma Theta Tau, Student Nurses' Association, nursing club.
Nursing Student Resources Academic advising; academic or career counseling; assistance for students with disabilities; bookstore; campus computer network; career placement assistance; computer lab; computer-assisted instruction; e-mail services; employment services for current students; housing assistance; interactive nursing skills videos; Internet; learning resource lab; library services; nursing audiovisuals; placement services for program completers; remedial services; resume preparation assistance; skills, simulation, or other laboratory; tutoring.

Library Facilities 4,793 volumes in health, 4,091 volumes in nursing; 4,367 periodical subscriptions health-care related.

BACCALAUREATE PROGRAMS

Degree BSN
Available Programs Accelerated Baccalaureate for Second Degree; Generic Baccalaureate.
Study Options Full-time.
Program Entrance Requirements Minimum overall college GPA of 2.5, transcript of college record, CPR certification, written essay, health insurance, immunizations, minimum GPA in nursing prerequisites of 3.0, professional liability insurance/malpractice insurance, prerequisite course work. Transfer students are accepted. *Application deadline:* 2/1 (fall), 8/1 (spring), 12/15 (summer). *Application fee:* $45.
Advanced Placement Credit given for nursing courses completed elsewhere dependent upon specific evaluations.
Contact *Telephone:* 210-567-5810. *Fax:* 210-567-3813.

GRADUATE PROGRAMS

Contact *Telephone:* 210-567-5810. *Fax:* 210-567-3813.

MASTER'S DEGREE PROGRAM
Degree MSN
Available Programs Master's; RN to Master's.
Concentrations Available Clinical nurse leader; nursing administration; nursing education. *Nurse practitioner programs in:* family health, gerontology, pediatric, psychiatric/mental health.
Study Options Full-time and part-time.
Program Entrance Requirements Computer literacy, minimum overall college GPA of 3.0, transcript of college record, CPR certification, written essay, immunizations, 3 letters of recommendation, professional liability insurance/malpractice insurance, statistics course. *Application deadline:* 2/1 (fall). *Application fee:* $45.
Advanced Placement Credit given for nursing courses completed elsewhere dependent upon specific evaluations.
Degree Requirements 50 total credit hours, thesis or project.

POST-MASTER'S PROGRAM
Areas of Study *Nurse practitioner programs in:* family health, pediatric, psychiatric/mental health.

DOCTORAL DEGREE PROGRAM
Degree PhD
Available Programs Doctorate; Post-Baccalaureate Doctorate.
Areas of Study Nursing research.
Program Entrance Requirements Clinical experience, minimum overall college GPA of 3.0, interview, 3 letters of recommendation, statistics course, vita, writing sample. Application deadline: 2/1 (fall). Application fee: $45.
Degree Requirements 80 total credit hours, dissertation.

CONTINUING EDUCATION PROGRAM

Contact *Telephone:* 210-567-0170. *Fax:* 210-567-5909.

The University of Texas Medical Branch

School of Nursing
Galveston, Texas

http://www.son.utmb.edu/
Founded in 1891
DEGREES • BSN • DNP • MSN
Nursing Program Faculty 60 (59% with doctorates).
Baccalaureate Enrollment 485 **Women** 87% **Men** 13% **Part-time** .5%
Graduate Enrollment 573 **Women** 87% **Men** 13% **Part-time** 71%
Distance Learning Courses Available.
Nursing Student Activities Nursing Honor Society, Sigma Theta Tau, Student Nurses' Association.
Nursing Student Resources Academic advising; academic or career counseling; assistance for students with disabilities; bookstore; campus computer network; career placement assistance; computer lab; computer-assisted instruction; e-mail services; employment services for current students; housing assistance; interactive nursing skills videos; Internet; learning resource lab; library services; nursing audiovisuals; resume preparation assistance; skills, simulation, or other laboratory; tutoring.

Library Facilities 28,598 volumes in health, 8,503 volumes in nursing; 12,438 periodical subscriptions health-care related.

BACCALAUREATE PROGRAMS

Degree BSN
Available Programs Accelerated Baccalaureate for Second Degree; Generic Baccalaureate; RN Baccalaureate.
Study Options Full-time.
Program Entrance Requirements Minimum overall college GPA of 2.75, transcript of college record, CPR certification, written essay, health insurance, high school chemistry, high school foreign language, high school math, immunizations, interview, minimum high school GPA, minimum GPA in nursing prerequisites of 2.75, professional liability insurance/malpractice insurance, prerequisite course work. Transfer students are accepted. *Application deadline:* 1/15 (fall), 6/15 (spring), 5/15 (summer). *Application fee:* $25.
Advanced Placement Credit by examination available. Credit given for nursing courses completed elsewhere dependent upon specific evaluations.
Expenses (2014–15) *Tuition, state resident:* full-time $8622; part-time $192 per credit hour. *Tuition, nonresident:* full-time $24,652; part-time $548 per credit hour. *International tuition:* $24,652 full-time. *Room and board:* $14,424; room only: $10,332 per academic year. *Required fees:* full-time $5197.
Financial Aid 95% of baccalaureate students in nursing programs received some form of financial aid in 2013–14.
Contact Dr. Patricia Richard, Associate Dean for Undergraduate Programs, School of Nursing, The University of Texas Medical Branch, 301 University Boulevard, Galveston, TX 77555-1132. *Telephone:* 409-772-8221. *Fax:* 409-772-5118. *E-mail:* plrichar@utmb.edu.

GRADUATE PROGRAMS

Expenses (2014–15) *Tuition, state resident:* full-time $8681; part-time $235 per credit hour. *Tuition, nonresident:* full-time $21,778; part-time $589 per credit hour. *International tuition:* $21,778 full-time. *Room and board:* $14,424; room only: $10,332 per academic year. *Required fees:* full-time $5664.
Financial Aid 46% of graduate students in nursing programs received some form of financial aid in 2013–14.
Contact Dr. Maureer Wilder, Associate Professor and Master's Program Director, School of Nursing, The University of Texas Medical Branch, 301 University Boulevard, Galveston, TX 77555-1029. *Telephone:* 409-772-8241. *Fax:* 409-772-8323. *E-mail:* mwilder@utmb.edu.

MASTER'S DEGREE PROGRAM
Degree MSN
Available Programs Master's.
Concentrations Available Clinical nurse leader; nursing administration; nursing education. *Nurse practitioner programs in:* family health, gerontology, neonatal health.
Study Options Full-time and part-time.
Online Degree Options Yes (online only).
Program Entrance Requirements Clinical experience, computer literacy, minimum overall college GPA of 3.0, transcript of college record, CPR certification, immunizations, interview, 3 letters of recommendation, professional liability insurance/malpractice insurance, prerequisite course work, statistics course. *Application deadline:* 3/1 (fall). *Application fee:* $60.
Advanced Placement Credit given for nursing courses completed elsewhere dependent upon specific evaluations.
Degree Requirements 46 total credit hours.

POST-MASTER'S PROGRAM
Areas of Study Clinical nurse leader; nursing administration; nursing education. *Nurse practitioner programs in:* family health, gerontology, neonatal health.

DOCTORAL DEGREE PROGRAM
Degree DNP
Available Programs Doctorate; Post-Baccalaureate Doctorate.
Areas of Study Health promotion/disease prevention.
Online Degree Options Yes (online only).
Program Entrance Requirements Clinical experience, minimum overall college GPA of 3.5, interview by faculty committee, interview, 3 letters of recommendation, MSN or equivalent, statistics course, vita, writing sample. Application deadline: 3/1 (fall). Application fee: $50.
Degree Requirements 63 total credit hours, residency.

The University of Texas Rio Grande Valley

School of Nursing
Edinburg, Texas

http://www.utpa.edu/
Founded in 1927

DEGREES • BSN • MSN

Baccalaureate Enrollment 295 **Women** 78% **Men** 22%
Graduate Enrollment 84 **Women** 88% **Men** 12% **Part-time** 75%
Distance Learning Courses Available.
Nursing Student Activities Sigma Theta Tau, Student Nurses' Association.
Nursing Student Resources Academic advising; academic or career counseling; assistance for students with disabilities; bookstore; campus computer network; career placement assistance; computer lab; computer-assisted instruction; daycare for children of students; e-mail services; employment services for current students; housing assistance; interactive nursing skills videos; Internet; learning resource lab; library services; nursing audiovisuals; remedial services; skills, simulation, or other laboratory; tutoring.
Library Facilities 230 volumes in health, 200 volumes in nursing; 300 periodical subscriptions health-care related.

BACCALAUREATE PROGRAMS

Degree BSN

Available Programs ADN to Baccalaureate; Generic Baccalaureate.
Study Options Full-time and part-time.
Online Degree Options Yes.
Program Entrance Requirements Transcript of college record, CPR certification, immunizations, minimum GPA in nursing prerequisites of 2.5, professional liability insurance/malpractice insurance, prerequisite course work. Transfer students are accepted. *Application deadline:* 3/1 (fall).
Contact Dr. Sandy M. Sánchez, BSN Program Coordinator, School of Nursing, The University of Texas Rio Grande Valley, 1201 West University Drive, Edinburg, TX 78539. *Telephone:* 956-665-3491. *Fax:* 956-665-2875. *E-mail:* sandy@utrgv.edu.

GRADUATE PROGRAMS

Financial Aid Scholarships and traineeships available.
Contact Dr. Lilia A. Fuentes, MSN Coordinator, School of Nursing, The University of Texas Rio Grande Valley, 1201 West University Drive, Edinburg, TX 78539. *Telephone:* 956-665-3491. *Fax:* 956-665-2875. *E-mail:* Lafuentes@utrgv.edu.

MASTER'S DEGREE PROGRAM
Degree MSN

Available Programs Master's.
Concentrations Available Nursing administration; nursing education. *Nurse practitioner programs in:* family health.
Study Options Full-time and part-time.
Online Degree Options Yes.
Program Entrance Requirements Minimum overall college GPA of 3.0, transcript of college record, CPR certification, written essay, immunizations, 3 letters of recommendation, resume, statistics course. *Application deadline:* 4/1 (fall). *Application fee:* $50.
Advanced Placement Credit given for nursing courses completed elsewhere dependent upon specific evaluations.
Degree Requirements 48 total credit hours, thesis or project.

POST-MASTER'S PROGRAM
Areas of Study *Nurse practitioner programs in:* family health, psychiatric/mental health.

University of the Incarnate Word

Program in Nursing
San Antonio, Texas

http://www.uiw.edu/snhp
Founded in 1881

DEGREES • BSN • DNP • MSN

Nursing Program Faculty 39 (41% with doctorates).
Baccalaureate Enrollment 251 **Women** 87% **Men** 13%
Graduate Enrollment 66 **Women** 76% **Men** 24% **Part-time** 91%
Distance Learning Courses Available.
Nursing Student Activities Sigma Theta Tau, Student Nurses' Association.
Nursing Student Resources Academic advising; academic or career counseling; assistance for students with disabilities; bookstore; campus computer network; career placement assistance; computer lab; computer-assisted instruction; e-mail services; employment services for current students; externships; housing assistance; interactive nursing skills videos; Internet; learning resource lab; library services; nursing audiovisuals; paid internships; placement services for program completers; remedial services; resume preparation assistance; skills, simulation, or other laboratory; tutoring; unpaid internships.
Library Facilities 6,000 volumes in health, 6,000 volumes in nursing; 3,048 periodical subscriptions health-care related.

BACCALAUREATE PROGRAMS

Degree BSN

Available Programs ADN to Baccalaureate; Baccalaureate for Second Degree; Generic Baccalaureate.
Study Options Full-time.
Online Degree Options Yes.
Program Entrance Requirements Minimum overall college GPA of 2.5, transcript of college record, CPR certification, health exam, health insurance, immunizations, minimum GPA in nursing prerequisites of 2.5, professional liability insurance/malpractice insurance, prerequisite course work. Transfer students are accepted. *Application deadline:* 2/1 (fall), 9/1 (spring). *Application fee:* $20.
Advanced Placement Credit given for nursing courses completed elsewhere dependent upon specific evaluations.
Contact *Telephone:* 210-829-6005.

GRADUATE PROGRAMS

Contact *Telephone:* 210-829-3977. *Fax:* 210-829-3174.

MASTER'S DEGREE PROGRAM
Degree MSN

Available Programs Accelerated AD/RN to Master's; Master's.
Concentrations Available Clinical nurse leader. *Clinical nurse specialist programs in:* adult health.
Study Options Full-time and part-time.
Program Entrance Requirements Clinical experience, minimum overall college GPA of 3.0, transcript of college record, CPR certification, immunizations, 3 letters of recommendation, physical assessment course, professional liability insurance/malpractice insurance, statistics course. *Application deadline:* Applications may be processed on a rolling basis for some programs. *Application fee:* $20.
Advanced Placement Credit given for nursing courses completed elsewhere dependent upon specific evaluations.
Degree Requirements 42 total credit hours.

POST-MASTER'S PROGRAM
Areas of Study Clinical nurse leader. *Clinical nurse specialist programs in:* adult health.

DOCTORAL DEGREE PROGRAM
Degree DNP

Available Programs Doctorate.
Areas of Study Advanced practice nursing.
Online Degree Options Yes (online only).
Program Entrance Requirements Minimum overall college GPA of 3.0, interview, 3 letters of recommendation, MSN or equivalent, statistics course. Application deadline: Applications may be processed on a rolling basis for some programs. Application fee: $20.
Degree Requirements 33 total credit hours.

Wayland Baptist University
Bachelor of Science in Nursing Program
Plainview, Texas

http://www.sa.wbu.edu
Founded in 1908
DEGREE • BSN

BACCALAUREATE PROGRAMS

Degree BSN
Available Programs RN Baccalaureate.
Contact *Telephone:* 210-826-7595 Ext. 228.

West Texas A&M University
Department of Nursing
Canyon, Texas

http://www.wtamu.edu/nursing
Founded in 1909
DEGREES • BSN • MSN
Nursing Program Faculty 30 (23% with doctorates).
Baccalaureate Enrollment 380 **Women** 84% **Men** 16% **Part-time** 35%
Graduate Enrollment 54 **Women** 85% **Men** 15% **Part-time** 52%
Nursing Student Activities Sigma Theta Tau, Student Nurses' Association.
Nursing Student Resources Academic advising; academic or career counseling; assistance for students with disabilities; bookstore; campus computer network; career placement assistance; computer lab; computer-assisted instruction; daycare for children of students; e-mail services; employment services for current students; housing assistance; interactive nursing skills videos; Internet; learning resource lab; library services; nursing audiovisuals; placement services for program completers; remedial services; resume preparation assistance; skills, simulation, or other laboratory; tutoring.
Library Facilities 17,000 volumes in health, 10,000 volumes in nursing; 75 periodical subscriptions health-care related.

BACCALAUREATE PROGRAMS

Degree BSN
Available Programs ADN to Baccalaureate; Generic Baccalaureate; LPN to Baccalaureate.
Study Options Full-time and part-time.
Program Entrance Requirements Minimum overall college GPA of 2.5, transcript of college record, CPR certification, immunizations, minimum GPA in nursing prerequisites of 2.0, prerequisite course work. Transfer students are accepted.
Advanced Placement Credit given for nursing courses completed elsewhere dependent upon specific evaluations.
Contact *Telephone:* 806-651-2661. *Fax:* 806-651-2632.

GRADUATE PROGRAMS

Contact *Telephone:* 806-651-2637. *Fax:* 806-651-2632.

MASTER'S DEGREE PROGRAM
Degree MSN
Available Programs Master's; RN to Master's.
Concentrations Available Nursing administration; nursing education. *Nurse practitioner programs in:* family health.
Study Options Full-time and part-time.
Program Entrance Requirements Clinical experience, computer literacy, minimum overall college GPA of 3.0, transcript of college record, CPR certification, immunizations, nursing research course, prerequisite course work, statistics course, GRE General Test.
Advanced Placement Credit given for nursing courses completed elsewhere dependent upon specific evaluations.
Degree Requirements 39 total credit hours, thesis or project.

POST-MASTER'S PROGRAM
Areas of Study *Nurse practitioner programs in:* family health.

UTAH

Brigham Young University
College of Nursing
Provo, Utah

http://nursing.byu.edu/
Founded in 1875
DEGREES • BS • MS
Nursing Program Faculty 52 (42% with doctorates).
Baccalaureate Enrollment 352 **Women** 90% **Men** 10%
Graduate Enrollment 30 **Women** 74% **Men** 26%
Nursing Student Activities Nursing Honor Society, Sigma Theta Tau, Student Nurses' Association.
Nursing Student Resources Academic advising; academic or career counseling; assistance for students with disabilities; bookstore; campus computer network; career placement assistance; computer lab; computer-assisted instruction; e-mail services; employment services for current students; housing assistance; interactive nursing skills videos; Internet; learning resource lab; library services; nursing audiovisuals; other; paid internships; resume preparation assistance; skills, simulation, or other laboratory; tutoring.
Library Facilities 72,332 volumes in health, 5,217 volumes in nursing; 10,500 periodical subscriptions health-care related.

BACCALAUREATE PROGRAMS

Degree BS
Available Programs RN Baccalaureate.
Study Options Full-time.
Program Entrance Requirements Minimum overall college GPA, transcript of college record, CPR certification, written essay, 2 letters of recommendation, minimum GPA in nursing prerequisites of 3.0, prerequisite course work. Transfer students are accepted. *Application deadline:* 5/31 (fall), 9/30 (winter).
Advanced Placement Credit given for nursing courses completed elsewhere dependent upon specific evaluations.
Expenses (2015–16) *Tuition:* full-time $7725; part-time $270 per credit. *International tuition:* $7725 full-time. *Room and board:* $10,995 per academic year.
Financial Aid 70% of baccalaureate students in nursing programs received some form of financial aid in 2014–15. *Gift aid (need-based):* Federal Pell, private, college/university gift aid from institutional funds. *Loans:* Federal Direct (Subsidized and Unsubsidized Stafford PLUS). *Work-study:* part-time campus jobs. *Financial aid application deadline (priority):* 4/15.
Contact Dr. Mark E. White, Advisement Center Supervisor, College of Nursing, Brigham Young University, 550 SWKT, Provo, UT 84602-5532. *Telephone:* 801-422-7211. *Fax:* 801-422-0536. *E-mail:* mark_white@byu.edu.

GRADUATE PROGRAMS

Expenses (2015–16) *Tuition:* full-time $9750; part-time $382 per credit. *International tuition:* $9750 full-time. *Room and board:* $21,990 per academic year.
Financial Aid 100% of graduate students in nursing programs received some form of financial aid in 2014–15. 2 research assistantships with full and partial tuition reimbursements available (averaging $10,000 per year), 3 teaching assistantships with full and partial tuition reimbursements available (averaging $10,000 per year) were awarded; institutionally sponsored loans, scholarships, tuition waivers (full), and unspecified assistantships also available. Aid available to part-time students. *Financial aid application deadline:* 2/1.
Contact Mrs. Cherie Top, Research Center and Graduate Program Secretary, College of Nursing, Brigham Young University, 400 SWKT, Provo, UT 84602-5532. *Telephone:* 801-422-4142. *Fax:* 801-422-0536. *E-mail:* nursing_graduate@byu.edu.

MASTER'S DEGREE PROGRAM
Degree MS
Available Programs Master's.
Concentrations Available *Nurse practitioner programs in:* family health.
Study Options Full-time.
Program Entrance Requirements Clinical experience, minimum overall college GPA of 3.0, transcript of college record, CPR certification, written essay, immunizations, interview, 3 letters of recommen-

dation, prerequisite course work, resume, statistics course, GRE. *Application deadline:* 12/1 (spring). *Application fee:* $50.
Advanced Placement Credit given for nursing courses completed elsewhere dependent upon specific evaluations.
Degree Requirements 59 total credit hours, thesis or project.

Dixie State University
Nursing Department
St. George, Utah

Founded in 1911
DEGREE • BSN

BACCALAUREATE PROGRAMS

Degree BSN
Available Programs RN Baccalaureate.
Program Entrance Requirements Written essay, immunizations, RN licensure. *Application deadline:* 3/15 (fall), 9/15 (spring).
Contact *Telephone:* 435-879-4802.

Southern Utah University
Department of Nursing
Cedar City, Utah

http://www.suu.edu/cose/nursing/
Founded in 1897
DEGREE • BSN
Nursing Program Faculty 9 (4% with doctorates).
Baccalaureate Enrollment 105 **Women** 70% **Men** 30%
Nursing Student Activities Nursing Honor Society, Student Nurses' Association, nursing club.
Nursing Student Resources Academic advising; academic or career counseling; assistance for students with disabilities; bookstore; campus computer network; career placement assistance; computer lab; computer-assisted instruction; daycare for children of students; e-mail services; employment services for current students; externships; housing assistance; interactive nursing skills videos; Internet; learning resource lab; library services; nursing audiovisuals; remedial services; resume preparation assistance; skills, simulation, or other laboratory; tutoring.
Library Facilities 1,000 volumes in health, 1,000 volumes in nursing; 5,000 periodical subscriptions health-care related.

BACCALAUREATE PROGRAMS

Degree BSN
Available Programs Generic Baccalaureate; RN Baccalaureate.
Study Options Full-time.
Program Entrance Requirements Minimum overall college GPA of 3.0, transcript of college record, written essay, health insurance, immunizations, 3 letters of recommendation, minimum GPA in nursing prerequisites of 3.0, prerequisite course work. Transfer students are accepted. *Application deadline:* 2/13 (fall), 9/11 (spring). *Application fee:* $20.
Advanced Placement Credit given for nursing courses completed elsewhere dependent upon specific evaluations.
Expenses (2015–16) *Tuition, state resident:* full-time $5578. *Tuition, nonresident:* full-time $23,988. *International tuition:* $36,820 full-time. *Required fees:* full-time $800.
Financial Aid 60% of baccalaureate students in nursing programs received some form of financial aid in 2014–15.
Contact Vikki Robertson, Department Secretary, Department of Nursing, Southern Utah University, 351 West University Boulevard, SCA 108A, Cedar City, UT 84720. *Telephone:* 435-586-1906. *Fax:* 435-586-1984. *E-mail:* robertsonv@suu.edu.

University of Phoenix–Utah Campus
College of Health and Human Services
Salt Lake City, Utah

Founded in 1984
Nursing Program Faculty 2

Nursing Student Activities Sigma Theta Tau.
Nursing Student Resources Academic advising; academic or career counseling; assistance for students with disabilities; bookstore; campus computer network; computer lab; computer-assisted instruction; e-mail services; interactive nursing skills videos; Internet; learning resource lab; library services; nursing audiovisuals; remedial services; skills, simulation, or other laboratory; tutoring.
Library Facilities 1,300 periodical subscriptions health-care related.

University of Utah
College of Nursing
Salt Lake City, Utah

http://www.nursing.utah.edu/
Founded in 1850
DEGREES • BS • MS • PHD
Nursing Program Faculty 119 (85% with doctorates).
Baccalaureate Enrollment 245 **Women** 81% **Men** 19% **Part-time** 35%
Graduate Enrollment 348 **Women** 78% **Men** 22% **Part-time** 18%
Distance Learning Courses Available.
Nursing Student Activities Sigma Theta Tau, Student Nurses' Association.
Nursing Student Resources Academic advising; academic or career counseling; assistance for students with disabilities; bookstore; campus computer network; career placement assistance; computer lab; computer-assisted instruction; e-mail services; employment services for current students; interactive nursing skills videos; Internet; learning resource lab; library services; nursing audiovisuals; remedial services; resume preparation assistance; skills, simulation, or other laboratory.
Library Facilities 212,579 volumes in health, 6,603 volumes in nursing; 5,201 periodical subscriptions health-care related.

BACCALAUREATE PROGRAMS

Degree BS
Available Programs ADN to Baccalaureate; Baccalaureate for Second Degree; Generic Baccalaureate; RN Baccalaureate.
Study Options Full-time.
Online Degree Options Yes.
Program Entrance Requirements Minimum overall college GPA of 2.8, transcript of college record, CPR certification, written essay, health exam, immunizations, interview, 3 letters of recommendation, minimum GPA in nursing prerequisites of 3.0, prerequisite course work. Transfer students are accepted. *Application deadline:* 1/15 (fall), 6/10 (spring). *Application fee:* $15.
Expenses (2015–16) *Tuition, state resident:* full-time $9721; part-time $2177 per term. *Tuition, nonresident:* full-time $28,762; part-time $6358 per term. *International tuition:* $28,762 full-time. *Room and board:* $7460; room only: $3853 per academic year. *Required fees:* full-time $1200; part-time $476 per term.
Financial Aid 54% of baccalaureate students in nursing programs received some form of financial aid in 2014–15.
Contact Ms. Jennifer Van Cott, Director, Student Services, College of Nursing, University of Utah, 10 South 2000 East, Salt Lake City, UT 84112-5880. *Telephone:* 801-585-6658. *Fax:* 801-581-3414. *E-mail:* jennifer.vancott@nurs.utah.edu.

GRADUATE PROGRAMS

Expenses (2015–16) *Tuition, state resident:* full-time $16,259. *Tuition, nonresident:* full-time $41,680. *International tuition:* $41,680 full-time. *Room and board:* $7460; room only: $3853 per academic year. *Required fees:* full-time $1022.
Financial Aid 46% of graduate students in nursing programs received some form of financial aid in 2014–15. 77 fellowships with full and partial tuition reimbursements available, 4 research assistantships with full and partial tuition reimbursements available, 9 teaching assistantships with partial tuition reimbursements available were awarded; scholarships, traineeships, and unspecified assistantships also available. Aid available to part-time students. *Financial aid application deadline:* 1/15.
Contact Jennifer Van Cott, Director, Student Services, College of Nursing, University of Utah, 10 South 2000 East, Salt Lake City, UT 84112-5880. *Telephone:* 801-581-2414 Ext. 1. *Fax:* 801-585-9705. *E-mail:* jennifer.vancott@nurs.utah.edu.

MASTER'S DEGREE PROGRAM
Degree MS

Available Programs Master's; Master's for Non-Nursing College Graduates; RN to Master's.
Concentrations Available Nurse case management; nursing education; nursing informatics.
Study Options Full-time and part-time.
Online Degree Options Yes.
Program Entrance Requirements Clinical experience, minimum overall college GPA of 3.0, transcript of college record, CPR certification, written essay, immunizations, interview, 2 letters of recommendation, resume, statistics course, GRE General Test (if cumulative GPA is less than 3.2). *Application deadline:* 1/15 (fall). *Application fee:* $55.
Degree Requirements 38 total credit hours, thesis or project, comprehensive exam.

POST-MASTER'S PROGRAM

Areas of Study Nurse-midwifery; nursing education; nursing informatics. *Nurse practitioner programs in:* acute care, adult-gerontology acute care, family health, gerontology, primary care, women's health.

DOCTORAL DEGREE PROGRAM

Degree PhD
Available Programs Doctorate; Doctorate for Nurses with Non-Nursing Degrees; Post-Baccalaureate Doctorate.
Areas of Study Advanced practice nursing, aging, bio-behavioral research, community health, critical care, ethics, family health, gerontology, health policy, health promotion/disease prevention, health-care systems, human health and illness, illness and transition, individualized study, information systems, nursing education, nursing policy, nursing research, nursing science, oncology, women's health.
Program Entrance Requirements Minimum overall college GPA of 3.3, interview by faculty committee, interview, 3 letters of recommendation, statistics course, vita, writing sample, GRE General Test. Application deadline: 1/15 (fall). Application fee: $55.
Degree Requirements 63 total credit hours, dissertation, oral exam, written exam.

POSTDOCTORAL PROGRAM

Areas of Study Aging, cancer care, chronic illness, community health, gerontology, information systems, nursing informatics, nursing interventions, nursing research, nursing science, women's health.
Postdoctoral Program Contact Dr. Ginette A. Pepper, Associate Dean for Research and PhD Program, College of Nursing, University of Utah, 10 South 2000 East, Salt Lake City, UT 84112-5880. *Telephone:* 801-585-7872. *Fax:* 801-585-9705. *E-mail:* ginny.pepper@nurs.utah.edu.

Utah Valley University
Department of Nursing
Orem, Utah

http://www.uvu.edu/
Founded in 1941
DEGREE • BSN
Nursing Program Faculty 22 (25% with doctorates).
Baccalaureate Enrollment 100 **Women** 60% **Men** 40% **Part-time** 99%
Nursing Student Activities Student Nurses' Association.
Nursing Student Resources Academic advising; academic or career counseling; assistance for students with disabilities; bookstore; campus computer network; career placement assistance; computer lab; computer-assisted instruction; daycare for children of students; e-mail services; employment services for current students; interactive nursing skills videos; Internet; learning resource lab; library services; nursing audiovisuals; resume preparation assistance; skills, simulation, or other laboratory; tutoring; unpaid internships.
Library Facilities 4,640 volumes in health, 361 volumes in nursing; 200 periodical subscriptions health-care related.

BACCALAUREATE PROGRAMS

Degree BSN
Available Programs ADN to Baccalaureate.
Study Options Part-time.
Program Entrance Requirements CPR certification, health exam, health insurance, immunizations, minimum GPA in nursing prerequisites of 2.5, prerequisite course work, RN licensure. Transfer students are accepted.
Advanced Placement Credit by examination available.
Contact *Telephone:* 801-863-8199. *Fax:* 801-863-6093.

Weber State University
Program in Nursing
Ogden, Utah

http://www.weber.edu/nursing
Founded in 1889
DEGREES • BSN • MSN
Nursing Program Faculty 48
Baccalaureate Enrollment 450 **Women** 82% **Men** 18% **Part-time** 10%
Graduate Enrollment 46 **Women** 84% **Men** 16%
Distance Learning Courses Available.
Nursing Student Activities Nursing Honor Society, Sigma Theta Tau, Student Nurses' Association.
Nursing Student Resources Academic advising; academic or career counseling; assistance for students with disabilities; bookstore; campus computer network; career placement assistance; computer lab; computer-assisted instruction; daycare for children of students; e-mail services; employment services for current students; housing assistance; interactive nursing skills videos; Internet; learning resource lab; library services; nursing audiovisuals; placement services for program completers; resume preparation assistance; skills, simulation, or other laboratory; tutoring; unpaid internships.
Library Facilities 800 volumes in health, 800 volumes in nursing; 1,200 periodical subscriptions health-care related.

BACCALAUREATE PROGRAMS

Degree BSN
Available Programs ADN to Baccalaureate.
Site Options Layton, UT.
Study Options Full-time and part-time.
Program Entrance Requirements Minimum overall college GPA of 3.0, transcript of college record, CPR certification, health insurance, minimum GPA in nursing prerequisites of 3.0, prerequisite course work, RN licensure. Transfer students are accepted. *Application deadline:* 3/10 (fall), 10/10 (spring). *Application fee:* $25.
Expenses (2015–16) *Tuition, state resident:* full-time $4456; part-time $370 per credit hour. *Tuition, nonresident:* full-time $13,369; part-time $1114 per credit hour. *International tuition:* $13,369 full-time. *Room and board:* $8638; room only: $4219 per academic year. *Required fees:* full-time $883; part-time $73 per credit; part-time $400 per term.
Financial Aid 50% of baccalaureate students in nursing programs received some form of financial aid in 2014–15. *Gift aid (need-based):* Federal Pell, FSEOG, state, private, college/university gift aid from institutional funds. *Loans:* Federal Direct (Subsidized and Unsubsidized Stafford PLUS), Perkins, college/university. *Work-study:* Federal Work-Study, part-time campus jobs. *Financial aid application deadline (priority):* 3/1.
Contact Ms. Tiffany Bennett, RN to BSN Advisor/Secretary, Program in Nursing, Weber State University, 3875 Stadium Way, Department 3903, Ogden, UT 84408-3903. *Telephone:* 801-626-6122. *Fax:* 801-626-6397. *E-mail:* tiffanybennett@weber.edu.

GRADUATE PROGRAMS

Expenses (2015–16) *Tuition, state resident:* full-time $4901; part-time $408 per credit hour. *Tuition, nonresident:* full-time $4901; part-time $408 per credit hour. *Room and board:* $8638; room only: $4219 per academic year. *Required fees:* part-time $36 per credit; part-time $215 per term.
Financial Aid 20% of graduate students in nursing programs received some form of financial aid in 2014–15.
Contact Mr. Robert W. Holt, Enrollment Director, Program in Nursing, Weber State University, 3903 University Circle, Ogden, UT 84408-3903. *Telephone:* 801-626-7774. *Fax:* 801-626-6397. *E-mail:* rholt@weber.edu.

MASTER'S DEGREE PROGRAM

Degree MSN
Available Programs Master's.
Concentrations Available Nursing administration; nursing education. *Nurse practitioner programs in:* family health.
Study Options Full-time.
Online Degree Options Yes.
Program Entrance Requirements Clinical experience, minimum overall college GPA of 3.0, transcript of college record, CPR certification, written essay, immunizations, interview, 2 letters of recommendation, nursing research course, professional liability insurance/malpractice insurance, prerequisite course work, resume, sta-

tistics course. *Application deadline:* 3/1 (fall), 9/1 (spring). *Application fee:* $100.
Degree Requirements 40 total credit hours, thesis or project.

POST-MASTER'S PROGRAM
Areas of Study Nursing administration; nursing education.

Western Governors University
Online College of Health Professions
Salt Lake City, Utah

Founded in 1998
DEGREES • BS • MS
Baccalaureate Enrollment 3,962
Graduate Enrollment 2,982
Distance Learning Courses Available.
Nursing Student Resources Academic advising; academic or career counseling; assistance for students with disabilities; campus computer network; computer lab; computer-assisted instruction; e-mail services; employment services for current students; interactive nursing skills videos; Internet; learning resource lab; library services; nursing audiovisuals; resume preparation assistance; skills, simulation, or other laboratory; tutoring.

BACCALAUREATE PROGRAMS

Degree BS
Available Programs Accelerated Baccalaureate; Accelerated RN Baccalaureate; Generic Baccalaureate; LPN to RN Baccalaureate; RN Baccalaureate.
Site Options Houston, TX; Indianapolis, IN; Los Angeles, CA.
Study Options Full-time.
Online Degree Options Yes (online only).
Program Entrance Requirements Transfer students are accepted. *Application deadline:* Applications may be processed on a rolling basis for some programs. *Application fee:* $65.
Advanced Placement Credit by examination available.
Contact *Telephone:* 801-274-3280. *Fax:* 801-274-3305.

GRADUATE PROGRAMS

Contact *Telephone:* 801-274-3280. *Fax:* 801-274-3305.

MASTER'S DEGREE PROGRAM
Degree MS
Available Programs Accelerated Master's; Accelerated RN to Master's; Master's; RN to Master's.
Concentrations Available Clinical nurse leader; health-care administration; nursing administration; nursing education.
Study Options Full-time.
Online Degree Options Yes (online only).
Program Entrance Requirements Computer literacy, transcript of college record, interview. *Application deadline:* Applications may be processed on a rolling basis for some programs. *Application fee:* $65.
Advanced Placement Credit by examination available.
Degree Requirements 30 total credit hours, thesis or project.

Westminster College
School of Nursing and Health Sciences
Salt Lake City, Utah

http://www.westminstercollege.edu/nursing/
Founded in 1875
DEGREES • BSN • MSN
Nursing Student Activities Sigma Theta Tau, Student Nurses' Association, nursing club.
Nursing Student Resources Academic advising; academic or career counseling; assistance for students with disabilities; bookstore; campus computer network; career placement assistance; computer lab; computer-assisted instruction; e-mail services; employment services for current students; housing assistance; interactive nursing skills videos; Internet; learning resource lab; library services; nursing audiovisuals; placement services for program completers; remedial services; resume preparation assistance; skills, simulation, or other laboratory; tutoring.

BACCALAUREATE PROGRAMS

Degree BSN
Available Programs Baccalaureate for Second Degree; Generic Baccalaureate; RN Baccalaureate.
Study Options Full-time.
Program Entrance Requirements Transcript of college record, written essay, 3 letters of recommendation, minimum GPA in nursing prerequisites of 2.5, prerequisite course work. Transfer students are accepted.
Contact *Telephone:* 801-832-2150. *Fax:* 801-832-3110.

GRADUATE PROGRAMS

Contact *Telephone:* 801-832-2150. *Fax:* 801-832-3110.

MASTER'S DEGREE PROGRAM
Degree MSN
Available Programs Master's.
Concentrations Available Nursing education. *Nurse practitioner programs in:* family health.
Program Entrance Requirements Transcript of college record, written essay, 3 letters of recommendation, resume, GRE.
Advanced Placement Credit given for nursing courses completed elsewhere dependent upon specific evaluations.
Degree Requirements 42 total credit hours, thesis or project.

POST-MASTER'S PROGRAM
Areas of Study *Nurse practitioner programs in:* family health.

VERMONT

Castleton State College
Baccalaureate Nursing Program
Castleton, Vermont

http://www.castleton.edu/academics/undergraduate-programs/nursing/
Founded in 1787
DEGREE • BS
Nursing Program Faculty 6 (13% with doctorates).
Baccalaureate Enrollment 110 **Women** 90% **Men** 10% **Part-time** 10%
Distance Learning Courses Available.
Nursing Student Activities Student Nurses' Association.
Nursing Student Resources Academic advising; academic or career counseling; assistance for students with disabilities; bookstore; campus computer network; career placement assistance; computer lab; computer-assisted instruction; e-mail services; employment services for current students; externships; housing assistance; interactive nursing skills videos; Internet; learning resource lab; library services; nursing audiovisuals; paid internships; placement services for program completers; remedial services; resume preparation assistance; skills, simulation, or other laboratory; tutoring; unpaid internships.
Library Facilities 4,234 volumes in health, 1,471 volumes in nursing; 4,031 periodical subscriptions health-care related.

BACCALAUREATE PROGRAMS

Degree BS
Available Programs Generic Baccalaureate; RN Baccalaureate.
Study Options Full-time and part-time.
Program Entrance Requirements Minimum overall college GPA, transcript of college record, CPR certification, written essay, health exam, health insurance, high school transcript, immunizations, letters of recommendation, minimum high school GPA of 3.0, minimum GPA in nursing prerequisites, RN licensure. Transfer students are accepted. *Application deadline:* Applications may be processed on a rolling basis for some programs.
Advanced Placement Credit given for nursing courses completed elsewhere dependent upon specific evaluations.
Expenses (2015–16) *Tuition, state resident:* full-time $13,320; part-time $555 per credit. *Tuition, nonresident:* full-time $28,728; part-time $1197 per credit. *Room and board:* $10,000; room only: $5000 per academic year. *Required fees:* full-time $700; part-time $50 per credit; part-time $300 per term.

Financial Aid 80% of baccalaureate students in nursing programs received some form of financial aid in 2014–15.
Contact Ms. Stephanie Cleveland, Nursing Department, Baccalaureate Nursing Program, Castleton State College, 251 South Street, Castleton, VT 05735. *Telephone:* 802-468-1230. *Fax:* 802-468-1442.
E-mail: stephanie.cleveland@castleton.edu.

Norwich University
Department of Nursing
Northfield, Vermont

http://profschools.norwich.edu/nursing/
Founded in 1819

DEGREE • BSN
Nursing Program Faculty 8 (10% with doctorates).
Baccalaureate Enrollment 90 **Women** 90% **Men** 10% **Part-time** 20%
Nursing Student Activities Student Nurses' Association, nursing club.
Nursing Student Resources Academic advising; academic or career counseling; assistance for students with disabilities; bookstore; campus computer network; career placement assistance; computer lab; e-mail services; employment services for current students; externships; housing assistance; interactive nursing skills videos; Internet; learning resource lab; library services; nursing audiovisuals; placement services for program completers; remedial services; resume preparation assistance; skills, simulation, or other laboratory; tutoring; unpaid internships.

BACCALAUREATE PROGRAMS

Degree BSN
Available Programs ADN to Baccalaureate; Generic Baccalaureate; RN Baccalaureate.
Site Options Rutland, VT.
Study Options Full-time and part-time.
Program Entrance Requirements Minimum overall college GPA of 2.5, transcript of college record, CPR certification, written essay, health exam, health insurance, high school biology, high school chemistry, 2 years high school math, 2 years high school science, high school transcript, immunizations, interview, 2 letters of recommendation, minimum GPA in nursing prerequisites of 2.5. Transfer students are accepted.
Advanced Placement Credit given for nursing courses completed elsewhere dependent upon specific evaluations.
Contact *Telephone:* 802-485-2008. *Fax:* 802-485-2032.

Southern Vermont College
Department of Nursing
Bennington, Vermont

http://www.svc.edu/academics/divisions/nursing/index.html
Founded in 1926

DEGREE • BSN
Nursing Program Faculty 9 (33% with doctorates).
Baccalaureate Enrollment 43 **Women** 88% **Men** 12% **Part-time** 14%
Distance Learning Courses Available.
Nursing Student Activities Student Nurses' Association.
Nursing Student Resources Academic advising; academic or career counseling; assistance for students with disabilities; bookstore; campus computer network; career placement assistance; computer lab; e-mail services; employment services for current students; interactive nursing skills videos; Internet; learning resource lab; library services; nursing audiovisuals; remedial services; resume preparation assistance; skills, simulation, or other laboratory; tutoring.
Library Facilities 360 volumes in health, 140 volumes in nursing; 100 periodical subscriptions health-care related.

BACCALAUREATE PROGRAMS

Degree BSN
Available Programs ADN to Baccalaureate; Generic Baccalaureate; RN Baccalaureate.
Site Options Bennington, VT.
Study Options Full-time and part-time.
Program Entrance Requirements Minimum overall college GPA of 2.8, transcript of college record, CPR certification, health exam, health insurance, high school biology, high school chemistry, high school transcript, immunizations, minimum high school GPA of 2.8, minimum GPA

in nursing prerequisites of 2.8. Transfer students are accepted. *Application deadline:* Applications may be processed on a rolling basis for some programs.
Expenses (2015–16) *Tuition:* full-time $22,985; part-time $960 per credit. *Room and board:* $10,700 per academic year. *Required fees:* full-time $445.
Contact Dr. Mary L. Botter, Chair, Division of Nursing, Department of Nursing, Southern Vermont College, 982 Mansion Drive, Bennington, VT 05201. *Telephone:* 802-447-6347. *E-mail:* mbotter@svc.edu.

University of Vermont
Department of Nursing
Burlington, Vermont

http://www.uvm.edu/~cnhs/nursing
Founded in 1791

DEGREES • BS • DNP • MS
Nursing Program Faculty 27 (67% with doctorates).
Baccalaureate Enrollment 412 **Women** 90% **Men** 10% **Part-time** 9%
Graduate Enrollment 91 **Women** 86% **Men** 14% **Part-time** 11%
Distance Learning Courses Available.
Nursing Student Activities Nursing Honor Society, Sigma Theta Tau, Student Nurses' Association.
Nursing Student Resources Academic advising; academic or career counseling; assistance for students with disabilities; bookstore; campus computer network; career placement assistance; computer-assisted instruction; e-mail services; Internet; learning resource lab; library services; resume preparation assistance; skills, simulation, or other laboratory; tutoring.

BACCALAUREATE PROGRAMS

Degree BS
Available Programs ADN to Baccalaureate; Generic Baccalaureate.
Study Options Full-time and part-time.
Program Entrance Requirements Minimum overall college GPA of 3.0, transcript of college record, written essay, health insurance, high school biology, high school chemistry, high school foreign language, 4 years high school math, 2 years high school science, high school transcript, immunizations, letters of recommendation, minimum GPA in nursing prerequisites of 2.5. *Application deadline:* 1/15 (fall). *Application fee:* $55.
Advanced Placement Credit given for nursing courses completed elsewhere dependent upon specific evaluations.
Expenses (2014–15) *Tuition, state resident:* full-time $14,184; part-time $591 per credit hour. *Tuition, nonresident:* part-time $1493 per credit hour. *Room and board:* $10,810 per academic year. *Required fees:* full-time $2042.
Financial Aid 89% of baccalaureate students in nursing programs received some form of financial aid in 2013–14. *Gift aid (need-based):* Federal Pell, FSEOG, state, private, college/university gift aid from institutional funds, Federal Nursing. *Loans:* Federal Nursing Student Loans, Federal Direct (Subsidized and Unsubsidized Stafford PLUS), Perkins, college/university. *Work-study:* Federal Work-Study. *Financial aid application deadline (priority):* 2/10.
Contact Ms. Erica S. Caloiero, Director, Student Services, Department of Nursing, University of Vermont, Rowell Building, Room 106, Burlington, VT 05405-0068. *Telephone:* 802-656-0968.
E-mail: erica.caloiero@uvm.edu.

GRADUATE PROGRAMS

Expenses (2014–15) *Tuition, state resident:* full-time $12,411; part-time $591 per credit hour. *Tuition, nonresident:* full-time $31,353; part-time $1493 per credit hour. *Required fees:* full-time $1804.
Financial Aid 50% of graduate students in nursing programs received some form of financial aid in 2013–14. *Application deadline:* 3/1.
Contact Ms. Kristen Cella, Graduate Nursing Admissions Specialist, Department of Nursing, University of Vermont, 002 Rowell Building, 106 Carrigan Drive, Burlington, VT 05405. *Telephone:* 802-656-3858.
E-mail: cnhsgrad@uvm.edu.

MASTER'S DEGREE PROGRAM
Degree MS
Available Programs Master's; Master's for Non-Nursing College Graduates; Master's for Nurses with Non-Nursing Degrees; RN to Master's.
Concentrations Available Clinical nurse leader. *Nurse practitioner programs in:* adult health, family health, primary care.

Study Options Full-time and part-time.

Program Entrance Requirements Minimum overall college GPA of 3.0, transcript of college record, written essay, 3 letters of recommendation, physical assessment course, prerequisite course work, statistics course, GRE General Test. *Application deadline:* Applications may be processed on a rolling basis for some programs. *Application fee:* $130.

Advanced Placement Credit by examination available. Credit given for nursing courses completed elsewhere dependent upon specific evaluations.

Degree Requirements Thesis or project, comprehensive exam.

POST-MASTER'S PROGRAM

Areas of Study *Nurse practitioner programs in:* adult health, family health, primary care.

DOCTORAL DEGREE PROGRAM

Degree DNP

Available Programs Doctorate; Doctorate for Nurses with Non-Nursing Degrees; Post-Baccalaureate Doctorate.

Areas of Study Advanced practice nursing.

Program Entrance Requirements Minimum overall college GPA of 3.0, 3 letters of recommendation, MSN or equivalent, statistics course, vita. Application deadline: Applications may be processed on a rolling basis for some programs. Application fee: $130.

Degree Requirements Oral exam, residency.

VIRGIN ISLANDS

University of the Virgin Islands
Division of Nursing
Saint Thomas, Virgin Islands

http://www.uvi.edu/
Founded in 1962

DEGREE • BSN

Nursing Program Faculty 8 (15% with doctorates).

Baccalaureate Enrollment 51 **Women** 98% **Men** 2% **Part-time** 20%

Nursing Student Activities Student Nurses' Association.

Nursing Student Resources Academic advising; academic or career counseling; assistance for students with disabilities; bookstore; campus computer network; career placement assistance; computer lab; computer-assisted instruction; e-mail services; employment services for current students; externships; housing assistance; interactive nursing skills videos; Internet; learning resource lab; library services; nursing audiovisuals; paid internships; remedial services; resume preparation assistance; skills, simulation, or other laboratory; tutoring.

Library Facilities 95,000 volumes in health, 600 volumes in nursing; 15 periodical subscriptions health-care related.

BACCALAUREATE PROGRAMS

Degree BSN

Available Programs ADN to Baccalaureate; Generic Baccalaureate; LPN to Baccalaureate; RN Baccalaureate.

Site Options St. Croix, VI.

Study Options Full-time and part-time.

Program Entrance Requirements Minimum overall college GPA of 2.5, transcript of college record, CPR certification, health exam, 2 years high school math, high school transcript, immunizations, minimum GPA in nursing prerequisites of 2.5, professional liability insurance/malpractice insurance, prerequisite course work. Transfer students are accepted. *Application deadline:* 10/15 (fall). Applications may be processed on a rolling basis for some programs. *Application fee:* $25.

Advanced Placement Credit by examination available. Credit given for nursing courses completed elsewhere dependent upon specific evaluations.

Contact *Telephone:* 340-778-1620 Ext. 4117. *Fax:* 340-693-1285.

VIRGINIA

Bluefield College
School of Nursing
Bluefield, Virginia

http://www.bluefield.edu/school-of-nursing/
Founded in 1922

DEGREE • BSN

BACCALAUREATE PROGRAMS

Degree BSN

Available Programs RN Baccalaureate.

Online Degree Options Yes (online only).

Contact School of Nursing, School of Nursing, Bluefield College, 3000 College Drive, Bluefield, VA 24605. *Telephone:* 276-326-4472. *E-mail:* jsharp@bluefield.edu.

Bon Secours Memorial College of Nursing
Bon Secours Memorial College of Nursing
Richmond, Virginia

DEGREE • BSN

BACCALAUREATE PROGRAMS

Degree BSN

Available Programs Generic Baccalaureate; RN Baccalaureate.

Online Degree Options Yes.

Program Entrance Requirements Minimum overall college GPA of 2.5, prerequisite course work.

Contact *Telephone:* 804-627-5300.

Eastern Mennonite University
Department of Nursing
Harrisonburg, Virginia

Founded in 1917

DEGREES • BS • MSN

Nursing Program Faculty 12 (25% with doctorates).

Baccalaureate Enrollment 374 **Women** 92% **Men** 8% **Part-time** 36%

Graduate Enrollment 57 **Women** 93% **Men** 7% **Part-time** 60%

Distance Learning Courses Available.

Nursing Student Activities Sigma Theta Tau, Student Nurses' Association.

Nursing Student Resources Academic advising; academic or career counseling; assistance for students with disabilities; bookstore; campus computer network; career placement assistance; computer lab; computer-assisted instruction; e-mail services; employment services for current students; externships; housing assistance; interactive nursing skills videos; Internet; learning resource lab; library services; nursing audiovisuals; placement services for program completers; remedial services; resume preparation assistance; skills, simulation, or other laboratory; tutoring.

Library Facilities 444 volumes in health, 3,091 volumes in nursing; 7,313 periodical subscriptions health-care related.

BACCALAUREATE PROGRAMS

Degree BS

Available Programs ADN to Baccalaureate; Accelerated Baccalaureate; Baccalaureate for Second Degree; Generic Baccalaureate; LPN to Baccalaureate; RN Baccalaureate.

Site Options Lancaster , PA.

Study Options Full-time and part-time.

Program Entrance Requirements Minimum overall college GPA of 2.8, transcript of college record, CPR certification, written essay, health exam, health insurance, high school chemistry, high school transcript, immunizations, 3 letters of recommendation, minimum high school GPA of 2.0, minimum GPA in nursing prerequisites of 2.8, professional liability insurance/malpractice insurance, prerequisite course work. Transfer students are accepted. *Application deadline:* 2/15 (fall), 6/15 (spring), 1/15 (summer). *Application fee:* $100.

Advanced Placement Credit by examination available. Credit given for nursing courses completed elsewhere dependent upon specific evaluations.

Expenses (2014–15) *Tuition:* full-time $15,330; part-time $1275 per credit hour. *International tuition:* $15,330 full-time. *Room and board:* $9860 per academic year. *Required fees:* full-time $550; part-time $250 per term.

Financial Aid 99% of baccalaureate students in nursing programs received some form of financial aid in 2013–14.

Contact Dr. Jason Good, Director of Admissions, Department of Nursing, Eastern Mennonite University, 1200 Park Road, Harrisonburg, VA 22802. *Telephone:* 800-368-2665. *Fax:* 540-432-4118. *E-mail:* jason.good@emu.edu.

GRADUATE PROGRAMS

Financial Aid 58% of graduate students in nursing programs received some form of financial aid in 2013–14.

Contact Dr. Don L. Tyson, Director, Department of Nursing, Eastern Mennonite University, 1200 Park Road, Harrisonburg, VA 22802. *Telephone:* 540-432-4000 Ext. 4194. *Fax:* 540-432-4000 Ext. 4444. *E-mail:* tysond@emu.edu.

MASTER'S DEGREE PROGRAM

Degree MSN

Available Programs Master's; Master's for Nurses with Non-Nursing Degrees.

Concentrations Available Nursing administration.

Study Options Full-time and part-time.

Online Degree Options Yes (online only).

Program Entrance Requirements Clinical experience, computer literacy, minimum overall college GPA of 3.0, transcript of college record, written essay, 2 letters of recommendation, nursing research course. *Application deadline:* 6/1 (winter). Applications may be processed on a rolling basis for some programs. *Application fee:* $25.

Advanced Placement Credit given for nursing courses completed elsewhere dependent upon specific evaluations.

Degree Requirements 37 total credit hours, thesis or project.

ECPI University

BSN Program
Virginia Beach, Virginia

http://www.ecpi.edu/medical/program/nursing-bachelor-degree/
Founded in 1966

DEGREE • BSN
Nursing Program Faculty 5 (60% with doctorates).
Baccalaureate Enrollment 30
Distance Learning Courses Available.
Nursing Student Resources Academic advising; academic or career counseling; assistance for students with disabilities; campus computer network; computer lab; e-mail services; Internet; library services; placement services for program completers; resume preparation assistance; tutoring.

BACCALAUREATE PROGRAMS

Degree BSN

Available Programs RN Baccalaureate.

Study Options Full-time and part-time.

Online Degree Options Yes.

Program Entrance Requirements CPR certification, health exam, immunizations, interview, minimum GPA in nursing prerequisites of 2.5, prerequisite course work, RN licensure. Transfer students are accepted. *Application deadline:* Applications may be processed on a rolling basis for some programs.

Advanced Placement Credit given for nursing courses completed elsewhere dependent upon specific evaluations.

Contact *Telephone:* 757-497-8400.

George Mason University

College of Health and Human Services
Fairfax, Virginia

http://chhs.gmu.edu/
Founded in 1957

DEGREES • BSN • MSN • PHD
Nursing Program Faculty 72 (53% with doctorates).
Baccalaureate Enrollment 317 **Women** 82% **Men** 18% **Part-time** 18%
Graduate Enrollment 136 **Women** 89% **Men** 11% **Part-time** 63%
Distance Learning Courses Available.
Nursing Student Activities Nursing Honor Society, Sigma Theta Tau, Student Nurses' Association.
Nursing Student Resources Academic advising; academic or career counseling; assistance for students with disabilities; bookstore; campus computer network; career placement assistance; computer lab; computer-assisted instruction; e-mail services; employment services for current students; housing assistance; interactive nursing skills videos; Internet; library services; nursing audiovisuals; remedial services; resume preparation assistance; skills, simulation, or other laboratory; tutoring.
Library Facilities 16,200 volumes in nursing; 700 periodical subscriptions health-care related.

BACCALAUREATE PROGRAMS

Degree BSN

Available Programs Accelerated Baccalaureate for Second Degree; Generic Baccalaureate; RN Baccalaureate.

Site Options Prince William County, VA.

Study Options Full-time.

Online Degree Options Yes.

Program Entrance Requirements Minimum overall college GPA of 2.85, transcript of college record, CPR certification, written essay, health exam, health insurance, immunizations, minimum GPA in nursing prerequisites of 3.0, professional liability insurance/malpractice insurance, prerequisite course work. Transfer students are accepted. *Application deadline:* 1/15 (fall). *Application fee:* $65.

Expenses (2014–15) *Tuition, state resident:* full-time $10,182; part-time $424 per credit. *Tuition, nonresident:* full-time $29,776; part-time $1240 per credit. *International tuition:* $29,776 full-time. *Room and board:* $16,710 per academic year. *Required fees:* full-time $2878.

Financial Aid 50% of baccalaureate students in nursing programs received some form of financial aid in 2013–14.

Contact Office of Student Affairs, BSN Programs, School of Nursing, College of Health and Human Services, George Mason University, Mailstop 3C4, 4400 University Drive, Fairfax, VA 22030-4444. *Telephone:* 703-993-8896. *Fax:* 703-993-3606. *E-mail:* bsnapps@gmu.edu.

GRADUATE PROGRAMS

Expenses (2014–15) *Tuition, state resident:* full-time $5796; part-time $483 per credit. *Tuition, nonresident:* full-time $14,388; part-time $1199 per credit. *International tuition:* $14,388 full-time. *Room and board:* $16,710 per academic year. *Required fees:* part-time $118 per credit.

Financial Aid 50% of graduate students in nursing programs received some form of financial aid in 2013–14. 11 fellowships (averaging $12,909 per year), 40 research assistantships with full and partial tuition reimbursements available (averaging $16,900 per year), 2 teaching assistantships with full and partial tuition reimbursements available (averaging $16,250 per year) were awarded; career-related internships or fieldwork, Federal Work-Study, scholarships, unspecified assistantships, and health care benefits (for full-time research or teaching assistantship recipients) also available. Aid available to part-time students. *Financial aid application deadline:* 3/1.

Contact Ms. Janice Lee-Beverly, Administrative Assistant, MSN Programs, School of Nursing, College of Health and Human Services, George Mason University, Mailstop 3C4, 4400 University Drive, Fairfax, VA 22030-4444. *Telephone:* 703-993-1947. *Fax:* 703-993-1949. *E-mail:* jleebev1@gmu.edu.

MASTER'S DEGREE PROGRAM

Degree MSN

Available Programs Master's.

Concentrations Available Nursing administration; nursing education. *Nurse practitioner programs in:* adult health, family health, gerontology, psychiatric/mental health.

Site Options Prince William County, VA.

Study Options Full-time and part-time.

Program Entrance Requirements Clinical experience, computer literacy, minimum overall college GPA of 3.0, CPR certification, written essay, immunizations, 2 letters of recommendation, physical assessment course, professional liability insurance/malpractice insurance, statistics course, GRE or GMAT (depending on program). *Application deadline:* 2/1 (fall), 2/1 (spring). *Application fee:* $65.
Degree Requirements 30 total credit hours.

POST-MASTER'S PROGRAM

Areas of Study Nursing administration; nursing education. *Nurse practitioner programs in:* psychiatric/mental health.

DOCTORAL DEGREE PROGRAM

Degree PhD
Available Programs Doctorate.
Areas of Study Individualized study.
Site Options Prince William County, VA.
Program Entrance Requirements Clinical experience, minimum overall college GPA of 3.5, interview, 3 letters of recommendation, MSN or equivalent, statistics course, writing sample, GRE or GMAT (depending on program). Application deadline: 2/1 (fall), 2/1 (spring). Application fee: $65.
Degree Requirements 48 total credit hours, dissertation, written exam.

POSTDOCTORAL PROGRAM

Postdoctoral Program Contact Jean Sorrell, Coordinator, College of Health and Human Services, George Mason University, Mailstop 3C4, 4400 University Drive, Fairfax, VA 22030-4444. *Telephone:* 703-993-1944. *Fax:* 703-993-1942. *E-mail:* jsorrell@gmu.edu.

CONTINUING EDUCATION PROGRAM

Contact Ms. Sandy Kellerhals, Administrative Assistant for Academic Outreach, College of Health and Human Services, George Mason University, Mailstop 1B8, 4400 University Drive, Fairfax, VA 22030-4444. *Telephone:* 703-993-2120. *Fax:* 703-993-1622. *E-mail:* skellerh@gmu.edu.

Hampton University
School of Nursing
Hampton, Virginia

http://nursing.hamptonu.edu/
Founded in 1868
DEGREES • BS • MS • PHD
Nursing Program Faculty 26 (51% with doctorates).
Baccalaureate Enrollment 470 **Women** 93% **Men** 7% **Part-time** 4%
Graduate Enrollment 66 **Women** 100% **Part-time** 25%
Distance Learning Courses Available.
Nursing Student Activities Sigma Theta Tau, Student Nurses' Association.
Nursing Student Resources Academic advising; bookstore; computer lab; e-mail services; interactive nursing skills videos; Internet; library services; skills, simulation, or other laboratory; tutoring.
Library Facilities 4,000 volumes in health, 2,000 volumes in nursing; 500 periodical subscriptions health-care related.

BACCALAUREATE PROGRAMS

Degree BS
Available Programs Accelerated Baccalaureate; Generic Baccalaureate; LPN to Baccalaureate; LPN to RN Baccalaureate; RN Baccalaureate.
Site Options Virginia Beach, VA.
Study Options Full-time and part-time.
Program Entrance Requirements Minimum overall college GPA of 2.3, transcript of college record, CPR certification, written essay, health exam, health insurance, high school biology, high school chemistry, 3 years high school math, 2 years high school science, high school transcript, immunizations, 2 letters of recommendation, minimum high school GPA of 2.0, minimum high school rank 50%, minimum GPA in nursing prerequisites of 2.0, professional liability insurance/malpractice insurance. Transfer students are accepted. *Application deadline:* 3/1 (fall), 12/1 (spring).
Advanced Placement Credit by examination available. Credit given for nursing courses completed elsewhere dependent upon specific evaluations.
Contact *Telephone:* 757-727-5251.

GRADUATE PROGRAMS

Contact *Telephone:* 757-727-5251. *Fax:* 757-727-5423.

MASTER'S DEGREE PROGRAM

Degree MS
Available Programs Master's; RN to Master's.
Concentrations Available Health-care administration; nursing administration; nursing education. *Nurse practitioner programs in:* family health, gerontology, pediatric, primary care, women's health.
Study Options Full-time and part-time.
Online Degree Options Yes.
Program Entrance Requirements Clinical experience, computer literacy, minimum overall college GPA of 2.5, transcript of college record, written essay, interview, 2 letters of recommendation, nursing research course, physical assessment course, resume, statistics course, GRE General Test. *Application deadline:* 3/30 (fall), 11/1 (spring).
Advanced Placement Credit given for nursing courses completed elsewhere dependent upon specific evaluations.
Degree Requirements 46 total credit hours, thesis or project, comprehensive exam.

DOCTORAL DEGREE PROGRAM

Degree PhD
Available Programs Doctorate.
Areas of Study Family health.
Online Degree Options Yes (online only).
Program Entrance Requirements Minimum overall college GPA of 3.5, interview by faculty committee, interview, 3 letters of recommendation, MSN or equivalent, statistics course, vita, writing sample. Application deadline: 3/30 (fall).
Degree Requirements 44 total credit hours, dissertation, oral exam, written exam, residency.

James Madison University
Department of Nursing
Harrisonburg, Virginia

http://www.nursing.jmu.edu/
Founded in 1908
DEGREES • BSN • DNP • MSN
Nursing Program Faculty 49 (40% with doctorates).
Baccalaureate Enrollment 345 **Women** 94% **Men** 6%
Graduate Enrollment 88 **Women** 84% **Men** 16% **Part-time** 84%
Distance Learning Courses Available.
Nursing Student Activities Sigma Theta Tau, Student Nurses' Association.
Nursing Student Resources Academic advising; academic or career counseling; assistance for students with disabilities; bookstore; campus computer network; career placement assistance; computer lab; computer-assisted instruction; e-mail services; employment services for current students; housing assistance; interactive nursing skills videos; Internet; learning resource lab; library services; nursing audiovisuals; remedial services; resume preparation assistance; skills, simulation, or other laboratory; tutoring; unpaid internships.
Library Facilities 29,418 volumes in health, 1,515 volumes in nursing; 11,236 periodical subscriptions health-care related.

BACCALAUREATE PROGRAMS

Degree BSN
Available Programs Generic Baccalaureate; RN Baccalaureate.
Study Options Full-time.
Program Entrance Requirements Minimum overall college GPA of 3.0, transcript of college record, CPR certification, written essay, health exam, health insurance, immunizations, minimum GPA in nursing prerequisites of 2.0, prerequisite course work. Transfer students are accepted. *Application deadline:* 12/1 (fall), 7/1 (spring).
Advanced Placement Credit given for nursing courses completed elsewhere dependent upon specific evaluations.
Expenses (2015–16) *Tuition, state resident:* full-time $10,066. *Tuition, nonresident:* full-time $25,200. *Room and board:* $9018 per academic year.
Financial Aid 56% of baccalaureate students in nursing programs received some form of financial aid in 2014–15. *Gift aid (need-based):* Federal Pell, FSEOG, state, private, college/university gift aid from institutional funds. *Loans:* Federal Direct (Subsidized and Unsubsidized

Stafford PLUS), Perkins. *Work-study:* Federal Work-Study, part-time campus jobs. *Financial aid application deadline (priority):* 3/1.
Contact Ms. Becky Meadows, Administrative Assistant, Department of Nursing, James Madison University, 820 Madison Drive, Burruss Hall, MSC 4305, Harrisonburg, VA 22807. *Telephone:* 540-568-6314. *Fax:* 540-568-5613. *E-mail:* meadowra@jmu.edu.

GRADUATE PROGRAMS

Expenses (2015–16) *Tuition, state resident:* part-time $434 per credit hour. *Tuition, nonresident:* part-time $1135 per credit hour.
Contact Dr. Patty Hale, Program Director, Department of Nursing, James Madison University, 820 Madison Drive, Burruss Hall, MSC 4305, Harrisonburg, VA 22807. *Telephone:* 540-568-6314. *Fax:* 540-568-7896. *E-mail:* halepj@jmu.edu.

MASTER'S DEGREE PROGRAM

Degree MSN
Available Programs Master's.
Concentrations Available Clinical nurse leader; nurse-midwifery; nursing administration. *Nurse practitioner programs in:* family health.
Study Options Full-time and part-time.
Online Degree Options Yes.
Program Entrance Requirements Clinical experience, computer literacy, minimum overall college GPA of 2.8, transcript of college record, CPR certification, written essay, immunizations, 2 letters of recommendation, prerequisite course work, resume, statistics course. *Application deadline:* 4/1 (fall), 10/1 (spring). Applications may be processed on a rolling basis for some programs. *Application fee:* $55.
Advanced Placement Credit given for nursing courses completed elsewhere dependent upon specific evaluations.
Degree Requirements 32 total credit hours.

DOCTORAL DEGREE PROGRAM

Degree DNP
Available Programs Doctorate.
Areas of Study Advanced practice nursing, clinical practice, clinical research, ethics, health policy, health promotion/disease prevention, health-care systems, individualized study, information systems, nursing administration, nursing policy, nursing research.
Online Degree Options Yes (online only).
Program Entrance Requirements Clinical experience, minimum overall college GPA of 3.2, interview, 3 letters of recommendation, MSN or equivalent, statistics course, vita, writing sample. Application deadline: 8/1 (spring). Applications may be processed on a rolling basis for some programs.
Degree Requirements 31 total credit hours, residency.

Jefferson College of Health Sciences

Nursing Education Program
Roanoke, Virginia

http://www.jchs.edu/
Founded in 1982
DEGREES • BSN • MSN
Nursing Program Faculty 24 (17% with doctorates).
Baccalaureate Enrollment 260 **Women** 93% **Men** 7% **Part-time** 47%
Graduate Enrollment 32 **Women** 91% **Men** 9% **Part-time** 3%
Distance Learning Courses Available.
Nursing Student Activities Nursing Honor Society, Sigma Theta Tau, Student Nurses' Association.
Nursing Student Resources Academic advising; academic or career counseling; assistance for students with disabilities; bookstore; campus computer network; computer lab; computer-assisted instruction; e-mail services; externships; housing assistance; interactive nursing skills videos; Internet; learning resource lab; library services; nursing audiovisuals; skills, simulation, or other laboratory; tutoring.
Library Facilities 4,403 volumes in health, 1,422 volumes in nursing; 277 periodical subscriptions health-care related.

BACCALAUREATE PROGRAMS

Degree BSN
Available Programs ADN to Baccalaureate; Generic Baccalaureate; RN Baccalaureate.
Site Options Roanoke, VA.

Study Options Full-time and part-time.
Program Entrance Requirements Minimum overall college GPA of 2.0, transcript of college record, CPR certification, health exam, health insurance, high school biology, high school chemistry, 2 years high school math, 2 years high school science, high school transcript, immunizations, minimum high school GPA of 2.0, prerequisite course work. Transfer students are accepted.
Advanced Placement Credit by examination available. Credit given for nursing courses completed elsewhere dependent upon specific evaluations.
Contact *Telephone:* 540-985-9083. *Fax:* 540-224-6703.

GRADUATE PROGRAMS

Contact *Telephone:* 540-985-9083. *Fax:* 540-224-6703.

MASTER'S DEGREE PROGRAM

Degree MSN
Available Programs Master's; Master's for Nurses with Non-Nursing Degrees.
Concentrations Available Nursing administration; nursing education.
Site Options Roanoke, VA.
Study Options Full-time.
Program Entrance Requirements Clinical experience, computer literacy, transcript of college record, 2 letters of recommendation, nursing research course, resume, statistics course.
Degree Requirements 37 total credit hours, thesis or project.

CONTINUING EDUCATION PROGRAM

Contact *Telephone:* 540-767-6072.

Liberty University

Department of Nursing
Lynchburg, Virginia

http://www.liberty.edu/
Founded in 1971
DEGREES • BSN • MSN
Nursing Program Faculty 25 (25% with doctorates).
Baccalaureate Enrollment 358 **Women** 93% **Men** 7%
Graduate Enrollment 280 **Women** 89% **Men** 11% **Part-time** 99%
Distance Learning Courses Available.
Nursing Student Activities Student Nurses' Association.
Nursing Student Resources Academic advising; academic or career counseling; assistance for students with disabilities; bookstore; campus computer network; career placement assistance; computer lab; e-mail services; externships; interactive nursing skills videos; Internet; learning resource lab; library services; nursing audiovisuals; resume preparation assistance; skills, simulation, or other laboratory; tutoring.
Library Facilities 3,632 volumes in health, 3,000 volumes in nursing; 46 periodical subscriptions health-care related.

BACCALAUREATE PROGRAMS

Degree BSN
Available Programs Generic Baccalaureate; RN Baccalaureate.
Site Options Lynchburg, VA.
Study Options Full-time and part-time.
Program Entrance Requirements Minimum overall college GPA of 3.0, transcript of college record, CPR certification, written essay, immunizations, 2 letters of recommendation, minimum GPA in nursing prerequisites of 3.0, professional liability insurance/malpractice insurance, prerequisite course work. Transfer students are accepted. *Application deadline:* 2/11 (spring).
Advanced Placement Credit given for nursing courses completed elsewhere dependent upon specific evaluations.
Contact *Telephone:* 804-582-2519. *Fax:* 804-582-7035.

GRADUATE PROGRAMS

Contact *Telephone:* 804-582-2519.

MASTER'S DEGREE PROGRAM

Degree MSN
Available Programs Master's.
Concentrations Available Nursing education. *Clinical nurse specialist programs in:* acute care.
Site Options Lynchburg, VA.

Study Options Full-time and part-time.
Online Degree Options Yes (online only).
Program Entrance Requirements Clinical experience, computer literacy, minimum overall college GPA of 3.0, transcript of college record, CPR certification, written essay, immunizations, interview, 3 letters of recommendation, nursing research course, physical assessment course, prerequisite course work, resume, statistics course. *Application deadline:* Applications may be processed on a rolling basis for some programs. *Application fee:* $50.
Degree Requirements 36 total credit hours, thesis or project.

Longwood University

Nursing Program
Farmville, Virginia

Founded in 1839
DEGREE • BSN

BACCALAUREATE PROGRAMS

Degree BSN
Available Programs RN Baccalaureate.
Contact *Telephone:* 434-395-2936. *Fax:* 434-395-2006.

Lynchburg College

School of Health Sciences and Human Performance
Lynchburg, Virginia

http://www.lynchburg.edu/nursing
Founded in 1903
DEGREES • BS • MSN
Nursing Program Faculty 11 (33% with doctorates).
Baccalaureate Enrollment 216 **Women** 91% **Men** 9% **Part-time** 3%
Graduate Enrollment 34 **Women** 94% **Men** 6% **Part-time** 94%
Distance Learning Courses Available.
Nursing Student Activities Nursing Honor Society, Sigma Theta Tau, Student Nurses' Association.
Nursing Student Resources Academic advising; academic or career counseling; assistance for students with disabilities; bookstore; campus computer network; career placement assistance; computer lab; computer-assisted instruction; e-mail services; employment services for current students; externships; housing assistance; interactive nursing skills videos; Internet; learning resource lab; library services; nursing audiovisuals; remedial services; resume preparation assistance; skills, simulation, or other laboratory; tutoring; unpaid internships.
Library Facilities 6,300 volumes in health, 2,000 volumes in nursing; 100 periodical subscriptions health-care related.

BACCALAUREATE PROGRAMS

Degree BS
Available Programs Accelerated Baccalaureate for Second Degree; Generic Baccalaureate.
Study Options Full-time and part-time.
Program Entrance Requirements Transcript of college record, high school biology, high school chemistry, 3 years high school math, 2 years high school science, high school transcript, minimum GPA in nursing prerequisites of 3.0, prerequisite course work. Transfer students are accepted. *Application deadline:* 4/1 (fall), 1/1 (summer). *Application fee:* $30.
Advanced Placement Credit given for nursing courses completed elsewhere dependent upon specific evaluations.
Expenses (2015–16) *Tuition:* full-time $34,610. *Room and board:* $8790; room only: $4870 per academic year. *Required fees:* full-time $705.
Financial Aid *Gift aid (need-based):* Federal Pell, FSEOG, state, private, college/university gift aid from institutional funds. *Loans:* Federal Direct (Subsidized and Unsubsidized Stafford PLUS), Perkins. *Work-study:* Federal Work-Study, part-time campus jobs. *Financial aid application deadline (priority):* 3/5.
Contact Dr. Jennifer Kaye Lloyd-Fitzgerald, Director of Nursing Program and Professor of Nursing, School of Health Sciences and Human Performance, Lynchburg College, 1501 Lakeside Drive,

McMillan Nursing Building, Lynchburg, VA 24501-3199. *Telephone:* 434-544-8461. *Fax:* 434-544-8323. *E-mail:* lloyd.j@lynchburg.edu.

GRADUATE PROGRAMS

Contact Dr. Nancy Overstreet, Director of Nursing Graduate Programs, School of Health Sciences and Human Performance, Lynchburg College, 1501 Lakeside Drive, Lynchburg, VA 24501. *Telephone:* 434-544-8340. *Fax:* 434-544-8323. *E-mail:* overstreet.n@lynchburg.edu.

MASTER'S DEGREE PROGRAM

Degree MSN
Available Programs Master's.
Concentrations Available Clinical nurse leader.
Study Options Full-time and part-time.
Online Degree Options Yes (online only).
Program Entrance Requirements Clinical experience, minimum overall college GPA of 3.0, transcript of college record, 3 letters of recommendation, physical assessment course, statistics course. *Application deadline:* 4/1 (fall), 10/1 (winter), 12/1 (spring), 4/1 (summer). Applications may be processed on a rolling basis for some programs. *Application fee:* $30.
Advanced Placement Credit given for nursing courses completed elsewhere dependent upon specific evaluations.
Degree Requirements 37 total credit hours, thesis or project.

Marymount University

School of Health Professions
Arlington, Virginia

http://www.marymount.edu/Academics/Malek-School-of-Health-Professions/Undergraduate-Programs/Nursing-%28B-S-N-%29
Founded in 1950
DEGREES • BSN • DNP • MSN
Nursing Program Faculty 20 (60% with doctorates).
Baccalaureate Enrollment 389 **Women** 90% **Men** 10% **Part-time** 17%
Graduate Enrollment 70 **Women** 91% **Men** 9% **Part-time** 84%
Distance Learning Courses Available.
Nursing Student Activities Sigma Theta Tau, Student Nurses' Association.
Nursing Student Resources Academic advising; academic or career counseling; assistance for students with disabilities; bookstore; campus computer network; career placement assistance; computer lab; computer-assisted instruction; e-mail services; externships; housing assistance; interactive nursing skills videos; Internet; learning resource lab; library services; nursing audiovisuals; paid internships; remedial services; resume preparation assistance; skills, simulation, or other laboratory; tutoring; unpaid internships.
Library Facilities 12,204 volumes in health, 1,623 volumes in nursing; 2,906 periodical subscriptions health-care related.

BACCALAUREATE PROGRAMS

Degree BSN
Available Programs ADN to Baccalaureate; Accelerated Baccalaureate for Second Degree; Generic Baccalaureate; RN Baccalaureate.
Site Options Arlington, VA.
Study Options Full-time and part-time.
Program Entrance Requirements Minimum overall college GPA of 2.5, transcript of college record, written essay, health exam, health insurance, high school transcript, 1 letter of recommendation, minimum high school GPA of 2.6. Transfer students are accepted. *Application deadline:* 5/29 (fall), 11/15 (spring). *Application fee:* $40.
Advanced Placement Credit by examination available. Credit given for nursing courses completed elsewhere dependent upon specific evaluations.
Expenses (2015–16) *Tuition:* full-time $27,900; part-time $885 per credit hour. *Required fees:* full-time $410; part-time $10 per credit.
Financial Aid *Gift aid (need-based):* Federal Pell, FSEOG, state, private, college/university gift aid from institutional funds. *Loans:* Federal Direct (Subsidized and Unsubsidized Stafford PLUS), Perkins. *Work-study:* Federal Work-Study. *Financial aid application deadline (priority):* 3/1.
Contact Admissions Counselor, Undergraduate Admissions, School of Health Professions, Marymount University, 2807 North Glebe Road, Arlington, VA 22207-4299. *Telephone:* 800-548-7638. *Fax:* 703-522-0349. *E-mail:* admissions@marymount.edu.

GRADUATE PROGRAMS

Expenses (2015–16) *Tuition:* part-time $910 per credit hour. *Required fees:* part-time $10 per credit.
Financial Aid 5 research assistantships, 16 teaching assistantships were awarded; career-related internships or fieldwork, Federal Work-Study, scholarships, and unspecified assistantships also available.
Contact Graduate Admissions Coordinator, School of Health Professions, Marymount University, 2807 North Glebe Road, Arlington, VA 22207-4299. *Telephone:* 703-284-5906. *E-mail:* grad.admissions@ marymount.edu.

MASTER'S DEGREE PROGRAM

Degree MSN
Available Programs Master's.
Concentrations Available *Nurse practitioner programs in:* family health.
Site Options Arlington, VA.
Study Options Full-time and part-time.
Program Entrance Requirements Clinical experience, minimum overall college GPA of 3.0, transcript of college record, CPR certification, written essay, immunizations, interview, 2 letters of recommendation, professional liability insurance/malpractice insurance, prerequisite course work, resume, statistics course, GRE, MAT. *Application deadline:* 9/15 (fall), 4/1 (spring). Applications may be processed on a rolling basis for some programs. *Application fee:* $40.
Advanced Placement Credit given for nursing courses completed elsewhere dependent upon specific evaluations.
Degree Requirements 45 total credit hours, comprehensive exam.

POST-MASTER'S PROGRAM

Areas of Study *Nurse practitioner programs in:* family health.

DOCTORAL DEGREE PROGRAM

Degree DNP
Available Programs Doctorate; Post-Baccalaureate Doctorate.
Areas of Study Advanced practice nursing.
Site Options Arlington, VA.
Program Entrance Requirements Clinical experience, minimum overall college GPA of 3.3, interview by faculty committee, interview, 2 letters of recommendation, MSN or equivalent, vita, writing sample, GRE. Application deadline: 4/1 (fall). Application fee: $40.
Degree Requirements 32 total credit hours, residency.

Norfolk State University
Department of Nursing
Norfolk, Virginia

http://cset.nsu.edu/nursing/
Founded in 1935
DEGREE • BSN
Nursing Program Faculty 26 (40% with doctorates).
Baccalaureate Enrollment 133 **Women** 90% **Men** 10% **Part-time** 45%
Distance Learning Courses Available.
Nursing Student Activities Nursing Honor Society, Student Nurses' Association, nursing club.
Nursing Student Resources Academic advising; academic or career counseling; assistance for students with disabilities; bookstore; campus computer network; career placement assistance; computer lab; computer-assisted instruction; daycare for children of students; e-mail services; employment services for current students; externships; housing assistance; interactive nursing skills videos; Internet; learning resource lab; library services; nursing audiovisuals; paid internships; remedial services; resume preparation assistance; skills, simulation, or other laboratory; tutoring; unpaid internships.
Library Facilities 600 volumes in health, 300 volumes in nursing; 125 periodical subscriptions health-care related.

BACCALAUREATE PROGRAMS

Degree BSN
Available Programs Accelerated Baccalaureate for Second Degree; Accelerated LPN to Baccalaureate; RN Baccalaureate.
Site Options Virginia Beach , VA.
Study Options Full-time and part-time.
Program Entrance Requirements Minimum overall college GPA of 2.5, transcript of college record, CPR certification, health exam, health insurance, high school biology, high school chemistry, 2 years high school math, high school transcript, immunizations, minimum high school GPA of 2.5, minimum GPA in nursing prerequisites of 2.5, professional liability insurance/malpractice insurance, prerequisite course work. Transfer students are accepted. *Application deadline:* 8/1 (fall), 12/1 (winter), 2/1 (spring), 8/1 (summer).
Advanced Placement Credit by examination available. Credit given for nursing courses completed elsewhere dependent upon specific evaluations.
Contact *Telephone:* 757-823-9015. *Fax:* 757-823-2131.

Old Dominion University
Department of Nursing
Norfolk, Virginia

http://www.odu.edu/nursing
Founded in 1930
DEGREES • BSN • DNP • MSN
Nursing Program Faculty 37 (46% with doctorates).
Baccalaureate Enrollment 598 **Women** 89% **Men** 11% **Part-time** 46%
Graduate Enrollment 194 **Women** 93% **Men** 7% **Part-time** 47%
Distance Learning Courses Available.
Nursing Student Activities Sigma Theta Tau, Student Nurses' Association.
Nursing Student Resources Academic advising; academic or career counseling; assistance for students with disabilities; bookstore; campus computer network; career placement assistance; computer lab; computer-assisted instruction; e-mail services; employment services for current students; externships; housing assistance; interactive nursing skills videos; Internet; learning resource lab; library services; nursing audiovisuals; paid internships; placement services for program completers; remedial services; resume preparation assistance; skills, simulation, or other laboratory; tutoring; unpaid internships.
Library Facilities 44,144 volumes in health, 3,622 volumes in nursing; 3,035 periodical subscriptions health-care related.

BACCALAUREATE PROGRAMS

Degree BSN
Available Programs Generic Baccalaureate; RN Baccalaureate.
Study Options Full-time.
Program Entrance Requirements Transcript of college record, CPR certification, health exam, immunizations, minimum GPA in nursing prerequisites of 3.0, prerequisite course work. Transfer students are accepted. *Application deadline:* 2/15 (fall). *Application fee:* $50.
Expenses (2015–16) *Tuition, state resident:* part-time $316 per contact hour. *Tuition, nonresident:* part-time $874 per contact hour. *International tuition:* $874 full-time. *Room and board:* $10,233; room only: $6500 per academic year.
Financial Aid 65% of baccalaureate students in nursing programs received some form of financial aid in 2014–15. *Gift aid (need-based):* Federal Pell, FSEOG, state, private, college/university gift aid from institutional funds, United Negro College Fund, Federal Nursing. *Loans:* Federal Nursing Student Loans, Federal Direct (Subsidized and Unsubsidized Stafford PLUS), Perkins, college/university. *Work-study:* Federal Work-Study. *Financial aid application deadline:* 3/15(priority: 2/15).
Contact Ms. Janice Hawkins, Chief Academic Advisor, Department of Nursing, Old Dominion University, 4608 Hampton Boulevard, Health Sciences Building, Norfolk, VA 23529-0500. *Telephone:* 757-683-5245. *Fax:* 757-683-5253. *E-mail:* jhawkins@odu.edu.

GRADUATE PROGRAMS

Expenses (2015–16) *Tuition, state resident:* part-time $464 per credit hour. *Tuition, nonresident:* part-time $1160 per credit hour.
Contact Dr. Carolyn Rutledge, Associate Chair for Graduate Nursing, Department of Nursing, Old Dominion University, 4608 Hampton Boulevard, 3122 Health Science Building, Norfolk, VA 23529-0500. *Telephone:* 757-683-5009. *Fax:* 757-683-5253. *E-mail:* crutledg@ odu.edu.

MASTER'S DEGREE PROGRAM

Degree MSN
Available Programs Master's; Master's for Nurses with Non-Nursing Degrees.
Concentrations Available Nurse anesthesia; nurse-midwifery; nursing administration. *Clinical nurse specialist programs in:* adult-gerontology acute care. *Nurse practitioner programs in:* family health, pediatric.
Study Options Full-time.

Online Degree Options Yes (online only).
Program Entrance Requirements Clinical experience, computer literacy, minimum overall college GPA of 3.0, transcript of college record, CPR certification, written essay, immunizations, interview, 3 letters of recommendation, physical assessment course, resume, statistics course. *Application deadline:* 5/1 (fall). *Application fee:* $50.
Advanced Placement Credit given for nursing courses completed elsewhere dependent upon specific evaluations.
Degree Requirements 47 total credit hours, comprehensive exam.

POST-MASTER'S PROGRAM

Areas of Study Nursing administration; nursing education.

DOCTORAL DEGREE PROGRAM

Degree DNP
Available Programs Doctorate.
Areas of Study Advanced practice nursing, nursing administration.
Online Degree Options Yes (online only).
Program Entrance Requirements Clinical experience, minimum overall college GPA of 3.0, 3 letters of recommendation, MSN or equivalent, statistics course, vita, writing sample. Application deadline: 9/15 (spring). Application fee: $50.
Degree Requirements 36 total credit hours.

Radford University
Program in Nursing Practice
Radford, Virginia

http://www.radford.edu/nurs-web
Founded in 1910
DEGREES • BSN • DNP • MSN
Nursing Program Faculty 42 (31% with doctorates).
Baccalaureate Enrollment 227
Graduate Enrollment 58
Distance Learning Courses Available.
Nursing Student Activities Nursing Honor Society, Sigma Theta Tau, Student Nurses' Association.
Nursing Student Resources Academic advising; academic or career counseling; assistance for students with disabilities; bookstore; campus computer network; career placement assistance; computer lab; computer-assisted instruction; e-mail services; employment services for current students; externships; housing assistance; interactive nursing skills videos; Internet; learning resource lab; library services; nursing audiovisuals; resume preparation assistance; skills, simulation, or other laboratory; tutoring; unpaid internships.

BACCALAUREATE PROGRAMS

Degree BSN
Available Programs Baccalaureate for Second Degree; Generic Baccalaureate; RN Baccalaureate.
Site Options Roanoke, VA.
Study Options Full-time.
Online Degree Options Yes.
Program Entrance Requirements Minimum overall college GPA of 2.8, transcript of college record, CPR certification, written essay, health exam, health insurance, immunizations, prerequisite course work. Transfer students are accepted. *Application deadline:* 11/15 (fall), 8/1 (spring).
Advanced Placement Credit given for nursing courses completed elsewhere dependent upon specific evaluations.
Contact *Telephone:* 540-831-7700. *Fax:* 540-831-7716.

GRADUATE PROGRAMS

Contact *Telephone:* 540-831-7714. *Fax:* 540-831-7716.

MASTER'S DEGREE PROGRAM

Degree MSN
Available Programs Master's.
Concentrations Available Nurse-midwifery. *Nurse practitioner programs in:* family health.
Study Options Full-time and part-time.
Program Entrance Requirements Clinical experience, computer literacy, transcript of college record, CPR certification, written essay, immunizations, interview, letters of recommendation, nursing research course, physical assessment course, professional liability insurance/mal-

practice insurance, resume, statistics course. *Application deadline:* Applications may be processed on a rolling basis for some programs.
Degree Requirements Thesis or project.

POST-MASTER'S PROGRAM

Areas of Study Nurse-midwifery. *Nurse practitioner programs in:* family health.

DOCTORAL DEGREE PROGRAM

Degree DNP
Available Programs Doctorate; Post-Baccalaureate Doctorate.
Areas of Study Advanced practice nursing, clinical practice, faculty preparation, family health, gerontology, maternity-newborn.
Online Degree Options Yes (online only).
Program Entrance Requirements Clinical experience, minimum overall college GPA of 3.0, interview by faculty committee, interview, 3 letters of recommendation, statistics course, vita, writing sample, GRE. Application deadline: Applications may be processed on a rolling basis for some programs.
Degree Requirements Residency.

Sentara College of Health Sciences
Bachelor of Science in Nursing Program
Chesapeake, Virginia

DEGREE • BSN

BACCALAUREATE PROGRAMS

Degree BSN
Available Programs Generic Baccalaureate; LPN to Baccalaureate; RN Baccalaureate.
Study Options Full-time and part-time.
Online Degree Options Yes.
Program Entrance Requirements Prerequisite course work.
Contact *Telephone:* 757-388-2862.

Shenandoah University
Eleanor Wade Custer School of Nursing
Winchester, Virginia

http://www.nursing.su.edu/
Founded in 1875
DEGREES • BS • DNP • MSN
Nursing Program Faculty 34 (62% with doctorates).
Baccalaureate Enrollment 335 **Women** 88% **Men** 12% **Part-time** 4%
Graduate Enrollment 66 **Women** 91% **Men** 9% **Part-time** 58%
Distance Learning Courses Available.
Nursing Student Activities Nursing Honor Society, Sigma Theta Tau, Student Nurses' Association.
Nursing Student Resources Academic advising; academic or career counseling; assistance for students with disabilities; bookstore; campus computer network; computer lab; computer-assisted instruction; daycare for children of students; e-mail services; externships; interactive nursing skills videos; Internet; learning resource lab; library services; nursing audiovisuals; resume preparation assistance; skills, simulation, or other laboratory; tutoring.
Library Facilities 2,300 volumes in health, 738 volumes in nursing; 6,900 periodical subscriptions health-care related.

BACCALAUREATE PROGRAMS

Degree BS
Available Programs ADN to Baccalaureate; Accelerated Baccalaureate for Second Degree; Baccalaureate for Second Degree; Generic Baccalaureate; RN Baccalaureate.
Site Options Leesburg, VA.
Study Options Full-time and part-time.
Online Degree Options Yes.
Program Entrance Requirements Minimum overall college GPA of 3.0, transcript of college record, CPR certification, health exam, health insurance, high school biology, high school chemistry, 2 years high school math, 2 years high school science, high school transcript, immunizations, minimum high school GPA of 3.0, minimum GPA in nursing pre-

requisites of 3.0, prerequisite course work. Transfer students are accepted. *Application deadline:* Applications may be processed on a rolling basis for some programs. *Application fee:* $30.

Advanced Placement Credit by examination available. Credit given for nursing courses completed elsewhere dependent upon specific evaluations.

Expenses (2015–16) *Tuition:* full-time $30,132; part-time $860 per credit hour. *Room and board:* $9920 per academic year. *Required fees:* full-time $1640; part-time $820 per term.

Financial Aid 94% of baccalaureate students in nursing programs received some form of financial aid in 2014–15. *Gift aid (need-based):* Federal Pell, FSEOG, state, college/university gift aid from institutional funds. *Loans:* Federal Nursing Student Loans, Federal Direct (Subsidized and Unsubsidized Stafford PLUS), Perkins. *Work-study:* Federal Work-Study, part-time campus jobs. *Financial aid application deadline:* Continuous.

Contact Kathryn Ganske, PhD, Dean, Eleanor Wade Custer School of Nursing, Shenandoah University, 1460 University Drive, Winchester, VA 22601-5195. *Telephone:* 540-665-4581. *Fax:* 540-665-4627. *E-mail:* kganske@su.edu.

GRADUATE PROGRAMS

Expenses (2015–16) *Tuition:* full-time $22,410; part-time $830 per credit hour. *Room and board:* $9920 per academic year. *Required fees:* full-time $1365; part-time $455 per term.

Financial Aid 88% of graduate students in nursing programs received some form of financial aid in 2014–15. 3 teaching assistantships with partial tuition reimbursements available (averaging $1,084 per year) were awarded; career-related internships or fieldwork, scholarships, and unspecified assistantships also available. Aid available to part-time students. *Financial aid application deadline:* 3/15.

Contact Elizabeth Courts, DNP, RN, FNP-BC, Director, Graduate Program, Eleanor Wade Custer School of Nursing, Shenandoah University, Health and Life Sciences Building, Winchester, VA 22601-5195. *Telephone:* 540-665-5502. *Fax:* 540-665-5519. *E-mail:* ecourts@su.edu.

MASTER'S DEGREE PROGRAM

Degree MSN

Available Programs Master's; RN to Master's.

Concentrations Available Nurse-midwifery. *Clinical nurse specialist programs in:* family health, psychiatric/mental health. *Nurse practitioner programs in:* family health, psychiatric/mental health.

Study Options Full-time and part-time.

Program Entrance Requirements Clinical experience, computer literacy, minimum overall college GPA of 3.0, transcript of college record, CPR certification, immunizations, interview, 3 letters of recommendation, nursing research course, physical assessment course, professional liability insurance/malpractice insurance, prerequisite course work, resume, statistics course. *Application deadline:* Applications may be processed on a rolling basis for some programs. *Application fee:* $30.

Advanced Placement Credit given for nursing courses completed elsewhere dependent upon specific evaluations.

Degree Requirements 48 total credit hours, thesis or project.

POST-MASTER'S PROGRAM

Areas of Study Nurse-midwifery. *Clinical nurse specialist programs in:* family health, psychiatric/mental health. *Nurse practitioner programs in:* family health, psychiatric/mental health.

DOCTORAL DEGREE PROGRAM

Degree DNP

Available Programs Doctorate; Post-Baccalaureate Doctorate.

Areas of Study Family health.

Program Entrance Requirements Clinical experience, minimum overall college GPA of 3.0, interview by faculty committee, letters of recommendation, MSN or equivalent, statistics course, vita. Application deadline: Applications may be processed on a rolling basis for some programs. Application fee: $30.

Degree Requirements 80 total credit hours.

CONTINUING EDUCATION PROGRAM

Contact Amy Brown, MSN, RN, Continuing Education Coordinator, Eleanor Wade Custer School of Nursing, Shenandoah University, 1460 University Drive, Winchester, VA 22601. *Telephone:* 540-678-4374. *Fax:* 540-665-5519. *E-mail:* abrown3@su.edu.

Stratford University
School of Nursing
Falls Church, Virginia

http://www.stratford.edu/
Founded in 1976

DEGREE • BSN

Nursing Program Faculty 14 (10% with doctorates).
Baccalaureate Enrollment 160 **Women** 90% **Men** 10% **Part-time** 90%
Distance Learning Courses Available.
Nursing Student Activities Nursing Honor Society, Student Nurses' Association, nursing club.
Nursing Student Resources Academic advising; academic or career counseling; assistance for students with disabilities; campus computer network; career placement assistance; computer lab; computer-assisted instruction; e-mail services; employment services for current students; externships; interactive nursing skills videos; Internet; learning resource lab; library services; nursing audiovisuals; placement services for program completers; resume preparation assistance; skills, simulation, or other laboratory; tutoring.
Library Facilities 237 volumes in health, 145 volumes in nursing; 400 periodical subscriptions health-care related.

BACCALAUREATE PROGRAMS

Degree BSN

Available Programs Generic Baccalaureate; RN Baccalaureate.
Site Options Woodbridge, VA; Glen Allen, VA.
Study Options Full-time and part-time.
Program Entrance Requirements Transcript of college record, written essay, high school transcript, 2 letters of recommendation, minimum high school GPA of 2.8, minimum GPA in nursing prerequisites of 2.0. Transfer students are accepted. *Application deadline:* 8/30 (fall), 11/30 (winter), 2/28 (spring), 5/10 (summer). *Application fee:* $50.
Advanced Placement Credit by examination available.
Expenses (2014–15) *Tuition:* full-time $18,450; part-time $410 per credit. *Required fees:* full-time $3400.
Financial Aid 92% of baccalaureate students in nursing programs received some form of financial aid in 2013–14.
Contact Bachelor of Science in Nursing, School of Nursing, Stratford University, 7777 Leesburg Pike, Falls Church, VA 22043. *Telephone:* 703-821-8570.

University of Virginia
School of Nursing
Charlottesville, Virginia

http://www.nursing.virginia.edu/
Founded in 1819

DEGREES • BSN • MSN • MSN/PHD • PHD

Nursing Program Faculty 133 (65% with doctorates).
Baccalaureate Enrollment 408 **Women** 95% **Men** 5% **Part-time** 5%
Graduate Enrollment 381 **Women** 88% **Men** 12% **Part-time** 50%
Nursing Student Activities Nursing Honor Society, Sigma Theta Tau, Student Nurses' Association, nursing club.
Nursing Student Resources Academic advising; academic or career counseling; assistance for students with disabilities; bookstore; campus computer network; career placement assistance; computer-assisted instruction; e-mail services; employment services for current students; housing assistance; interactive nursing skills videos; Internet; learning resource lab; library services; nursing audiovisuals; placement services for program completers; remedial services; resume preparation assistance; skills, simulation, or other laboratory; tutoring.
Library Facilities 200,000 volumes in health; 1,000 periodical subscriptions health-care related.

BACCALAUREATE PROGRAMS

Degree BSN

Available Programs ADN to Baccalaureate; Generic Baccalaureate; RN Baccalaureate.
Study Options Full-time.
Program Entrance Requirements Transcript of college record, written essay, 3 years high school math, 2 years high school science, high school transcript, 1 letter of recommendation, minimum high school GPA.

Transfer students are accepted. *Application deadline:* 1/1 (fall). *Application fee:* $75.

Advanced Placement Credit by examination available.

Contact Ms. Austin Stajduhar, Assistant Director for Undergraduate Admissions and Financial Aid, School of Nursing, University of Virginia, Claude Moore Nursing Education Building, PO Box 800826, Charlottesville, VA 22908. *Telephone:* 888-283-8703. *Fax:* 434-924-0528. *E-mail:* nursing-admissions@virginia.edu.

GRADUATE PROGRAMS

Financial Aid Fellowships, research assistantships, teaching assistantships, Federal Work-Study and scholarships available.

Contact Mr. Christopher De La Cerda, Assistant Director for Graduate Admissions and Financial Aid, School of Nursing, University of Virginia, Claude Moore Nursing Education Building, PO Box 800826, Charlottesville, VA 22908. *Telephone:* 888-283-8703. *Fax:* 434-924-0528. *E-mail:* nursing-admissions@virginia.edu.

MASTER'S DEGREE PROGRAM

Degrees MSN; MSN/PhD

Available Programs Master's; Master's for Non-Nursing College Graduates; Master's for Nurses with Non-Nursing Degrees; RN to Master's.

Concentrations Available Clinical nurse leader. *Clinical nurse specialist programs in:* adult-gerontology acute care. *Nurse practitioner programs in:* adult-gerontology acute care, family health, pediatric, psychiatric/mental health.

Study Options Full-time and part-time.

Program Entrance Requirements Clinical experience, minimum overall college GPA of 3.0, transcript of college record, written essay, interview, 3 letters of recommendation, resume, statistics course, GRE General Test, MAT. *Application deadline:* 11/1 (fall). *Application fee:* $75.

Advanced Placement Credit given for nursing courses completed elsewhere dependent upon specific evaluations.

Degree Requirements 34 total credit hours.

POST-MASTER'S PROGRAM

Areas of Study *Clinical nurse specialist programs in:* adult-gerontology acute care. *Nurse practitioner programs in:* adult-gerontology acute care, family health, pediatric, psychiatric/mental health.

DOCTORAL DEGREE PROGRAM

Degree PhD

Available Programs Doctorate; Post-Baccalaureate Doctorate.

Areas of Study Advanced practice nursing, aging, bio-behavioral research, clinical practice, clinical research, community health, critical care, ethics, faculty preparation, family health, forensic nursing, gerontology, health policy, health promotion/disease prevention, health-care systems, human health and illness, information systems, maternity-newborn, neuro-behavior, nursing administration, nursing education, nursing policy, nursing research, nursing science, oncology, palliative care, urban health, women's health.

Program Entrance Requirements Minimum overall college GPA of 3.0, interview by faculty committee, interview, 3 letters of recommendation, statistics course, vita, GRE General Test. Application deadline: 11/1 (fall). Applications may be processed on a rolling basis for some programs. Application fee: $75.

Degree Requirements 46 total credit hours, dissertation, written exam, residency.

POSTDOCTORAL PROGRAM

Areas of Study Nursing research, nursing science.

Postdoctoral Program Contact Mr. Christopher De La Cerda, Assistant Director for Graduate Admissions and Financial Aid, School of Nursing, University of Virginia, Claude Moore Nursing Education Building, PO Box 800826, Charlottesville, VA 22908. *Telephone:* 434-924-0141. *Fax:* 434-924-0528. *E-mail:* nursing-admissions@virginia.edu.

The University of Virginia's College at Wise
Department of Nursing
Wise, Virginia

http://www.uvawise.edu/
Founded in 1954

DEGREE • BSN

Nursing Program Faculty 10 (30% with doctorates).
Baccalaureate Enrollment 47 **Women** 79% **Men** 21% **Part-time** 5%
Nursing Student Activities Sigma Theta Tau, Student Nurses' Association.
Nursing Student Resources Academic advising; academic or career counseling; assistance for students with disabilities; bookstore; campus computer network; career placement assistance; computer lab; computer-assisted instruction; e-mail services; employment services for current students; externships; housing assistance; interactive nursing skills videos; Internet; learning resource lab; library services; nursing audiovisuals; resume preparation assistance; skills, simulation, or other laboratory; tutoring.
Library Facilities 4,654 volumes in health, 2,761 volumes in nursing; 40 periodical subscriptions health-care related.

BACCALAUREATE PROGRAMS

Degree BSN
Available Programs ADN to Baccalaureate; Generic Baccalaureate; RN Baccalaureate.
Study Options Full-time.
Program Entrance Requirements Minimum overall college GPA of 2.75, transcript of college record, CPR certification, written essay, health exam, health insurance, immunizations, minimum GPA in nursing prerequisites of 2.75, professional liability insurance/malpractice insurance, prerequisite course work. Transfer students are accepted. *Application deadline:* 11/1 (spring). *Application fee:* $25.
Advanced Placement Credit given for nursing courses completed elsewhere dependent upon specific evaluations.
Contact *Telephone:* 276-328-0275. *Fax:* 276-376-4589.

Virginia Commonwealth University
School of Nursing
Richmond, Virginia

http://www.nursing.vcu.edu/
Founded in 1838

DEGREES • BS • DNP • MS • PHD

Nursing Program Faculty 91 (73% with doctorates).
Baccalaureate Enrollment 613 **Women** 85% **Men** 15% **Part-time** 39%
Graduate Enrollment 222 **Women** 94% **Men** 6% **Part-time** 66%
Distance Learning Courses Available.
Nursing Student Activities Sigma Theta Tau, Student Nurses' Association, nursing club.
Nursing Student Resources Academic advising; academic or career counseling; assistance for students with disabilities; bookstore; campus computer network; career placement assistance; computer lab; computer-assisted instruction; daycare for children of students; e-mail services; employment services for current students; externships; housing assistance; interactive nursing skills videos; Internet; learning resource lab; library services; nursing audiovisuals; placement services for program completers; remedial services; resume preparation assistance; skills, simulation, or other laboratory; tutoring.
Library Facilities 458,650 volumes in health, 13,536 volumes in nursing; 14,436 periodical subscriptions health-care related.

BACCALAUREATE PROGRAMS

Degree BS
Available Programs ADN to Baccalaureate; Accelerated Baccalaureate for Second Degree; Generic Baccalaureate.
Study Options Full-time.
Program Entrance Requirements Minimum overall college GPA of 2.5, transcript of college record, CPR certification, written essay, immunizations, 3 letters of recommendation, minimum GPA in nursing prereq-

uisites of 2.5, prerequisite course work. Transfer students are accepted. *Application deadline:* 2/1 (fall). *Application fee:* $50.

Advanced Placement Credit by examination available. Credit given for nursing courses completed elsewhere dependent upon specific evaluations.

Expenses (2015–16) *Tuition, state resident:* full-time $8765; part-time $365 per credit hour. *Tuition, nonresident:* full-time $23,724; part-time $988 per credit hour. *International tuition:* $23,724 full-time. *Room and board:* $8950; room only: $5430 per academic year. *Required fees:* full-time $2562.

Contact Mrs. Susan L. Lipp, Assistant Dean of Enrollment and Student Services, School of Nursing, Virginia Commonwealth University, 1100 East Leigh Street, PO Box 980567, Richmond, VA 23298-0567. *Telephone:* 804-828-5171. *Fax:* 804-828-7743. *E-mail:* slipp@vcu.edu.

GRADUATE PROGRAMS

Expenses (2015–16) *Tuition, state resident:* full-time $10,627; part-time $487 per credit hour. *Tuition, nonresident:* full-time $21,850; part-time $1038 per credit hour. *International tuition:* $21,850 full-time. *Room and board:* $10,518; room only: $6998 per academic year. *Required fees:* full-time $2362; part-time $87 per credit; part-time $115 per term.

Financial Aid Fellowships, research assistantships, teaching assistantships, career-related internships or fieldwork and institutionally sponsored loans available.

Contact Mrs. Susan L. Lipp, Assistant Dean of Enrollment and Student Services, School of Nursing, Virginia Commonwealth University, 1100 East Leigh Street, PO Box 980567, Richmond, VA 23298-0567. *Telephone:* 804-828-5171. *Fax:* 804-828-7743. *E-mail:* slipp@vcu.edu.

MASTER'S DEGREE PROGRAM

Degree MS
Available Programs Master's.
Concentrations Available Nursing administration. *Nurse practitioner programs in:* adult health, adult-gerontology acute care, family health, psychiatric/mental health.
Study Options Full-time and part-time.
Program Entrance Requirements Computer literacy, minimum overall college GPA of 3.0, transcript of college record, CPR certification, written essay, immunizations, 3 letters of recommendation, prerequisite course work, resume, statistics course, GRE General Test. *Application deadline:* 3/15 (fall). *Application fee:* $130.
Advanced Placement Credit given for nursing courses completed elsewhere dependent upon specific evaluations.
Degree Requirements 55 total credit hours.

POST-MASTER'S PROGRAM

Areas of Study Nursing administration. *Nurse practitioner programs in:* adult health, adult-gerontology acute care, family health, psychiatric/mental health.

DOCTORAL DEGREE PROGRAM

Degree DNP
Available Programs Doctorate.
Areas of Study Bio-behavioral research.
Online Degree Options Yes (online only).
Program Entrance Requirements Minimum overall college GPA of 3.0, interview, interview by faculty committee, 3 letters of recommendation, MSN or equivalent, statistics course, vita, writing sample. Application deadline: 2/1 (fall), 1/1 (spring), 1/1 (summer), 1/1 (winter). Application fee: $130.
Degree Requirements 61 total credit hours, dissertation, written exam.

Degree PhD
Available Programs Doctorate.
Areas of Study Bio-behavioral research, Quality and Safety.
Online Degree Options Yes (online only).
Program Entrance Requirements Minimum overall college GPA of 3.0, interview by faculty committee, interview, 3 letters of recommendation, MSN or equivalent, statistics course, vita, writing sample, GRE General Test. Application deadline: 2/1 (fall). Application fee: $130.
Degree Requirements 61 total credit hours, dissertation, written exam.

POSTDOCTORAL PROGRAM

Postdoctoral Program Contact Ms. Susan L. Lipp, Assistant Dean of Enrollment and Student Services, School of Nursing, Virginia Commonwealth University, 1100 East Leigh Street, PO Box 980567, Richmond, VA 23298-0567. *Telephone:* 804-828-5171. *Fax:* 804-828-7743. *E-mail:* slipp@vcu.edu.

WASHINGTON

Bellevue College
Nursing Program
Bellevue, Washington

http://www.bellevuecollege.edu/
Founded in 1966
DEGREE • BSN

BACCALAUREATE PROGRAMS

Degree BSN
Available Programs RN Baccalaureate.
Study Options Full-time and part-time.
Program Entrance Requirements *Application deadline:* 3/4 (fall).
Contact Chie McCaughey, BSN Program Manager. *Telephone:* 425-564-5078. *E-mail:* CMcCaugh@bellevuecollege.edu.

Eastern Washington University
WSU College of Nursing
Cheney, Washington

See description of programs under WSU College of Nursing (Spokane, Washington).

Gonzaga University
School of Nursing and Human Psychology
Spokane, Washington

http://online.gonzaga.edu/online-nursing-programs
Founded in 1887
DEGREES • BSN • DNP • MSN
Nursing Program Faculty 17 (71% with doctorates).
Baccalaureate Enrollment 299 **Women** 79% **Men** 21%
Graduate Enrollment 582 **Women** 89% **Men** 11% **Part-time** 14%
Distance Learning Courses Available.
Nursing Student Activities Sigma Theta Tau, Student Nurses' Association, nursing club.
Nursing Student Resources Academic advising; academic or career counseling; assistance for students with disabilities; bookstore; campus computer network; career placement assistance; computer lab; computer-assisted instruction; e-mail services; employment services for current students; housing assistance; interactive nursing skills videos; Internet; learning resource lab; library services; nursing audiovisuals; resume preparation assistance; skills, simulation, or other laboratory; tutoring.
Library Facilities 35,000 volumes in health, 950 volumes in nursing; 206 periodical subscriptions health-care related.

BACCALAUREATE PROGRAMS

Degree BSN
Available Programs Generic Baccalaureate.
Study Options Full-time.
Program Entrance Requirements Transcript of college record, written essay, high school biology, high school chemistry, high school foreign language, 4 years high school math, 4 years high school science, high school transcript, 2 letters of recommendation, minimum high school GPA of 3.4, minimum GPA in nursing prerequisites of 2.0, prerequisite course work. *Application deadline:* 11/15 (fall), 2/1 (winter), 2/1 (spring), 11/15 (summer). *Application fee:* $50.
Advanced Placement Credit given for nursing courses completed elsewhere dependent upon specific evaluations.
Expenses (2014–15) *Tuition:* full-time $18,020; part-time $1010 per credit. *International tuition:* $18,020 full-time. *Room and board:* $10,000 per academic year. *Required fees:* full-time $550.
Financial Aid 90% of baccalaureate students in nursing programs received some form of financial aid in 2013–14. *Gift aid (need-based):* Federal Pell, FSEOG, state, private, college/university gift aid from institutional funds, Federal Nursing. *Loans:* Federal Nursing Student Loans, Federal Direct (Subsidized and Unsubsidized Stafford PLUS), Perkins,

state, college/university. *Work-study:* Federal Work-Study, part-time campus jobs. *Financial aid application deadline (priority):* 2/1.

Contact Marcy Heldt, Program Assistant, School of Nursing and Human Psychology, Gonzaga University, 502 East Boone Avenue, Spokane, WA 99258-0038. *Telephone:* 509-313-3580. *Fax:* 509-313-5827. *E-mail:* heldt@gonzaga.edu.

GRADUATE PROGRAMS

Expenses (2014–15) *Tuition:* part-time $900 per credit. *International tuition:* $900 full-time. *Required fees:* full-time $1200; part-time $600 per term.

Financial Aid 78% of graduate students in nursing programs received some form of financial aid in 2013–14. *Application deadline:* 2/1.

Contact Mrs. Molly Woof, Program Assistant, School of Nursing and Human Psychology, Gonzaga University, 502 East Boone Avenue, Spokane, WA 99258-0038. *Telephone:* 509-313-6640. *Fax:* 509-323-5827. *E-mail:* woodm@gonzaga.edu.

MASTER'S DEGREE PROGRAM

Degree MSN
Available Programs Accelerated RN to Master's; Master's; Master's for Nurses with Non-Nursing Degrees.
Concentrations Available Health-care administration; nursing administration; nursing education. *Clinical nurse specialist programs in:* psychiatric/mental health. *Nurse practitioner programs in:* adult-gerontology acute care, family health, primary care, psychiatric/mental health.
Study Options Full-time and part-time.
Online Degree Options Yes (online only).
Program Entrance Requirements Computer literacy, minimum overall college GPA of 3.0, transcript of college record, written essay, 2 letters of recommendation, resume, statistics course, MAT. *Application deadline:* 8/10 (fall), 12/10 (winter), 2/10 (spring), 4/10 (summer). Applications may be processed on a rolling basis for some programs. *Application fee:* $50.
Advanced Placement Credit given for nursing courses completed elsewhere dependent upon specific evaluations.
Degree Requirements 47 total credit hours.

POST-MASTER'S PROGRAM

Areas of Study Health-care administration; nursing administration; nursing education. *Clinical nurse specialist programs in:* psychiatric/mental health. *Nurse practitioner programs in:* adult-gerontology acute care, family health, primary care, psychiatric/mental health.

DOCTORAL DEGREE PROGRAM

Degree DNP
Available Programs Doctorate; Post-Baccalaureate Doctorate.
Areas of Study Aging, family health, gerontology, health-care systems, individualized study, nursing administration.
Online Degree Options Yes (online only).
Program Entrance Requirements Minimum overall college GPA of 3.3, 3 letters of recommendation, MSN or equivalent, statistics course, vita, writing sample, MAT or GRE within the last 5 years. Application deadline: 8/10 (fall), 11/10 (winter), 1/10 (spring), 4/10 (summer). Applications may be processed on a rolling basis for some programs. Application fee: $50.
Degree Requirements 31 total credit hours, dissertation, residency.

Northwest University
The Mark and Huldah Buntain School of Nursing
Kirkland, Washington

http://www.northwestu.edu/schools/nursing/
Founded in 1934
DEGREE • BS
Nursing Program Faculty 36 (3% with doctorates).
Baccalaureate Enrollment 92 **Women** 92% **Men** 8%
Nursing Student Resources Academic advising; academic or career counseling; assistance for students with disabilities; bookstore; campus computer network; computer lab; computer-assisted instruction; e-mail services; employment services for current students; housing assistance; interactive nursing skills videos; Internet; learning resource lab; library services; nursing audiovisuals; other; remedial services; resume preparation assistance; skills, simulation, or other laboratory; tutoring; unpaid internships.

Library Facilities 1,954 volumes in health; 815 periodical subscriptions health-care related.

BACCALAUREATE PROGRAMS

Degree BS
Available Programs Generic Baccalaureate; RN Baccalaureate.
Study Options Full-time.
Program Entrance Requirements Minimum overall college GPA of 3.0, transcript of college record, CPR certification, written essay, health exam, health insurance, high school transcript, immunizations, 2 letters of recommendation, minimum GPA in nursing prerequisites of 3.0, prerequisite course work. Transfer students are accepted. *Application deadline:* 1/30 (fall). *Application fee:* $35.
Expenses (2015–16) *Tuition:* full-time $27,700; part-time $1150 per credit. *Room and board:* $7790; room only: $4660 per academic year. *Required fees:* full-time $4022.
Financial Aid 98% of baccalaureate students in nursing programs received some form of financial aid in 2014–15. *Gift aid (need-based):* Federal Pell, FSEOG, state, private, college/university gift aid from institutional funds. *Loans:* Federal Direct (Subsidized and Unsubsidized Stafford PLUS), Perkins, state, alternative loans. *Work-study:* Federal Work-Study, part-time campus jobs. *Financial aid application deadline:* 8/1(priority: 2/15).
Contact Dr. Carl N. Christensen, Dean, The Mark and Huldah Buntain School of Nursing, Northwest University, PO Box 579, 5520 108th Avenue NE, Kirkland, WA 98083. *Telephone:* 800-669-3781 Ext. 7822. *Fax:* 425-889-7822. *E-mail:* nursing@northwestu.edu.

Olympic College
Nursing Programs
Bremerton, Washington

Founded in 1946
DEGREE • BSN

BACCALAUREATE PROGRAMS

Degree BSN
Available Programs RN Baccalaureate.
Study Options Full-time and part-time.
Program Entrance Requirements Minimum overall college GPA of 2.5, minimum GPA in nursing prerequisites of 2.0, RN licensure.
Contact *Telephone:* 360-475-7748. *Fax:* 360-475-7628.

Pacific Lutheran University
School of Nursing
Tacoma, Washington

http://www.plu.edu/nursing/
Founded in 1890
DEGREES • BSN • DNP • MSN • MSN/MBA
Nursing Program Faculty 36 (40% with doctorates).
Baccalaureate Enrollment 234 **Women** 89% **Men** 11%
Graduate Enrollment 75 **Women** 85% **Men** 15%
Nursing Student Activities Nursing Honor Society, Sigma Theta Tau, Student Nurses' Association, nursing club.
Nursing Student Resources Academic advising; academic or career counseling; assistance for students with disabilities; bookstore; campus computer network; career placement assistance; computer lab; computer-assisted instruction; e-mail services; employment services for current students; housing assistance; interactive nursing skills videos; Internet; learning resource lab; library services; nursing audiovisuals; other; resume preparation assistance; skills, simulation, or other laboratory; tutoring; unpaid internships.
Library Facilities 15,000 volumes in health, 6,500 volumes in nursing; 150 periodical subscriptions health-care related.

BACCALAUREATE PROGRAMS

Degree BSN
Available Programs Generic Baccalaureate; LPN to Baccalaureate.
Study Options Full-time.
Program Entrance Requirements Minimum overall college GPA of 3.0, transcript of college record, CPR certification, written essay, health exam, health insurance, high school foreign language, 2 years high

school math, high school transcript, immunizations, 2 letters of recommendation, minimum GPA in nursing prerequisites of 2.75, professional liability insurance/malpractice insurance, prerequisite course work. Transfer students are accepted. *Application deadline:* 2/1 (fall), 2/1 (spring). Applications may be processed on a rolling basis for some programs.

Advanced Placement Credit given for nursing courses completed elsewhere dependent upon specific evaluations.

Expenses (2015–16) *Tuition:* full-time $37,950. *International tuition:* $37,950 full-time. *Room and board:* $10,330; room only: $7000 per academic year. *Required fees:* full-time $2000.

Financial Aid 97% of baccalaureate students in nursing programs received some form of financial aid in 2014–15. *Gift aid (need-based):* Federal Pell, FSEOG, state, private, college/university gift aid from institutional funds, Federal Nursing. *Loans:* Federal Nursing Student Loans, Federal Direct (Subsidized and Unsubsidized Stafford PLUS), Perkins, state. *Work-study:* Federal Work-Study, part-time campus jobs. *Financial aid application deadline (priority):* 3/1.

Contact Admissions Coordinator, School of Nursing, Pacific Lutheran University, 12180 Park Avenue South, Tacoma, WA 98447-0029. *Telephone:* 253-535-7672. *Fax:* 253-535-7590.

GRADUATE PROGRAMS

Expenses (2015–16) *Tuition:* full-time $34,250. *International tuition:* $34,250 full-time. *Room and board:* $10,330; room only: $7000 per academic year. *Required fees:* full-time $2000.

Financial Aid 8 fellowships (averaging $827 per year) were awarded; Federal Work-Study and scholarships also available.

Contact Dr. Teri M. Woo, Associate Dean for Graduate Nursing Programs, School of Nursing, Pacific Lutheran University, 12180 Park Avenue South, Tacoma, WA 98447-0029. *Telephone:* 253-535-7672. *Fax:* 253-535-7590. *E-mail:* gradnurs@plu.edu.

MASTER'S DEGREE PROGRAM

Degrees MSN; MSN/MBA

Available Programs Accelerated Master's for Non-Nursing College Graduates; Master's; Master's for Nurses with Non-Nursing Degrees.

Concentrations Available Clinical nurse leader; health-care administration; nurse case management; nursing administration; nursing education. *Nurse practitioner programs in:* family health.

Study Options Full-time.

Program Entrance Requirements Clinical experience, minimum overall college GPA of 3.0, transcript of college record, CPR certification, written essay, immunizations, 2 letters of recommendation, professional liability insurance/malpractice insurance, prerequisite course work, resume, statistics course, GRE General Test. *Application deadline:* 11/15 (summer). Applications may be processed on a rolling basis for some programs. *Application fee:* $40.

Advanced Placement Credit given for nursing courses completed elsewhere dependent upon specific evaluations.

Degree Requirements 33 total credit hours, thesis or project.

DOCTORAL DEGREE PROGRAM

Degree DNP

Available Programs Doctorate; Post-Baccalaureate Doctorate.

Areas of Study Advanced practice nursing, family health.

Program Entrance Requirements Clinical experience, minimum overall college GPA of 3.0, interview by faculty committee, 2 letters of recommendation, statistics course, vita. Application deadline: 11/1 (winter), 11/15 (summer). Applications may be processed on a rolling basis for some programs. Application fee: $40.

Degree Requirements 79 total credit hours.

CONTINUING EDUCATION PROGRAM

Contact Ms. Louise Reulbach, Coordinator for Continuing Nursing Education, School of Nursing, Pacific Lutheran University, 12180 Park Avenue South, Tacoma, WA 98447-0029. *Telephone:* 253-535-7683. *Fax:* 253-535-7590. *E-mail:* lmr@plu.edu.

Saint Martin's University
Nursing Program
Lacey, Washington

http://www.stmartin.edu/nursing
Founded in 1895
DEGREE • BSN
Nursing Program Faculty 2 (100% with doctorates).
Baccalaureate Enrollment 22 **Women** 85% **Men** 15% **Part-time** 75%
Distance Learning Courses Available.
Nursing Student Resources Academic advising; assistance for students with disabilities; bookstore; campus computer network; computer lab; e-mail services; Internet; library services.

BACCALAUREATE PROGRAMS

Degree BSN
Available Programs ADN to Baccalaureate.
Study Options Full-time and part-time.
Program Entrance Requirements Transfer students are accepted. *Application deadline:* 7/31 (fall), 12/1 (spring), 4/1 (summer). Applications may be processed on a rolling basis for some programs.
Expenses (2015–16) *Tuition:* full-time $16,000; part-time $5500 per semester. *International tuition:* $25,000 full-time. *Required fees:* full-time $1500; part-time $60 per credit; part-time $200 per term.
Financial Aid 100% of baccalaureate students in nursing programs received some form of financial aid in 2014–15.
Contact Dr. Louise Kapla, Director, Nursing Program, Nursing Program, Saint Martin's University, 5000 Abbey Way SE, Lacey, WA 98503. *Telephone:* 360-412-6129. *E-mail:* lkaplan@stmartin.edu.

Seattle Pacific University
School of Health Sciences
Seattle, Washington

http://www.spu.edu/depts/hsc
Founded in 1891
DEGREES • BS • MSN
Nursing Program Faculty 23 (39% with doctorates).
Baccalaureate Enrollment 98 **Women** 91% **Men** 9%
Graduate Enrollment 61 **Women** 89% **Men** 11% **Part-time** 49%
Nursing Student Activities Nursing Honor Society, Sigma Theta Tau, Student Nurses' Association, nursing club.
Nursing Student Resources Academic advising; academic or career counseling; assistance for students with disabilities; bookstore; campus computer network; career placement assistance; computer lab; computer-assisted instruction; e-mail services; employment services for current students; housing assistance; Internet; learning resource lab; library services; nursing audiovisuals; placement services for program completers; remedial services; resume preparation assistance; skills, simulation, or other laboratory; tutoring; unpaid internships.
Library Facilities 11,539 volumes in health, 1,791 volumes in nursing; 274 periodical subscriptions health-care related.

BACCALAUREATE PROGRAMS

Degree BS
Available Programs Generic Baccalaureate; RN Baccalaureate.
Study Options Full-time.
Program Entrance Requirements Minimum overall college GPA of 2.75, transcript of college record, CPR certification, written essay, health exam, health insurance, high school transcript, immunizations, 1 letter of recommendation, minimum GPA in nursing prerequisites of 2.75, prerequisite course work. Transfer students are accepted. *Application deadline:* 1/15 (fall).
Advanced Placement Credit given for nursing courses completed elsewhere dependent upon specific evaluations.
Contact *Telephone:* 206-281-2612. *Fax:* 206-281-2767.

GRADUATE PROGRAMS

Contact *Telephone:* 206-281-2888. *Fax:* 206-378-5480.

MASTER'S DEGREE PROGRAM
Degree MSN
Available Programs Master's; Master's for Nurses with Non-Nursing Degrees.

Concentrations Available Nursing administration; nursing education. *Clinical nurse specialist programs in:* acute care, adult health, community health, critical care, gerontology, medical-surgical, oncology, palliative care, parent-child, pediatric, women's health. *Nurse practitioner programs in:* adult health, family health.

Study Options Full-time and part-time.

Program Entrance Requirements Clinical experience, computer literacy, minimum overall college GPA of 3.0, transcript of college record, CPR certification, written essay, immunizations, interview, 3 letters of recommendation, nursing research course, professional liability insurance/malpractice insurance, prerequisite course work, resume, statistics course, GRE General Test. *Application deadline:* 5/1 (fall). *Application fee:* $50.

Advanced Placement Credit given for nursing courses completed elsewhere dependent upon specific evaluations.

Degree Requirements 59 total credit hours, thesis or project, comprehensive exam.

POST-MASTER'S PROGRAM

Areas of Study Nursing education. *Nurse practitioner programs in:* adult health, family health.

Seattle University
College of Nursing
Seattle, Washington

http://www.seattleu.edu/nursing
Founded in 1891

DEGREES • BSN • DNP • MSN
Nursing Program Faculty 79 (42% with doctorates).
Baccalaureate Enrollment 464 **Women** 90% **Men** 10%
Graduate Enrollment 110 **Women** 89% **Men** 11%
Distance Learning Courses Available.
Nursing Student Activities Sigma Theta Tau, Student Nurses' Association.
Nursing Student Resources Academic advising; academic or career counseling; assistance for students with disabilities; bookstore; campus computer network; career placement assistance; computer lab; computer-assisted instruction; e-mail services; employment services for current students; housing assistance; interactive nursing skills videos; Internet; learning resource lab; library services; nursing audiovisuals; paid internships; remedial services; resume preparation assistance; skills, simulation, or other laboratory; tutoring.

BACCALAUREATE PROGRAMS

Degree BSN
Available Programs Baccalaureate for Second Degree; Generic Baccalaureate.
Study Options Full-time.
Program Entrance Requirements Minimum overall college GPA of 2.75, transcript of college record, written essay, health insurance, high school biology, high school chemistry, high school foreign language, 3 years high school math, 2 years high school science, high school transcript, minimum GPA in nursing prerequisites of 3.0, prerequisite course work. Transfer students are accepted. *Application deadline:* 1/5 (winter). *Application fee:* $50.
Contact *Telephone:* 206-296-2242. *Fax:* 206-296-5544.

GRADUATE PROGRAMS

Contact *Telephone:* 206-296-5660. *Fax:* 206-296-5544.

MASTER'S DEGREE PROGRAM

Degree MSN
Available Programs Accelerated Master's for Nurses with Non-Nursing Degrees; Master's.
Concentrations Available *Clinical nurse specialist programs in:* community health. *Nurse practitioner programs in:* family health, gerontology, psychiatric/mental health.
Study Options Full-time.
Program Entrance Requirements Clinical experience, computer literacy, minimum overall college GPA of 3.0, transcript of college record, CPR certification, written essay, immunizations, interview, 2 letters of recommendation, professional liability insurance/malpractice insurance, prerequisite course work, resume, statistics course, GRE General Test. *Application deadline:* 12/1 (fall). *Application fee:* $55.

Advanced Placement Credit given for nursing courses completed elsewhere dependent upon specific evaluations.
Degree Requirements 110 total credit hours, thesis or project.

POST-MASTER'S PROGRAM

Areas of Study *Clinical nurse specialist programs in:* community health. *Nurse practitioner programs in:* family health, gerontology, psychiatric/mental health.

DOCTORAL DEGREE PROGRAM

Degree DNP
Available Programs Doctorate.
Areas of Study Advanced practice nursing, clinical practice, community health, critical care, family health, health policy, individualized study, information systems, nursing education, nursing policy, nursing research.
Program Entrance Requirements Clinical experience, minimum overall college GPA of 3.25, interview by faculty committee, 2 letters of recommendation, MSN or equivalent, writing sample. Application deadline: 5/1 (fall). Applications may be processed on a rolling basis for some programs. Application fee: $55.
Degree Requirements 40 total credit hours.

University of Washington
School of Nursing
Seattle, Washington

http://www.nursing.uw.edu/
Founded in 1861

DEGREES • BSN • DNP • MN • MN/MPH • PHD
Nursing Program Faculty 92 (74% with doctorates).
Baccalaureate Enrollment 231 **Women** 84% **Men** 16% **Part-time** 13%
Graduate Enrollment 407 **Women** 86% **Men** 14% **Part-time** 59%
Distance Learning Courses Available.
Nursing Student Activities Nursing Honor Society, Sigma Theta Tau, Student Nurses' Association, nursing club.
Nursing Student Resources Academic advising; academic or career counseling; assistance for students with disabilities; bookstore; campus computer network; computer lab; computer-assisted instruction; daycare for children of students; e-mail services; employment services for current students; housing assistance; interactive nursing skills videos; Internet; learning resource lab; library services; nursing audiovisuals; resume preparation assistance; skills, simulation, or other laboratory; tutoring.
Library Facilities 350,000 volumes in health; 2,400 periodical subscriptions health-care related.

BACCALAUREATE PROGRAMS

Degree BSN
Available Programs ADN to Baccalaureate; Accelerated Baccalaureate for Second Degree; Generic Baccalaureate.
Site Options Tacoma, WA; Bothell, WA.
Study Options Full-time.
Program Entrance Requirements Minimum overall college GPA of 2.0, transcript of college record, written essay, 1 letter of recommendation, minimum GPA in nursing prerequisites of 2.0, prerequisite course work. *Application deadline:* 1/15 (fall).
Financial Aid *Gift aid (need-based):* Federal Pell, FSEOG, state, private, college/university gift aid from institutional funds, Federal Nursing. *Loans:* Federal Nursing Student Loans, Federal Direct (Subsidized and Unsubsidized Stafford PLUS), Perkins. *Work-study:* Federal Work-Study, part-time campus jobs. *Financial aid application deadline (priority):* 2/28.
Contact Student and Academic Services, School of Nursing, University of Washington, Box 357260, Health Sciences Building, Room T301, Seattle, WA 98195. *Telephone:* 206-543-8736. *Fax:* 206-543-3624. *E-mail:* sonsas@u.washington.edu.

GRADUATE PROGRAMS

Financial Aid Fellowships, research assistantships, teaching assistantships, Federal Work-Study, institutionally sponsored loans, scholarships, and traineeships available.
Contact Student and Academic Services, School of Nursing, University of Washington, Box 357260, Health Sciences Building, Room T301, Seattle, WA 98195. *Telephone:* 206-543-8736. *Fax:* 206-543-3624. *E-mail:* sonsas@u.washington.edu.

MASTER'S DEGREE PROGRAM
Degrees MN; MN/MPH
Available Programs Master's; Master's for Nurses with Non-Nursing Degrees.
Concentrations Available *Clinical nurse specialist programs in:* community health.
Site Options Tacoma, WA; Bothell, WA.
Study Options Full-time and part-time.
Program Entrance Requirements Minimum overall college GPA of 3.0, transcript of college record, written essay, 3 letters of recommendation, resume, statistics course, GRE. *Application deadline:* 1/15 (fall). *Application fee:* $85.
Advanced Placement Credit given for nursing courses completed elsewhere dependent upon specific evaluations.
Degree Requirements 38 total credit hours, thesis or project.

POST-MASTER'S PROGRAM
Areas of Study Nurse-midwifery. *Clinical nurse specialist programs in:* adult health, community health, pediatric, perinatal. *Nurse practitioner programs in:* adult health, adult-gerontology acute care, family health, neonatal health, pediatric, psychiatric/mental health.

DOCTORAL DEGREE PROGRAM
Degree DNP
Available Programs Doctorate; Doctorate for Nurses with Non-Nursing Degrees; Post-Baccalaureate Doctorate.
Areas of Study Advanced practice nursing.
Program Entrance Requirements Minimum overall college GPA of 3.0, 3 letters of recommendation, statistics course, vita, GRE. Application deadline: 1/15 (fall). Application fee: $85.
Degree Requirements 93 total credit hours.

Degree PhD
Available Programs Doctorate, Doctorate for Nurses with Non-Nursing Degrees, Post-Baccalaureate Doctorate.
Areas of Study Clinical research, health policy, nursing education, nursing research, nursing science.
Program Entrance Requirements Minimum overall college GPA of 3.0, 3 letters of recommendation, statistics course, vita, writing sample. Application deadline: 1/15 (fall). Application fee: $85.
Degree Requirements 93 total credit hours, dissertation, oral exam, written exam.

POSTDOCTORAL PROGRAM
Areas of Study Aging, nursing informatics, nursing research, vulnerable population.
Postdoctoral Program Contact Student and Academic Services, School of Nursing, University of Washington, Box 357260, Health Sciences Building, Room T310, Seattle, WA 98195. *Telephone:* 206-543-8736. *Fax:* 206-685-1613. *E-mail:* sonsas@uw.edu.

CONTINUING EDUCATION PROGRAM
Contact Continuing Nursing Education, School of Nursing, University of Washington, Box 359440, Seattle, WA 98195-9440. *Telephone:* 206-543-1047. *Fax:* 206-543-6953. *E-mail:* cne@uw.edu.

Walla Walla University
School of Nursing
College Place, Washington

http://www.wallawalla.edu/nursing
Founded in 1892
DEGREE • BS
Nursing Program Faculty 25 (12% with doctorates).
Baccalaureate Enrollment 182 **Women** 80% **Men** 20% **Part-time** 1%
Nursing Student Activities Nursing Honor Society, nursing club.
Nursing Student Resources Academic advising; academic or career counseling; assistance for students with disabilities; bookstore; campus computer network; computer lab; e-mail services; Internet; learning resource lab; library services; nursing audiovisuals; skills, simulation, or other laboratory; tutoring.
Library Facilities 10,000 volumes in health, 7,000 volumes in nursing; 450 periodical subscriptions health-care related.

BACCALAUREATE PROGRAMS
Degree BS

Available Programs ADN to Baccalaureate; Generic Baccalaureate; LPN to Baccalaureate; RN Baccalaureate.
Site Options Portland, OR.
Study Options Full-time.
Program Entrance Requirements Minimum overall college GPA of 2.75, transcript of college record, CPR certification, written essay, health exam, health insurance, high school biology, 3 years high school math, 2 years high school science, high school transcript, immunizations, 3 letters of recommendation, minimum high school GPA of 2.75, minimum GPA in nursing prerequisites of 2.75, prerequisite course work. Transfer students are accepted. *Application deadline:* 4/15 (fall), 2/1 (summer). *Application fee:* $200.
Advanced Placement Credit given for nursing courses completed elsewhere dependent upon specific evaluations.
Expenses (2015–16) *Tuition:* full-time $25,587; part-time $669 per quarter hour. *International tuition:* $25,587 full-time. *Room and board:* $6840; room only: $4035 per academic year. *Required fees:* full-time $795; part-time $265 per term.
Financial Aid 95% of baccalaureate students in nursing programs received some form of financial aid in 2014–15.
Contact Jan Vigil, Student Program Advisor, School of Nursing, Walla Walla University, 10345 SE Market Street, Portland, OR 97216. *Telephone:* 503-251-6115. *Fax:* 503-251-6249. *E-mail:* Portland.Advising@wallawalla.edu.

Washington State University
WSU College of Nursing
Pullman, Washington

See description of programs under WSU College of Nursing (Spokane, Washington).

Western Washington University
RN-to-BSN Program
Bellingham, Washington

http://www.wwu.edu/
Founded in 1893
DEGREE • BSN

BACCALAUREATE PROGRAMS
Degree BSN
Available Programs RN Baccalaureate.
Program Entrance Requirements *Application deadline:* 3/1 (fall), 1/10 (spring).
Contact Dr. Christine Espina, Interim Director, RN-to-BSN Program, Western Washington University, 516 High Street, Bellingham, WA 98225. *Telephone:* 360-650-6631. *E-mail:* christine.espina@wwu.edu.

Whitworth College
WSU College of Nursing
Spokane, Washington

See description of programs under WSU College of Nursing (Spokane, Washington).

WSU College of Nursing
Spokane, Washington

http://www.nursing.wsu.edu/
DEGREES • BSN • MN • PHD
Nursing Program Faculty 114 (39% with doctorates).
Baccalaureate Enrollment 759 **Women** 84% **Men** 16% **Part-time** 29%
Graduate Enrollment 274 **Women** 89% **Men** 11% **Part-time** 83%
Distance Learning Courses Available.
Nursing Student Activities Nursing Honor Society, Sigma Theta Tau, Student Nurses' Association, nursing club.

Nursing Student Resources Academic advising; academic or career counseling; assistance for students with disabilities; bookstore; campus computer network; computer lab; computer-assisted instruction; e-mail services; interactive nursing skills videos; Internet; learning resource lab; library services; nursing audiovisuals; other; remedial services; resume preparation assistance; skills, simulation, or other laboratory; tutoring; unpaid internships.

Library Facilities 15,000 volumes in health, 7,000 volumes in nursing; 2,000 periodical subscriptions health-care related.

BACCALAUREATE PROGRAMS

Degree BSN

Available Programs Generic Baccalaureate; RN Baccalaureate.

Site Options Richland, WA; Yakima, WA; Vancouver, WA.

Study Options Full-time.

Program Entrance Requirements Minimum overall college GPA of 2.8, transcript of college record, CPR certification, health insurance, immunizations, interview, minimum GPA in nursing prerequisites of 2.8, professional liability insurance/malpractice insurance, prerequisite course work. Transfer students are accepted. *Application deadline:* 1/15 (fall), 8/5 (spring). *Application fee:* $45.

Advanced Placement Credit given for nursing courses completed elsewhere dependent upon specific evaluations.

Contact *Telephone:* 509-324-7337. *Fax:* 509-324-7336.

GRADUATE PROGRAMS

Contact *Telephone:* 509-324-7334. *Fax:* 509-324-7336.

MASTER'S DEGREE PROGRAM

Degree MN

Available Programs Accelerated Master's for Nurses with Non-Nursing Degrees; Accelerated RN to Master's; Master's.

Concentrations Available Nurse case management; nursing administration; nursing education. *Clinical nurse specialist programs in:* community health. *Nurse practitioner programs in:* family health, psychiatric/mental health.

Site Options Richland, WA; Yakima, WA; Vancouver, WA.

Study Options Full-time and part-time.

Program Entrance Requirements Computer literacy, minimum overall college GPA of 3.0, transcript of college record, CPR certification, written essay, immunizations, interview, 3 letters of recommendation, physical assessment course, professional liability insurance/malpractice insurance, prerequisite course work, statistics course. *Application deadline:* 2/1 (fall), 10/1 (spring).

Advanced Placement Credit given for nursing courses completed elsewhere dependent upon specific evaluations.

Degree Requirements 45 total credit hours, thesis or project.

POST-MASTER'S PROGRAM

Areas of Study *Nurse practitioner programs in:* family health, psychiatric/mental health.

DOCTORAL DEGREE PROGRAM

Degree PhD

Available Programs Doctorate.

Areas of Study Nursing education, nursing research.

Program Entrance Requirements Minimum overall college GPA of 3.5, interview by faculty committee, 3 letters of recommendation, MSN or equivalent, scholarly papers, statistics course, vita. Application deadline: 1/10 (summer).

Degree Requirements 72 total credit hours, dissertation.

CONTINUING EDUCATION PROGRAM

Contact *Telephone:* 509-324-7354. *Fax:* 509-324-7341.

WEST VIRGINIA

Alderson Broaddus University
Department of Nursing
Philippi, West Virginia

http://www.ab.edu/
Founded in 1871

DEGREE • BSN

Nursing Program Faculty 13 (1% with doctorates).

Baccalaureate Enrollment 96 **Women** 94% **Men** 6% **Part-time** 2%

Nursing Student Activities Student Nurses' Association.

Nursing Student Resources Academic advising; academic or career counseling; assistance for students with disabilities; bookstore; campus computer network; career placement assistance; computer lab; computer-assisted instruction; e-mail services; employment services for current students; Internet; learning resource lab; library services; nursing audiovisuals; remedial services; resume preparation assistance; skills, simulation, or other laboratory; tutoring.

Library Facilities 6,000 volumes in health, 1,000 volumes in nursing; 172 periodical subscriptions health-care related.

BACCALAUREATE PROGRAMS

Degree BSN

Available Programs Generic Baccalaureate; LPN to RN Baccalaureate; RN Baccalaureate.

Study Options Full-time.

Program Entrance Requirements Minimum overall college GPA of 2.0, transcript of college record, CPR certification, health exam, high school chemistry, high school transcript, immunizations, minimum GPA in nursing prerequisites of 2.25, professional liability insurance/malpractice insurance, prerequisite course work. Transfer students are accepted. *Application deadline:* 7/30 (fall), 1/5 (winter). Applications may be processed on a rolling basis for some programs. *Application fee:* $25.

Advanced Placement Credit by examination available. Credit given for nursing courses completed elsewhere dependent upon specific evaluations.

Contact *Telephone:* 304-457-6384. *Fax:* 304-457-6293.

American Public University System
Bachelor of Science in Nursing
Charles Town, West Virginia

http://www.apus.edu/
Founded in 1991

DEGREE • BSN

Nursing Program Faculty 45

Baccalaureate Enrollment 187 **Women** 91% **Men** 9% **Part-time** 100%

Distance Learning Courses Available.

Nursing Student Resources Academic advising; academic or career counseling; assistance for students with disabilities; career placement assistance; e-mail services; Internet; library services; nursing audiovisuals; placement services for program completers; resume preparation assistance; tutoring.

BACCALAUREATE PROGRAMS

Degree BSN

Available Programs RN Baccalaureate.

Study Options Full-time and part-time.

Online Degree Options Yes (online only).

Program Entrance Requirements Prerequisite course work, RN licensure. Transfer students are accepted. *Application deadline:* Applications may be processed on a rolling basis for some programs.

Expenses (2014–15) *Tuition:* part-time $250 per credit hour.

Contact Valerie Ellington, Nursing Program Admissions, Bachelor of Science in Nursing, American Public University System, 111 West Congress Street, Charles Town, WV 25414. *Telephone:* 304-885-5239. *E-mail:* vellington@apus.edu.

Bluefield State College
Program in Nursing
Bluefield, West Virginia

http://www.bluefieldstate.edu/
Founded in 1895

DEGREE • BSN

Nursing Program Faculty 15
Baccalaureate Enrollment 18 **Women** 93% **Men** 7% **Part-time** 20%
Distance Learning Courses Available.
Nursing Student Activities Nursing Honor Society, Sigma Theta Tau, Student Nurses' Association.
Nursing Student Resources Academic advising; academic or career counseling; assistance for students with disabilities; bookstore; campus computer network; career placement assistance; computer lab; computer-assisted instruction; e-mail services; interactive nursing skills videos; Internet; learning resource lab; library services; nursing audiovisuals; resume preparation assistance; skills, simulation, or other laboratory; tutoring.
Library Facilities 5,649 volumes in health, 1,250 volumes in nursing; 200 periodical subscriptions health-care related.

BACCALAUREATE PROGRAMS

Degree BSN
Available Programs ADN to Baccalaureate; RN Baccalaureate.
Site Options Beckley, WV; Bluefield, WV.
Study Options Full-time and part-time.
Online Degree Options Yes (online only).
Program Entrance Requirements Minimum overall college GPA of 2.5, transcript of college record, CPR certification, health exam, health insurance, high school chemistry, immunizations, 1 letter of recommendation, minimum high school GPA of 2.8, minimum GPA in nursing pre-requisites of 2.5, prerequisite course work, RN licensure. Transfer students are accepted. *Application deadline:* 3/1 (fall), 4/15 (spring).
Advanced Placement Credit given for nursing courses completed elsewhere dependent upon specific evaluations.
Expenses (2015–16) *Tuition, area resident:* full-time $2710; part-time $134 per credit hour. *Tuition, state resident:* full-time $3320; part-time $198 per credit hour. *Tuition, nonresident:* full-time $5400; part-time $336 per credit hour. *Required fees:* full-time $150; part-time $40 per credit.
Financial Aid 78% of baccalaureate students in nursing programs received some form of financial aid in 2014–15. *Gift aid (need-based):* Federal Pell, FSEOG, state. *Loans:* Federal Direct (Subsidized and Unsubsidized Stafford PLUS). *Work-study:* Federal Work-Study, part-time campus jobs. *Financial aid application deadline (priority):* 3/1.
Contact Mrs. Carol Cofer, Director, Program in Nursing, Bluefield State College, 219 Rock Street, Bluefield, WV 24701. *Telephone:* 304-327-4144. *Fax:* 304-327-4144. *E-mail:* ccofer@bluefieldstate.edu.

Fairmont State University
School of Nursing and Allied Health Administration
Fairmont, West Virginia

http://www.fairmontstate.edu/
Founded in 1865

DEGREE • BSN

Nursing Program Faculty 4 (75% with doctorates).
Baccalaureate Enrollment 150 **Women** 96% **Men** 4% **Part-time** 40%
Distance Learning Courses Available.
Nursing Student Activities Sigma Theta Tau, Student Nurses' Association.
Nursing Student Resources Academic advising; academic or career counseling; assistance for students with disabilities; bookstore; campus computer network; career placement assistance; computer lab; computer-assisted instruction; e-mail services; housing assistance; interactive nursing skills videos; Internet; learning resource lab; library services; nursing audiovisuals; placement services for program completers; remedial services; resume preparation assistance; skills, simulation, or other laboratory; tutoring.
Library Facilities 9,000 volumes in health, 1,100 volumes in nursing; 50 periodical subscriptions health-care related.

BACCALAUREATE PROGRAMS

Degree BSN
Available Programs ADN to Baccalaureate; Accelerated RN Baccalaureate; RN Baccalaureate.
Study Options Full-time and part-time.
Program Entrance Requirements Minimum overall college GPA of 2.0, transcript of college record, CPR certification, health exam, high school transcript, immunizations, minimum high school GPA of 2.0, RN licensure. Transfer students are accepted. *Application deadline:* 8/15 (fall), 8/15 (winter), 1/2 (spring), 5/15 (summer). Applications may be processed on a rolling basis for some programs.
Advanced Placement Credit by examination available. Credit given for nursing courses completed elsewhere dependent upon specific evaluations.
Contact *Telephone:* 304-367-4074. *Fax:* 304-367-4268.

CONTINUING EDUCATION PROGRAM

Contact *Telephone:* 304-367-4074. *Fax:* 304-367-4268.

Marshall University
College of Health Professions
Huntington, West Virginia

http://www.marshall.edu/cohp
Founded in 1837

DEGREES • BSN • MSN

Nursing Program Faculty 32 (56% with doctorates).
Baccalaureate Enrollment 345 **Women** 80% **Men** 20% **Part-time** 35%
Graduate Enrollment 100 **Women** 90% **Men** 10% **Part-time** 60%
Distance Learning Courses Available.
Nursing Student Activities Nursing Honor Society, Sigma Theta Tau, Student Nurses' Association, nursing club.
Nursing Student Resources Academic advising; academic or career counseling; assistance for students with disabilities; bookstore; campus computer network; career placement assistance; computer lab; computer-assisted instruction; daycare for children of students; e-mail services; employment services for current students; externships; housing assistance; interactive nursing skills videos; Internet; learning resource lab; library services; nursing audiovisuals; placement services for program completers; remedial services; resume preparation assistance; skills, simulation, or other laboratory; tutoring.
Library Facilities 20,200 volumes in health, 6,400 volumes in nursing; 500 periodical subscriptions health-care related.

BACCALAUREATE PROGRAMS

Degree BSN
Available Programs Generic Baccalaureate; RN Baccalaureate.
Site Options Point Pleasant, WV.
Study Options Full-time and part-time.
Online Degree Options Yes.
Program Entrance Requirements Minimum overall college GPA of 2.5, transcript of college record, high school transcript, minimum high school GPA of 2.5. Transfer students are accepted. *Application deadline:* 1/15 (fall). *Application fee:* $30.
Advanced Placement Credit given for nursing courses completed elsewhere dependent upon specific evaluations.
Expenses (2014–15) *Tuition, area resident:* full-time $8628; part-time $285 per credit hour. *Tuition, state resident:* full-time $12,406; part-time $571 per credit hour. *Tuition, nonresident:* full-time $15,926; part-time $664 per credit hour. *Room and board:* $9546; room only: $6000 per academic year.
Financial Aid 52% of baccalaureate students in nursing programs received some form of financial aid in 2013–14.
Contact Dr. Denise Landry, Chairperson, College of Health Professions, Marshall University, One John Marshall Drive, Huntington, WV 25755-9500. *Telephone:* 304-696-2630. *Fax:* 304-696-6739. *E-mail:* landry@marshall.edu.

GRADUATE PROGRAMS

Expenses (2014–15) *Tuition, area resident:* full-time $7566; part-time $413 per credit hour. *Tuition, state resident:* full-time $13,710; part-time $762 per credit hour. *Tuition, nonresident:* full-time $17,858; part-time $993 per credit hour.
Financial Aid 51% of graduate students in nursing programs received some form of financial aid in 2013–14.

Contact Dr. Denise Landry, Chairperson, College of Health Professions, Marshall University, One John Marshall Drive, Huntington, WV 25755-9500. *Telephone:* 304-696-2630. *Fax:* 304-696-6739. *E-mail:* landry@marshall.edu.

MASTER'S DEGREE PROGRAM

Degree MSN

Available Programs Master's.

Concentrations Available Nurse-midwifery; nursing administration; nursing education. *Nurse practitioner programs in:* family health, psychiatric/mental health.

Site Options Bluefield, WV; South Charleston, WV; Point Pleasant, WV.

Study Options Full-time and part-time.

Online Degree Options Yes.

Program Entrance Requirements Minimum overall college GPA of 3.0, transcript of college record, CPR certification, immunizations, nursing research course, statistics course, GRE General Test.

Advanced Placement Credit given for nursing courses completed elsewhere dependent upon specific evaluations.

Degree Requirements 36 total credit hours.

POST-MASTER'S PROGRAM

Areas of Study Nurse-midwifery; nursing administration; nursing education. *Nurse practitioner programs in:* family health, psychiatric/mental health.

Shepherd University
Department of Nursing Education
Shepherdstown, West Virginia

http://www.shepherd.edu/nurseweb/
Founded in 1871

DEGREE • BSN

Nursing Program Faculty 8 (50% with doctorates).

Baccalaureate Enrollment 144 **Women** 92% **Men** 8%

Nursing Student Activities Nursing Honor Society, Student Nurses' Association.

Nursing Student Resources Academic advising; academic or career counseling; assistance for students with disabilities; bookstore; campus computer network; career placement assistance; computer lab; computer-assisted instruction; e-mail services; interactive nursing skills videos; Internet; learning resource lab; library services; nursing audiovisuals; remedial services; resume preparation assistance; skills, simulation, or other laboratory; tutoring.

Library Facilities 4,997 volumes in health, 462 volumes in nursing; 1,956 periodical subscriptions health-care related.

BACCALAUREATE PROGRAMS

Degree BSN

Available Programs ADN to Baccalaureate; Generic Baccalaureate; RN Baccalaureate.

Study Options Full-time.

Program Entrance Requirements Minimum overall college GPA of 2.5, transcript of college record, CPR certification, written essay, health exam, health insurance, immunizations, interview, minimum GPA in nursing prerequisites of 2.0, professional liability insurance/malpractice insurance, prerequisite course work. Transfer students are accepted. *Application deadline:* 3/1 (fall), 10/1 (spring).

Advanced Placement Credit by examination available. Credit given for nursing courses completed elsewhere dependent upon specific evaluations.

Contact *Telephone:* 304-876-5341. *Fax:* 304-876-5169.

CONTINUING EDUCATION PROGRAM

Contact *Telephone:* 304-876-5341. *Fax:* 304-876-5169.

University of Charleston
Department of Nursing
Charleston, West Virginia

http://www.ucwv.edu/majors/nursing/
Founded in 1888

DEGREE • BSN

Nursing Program Faculty 6 (33% with doctorates).

Baccalaureate Enrollment 65 **Women** 97% **Men** 3% **Part-time** 1%

Nursing Student Activities Nursing Honor Society, Sigma Theta Tau, Student Nurses' Association, nursing club.

Nursing Student Resources Academic advising; academic or career counseling; assistance for students with disabilities; bookstore; campus computer network; career placement assistance; computer lab; computer-assisted instruction; e-mail services; employment services for current students; externships; housing assistance; interactive nursing skills videos; Internet; learning resource lab; library services; nursing audiovisuals; paid internships; placement services for program completers; remedial services; resume preparation assistance; skills, simulation, or other laboratory; tutoring; unpaid internships.

Library Facilities 3,900 volumes in health, 1,550 volumes in nursing; 75 periodical subscriptions health-care related.

BACCALAUREATE PROGRAMS

Degree BSN

Available Programs Generic Baccalaureate.

Study Options Full-time and part-time.

Program Entrance Requirements Minimum overall college GPA of 2.75, transcript of college record, CPR certification, health exam, high school biology, 1 year of high school math, high school transcript, immunizations, minimum high school GPA of 2.25, minimum GPA in nursing prerequisites of 2.75, professional liability insurance/malpractice insurance, prerequisite course work. Transfer students are accepted. *Application deadline:* Applications may be processed on a rolling basis for some programs.

Advanced Placement Credit given for nursing courses completed elsewhere dependent upon specific evaluations.

Contact *Telephone:* 304-357-4750. *Fax:* 304-357-4781.

West Liberty University
Department of Health Sciences
West Liberty, West Virginia

http://westliberty.edu/health-sciences/academics/nursing/
Founded in 1837

DEGREE • BSN

Nursing Program Faculty 8 (50% with doctorates).

Baccalaureate Enrollment 105 **Women** 90% **Men** 10%

Distance Learning Courses Available.

Nursing Student Activities Student Nurses' Association.

Nursing Student Resources Academic advising; academic or career counseling; assistance for students with disabilities; bookstore; campus computer network; career placement assistance; computer lab; computer-assisted instruction; e-mail services; externships; housing assistance; interactive nursing skills videos; Internet; learning resource lab; library services; nursing audiovisuals; placement services for program completers; remedial services; resume preparation assistance; skills, simulation, or other laboratory; tutoring; unpaid internships.

Library Facilities 2,500 volumes in health, 750 volumes in nursing; 350 periodical subscriptions health-care related.

BACCALAUREATE PROGRAMS

Degree BSN

Available Programs Accelerated RN Baccalaureate; Generic Baccalaureate.

Site Options Triadelphia, WV.

Study Options Full-time.

Program Entrance Requirements Minimum overall college GPA of 3.0, transcript of college record, health exam, immunizations, minimum high school GPA of 3.0, minimum GPA in nursing prerequisites of 2.0, prerequisite course work. Transfer students are accepted. *Application deadline:* 3/31 (fall).

Advanced Placement Credit by examination available. Credit given for nursing courses completed elsewhere dependent upon specific evaluations.

Expenses (2015–16) *Tuition, state resident:* full-time $6702; part-time $273 per credit hour. *Tuition, nonresident:* full-time $14,112; part-time $582 per credit hour. *Room and board:* $8810; room only: $4860 per academic year. *Required fees:* full-time $950.

Financial Aid 96% of baccalaureate students in nursing programs received some form of financial aid in 2014–15.

Contact Dr. Rose Kutlenios, Interim Program Director, Nursing, Department of Health Sciences, West Liberty University, 208 University Drive, College Union Box 140, West Liberty, WV 26074. *Telephone:* 304-336-8911. *Fax:* 304-336-5104. *E-mail:* rose.kutlenios@ westliberty.edu.

West Virginia University

School of Nursing
Morgantown, West Virginia

http://www.nursing.hsc.wvu.edu/
Founded in 1867

DEGREES • BSN • DNP • MSN • PHD

Nursing Program Faculty 81 (43% with doctorates).

Baccalaureate Enrollment 570 **Women** 86% **Men** 14% **Part-time** 19%

Graduate Enrollment 152 **Women** 91% **Men** 9% **Part-time** 80%

Distance Learning Courses Available.

Nursing Student Activities Nursing Honor Society, Sigma Theta Tau, Student Nurses' Association.

Nursing Student Resources Academic advising; academic or career counseling; assistance for students with disabilities; bookstore; campus computer network; career placement assistance; computer lab; computer-assisted instruction; daycare for children of students; e-mail services; employment services for current students; externships; housing assistance; interactive nursing skills videos; Internet; learning resource lab; library services; nursing audiovisuals; other; paid internships; remedial services; resume preparation assistance; skills, simulation, or other laboratory; tutoring.

Library Facilities 80,034 volumes in health, 4,564 volumes in nursing; 73,528 periodical subscriptions health-care related.

BACCALAUREATE PROGRAMS

Degree BSN

Available Programs ADN to Baccalaureate; Accelerated Baccalaureate; Accelerated Baccalaureate for Second Degree; Generic Baccalaureate; RN Baccalaureate.

Site Options Montgomery, WV; Glenville, WV.

Study Options Full-time.

Program Entrance Requirements Minimum overall college GPA of 3.0, transcript of college record, CPR certification, health insurance, high school biology, high school chemistry, 3 years high school math, 3 years high school science, high school transcript, immunizations, minimum high school GPA of 3.0, minimum GPA in nursing prerequisites of 3.0, prerequisite course work. Transfer students are accepted. *Application deadline:* 1/15 (fall), 5/15 (spring). *Application fee:* $45.

Advanced Placement Credit by examination available. Credit given for nursing courses completed elsewhere dependent upon specific evaluations.

Expenses (2015–16) *Tuition, state resident:* full-time $8736; part-time $364 per credit. *Tuition, nonresident:* full-time $22,008; part-time $917 per credit. *Room and board:* $9286 per academic year. *Required fees:* full-time $1248; part-time $52 per credit.

Financial Aid *Gift aid (need-based):* Federal Pell, FSEOG, state, private, college/university gift aid from institutional funds. *Loans:* Federal Nursing Student Loans, Federal Direct (Subsidized and Unsubsidized Stafford PLUS), Perkins, college/university. *Work-study:* Federal Work-Study, part-time campus jobs. *Financial aid application deadline:* 3/1.

Contact Mrs. Kim McCourt, Recruiting and Outreach Coordinator, School of Nursing, West Virginia University, PO Box 9600, 6700 Health Sciences Center South, Morgantown, WV 26506-9600. *Telephone:* 304-293-1386. *Fax:* 304-293-2546. *E-mail:* kmccourt@hsc.wvu.edu.

GRADUATE PROGRAMS

Expenses (2015–16) *Tuition, state resident:* full-time $9054; part-time $503 per credit hour. *Tuition, nonresident:* full-time $21,996; part-time $1222 per credit hour. *Room and board:* $9000 per academic year. *Required fees:* full-time $1260; part-time $70 per credit.

Financial Aid 88% of graduate students in nursing programs received some form of financial aid in 2014–15. 1 teaching assistantship with tuition reimbursement available (averaging $10,000 per year) was awarded; institutionally sponsored loans, tuition waivers (partial), and graduate administrative assistantships also available. *Financial aid application deadline:* 2/1.

Contact Mrs. Kim McCourt, Recruiting and Outreach Coordinator, School of Nursing, West Virginia University, PO Box 9600, 6700 RCB Health Sciences Center South, Morgantown, WV 26506-9600. *Telephone:* 304-293-1386. *Fax:* 304-293-2546. *E-mail:* kmccourt@ hsc.wvu.edu.

MASTER'S DEGREE PROGRAM

Degree MSN

Available Programs Accelerated AD/RN to Master's; Accelerated Master's; Accelerated RN to Master's; Master's; RN to Master's.

Concentrations Available Nursing administration. *Nurse practitioner programs in:* family health, neonatal health, pediatric, women's health.

Site Options Charleston, WV.

Study Options Full-time and part-time.

Online Degree Options Yes (online only).

Program Entrance Requirements Computer literacy, minimum overall college GPA of 3.0, transcript of college record, CPR certification, written essay, immunizations, 3 letters of recommendation, nursing research course, physical assessment course, resume, statistics course. *Application deadline:* 2/1 (fall). *Application fee:* $60.

Advanced Placement Credit by examination available. Credit given for nursing courses completed elsewhere dependent upon specific evaluations.

Degree Requirements 44 total credit hours.

POST-MASTER'S PROGRAM

Areas of Study Nursing administration. *Nurse practitioner programs in:* family health, neonatal health, pediatric, women's health.

DOCTORAL DEGREE PROGRAM

Degree DNP

Available Programs Doctorate.

Areas of Study Addiction/substance abuse, advanced practice nursing, aging, bio-behavioral research, clinical practice, community health, ethics, family health, gerontology, health promotion/disease prevention, human health and illness, individualized study, maternity-newborn, neuro-behavior, nursing administration, oncology, women's health.

Online Degree Options Yes (online only).

Program Entrance Requirements Minimum overall college GPA of 3.0, 3 letters of recommendation, MSN or equivalent, statistics course, vita, writing sample. Application deadline: 3/1 (summer). Application fee: $50.

Degree Requirements 44 total credit hours, Capstone project, oral exam.

Degree PhD

Available Programs Doctorate.

Areas of Study Addiction/substance abuse, aging, bio-behavioral research, community health, ethics, gerontology, health promotion/disease prevention, human health and illness, individualized study, maternity-newborn, nursing research, oncology, women's health.

Site Options Charleston, WV.

Program Entrance Requirements Minimum overall college GPA of 3.0, interview by faculty committee, interview, 3 letters of recommendation, MSN or equivalent, statistics course, vita, writing sample, GRE General Test (PhD). Application deadline: 3/1 (summer). Application fee: $60.

Degree Requirements 55 total credit hours, dissertation, oral exam, written exam, residency.

CONTINUING EDUCATION PROGRAM

Contact Academic Innovations, School of Nursing, West Virginia University, PO Box 6800, 150 Clay Street, Morgantown, WV 26506-6800. *Telephone:* 800-253-2762. *Fax:* 304-293-4899. *E-mail:* elearn@ mail.wvu.edu.

West Virginia Wesleyan College
School of Nursing
Buckhannon, West Virginia

http://www.wvwc.edu/
Founded in 1890
DEGREES • BSN • MSN
Nursing Program Faculty 11 (36% with doctorates).
Baccalaureate Enrollment 140 **Women** 94% **Men** 6%
Graduate Enrollment 20 **Women** 97% **Men** 3%
Nursing Student Activities Nursing Honor Society, Sigma Theta Tau, Student Nurses' Association.
Nursing Student Resources Academic advising; academic or career counseling; assistance for students with disabilities; bookstore; campus computer network; career placement assistance; computer-assisted instruction; e-mail services; employment services for current students; externships; interactive nursing skills videos; Internet; learning resource lab; library services; nursing audiovisuals; placement services for program completers; remedial services; resume preparation assistance; skills, simulation, or other laboratory; tutoring.
Library Facilities 4,000 volumes in health, 600 volumes in nursing; 90 periodical subscriptions health-care related.

BACCALAUREATE PROGRAMS

Degree BSN
Available Programs Generic Baccalaureate.
Study Options Full-time and part-time.
Program Entrance Requirements Minimum overall college GPA of 3.0, transcript of college record, CPR certification, health exam, health insurance, high school transcript, immunizations, interview, minimum high school GPA of 2.5, minimum GPA in nursing prerequisites of 2.0, prerequisite course work. Transfer students are accepted. *Application deadline:* 6/15 (fall), 12/15 (spring). Applications may be processed on a rolling basis for some programs.
Advanced Placement Credit by examination available. Credit given for nursing courses completed elsewhere dependent upon specific evaluations.
Contact *Telephone:* 304-473-8224. *Fax:* 304-473-8435.

GRADUATE PROGRAMS

Contact *Telephone:* 304-473-8228.

MASTER'S DEGREE PROGRAM
Degree MSN
Available Programs Master's.
Concentrations Available Nurse-midwifery; nursing administration; nursing education. *Nurse practitioner programs in:* psychiatric/mental health.
Study Options Full-time and part-time.
Program Entrance Requirements Minimum overall college GPA of 3.0, transcript of college record, CPR certification, immunizations, interview, letters of recommendation, physical assessment course, professional liability insurance/malpractice insurance, resume, statistics course. *Application deadline:* 8/1 (fall), 12/10 (spring), 5/1 (summer). Applications may be processed on a rolling basis for some programs. *Application fee:* $50.
Degree Requirements 36 total credit hours, thesis or project.

Wheeling Jesuit University
Department of Nursing
Wheeling, West Virginia

http://www.wju.edu/
Founded in 1954
DEGREES • BSN • MSN
Nursing Program Faculty 26 (35% with doctorates).
Baccalaureate Enrollment 133 **Women** 93% **Men** 7% **Part-time** 52%
Graduate Enrollment 177 **Women** 94% **Men** 6% **Part-time** 88%
Distance Learning Courses Available.
Nursing Student Activities Sigma Theta Tau, Student Nurses' Association.
Nursing Student Resources Academic advising; academic or career counseling; assistance for students with disabilities; bookstore; campus computer network; career placement assistance; computer lab; computer-assisted instruction; e-mail services; employment services for current students; externships; housing assistance; Internet; learning resource lab; library services; nursing audiovisuals; placement services for program completers; remedial services; resume preparation assistance; skills, simulation, or other laboratory; tutoring.
Library Facilities 5,065 volumes in nursing; 90 periodical subscriptions health-care related.

BACCALAUREATE PROGRAMS

Degree BSN
Available Programs Accelerated Baccalaureate for Second Degree; Generic Baccalaureate; RN Baccalaureate.
Study Options Full-time and part-time.
Online Degree Options Yes.
Program Entrance Requirements Minimum overall college GPA of 2.75, transcript of college record, CPR certification, health exam, health insurance, high school transcript, immunizations, minimum GPA in nursing prerequisites of 2.0, prerequisite course work. Transfer students are accepted. *Application deadline:* Applications may be processed on a rolling basis for some programs.
Advanced Placement Credit by examination available. Credit given for nursing courses completed elsewhere dependent upon specific evaluations.
Contact *Telephone:* 304-243-2359. *Fax:* 304-243-2397.

GRADUATE PROGRAMS

Contact *Telephone:* 304-243-2344. *Fax:* 304-243-2608.

MASTER'S DEGREE PROGRAM
Degree MSN
Available Programs Master's; RN to Master's.
Concentrations Available Nursing administration; nursing education. *Nurse practitioner programs in:* family health.
Site Options Charleston, WV.
Study Options Full-time and part-time.
Online Degree Options Yes (online only).
Program Entrance Requirements Computer literacy, minimum overall college GPA of 3.0, 3 letters of recommendation, statistics course, GRE General Test or MAT. *Application deadline:* Applications may be processed on a rolling basis for some programs.
Advanced Placement Credit given for nursing courses completed elsewhere dependent upon specific evaluations.
Degree Requirements 42 total credit hours, thesis or project, comprehensive exam.

POST-MASTER'S PROGRAM
Areas of Study Nursing administration; nursing education. *Nurse practitioner programs in:* family health.

WISCONSIN

Alverno College
Division of Nursing
Milwaukee, Wisconsin

http://www.alverno.edu/
Founded in 1887
DEGREES • BSN • MSN
Nursing Program Faculty 39 (5% with doctorates).
Baccalaureate Enrollment 763 **Women** 100% **Part-time** 22%
Graduate Enrollment 43 **Women** 96% **Men** 4% **Part-time** 62%
Nursing Student Activities Student Nurses' Association.
Nursing Student Resources Academic advising; academic or career counseling; assistance for students with disabilities; bookstore; campus computer network; career placement assistance; computer lab; computer-assisted instruction; daycare for children of students; e-mail services; employment services for current students; externships; housing assistance; interactive nursing skills videos; Internet; learning resource lab; library services; nursing audiovisuals; remedial services; resume preparation assistance; skills, simulation, or other laboratory; tutoring; unpaid internships.

BACCALAUREATE PROGRAMS

Degree BSN

Available Programs ADN to Baccalaureate; Baccalaureate for Second Degree; Generic Baccalaureate; LPN to Baccalaureate; RN Baccalaureate.

Study Options Full-time and part-time.

Program Entrance Requirements Minimum overall college GPA of 2.5, transcript of college record, written essay, high school biology, high school chemistry, 3 years high school math, 2 years high school science, high school transcript, minimum high school GPA of 2.0, prerequisite course work. Transfer students are accepted.

Advanced Placement Credit by examination available. Credit given for nursing courses completed elsewhere dependent upon specific evaluations.

Contact *Telephone:* 414-382-6276. *Fax:* 414-382-6279.

GRADUATE PROGRAMS

Contact *Telephone:* 414-382-6278. *Fax:* 414-382-6279.

MASTER'S DEGREE PROGRAM

Degree MSN

Available Programs Master's.

Concentrations Available Nursing education. *Clinical nurse specialist programs in:* adult health, gerontology, medical-surgical.

Study Options Full-time and part-time.

Program Entrance Requirements Clinical experience, transcript of college record, CPR certification, written essay, immunizations, 3 letters of recommendation, physical assessment course, statistics course.

Advanced Placement Credit given for nursing courses completed elsewhere dependent upon specific evaluations.

Degree Requirements 39 total credit hours, thesis or project.

CONTINUING EDUCATION PROGRAM

Contact *Telephone:* 414-382-6177. *Fax:* 414-382-6354.

Bellin College

Nursing Program
Green Bay, Wisconsin

http://www.bellincollege.edu/
Founded in 1909

DEGREES • BSN • MSN

Nursing Program Faculty 20 (21% with doctorates).

Baccalaureate Enrollment 274 **Women** 92% **Men** 8% **Part-time** 9%

Graduate Enrollment 32 **Women** 93% **Men** 7% **Part-time** 81%

Distance Learning Courses Available.

Nursing Student Activities Sigma Theta Tau, Student Nurses' Association.

Nursing Student Resources Academic advising; academic or career counseling; assistance for students with disabilities; career placement assistance; computer lab; computer-assisted instruction; e-mail services; interactive nursing skills videos; Internet; learning resource lab; library services; nursing audiovisuals; resume preparation assistance; skills, simulation, or other laboratory; tutoring.

Library Facilities 7,000 volumes in health, 4,000 volumes in nursing; 190 periodical subscriptions health-care related.

BACCALAUREATE PROGRAMS

Degree BSN

Available Programs Accelerated Baccalaureate; Accelerated Baccalaureate for Second Degree; Baccalaureate for Second Degree; Generic Baccalaureate.

Study Options Full-time and part-time.

Program Entrance Requirements Minimum overall college GPA of 2.7, transcript of college record, CPR certification, health exam, health insurance, high school biology, high school chemistry, 3 years high school math, 3 years high school science, high school transcript, immunizations, interview, 3 letters of recommendation, minimum high school GPA of 3.25, minimum GPA in nursing prerequisites of 2.7. Transfer students are accepted. *Application deadline:* Applications may be processed on a rolling basis for some programs. *Application fee:* $30.

Advanced Placement Credit by examination available. Credit given for nursing courses completed elsewhere dependent upon specific evaluations.

Contact *Telephone:* 920-433-6651. *Fax:* 920-433-1922.

GRADUATE PROGRAMS

Contact *Telephone:* 920-433-3624. *Fax:* 920-433-1922.

MASTER'S DEGREE PROGRAM

Degree MSN

Available Programs Master's.

Concentrations Available Nursing administration; nursing education.

Study Options Full-time and part-time.

Online Degree Options Yes.

Program Entrance Requirements Computer literacy, minimum overall college GPA of 3.0, transcript of college record, written essay, interview, 3 letters of recommendation, nursing research course, resume, statistics course. *Application deadline:* Applications may be processed on a rolling basis for some programs. *Application fee:* $50.

Advanced Placement Credit given for nursing courses completed elsewhere dependent upon specific evaluations.

Degree Requirements 38 total credit hours, thesis or project.

Cardinal Stritch University

Ruth S. Coleman College of Nursing and Health Sciences
Milwaukee, Wisconsin

http://www.stritch.edu/nursing
Founded in 1937

DEGREES • BSN • MSN

Nursing Program Faculty 23

Baccalaureate Enrollment 255 **Women** 87.8% **Men** 12.2% **Part-time** 8.6%

Graduate Enrollment 18 **Women** 100% **Part-time** 50%

Distance Learning Courses Available.

Nursing Student Activities Sigma Theta Tau, Student Nurses' Association.

Nursing Student Resources Academic advising; academic or career counseling; assistance for students with disabilities; bookstore; campus computer network; career placement assistance; computer lab; e-mail services; employment services for current students; interactive nursing skills videos; Internet; learning resource lab; library services; nursing audiovisuals; other; remedial services; resume preparation assistance; skills, simulation, or other laboratory; tutoring.

BACCALAUREATE PROGRAMS

Degree BSN

Available Programs ADN to Baccalaureate; Accelerated RN Baccalaureate; Generic Baccalaureate.

Site Options Milwaukee, WI; West Allis, WI; Hartford, WI.

Study Options Full-time and part-time.

Online Degree Options Yes.

Program Entrance Requirements Minimum overall college GPA of 2.75, transcript of college record, high school transcript, minimum high school GPA of 2.75. Transfer students are accepted. *Application deadline:* Applications may be processed on a rolling basis for some programs.

Advanced Placement Credit by examination available. Credit given for nursing courses completed elsewhere dependent upon specific evaluations.

Expenses (2015–16) *Tuition:* full-time $13,445; part-time $880 per credit. *International tuition:* $13,445 full-time. *Room and board:* $7700 per academic year. *Required fees:* full-time $750; part-time $325 per term.

Financial Aid *Gift aid (need-based):* Federal Pell, FSEOG, state, private, college/university gift aid from institutional funds. *Loans:* Federal Direct (Subsidized and Unsubsidized Stafford PLUS), Perkins, state. *Work-study:* Federal Work-Study, part-time campus jobs. *Financial aid application deadline:* Continuous.

Contact Ms. Elyse Eggers, Nursing Admissions Counselor, Ruth S. Coleman College of Nursing and Health Sciences, Cardinal Stritch University, 6801 North Yates Road, Milwaukee, WI 53217-3985. *Telephone:* 414-410-4966. *Fax:* 414-410-4049. *E-mail:* ekeggers@stritch.edu.

GRADUATE PROGRAMS

Expenses (2015–16) *Tuition:* part-time $705 per credit. *Room and board:* $6518 per academic year.

Financial Aid 47% of graduate students in nursing programs received some form of financial aid in 2014–15.

Contact Alexandra Trumbull-Holper, Graduate Admissions Counselor, Ruth S. Coleman College of Nursing and Health Sciences, Cardinal Stritch University, 6801 North Yates Road, Milwaukee, WI 53217-3985. *Telephone:* 414-410-4093. *Fax:* 414-410-4049. *E-mail:* amtrumbull-holper@stritch.edu.

MASTER'S DEGREE PROGRAM
Degree MSN
Available Programs Master's.
Concentrations Available Nursing administration; nursing education.
Study Options Full-time and part-time.
Program Entrance Requirements Computer literacy, minimum overall college GPA of 3.0, transcript of college record, written essay, interview, 2 letters of recommendation, nursing research course, resume. *Application deadline:* Applications may be processed on a rolling basis for some programs.
Advanced Placement Credit given for nursing courses completed elsewhere dependent upon specific evaluations.
Degree Requirements 29 total credit hours, thesis or project.

Carroll University
Nursing Program
Waukesha, Wisconsin

http://www.carrollu.edu/programs/nursing/
Founded in 1846
DEGREE • BSN
Nursing Program Faculty 15
Baccalaureate Enrollment 372 **Women** 92.5% **Men** 7.5% **Part-time** 2.2%
Nursing Student Activities Nursing Honor Society, Sigma Theta Tau, Student Nurses' Association.
Nursing Student Resources Academic advising; academic or career counseling; assistance for students with disabilities; bookstore; campus computer network; computer lab; computer-assisted instruction; e-mail services; housing assistance; interactive nursing skills videos; Internet; learning resource lab; library services; nursing audiovisuals; resume preparation assistance; skills, simulation, or other laboratory; tutoring.

BACCALAUREATE PROGRAMS
Degree BSN
Available Programs ADN to Baccalaureate; Generic Baccalaureate.
Study Options Full-time.
Program Entrance Requirements Minimum overall college GPA of 2.75, transcript of college record, written essay, health exam, health insurance, high school biology, high school chemistry, 3 years high school math, high school transcript, minimum high school GPA of 2.75, minimum GPA in nursing prerequisites of 2.75, prerequisite course work. Transfer students are accepted. *Application deadline:* Applications may be processed on a rolling basis for some programs.
Expenses (2015–16) *Tuition:* full-time $29,660; part-time $469 per credit. *International tuition:* $29,660 full-time. *Room and board:* $9300; room only: $4936 per academic year. *Required fees:* full-time $775.
Financial Aid 98% of baccalaureate students in nursing programs received some form of financial aid in 2014–15.
Contact Ms. Angela Rose Brindowski, Chair, Department of Nursing, Nursing Program, Carroll University, 100 North East Avenue, Waukesha, WI 53186. *Telephone:* 262-524-4927. *E-mail:* abrindow@carrollu.edu.

Columbia College of Nursing
Milwaukee, Wisconsin

http://www.ccon.edu/
Founded in 2002
DEGREES • BSN • MSN
Nursing Program Faculty 25 (24% with doctorates).
Baccalaureate Enrollment 147 **Women** 91% **Men** 9% **Part-time** 1%
Graduate Enrollment 4 **Women** 100%
Nursing Student Activities Sigma Theta Tau, Student Nurses' Association.
Nursing Student Resources Academic advising; academic or career counseling; bookstore; campus computer network; career placement assistance; computer lab; computer-assisted instruction; e-mail services; employment services for current students; housing assistance; interactive nursing skills videos; Internet; learning resource lab; library services; nursing audiovisuals; resume preparation assistance; skills, simulation, or other laboratory; tutoring.
Library Facilities 2,500 volumes in health, 1,400 volumes in nursing; 69,950 periodical subscriptions health-care related.

BACCALAUREATE PROGRAMS
Degree BSN
Available Programs Baccalaureate for Second Degree; Generic Baccalaureate; RN Baccalaureate.
Site Options Mequon, WI; Milwaukee, WI.
Study Options Full-time and part-time.
Program Entrance Requirements Minimum overall college GPA of 2.8, transcript of college record, health exam, health insurance, high school transcript, minimum GPA in nursing prerequisites of 2.5, prerequisite course work. Transfer students are accepted. *Application deadline:* 3/1 (fall), 10/1 (spring). Applications may be processed on a rolling basis for some programs. *Application fee:* $50.
Expenses (2015–16) *Tuition:* full-time $26,230; part-time $795 per credit. *Required fees:* full-time $550; part-time $50 per credit.
Contact Mr. Tyler Lorenz, Academic Advisor, Columbia College of Nursing, 4425 North Port Washington Road, Glendale, WI 53129. *Telephone:* 414-326-1797. *Fax:* 414-326-2362. *E-mail:* admissions@ccon.edu.

GRADUATE PROGRAMS
Expenses (2015–16) *Tuition:* full-time $20,400; part-time $850 per credit. *Required fees:* full-time $450.
Contact Mr. Tyler Lorenz, Academic Advisor, Columbia College of Nursing, 4425 North Port Washington Road, Glendale, WI 53212. *Telephone:* 414-326-1797. *E-mail:* admissions@ccon.edu.

MASTER'S DEGREE PROGRAM
Degree MSN
Available Programs Master's.
Concentrations Available Clinical nurse leader.
Site Options Mequon, WI; Milwaukee, WI.
Study Options Full-time and part-time.
Program Entrance Requirements Minimum overall college GPA of 3.0, transcript of college record, written essay, interview, 3 letters of recommendation, nursing research course, physical assessment course, resume, statistics course. *Application deadline:* 4/20 (spring). Applications may be processed on a rolling basis for some programs. *Application fee:* $25.
Advanced Placement Credit given for nursing courses completed elsewhere dependent upon specific evaluations.
Degree Requirements 34 total credit hours, thesis or project.

Concordia University Wisconsin
Program in Nursing
Mequon, Wisconsin

http://www.cuw.edu/
Founded in 1881
DEGREES • BSN • DNP • MSN
Nursing Program Faculty 12 (3% with doctorates).
Baccalaureate Enrollment 291 **Women** 92% **Men** 8% **Part-time** 32%
Graduate Enrollment 787 **Women** 93% **Men** 7% **Part-time** 52%
Distance Learning Courses Available.
Nursing Student Activities Nursing Honor Society, Sigma Theta Tau, Student Nurses' Association.
Nursing Student Resources Academic advising; academic or career counseling; assistance for students with disabilities; bookstore; campus computer network; career placement assistance; computer lab; computer-assisted instruction; e-mail services; employment services for current students; externships; interactive nursing skills videos; Internet; learning resource lab; library services; nursing audiovisuals; paid internships; placement services for program completers; resume preparation assistance; skills, simulation, or other laboratory; tutoring.
Library Facilities 3,893 volumes in health, 1,011 volumes in nursing; 922 periodical subscriptions health-care related.

BACCALAUREATE PROGRAMS
Degree BSN

Available Programs ADN to Baccalaureate; Generic Baccalaureate; LPN to RN Baccalaureate; RN Baccalaureate.

Site Options Mequon, WI; Milwaukee, WI.

Study Options Full-time.

Program Entrance Requirements Transcript of college record, CPR certification, health exam, health insurance, high school transcript, immunizations, minimum high school GPA of 2.75, minimum GPA in nursing prerequisites of 2.75, RN licensure. Transfer students are accepted. *Application deadline:* 7/15 (fall), 7/15 (winter), 10/15 (spring), 3/15 (summer). *Application fee:* $50.

Advanced Placement Credit given for nursing courses completed elsewhere dependent upon specific evaluations.

Expenses (2014–15) *Tuition:* full-time $35,970; part-time $1080 per credit. *Room and board:* $9780 per academic year. *Required fees:* full-time $260; part-time $130 per term.

Financial Aid 98% of baccalaureate students in nursing programs received some form of financial aid in 2013–14. *Gift aid (need-based):* Federal Pell, FSEOG, state, private, college/university gift aid from institutional funds. *Loans:* Federal Direct (Subsidized and Unsubsidized Stafford PLUS), state. *Work-study:* Federal Work-Study. *Financial aid application deadline (priority):* 3/15.

Contact Dr. April Folgert, Chair of Traditional Undergraduate Department, Program in Nursing, Concordia University Wisconsin, 12800 North Lake Shore Drive, Mequon, WI 53097-2402. *Telephone:* 262-243-4452. *Fax:* 262-243-4466. *E-mail:* april.folgert@cuw.edu.

GRADUATE PROGRAMS

Expenses (2014–15) *Tuition:* part-time $640 per credit. *Required fees:* part-time $30 per term.

Financial Aid 91% of graduate students in nursing programs received some form of financial aid in 2013–14. *Application deadline:* 8/1.

Contact Dr. Sharon Chappy, Dean of the School of Nursing, Program in Nursing, Concordia University Wisconsin, 12800 North Lake Shore Drive, Mequon, WI 53097. *Telephone:* 262-243-4246. *Fax:* 262-243-4466. *E-mail:* sharon.chappy@cuw.edu.

MASTER'S DEGREE PROGRAM

Degree MSN

Available Programs Accelerated RN to Master's; Master's.

Concentrations Available Nursing education. *Nurse practitioner programs in:* adult health, family health.

Site Options Mequon, WI; Milwaukee, WI; multiple cities and states.

Study Options Full-time and part-time.

Online Degree Options Yes (online only).

Program Entrance Requirements Clinical experience, computer literacy, minimum overall college GPA of 3.0, transcript of college record, CPR certification, written essay, immunizations, interview, 3 letters of recommendation, physical assessment course, professional liability insurance/malpractice insurance, resume, statistics course. *Application deadline:* 5/1 (fall), 10/1 (spring). *Application fee:* $50.

Advanced Placement Credit given for nursing courses completed elsewhere dependent upon specific evaluations.

Degree Requirements 44 total credit hours, thesis or project.

POST-MASTER'S PROGRAM

Areas of Study *Nurse practitioner programs in:* adult health, family health.

DOCTORAL DEGREE PROGRAM

Degree DNP

Available Programs Doctorate.

Areas of Study Family health, gerontology, nursing administration, nursing education.

Site Options Mequon, WI; Milwaukee, WI; multiple cities and states.

Online Degree Options Yes (online only).

Program Entrance Requirements Clinical experience, minimum overall college GPA of 3.0, interview, 2 letters of recommendation, MSN or equivalent, statistics course, vita, writing sample. Application deadline: 4/1 (spring). Application fee: $50.

Degree Requirements 36 total credit hours, dissertation.

Edgewood College
Henry Predolin School of Nursing
Madison, Wisconsin

http://www.edgewood.edu/
Founded in 1927

DEGREES • BS • MS • MSN/MBA

Nursing Program Faculty 36 (25% with doctorates).

Baccalaureate Enrollment 220 **Women** 90% **Men** 10% **Part-time** 35%

Graduate Enrollment 45 **Women** 86% **Men** 14% **Part-time** 100%

Distance Learning Courses Available.

Nursing Student Activities Sigma Theta Tau, Student Nurses' Association.

Nursing Student Resources Academic advising; academic or career counseling; assistance for students with disabilities; bookstore; campus computer network; career placement assistance; computer lab; computer-assisted instruction; e-mail services; employment services for current students; externships; housing assistance; interactive nursing skills videos; Internet; learning resource lab; library services; nursing audiovisuals; paid internships; remedial services; resume preparation assistance; skills, simulation, or other laboratory; tutoring; unpaid internships.

Library Facilities 4,500 volumes in health, 1,000 volumes in nursing; 45 periodical subscriptions health-care related.

BACCALAUREATE PROGRAMS

Degree BS

Available Programs Accelerated Baccalaureate for Second Degree; Baccalaureate for Second Degree; Generic Baccalaureate.

Site Options Madison, WI.

Study Options Full-time and part-time.

Program Entrance Requirements Minimum overall college GPA of 2.75, transcript of college record, CPR certification, written essay, health exam, high school biology, high school chemistry, high school foreign language, high school math, high school transcript, immunizations, interview, minimum high school GPA of 2.75, minimum GPA in nursing prerequisites of 2.75, prerequisite course work. Transfer students are accepted. *Application deadline:* 1/15 (fall), 9/15 (spring). *Application fee:* $40.

Advanced Placement Credit given for nursing courses completed elsewhere dependent upon specific evaluations.

Contact *Telephone:* 608-663-2280. *Fax:* 608-663-2863.

GRADUATE PROGRAMS

Contact *Telephone:* 608-663-2280. *Fax:* 608-663-2863.

MASTER'S DEGREE PROGRAM

Degrees MS; MSN/MBA

Available Programs Master's.

Concentrations Available Nursing administration; nursing education.

Site Options Madison, WI.

Study Options Full-time and part-time.

Program Entrance Requirements Clinical experience, computer literacy, minimum overall college GPA of 3.0, transcript of college record, CPR certification, written essay, immunizations, interview, 2 letters of recommendation, nursing research course, prerequisite course work, resume, statistics course. *Application deadline:* Applications may be processed on a rolling basis for some programs.

Advanced Placement Credit given for nursing courses completed elsewhere dependent upon specific evaluations.

Degree Requirements 36 total credit hours, thesis or project.

Herzing University Online
Program in Nursing
Menomonee Falls, Wisconsin

http://www.herzing.edu

DEGREES • BSN • MSN

Nursing Program Faculty 27 (93% with doctorates).

Baccalaureate Enrollment 100 **Women** 85% **Men** 15% **Part-time** 55%

Graduate Enrollment 197 **Women** 75% **Men** 25% **Part-time** 47%

Distance Learning Courses Available.

Nursing Student Resources Academic advising; academic or career counseling; assistance for students with disabilities; bookstore; campus computer network; career placement assistance; computer-assisted instruction; e-mail services; employment services for current students; interactive nursing skills videos; learning resource lab; library services; nursing audiovisuals; other; paid internships; placement services for program completers; remedial services; resume preparation assistance; skills, simulation, or other laboratory; tutoring.

Library Facilities 300 volumes in health, 225 volumes in nursing; 4,274 periodical subscriptions health-care related.

BACCALAUREATE PROGRAMS

Degree BSN

Available Programs RN Baccalaureate.

Study Options Full-time and part-time.

Online Degree Options Yes (online only).

Program Entrance Requirements CPR certification, health exam, immunizations, prerequisite course work, RN licensure. Transfer students are accepted. *Application deadline:* Applications may be processed on a rolling basis for some programs. *Application fee:* $50.

Advanced Placement Credit given for nursing courses completed elsewhere dependent upon specific evaluations.

Contact Mr. Fred Ortiz, Nursing Admissions Director, Program in Nursing, Herzing University Online, Administrative Offices, W140 N8917 Lilly Road, Menomonee Falls, WI 53051. *Telephone:* 866-508-0748. *Fax:* 414-727-7090. *E-mail:* admissions@onl.herzing.edu.

GRADUATE PROGRAMS

Contact Dr. Catherine N. Kotecki, Department Chair of Nursing, Program in Nursing, Herzing University Online, W140 N8917 Lilly Road, Menomonee Falls, WI 53051. *Telephone:* 866-508-0748 Ext. 66815. *E-mail:* Ckotecki@herzing.edu.

MASTER'S DEGREE PROGRAM

Degree MSN

Available Programs Master's.

Concentrations Available Nursing education. *Nurse practitioner programs in:* family health.

Study Options Full-time and part-time.

Online Degree Options Yes (online only).

Program Entrance Requirements Computer literacy, minimum overall college GPA of 3.0, transcript of college record, CPR certification, written essay, immunizations, interview, 3 letters of recommendation, nursing research course, statistics course. *Application deadline:* Applications may be processed on a rolling basis for some programs. *Application fee:* $50.

Degree Requirements 36 total credit hours.

Maranatha Baptist University
Nursing Department
Watertown, Wisconsin

http://www.mbu.edu/academics/majors/nursing/
Founded in 1968

DEGREE • BSN

Baccalaureate Enrollment 58

Nursing Student Activities Student Nurses' Association.

Nursing Student Resources Academic advising; academic or career counseling; assistance for students with disabilities; bookstore; campus computer network; career placement assistance; computer lab; computer-assisted instruction; e-mail services; employment services for current students; housing assistance; interactive nursing skills videos; Internet; learning resource lab; library services; nursing audiovisuals; skills, simulation, or other laboratory; tutoring.

BACCALAUREATE PROGRAMS

Degree BSN

Available Programs RN Baccalaureate.

Program Entrance Requirements Minimum overall college GPA of 2.5, CPR certification, written essay, health exam, immunizations, interview, minimum high school GPA, minimum GPA in nursing prerequisites of 2.5, prerequisite course work. Transfer students are accepted. *Application deadline:* Applications may be processed on a rolling basis for some programs.

Contact *Telephone:* 920-206-4050.

Marian University
School of Nursing
Fond du Lac, Wisconsin

http://www.mariancollege.edu/
Founded in 1936

DEGREES • BSN • MSN

Baccalaureate Enrollment 221 **Women** 95% **Men** 5% **Part-time** 7%

Graduate Enrollment 39 **Women** 97% **Men** 3% **Part-time** 15%

Nursing Student Activities Student Nurses' Association.

Nursing Student Resources Academic advising; academic or career counseling; assistance for students with disabilities; bookstore; career placement assistance; computer lab; daycare for children of students; e-mail services; externships; interactive nursing skills videos; Internet; learning resource lab; library services; nursing audiovisuals.

Library Facilities 3,000 volumes in health, 2,500 volumes in nursing; 91 periodical subscriptions health-care related.

BACCALAUREATE PROGRAMS

Degree BSN

Available Programs ADN to Baccalaureate; Generic Baccalaureate.

Site Options Appleton, WI; Beaver Dam, WI.

Study Options Full-time and part-time.

Program Entrance Requirements Transcript of college record, high school biology, high school chemistry, 3 years high school math, high school science, high school transcript, minimum high school GPA of 2.5. Transfer students are accepted.

Advanced Placement Credit given for nursing courses completed elsewhere dependent upon specific evaluations.

Contact *Telephone:* 920-923-8732. *Fax:* 920-923-8770.

GRADUATE PROGRAMS

Contact *Telephone:* 920-923-8094. *Fax:* 920-923-8094.

MASTER'S DEGREE PROGRAM

Degree MSN

Available Programs Master's.

Concentrations Available Nursing education. *Nurse practitioner programs in:* adult health.

Study Options Full-time and part-time.

Program Entrance Requirements Clinical experience, minimum overall college GPA of 3.0, transcript of college record, CPR certification, written essay, immunizations, 3 letters of recommendation, nursing research course, professional liability insurance/malpractice insurance, resume, statistics course.

Advanced Placement Credit given for nursing courses completed elsewhere dependent upon specific evaluations.

Degree Requirements 39 total credit hours, thesis or project.

POST-MASTER'S PROGRAM

Areas of Study Nursing education.

Marquette University
College of Nursing
Milwaukee, Wisconsin

http://www.marquette.edu/nursing
Founded in 1881

DEGREES • BSN • DNP • MSN • MSN/MBA • PHD

Nursing Program Faculty 70 (51% with doctorates).

Baccalaureate Enrollment 565 **Women** 95% **Men** 5% **Part-time** 2%

Graduate Enrollment 304 **Women** 87.5% **Men** 12.5% **Part-time** 56%

Distance Learning Courses Available.

Nursing Student Activities Nursing Honor Society, Sigma Theta Tau, Student Nurses' Association.

Nursing Student Resources Academic advising; academic or career counseling; assistance for students with disabilities; bookstore; campus computer network; career placement assistance; computer-assisted instruction; daycare for children of students; e-mail services; employment services for current students; housing assistance; interactive nursing skills videos; Internet; learning resource lab; library services; nursing audiovisuals; remedial services; resume preparation assistance; skills, simulation, or other laboratory; tutoring.

Library Facilities 66,103 volumes in health, 7,866 volumes in nursing; 6,300 periodical subscriptions health-care related.

BACCALAUREATE PROGRAMS

Degree BSN
Available Programs Generic Baccalaureate.
Study Options Full-time and part-time.
Program Entrance Requirements Minimum overall college GPA of 3.0, transcript of college record, written essay, high school biology, high school chemistry, 3 years high school math, high school transcript, 1 letter of recommendation, minimum high school GPA of 2.5, minimum high school rank 25%. *Application deadline:* 12/1 (fall).
Advanced Placement Credit given for nursing courses completed elsewhere dependent upon specific evaluations.
Expenses (2015–16) *Tuition:* full-time $36,720; part-time $995 per credit hour. *International tuition:* $36,720 full-time. *Room and board:* $11,220; room only: $7230 per academic year. *Required fees:* full-time $450.
Financial Aid 100% of baccalaureate students in nursing programs received some form of financial aid in 2014–15. *Gift aid (need-based):* Federal Pell, FSEOG, state, private, college/university gift aid from institutional funds, Veterans Benefits. *Loans:* Federal Nursing Student Loans, Federal Direct (Subsidized and Unsubsidized Stafford PLUS), Perkins, state, college/university, private loans. *Work-study:* Federal Work-Study, part-time campus jobs. *Financial aid application deadline:* Continuous.
Contact Dr. Kerry Kosmoski-Goepfert, Associate Dean for Undergraduate Programs, College of Nursing, Marquette University, Clark Hall, PO Box 1881, Milwaukee, WI 53201-1881. *Telephone:* 414-288-3809. *Fax:* 414-288-1597. *E-mail:* kerry.goepfert@marquette.edu.

GRADUATE PROGRAMS

Expenses (2015–16) *Tuition:* part-time $1050 per credit.
Financial Aid 64% of graduate students in nursing programs received some form of financial aid in 2014–15. 1 fellowship with partial tuition reimbursement available (averaging $17,500 per year), 2 research assistantships with full tuition reimbursements available (averaging $13,285 per year), 8 teaching assistantships with full tuition reimbursements available (averaging $13,912 per year) were awarded; career-related internships or fieldwork, Federal Work-Study, scholarships, tuition waivers (partial), and unspecified assistantships also available. Aid available to part-time students. *Financial aid application deadline:* 2/15.
Contact Dr. Maureen O'Brien, Associate Dean for Graduate Programs, College of Nursing, Marquette University, Clark Hall, PO Box 1881, Milwaukee, WI 53201-1881. *Telephone:* 414-288-3869. *Fax:* 414-288-1597. *E-mail:* maureen.obrien@marquette.edu.

MASTER'S DEGREE PROGRAM

Degrees MSN; MSN/MBA
Available Programs Master's; Master's for Non-Nursing College Graduates; Master's for Nurses with Non-Nursing Degrees.
Concentrations Available Clinical nurse leader; nurse-midwifery; nursing administration. *Clinical nurse specialist programs in:* adult health. *Nurse practitioner programs in:* adult health, adult-gerontology acute care, pediatric, pediatric primary care.
Study Options Full-time and part-time.
Program Entrance Requirements Minimum overall college GPA of 3.0, transcript of college record, CPR certification, written essay, immunizations, 3 letters of recommendation, nursing research course, physical assessment course, prerequisite course work, resume, statistics course, GRE General Test. *Application deadline:* 2/15 (fall), 11/15 (spring). Applications may be processed on a rolling basis for some programs. *Application fee:* $65.
Advanced Placement Credit given for nursing courses completed elsewhere dependent upon specific evaluations.
Degree Requirements 42 total credit hours, comprehensive exam.

POST-MASTER'S PROGRAM

Areas of Study Nurse-midwifery; nursing administration. *Clinical nurse specialist programs in:* adult health. *Nurse practitioner programs in:* adult health, adult-gerontology acute care, family health, pediatric, pediatric primary care.

DOCTORAL DEGREE PROGRAM

Degree DNP
Available Programs Doctorate, Post-Baccalaureate Doctorate.
Areas of Study Advanced practice nursing, health-care systems, nursing administration.

Program Entrance Requirements Minimum overall college GPA of 3.0, 3 letters of recommendation, statistics course, vita. Application deadline: 2/15 (fall).
Degree Requirements 69 total credit hours, residency.

Degree PhD
Available Programs Doctorate; Post-Baccalaureate Doctorate.
Areas of Study Aging, faculty preparation, health promotion/disease prevention, health-care systems, human health and illness, illness and transition, nursing administration, nursing education, nursing research, nursing science.
Program Entrance Requirements Minimum overall college GPA of 3.2, interview, 3 letters of recommendation, MSN or equivalent, statistics course, vita, writing sample, GRE General Test. Application deadline: 2/15 (fall), 11/15 (spring). Applications may be processed on a rolling basis for some programs. Application fee: $65.
Degree Requirements 51 total credit hours, dissertation, oral exam, written exam, residency.

Milwaukee School of Engineering
School of Nursing
Milwaukee, Wisconsin

http://www.msoe.edu/nursing
Founded in 1903
DEGREES • BSN • MSN
Nursing Program Faculty 39 (27% with doctorates).
Baccalaureate Enrollment 239 **Women** 87% **Men** 13% **Part-time** .5%
Graduate Enrollment 10
Distance Learning Courses Available.
Nursing Student Activities Nursing Honor Society, Student Nurses' Association.
Nursing Student Resources Academic advising; academic or career counseling; assistance for students with disabilities; bookstore; campus computer network; career placement assistance; computer lab; computer-assisted instruction; e-mail services; employment services for current students; externships; housing assistance; interactive nursing skills videos; Internet; learning resource lab; library services; nursing audiovisuals; placement services for program completers; remedial services; resume preparation assistance; skills, simulation, or other laboratory; tutoring.
Library Facilities 2,528 volumes in health, 2,528 volumes in nursing; 8,625 periodical subscriptions health-care related.

BACCALAUREATE PROGRAMS

Degree BSN
Available Programs Accelerated Baccalaureate; Accelerated Baccalaureate for Second Degree; Accelerated RN Baccalaureate; Baccalaureate for Second Degree; Generic Baccalaureate; RN Baccalaureate.
Study Options Full-time and part-time.
Program Entrance Requirements Minimum overall college GPA of 3.0, transcript of college record, CPR certification, health exam, health insurance, high school biology, high school chemistry, 3 years high school math, 2 years high school science, high school transcript, immunizations, minimum high school GPA of 2.75. Transfer students are accepted. *Application deadline:* 9/1 (fall), 11/20 (winter), 3/1 (spring), 4/20 (summer). Applications may be processed on a rolling basis for some programs.
Advanced Placement Credit by examination available. Credit given for nursing courses completed elsewhere dependent upon specific evaluations.
Expenses (2015–16) *Tuition:* full-time $34,890; part-time $605 per credit. *International tuition:* $34,890 full-time. *Room and board:* $86,013; room only: $5439 per academic year. *Required fees:* full-time $1650.
Financial Aid 97% of baccalaureate students in nursing programs received some form of financial aid in 2014–15. *Gift aid (need-based):* Federal Pell, FSEOG, state, private, college/university gift aid from institutional funds. *Loans:* Federal Direct (Subsidized and Unsubsidized Stafford PLUS), Perkins, state, college/university. *Work-study:* Federal Work-Study. *Financial aid application deadline (priority):* 3/15.
Contact Dr. Debra L. Jenks, Chair, School of Nursing, Milwaukee School of Engineering, 1025 North Broadway Street, Milwaukee, WI 53202-3109. *Telephone:* 414-277-4516. *Fax:* 414-277-4540. *E-mail:* jenks@msoe.edu.

GRADUATE PROGRAMS

Expenses (2015–16) *Tuition:* part-time $732 per credit. *Room and board:* $8613; room only: $5439 per academic year.

Financial Aid 100% of graduate students in nursing programs received some form of financial aid in 2014–15.

Contact Dr. Debra Jenks, Department Chair, School of Nursing, Milwaukee School of Engineering, 1025 North Broadway, Milwaukee, WI 53202. *Telephone:* 414-277-4516. *Fax:* 414-277-4540. *E-mail:* jenks@msoe.edu.

MASTER'S DEGREE PROGRAM

Degree MSN

Available Programs Master's.

Concentrations Available Health-care administration; nursing administration.

Study Options Part-time.

Program Entrance Requirements Minimum overall college GPA of 3.0, transcript of college record, CPR certification, written essay, 3 letters of recommendation, nursing research course, statistics course. *Application deadline:* 9/1 (fall), 11/20 (winter), 3/1 (spring), 4/20 (summer). Applications may be processed on a rolling basis for some programs.

Advanced Placement Credit by examination available. Credit given for nursing courses completed elsewhere dependent upon specific evaluations.

Degree Requirements 47 total credit hours, thesis or project.

CONTINUING EDUCATION PROGRAM

Contact Dr. Debra L. Jenks, Department Chair, School of Nursing, Milwaukee School of Engineering, 1025 North Broadway, Milwaukee, WI 53202. *Telephone:* 414-277-4516. *Fax:* 414-277-4540. *E-mail:* jenks@msoe.edu.

Silver Lake College of the Holy Family

Nursing Program
Manitowoc, Wisconsin

http://www.sl.edu/
Founded in 1869

DEGREE • BSN
Nursing Program Faculty 1
Baccalaureate Enrollment 7 **Women** 100% **Part-time** 100%
Distance Learning Courses Available.
Nursing Student Resources Academic advising; academic or career counseling; assistance for students with disabilities; bookstore; campus computer network; computer lab; computer-assisted instruction; e-mail services; interactive nursing skills videos; Internet; learning resource lab; library services; nursing audiovisuals; tutoring.

BACCALAUREATE PROGRAMS

Degree BSN

Available Programs ADN to Baccalaureate.

Study Options Part-time.

Online Degree Options Yes.

Program Entrance Requirements Minimum overall college GPA of 2.0, transcript of college record, health insurance, immunizations, 1 letter of recommendation, minimum GPA in nursing prerequisites, prerequisite course work, RN licensure. Transfer students are accepted. *Application deadline:* Applications may be processed on a rolling basis for some programs.

Advanced Placement Credit given for nursing courses completed elsewhere dependent upon specific evaluations.

Expenses (2015–16) *Tuition:* part-time $500 per credit.

Contact Brianna Neuser, BSN Completion Program Director, Nursing Program, Silver Lake College of the Holy Family, 2406 South Alverno Road, Manitowoc, WI 54220. *Telephone:* 920-686-6213. *E-mail:* brianna.neuser@sl.edu.

University of Phoenix–Milwaukee Campus

College of Health and Human Services
Milwaukee, Wisconsin

http://www.phoenix.edu/campus-locations/wi/milwaukee-campus/milwaukee-campus.html
DEGREES • BSN • MSN • PHD

BACCALAUREATE PROGRAMS

Degree BSN

Available Programs RN Baccalaureate.

Contact *Telephone:* 262-785-0608.

GRADUATE PROGRAMS

Contact *Telephone:* 262-785-0608.

MASTER'S DEGREE PROGRAM

Degree MSN

Available Programs Master's.

DOCTORAL DEGREE PROGRAM

Degree PhD

Available Programs Doctorate.

University of Wisconsin– Eau Claire

College of Nursing and Health Sciences
Eau Claire, Wisconsin

http://www.uwec.edu/conhs/index.htm
Founded in 1916

DEGREES • BSN • DNP • MSN
Nursing Program Faculty 47 (28% with doctorates).
Baccalaureate Enrollment 401 **Women** 91% **Men** 9% **Part-time** 20%
Graduate Enrollment 102 **Women** 96% **Men** 4% **Part-time** 61%
Distance Learning Courses Available.
Nursing Student Activities Sigma Theta Tau, Student Nurses' Association.
Nursing Student Resources Academic advising; academic or career counseling; assistance for students with disabilities; bookstore; campus computer network; career placement assistance; computer lab; computer-assisted instruction; daycare for children of students; e-mail services; employment services for current students; housing assistance; interactive nursing skills videos; Internet; learning resource lab; library services; nursing audiovisuals; other; placement services for program completers; remedial services; resume preparation assistance; skills, simulation, or other laboratory; tutoring.
Library Facilities 17,256 volumes in health, 1,984 volumes in nursing; 3,893 periodical subscriptions health-care related.

BACCALAUREATE PROGRAMS

Degree BSN

Available Programs ADN to Baccalaureate; Accelerated Baccalaureate for Second Degree; Generic Baccalaureate; RN Baccalaureate.

Site Options Marshfield, WI.

Study Options Full-time.

Program Entrance Requirements Minimum overall college GPA of 3.0, transcript of college record, CPR certification, written essay, health exam, high school biology, high school chemistry, high school foreign language, 3 years high school math, 3 years high school science, high school transcript, immunizations, minimum GPA in nursing prerequisites of 2.5, prerequisite course work. Transfer students are accepted. *Application deadline:* 5/1 (fall), 12/1 (spring). *Application fee:* $86.

Advanced Placement Credit given for nursing courses completed elsewhere dependent upon specific evaluations.

Contact *Telephone:* 715-836-5287. *Fax:* 715-836-5925.

GRADUATE PROGRAMS

Contact *Telephone:* 715-836-5287. *Fax:* 715-836-5925.

MASTER'S DEGREE PROGRAM

Degree MSN

Available Programs Master's; RN to Master's.

Concentrations Available Nursing administration; nursing education. *Clinical nurse specialist programs in:* adult health. *Nurse practitioner programs in:* adult health, family health, gerontology.

Site Options Marshfield, WI.

Study Options Full-time and part-time.

Program Entrance Requirements Clinical experience, minimum overall college GPA of 3.0, transcript of college record, CPR certification, written essay, immunizations, 3 letters of recommendation, physical assessment course, professional liability insurance/malpractice insurance, statistics course. *Application deadline:* 1/15 (summer). Applications may be processed on a rolling basis for some programs. *Application fee:* $86.

Advanced Placement Credit given for nursing courses completed elsewhere dependent upon specific evaluations.

Degree Requirements 42 total credit hours, thesis or project.

POST-MASTER'S PROGRAM

Areas of Study Nursing administration; nursing education. *Clinical nurse specialist programs in:* adult health. *Nurse practitioner programs in:* adult health, family health, gerontology.

DOCTORAL DEGREE PROGRAM

Degree DNP

Available Programs Doctorate; Post-Baccalaureate Doctorate.

Areas of Study Family health, gerontology, nursing administration.

Program Entrance Requirements Clinical experience, minimum overall college GPA of 3.00, 3 letters of recommendation, statistics course, vita, writing sample. Application deadline: 1/4 (summer). Applications may be processed on a rolling basis for some programs. Application fee: $86.

Degree Requirements 72 total credit hours.

CONTINUING EDUCATION PROGRAM

Contact *Telephone:* 715-836-5645. *Fax:* 715-836-5263.

University of Wisconsin– Green Bay

Online Nursing and Health Programs
Green Bay, Wisconsin

http://www.uwgb.edu/nursing/
Founded in 1968

DEGREES • BSN • MSN

Nursing Program Faculty 12 (92% with doctorates).
Baccalaureate Enrollment 401 **Women** 92% **Men** 8% **Part-time** 97%
Graduate Enrollment 32 **Women** 84% **Men** 16% **Part-time** 100%
Distance Learning Courses Available.
Nursing Student Activities Sigma Theta Tau, Student Nurses' Association.
Nursing Student Resources Academic advising; academic or career counseling; assistance for students with disabilities; bookstore; campus computer network; career placement assistance; computer lab; computer-assisted instruction; e-mail services; employment services for current students; Internet; learning resource lab; library services; nursing audiovisuals; resume preparation assistance; skills, simulation, or other laboratory; tutoring.
Library Facilities 1,000 volumes in health, 675 volumes in nursing; 100 periodical subscriptions health-care related.

BACCALAUREATE PROGRAMS

Degree BSN

Available Programs ADN to Baccalaureate.

Site Options Marinette, WI; Rhinelander, WI.

Study Options Full-time and part-time.

Online Degree Options Yes.

Program Entrance Requirements Minimum overall college GPA of 2.5, transcript of college record, RN licensure. Transfer students are accepted. *Application fee:* $44.

Expenses (2015–16) *Tuition, area resident:* part-time $323 per credit hour. *Tuition, state resident:* part-time $452 per credit hour. *Tuition, nonresident:* part-time $415 per credit hour.

Financial Aid 42% of baccalaureate students in nursing programs received some form of financial aid in 2014–15.

Contact Ms. Ruth Pearson, Student Services Specialist, Online Nursing and Health Programs, University of Wisconsin–Green Bay, 2420 Nicolet Drive, Green Bay, WI 54311-7001. *Telephone:* 920-465-2818. *Fax:* 920-465-2854. *E-mail:* pearsonr@uwgb.edu.

GRADUATE PROGRAMS

Expenses (2015–16) *Tuition, state resident:* part-time $571 per credit hour. *Tuition, nonresident:* part-time $571 per credit hour.

Financial Aid 33% of graduate students in nursing programs received some form of financial aid in 2014–15.

Contact Dr. Janet Reilly, Director of MSN-LINC, Online Nursing and Health Programs, University of Wisconsin–Green Bay, 2420 Nicolet Drive, RH 325, Green Bay, WI 54311-7001. *Telephone:* 920-465-2365. *Fax:* 920-465-2854. *E-mail:* reillyj@uwgb.edu.

MASTER'S DEGREE PROGRAM

Degree MSN

Available Programs Master's.

Concentrations Available Nursing administration.

Study Options Part-time.

Online Degree Options Yes (online only).

Program Entrance Requirements Minimum overall college GPA of 3.0, transcript of college record, written essay, 3 letters of recommendation, resume, statistics course. *Application deadline:* 7/1 (fall), 12/1 (spring). *Application fee:* $54.

Advanced Placement Credit given for nursing courses completed elsewhere dependent upon specific evaluations.

Degree Requirements 34 total credit hours, thesis or project.

University of Wisconsin–Madison

School of Nursing
Madison, Wisconsin

http://www.son.wisc.edu/
Founded in 1848

DEGREES • BS • PHD

Nursing Program Faculty 52 (35% with doctorates).
Baccalaureate Enrollment 384 **Women** 86% **Men** 14% **Part-time** 25%
Graduate Enrollment 164 **Women** 95% **Men** 5% **Part-time** 60%
Distance Learning Courses Available.
Nursing Student Activities Nursing Honor Society, Sigma Theta Tau, Student Nurses' Association, nursing club.
Nursing Student Resources Academic advising; academic or career counseling; assistance for students with disabilities; bookstore; campus computer network; career placement assistance; computer lab; computer-assisted instruction; e-mail services; externships; interactive nursing skills videos; Internet; learning resource lab; library services; nursing audiovisuals; resume preparation assistance; skills, simulation, or other laboratory; tutoring.
Library Facilities 334,000 volumes in health, 8,300 volumes in nursing; 1,500 periodical subscriptions health-care related.

BACCALAUREATE PROGRAMS

Degree BS

Available Programs ADN to Baccalaureate; Generic Baccalaureate; RN Baccalaureate.

Study Options Full-time.

Program Entrance Requirements Minimum overall college GPA of 2.75, transcript of college record, CPR certification, written essay, high school chemistry, high school foreign language, 3 years high school math, 3 years high school science, high school transcript, immunizations, minimum GPA in nursing prerequisites of 2.75, prerequisite course work. Transfer students are accepted. *Application deadline:* 2/1 (fall). *Application fee:* $50.

Advanced Placement Credit by examination available. Credit given for nursing courses completed elsewhere dependent upon specific evaluations.

Expenses (2015–16) *Tuition, state resident:* full-time $10,416; part-time $481 per credit. *Tuition, nonresident:* full-time $29,665; part-time $1283 per credit. *International tuition:* $30,666 full-time. *Required fees:* full-time $1142; part-time $94 per credit.

Financial Aid *Gift aid (need-based):* Federal Pell, FSEOG, state, private, college/university gift aid from institutional funds. *Loans:* Federal Nursing Student Loans, Federal Direct (Subsidized and Unsubsidized

Stafford PLUS), Perkins. *Work-study:* Federal Work-Study, part-time campus jobs. *Financial aid application deadline:* Continuous.

Contact Nursing Admissions, School of Nursing, University of Wisconsin–Madison, 701 Highland Avenue, Madison, WI 53705. *Telephone:* 608-263-5202. *Fax:* 608-263-5296. *E-mail:* ugadmit@son.wisc.edu.

GRADUATE PROGRAMS

Expenses (2015–16) *Tuition, state resident:* full-time $12,989; part-time $856 per credit. *Tuition, nonresident:* full-time $26,796; part-time $1719 per credit. *Required fees:* full-time $1142.

Financial Aid 8 fellowships (averaging $26,900 per year), 8 research assistantships (averaging $18,000 per year), 5 teaching assistantships (averaging $11,000 per year) were awarded; career-related internships or fieldwork, Federal Work-Study, institutionally sponsored loans, scholarships, traineeships, and unspecified assistantships also available.

Contact Kristi Hammond, Graduate Program Coordinator, School of Nursing, University of Wisconsin–Madison, 701 Highland Avenue, Madison, WI 53705. *Telephone:* 608-263-5258. *Fax:* 608-263-5296. *E-mail:* khammond@wisc.edu.

DOCTORAL DEGREE PROGRAM

Degree PhD

Available Programs Doctorate; Post-Baccalaureate Doctorate.

Areas of Study Aging, bio-behavioral research, biology of health and illness, community health, faculty preparation, family health, gerontology, health policy, health promotion/disease prevention, human health and illness, information systems, nursing education, nursing research, oncology, women's health.

Program Entrance Requirements Minimum overall college GPA of 3.0, interview, 3 letters of recommendation, scholarly papers, vita, writing sample, GRE General Test. Application deadline: 1/15 (fall), 9/15 (spring). Application fee: $56.

Degree Requirements 60 total credit hours, dissertation, written exam, residency.

POSTDOCTORAL PROGRAM

Areas of Study Adolescent health, aging, cancer care, chronic illness, community health, family health, gerontology, health promotion/disease prevention, individualized study, nursing informatics, nursing interventions, nursing research, vulnerable population, women's health.

Postdoctoral Program Contact Carol Aspinwall, Student Services Coordinator, School of Nursing, University of Wisconsin–Madison, 701 Highland Avenue, Madison, WI 53705. *Telephone:* 608-263-9109. *Fax:* 608-263-5296. *E-mail:* caaspinwall@wisc.edu.

CONTINUING EDUCATION PROGRAM

Contact Ms. Sandra Galles, Senior Outreach Specialist, School of Nursing, University of Wisconsin–Madison, 701 Highland Avenue, Madison, WI 53705. *Telephone:* 608-265-9003. *Fax:* 608-262-0053. *E-mail:* slgalles@wisc.edu.

University of Wisconsin–Milwaukee

College of Nursing
Milwaukee, Wisconsin

http://www.nursing.uwm.edu/
Founded in 1956

DEGREES • BSN • DNP • MN • PHD

Nursing Program Faculty 26 (100% with doctorates).
Baccalaureate Enrollment 1,243 **Women** 85% **Men** 15% **Part-time** 30%
Graduate Enrollment 293 **Women** 89% **Men** 11% **Part-time** 54%
Distance Learning Courses Available.
Nursing Student Activities Sigma Theta Tau, Student Nurses' Association.
Nursing Student Resources Academic advising; academic or career counseling; assistance for students with disabilities; bookstore; campus computer network; career placement assistance; computer lab; computer-assisted instruction; e-mail services; interactive nursing skills videos; Internet; learning resource lab; library services; nursing audiovisuals; remedial services; skills, simulation, or other laboratory; tutoring.
Library Facilities 330,089 volumes in health, 179,089 volumes in nursing; 926 periodical subscriptions health-care related.

BACCALAUREATE PROGRAMS

Degree BSN
Available Programs ADN to Baccalaureate; Generic Baccalaureate; RN Baccalaureate.
Site Options West Bend, WI; Kenosha, WI.
Study Options Full-time and part-time.
Program Entrance Requirements Minimum overall college GPA of 2.75, transcript of college record, written essay, high school biology, high school chemistry, high school foreign language, 3 years high school math, 3 years high school science, high school transcript, minimum high school GPA of 2.0, minimum GPA in nursing prerequisites of 2.75, prerequisite course work. Transfer students are accepted. *Application deadline:* 1/15 (fall), 8/15 (spring). *Application fee:* $44.
Advanced Placement Credit given for nursing courses completed elsewhere dependent upon specific evaluations.
Expenses (2015–16) *Tuition, state resident:* full-time $8091; part-time $337 per credit. *Tuition, nonresident:* full-time $18,265; part-time $761 per credit. *Room and board:* $6290 per academic year. *Required fees:* part-time $32 per credit.
Financial Aid *Gift aid (need-based):* Federal Pell, FSEOG, state, private, college/university gift aid from institutional funds, Federal Nursing. *Loans:* Federal Nursing Student Loans, Federal Direct (Subsidized and Unsubsidized Stafford PLUS), Perkins, state, alternative loans. *Work-study:* Federal Work-Study. *Financial aid application deadline (priority):* 3/1.
Contact Ms. Donna Wier, Senior Advisor, College of Nursing, University of Wisconsin–Milwaukee, PO Box 413, Student Affairs, Milwaukee, WI 53201. *Telephone:* 414-229-5481. *Fax:* 414-229-5554. *E-mail:* ddw@uwm.edu.

GRADUATE PROGRAMS

Expenses (2015–16) *Tuition, state resident:* full-time $11,748; part-time $1196 per credit. *Tuition, nonresident:* full-time $24,784; part-time $1464 per credit. *Room and board:* $6290 per academic year.
Financial Aid Fellowships, research assistantships, teaching assistantships, career-related internships or fieldwork, Federal Work-Study, unspecified assistantships, and project assistantships available.
Contact Ms. Robin Jens, Director, Student Services, College of Nursing, University of Wisconsin–Milwaukee, PO Box 413, Student Affairs, Milwaukee, WI 53201. *Telephone:* 414-229-2494. *Fax:* 414-229-5554. *E-mail:* rjens@uwm.edu.

MASTER'S DEGREE PROGRAM

Degree MN
Available Programs Master's; Master's for Non-Nursing College Graduates.
Concentrations Available Clinical nurse leader.
Study Options Full-time and part-time.
Program Entrance Requirements Minimum overall college GPA of 3.0, transcript of college record, written essay, 3 letters of recommendation, prerequisite course work, resume, statistics course, GRE General Test or MAT. *Application deadline:* 1/1 (fall), 9/1 (spring). *Application fee:* $56.
Advanced Placement Credit given for nursing courses completed elsewhere dependent upon specific evaluations.
Degree Requirements 33 total credit hours.

DOCTORAL DEGREE PROGRAM

Degree DNP
Available Programs Doctorate, Post-Baccalaureate Doctorate.
Areas of Study Advanced practice nursing, clinical practice, community health, family health, gerontology, health-care systems, human health and illness, individualized study, maternity-newborn, neuro-behavior, women's health.
Program Entrance Requirements Minimum overall college GPA of 3.2, interview, 3 letters of recommendation, scholarly papers, statistics course, vita, writing sample. Application deadline: 1/1 (fall), 9/1 (spring), 11/1 (summer). Applications may be processed on a rolling basis for some programs. Application fee: $56.
Degree Requirements 64 total credit hours, residency.

Degrees DNP; PhD
Available Programs Doctorate; Post-Baccalaureate Doctorate.
Areas of Study Health-care systems, individualized study, neuro-behavior, nursing research, women's health.
Program Entrance Requirements Minimum overall college GPA of 3.2, interview, 3 letters of recommendation, scholarly papers, statistics course, vita, writing sample, GRE. Application deadline: 1/1 (fall), 9/1

(spring), 11/1 (summer). Applications may be processed on a rolling basis for some programs. Application fee: $56.

Degree Requirements 64 total credit hours, dissertation, oral exam, written exam.

See display below and full description on page 512.

University of Wisconsin–Oshkosh
College of Nursing
Oshkosh, Wisconsin

http://www.uwosh.edu/con
Founded in 1871
DEGREES • BSN • DNP • MSN
Nursing Program Faculty 87 (28% with doctorates).
Baccalaureate Enrollment 559 **Women** 91% **Men** 9% **Part-time** 24%
Graduate Enrollment 124 **Women** 94% **Men** 6% **Part-time** 58%
Distance Learning Courses Available.
Nursing Student Activities Sigma Theta Tau, Student Nurses' Association, nursing club.
Nursing Student Resources Academic advising; academic or career counseling; assistance for students with disabilities; bookstore; campus computer network; career placement assistance; computer lab; computer-assisted instruction; daycare for children of students; e-mail services; employment services for current students; externships; housing assistance; interactive nursing skills videos; Internet; learning resource lab; library services; nursing audiovisuals; other; paid internships; placement services for program completers; remedial services; resume preparation assistance; skills, simulation, or other laboratory; tutoring; unpaid internships.

BACCALAUREATE PROGRAMS

Degree BSN
Available Programs ADN to Baccalaureate; Accelerated Baccalaureate for Second Degree; RN Baccalaureate.
Site Options Janesville, WI; Wausau, WI; Sheboygan/Manitowoc, WI.
Study Options Full-time and part-time.
Online Degree Options Yes.

Program Entrance Requirements Minimum overall college GPA of 2.75, transcript of college record, CPR certification, written essay, interview, minimum GPA in nursing prerequisites of 3.0, prerequisite course work. Transfer students are accepted. *Application deadline:* 1/30 (fall), 8/30 (spring).
Financial Aid 60% of baccalaureate students in nursing programs received some form of financial aid in 2014–15. *Gift aid (need-based):* Federal Pell, FSEOG, state, private, college/university gift aid from institutional funds, United Negro College Fund, Federal Nursing. *Loans:* Federal Nursing Student Loans, Federal Direct (Subsidized and Unsubsidized Stafford PLUS), Perkins, state, college/university. *Work-study:* Federal Work-Study, part-time campus jobs. *Financial aid application deadline (priority):* 3/15.
Contact Mrs. Sarah White, Pre-Licensure Program Associate, College of Nursing, University of Wisconsin–Oshkosh, 800 Algoma Boulevard, Oshkosh, WI 54901-8660. *Telephone:* 920-424-1028. *Fax:* 920-424-0123. *E-mail:* undergradnrs@uwosh.edu.

GRADUATE PROGRAMS

Financial Aid 53% of graduate students in nursing programs received some form of financial aid in 2014–15. Fellowships, research assistantships with partial tuition reimbursements available, institutionally sponsored loans, scholarships, traineeships, tuition waivers (partial), and unspecified assistantships available. *Financial aid application deadline:* 3/15.
Contact Ms. Katrina Helmer, Graduate Program Assistant, College of Nursing, University of Wisconsin–Oshkosh, College of Nursing, 800 Algoma Boulevard, Oshkosh, WI 54901-8660. *Telephone:* 920-424-2106. *Fax:* 920-424-0123. *E-mail:* congrad@uwosh.edu.

MASTER'S DEGREE PROGRAM
Degree MSN
Available Programs Master's; RN to Master's.
Concentrations Available Clinical nurse leader; nursing education.
Study Options Full-time and part-time.
Online Degree Options Yes (online only).
Program Entrance Requirements Computer literacy, minimum overall college GPA of 3.0, transcript of college record, CPR certification, written essay, immunizations, interview, 3 letters of recommendation, resume, statistics course. *Application deadline:* 4/1 (fall). *Application fee:* $56.

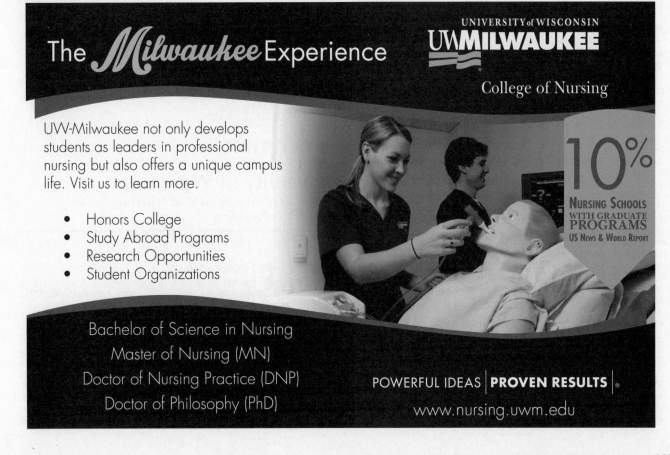

The *Milwaukee* Experience

UNIVERSITY of WISCONSIN
UWMILWAUKEE
College of Nursing

UW-Milwaukee not only develops students as leaders in professional nursing but also offers a unique campus life. Visit us to learn more.

- Honors College
- Study Abroad Programs
- Research Opportunities
- Student Organizations

10%
NURSING SCHOOLS
WITH GRADUATE
PROGRAMS
US NEWS & WORLD REPORT

Bachelor of Science in Nursing
Master of Nursing (MN)
Doctor of Nursing Practice (DNP)
Doctor of Philosophy (PhD)

POWERFUL IDEAS | **PROVEN RESULTS**

www.nursing.uwm.edu

Advanced Placement Credit given for nursing courses completed elsewhere dependent upon specific evaluations.
Degree Requirements 37 total credit hours, thesis or project.

POST-MASTER'S PROGRAM
Areas of Study Clinical nurse leader; nursing education; nursing informatics.

DOCTORAL DEGREE PROGRAM
Degree DNP
Available Programs Doctorate; Post-Baccalaureate Doctorate.
Areas of Study Advanced practice nursing.
Program Entrance Requirements Minimum overall college GPA of 3.0, interview, 3 letters of recommendation, statistics course, vita, writing sample. Application deadline: 4/1 (fall). Application fee: $56.
Degree Requirements 74 total credit hours, residency.

CONTINUING EDUCATION PROGRAM
Contact Dr. Charles Hill, Director, Lifelong Learning and Community Engagement, College of Nursing, University of Wisconsin–Oshkosh, 800 Algoma Boulevard, Oshkosh, WI 54901-8660. *Telephone:* 920-424-1255. *E-mail:* hill@uwosh.edu.

Viterbo University
School of Nursing
La Crosse, Wisconsin

http://www.viterbo.edu/
Founded in 1890
DEGREES • BSN • DNP
Nursing Program Faculty 36 (15% with doctorates).
Baccalaureate Enrollment 876 **Women** 94% **Men** 6% **Part-time** 20%
Graduate Enrollment 60 **Women** 99% **Men** 1% **Part-time** 15%
Distance Learning Courses Available.
Nursing Student Activities Sigma Theta Tau, Student Nurses' Association.
Nursing Student Resources Academic advising; academic or career counseling; assistance for students with disabilities; bookstore; campus computer network; career placement assistance; computer lab; computer-assisted instruction; e-mail services; employment services for current students; interactive nursing skills videos; Internet; learning resource lab; library services; nursing audiovisuals; remedial services; resume preparation assistance; skills, simulation, or other laboratory; tutoring.
Library Facilities 5,200 volumes in health, 3,398 volumes in nursing; 312 periodical subscriptions health-care related.

BACCALAUREATE PROGRAMS
Degree BSN
Available Programs Generic Baccalaureate; RN Baccalaureate.
Site Options Madison, WI; Rochester, MN; Janesville, WI.
Study Options Full-time and part-time.
Program Entrance Requirements Minimum overall college GPA of 2.75, transcript of college record, CPR certification, health exam, high school chemistry, 2 years high school math, 2 years high school science, high school transcript, immunizations, minimum high school GPA of 3.0, minimum high school rank 55%, minimum GPA in nursing prerequisites of 2.75, prerequisite course work. Transfer students are accepted. *Application deadline:* Applications may be processed on a rolling basis for some programs.
Advanced Placement Credit given for nursing courses completed elsewhere dependent upon specific evaluations.
Expenses (2015–16) *Tuition:* full-time $24,360; part-time $720 per credit. *Room and board:* $5955; room only: $3650 per academic year. *Required fees:* part-time $280 per credit; part-time $95 per term.
Financial Aid 98% of baccalaureate students in nursing programs received some form of financial aid in 2014–15.
Contact Eric Schmidt, Associate Director for Admissions, School of Nursing, Viterbo University, 900 Viterbo Drive, La Crosse, WI 54601. *Telephone:* 608-796-3017. *Fax:* 608-796-3050. *E-mail:* eschmidt@viterbo.edu.

GRADUATE PROGRAMS
Expenses (2015–16) *Tuition:* part-time $750 per credit.
Financial Aid 15% of graduate students in nursing programs received some form of financial aid in 2014–15.

Contact Dr. Mary Ellen Stolder, Director, School of Nursing, Viterbo University, 900 Viterbo Drive, La Crosse, WI 54601. *Telephone:* 608-796-3688. *Fax:* 608-796-3668. *E-mail:* mestolder@viterbo.edu.

MASTER'S DEGREE PROGRAM
Program Entrance Requirements *Application deadline:* 2/15 (fall). *Application fee:* $50.

DOCTORAL DEGREE PROGRAM
Degree DNP
Available Programs Doctorate.
Areas of Study Advanced practice nursing.
Program Entrance Requirements Clinical experience, minimum overall college GPA of 3.0, interview by faculty committee, 2 letters of recommendation, statistics course, vita, writing sample. Application deadline: 2/15 (fall). Application fee: $50.
Degree Requirements 66 total credit hours, residency.

Wisconsin Lutheran College
Nursing Program
Milwaukee, Wisconsin

Founded in 1973
DEGREE • BSN
Nursing Program Faculty 2
Baccalaureate Enrollment 14
Nursing Student Activities Student Nurses' Association.
Nursing Student Resources Academic advising; academic or career counseling; assistance for students with disabilities; bookstore; campus computer network; career placement assistance; computer lab; computer-assisted instruction; e-mail services; externships; housing assistance; interactive nursing skills videos; Internet; learning resource lab; library services; nursing audiovisuals; skills, simulation, or other laboratory; tutoring.

BACCALAUREATE PROGRAMS
Degree BSN
Available Programs Generic Baccalaureate.
Study Options Full-time.
Program Entrance Requirements Minimum overall college GPA of 2.75, transcript of college record, written essay, high school foreign language, interview, 3 letters of recommendation, minimum GPA in nursing prerequisites of 2.0, prerequisite course work. Transfer students are accepted. *Application deadline:* 3/15 (spring).
Contact *Telephone:* 414-443-8800.

CONTINUING EDUCATION PROGRAM
Contact *Telephone:* 414-443-8800.

WYOMING

University of Wyoming
Fay W. Whitney School of Nursing
Laramie, Wyoming

http://www.uwyo.edu/nursing
Founded in 1886
DEGREES • BSN • DNP • MS
Nursing Program Faculty 52 (33% with doctorates).
Baccalaureate Enrollment 364 **Women** 87% **Men** 13% **Part-time** 70%
Graduate Enrollment 62 **Women** 87% **Men** 13% **Part-time** 24%
Distance Learning Courses Available.
Nursing Student Activities Sigma Theta Tau, Student Nurses' Association.
Nursing Student Resources Academic advising; academic or career counseling; assistance for students with disabilities; bookstore; campus computer network; career placement assistance; computer lab; computer-assisted instruction; e-mail services; employment services for current students; externships; housing assistance; interactive nursing skills videos; Internet; learning resource lab; library services; nursing audiovisuals; paid internships; placement services for program completers; remedial

services; resume preparation assistance; skills, simulation, or other laboratory; tutoring; unpaid internships.

Library Facilities 56,231 volumes in health; 1,689 periodical subscriptions health-care related.

BACCALAUREATE PROGRAMS

Degree BSN

Available Programs ADN to Baccalaureate; Accelerated Baccalaureate for Second Degree; Generic Baccalaureate.

Study Options Full-time.

Online Degree Options Yes.

Program Entrance Requirements Transcript of college record, CPR certification, written essay, immunizations, interview, minimum GPA in nursing prerequisites of 2.75, professional liability insurance/malpractice insurance, prerequisite course work. Transfer students are accepted. *Application deadline:* 2/1 (fall). *Application fee:* $68.

Expenses (2015–16) *Tuition, state resident:* part-time $119 per credit hour. *Tuition, nonresident:* part-time $477 per credit hour.

Contact Ms. Debbie A. Shoefelt, Credentials Analyst/Academic Advisor, Fay W. Whitney School of Nursing, University of Wyoming, Department 3065, 1000 East University Avenue, Laramie, WY 82071. *Telephone:* 307-766-4292. *Fax:* 307-766-4294. *E-mail:* basicbsn@uwyo.edu.

GRADUATE PROGRAMS

Financial Aid Research assistantships (averaging $10,062 per year), teaching assistantships (averaging $10,062 per year) were awarded; career-related internships or fieldwork, institutionally sponsored loans, scholarships, traineeships, and unspecified assistantships also available.

Contact Ms. Crystal McFadden, Office Associate, Fay W. Whitney School of Nursing, University of Wyoming, Department 3065, 1000 East University Avenue, Laramie, WY 82071. *Telephone:* 307-766-6568. *Fax:* 307-766-4294. *E-mail:* gradnurse@uwyo.edu.

MASTER'S DEGREE PROGRAM

Degree MS

Available Programs Master's.

Concentrations Available Nursing education.

Study Options Full-time.

Online Degree Options Yes (online only).

Program Entrance Requirements Clinical experience, minimum overall college GPA of 3.0, transcript of college record, CPR certification, written essay, immunizations, 3 letters of recommendation, professional liability insurance/malpractice insurance, resume, statistics course, GRE General Test. *Application deadline:* 2/1 (fall). *Application fee:* $50.

Degree Requirements 36 total credit hours.

POST-MASTER'S PROGRAM

Areas of Study Nursing education.

DOCTORAL DEGREE PROGRAM

Degree DNP

Available Programs Doctorate.

Areas of Study Advanced practice nursing, clinical practice, ethics, family health, health policy, health promotion/disease prevention, human health and illness, individualized study, information systems, nursing policy, women's health.

Program Entrance Requirements Clinical experience, minimum overall college GPA of 3.5, interview by faculty committee, interview, 3 letters of recommendation, vita, writing sample. Application deadline: 2/1 (fall). Application fee: $50.

Degree Requirements 84 total credit hours.

CANADA

ALBERTA

Athabasca University

Centre for Nursing and Health Studies
Athabasca, Alberta

http://www.athabascau.ca/cnhs/
Founded in 1970

DEGREES • BN • MN • MN/MHSA

Nursing Program Faculty 130 (45% with doctorates).

Baccalaureate Enrollment 3,665

Graduate Enrollment 1,517

Distance Learning Courses Available.

Nursing Student Activities Student Nurses' Association.

Nursing Student Resources Academic advising; academic or career counseling; assistance for students with disabilities; bookstore; campus computer network; computer lab; computer-assisted instruction; e-mail services; interactive nursing skills videos; Internet; library services; nursing audiovisuals; remedial services; skills, simulation, or other laboratory; tutoring.

BACCALAUREATE PROGRAMS

Degree BN

Available Programs Generic Baccalaureate; LPN to RN Baccalaureate; RN Baccalaureate.

Site Options Athabasca, AB.

Study Options Full-time and part-time.

Program Entrance Requirements CPR certification, immunizations, RN licensure. Transfer students are accepted. *Application deadline:* Applications may be processed on a rolling basis for some programs.

Advanced Placement Credit by examination available. Credit given for nursing courses completed elsewhere dependent upon specific evaluations.

Expenses (2014–15) *Tuition, area resident:* part-time CAN$667 per course. *Tuition, state resident:* part-time CAN$781 per course. *Tuition, nonresident:* part-time CAN$1001 per course.

Contact Gayle Deren-Purdy, Undergraduate Student Advisor, Centre for Nursing and Health Studies, Athabasca University, 1 University Drive, Athabasca, AB T9S 3A3. *Telephone:* 800-788-9041 Ext. 6446. *Fax:* 780-675-6468. *E-mail:* gayled@athabascau.ca.

GRADUATE PROGRAMS

Expenses (2014–15) *Tuition, area resident:* part-time CAN$1425 per course. *Tuition, state resident:* part-time CAN$1625 per course.

Contact Ms. Donna Dunn Hart, Graduate Student Advisor, Centre for Nursing and Health Studies, Athabasca University, 1 University Drive, Athabasca, AB T9S 3A3. *Telephone:* 800-788-9041 Ext. 6300. *Fax:* 780-675-6468. *E-mail:* donnad@athabascau.ca.

MASTER'S DEGREE PROGRAM

Degrees MN; MN/MHSA

Available Programs Master's; Master's for Nurses with Non-Nursing Degrees.

Concentrations Available Nursing administration; nursing education. *Nurse practitioner programs in:* community health, family health, primary care.

Site Options Athabasca, AB.

Study Options Full-time and part-time.

Online Degree Options Yes.

Program Entrance Requirements Clinical experience, computer literacy, minimum overall college GPA of 3.0, transcript of college record, written essay, 3 letters of recommendation, resume. *Application deadline:* 6/1 (fall), 10/1 (winter), 2/1 (spring). *Application fee:* CAN$150.

Advanced Placement Credit given for nursing courses completed elsewhere dependent upon specific evaluations.
Degree Requirements 33 total credit hours, thesis or project, comprehensive exam.

POST-MASTER'S PROGRAM
Areas of Study *Nurse practitioner programs in:* community health, family health.

University of Alberta
Faculty of Nursing
Edmonton, Alberta

http://uofa.ualberta.ca/nursing
Founded in 1906
DEGREES • BSCN • MN • PHD
Nursing Program Faculty 106 (50% with doctorates).
Baccalaureate Enrollment 1,497 **Women** 92% **Men** 8% **Part-time** 7%
Graduate Enrollment 171 **Women** 90% **Men** 10% **Part-time** 60%
Distance Learning Courses Available.
Nursing Student Activities Nursing Honor Society, Sigma Theta Tau, Student Nurses' Association.
Nursing Student Resources Academic advising; academic or career counseling; assistance for students with disabilities; bookstore; campus computer network; career placement assistance; computer lab; computer-assisted instruction; daycare for children of students; e-mail services; employment services for current students; housing assistance; interactive nursing skills videos; Internet; learning resource lab; library services; nursing audiovisuals; other; paid internships; remedial services; resume preparation assistance; skills, simulation, or other laboratory; tutoring; unpaid internships.
Library Facilities 115,000 volumes in health, 19,000 volumes in nursing; 2,400 periodical subscriptions health-care related.

BACCALAUREATE PROGRAMS
Degree BScN
Available Programs Accelerated Baccalaureate for Second Degree; Baccalaureate for Second Degree; Generic Baccalaureate; RN Baccalaureate; RPN to Baccalaureate.
Site Options Red Deer, AB; Grande Prairie, AB; Fort McMurray, AB.
Study Options Full-time.
Program Entrance Requirements Minimum overall college GPA, transcript of college record, CPR certification, health exam, high school biology, high school chemistry, 3 years high school math, 3 years high school science, high school transcript, immunizations, minimum high school GPA, minimum high school rank, minimum GPA in nursing prerequisites. Transfer students are accepted. *Application deadline:* 3/1 (fall). Applications may be processed on a rolling basis for some programs. *Application fee:* CAN$125.
Advanced Placement Credit given for nursing courses completed elsewhere dependent upon specific evaluations.
Contact Undergraduate Student Inquiries, Faculty of Nursing, University of Alberta, Level 3, Edmonton Clinic Health Academy, 11405-87 Avenue, Edmonton, AB T6G 1C9. *Telephone:* 780-492-5300. *Fax:* 780-492-2551. *E-mail:* nursing.undergraduate@ualberta.ca.

GRADUATE PROGRAMS
Financial Aid 12 fellowships (averaging $23,868 per year), 27 research assistantships (averaging $6,186 per year), 12 teaching assistantships (averaging $2,365 per year) were awarded; institutionally sponsored loans and scholarships also available.
Contact Graduate Services Administrator, Faculty of Nursing, University of Alberta, 4-171 Edmonton Clinic Health Academy, 11405 87 Avenue, Edmonton, AB T6G 1C9. *Telephone:* 780-492-9546. *Fax:* 780-492-2551. *E-mail:* nursing.graduate@ualberta.ca.

MASTER'S DEGREE PROGRAM
Degree MN
Available Programs Master's.
Concentrations Available *Nurse practitioner programs in:* adult health, gerontology.
Study Options Full-time and part-time.
Program Entrance Requirements Clinical experience, computer literacy, minimum overall college GPA of 3.0, transcript of college record, CPR certification, 3 letters of recommendation, nursing research course,

physical assessment course, resume, statistics course. *Application deadline:* 2/1 (fall). *Application fee:* CAN$100.
Advanced Placement Credit given for nursing courses completed elsewhere dependent upon specific evaluations.
Degree Requirements 39 total credit hours, thesis or project.

POST-MASTER'S PROGRAM
Areas of Study *Nurse practitioner programs in:* adult health, gerontology.

DOCTORAL DEGREE PROGRAM
Degree PhD
Available Programs Doctorate.
Areas of Study Aging, community health, ethics, family health, gerontology, health policy, health promotion/disease prevention, health-care systems, nursing education, nursing policy, nursing research.
Online Degree Options Yes.
Program Entrance Requirements Clinical experience, minimum overall college GPA of 3.0, 3 letters of recommendation, MSN or equivalent, scholarly papers, statistics course, vita, writing sample. Application deadline: 2/1 (fall). Application fee: CAN$100.
Degree Requirements 36 total credit hours, dissertation, oral exam, written exam, residency.

POSTDOCTORAL PROGRAM
Postdoctoral Program Contact Dr. Phyllis Giovannetti, Associate Dean, Graduate Education, Faculty of Nursing, University of Alberta, Clinical Sciences Building, 3rd Floor, Edmonton, AB T6G 2G3. *Telephone:* 780-492-6764. *Fax:* 780-492-2551. *E-mail:* phyllis.giovannetti@ualberta.ca.

University of Calgary
Faculty of Nursing
Calgary, Alberta

http://www.ucalgary.ca/nu
Founded in 1945
DEGREES • BN • MN • PHD
Nursing Program Faculty 50 (85% with doctorates).
Baccalaureate Enrollment 930 **Women** 90% **Men** 10%
Graduate Enrollment 110 **Women** 95% **Men** 5% **Part-time** 21%
Nursing Student Activities Student Nurses' Association.
Nursing Student Resources Academic advising; academic or career counseling; assistance for students with disabilities; bookstore; campus computer network; career placement assistance; computer lab; computer-assisted instruction; daycare for children of students; e-mail services; externships; housing assistance; interactive nursing skills videos; Internet; learning resource lab; library services; nursing audiovisuals; remedial services; resume preparation assistance; skills, simulation, or other laboratory; tutoring.

BACCALAUREATE PROGRAMS
Degree BN
Available Programs Accelerated Baccalaureate; Accelerated Baccalaureate for Second Degree; Baccalaureate for Second Degree; Generic Baccalaureate; RN Baccalaureate.
Site Options Medicine Hat, AB.
Study Options Full-time.
Program Entrance Requirements Minimum overall college GPA of 3.3, transcript of college record, CPR certification, health exam, high school biology, high school chemistry, 3 years high school math, high school transcript, immunizations, minimum high school rank 78%. Transfer students are accepted.
Advanced Placement Credit by examination available. Credit given for nursing courses completed elsewhere dependent upon specific evaluations.
Contact *Telephone:* 403-220-4636. *Fax:* 403-284-4803.

GRADUATE PROGRAMS
Contact *Telephone:* 403-220-6241. *Fax:* 403-284-4803.

MASTER'S DEGREE PROGRAM
Degree MN
Available Programs Master's; RN to Master's.
Concentrations Available *Clinical nurse specialist programs in:* acute care, adult health, cardiovascular, community health, critical care, family

health, gerontology, maternity-newborn, medical-surgical, parent-child, pediatric, perinatal, psychiatric/mental health, public health, rehabilitation, women's health. *Nurse practitioner programs in:* acute care, adult health, neonatal health.

Study Options Full-time and part-time.

Program Entrance Requirements Clinical experience, computer literacy, minimum overall college GPA of 3.0, transcript of college record, CPR certification, written essay, 3 letters of recommendation, nursing research course, statistics course.

Advanced Placement Credit given for nursing courses completed elsewhere dependent upon specific evaluations.

Degree Requirements 30 total credit hours, thesis or project, comprehensive exam.

POST-MASTER'S PROGRAM

Areas of Study *Nurse practitioner programs in:* acute care, adult health, neonatal health.

DOCTORAL DEGREE PROGRAM

Degree PhD

Available Programs Doctorate; Doctorate for Nurses with Non-Nursing Degrees.

Areas of Study Advanced practice nursing, aging, clinical practice, community health, critical care, ethics, family health, gerontology, health promotion/disease prevention, health-care systems, human health and illness, illness and transition, individualized study, maternity-newborn, neuro-behavior, nursing research, women's health.

Program Entrance Requirements Clinical experience, minimum overall college GPA of 3.0, 3 letters of recommendation, MSN or equivalent, scholarly papers, statistics course, vita, writing sample.

Degree Requirements Dissertation, oral exam, written exam.

University of Lethbridge
Faculty of Health Sciences
Lethbridge, Alberta

http://www.uleth.ca/healthsciences
Founded in 1967

DEGREES • BN • MN

Nursing Program Faculty 32 (28% with doctorates).

Baccalaureate Enrollment 580 **Women** 89% **Men** 11%

Graduate Enrollment 11 **Women** 90% **Men** 10% **Part-time** 64%

Nursing Student Activities Nursing club.

Nursing Student Resources Academic advising; academic or career counseling; assistance for students with disabilities; bookstore; campus computer network; career placement assistance; computer lab; computer-assisted instruction; daycare for children of students; e-mail services; employment services for current students; housing assistance; interactive nursing skills videos; Internet; learning resource lab; library services; nursing audiovisuals; other; remedial services; resume preparation assistance; skills, simulation, or other laboratory; tutoring; unpaid internships.

Library Facilities 14,743 volumes in health, 2,554 volumes in nursing; 11,168 periodical subscriptions health-care related.

BACCALAUREATE PROGRAMS

Degree BN

Available Programs Accelerated Baccalaureate; Baccalaureate for Second Degree; Generic Baccalaureate.

Site Options Lethbridge, AB.

Study Options Full-time.

Program Entrance Requirements CPR certification, high school biology, high school chemistry, 3 years high school math, 3 years high school science, high school transcript, immunizations. Transfer students are accepted. *Application deadline:* 3/1 (fall). *Application fee:* CAN$125.

Advanced Placement Credit given for nursing courses completed elsewhere dependent upon specific evaluations.

Financial Aid *Gift aid (need-based):* private, college/university gift aid from institutional funds. *Financial aid application deadline:* Continuous.

Contact Sherry Hogeweide, Academic Advisor, Faculty of Health Sciences, University of Lethbridge, 4401 University Drive, Lethbridge, AB T1K 3M4. *Telephone:* 403-329-2220. *Fax:* 403-329-2668. *E-mail:* nursing@uleth.ca.

GRADUATE PROGRAMS

Contact Sherry Hogeweide, Academic Advisor, Faculty of Health Sciences, University of Lethbridge, 4401 University Drive, Lethbridge, AB T1K 3M4. *Telephone:* 403-329-2699. *Fax:* 403-329-2668. *E-mail:* masternursing@uleth.ca.

MASTER'S DEGREE PROGRAM

Degree MN

Available Programs Master's.

Study Options Full-time and part-time.

Online Degree Options Yes (online only).

Program Entrance Requirements Clinical experience, computer literacy, minimum overall college GPA of 3.0, transcript of college record, CPR certification, written essay, immunizations, 3 letters of recommendation, resume. *Application deadline:* 2/1 (fall).

Degree Requirements Thesis or project.

BRITISH COLUMBIA

British Columbia Institute of Technology
School of Health Sciences
Burnaby, British Columbia

http://www.bcit.ca/health/
Founded in 1964

DEGREE • BSN

Nursing Program Faculty 95

Baccalaureate Enrollment 540 **Women** 90% **Men** 10%

Distance Learning Courses Available.

Nursing Student Activities Student Nurses' Association.

Nursing Student Resources Academic advising; academic or career counseling; assistance for students with disabilities; bookstore; campus computer network; computer lab; computer-assisted instruction; daycare for children of students; e-mail services; housing assistance; interactive nursing skills videos; Internet; learning resource lab; library services; nursing audiovisuals; paid internships; remedial services; resume preparation assistance; skills, simulation, or other laboratory; tutoring; unpaid internships.

Library Facilities 10,000 volumes in health, 2,600 volumes in nursing; 110 periodical subscriptions health-care related.

BACCALAUREATE PROGRAMS

Degree BSN

Available Programs RN Baccalaureate.

Study Options Full-time.

Program Entrance Requirements Transcript of college record, CPR certification, high school chemistry, 11 years high school math, high school transcript, immunizations, prerequisite course work. Transfer students are accepted. *Application deadline:* 2/28 (fall), 8/31 (winter). *Application fee:* CAN$90.

Advanced Placement Credit given for nursing courses completed elsewhere dependent upon specific evaluations.

Expenses (2015–16) *Tuition, area resident:* full-time CAN$6080; part-time CAN$220 per credit. *Required fees:* full-time CAN$1050.

Financial Aid 70% of baccalaureate students in nursing programs received some form of financial aid in 2014–15. *Financial aid application deadline:* Continuous.

Contact Ms. Loreen Martin, Administrative Coordinator, School of Health Sciences, British Columbia Institute of Technology, 3700 Willingdon Avenue, SE12, Room 418, Burnaby, BC V5G 3H2. *Telephone:* 604-432-8884. *Fax:* 604-436-9590. *E-mail:* loreen_martin@bcit.ca.

CONTINUING EDUCATION PROGRAM

Contact Ms. Pauline O'Reilly, Program Head, School of Health Sciences, British Columbia Institute of Technology, 3700 Willingdon Avenue, SE12, Room 328, Burnaby, BC V5G 3H2. *Telephone:* 604-451-7115. *E-mail:* pauline_o'reilly@bcit.ca.

Kwantlen Polytechnic University
Faculty of Community and Health Sciences
Surrey, British Columbia

http://www.kwantlen.ca/
Founded in 1981
DEGREE • BSN
Nursing Program Faculty 60 (13% with doctorates).
Baccalaureate Enrollment 360 **Women** 90% **Men** 10% **Part-time** 13%
Nursing Student Activities Student Nurses' Association.
Nursing Student Resources Academic advising; academic or career counseling; assistance for students with disabilities; bookstore; campus computer network; career placement assistance; computer lab; computer-assisted instruction; e-mail services; employment services for current students; interactive nursing skills videos; Internet; learning resource lab; library services; nursing audiovisuals; remedial services; resume preparation assistance; skills, simulation, or other laboratory.

BACCALAUREATE PROGRAMS

Degree BSN
Available Programs Accelerated Baccalaureate for Second Degree; Generic Baccalaureate; RN Baccalaureate.
Study Options Full-time.
Program Entrance Requirements CPR certification, health insurance, high school biology, high school chemistry, high school math, 2 years high school science, high school transcript, immunizations. Transfer students are accepted.
Advanced Placement Credit given for nursing courses completed elsewhere dependent upon specific evaluations.
Contact *Telephone:* 604-599-2141.

Thompson Rivers University
School of Nursing
Kamloops, British Columbia

http://www.tru.ca/nursing.html
Founded in 1970
DEGREE • BSN
Nursing Program Faculty 56
Library Facilities 7,326 volumes in health, 2,275 volumes in nursing; 89 periodical subscriptions health-care related.

BACCALAUREATE PROGRAMS

Degree BSN
Study Options Full-time and part-time.
Program Entrance Requirements Minimum overall college GPA of 2.7, transcript of college record, CPR certification, health exam, high school biology, high school chemistry, high school foreign language, high school math, high school science, high school transcript, immunizations, interview, 2 letters of recommendation, minimum high school GPA of 2.3, minimum GPA in nursing prerequisites of 2.3. Transfer students are accepted.
Advanced Placement Credit given for nursing courses completed elsewhere dependent upon specific evaluations.
Contact *Telephone:* 250-828-5435. *Fax:* 250-828-5450.

CONTINUING EDUCATION PROGRAM

Contact *Telephone:* 250-828-5210. *Fax:* 250-371-5510.

Trinity Western University
Department of Nursing
Langley, British Columbia

http://www.twu.ca/nursing
Founded in 1962
DEGREES • BSCN • MSN
Nursing Program Faculty 15 (47% with doctorates).
Baccalaureate Enrollment 200 **Women** 93% **Men** 7%
Graduate Enrollment 45 **Women** 100% **Part-time** 6%
Nursing Student Activities Student Nurses' Association, nursing club.

Nursing Student Resources Academic advising; academic or career counseling; assistance for students with disabilities; bookstore; campus computer network; computer lab; computer-assisted instruction; e-mail services; employment services for current students; housing assistance; interactive nursing skills videos; Internet; learning resource lab; library services; nursing audiovisuals; remedial services; resume preparation assistance; skills, simulation, or other laboratory; tutoring.
Library Facilities 2,500 volumes in health, 800 volumes in nursing; 369 periodical subscriptions health-care related.

BACCALAUREATE PROGRAMS

Degree BScN
Available Programs Generic Baccalaureate.
Study Options Full-time.
Program Entrance Requirements Minimum overall college GPA of 2.0, CPR certification, health insurance, high school biology, high school chemistry, 2 years high school math, 2 years high school science, high school transcript, immunizations, 2 letters of recommendation, minimum high school GPA of 2.7, minimum GPA in nursing prerequisites of 2.3. Transfer students are accepted. *Application deadline:* 2/28 (fall).
Advanced Placement Credit given for nursing courses completed elsewhere dependent upon specific evaluations.
Financial Aid *Gift aid (need-based):* private, college/university gift aid from institutional funds. *Loans:* federal and provincial loans. *Financial aid application deadline (priority):* 2/28.
Contact Dr. Sonya Grypma, Dean, Department of Nursing, Trinity Western University, 7600 Glover Road, Langley, BC V2Y 1Y1. *Telephone:* 604-513-2121 Ext. 3283. *Fax:* 604-513-2012. *E-mail:* sonya.grypma@twu.ca.

GRADUATE PROGRAMS

Contact Ms. Guelda Redman, MSN Administrative Assistant, Department of Nursing, Trinity Western University, 7600 Glover Road, Langley, BC V2Y 1Y1. *Telephone:* 604-888-7511 Ext. 3270. *Fax:* 604-513-2012. *E-mail:* guelda.redman@twu.ca.

MASTER'S DEGREE PROGRAM
Degree MSN
Available Programs Master's.
Study Options Part-time.
Program Entrance Requirements Minimum overall college GPA of 3.0, transcript of college record, 2 letters of recommendation, statistics course. *Application deadline:* 5/1 (summer).
Advanced Placement Credit given for nursing courses completed elsewhere dependent upon specific evaluations.
Degree Requirements 30 total credit hours, thesis or project.

The University of British Columbia
Program in Nursing
Vancouver, British Columbia

http://www.nursing.ubc.ca/
Founded in 1915
DEGREES • BSN • MSN • MSN/MPH • PHD
Nursing Program Faculty 55 (51% with doctorates).
Baccalaureate Enrollment 237 **Women** 83.5% **Men** 16.5%
Graduate Enrollment 210 **Women** 91.4% **Men** 8.6% **Part-time** 25.7%
Distance Learning Courses Available.
Nursing Student Activities Sigma Theta Tau, Student Nurses' Association, nursing club.
Nursing Student Resources Academic advising; academic or career counseling; assistance for students with disabilities; bookstore; campus computer network; career placement assistance; computer lab; computer-assisted instruction; e-mail services; employment services for current students; housing assistance; interactive nursing skills videos; Internet; learning resource lab; library services; nursing audiovisuals; remedial services; resume preparation assistance; skills, simulation, or other laboratory.
Library Facilities 160,000 volumes in health, 11,000 volumes in nursing; 17,000 periodical subscriptions health-care related.

BACCALAUREATE PROGRAMS

Degree BSN

Available Programs Accelerated Baccalaureate; Accelerated Baccalaureate for Second Degree.
Study Options Full-time.
Program Entrance Requirements Minimum overall college GPA of 2.8, transcript of college record, CPR certification, written essay, immunizations, interview, professional liability insurance/malpractice insurance, prerequisite course work. *Application deadline:* 12/1 (winter). *Application fee:* CAN$238.
Expenses (2015–16) *Tuition, state resident:* full-time CAN$7981. *Tuition, nonresident:* full-time CAN$7981. *International tuition:* CAN$42,239 full-time. *Room and board:* CAN$10,760; room only: CAN$6200 per academic year. *Required fees:* full-time CAN$960.
Financial Aid *Gift aid (need-based):* state, private, college/university gift aid from institutional funds, Canadian Federal and Provincial Grants. *Loans:* college/university, Canadian federal and provincial loans. *Work-study:* part-time campus jobs. *Financial aid application deadline:* 9/15(priority: 4/15).
Contact Ruxandra Vasiljevic, Undergraduate Admissions Assistant, Program in Nursing, The University of British Columbia, T201-2211 Wesbrook Mall, Vancouver, BC V6T 2B5. *Telephone:* 604-822-9754. *Fax:* 604-822-7466. *E-mail:* information@nursing.ubc.ca.

GRADUATE PROGRAMS

Expenses (2015–16) *Tuition, area resident:* full-time CAN$4615. *International tuition:* CAN$8108 full-time. *Required fees:* full-time CAN$373.
Financial Aid 4 fellowships (averaging $8,000 per year), 14 research assistantships (averaging $800 per year), 3 teaching assistantships were awarded.
Contact Mr. Drew St. Laurent, Recruitment and Graduate Admissions Officer, Program in Nursing, The University of British Columbia, T201-2211 Wesbrook Mall, Vancouver, BC V6T 2B5. *Telephone:* 604-822-7446. *E-mail:* student.services@nursing.ubc.ca.

MASTER'S DEGREE PROGRAM
Degrees MSN; MSN/MPH
Available Programs Master's.
Concentrations Available Nursing administration; nursing education. *Clinical nurse specialist programs in:* adult health, cardiovascular, community health, family health, gerontology, maternity-newborn, oncology, parent-child, pediatric, perinatal, psychiatric/mental health, public health, women's health. *Nurse practitioner programs in:* community health, family health, primary care.
Study Options Full-time and part-time.
Program Entrance Requirements Computer literacy, minimum overall college GPA of 3.3, transcript of college record, 3 letters of recommendation, resume, GRE. *Application deadline:* 12/1 (fall). *Application fee:* CAN$93.
Advanced Placement Credit given for nursing courses completed elsewhere dependent upon specific evaluations.
Degree Requirements 33 total credit hours, thesis or project.

DOCTORAL DEGREE PROGRAM
Degree PhD
Available Programs Doctorate.
Areas of Study Addiction/substance abuse, advanced practice nursing, aging, clinical practice, clinical research, community health, ethics, faculty preparation, family health, gerontology, health policy, health promotion/disease prevention, health-care systems, human health and illness, illness and transition, individualized study, information systems, maternity-newborn, nursing administration, nursing education, nursing policy, nursing research, nursing science, oncology, palliative care, urban health, women's health.
Program Entrance Requirements 3 letters of recommendation, MSN or equivalent, vita, writing sample, GRE. Application deadline: 12/1 (fall). Applications may be processed on a rolling basis for some programs. Application fee: CAN$153.
Degree Requirements 18 total credit hours, dissertation, oral exam, written exam, residency.

POSTDOCTORAL PROGRAM
Areas of Study Addiction/substance abuse, adolescent health, aging, cancer care, chronic illness, community health, family health, gerontology, health promotion/disease prevention, individualized study, information systems, neonatal health, neuro-behavior, nursing informatics, nursing interventions, nursing research, nursing science, outcomes, self-care, vulnerable population, women's health.

Postdoctoral Program Contact Dr. Elizabeth Saewyc, Associate Director, Research, Program in Nursing, The University of British Columbia, T201-2211 Wesbrook Mall, Vancouver, BC V6T 2B5. *Telephone:* 604-822-7505. *Fax:* 604-822-7466. *E-mail:* elizabeth.saewyc@nursing.ubc.ca.

University of Northern British Columbia
Nursing Programme
Prince George, British Columbia

http://www.unbc.ca/nursing/
Founded in 1994
DEGREES • BSCN • M SC N
Nursing Program Faculty 40 (18% with doctorates).
Baccalaureate Enrollment 600
Graduate Enrollment 60
Distance Learning Courses Available.
Nursing Student Activities Student Nurses' Association.
Nursing Student Resources Academic advising; academic or career counseling; assistance for students with disabilities; bookstore; campus computer network; computer lab; computer-assisted instruction; e-mail services; employment services for current students; externships; Internet; learning resource lab; library services; nursing audiovisuals; skills, simulation, or other laboratory.
Library Facilities 4,000 volumes in health, 2,000 volumes in nursing; 300 periodical subscriptions health-care related.

BACCALAUREATE PROGRAMS

Degree BScN
Available Programs Generic Baccalaureate; RN Baccalaureate.
Site Options Prince George, BC; Quesnel, BC; Terrace, BC.
Study Options Full-time.
Program Entrance Requirements Minimum overall college GPA of 2.33, transcript of college record, CPR certification, health exam, high school biology, high school chemistry, 1 year of high school math, 4 years high school science, high school transcript, immunizations, minimum high school GPA of 2.3, minimum high school rank 65%, minimum GPA in nursing prerequisites of 2.0, professional liability insurance/malpractice insurance. Transfer students are accepted. *Application deadline:* 3/31 (fall). *Application fee:* CAN$35.
Advanced Placement Credit given for nursing courses completed elsewhere dependent upon specific evaluations.
Contact *Telephone:* 250-960-5645.

GRADUATE PROGRAMS
Contact *Telephone:* 250-960-5848. *Fax:* 250-960-6410.

MASTER'S DEGREE PROGRAM
Degree M Sc N
Available Programs Master's.
Concentrations Available *Nurse practitioner programs in:* family health.
Study Options Full-time and part-time.
Program Entrance Requirements Clinical experience, minimum overall college GPA of 3.0, transcript of college record, CPR certification, written essay, 3 letters of recommendation, nursing research course, professional liability insurance/malpractice insurance, prerequisite course work. *Application deadline:* 2/15 (fall). *Application fee:* CAN$75.
Advanced Placement Credit given for nursing courses completed elsewhere dependent upon specific evaluations.
Degree Requirements 51 total credit hours, thesis or project.

POSTDOCTORAL PROGRAM
Areas of Study Chronic illness, community health, family health, health promotion/disease prevention, individualized study, nursing interventions, nursing research, nursing science, outcomes, vulnerable population.
Postdoctoral Program Contact *Telephone:* 250-960-6507. *Fax:* 250-960-6410.

University of Victoria
School of Nursing
Victoria, British Columbia

http://www.web.uvic.ca/nurs/
Founded in 1963
DEGREES • BSN • MN • PHD
Nursing Program Faculty 21 (95% with doctorates).
Baccalaureate Enrollment 1,100 **Women** 95% **Men** 5% **Part-time** 50%
Nursing Student Activities Student Nurses' Association.
Nursing Student Resources Academic advising; assistance for students with disabilities; bookstore; campus computer network; computer lab; e-mail services; employment services for current students; interactive nursing skills videos; Internet; library services; nursing audiovisuals; remedial services; resume preparation assistance; unpaid internships.

BACCALAUREATE PROGRAMS

Degree BSN
Site Options Vancouver, BC.
Program Entrance Requirements Minimum overall college GPA of 3.5, transcript of college record, CPR certification, high school transcript, immunizations, prerequisite course work. Transfer students are accepted.
Contact *Telephone:* 250-721-7961. *Fax:* 250-721-6231.

GRADUATE PROGRAMS

Contact *Telephone:* 250-721-7961. *Fax:* 250-721-6231.

MASTER'S DEGREE PROGRAM
Degree MN
Available Programs Master's.
Site Options Victoria.
Study Options Full-time and part-time.
Program Entrance Requirements Clinical experience, transcript of college record, letters of recommendation.
Advanced Placement Credit given for nursing courses completed elsewhere dependent upon specific evaluations.
Degree Requirements 18 total credit hours, thesis or project.

DOCTORAL DEGREE PROGRAM
Degree PhD
Program Entrance Requirements Clinical experience, MSN or equivalent.
Degree Requirements Dissertation.

Vancouver Island University
Department of Nursing
Nanaimo, British Columbia

http://www.viu.ca/calendar/Health/bscnursing.asp
Founded in 1969
DEGREE • BSCN
Nursing Program Faculty 36 (2% with doctorates).
Baccalaureate Enrollment 279 **Women** 92% **Men** 8%
Distance Learning Courses Available.
Nursing Student Activities Student Nurses' Association.
Nursing Student Resources Academic advising; academic or career counseling; assistance for students with disabilities; bookstore; campus computer network; computer lab; computer-assisted instruction; e-mail services; employment services for current students; housing assistance; interactive nursing skills videos; Internet; learning resource lab; library services; nursing audiovisuals; remedial services; resume preparation assistance; skills, simulation, or other laboratory; tutoring; unpaid internships.
Library Facilities 9,475 volumes in health, 1,299 volumes in nursing; 800 periodical subscriptions health-care related.

BACCALAUREATE PROGRAMS

Degree BScN
Available Programs Generic Baccalaureate; LPN to RN Baccalaureate.
Study Options Full-time.
Program Entrance Requirements CPR certification, health insurance, high school biology, high school chemistry, 11 years high school math,

high school transcript, immunizations, minimum GPA in nursing prerequisites of 3.0, prerequisite course work. Transfer students are accepted.
Application deadline: 2/28 (fall). *Application fee:* CAN$35.
Advanced Placement Credit given for nursing courses completed elsewhere dependent upon specific evaluations.
Contact *Telephone:* 250-740-6260. *Fax:* 250-740-6468.

CONTINUING EDUCATION PROGRAM

Contact *Telephone:* 250-740-6327.

MANITOBA

Brandon University
School of Health Studies
Brandon, Manitoba

http://www.brandonu.ca/health-studies/
Founded in 1899
DEGREES • BN • MN
Nursing Program Faculty 20 (40% with doctorates).
Baccalaureate Enrollment 480 **Women** 95% **Men** 5% **Part-time** 25%
Graduate Enrollment 45
Distance Learning Courses Available.
Nursing Student Activities Nursing Honor Society, Sigma Theta Tau, Student Nurses' Association.
Nursing Student Resources Academic advising; academic or career counseling; assistance for students with disabilities; bookstore; campus computer network; career placement assistance; computer lab; computer-assisted instruction; e-mail services; employment services for current students; housing assistance; interactive nursing skills videos; Internet; library services; resume preparation assistance; skills, simulation, or other laboratory; tutoring.

BACCALAUREATE PROGRAMS

Degree BN
Available Programs Baccalaureate for Second Degree; Generic Baccalaureate; LPN to Baccalaureate; RN Baccalaureate.
Site Options Winnipeg, MB.
Study Options Full-time and part-time.
Program Entrance Requirements Minimum overall college GPA of 2.0, CPR certification, immunizations, minimum GPA in nursing prerequisites of 2.0, prerequisite course work. Transfer students are accepted.
Application deadline: 5/1 (fall).
Advanced Placement Credit given for nursing courses completed elsewhere dependent upon specific evaluations.
Financial Aid *Gift aid (need-based):* college/university gift aid from institutional funds. *Loans:* provincial and federal student loans. *Financial aid application deadline (priority):* 6/30.
Contact Ms. Tracey Collyer, Instructional Associate/Student Advisor, School of Health Studies, Brandon University, 270 18th Street, Brandon, MB R7A 6A9. *Telephone:* 204-571-8567. *Fax:* 204-571-8568. *E-mail:* collyert@brandonu.ca.

GRADUATE PROGRAMS

MASTER'S DEGREE PROGRAM
Degree MN
Available Programs Master's.
Concentrations Available *Clinical nurse specialist programs in:* psychiatric/mental health.
Site Options Winnipeg, MB.
Study Options Full-time and part-time.
Online Degree Options Yes (online only).
Program Entrance Requirements Clinical experience, minimum overall college GPA of 3.5, transcript of college record, written essay, 3 letters of recommendation, resume, statistics course. *Application deadline:* 3/1 (fall). *Application fee:* CAN$100.
Degree Requirements 33 total credit hours, thesis or project.

University of Manitoba
Faculty of Nursing
Winnipeg, Manitoba

http://www.umanitoba.ca/faculties/nursing/
Founded in 1877

DEGREES • BN • MN • PHD

Nursing Program Faculty 59 (50% with doctorates).
Baccalaureate Enrollment 807 **Women** 86% **Men** 14% **Part-time** 10%
Graduate Enrollment 98 **Women** 93% **Men** 7% **Part-time** 31%
Distance Learning Courses Available.
Nursing Student Activities Nursing Honor Society, Sigma Theta Tau, Student Nurses' Association.
Nursing Student Resources Academic advising; academic or career counseling; assistance for students with disabilities; bookstore; campus computer network; computer lab; computer-assisted instruction; daycare for children of students; e-mail services; employment services for current students; housing assistance; interactive nursing skills videos; Internet; learning resource lab; library services; skills, simulation, or other laboratory; unpaid internships.
Library Facilities 137,100 volumes in health, 5,000 volumes in nursing; 2,208 periodical subscriptions health-care related.

BACCALAUREATE PROGRAMS

Degree BN
Available Programs Generic Baccalaureate; RN Baccalaureate.
Site Options Thompson, MB; The Pas, MB.
Study Options Full-time and part-time.
Program Entrance Requirements Minimum overall college GPA of 2.5, transcript of college record, CPR certification, immunizations, prerequisite course work. Transfer students are accepted. *Application deadline:* 4/1 (fall), 8/1 (winter). *Application fee:* CAN$90.
Advanced Placement Credit given for nursing courses completed elsewhere dependent upon specific evaluations.
Financial Aid *Gift aid (need-based):* state, private, college/university gift aid from institutional funds. *Loans:* Federal Direct (Subsidized and Unsubsidized Stafford PLUS), Perkins, state, college/university, TERI Loans. *Work-study:* part-time campus jobs. *Financial aid application deadline (priority):* 10/1.
Contact Dr. Terri Ashcroft, Associate Dean, Undergraduate Program, Faculty of Nursing, University of Manitoba, 277 Helen Glass Centre for Nursing, Winnipeg, MB R3T 2N2. *Telephone:* 204-474-6220. *Fax:* 204-474-7682. *E-mail:* terri.ashcroft@umanitoba.ca.

GRADUATE PROGRAMS

Expenses (2014–15) *International tuition:* CAN$8911 full-time. *Required fees:* full-time CAN$4456.
Contact Dr. Jo-Ann Sawatzky, Associate Dean, Graduate Programs, Faculty of Nursing, University of Manitoba, 281-89 Curry Place, Winnipeg, MB R3T 2N2. *Telephone:* 204-474-9317. *Fax:* 204-474-7682. *E-mail:* joann.sawatzky@ad.umanitoba.ca.

MASTER'S DEGREE PROGRAM

Degree MN
Available Programs Master's.
Concentrations Available Clinical nurse leader; health-care administration; nurse case management; nursing education; nursing informatics. *Clinical nurse specialist programs in:* acute care, adult health, adult-gerontology acute care, adult-psychiatric mental health, cardiovascular, child/adolescent psychiatric-mental health, community health, critical care, family health, gerontology, home health care, maternity-newborn, medical-surgical, oncology, palliative care, parent-child, pediatric, perinatal, psychiatric/mental health, public health, public/community health, rehabilitation, school health, women's health. *Nurse practitioner programs in:* primary care.
Study Options Full-time and part-time.
Program Entrance Requirements Clinical experience, minimum overall college GPA of 3.0, transcript of college record, CPR certification, written essay, 3 letters of recommendation, nursing research course, prerequisite course work, resume, statistics course. *Application deadline:* 4/1 (fall). *Application fee:* CAN$100.
Advanced Placement Credit given for nursing courses completed elsewhere dependent upon specific evaluations.
Degree Requirements 27 total credit hours, thesis or project, comprehensive exam.

DOCTORAL DEGREE PROGRAM

Degree PhD
Available Programs Doctorate.
Areas of Study Advanced practice nursing, aging, clinical nurse leader, clinical practice, clinical research, community health, critical care, ethics, faculty preparation, family health, gerontology, health policy, health promotion/disease prevention, health-care systems, human health and illness, illness and transition, individualized study, information systems, maternity-newborn, nurse case management, nursing administration, nursing education, nursing policy, nursing research, nursing science, oncology, palliative care, urban health, women's health.
Program Entrance Requirements Minimum overall college GPA of 3.5, 3 letters of recommendation, MSN or equivalent, scholarly papers, writing sample. Application deadline: 2/1 (fall). Application fee: CAN$100.
Degree Requirements 21 total credit hours, dissertation, oral exam, written exam.

NEW BRUNSWICK

Université de Moncton
School of Nursing
Moncton, New Brunswick

http://www.umoncton.ca/umcm-fsssc-scienceinfirmiere
Founded in 1963

DEGREES • BSCN • M SC N

Nursing Program Faculty 64 (17% with doctorates).
Baccalaureate Enrollment 548 **Women** 86% **Men** 14% **Part-time** 1%
Graduate Enrollment 56 **Women** 89% **Men** 11% **Part-time** 100%
Distance Learning Courses Available.
Nursing Student Activities Student Nurses' Association.
Nursing Student Resources Academic or career counseling; assistance for students with disabilities; bookstore; campus computer network; career placement assistance; computer lab; computer-assisted instruction; daycare for children of students; e-mail services; employment services for current students; externships; housing assistance; Internet; library services; nursing audiovisuals; placement services for program completers; resume preparation assistance; skills, simulation, or other laboratory; tutoring; unpaid internships.
Library Facilities 10,757 volumes in health, 3,807 volumes in nursing; 210 periodical subscriptions health-care related.

BACCALAUREATE PROGRAMS

Degree BScN
Available Programs RN Baccalaureate.
Site Options Edmundston, NB; Bathurst, NB; Moncton, NB.
Study Options Full-time.
Program Entrance Requirements Transcript of college record, CPR certification, high school biology, high school chemistry, 30411 years high school math, high school science, high school transcript, immunizations, minimum high school rank 65%. Transfer students are accepted. *Application deadline:* 4/1 (winter). *Application fee:* CAN$50.
Advanced Placement Credit given for nursing courses completed elsewhere dependent upon specific evaluations.
Contact *Telephone:* 506-858-4443. *Fax:* 506-858-4538.

GRADUATE PROGRAMS

Contact *Telephone:* 506-858-4443. *Fax:* 506-858-4538.

MASTER'S DEGREE PROGRAM

Degree M Sc N
Available Programs Master's; RN to Master's.
Concentrations Available Health-care administration; nurse case management; nursing administration; nursing education. *Clinical nurse specialist programs in:* community health, family health, home health care, occupational health, pediatric, psychiatric/mental health, public health, school health. *Nurse practitioner programs in:* adult health, community health, family health, oncology, primary care.
Site Options Moncton, NB.
Study Options Full-time and part-time.
Program Entrance Requirements Minimum overall college GPA of 3.0, transcript of college record, CPR certification, written essay, immu-

nizations, 2 letters of recommendation, resume, statistics course. *Application deadline:* 6/1 (summer). *Application fee:* CAN$50.

Advanced Placement Credit given for nursing courses completed elsewhere dependent upon specific evaluations.

Degree Requirements 45 total credit hours, thesis or project.

CONTINUING EDUCATION PROGRAM

Contact *Telephone:* 506-858-4621. *Fax:* 506-858-4480.

University of New Brunswick Fredericton

Faculty of Nursing
Fredericton, New Brunswick

http://www.unbf.ca/nursing/
Founded in 1785

DEGREES • BN • MN

Nursing Program Faculty 75 (17% with doctorates).
Baccalaureate Enrollment 706 **Women** 94% **Men** 6%
Graduate Enrollment 53 **Women** 96% **Men** 4% **Part-time** 30%
Distance Learning Courses Available.
Nursing Student Activities Student Nurses' Association, nursing club.
Nursing Student Resources Academic advising; academic or career counseling; assistance for students with disabilities; bookstore; campus computer network; computer lab; computer-assisted instruction; daycare for children of students; e-mail services; employment services for current students; interactive nursing skills videos; Internet; learning resource lab; library services; nursing audiovisuals; resume preparation assistance; skills, simulation, or other laboratory; tutoring.
Library Facilities 12,547 volumes in health, 1,910 volumes in nursing; 250 periodical subscriptions health-care related.

BACCALAUREATE PROGRAMS

Degree BN
Available Programs Accelerated Baccalaureate; Generic Baccalaureate.
Site Options Bathurst, NB; Moncton, NB; Fredericton, NB.
Study Options Full-time.
Program Entrance Requirements Minimum overall college GPA of 3.0, transcript of college record, CPR certification, written essay, health exam, high school biology, high school chemistry, 70 years high school math, high school transcript, immunizations, interview, minimum high school rank 75%, prerequisite course work. Transfer students are accepted. *Application deadline:* 3/31 (fall). *Application fee:* CAN$55.
Advanced Placement Credit given for nursing courses completed elsewhere dependent upon specific evaluations.
Contact Ms. Pam Wiebe, Administrative Assistant, Faculty of Nursing, University of New Brunswick Fredericton, PO Box 4400, Fredericton, NB E3B 5A3. *Telephone:* 506-458-7670. *Fax:* 506-453-3512. *E-mail:* pwiebe@unb.ca.

GRADUATE PROGRAMS

Contact Mr. Francis Perry, Graduate Assistant, Faculty of Nursing, University of New Brunswick Fredericton, PO Box 4400, Fredericton, NB E3B 5A3. *Telephone:* 506-451-6844. *Fax:* 506-453-4503. *E-mail:* fperry@unb.ca.

MASTER'S DEGREE PROGRAM

Degree MN
Available Programs Master's.
Concentrations Available Nurse case management; nursing administration; nursing education; nursing informatics. *Clinical nurse specialist programs in:* acute care, adult health, cardiovascular, community health, critical care, family health, gerontology, maternity-newborn, medical-surgical, oncology, parent-child, pediatric, psychiatric/mental health, public health, school health, women's health. *Nurse practitioner programs in:* acute care, adult health, community health, family health, gerontology, neonatal health, pediatric, primary care, psychiatric/mental health, women's health.
Site Options Fredericton, NB.
Study Options Full-time and part-time.
Program Entrance Requirements Clinical experience, computer literacy, minimum overall college GPA of 3.3, transcript of college record, CPR certification, written essay, immunizations, 3 letters of recommendation, nursing research course, physical assessment course, prerequisite

course work, statistics course. *Application deadline:* 1/15 (winter). *Application fee:* CAN$50.
Advanced Placement Credit given for nursing courses completed elsewhere dependent upon specific evaluations.
Degree Requirements 27 total credit hours, thesis or project.

CONTINUING EDUCATION PROGRAM

Contact Mr. Lee Heenan, Administrative Assistant, Faculty of Nursing, University of New Brunswick Fredericton, PO Box 4400, Fredericton, NB E3B 5A3. *Telephone:* 506-458-7625. *Fax:* 506-447-3057. *E-mail:* nursing@unb.ca.

NEWFOUNDLAND AND LABRADOR

Memorial University of Newfoundland

School of Nursing
St. John's, Newfoundland and Labrador

http://www.nurs.mun.ca/
Founded in 1925

DEGREES • BN • MN • PHD

Nursing Program Faculty 42 (30% with doctorates).
Baccalaureate Enrollment 642 **Women** 92% **Men** 8% **Part-time** 50%
Graduate Enrollment 100 **Women** 91% **Men** 9% **Part-time** 82%
Distance Learning Courses Available.
Nursing Student Activities Student Nurses' Association.
Nursing Student Resources Academic advising; academic or career counseling; assistance for students with disabilities; bookstore; campus computer network; computer lab; computer-assisted instruction; daycare for children of students; e-mail services; employment services for current students; externships; interactive nursing skills videos; Internet; learning resource lab; library services; nursing audiovisuals; remedial services; skills, simulation, or other laboratory; tutoring.
Library Facilities 40,000 volumes in health, 5,000 volumes in nursing; 3,800 periodical subscriptions health-care related.

BACCALAUREATE PROGRAMS

Degree BN
Available Programs Accelerated Baccalaureate; Generic Baccalaureate; LPN to Baccalaureate.
Study Options Full-time.
Program Entrance Requirements Minimum overall college GPA of 3.0, transcript of college record, written essay, high school biology, high school chemistry, high school foreign language, high school math, high school science, high school transcript, 1 letter of recommendation, minimum high school rank 80%. Transfer students are accepted. *Application deadline:* 3/1 (fall).
Financial Aid *Loans:* college/university. *Financial aid application deadline:* Continuous.
Contact Ms. Penny-Lynn White, Nursing Consortium Coordinator, School of Nursing, Memorial University of Newfoundland, Registrar's Office, PO Box 4200, St. John's, NF A1C 5S7. *Telephone:* 709-864-6871. *Fax:* 709-864-2337. *E-mail:* nursingadmissions@mun.ca.

GRADUATE PROGRAMS

Financial Aid 25% of graduate students in nursing programs received some form of financial aid in 2013–14. Fellowships, research assistantships, teaching assistantships available. *Financial aid application deadline:* 12/31.
Contact Dr. Donna Moralejo, Associate Director, Graduate Program, School of Nursing, Memorial University of Newfoundland, 300 Prince Philip Drive, St. John's, NF A1B 3V6. *Telephone:* 709-777-6679. *Fax:* 709-777-7037. *E-mail:* moralejo@mun.ca.

MASTER'S DEGREE PROGRAM

Degree MN
Available Programs Master's.

Concentrations Available *Nurse practitioner programs in:* adult health, family health.
Study Options Full-time and part-time.
Online Degree Options Yes (online only).
Program Entrance Requirements Clinical experience, minimum overall college GPA of 3.0, transcript of college record, written essay, 2 letters of recommendation, nursing research course, professional liability insurance/malpractice insurance, prerequisite course work, resume, statistics course. *Application deadline:* 2/15 (fall). *Application fee:* CAN$40.
Advanced Placement Credit given for nursing courses completed elsewhere dependent upon specific evaluations.
Degree Requirements 27 total credit hours, thesis or project.

POST-MASTER'S PROGRAM

Areas of Study *Nurse practitioner programs in:* adult health, family health.

DOCTORAL DEGREE PROGRAM

Degree PhD
Available Programs Doctorate.
Program Entrance Requirements interview, letters of recommendation, MSN or equivalent, vita, writing sample. Application deadline: 1/31 (fall).
Degree Requirements Dissertation, oral exam, written exam, residency.

NOVA SCOTIA

St. Francis Xavier University
Department of Nursing
Antigonish, Nova Scotia

http://www.stfx.ca/
Founded in 1853
DEGREE • BSCN
Nursing Program Faculty 67 (10% with doctorates).
Baccalaureate Enrollment 1,067 **Women** 90% **Men** 10% **Part-time** 40%
Nursing Student Activities Student Nurses' Association, nursing club.
Nursing Student Resources Academic advising; academic or career counseling; assistance for students with disabilities; bookstore; campus computer network; career placement assistance; computer lab; computer-assisted instruction; daycare for children of students; e-mail services; employment services for current students; externships; housing assistance; interactive nursing skills videos; Internet; learning resource lab; library services; nursing audiovisuals; other; paid internships; placement services for program completers; remedial services; resume preparation assistance; skills, simulation, or other laboratory; tutoring; unpaid internships.
Library Facilities 4,000 volumes in health, 4,000 volumes in nursing; 1,015 periodical subscriptions health-care related.

BACCALAUREATE PROGRAMS

Degree BScN
Available Programs Accelerated Baccalaureate; Accelerated Baccalaureate for Second Degree; Accelerated LPN to Baccalaureate; Generic Baccalaureate; RN Baccalaureate.
Site Options Sydney, NS.
Study Options Full-time.
Program Entrance Requirements Transcript of college record, CPR certification, health exam, high school biology, high school chemistry, 2 years high school math, 2 years high school science, high school transcript, immunizations, minimum high school GPA, prerequisite course work. Transfer students are accepted.
Advanced Placement Credit given for nursing courses completed elsewhere dependent upon specific evaluations.
Contact *Telephone:* 902-867-5386. *Fax:* 902-867-2329.

CONTINUING EDUCATION PROGRAM

Contact *Telephone:* 902-867-5186. *Fax:* 902-867-5154.

ONTARIO

Brock University
Department of Nursing
St. Catharines, Ontario

http://www.brocku.ca/nursing/
Founded in 1964
DEGREE • BSCN
Nursing Program Faculty 9 (100% with doctorates).
Baccalaureate Enrollment 380 **Women** 98% **Men** 2%
Nursing Student Activities Student Nurses' Association, nursing club.
Nursing Student Resources Academic advising; academic or career counseling; assistance for students with disabilities; bookstore; campus computer network; computer lab; computer-assisted instruction; daycare for children of students; e-mail services; employment services for current students; housing assistance; interactive nursing skills videos; Internet; learning resource lab; library services; nursing audiovisuals; other; resume preparation assistance; skills, simulation, or other laboratory; tutoring.

BACCALAUREATE PROGRAMS

Degree BScN
Available Programs Generic Baccalaureate.
Study Options Full-time.
Program Entrance Requirements High school biology, high school chemistry. *Application deadline:* 1/15 (winter).
Financial Aid *Gift aid (need-based):* private, college/university gift aid from institutional funds. *Loans:* Federal Direct (Subsidized and Unsubsidized Stafford), state. *Work-study:* part-time campus jobs. *Financial aid application deadline (priority):* 3/15.
Contact Dr. Dawn Prentice, Chair and Associate Professor, Department of Nursing, Brock University, 1812 Sir Isaac Brock Way, St. Catharines, ON L2S 3A1. *Telephone:* 905-688-5550 Ext. 5161. *E-mail:* dprentice@brocku.ca.

GRADUATE PROGRAMS

Contact Graduate Studies Brock Univesity, Department of Nursing, Brock University, 1812 Sir Isaac Brock Way, St. Catharines, ON L2S 3A1. *Telephone:* 905-688-5550 Ext. 4490. *E-mail:* gradadmissions@brocku.ca.

MASTER'S DEGREE PROGRAM

Program Entrance Requirements *Application deadline:* 2/15 (winter).

Lakehead University
School of Nursing
Thunder Bay, Ontario

http://www.lakeheadu.ca/
Founded in 1965
DEGREE • BSCN
Nursing Program Faculty 15 (20% with doctorates).
Baccalaureate Enrollment 575 **Women** 82% **Men** 18%
Distance Learning Courses Available.
Nursing Student Activities Student Nurses' Association.
Nursing Student Resources Academic advising; academic or career counseling; assistance for students with disabilities; bookstore; campus computer network; career placement assistance; computer lab; daycare for children of students; e-mail services; employment services for current students; externships; housing assistance; interactive nursing skills videos; Internet; library services; nursing audiovisuals; resume preparation assistance; skills, simulation, or other laboratory; tutoring; unpaid internships.

BACCALAUREATE PROGRAMS

Degree BScN
Available Programs Accelerated Baccalaureate; Generic Baccalaureate; RN Baccalaureate.
Study Options Full-time and part-time.
Online Degree Options Yes.
Program Entrance Requirements Transcript of college record, CPR certification, health insurance, high school biology, high school chem-

istry, 4 years high school math, high school transcript, immunizations, minimum high school GPA. Transfer students are accepted. *Application deadline:* 1/12 (winter). Applications may be processed on a rolling basis for some programs.

Advanced Placement Credit given for nursing courses completed elsewhere dependent upon specific evaluations.

Contact *Telephone:* 807-343-8439. *Fax:* 807-343-8246.

Laurentian University
School of Nursing
Sudbury, Ontario

http://www.laurentian.ca/
Founded in 1960
DEGREES • BSCN • M SC N
Nursing Program Faculty 15 (10% with doctorates).
Baccalaureate Enrollment 260 **Women** 90% **Men** 10%
Distance Learning Courses Available.
Nursing Student Activities Student Nurses' Association.
Nursing Student Resources Academic advising; academic or career counseling; assistance for students with disabilities; bookstore; campus computer network; career placement assistance; computer lab; computer-assisted instruction; daycare for children of students; e-mail services; employment services for current students; externships; housing assistance; interactive nursing skills videos; Internet; learning resource lab; library services; nursing audiovisuals; placement services for program completers; remedial services; resume preparation assistance; skills, simulation, or other laboratory; tutoring; unpaid internships.

BACCALAUREATE PROGRAMS

Degree BScN
Available Programs Generic Baccalaureate; RN Baccalaureate.
Study Options Full-time.
Program Entrance Requirements CPR certification, high school biology, high school chemistry, high school transcript, immunizations. Transfer students are accepted. *Application deadline:* Applications may be processed on a rolling basis for some programs.
Contact *Telephone:* 705-675-1151 Ext. 3800. *Fax:* 705-675-4861.

GRADUATE PROGRAMS

Contact *Telephone:* 705-675-1151 Ext. 3800. *Fax:* 705-675-4861.

MASTER'S DEGREE PROGRAM
Degree M Sc N
Available Programs Master's.
Study Options Full-time and part-time.
Program Entrance Requirements Clinical experience, written essay, letters of recommendation, resume.
Degree Requirements Thesis or project.

CONTINUING EDUCATION PROGRAM

Contact *Telephone:* 705-675-1151 Ext. 3800. *Fax:* 705-675-4861.

McMaster University
School of Nursing
Hamilton, Ontario

http://www.fhs.mcmaster.ca/nursing
Founded in 1887
DEGREES • BSCN • M SC • MSN/PHD • PHD
Nursing Program Faculty 53 (47% with doctorates).
Baccalaureate Enrollment 548 **Women** 90% **Men** 10% **Part-time** 20%
Nursing Student Activities Student Nurses' Association.
Nursing Student Resources Academic advising; academic or career counseling; assistance for students with disabilities; bookstore; campus computer network; career placement assistance; computer lab; daycare for children of students; e-mail services; employment services for current students; housing assistance; Internet; learning resource lab; library services; nursing audiovisuals; placement services for program completers; remedial services; resume preparation assistance; skills, simulation, or other laboratory; tutoring.
Library Facilities 150,446 volumes in health; 89,267 periodical subscriptions health-care related.

BACCALAUREATE PROGRAMS

Degree BScN
Available Programs Baccalaureate for Second Degree; Generic Baccalaureate; RN Baccalaureate.
Site Options Kitchener, ON.
Study Options Full-time and part-time.
Program Entrance Requirements CPR certification, health exam, high school biology, high school chemistry, 4 years high school math, 4 years high school science, high school transcript, immunizations, minimum high school GPA of 3.0, minimum high school rank 75%. Transfer students are accepted.
Advanced Placement Credit by examination available. Credit given for nursing courses completed elsewhere dependent upon specific evaluations.
Contact *Telephone:* 905-525-9140 Ext. 22232. *Fax:* 905-528-4727.

GRADUATE PROGRAMS

Contact *Telephone:* 905-525-9140 Ext. 22982. *Fax:* 905-546-1129.

MASTER'S DEGREE PROGRAM
Degrees M Sc; MSN/PhD
Available Programs Master's.
Concentrations Available *Clinical nurse specialist programs in:* perinatal. *Nurse practitioner programs in:* neonatal health.
Study Options Full-time and part-time.
Program Entrance Requirements Transcript of college record, written essay, 2 letters of recommendation.
Advanced Placement Credit given for nursing courses completed elsewhere dependent upon specific evaluations.
Degree Requirements Thesis or project.

DOCTORAL DEGREE PROGRAM
Degree PhD
Available Programs Doctorate.
Program Entrance Requirements 2 letters of recommendation, MSN or equivalent, vita.
Degree Requirements Dissertation, oral exam.

Nipissing University
Nursing Department
North Bay, Ontario

http://www.nipissingu.ca/nursing/
Founded in 1992
DEGREE • BSCN
Nursing Program Faculty 16
Baccalaureate Enrollment 1,400 **Women** 80% **Men** 20%
Distance Learning Courses Available.
Nursing Student Activities Student Nurses' Association, nursing club.
Nursing Student Resources Academic advising; academic or career counseling; assistance for students with disabilities; bookstore; campus computer network; career placement assistance; computer lab; computer-assisted instruction; e-mail services; employment services for current students; externships; housing assistance; interactive nursing skills videos; Internet; learning resource lab; library services; nursing audiovisuals; placement services for program completers; remedial services; resume preparation assistance; skills, simulation, or other laboratory; tutoring; unpaid internships.
Library Facilities 3,000 volumes in health, 1,820 volumes in nursing; 2,430 periodical subscriptions health-care related.

BACCALAUREATE PROGRAMS

Degree BScN
Available Programs RN Baccalaureate; RPN to Baccalaureate.
Site Options all Ontario, ON; Toronto, ON.
Study Options Full-time and part-time.
Online Degree Options Yes.
Program Entrance Requirements Minimum overall college GPA of 3.0, transcript of college record, CPR certification, written essay, high school biology, high school chemistry, high school transcript, immunizations, interview, letters of recommendation, minimum high school rank 80%. Transfer students are accepted. *Application deadline:* 4/1 (fall). Applications may be processed on a rolling basis for some programs. *Application fee:* CAN$130.
Advanced Placement Credit given for nursing courses completed elsewhere dependent upon specific evaluations.

Contact Registrar's Office, Nursing Department, Nipissing University, 100 College Drive, PO Box 5002, North Bay, ON P1B 8L7. *Telephone:* 705-474-3450 Ext. 4521. *E-mail:* registrar@nipssingu.ca.

Queen's University at Kingston
School of Nursing
Kingston, Ontario

http://www.nursing.queensu.ca/
Founded in 1841
DEGREES • BNSC • MN SC • PHD
Nursing Program Faculty 31 (80% with doctorates).
Baccalaureate Enrollment 453 **Women** 85% **Men** 15%
Graduate Enrollment 110 **Women** 87% **Men** 13%
Distance Learning Courses Available.
Nursing Student Activities Student Nurses' Association.
Nursing Student Resources Academic advising; academic or career counseling; assistance for students with disabilities; bookstore; campus computer network; career placement assistance; computer lab; computer-assisted instruction; e-mail services; employment services for current students; housing assistance; interactive nursing skills videos; Internet; learning resource lab; library services; nursing audiovisuals; resume preparation assistance; skills, simulation, or other laboratory; tutoring; unpaid internships.
Library Facilities 5,209 volumes in health, 3,652 volumes in nursing; 1,054 periodical subscriptions health-care related.

BACCALAUREATE PROGRAMS

Degree BNSc
Available Programs Accelerated Baccalaureate; Generic Baccalaureate.
Site Options Napanee, ON.
Study Options Full-time.
Program Entrance Requirements CPR certification, high school biology, high school chemistry, high school math, high school science, high school transcript, immunizations, minimum high school GPA, minimum high school rank 75%. Transfer students are accepted. *Application deadline:* 2/1 (fall). *Application fee:* CAN$150.
Advanced Placement Credit given for nursing courses completed elsewhere dependent upon specific evaluations.
Expenses (2015–16) *Tuition, area resident:* full-time CAN$7352; part-time CAN$206 per unit. *International tuition:* CAN$32,188 full-time. *Room and board:* CAN$13,242 per academic year. *Required fees:* full-time CAN$730.
Financial Aid 86% of baccalaureate students in nursing programs received some form of financial aid in 2014–15.
Contact Dr. Christina Godfrey, Chair, Admissions Committee, School of Nursing, Queen's University at Kingston, Cataraqui Building, 92 Barrie Street, Kingston, ON K7L 3N6. *Telephone:* 613-533-2668 Ext. 78760. *Fax:* 613-533-6770. *E-mail:* christina.godfrey@queensu.ca.

GRADUATE PROGRAMS

Financial Aid 25 fellowships (averaging $6,636 per year), 4 research assistantships, 9 teaching assistantships (averaging $2,592 per year) were awarded; institutionally sponsored loans and scholarships also available.
Contact Dr. Joan Almost, Associate Director, Graduate Nursing Programs, School of Nursing, Queen's University at Kingston, Cataraqui Building, 92 Barrie Street, Kingston, ON K7L 3N6. *Telephone:* 613-533-6000 Ext. 74748. *Fax:* 613-533-6770. *E-mail:* joan.almost@queensu.ca.

MASTER'S DEGREE PROGRAM
Degree MN Sc
Available Programs Master's.
Study Options Full-time.
Program Entrance Requirements Minimum overall college GPA of 3.0, transcript of college record, 2 letters of recommendation, nursing research course, professional liability insurance/malpractice insurance, resume, statistics course. *Application deadline:* 2/1 (fall). *Application fee:* CAN$107.
Advanced Placement Credit given for nursing courses completed elsewhere dependent upon specific evaluations.
Degree Requirements 21 total credit hours, thesis or project.

DOCTORAL DEGREE PROGRAM
Degree PhD
Available Programs Doctorate.
Areas of Study Illness and transition, nursing research, nursing science.

Program Entrance Requirements Minimum overall college GPA of 3.3, 2 letters of recommendation, MSN or equivalent, statistics course, vita. Application deadline: 2/1 (fall). Application fee: CAN$107.
Degree Requirements 21 total credit hours, dissertation, oral exam, written exam.

Ryerson University
Program in Nursing
Toronto, Ontario

http://www.ryerson.ca/nursing
Founded in 1948
DEGREES • BSCN • MN
Nursing Program Faculty 83 (94% with doctorates).
Baccalaureate Enrollment 1,953 **Women** 89% **Men** 11% **Part-time** 25.75%
Graduate Enrollment 168 **Women** 89% **Men** 11% **Part-time** 28%
Distance Learning Courses Available.
Nursing Student Activities Sigma Theta Tau, Student Nurses' Association, nursing club.
Nursing Student Resources Academic advising; academic or career counseling; assistance for students with disabilities; bookstore; campus computer network; career placement assistance; computer lab; computer-assisted instruction; daycare for children of students; e-mail services; employment services for current students; housing assistance; interactive nursing skills videos; Internet; learning resource lab; library services; nursing audiovisuals; other; remedial services; resume preparation assistance; skills, simulation, or other laboratory; tutoring.
Library Facilities 29,163 volumes in health, 4,963 volumes in nursing; 5,567 periodical subscriptions health-care related.

BACCALAUREATE PROGRAMS

Degree BScN
Available Programs International Nurse to Baccalaureate; RN Baccalaureate; RPN to Baccalaureate.
Study Options Full-time.
Online Degree Options Yes.
Program Entrance Requirements Transcript of college record, CPR certification, health exam, health insurance, high school biology, high school chemistry, 3 years high school math, 4 years high school science, high school transcript, immunizations, minimum GPA in nursing prerequisites of 3.0. Transfer students are accepted. *Application deadline:* 3/1 (fall). *Application fee:* CAN$240.
Financial Aid *Gift aid (need-based):* college/university gift aid from institutional funds. *Loans:* Federal Direct (Subsidized and Unsubsidized Stafford). *Financial aid application deadline:* 1/15.
Contact Heather Palmer-Saettone, Senior Admissions Officer, Program in Nursing, Ryerson University, 350 Victoria Street, Toronto, ON M5B 2K3. *Telephone:* 416-979-5000 Ext. 4122. *Fax:* 416-979-5221. *E-mail:* hpsaettone@ryerson.ca.

GRADUATE PROGRAMS

Contact Mr. Gerry Warner, Program Administrator, Program in Nursing, Ryerson University, 350 Victoria Street, Toronto, ON M5B 2K3. *Telephone:* 416-979-5000 Ext. 7852. *Fax:* 416-979-5332. *E-mail:* gerry.warner@ryerson.ca.

MASTER'S DEGREE PROGRAM
Degree MN
Available Programs Master's.
Concentrations Available *Clinical nurse specialist programs in:* adult health, community health, family health, public health. *Nurse practitioner programs in:* primary care.
Study Options Full-time and part-time.
Program Entrance Requirements Minimum overall college GPA of 3.33, transcript of college record, written essay, immunizations, 2 letters of recommendation, nursing research course, physical assessment course, resume. *Application deadline:* 1/19 (fall). Applications may be processed on a rolling basis for some programs. *Application fee:* CAN$110.
Advanced Placement Credit given for nursing courses completed elsewhere dependent upon specific evaluations.
Degree Requirements 10 total credit hours, thesis or project.

CONTINUING EDUCATION PROGRAM

Contact Rheney Castillo, Program Manager, Program in Nursing, Ryerson University, 380 Victoria Street, CED 512-O, Toronto, ON M5B

2K3. *Telephone:* 416-979-0000 Ext. 5178. *Fax:* 416-542-5878. *E-mail:* rcastillo@ryerson.ca.

Trent University
Nursing Program
Peterborough, Ontario

http://www.trentu.ca/nursing/
Founded in 1963
DEGREE • BSCN
Nursing Program Faculty 56 (10% with doctorates).
Baccalaureate Enrollment 852 **Part-time** 11%
Distance Learning Courses Available.
Nursing Student Activities Student Nurses' Association.
Nursing Student Resources Academic advising; academic or career counseling; assistance for students with disabilities; bookstore; campus computer network; career placement assistance; computer lab; computer-assisted instruction; e-mail services; employment services for current students; housing assistance; interactive nursing skills videos; Internet; learning resource lab; library services; nursing audiovisuals; remedial services; resume preparation assistance; skills, simulation, or other laboratory; tutoring.
Library Facilities 6,393 volumes in health, 1,281 volumes in nursing; 360 periodical subscriptions health-care related.

BACCALAUREATE PROGRAMS

Degree BScN
Available Programs Accelerated Baccalaureate; Generic Baccalaureate.
Site Options Peterborough, ON; Toronto, ON.
Study Options Full-time.
Program Entrance Requirements Minimum overall college GPA of 3.0, transcript of college record, CPR certification, health exam, high school biology, high school chemistry, 4 years high school math, high school transcript, immunizations, minimum high school GPA of 3.0, minimum high school rank 75%, minimum GPA in nursing prerequisites. Transfer students are accepted. *Application deadline:* Applications may be processed on a rolling basis for some programs. *Application fee:* CAN$220.
Advanced Placement Credit given for nursing courses completed elsewhere dependent upon specific evaluations.
Financial Aid *Loans:* Sallie Mae Smart Option Loans.
Contact Nursing Enrolment Advisor, Nursing Program, Trent University, 1600 West Bank Drive, Peterborough, ON K9L 0G2. *Telephone:* 705-748-1011 Ext. 7809. *Fax:* 705-748-1629. *E-mail:* nursingadmissions@trentu.ca.

University of Ottawa
School of Nursing
Ottawa, Ontario

http://www.health.uottawa.ca/sn/
Founded in 1848
DEGREES • BSCN • M SC N • PHD
Nursing Program Faculty 122 (34% with doctorates).
Baccalaureate Enrollment 1,542 **Women** 89.14% **Men** 10.86% **Part-time** 13.01%
Graduate Enrollment 224 **Women** 90.18% **Men** 9.82% **Part-time** 60.71%
Distance Learning Courses Available.
Nursing Student Activities Sigma Theta Tau, Student Nurses' Association.
Nursing Student Resources Academic advising; academic or career counseling; assistance for students with disabilities; bookstore; campus computer network; career placement assistance; computer lab; computer-assisted instruction; e-mail services; employment services for current students; housing assistance; interactive nursing skills videos; Internet; learning resource lab; library services; nursing audiovisuals; remedial services; resume preparation assistance; skills, simulation, or other laboratory; tutoring.
Library Facilities 46,081 volumes in health, 8,911 volumes in nursing; 8,304 periodical subscriptions health-care related.

BACCALAUREATE PROGRAMS

Degree BScN
Available Programs Accelerated Baccalaureate for Second Degree; Accelerated RN Baccalaureate; Generic Baccalaureate; International Nurse to Baccalaureate; RN Baccalaureate; RPN to Baccalaureate.
Site Options Pembroke, ON.
Study Options Full-time.
Program Entrance Requirements Transcript of college record, high school biology, high school chemistry, high school math, high school transcript, minimum high school GPA. Transfer students are accepted. *Application deadline:* 3/30 (fall). *Application fee:* CAN$130.
Advanced Placement Credit given for nursing courses completed elsewhere dependent upon specific evaluations.
Expenses (2014–15) *Tuition:* full-time CAN$3005; part-time CAN$238 per credit. *Room and board:* CAN$8845; room only: CAN$5545 per academic year. *Required fees:* part-time CAN$127 per credit; part-time CAN$432 per term.
Financial Aid *Gift aid (need-based):* state, private, college/university gift aid from institutional funds. *Loans:* Federal Direct (Subsidized and Unsubsidized Stafford PLUS). *Work-study:* part-time campus jobs. *Financial aid application deadline:* 1/31.
Contact Ms. Anne Racine, Undergraduate Studies Office, School of Nursing, University of Ottawa, 125 Université, Ottawa, ON K1N 6N5. *Telephone:* 613-562-5800 Ext. 4238. *Fax:* 613-562-5149. *E-mail:* esecr@uottawa.ca.

GRADUATE PROGRAMS

Expenses (2014–15) *Tuition, area resident:* full-time CAN$2726. *International tuition:* CAN$6233 full-time. *Required fees:* full-time CAN$664.
Financial Aid Fellowships, research assistantships, teaching assistantships, career-related internships or fieldwork, Federal Work-Study, scholarships, traineeships, tuition waivers (full and partial), and unspecified assistantships available.
Contact Dr. Wendy Peterson, Assistant Director of Graduate Program, School of Nursing, University of Ottawa, 451 Smyth Road, Ottawa, ON K1H 8M5. *Telephone:* 613-562-5800 Ext. 8422. *Fax:* 613-562-5443. *E-mail:* wendy.peterson@uottawa.ca.

MASTER'S DEGREE PROGRAM
Degree M Sc N
Available Programs Master's.
Concentrations Available *Clinical nurse specialist programs in:* acute care, adult health, cardiovascular, community health, critical care, family health, forensic nursing, gerontology, home health care, maternity-newborn, medical-surgical, occupational health, oncology, palliative care, parent-child, pediatric, perinatal, psychiatric/mental health, public health, rehabilitation, school health, women's health. *Nurse practitioner programs in:* primary care.
Study Options Full-time and part-time.
Program Entrance Requirements Clinical experience, minimum overall college GPA of 3.0, transcript of college record, written essay, immunizations, 3 letters of recommendation, nursing research course, physical assessment course, prerequisite course work, resume, statistics course. *Application deadline:* 2/1 (winter).
Advanced Placement Credit given for nursing courses completed elsewhere dependent upon specific evaluations.
Degree Requirements 24 total credit hours, thesis or project.

DOCTORAL DEGREE PROGRAM
Degree PhD
Available Programs Doctorate; Doctorate for Nurses with Non-Nursing Degrees.
Areas of Study Aging, community health, critical care, ethics, forensic nursing, gerontology, health policy, health promotion/disease prevention, health-care systems, human health and illness, illness and transition, maternity-newborn, nursing education, nursing policy, nursing research, nursing science, oncology, women's health.
Program Entrance Requirements Minimum overall college GPA of 3.5, 3 letters of recommendation, MSN or equivalent, statistics course, vita, writing sample. Application deadline: 2/1 (winter). Application fee: CAN$100.
Degree Requirements 18 total credit hours, dissertation, oral exam, written exam, residency.

POSTDOCTORAL PROGRAM
Areas of Study Addiction/substance abuse, aging, cancer care, chronic illness, community health, health promotion/disease prevention, infor-

mation systems, nursing interventions, nursing research, nursing science, outcomes, vulnerable population, women's health.

Postdoctoral Program Contact Dr. Wendy Peterson, Assistant Director of Graduate Program, School of Nursing, University of Ottawa, 451 Smyth Road, Ottawa, ON K1H 8M5. *Telephone:* 613-562-5800 Ext. 8422. *Fax:* 613-562-5443. *E-mail:* wendy.peterson@uottawa.ca.

University of Toronto
Faculty of Nursing
Toronto, Ontario

http://www.bloomberg.nursing.utoronto.ca/
Founded in 1827
DEGREES • BSCN • MN • PHD
Nursing Program Faculty 250 (50% with doctorates).
Baccalaureate Enrollment 340 **Women** 87% **Men** 13%
Graduate Enrollment 360
Distance Learning Courses Available.
Nursing Student Activities Sigma Theta Tau, Student Nurses' Association, nursing club.
Nursing Student Resources Academic advising; academic or career counseling; assistance for students with disabilities; bookstore; campus computer network; career placement assistance; computer lab; computer-assisted instruction; daycare for children of students; e-mail services; employment services for current students; externships; housing assistance; interactive nursing skills videos; Internet; learning resource lab; library services; nursing audiovisuals; paid internships; remedial services; resume preparation assistance; skills, simulation, or other laboratory; tutoring.

BACCALAUREATE PROGRAMS

Degree BScN
Available Programs Accelerated Baccalaureate; Accelerated Baccalaureate for Second Degree; Accelerated RN Baccalaureate; Baccalaureate for Second Degree.
Study Options Full-time.
Program Entrance Requirements Minimum overall college GPA of 3.0, CPR certification, written essay, immunizations, 2 letters of recommendation, minimum GPA in nursing prerequisites of 3.0, prerequisite course work. *Application deadline:* 2/1 (fall).
Contact *Telephone:* 416-978-2392. *Fax:* 416-978-8222.

GRADUATE PROGRAMS

Contact *Telephone:* 416-978-2392. *Fax:* 416-978-8222.

MASTER'S DEGREE PROGRAM
Degree MN
Available Programs Master's.
Concentrations Available Clinical nurse leader; health-care administration; nurse anesthesia; nursing administration; nursing education; nursing informatics. *Clinical nurse specialist programs in:* acute care, adult health, cardiovascular, community health, critical care, family health, gerontology, maternity-newborn, medical-surgical, occupational health, oncology, palliative care, parent-child, pediatric, perinatal, psychiatric/mental health, public health, rehabilitation, school health, women's health. *Nurse practitioner programs in:* acute care, adult health, family health, gerontology, neonatal health, oncology, pediatric, primary care.
Study Options Full-time.
Online Degree Options Yes.
Program Entrance Requirements Clinical experience, minimum overall college GPA of 3.0, transcript of college record, CPR certification, written essay, 2 letters of recommendation, prerequisite course work, resume, statistics course. *Application deadline:* 3/15 (fall).
Degree Requirements 9 total credit hours.

POST-MASTER'S PROGRAM
Areas of Study Nurse anesthesia. *Clinical nurse specialist programs in:* acute care, adult health, gerontology, maternity-newborn, pediatric. *Nurse practitioner programs in:* acute care, adult health, pediatric, primary care.

DOCTORAL DEGREE PROGRAM
Degree PhD
Available Programs Doctorate; Doctorate for Nurses with Non-Nursing Degrees; Post-Baccalaureate Doctorate.

Areas of Study Addiction/substance abuse, advanced practice nursing, aging, bio-behavioral research, biology of health and illness, community health, critical care, ethics, faculty preparation, family health, gerontology, health policy, health promotion/disease prevention, health-care systems, human health and illness, individualized study, information systems, maternity-newborn, neuro-behavior, nurse case management, nursing administration, nursing education, nursing policy, nursing research, nursing science, oncology, urban health, women's health.
Program Entrance Requirements Minimum overall college GPA of 3.3, interview by faculty committee, 2 letters of recommendation, MSN or equivalent, scholarly papers, statistics course, vita, writing sample. Application deadline: 2/1 (fall).
Degree Requirements 6 total credit hours, dissertation, oral exam.

POSTDOCTORAL PROGRAM
Postdoctoral Program Contact *Telephone:* 416-978-8069.

The University of Western Ontario
School of Nursing
London, Ontario

http://www.uwo.ca/fhs/nursing
Founded in 1878
DEGREES • BSCN • M SC N • PHD
Nursing Program Faculty 101 (18% with doctorates).
Baccalaureate Enrollment 1,153 **Women** 93.24% **Men** 6.76% **Part-time** 13.53%
Graduate Enrollment 54 **Women** 89% **Men** 11% **Part-time** 28%
Nursing Student Activities Nursing Honor Society, Sigma Theta Tau, Student Nurses' Association.
Nursing Student Resources Academic advising; academic or career counseling; assistance for students with disabilities; bookstore; campus computer network; computer lab; computer-assisted instruction; daycare for children of students; e-mail services; employment services for current students; housing assistance; interactive nursing skills videos; Internet; learning resource lab; library services; nursing audiovisuals; resume preparation assistance; unpaid internships.
Library Facilities 357,263 volumes in health, 40 volumes in nursing; 250 periodical subscriptions health-care related.

BACCALAUREATE PROGRAMS

Degree BScN
Available Programs Accelerated Baccalaureate; Generic Baccalaureate; RN Baccalaureate.
Study Options Full-time.
Program Entrance Requirements CPR certification, high school biology, high school chemistry, 4 years high school math, high school science, high school transcript, immunizations, minimum high school rank 80%. Transfer students are accepted.
Advanced Placement Credit given for nursing courses completed elsewhere dependent upon specific evaluations.
Contact *Telephone:* 519-661-2111 Ext. 86564. *Fax:* 519-661-3928.

GRADUATE PROGRAMS

Contact *Telephone:* 519-661-3409. *Fax:* 519-661-3928.

MASTER'S DEGREE PROGRAM
Degree M Sc N
Available Programs Master's.
Concentrations Available Health-care administration; nursing administration; nursing education. *Clinical nurse specialist programs in:* acute care, adult health, community health, psychiatric/mental health, public health, women's health. *Nurse practitioner programs in:* community health.
Study Options Full-time and part-time.
Program Entrance Requirements Minimum overall college GPA of 3.5, transcript of college record, written essay, interview, 2 letters of recommendation, nursing research course, prerequisite course work, resume, statistics course.
Advanced Placement Credit given for nursing courses completed elsewhere dependent upon specific evaluations.
Degree Requirements 7 total credit hours, thesis or project.

DOCTORAL DEGREE PROGRAM

Degree PhD

Available Programs Doctorate.

Areas of Study Addiction/substance abuse, advanced practice nursing, aging, clinical practice, community health, faculty preparation, health policy, health promotion/disease prevention, health-care systems, human health and illness, individualized study, nurse case management, nursing administration, nursing education, nursing research, nursing science, women's health.

Program Entrance Requirements Clinical experience, minimum overall college GPA of 3.5, interview by faculty committee, interview, 2 letters of recommendation, MSN or equivalent, scholarly papers, statistics course, vita, writing sample.

Degree Requirements 4 total credit hours, dissertation, written exam.

POSTDOCTORAL PROGRAM

Areas of Study Addiction/substance abuse, community health, health promotion/disease prevention, vulnerable population, women's health.

Postdoctoral Program Contact *Telephone:* 519-661-2111 Ext. 86573.

University of Windsor

Faculty of Nursing
Windsor, Ontario

http://www.uwindsor.ca/nursing

Founded in 1857

DEGREES • BSCN • M SC N

Nursing Program Faculty 204 (7% with doctorates).

Baccalaureate Enrollment 924 **Women** 82% **Men** 18% **Part-time** 3%

Graduate Enrollment 102 **Women** 86% **Men** 14% **Part-time** 39%

Distance Learning Courses Available.

Nursing Student Activities Nursing Honor Society, Sigma Theta Tau, Student Nurses' Association, nursing club.

Nursing Student Resources Academic advising; academic or career counseling; assistance for students with disabilities; bookstore; campus computer network; career placement assistance; computer lab; computer-assisted instruction; e-mail services; employment services for current students; interactive nursing skills videos; Internet; learning resource lab; library services; nursing audiovisuals; placement services for program completers; remedial services; resume preparation assistance; skills, simulation, or other laboratory; tutoring.

Library Facilities 65,200 volumes in health, 9,160 volumes in nursing; 9,807 periodical subscriptions health-care related.

BACCALAUREATE PROGRAMS

Degree BScN

Available Programs Generic Baccalaureate.

Study Options Full-time.

Program Entrance Requirements CPR certification, health insurance, high school biology, high school chemistry, high school math, 4 years high school science, high school transcript, immunizations, minimum high school rank 82%. Transfer students are accepted. *Application deadline:* 1/13 (fall). *Application fee:* CAN$150.

Advanced Placement Credit given for nursing courses completed elsewhere dependent upon specific evaluations.

Expenses (2015–16) *Tuition, area resident:* full-time CAN$6014; part-time CAN$601 per course. *International tuition:* CAN$22,580 full-time. *Room and board:* CAN$11,092; room only: CAN$6942 per academic year. *Required fees:* full-time CAN$1036; part-time CAN$18 per credit; part-time CAN$449 per term.

Financial Aid 29% of baccalaureate students in nursing programs received some form of financial aid in 2014–15.

Contact Nursing Contact, Faculty of Nursing, University of Windsor, 401 Sunset Avenue, Windsor, ON N9B 3P4. *Telephone:* 519-253-3000 Ext. 2258. *Fax:* 519-973-7084. *E-mail:* nurse@uwindsor.ca.

GRADUATE PROGRAMS

Expenses (2015–16) *Tuition, area resident:* full-time CAN$5162; part-time CAN$1290 per term. *International tuition:* CAN$13,130 full-time.

Room and board: CAN$11,092; room only: CAN$6942 per academic year. *Required fees:* full-time CAN$803; part-time CAN$14 per credit; part-time CAN$91 per term.

Financial Aid 20% of graduate students in nursing programs received some form of financial aid in 2014–15.

Contact Dr. Michelle Freeman, Graduate Coordinator, Faculty of Nursing, University of Windsor, 401 Sunset Avenue, Windsor, ON N9B 3P4. *Telephone:* 519-253-3000 Ext. 4812. *Fax:* 519-973-7084. *E-mail:* mfreeman@uwindsor.ca.

MASTER'S DEGREE PROGRAM

Degree M Sc N

Available Programs Master's.

Concentrations Available Clinical nurse leader; nursing administration. *Nurse practitioner programs in:* primary care.

Study Options Full-time and part-time.

Program Entrance Requirements Minimum overall college GPA of 3.0, transcript of college record, written essay, 3 letters of recommendation, nursing research course, physical assessment course, prerequisite course work, statistics course. *Application deadline:* 2/15 (fall). *Application fee:* CAN$105.

Advanced Placement Credit given for nursing courses completed elsewhere dependent upon specific evaluations.

Degree Requirements 6 total credit hours, thesis or project.

POST-MASTER'S PROGRAM

Areas of Study *Nurse practitioner programs in:* primary care.

CONTINUING EDUCATION PROGRAM

Contact Nursing Main Office, Faculty of Nursing, University of Windsor, 401 Sunset Avenue, Windsor, ON N9B 3P4. *Telephone:* 519-253-3000 Ext. 2258. *Fax:* 519-973-7084. *E-mail:* nurse@uwindsor.ca.

York University

School of Nursing
Toronto, Ontario

Founded in 1959

DEGREE • BSCN

Nursing Program Faculty 19 (79% with doctorates).

Baccalaureate Enrollment 850 **Women** 96% **Men** 4% **Part-time** 15%

Nursing Student Resources Academic advising; academic or career counseling; assistance for students with disabilities; bookstore; campus computer network; career placement assistance; computer lab; computer-assisted instruction; daycare for children of students; e-mail services; employment services for current students; housing assistance; interactive nursing skills videos; Internet; learning resource lab; library services; nursing audiovisuals; skills, simulation, or other laboratory; unpaid internships.

BACCALAUREATE PROGRAMS

Degree BScN

Available Programs Generic Baccalaureate; RN Baccalaureate.

Site Options King City, ON; Barrie, ON; Oshawa, ON.

Study Options Full-time and part-time.

Program Entrance Requirements CPR certification, written essay, health exam, high school biology, high school chemistry, high school math, high school science, high school transcript, immunizations, 1 letter of recommendation, minimum high school GPA, minimum GPA in nursing prerequisites. Transfer students are accepted.

Advanced Placement Credit by examination available. Credit given for nursing courses completed elsewhere dependent upon specific evaluations.

Contact *Telephone:* 416-736-5271 Ext. 66351. *Fax:* 416-736-5714.

CONTINUING EDUCATION PROGRAM

Contact *Telephone:* 416-736-5271. *Fax:* 416-736-5714.

PRINCE EDWARD ISLAND

University of Prince Edward Island

School of Nursing
Charlottetown, Prince Edward Island

Founded in 1834

DEGREE • BSCN

Nursing Program Faculty 10 (2% with doctorates).
Baccalaureate Enrollment 211 **Women** 97% **Men** 3%
Nursing Student Activities Nursing Honor Society, Student Nurses' Association, nursing club.
Nursing Student Resources Academic advising; academic or career counseling; assistance for students with disabilities; bookstore; campus computer network; career placement assistance; computer lab; computer-assisted instruction; daycare for children of students; e-mail services; employment services for current students; housing assistance; interactive nursing skills videos; Internet; learning resource lab; library services; nursing audiovisuals; placement services for program completers; remedial services; resume preparation assistance; skills, simulation, or other laboratory; tutoring.

BACCALAUREATE PROGRAMS

Degree BScN
Available Programs Generic Baccalaureate.
Study Options Full-time and part-time.
Program Entrance Requirements Transcript of college record, CPR certification, high school chemistry, high school math, high school science, high school transcript, immunizations, minimum high school GPA of 3.0, minimum high school rank 75%, minimum GPA in nursing prerequisites of 3.0, prerequisite course work. Transfer students are accepted.
Advanced Placement Credit given for nursing courses completed elsewhere dependent upon specific evaluations.
Contact *Telephone:* 902-566-0733. *Fax:* 902-566-0777.

QUEBEC

McGill University

School of Nursing
Montréal, Quebec

http://www.mcgill.ca/
Founded in 1821

DEGREES • BSCN • M SC • PHD

Nursing Program Faculty 163 (13% with doctorates).
Baccalaureate Enrollment 438 **Women** 90% **Men** 10% **Part-time** 25%
Graduate Enrollment 93 **Women** 90% **Men** 10% **Part-time** 26%
Nursing Student Activities Student Nurses' Association.
Nursing Student Resources Academic advising; academic or career counseling; assistance for students with disabilities; bookstore; campus computer network; career placement assistance; computer lab; e-mail services; Internet; learning resource lab; library services; nursing audiovisuals; skills, simulation, or other laboratory; tutoring; unpaid internships.

BACCALAUREATE PROGRAMS

Degree BScN
Available Programs Accelerated RN Baccalaureate; Generic Baccalaureate; RN Baccalaureate.
Study Options Full-time.
Program Entrance Requirements Minimum overall college GPA of 3.0, transcript of college record, high school chemistry, 4 years high school math, 4 years high school science, high school transcript, minimum high school GPA of 3.3, minimum high school rank 25%. Transfer students are accepted. *Application deadline:* 1/15 (fall), 11/1 (winter). *Application fee:* CAN$85.

Advanced Placement Credit given for nursing courses completed elsewhere dependent upon specific evaluations.
Contact *Telephone:* 514-398-3784. *Fax:* 514-398-8455.

GRADUATE PROGRAMS

Contact *Telephone:* 514-398-4151. *Fax:* 514-398-8455.

MASTER'S DEGREE PROGRAM

Degree M Sc
Available Programs Master's; Master's for Non-Nursing College Graduates.
Concentrations Available Nursing administration. *Clinical nurse specialist programs in:* acute care, adult health, cardiovascular, community health, critical care, family health, gerontology, home health care, maternity-newborn, medical-surgical, oncology, parent-child, pediatric, perinatal, psychiatric/mental health, public health, rehabilitation, women's health. *Nurse practitioner programs in:* neonatal health, primary care.
Study Options Full-time.
Program Entrance Requirements Clinical experience, minimum overall college GPA of 3.0, transcript of college record, CPR certification, written essay, immunizations, interview, 3 letters of recommendation, resume, statistics course. *Application deadline:* 1/15 (fall). *Application fee:* CAN$85.
Degree Requirements 53 total credit hours, thesis or project.

DOCTORAL DEGREE PROGRAM

Degree PhD
Available Programs Doctorate; Post-Baccalaureate Doctorate.
Areas of Study Family health, health-care systems, human health and illness, nursing administration, nursing research, oncology.
Program Entrance Requirements Minimum overall college GPA of 3.3, interview, 2 letters of recommendation, MSN or equivalent, statistics course, vita, writing sample. Application deadline: 1/15 (fall). Application fee: CAN$85.
Degree Requirements 90 total credit hours, dissertation, oral exam, written exam, residency.

POSTDOCTORAL PROGRAM

Areas of Study Cancer care, chronic illness.
Postdoctoral Program Contact *Telephone:* 514-398-4157. *Fax:* 514-398-8455.

Université de Montréal

Faculty of Nursing
Montréal, Quebec

http://www.scinf.umontreal.ca/
Founded in 1920

DEGREES • BSCN • M SC • PHD

Nursing Program Faculty 43 (93% with doctorates).
Baccalaureate Enrollment 1,100 **Women** 80% **Men** 20% **Part-time** 10%
Graduate Enrollment 300 **Women** 75% **Men** 25% **Part-time** 60%
Distance Learning Courses Available.
Nursing Student Activities Student Nurses' Association.
Nursing Student Resources Academic advising; academic or career counseling; assistance for students with disabilities; bookstore; campus computer network; career placement assistance; computer lab; computer-assisted instruction; daycare for children of students; e-mail services; employment services for current students; externships; housing assistance; interactive nursing skills videos; Internet; learning resource lab; library services; nursing audiovisuals; other; placement services for program completers; remedial services; resume preparation assistance; skills, simulation, or other laboratory; tutoring; unpaid internships.
Library Facilities 32,536 volumes in health, 32,536 volumes in nursing; 1,319 periodical subscriptions health-care related.

BACCALAUREATE PROGRAMS

Degree BScN
Available Programs Generic Baccalaureate; RN Baccalaureate.
Site Options Laval, QC.
Study Options Full-time.
Program Entrance Requirements Minimum overall college GPA, transcript of college record, CPR certification, high school biology, high school chemistry, immunizations, minimum GPA in nursing prerequi-

sites. Transfer students are accepted. *Application deadline:* 2/1 (fall), 10/3 (winter). *Application fee:* CAN$95.

Advanced Placement Credit given for nursing courses completed elsewhere dependent upon specific evaluations.

Expenses (2015–16) *Tuition, state resident:* full-time CAN$4500. *Tuition, nonresident:* full-time CAN$7000. *International tuition:* CAN$10,000 full-time. *Room and board:* CAN$14,000; room only: CAN$10,000 per academic year.

Contact Catherine Sarrazin, Assistant to Vice Dean, Faculty of Nursing, Université de Montréal, Pav. Marg. d'Youville, CP 6128 Succursale Centre-Ville, Montreal, QC H3C 3J7. *Telephone:* 514-343-6439. *Fax:* 514-343-2306. *E-mail:* catherine.sarrazin@umontreal.ca.

GRADUATE PROGRAMS

Expenses (2015–16) *Tuition, state resident:* full-time CAN$2000. *Tuition, nonresident:* full-time CAN$4000. *International tuition:* CAN$10,000 full-time.

Financial Aid Fellowships, research assistantships, teaching assistantships, career-related internships or fieldwork, Federal Work-Study, and institutionally sponsored loans available.

Contact Rejean Goulet, Program Administrator, Faculty of Nursing, Université de Montréal, Pav. Marg. d'Youville, CP 6128 Succursale Centre-Ville, Montreal, QC H3C 3J7. *Telephone:* 514-343-6111 Ext. 34290. *E-mail:* rejean.gouletl@umontreal.ca.

MASTER'S DEGREE PROGRAM

Degree M Sc

Available Programs Accelerated RN to Master's; Master's; RN to Master's.

Concentrations Available Clinical nurse leader; nursing administration; nursing education. *Clinical nurse specialist programs in:* acute care, adult health, cardiovascular, community health, family health, gerontology, maternity-newborn, medical-surgical, occupational health, oncology, palliative care, parent-child, psychiatric/mental health, public health, rehabilitation, women's health. *Nurse practitioner programs in:* acute care, adult health, community health, family health, primary care.

Study Options Full-time and part-time.

Program Entrance Requirements Minimum overall college GPA of 3.0, transcript of college record, CPR certification, written essay, immunizations, nursing research course, resume, statistics course. *Application deadline:* 3/1 (fall). *Application fee:* CAN$95.

Degree Requirements 45 total credit hours, thesis or project.

POST-MASTER'S PROGRAM

Areas of Study *Nurse practitioner programs in:* acute care, adult health, community health, family health, primary care.

DOCTORAL DEGREE PROGRAM

Degree PhD

Available Programs Doctorate.

Areas of Study Addiction/substance abuse, aging, bio-behavioral research, clinical practice, community health, critical care, family health, gerontology, health policy, health promotion/disease prevention, healthcare systems, human health and illness, illness and transition, maternity-newborn, neuro-behavior, nursing administration, nursing education, nursing policy, nursing research, nursing science, oncology, urban health, women's health.

Program Entrance Requirements Minimum overall college GPA of 3.4, interview by faculty committee, interview, 2 letters of recommendation, MSN or equivalent, statistics course, vita, writing sample. Application deadline: 3/1 (fall). Application fee: CAN$90.

Degree Requirements 90 total credit hours, dissertation, oral exam.

POSTDOCTORAL PROGRAM

Areas of Study Adolescent health, aging, cancer care, chronic illness, community health, family health, gerontology, health promotion/disease prevention, individualized study, neuro-behavior, nursing informatics, nursing interventions, nursing research, nursing science, outcomes, self-care, vulnerable population, women's health.

Postdoctoral Program Contact Ms. Caroline Larue, PhD, Vice Dean, Graduate studies, Faculty of Nursing, Université de Montréal, Faculte des sciences infirmieres, C.P. 6128, Succursale Centre-Ville, Montreal, QC H3C 3J7. *Telephone:* 514-343-5835. *E-mail:* caroline.larue@umontreal.ca.

CONTINUING EDUCATION PROGRAM

Contact Ms. Camille Sasseville, Program Coordinator, Faculty of Nursing, Université de Montréal, Pav. Marg. d'Youville, CP 6128 Succursale Centre-Ville, Montreal, QC H3C 3J7. *Telephone:* 514-343-6111 Ext. 84164. *E-mail:* camille.sasseville@umontreal.ca.

Université de Sherbrooke
Department of Nursing
Sherbrooke, Quebec

http://www.usherbrooke.ca/scinf/
Founded in 1954

DEGREES • BSCN • M SC • PHD
Nursing Program Faculty 17 (76% with doctorates).
Baccalaureate Enrollment 482 **Women** 90% **Men** 10% **Part-time** 30%
Graduate Enrollment 61 **Women** 95% **Men** 5% **Part-time** 50%
Nursing Student Activities Student Nurses' Association.
Nursing Student Resources Academic advising; academic or career counseling; assistance for students with disabilities; bookstore; computer lab; computer-assisted instruction; e-mail services; externships; housing assistance; Internet; learning resource lab; library services; nursing audiovisuals; tutoring.
Library Facilities 40,000 volumes in health, 4,000 volumes in nursing; 3,000 periodical subscriptions health-care related.

BACCALAUREATE PROGRAMS

Degree BScN
Available Programs RN Baccalaureate.
Site Options Longueuil, QC.
Study Options Full-time and part-time.
Program Entrance Requirements Transcript of college record, high school chemistry, 4 years high school math, immunizations, professional liability insurance/malpractice insurance, RN licensure. Transfer students are accepted.
Advanced Placement Credit given for nursing courses completed elsewhere dependent upon specific evaluations.
Contact *Telephone:* 819-563-5355. *Fax:* 819-820-6816.

GRADUATE PROGRAMS

Contact *Telephone:* 819-564-5354. *Fax:* 819-820-6816.

MASTER'S DEGREE PROGRAM

Degree M Sc
Available Programs Master's.
Concentrations Available *Clinical nurse specialist programs in:* acute care, community health, family health, gerontology.
Site Options Longueuil, QC.
Study Options Full-time and part-time.
Program Entrance Requirements Transcript of college record, interview, 3 letters of recommendation, nursing research course, professional liability insurance/malpractice insurance, resume.
Degree Requirements 45 total credit hours, thesis or project.

DOCTORAL DEGREE PROGRAM

Degree PhD
Available Programs Doctorate.
Areas of Study Advanced practice nursing, aging, biology of health and illness, clinical practice, community health, critical care, family health, gerontology, health promotion/disease prevention, human health and illness, illness and transition, information systems, maternity-newborn, neuro-behavior, nurse case management, nursing administration, nursing education, nursing policy, nursing research, nursing science, oncology, women's health.
Site Options Longueuil, QC.
Program Entrance Requirements Clinical experience, interview, 3 letters of recommendation, MSN or equivalent, statistics course, vita, writing sample.
Degree Requirements 90 total credit hours, dissertation, oral exam, written exam.

POSTDOCTORAL PROGRAM

Postdoctoral Program Contact *Telephone:* 819-564-5355. *Fax:* 819-820-6816.

Université du Québec à Chicoutimi

Program in Nursing
Chicoutimi, Quebec

http://programmes.uqac.ca/liste_prog.html?type=clarder&cl arder=1203

Founded in 1969

DEGREES • BNSC • MSN

Nursing Program Faculty 10 (3% with doctorates).
Baccalaureate Enrollment 537 **Women** 89% **Men** 11% **Part-time** 80%
Graduate Enrollment 50 **Women** 100% **Part-time** 100%
Distance Learning Courses Available.
Nursing Student Activities Student Nurses' Association.
Nursing Student Resources Academic advising; academic or career counseling; assistance for students with disabilities; bookstore; campus computer network; computer lab; computer-assisted instruction; e-mail services; employment services for current students; externships; housing assistance; interactive nursing skills videos; Internet; learning resource lab; library services; nursing audiovisuals; other; resume preparation assistance; skills, simulation, or other laboratory; tutoring; unpaid internships.
Library Facilities 8,000 volumes in health, 6,300 volumes in nursing; 5,250 periodical subscriptions health-care related.

BACCALAUREATE PROGRAMS

Degree BNSc
Available Programs Accelerated RN Baccalaureate; Generic Baccalaureate; RN Baccalaureate.
Site Options Sept-Iles, QC.
Study Options Full-time and part-time.
Program Entrance Requirements Transcript of college record, high school biology, 1 year of high school math, immunizations, interview, 1 letter of recommendation. Transfer students are accepted. *Application deadline:* 3/1 (fall), 3/1 (winter), 3/1 (spring), 3/1 (summer). *Application fee:* CAN$30.
Advanced Placement Credit given for nursing courses completed elsewhere dependent upon specific evaluations.
Expenses (2015–16) *Tuition, area resident:* full-time CAN$3475; part-time CAN$76 per credit. *Tuition, state resident:* full-time CAN$2950; part-time CAN$76 per credit. *Tuition, nonresident:* full-time CAN$7750; part-time CAN$234 per credit. *International tuition:* CAN$18,000 full-time. *Required fees:* full-time CAN$2750; part-time CAN$1376 per term.
Financial Aid 20% of baccalaureate students in nursing programs received some form of financial aid in 2014–15. *Gift aid (need-based):* private, college/university gift aid from institutional funds. *Loans:* college/university. *Work-study:* part-time campus jobs.
Contact Mme. Anna Gauthier, Secretary, Program in Nursing, Université du Québec à Chicoutimi, 555 Boulevard de l'Universite, Chicoutimi, QC G7H 2B1. *Telephone:* 418-545-5011 Ext. 5315. *Fax:* 418-615-1205. *E-mail:* anna_gauthier@uqac.ca.

GRADUATE PROGRAMS

Expenses (2015–16) *Tuition, area resident:* full-time CAN$1720; part-time CAN$76 per credit. *Tuition, state resident:* full-time CAN$1700; part-time CAN$76 per credit. *Tuition, nonresident:* full-time CAN$5271; part-time CAN$234 per credit. *International tuition:* CAN$11,780 full-time. *Required fees:* part-time CAN$286 per term.
Financial Aid 2% of graduate students in nursing programs received some form of financial aid in 2014–15.
Contact Ms. Marie Tremblay, RN, Director of Master's Degree Program, Program in Nursing, Université du Québec à Chicoutimi, 555 Boulevard de l'Université, Saguenay, QC G7H 2B1. *Telephone:* 418-545-5011 Ext. 5331. *Fax:* 418-615-1205. *E-mail:* Marie_Tremblay@uqac.ca.

MASTER'S DEGREE PROGRAM

Degree MSN
Available Programs Master's; RN to Master's.
Concentrations Available *Clinical nurse specialist programs in:* adult-psychiatric mental health, psychiatric/mental health. *Nurse practitioner programs in:* primary care.

Site Options Sept-Iles, QC.
Study Options Full-time and part-time.
Program Entrance Requirements Clinical experience, minimum overall college GPA of 3.2, transcript of college record, written essay, interview, 3 letters of recommendation, nursing research course, professional liability insurance/malpractice insurance, resume, statistics course. *Application deadline:* 3/1 (fall), 3/1 (winter), 3/1 (spring), 3/1 (summer). *Application fee:* CAN$30.
Advanced Placement Credit given for nursing courses completed elsewhere dependent upon specific evaluations.
Degree Requirements 45 total credit hours, thesis or project, comprehensive exam.

CONTINUING EDUCATION PROGRAM

Contact Ms. Annie Rioux, Secretary, Program in Nursing, Université du Québec à Chicoutimi, 555, boulevard de l'Université, Chicoutimi, QC G7H 2B1. *Telephone:* 418-545-5011 Ext. 2425. *E-mail:* cesam@uqac.ca.

Université du Québec à Rimouski

Program in Nursing
Rimouski, Quebec

http://www.uqar.ca/english/

Founded in 1973

DEGREES • BSCN • M SC N

Nursing Program Faculty 17 (53% with doctorates).
Baccalaureate Enrollment 750 **Women** 90% **Men** 10% **Part-time** 74%
Graduate Enrollment 24 **Women** 96% **Men** 4% **Part-time** 92%
Distance Learning Courses Available.
Nursing Student Activities Student Nurses' Association.
Nursing Student Resources Academic advising; academic or career counseling; assistance for students with disabilities; bookstore; campus computer network; career placement assistance; computer lab; daycare for children of students; e-mail services; employment services for current students; housing assistance; Internet; learning resource lab; library services; nursing audiovisuals; other; placement services for program completers; resume preparation assistance; skills, simulation, or other laboratory; tutoring.
Library Facilities 5,200 volumes in health, 1,100 volumes in nursing; 1,300 periodical subscriptions health-care related.

BACCALAUREATE PROGRAMS

Degree BScN
Available Programs RN Baccalaureate.
Site Options Rimouski, QC; Lévis, QC.
Study Options Full-time and part-time.
Program Entrance Requirements Transcript of college record, professional liability insurance/malpractice insurance, prerequisite course work. Transfer students are accepted.
Advanced Placement Credit by examination available.
Contact *Telephone:* 418-723-1986 Ext. 1568. *Fax:* 418-724-1450.

GRADUATE PROGRAMS

Contact *Telephone:* 418-723-1986 Ext. 1345. *Fax:* 418-724-1450.

MASTER'S DEGREE PROGRAM

Degree M Sc N
Available Programs Master's.
Concentrations Available *Clinical nurse specialist programs in:* community health, critical care, gerontology, psychiatric/mental health.
Site Options Rimouski, QC; Lévis, QC.
Study Options Full-time and part-time.
Program Entrance Requirements Clinical experience, transcript of college record, interview, 3 letters of recommendation, nursing research course, prerequisite course work, statistics course.
Advanced Placement Credit given for nursing courses completed elsewhere dependent upon specific evaluations.
Degree Requirements 45 total credit hours, thesis or project.

CONTINUING EDUCATION PROGRAM

Contact *Telephone:* 418-723-1986 Ext. 1818. *Fax:* 418-724-1525.

Université du Québec à Trois-Rivières

Program in Nursing
Trois-Rivières, Quebec

http://www.uqtr.ca/
Founded in 1969
DEGREES • BSN • MSN
Nursing Program Faculty 28 (30% with doctorates).
Baccalaureate Enrollment 180 **Women** 95% **Men** 5% **Part-time** 75%
Graduate Enrollment 50 **Women** 97% **Men** 3% **Part-time** 90%
Distance Learning Courses Available.
Nursing Student Activities Student Nurses' Association.
Nursing Student Resources Academic advising; academic or career counseling; assistance for students with disabilities; bookstore; campus computer network; career placement assistance; computer lab; computer-assisted instruction; daycare for children of students; e-mail services; employment services for current students; externships; interactive nursing skills videos; Internet; learning resource lab; library services; nursing audiovisuals; placement services for program completers; resume preparation assistance; skills, simulation, or other laboratory; tutoring; unpaid internships.
Library Facilities 2,000 volumes in health, 500 volumes in nursing; 2,000 periodical subscriptions health-care related.

BACCALAUREATE PROGRAMS

Degree BSN
Available Programs Generic Baccalaureate; RN Baccalaureate.
Study Options Full-time and part-time.
Program Entrance Requirements Transcript of college record, CPR certification, high school biology, high school chemistry, prerequisite course work, RN licensure. Transfer students are accepted. *Application deadline:* 3/1 (fall). Applications may be processed on a rolling basis for some programs. *Application fee:* CAN$30.
Advanced Placement Credit given for nursing courses completed elsewhere dependent upon specific evaluations.
Contact *Telephone:* 819-376-5011 Ext. 3471. *Fax:* 819-376-5048.

GRADUATE PROGRAMS

Contact *Telephone:* 819-376-5011 Ext. 3460.

MASTER'S DEGREE PROGRAM

Degree MSN
Available Programs Master's.
Concentrations Available *Clinical nurse specialist programs in:* acute care, adult health, community health, critical care, family health, home health care, maternity-newborn, medical-surgical, pediatric, perinatal, psychiatric/mental health, public health. *Nurse practitioner programs in:* primary care.
Study Options Full-time and part-time.
Program Entrance Requirements Minimum overall college GPA of 3, transcript of college record, CPR certification, immunizations, 3 letters of recommendation, nursing research course, physical assessment course, prerequisite course work, statistics course. *Application deadline:* 8/29 (fall), 11/29 (winter), 4/29 (spring). Applications may be processed on a rolling basis for some programs. *Application fee:* CAN$30.
Advanced Placement Credit by examination available.
Degree Requirements 45 total credit hours, thesis or project.

Université du Québec en Abitibi-Témiscamingue

Département des sciences sociales et de la santé
Rouyn-Noranda, Quebec

http://www.uqat.ca/en/
Founded in 1983
DEGREE • BN
Nursing Program Faculty 12
Baccalaureate Enrollment 78 **Women** 95% **Men** 5% **Part-time** 64%
Nursing Student Resources Academic advising; assistance for students with disabilities; bookstore; campus computer network; computer lab; computer-assisted instruction; housing assistance; Internet; library ser-

vices; resume preparation assistance; skills, simulation, or other laboratory.
Library Facilities 3,239 volumes in health, 715 volumes in nursing; 17 periodical subscriptions health-care related.

BACCALAUREATE PROGRAMS

Degree BN
Program Entrance Requirements Transfer students are accepted.
Contact *Telephone:* 819-762-0971 Ext. 2370. *Fax:* 819-797-4727.

Université du Québec en Outaouais

Département des Sciences Infirmières
Gatineau, Quebec

http://www.uqo.ca/
Founded in 1981
DEGREES • BSCN • M SC N
Nursing Program Faculty 23 (78% with doctorates).
Baccalaureate Enrollment 1,000 **Women** 90% **Men** 10% **Part-time** 40%
Graduate Enrollment 100 **Women** 95% **Men** 5% **Part-time** 90%
Nursing Student Activities Student Nurses' Association.
Nursing Student Resources Academic advising; academic or career counseling; assistance for students with disabilities; bookstore; campus computer network; career placement assistance; computer lab; daycare for children of students; e-mail services; employment services for current students; externships; housing assistance; Internet; learning resource lab; library services; nursing audiovisuals; placement services for program completers; skills, simulation, or other laboratory; unpaid internships.

BACCALAUREATE PROGRAMS

Degree BScN
Available Programs Generic Baccalaureate; RN Baccalaureate.
Site Options St. Jerome, QC.
Study Options Full-time and part-time.
Program Entrance Requirements CPR certification, immunizations. Transfer students are accepted. *Application deadline:* 3/1 (fall). *Application fee:* CAN$30.
Advanced Placement Credit by examination available. Credit given for nursing courses completed elsewhere dependent upon specific evaluations.
Expenses (2014–15) *International tuition:* CAN$8200 full-time.
Financial Aid 10% of baccalaureate students in nursing programs received some form of financial aid in 2013–14. *Loans:* college/university.
Contact Prof. Robert Bilterys, Directeur, Département des Sciences Infirmières, Université du Québec en Outaouais, 5, rue Saint-Joseph, Succursale Hull, Hull, QC J8X 3X7. *Telephone:* 819-595-3900 Ext. 4102. *Fax:* 819-595-3801. *E-mail:* robert.bilterys@uqo.ca.

GRADUATE PROGRAMS

Expenses (2014–15) *International tuition:* CAN$4900 full-time.
Financial Aid 50% of graduate students in nursing programs received some form of financial aid in 2013–14.
Contact Prof. Chantal St-Pierre, Director, Département des Sciences Infirmières, Université du Québec en Outaouais, CP 1250, Succursale Hull, Gatineau, QC J8X 3X7. *Telephone:* 819-595-3900 Ext. 2347. *E-mail:* chantal.saint-pierre@uqo.ca.

MASTER'S DEGREE PROGRAM

Degree M Sc N
Available Programs Master's; Master's for Nurses with Non-Nursing Degrees.
Concentrations Available *Clinical nurse specialist programs in:* acute care, adult health, adult-gerontology acute care, adult-psychiatric mental health, cardiovascular, child/adolescent psychiatric-mental health, community health, critical care, family health, forensic nursing, gerontology, home health care, maternity-newborn, medical-surgical, occupational health, oncology, palliative care, parent-child, pediatric, perinatal, psychiatric/mental health, public health, public/community health, rehabilitation, school health, women's health. *Nurse practitioner programs in:* primary care.
Site Options St. Jerome, QC.
Study Options Full-time and part-time.

Program Entrance Requirements Clinical experience, computer literacy, minimum overall college GPA of 3.0, transcript of college record, interview, 3 letters of recommendation, nursing research course, resume, statistics course. *Application deadline:* 5/1 (fall), 11/1 (winter), 3/1 (spring). *Application fee:* CAN$30.
Advanced Placement Credit given for nursing courses completed elsewhere dependent upon specific evaluations.
Degree Requirements 45 total credit hours, thesis or project.

POSTDOCTORAL PROGRAM

Areas of Study Family health.
Postdoctoral Program Contact Prof. Francne de Montigny, Professor, Département des Sciences Infirmières, Université du Québec en Outaouais, C.P. 1250 succ Hull, Gatineau, QC J8T 5K7. *Telephone:* 819-595-3900 Ext. 2257.

CONTINUING EDUCATION PROGRAM

Contact Ms. Sophie Godbout, Chargée de projet en formation continue, Département des Sciences Infirmières, Université du Québec en Outaouais, Décanat de la formation continue et des partenariats (DFCP), Gatineau, QC J8X 3X7. *Telephone:* 819-595-3900 Ext. 1805. *E-mail:* monique.fecteau@uqo.ca.

Université Laval
Faculty of Nursing
Québec, Quebec

http://www.fsi.ulaval.ca/
Founded in 1852
DEGREES • BSCN • MSN • PHD
Nursing Program Faculty 25 (64% with doctorates).
Baccalaureate Enrollment 798 **Women** 94% **Men** 6% **Part-time** 32%
Graduate Enrollment 116 **Women** 72% **Men** 28% **Part-time** 22%
Distance Learning Courses Available.
Nursing Student Activities Student Nurses' Association, nursing club.
Nursing Student Resources Academic advising; academic or career counseling; assistance for students with disabilities; bookstore; campus computer network; career placement assistance; computer lab; computer-assisted instruction; daycare for children of students; e-mail services; employment services for current students; externships; housing assistance; interactive nursing skills videos; Internet; learning resource lab; library services; nursing audiovisuals; placement services for program completers; resume preparation assistance; skills, simulation, or other laboratory; tutoring.
Library Facilities 118,994 volumes in health, 3,781 volumes in nursing; 624 periodical subscriptions health-care related.

BACCALAUREATE PROGRAMS

Degree BScN
Available Programs Accelerated Baccalaureate; Accelerated RN Baccalaureate; Generic Baccalaureate; RN Baccalaureate.
Study Options Full-time and part-time.
Program Entrance Requirements Transcript of college record, high school biology, high school chemistry, 5 years high school math, high school transcript, immunizations, minimum high school GPA. Transfer students are accepted.
Advanced Placement Credit given for nursing courses completed elsewhere dependent upon specific evaluations.
Contact *Telephone:* 418-656-2131 Ext. 7930. *Fax:* 418-656-7747.

GRADUATE PROGRAMS

Contact *Telephone:* 418-656-3356. *Fax:* 418-656-7304.

MASTER'S DEGREE PROGRAM

Degree MSN
Available Programs Accelerated Master's; Master's.
Concentrations Available Clinical nurse leader; health-care administration; nursing administration. *Clinical nurse specialist programs in:* acute care, adult health, cardiovascular, community health, critical care, family health, gerontology, oncology, palliative care, parent-child, pediatric, perinatal, psychiatric/mental health, public health, rehabilitation. *Nurse practitioner programs in:* adult health, primary care.
Study Options Full-time and part-time.
Program Entrance Requirements Clinical experience, transcript of college record, 2 letters of recommendation, nursing research course, resume, statistics course, French exam.
Advanced Placement Credit given for nursing courses completed elsewhere dependent upon specific evaluations.
Degree Requirements 45 total credit hours, thesis or project.

POST-MASTER'S PROGRAM

Areas of Study *Clinical nurse specialist programs in:* acute care, adult health, cardiovascular, community health, critical care, family health, gerontology, oncology, palliative care, parent-child, pediatric, perinatal, psychiatric/mental health, public health, rehabilitation. *Nurse practitioner programs in:* adult health, primary care.

DOCTORAL DEGREE PROGRAM

Degree PhD
Available Programs Doctorate.
Areas of Study Community health, nursing science.
Program Entrance Requirements Clinical experience, interview, 2 letters of recommendation, MSN or equivalent, scholarly papers, statistics course, vita, writing sample.
Degree Requirements 96 total credit hours, dissertation, oral exam, written exam.

POSTDOCTORAL PROGRAM

Areas of Study Aging, cancer care, community health, gerontology, health promotion/disease prevention, nursing interventions, nursing research, nursing science, outcomes.
Postdoctoral Program Contact *Telephone:* 418-656-3356. *Fax:* 418-656-7747. S

CONTINUING EDUCATION PROGRAM

Contact *Telephone:* 418-656-2131 Ext. 6712. *Fax:* 418-656-7747.

SASKATCHEWAN

University of Saskatchewan
College of Nursing
Saskatoon, Saskatchewan

http://www.usask.ca/nursing/
Founded in 1907
DEGREES • BSN • MN • PHD
Nursing Program Faculty 134 (20% with doctorates).
Baccalaureate Enrollment 1,678 **Women** 93% **Men** 7% **Part-time** 17%
Graduate Enrollment 50 **Women** 94% **Men** 6% **Part-time** 62%
Distance Learning Courses Available.
Nursing Student Activities Student Nurses' Association.
Nursing Student Resources Academic advising; academic or career counseling; assistance for students with disabilities; bookstore; campus computer network; computer lab; computer-assisted instruction; daycare for children of students; e-mail services; employment services for current students; interactive nursing skills videos; Internet; learning resource lab; library services; nursing audiovisuals; other; remedial services; resume preparation assistance; skills, simulation, or other laboratory; tutoring.
Library Facilities 92,505 volumes in health, 3,932 volumes in nursing; 3,069 periodical subscriptions health-care related.

BACCALAUREATE PROGRAMS

Degree BSN
Available Programs Accelerated Baccalaureate; Accelerated RN Baccalaureate; Baccalaureate for Second Degree; Generic Baccalaureate; RN Baccalaureate.
Site Options Regina , SK; Prince Albert, SK; Saskatoon , SK.
Study Options Full-time and part-time.
Program Entrance Requirements Transcript of college record, CPR certification, high school biology, high school chemistry, 4 years high school math, 4 years high school science, high school transcript, immunizations, minimum high school GPA of 2.0. Transfer students are accepted. *Application deadline:* 1/15 (fall). *Application fee:* CAN$90.
Advanced Placement Credit given for nursing courses completed elsewhere dependent upon specific evaluations.
Contact *Telephone:* 306-966-6231. *Fax:* 306-966-6621.

GRADUATE PROGRAMS

Contact *Telephone:* 306-966-1477. *Fax:* 306-966-6703.

MASTER'S DEGREE PROGRAM
Degree MN
Available Programs Master's.
Concentrations Available Nursing education. *Nurse practitioner programs in:* primary care.
Site Options Saskatoon , SK.
Study Options Full-time and part-time.
Program Entrance Requirements Minimum overall college GPA of 2.5, transcript of college record, 3 letters of recommendation, nursing research course, statistics course. *Application deadline:* 11/15 (fall). *Application fee:* CAN$75.
Advanced Placement Credit given for nursing courses completed elsewhere dependent upon specific evaluations.
Degree Requirements 24 total credit hours, thesis or project.

POST-MASTER'S PROGRAM
Areas of Study *Nurse practitioner programs in:* primary care.

DOCTORAL DEGREE PROGRAM
Degree PhD
Available Programs Doctorate.
Areas of Study Individualized study.
Site Options Saskatoon , SK.
Program Entrance Requirements Minimum overall college GPA of 4, 3 letters of recommendation, MSN or equivalent, statistics course, vita. Application deadline: 11/15 (fall). Application fee: CAN$75.
Degree Requirements 18 total credit hours, dissertation, oral exam, written exam.

CONTINUING EDUCATION PROGRAM

Contact *Telephone:* 306-966-6261. *Fax:* 306-966-7673.

TWO-PAGE DESCRIPTIONS

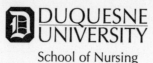

DUQUESNE UNIVERSITY
School of Nursing

The Duquesne University School of Nursing has a long history of innovation and excellence in undergraduate and graduate nursing education and remains at the forefront. Its location in Pittsburgh, Pennsylvania, a national leader in health care, provides students with unparalleled opportunities for learning and launching a professional career.

RANKINGS AND RECOGNITION

The School of Nursing was designated as a "Center for Excellence in Nursing Education" for the third consecutive year by the National League for Nursing, for creating environments that enhance student learning and professional development. The School has also been recognized consistently by *U.S. News & World Report* as follows:

- Number 75 among all graduate programs
- Number 9 among the Top 10 Best Online Graduate Nursing Programs
- Number 9 among the Best Online Graduate Programs for Veterans

Additional achievements include:

- Awarded a nearly $1 million federal grant that provides support for veterans who wish to earn B.S.N. degrees.
- Designated as a 2016 Military Friendly School.
- Received a major NIH grant to continue the investigation of the psychosocial effects of bariatric surgery.
- To improve the quality of life in neighboring communities, the School of Nursing operates the Community-Based Health & Wellness Center for Older Adults where students have opportunities for interdisciplinary care experiences and community service. The school is also home to the Center for Research for Underserved and Vulnerable Populations, a forum for networking, exchanging information, and fostering innovation.

UNDERGRADUATE PROGRAMS

Bachelor of Science in Nursing (B.S.N.)

Clinical experiences, which begin in the sophomore year, create a strong nursing practice foundation. Students complete over 810 clinical hours in local, nationally ranked hospitals and community health facilities. The clinical faculty-to-student ratio is 1:8. State-of-the-art facilities, such as Duquesne's new Learning and Simulation Lab, that includes vital technological resources, help students gain patient-care skills in a controlled environment designed to improve decision making and develop teamwork, communications, and

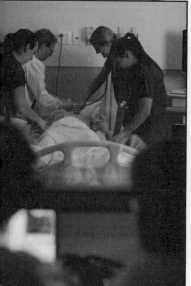

Undergraduate nursing students use e-textbooks for both classroom and clinical learning.

leadership skills. Nursing students can add international perspectives by participating in faculty-led, spring, summer, and semester-long study-abroad programs.

Biomedical Engineering / Bachelor of Science in Nursing

To meet emerging health care trends, the school has introduced a ground-breaking five-year B.M.E./B.S.N. program, the first of its kind in the nation. This interdisciplinary dual-degree program combines the science and art of patient care with principles of electrical, chemical, and mechanical engineering. Students develop expertise that is unique, timely, and essential to develop technological solutions to clinical problems and improve the health and quality of life for patients.

Second Degree B.S.N.

The Second Degree Bachelor of Science in Nursing (B.S.N.) program enables a student with any baccalaureate degree to obtain a B.S.N. in eleven months. The program requires full-time study; after three semesters of course work and over 630 hours of clinical experience, students are eligible to take the nursing licensure exam to become registered nurses.

RN–B.S.N.

This completely online program enables the RN with an ADN or diploma degree in nursing to obtain a B.S.N. degree. This program is structured to provide innovative and relevant course work and is offered full or part-time. Courses are eight weeks long and taught by experienced faculty who provide exceptional academic support and professional development.

GRADUATE PROGRAMS

All graduate nursing programs are offered exclusively online in a user-friendly, flexible format. Highly interactive course work allows students to communicate often with instructors and classmates. Online flexibility plus academic rigor make the Duquesne University School of Nursing the ideal choice for graduate nursing education.

Master of Science in Nursing (M.S.N.)

The M.S.N. program offers three areas of specialization:

- Family (Individual Across the Lifespan) Nurse Practitioner
- Forensic Nursing
- Nursing Education

Post-Master's Certificates

Duquesne's certificate programs enable nurses with M.S.N. degrees to acquire additional specialized skills in these areas:

- Family (Individual Across the Lifespan) Nurse Practitioner
- Forensic Nursing
- Nursing Education and Faculty Role

Ph.D. in Nursing

The Ph.D. in nursing degree is designed to nurture scholarship and research that will expand scientific knowledge and improve nursing practice. The curriculum is research focused and prepares graduate students for a lifetime of intellectual inquiry and creative scholarship. Students develop the knowledge and skills to obtain predoctoral research funding. Students may also obtain a post-master's certificate prior to, or while, pursuing the Ph.D. degree.

Doctor of Nursing Practice (D.N.P.)

The D.N.P. program is designed to improve patient care practice and is for nurses who seek an alternative to research-focused doctoral programs. This program provides a strong evidence-based foundation for learning, and students acquire the skills and knowledge needed for assessing health care policy, economic trends, and organizational competence so new, more effective patient care models can be designed.

Visit www.duq.edu/nursing or e-mail nursing@duq.edu for more information.

- *2015–16 FULL-TIME UNDERGRADUATE TUITION & FEES: $33,778 ($1,119 per credit)*
- *2015–16 FULL-TIME GRADUATE TUITION & FEES: $1,218 per credit*
- *APPLICATION DEADLINES:*

  B.S.N.: May 1

  B.S.N. (transfer students): April 1 (fall admission); October 1 (spring admission)

  Second Degree B.S.N.: April 1

  B.M.E./B.S.N.: December 1

  RN–B.S.N.: April 1, July 15, December 1

  M.S.N.: March 1

  Ph.D.: February 1

  D.N.P.: February 1

CONTACT INFORMATION
Susan Hardner, Nurse Recruiter, Graduate
   Programs
545-A Fisher Hall
Phone: 412-396-4945
Fax: 412-396-6346
E-mail: hardnersue@duq.edu

Gina Plocki, Nurse Recruiter, Undergraduate
   Programs
543 Fisher Hall
Phone: 412-396-6534
Fax: 412-396-6346
E-mail: plockir@duq.edu

Duquesne University
600 Forbes Avenue
Pittsburgh, Pennsylvania 15282
Website: duq.edu/nursing
Facebook: facebook.com/DUNursing
Twitter: twitter.com/dunursing
YouTube: youtube.com/dunursing
LinkedIn: linkedin.com/groups/Duquesne-
   University-School-Nursing-4803465
GooglePlus: plus.google.
   com/118445490080314869545/posts
Pinterest: pinterest.com/dunursing/
Instagram: instagram.com/dunursing#
NursesLounge: nurseslounge.com/lounges/
   profile/16193/duquesne-university

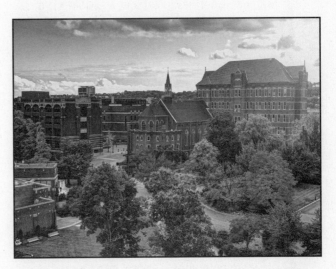

The School of Nursing encourages students to engage in international travel and study to explore global health issues. Since 1995, students and faculty have traveled to many locations, such as Nicaragua, in a spirit of service, learning, and international collaboration.

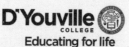

D'Youville
COLLEGE
Educating for life

School of Nursing

Educating competent, compassionate, knowledgeable, professional nurses.

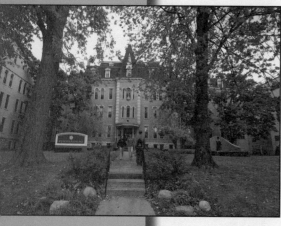

The Koessler Administration Building dates back to 1872 when it was the home of Holy Angels Academy, a private boarding school for young ladies in elementary and secondary grades. In 1908, a charter established D'Youville College and the Academy of the Holy Angels. As the College grew, the Academy moved to another location in Buffalo in 1930. Today, the landmark building houses the President's suite and other administrative offices.

D'Youville College is a private, co-educational liberal arts and professional college offering students a high-quality education in more than thirty undergraduate and graduate degree programs. Founded in 1908 by the Grey Nuns as the first college for women in western New York to offer baccalaureate degrees to women, it was named for their founder, Saint Marguerite D'Youville. The current enrollment is 3,000 men and women; the student-faculty ratio is 12:1, allowing for individual attention and student support by faculty. The College is committed to helping its students grow academically, socially, and personally throughout their college experience. The Learning Center and other college-wide support services are available to enhance students' opportunity for success. Many student organizations, including pre-professional student associations, expand the learning environment.

D'Youville College has been growing and attracting students from all over the world since 1908, particularly in the areas of professional health-related programs. D'Youville College has been educating and preparing professional nurses for careers since 1942; the first Bachelor of Science in Nursing (B.S.N.) class graduated in 1946. Since then, nursing education programs at D'Youville have continued to grow, and the school of nursing is now the largest single education entity on campus. D'Youville offers a four-year Bachelor of Science in Nursing. The B.S.N. program combines a liberal arts foundation with professional nursing classroom and clinical instruction. An active Student Nurses Association orients students to the role that professional organizations play in life-long

professional practice and promotion of health for populations.

Classroom instruction concentrates on preparing students for critical thinking and clinical decision making required for clinical practice. Students begin their clinical experiences at area hospitals, long-term care facilities, community agencies, and other health-related facilities and services. On-campus nursing laboratory instruction and practice with low-, mid-, and high-fidelity simulators; standardized patients; and inter-professional learning opportunities help to prepare students for actual clinical practice. Clinical practice begins in the sophomore year. Areas of clinical experience include geriatrics, pediatrics, obstetrics/gynecology, behavioral health, community health, and medical/surgical nursing. Some area hospital systems provide paid competitive internship opportunities for students between their junior and senior years. D'Youville enjoys partnerships and active affiliations with area healthcare facilities and agencies where students develop their clinical competencies. Within a narrow geographic area surrounding the college campus and its nearby suburbs are several institutions of the Catholic Health System; Erie County Medical Center (including WNY's Level 1 Trauma and Burn Center); Buffalo Psychiatric Center, Kaleida Health Care System (including Women and Children's Hospital of Buffalo and the Gates Vascular Institute); the Visiting Nurses Association of Western New York; the world-renowned Roswell Park Cancer Institute; Buffalo's VA hospital; and numerous community health agencies and services that provide for primary care and population health. Opportunity is available for service-learning locally and in third-world locations.

In 1957, the RN to B.S.N. program was initiated, offering a specialized curriculum for licensed professional nurses with nursing diplomas and associate degrees. Professional nurses can complete a two-year RN to B.S.N. online program. A special feature of this program is that all RN to B.S.N. online accepted students will receive 50 percent off net tuition.

Graduate programs offer several options for baccalaureate–prepared nurses to continue their professional development, including the M.S. in family nurse practitioner studies. Begun in fall 2012, D'Youville now offers a Doctor of Nursing Practice (DNP). The DNP can be taken as a post-baccalaureate degree or as a post-master's degree. Admission and progression in the program is individualized to the student's prior preparation.

All baccalaureate and masters programs offered by the School of Nursing are fully accredited by the Commission on Collegiate Nursing Education (CCNE) and approved by the New York State Education Department. The DNP program is approved by the New York State Education Department; the application for accreditation by CCNE will be made one year prior to the graduation of the first class, which is the standard procedure for new programs.

The nursing faculty members are committed, dedicated educators who pride themselves on providing individual attention to students. Faculty members represent diverse educational and clinical preparation and expertise. Their active practice in a variety of specialty practice areas, their research and other scholarly work, and their participation in professional organizations enrich the teaching/learning opportunities provided at D'Youville.

D'Youville College admits students on a rolling admissions basis but recommends students submit applications well before the start of the semester. Applications are reviewed as they are received by the Admissions Office. Freshman applicants must submit a completed application; official high school transcripts, and SAT or ACT scores. Transfer students must also submit official transcripts from all colleges previously attended. Graduate and doctorate applicants present evidence of their undergraduate education from an accredited college or university and their current unrestricted license to practice as a professional registered nurse and/or nurse practitioner.

- *2015–16 UNDERGRADUATE TUITION & FEES:*
  Full-time: $24,400
  Room and Board: $10,800 per year

- *2015–16 GRADUATE TUITION & FEES:*
  $880 per credit for master's program courses
  $955 per credit for doctoral courses

- *APPLICATION DEADLINES: Rolling admissions*

- *FACULTY: http://www.dyc.edu/academics/ nursing/faculty.asp*

CONTACT INFORMATION

Dr. Judith Lewis
School of Nursing
D'Youville College
320 Porter Avenue
Buffalo, New York 14201
Phone: 716-829-7600
**   800-777-3921 (toll-free)**
Fax: 716-829-7900
E-mail: admissions@dyc.edu
Web site: http://www.dyc.edu/academics/ nursing/

UNDERGRADUATE NURSING PROGRAM
Dr. Steve Smith, Director of Admissions
Phone: 716-829-7600
E-mail: admissions@dyc.edu

GRADUATE NURSING PROGRAM
Mark Pavone, Director of Graduate Admissions
Phone: 716-829-8400
E-mail: graduateadmissions@dyc.edu

Find us on Facebook®: http://www.dyc.edu/facebook
Follow us on Twitter™: http://twitter.com/uanursing

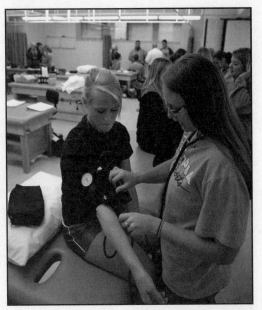

D'Youville College is internationally known for its wide array of health-care academic offerings. Majors include nursing, physician assistant, occupational and physical therapy, pharmacy, chiropractic, and dietetics. All majors include a strong liberal arts component.

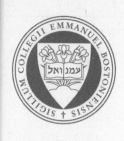

EMMANUEL COLLEGE

Graduate and Professional Programs

UNDERGRADUATE AND GRADUATE PROGRAMS IN NURSING FOR RNS

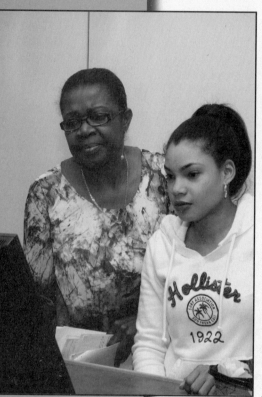

Students benefit from small, interactive classes.

Emmanuel College, located in the heart of the Longwood Medical and Academic Area (LMA) of Boston, offers a Bachelor of Science in Nursing (BSN), a Master of Science in Nursing (MSN), and Certificates of Graduate Study in nursing education and nursing management. The curriculum has been tailored to meet students' learning needs and career goals in an ever-changing health care environment. Faculty and advisors work one-on-one with students to develop individualized plans for nursing study and professional development.

The Bachelor of Science in Nursing (RN to BSN) program prepares students to think critically, appreciate diverse human experience, and use personal and professional values in everyday life. Emmanuel College's program is health promotion–based, enabling students to meet career goals. Teaching and learning strategies throughout Emmanuel College's nursing courses prepare graduates with the knowledge, skills, and attitudes necessary to continuously improve the quality and safety of the healthcare systems in which they work. The BSN and MSN programs are fully accredited by the Commission on Collegiate Nursing Education (CCNE).

The Master of Science in Nursing program prepares students for an advanced role as a nurse educator or nurse manager/administrator. These distinctive tracks offer students the knowledge and expertise to thrive in a wide variety of clinical settings and to work with diverse populations. Students who choose the education concentration are qualified to pursue roles in clinical education, staff development, and as nursing faculty members; graduates of the management track are prepared for management/administration positions such as nurse executive, administrator, manager, director, coordinator, and case manager.

Graduate Certificates in Nursing Education or Nursing Management at Emmanuel offer the opportunity for nurses who have completed a Master of Science in Nursing to further develop their skills in the nursing education and nursing management tracks. These certificate programs enable students to strengthen and broaden the advanced skills and knowledge needed to explore new professional directions.

As respected professionals with years of experience in nursing, Emmanuel College faculty members maintain a strong and up-to-date command in their areas of expertise in research and teaching. As understanding nurse educators, they cultivate lively dialogue so that students share first-hand perspectives on patient care, healthcare issues, and other key subjects. Emmanuel College professors are clinicians, researchers and teachers who serve as true advocates. Each student works directly with a full-time member of the nursing faculty as a dedicated advisor. This provides students with the individual attention necessary to get the most from their plan of study.

With an average class size of 15, students have the ability to engage in lively classroom discussions, to share their unique experiences as RNs, and to exchange views and clinical knowledge. Classes meet evenings or Saturday mornings every other week, enabling students to fit academics into their professional and personal schedules. All modified accelerated courses include independent study, and students can set their own pace with flexible program scheduling. Graduate nursing classes meet seven times during the semester and undergraduate nursing classes meet six times. All courses are offered at Emmanuel College's easy-to-reach Boston campus in the Longwood Medical and Academic Area. Emmanuel offers on-campus parking for visitors, as well as parking passes for purchase by Graduate and Professional Programs students.

The BSN program has enrollment and application opportunities multiple times per year and is also available by request at employer sites. The MSN and graduate certificate programs have new cohorts beginning each fall semester, and the preferred application deadline for the MSN is June 30. More information is available on the website at www.emmanuel.edu/nursing.

- *2015–16 TUITION & FEES*

Bachelor of Science in Nursing (BSN):

> *$1,816 per 4-credit course*

Master of Science (MSN) and Certificates in Graduate Study in Nursing:

> *$2,581 per 3-credit course*

There are no additional fees associated with these programs.

- *APPLICATION DEADLINES*

Bachelor of Science in Nursing (BSN):

There are enrollment opportunities multiple times per year. An application form must be submitted prior to enrollment.

Master of Science in Nursing (MSN) and Certificates in Graduate Study in Nursing:

The preferred application deadline is June 30 for enrollment in the fall semester. There is no application fee.

CONTACT INFORMATION

Helen Muterperl, Assistant Director
Graduate Admissions /Nursing Programs
Emmanuel College
Graduate and Professional Programs
400 The Fenway
Boston, Massachusetts 02115
Phone: 617-735-9700
E-mail: gpp@emmanuel.edu
Website: www.emmanuel.edu/nursing

Find us on Facebook®: http://www.facebook.com/emmanuelgpp

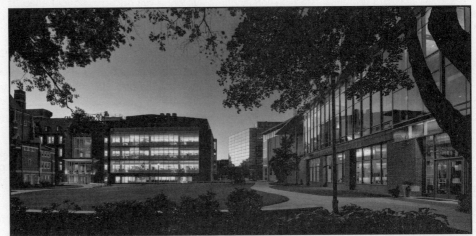

Emmanuel's Boston campus is located in the world-renowned Longwood Medical and Academic Area.

FRONTIER NURSING UNIVERSITY

School of Nursing

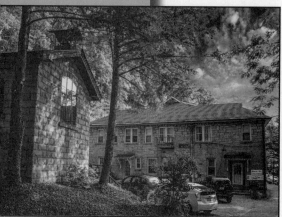

Frontier Nursing University provides distance education programs, so students can learn in their own communities, with only two or three brief visits to the historic campus in Hyden, Kentucky.

Complete your degree online and become a nurse-midwife or nurse practitioner

Graduate Distance Education at Frontier Nursing University

Established in 1939, Frontier Nursing University is a pioneer in graduate-level nursing and midwifery education. Today, it provides innovative distance education that allows students from around the world to complete didactic courses online and receive clinical education in their communities.

The University has received national recognition for its long tradition of providing innovation and excellence in education. U.S. News & World Report ranks Frontier Nursing University in the top 30 nursing graduate schools and #1 for its nurse-midwifery program.

Frontier Nursing University (FNU) is located in Hyden, Kentucky, in the southeastern region of the United States. Its historic campus provides a tranquil, picturesque environment in which to learn and connect with faculty and fellow students during the brief two to three required visits to campus.

Programs and Specialties

Frontier Nursing University offers evidence-based Master of Science in Nursing (M.S.N.) degree programs, post-master's certificates, and Doctor of Nursing Practice (D.N.P.) programs. Its curricula include three specialties: nurse-midwife, family nurse practitioner, and women's health care nurse practitioner.

The University also offers a dual M.S.N. and D.N.P. degree program that allows students to earn an M.S.N. degrees and then advance to the D.N.P. program with no additional admission requirements. When the M.S.N. is conferred, students are prepared for the national certification exam and careers as nurse-midwives or nurse practitioners.

MSN + Companion DNP Program of Study

The MSN + Companion DNP program offers students the option to complete the Master of Science in Nursing degree and continue on and seamlessly complete a companion Doctor of Nursing Practice degree without reapplying. The program begins with a 3-day "Frontier Bound Orientation" that takes place on FNU's campus; all course work and clinicals are completed in the student's own community. For registered nurses entering with a bachelor's degree, the M.S.N. program takes approximately two years to complete full-time (part-time option also available) with the Companion D.N.P. requiring an additional 17 credit hours. This means that the full MSN + Companion DNP program can be completed in about three years. Students also have the option to exit the program once the M.S.N. degree is conferred.

The program includes online course work that involves frequent interaction among faculty members and students via e-mail, forums, and other communications. Didactic course work is followed by a 5-day "Clinical Bound" session at FNU where students demonstrate their ability to begin community-based clinical practice.

Following the clinical session, students must complete a 675-hour clinical practicum in their own communities. Once the M.S.N. degree is conferred, students complete nine to twelve months of D.N.P. course work and clinical education if they choose to continue and complete the D.N.P.

Nurse-Midwife Specialty

The nurse-midwife curriculum trains students to become outstanding clinicians as well as leaders and entrepreneurs in maternal and infant health care. The program's strong primary care component ensures that students also gain the skills needed to care for women across their life spans.

Family Nurse Practitioner Specialty

Students who choose the family nurse practitioner specialty receive the training needed to become well-rounded clinicians, leaders, and entrepreneurs in primary health care.

Women's Health Care Nurse Practitioner Specialty

The women's health care nurse practitioner specialty prepares students for advanced nursing practice as well as leadership and entrepreneurial roles in women's health care. The curriculum's solid primary care component ensures that students receive the skills needed to care for women in all stages of life.

ADN Bridge Entry Option

Frontier Nursing University also offers the A.D.N. Bridge entry option that allows nurses with associate degrees in nursing (but no bachelor's degrees in any field) to enroll in the M.S.N. program with either the nurse-midwifery or the family nurse practitioner specialty. The curriculum includes approximately one year to complete the required Bridge course work, followed by approximately two years full-time to complete the M.S.N. (part-time option also available), and an additional nine to twelve months to complete the Companion D.N.P. (17 credit hours).

The program begins with "Bridge Bound," an on-campus orientation that allows students to connect with fellow students and faculty members and learn more about the program. Then students go back to their communities to complete Bridge courses online.

Upon completion of the Bridge course work, students return to FNU to participate in "Crossing the Bridge," an event that enables them to reconnect with FNU's community and present their community health projects. Upon successful completion of the Bridge courses, students begin the M.S.N. curriculum in the nurse-midwife or family nurse practitioner specialty, and they can opt to complete the D.N.P. program once they earn their M.S.N. degrees.

Financial Aid

FNU students may qualify for Federal Stafford Unsubsidized Loans, private loans, and external scholarships. In addition, Frontier offers several scholarships including the Kitty Ernst Scholarship, Alumni Scholarship, Family Nurse Practitioner Scholarship, and Student Scholarship.

Dedicated and Expert Faculty Members

FNU's faculty members are accomplished teachers, expert clinicians, and dedicated mentors. They create mutually-respectful relationships with students and support them in achieving their academic and professional goals.

They are also pioneers in distance nursing education who are highly accessible and skilled at supporting students in a virtual learning environment.

- *2015–16 TUITION & FEES:*
  Tuition ranges from $18,645–$54,570
  (Tuition fees are subject to change)

  Master of Science in Nursing + Companion Doctor of Nursing Practice program: $535/credit hour

  Post-Master's Doctor of Nursing Practice program: $565/credit hour

- *APPLICATION DEADLINES:*

  Multiple deadlines every quarter; varies by program

CONTACT INFORMATION
Frontier Nursing University
195 School Street
Hyden, Kentucky 41749
Phone: 606-672-2312
Fax: 606-672-3776
E-mail: admissionscounselor@frontier.edu

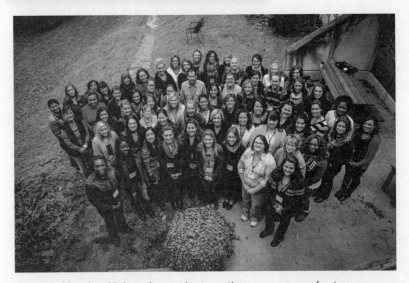

Frontier Nursing University students gather on campus for two or three brief visits, including a three-day orientation before beginning the program. During the orientation, they connect with other students as well as instructors and staff members before returning to their home communities to begin online course work.

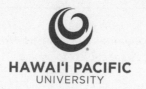

Hawai'i Pacific University

College of Nursing and Health Sciences

The College of Nursing and Health Sciences exemplifies the three values of Hawai'i Pacific University—*aloha, pono, and kuleana*—through its mission of educating competent and caring professionals in the practice of health promotion and health care.

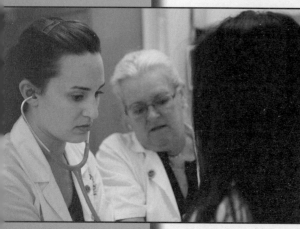

Hands-on experiences in HPU's Nursing Program.

Hawai'i Pacific University (HPU) is a private, nonprofit university with an international student population of approximately 8,200 students. The nursing program at HPU is the largest in the state, with more than 1,600 students in the baccalaureate and master's programs. The College maintains small class sizes, where faculty members provide individual attention to students. Students receive high-quality instruction in multicultural classrooms consisting of 24 to 32 students and clinical groups consisting of 8 to 10 students.

The students in the School of Nursing are representative of the global community in terms of age, ethnicity, citizenship, gender, and professional experience. Students may attend either full- or part-time, with a substantial number of students choosing to accelerate the completion of their degree by studying during summer sessions. Various nursing courses are offered during summer sessions. All nursing lecture and science laboratory classes are held on the suburban and residential windward Hawai'i Loa campus.

The program emphasizes the qualities of humanism, caring, and collaboration as a foundation for the comprehensive study of the art and science of nursing. The program provides students with experience in the physical, mental, emotional, and spiritual care of clients from varied age groups and multiple ethnic backgrounds.

Programs of Study

The baccalaureate nursing program offers four pathways toward a Bachelor of Science in Nursing (B.S.N.) degree. The first is the Basic Pathway for the beginning or transfer student with fewer than 45 college credits. Second is an LPN to B.S.N. Pathway for U.S. licensed practical nurses. Third, an RN to B.S.N. Pathway for licensed registered nurses from associate degree or diploma programs, and fourth, an International Nurse Pathway for persons who have graduated from a nursing program in another country and are not licensed in the United States.

HPU's graduate nursing program brings together theory and community-based practice. The M.S.N. program enables the registered nurse the opportunity to advance as a family nurse practitioner (FNP), or a community clinical nurse specialist (CNS). An RN to M.S.N. Pathway allows registered nurses without baccalaureate degrees in nursing to make the transition into the M.S.N. program. Students in the pathway are granted provisional admission status until all prerequisites are completed. Students interested in gaining a solid foundation in current business and management practice may pursue a joint M.S.N./M.B.A. degree program.

A post-master's certificate as a family nurse practitioner is also possible for nurses with master's degrees seeking to expand their practice. A certificate program in nursing education can be taken as part of the CNS concentration or as a stand-alone certificate.

Facilities and Student Services

The Nursing program at HPU chooses health-care facilities that give students the best experience possible. Within these facilities, the choice of clinical units is made based upon the learning needs of the students. The majority of clinical faculty members are actively employed in the clinical specialties and/or facilities where they teach.

The University has many services to meet student needs, including a professional staff of advisers to assist undergraduate students. Other services include career placement programs, the Student Nurses' Association, and many other student organizations. On-campus residence halls with cafeteria service are available on the windward Hawai'i Loa campus, while off-campus apartments are available in the Honolulu and Waikiki area for those seeking more independent living arrangements.

Financial Aid

The University provides financial aid for qualified students through institutional, state, and federal aid programs. Approximately 64 percent of students receive aid. To apply, students must submit the Free Application for Federal Student Aid (FAFSA); the priority deadline is March 1. Several local health-care agencies award low-interest loans to student nurses, which are forgiven for various lengths of service following successful completion of the NCLEX-RN examination.

• *2016–17 UNDERGRADUATE TUITION & FEES:*

Nursing/pre-nursing (12–16 credits per semester): $11,580

Nursing, Level 1 and above (12–16 credits per semester): $14,870

Additional fees include: $50 application; $120 fall new student orientation (one-time); $50 spring new student orientation (one-time); $50 technology fee (per semester); $25 activity fee (per semester); $40 transportation fee (per semester).

• *2016–17 GRADUATE TUITION & FEES:*

Nursing programs: $1,330 per credit

Additional fees include: $50 application, $35 new student orientation (one-time, optional), $25 activity fee (per semester, 9 credits or more), $13 activity fee (per semester, 8 credits or fewer), $40 transportation fee (per semester)

• *APPLICATION DEADLINES*

Undergraduate early action: November 15

Undergraduate priority: January 15

Undergraduate applications are reviewed on a rolling basis year-round.

Graduate: Applications are accepted and admissions decisions are made throughout the year.

FACULTY INFORMATION

http://www.hpu.edu/CNHS/CNHS_Faculty_and_Staff.html

CONTACT INFORMATION

Office of Admissions
Hawai'i Pacific University
1164 Bishop Street, Suite 200
Honolulu, Hawaii 96813
Phone: 808-544-0238
866-CALL-HPU (toll-free)
Fax: 808-544-1136
E-mail: admissions@hpu.edu
Website: http://www.hpu.edu/CNHS/index.html

Undergraduate Nursing Program:
Phone: 808-544-0238
866-CALL-HPU (toll-free)
E-mail: admissions@hpu.edu
Graduate Nursing Program:
Phone: 808-544-1135
866-GRAD-HPU (toll-free)
E-mail: graduate@hpu.edu

Facebook®: https://www.facebook.com/hawaiipacific/
Twittter™: https://twitter.com/hpu

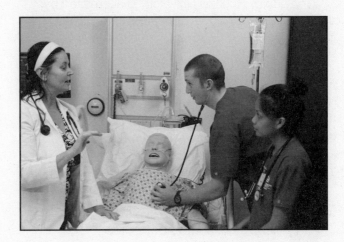

HPU Nursing Students use the latest in simulation rooms.

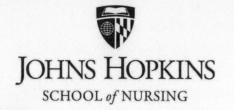

JOHNS HOPKINS
SCHOOL *of* NURSING

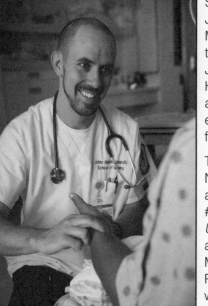

Standing with the top-ranked Johns Hopkins Schools of Medicine and Public Health and the internationally renowned Johns Hopkins Hospital, the Johns Hopkins School of Nursing offers an unmatched interprofessional environment to students and faculty.

The Johns Hopkins School of Nursing is a recognized leader among its peers and holds the #2 rank for graduate programs in *U.S. News & World Report's* annual survey. It was named the Most Innovative Nursing Graduate Program in the U.S. by the website Best Master of Science in Nursing Degrees. It is #1 among nursing schools in federal research grants and National Institutes of Health funding. The Johns Hopkins School of Nursing is also recognized as a Center of Excellence in Nursing Education by the National League of Nursing. More than 40 percent of its faculty members have been named Fellows of the American Academy of Nursing.

Johns Hopkins University is accredited by the Middle States Commission on Higher Education (MSCHE). The baccalaureate degree in nursing, master's degree in nursing, and Doctor of Nursing Practice at Johns Hopkins School of Nursing is accredited by the Commission on Collegiate Nursing Education. Additionally, the baccalaureate and master's programs are approved by the Maryland State Board of Examiners of Nurses. The baccalaureate, master's, and doctoral programs are endorsed by the Maryland State Board for Higher Education.

• PROGRAMS AND ACADEMICS

The Johns Hopkins School of Nursing offers a wide range of academic programs tailored to students' specialized needs, interests, and strengths.

Master of Science in Nursing: Entry into Nursing Practice

The power of choice defines the very best of career education. Students who have already earned a non-nursing bachelor's degree are familiar with their own unique learning style, professional goals, and scheduling needs. The Johns Hopkins School of Nursing offers one program that can accelerate the track to nursing practice, extend studies through a doctoral program, or provide clinical experience as students work toward advanced practice nursing.

Master of Science in Nursing: Advanced Nursing Practice

The advanced practice and master's specialty tracks prepare students for advanced practice, management, and/or public health nursing. The interdisciplinary approach provides students with the tools to address a variety of changing healthcare needs. Both full-time and part-time study are available with specialty tracks for nurse practitioners, clinical nurse specialists, health systems management, and public health nursing.

Doctoral

The Doctor of Nursing Practice (DNP) and Doctor of Philosophy in Nursing (PhD) programs prepare clinical and research leaders respectively to advance the practice of nursing and improve health locally and globally.

Post-Degree Certificates

Post-degree certificates allow for lifelong learning and offer an opportunity for further specialization in a field.

Visit nursing.jhu.edu/academics to view a full listing of the school's program offerings.

• FINANCIAL AID AND SCHOLARSHIPS

The Johns Hopkins School of Nursing offers a range of financial aid programs within each degree, including grants, fellowships, scholarships, loans, and work-study. All returned Peace Corps Volunteers in the pre-licensure program are offered the Coverdell Fellows scholarship. Qualified students interested in the PhD program may be eligible for 100 percent funding for their first two years. The school also has a number of fellowships for both pre- and post-doctoral students. Federal and supplemental (private) student loans are available to assist students in meeting their educational expenses.

• ADMISSIONS

A master's application consists of an application form and a nonrefundable $75 application fee. Doctoral applicants pay an application fee of $100. In general, applicants to the School of Nursing are required to submit official transcripts from all post-secondary schools attended, academic and professional letters of recommendation, essay(s) or a goal statement, and a resume or CV. The Master's Entry into Nursing, MSN/MPH, and PhD programs require submission of the GRE. The Test of English as a Foreign Language is required if English is not the applicant's first language. A grade point average above 3.0 (on a 4.0 scale) is recommended. Personal interviews may be requested. Application requirements vary by program. Applicants are encouraged to visit nursing.jhu.edu/academics to review specific program information and admissions requirements.

• TUITION & FEES (2015–16):

Master of Science in Nursing (MSN):
Tuition: $17,412 (full-time—12 credit hours/ semester); $1,451 per credit (part-time). Books/supplies: $1,856

Dual Master's Degree Program (MSN/MPH):
Tuition: $23,680 (full-time—16 credit hours/ semester); $1,480 per credit (part-time). Books/supplies: $2,320

Doctor of Nursing Practice (DNP):
Tuition: $27,436 (full-time—19 credits/first year); $1,444 per credit (part-time). Books/supplies: $2,320

Doctor of Philosophy in Nursing (PhD):
Tuition: $20,313 (full-time—9 credit hours/ semester); $2,257 per credit (part-time). Books/supplies: $1,856

• PRIORITY APPLICATION DEADLINES:

Master of Science in Nursing (MSN): Entry into Nursing Practice:
Fall entry (January 1); spring entry (July 1)

Doctor of Nursing Practice (DNP):
Summer entry (January 1)

Doctor of Philosophy in Nursing (PhD):
Fall entry (January 15)

Master of Science in Nursing: Advanced Nursing Practice:
Visit nursing.jhu.edu/deadlines for the most complete and up-to-date list of priority application deadlines by degree and specialty.

Post-Degree Certificates:
Fall entry (January 1)
Visit nursing.jhu.edu/deadlines for the most complete and up-to-date list of priority application deadlines by degree and specialty.

FACULTY INFORMATION:
nursing.jhu.edu/faculty

• MULTIMEDIA:
youtube.com/hopkinsnursing

CONTACT INFORMATION
Johns Hopkins School of Nursing
525 North Wolfe Street
Baltimore, Maryland 21205
Phone: 410-955-7548
Fax: 410-614-7086
E-mail: jhuson@jhu.edu
Website: nursing.jhu.edu

Find us on Facebook®: facebook.com/jhunursing
Follow us on Twitter™: twitter.com/jhunursing

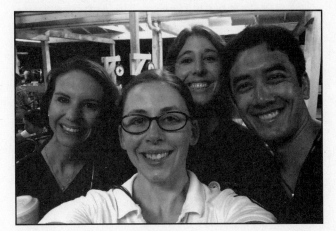

LUTHER COLLEGE

Department of Nursing

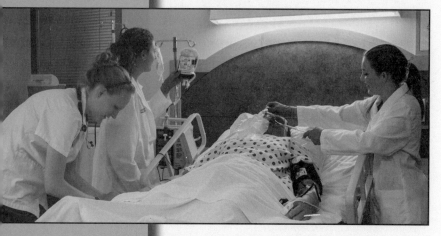

The nursing major at Luther College offers an integrated program of liberal arts and professional nursing courses, giving students a broad approach to nursing and providing a base for graduate study or immediate entry into the profession. Students gain clinical experience at healthcare sites such as Mayo Clinic in Rochester, Minnesota.

The goal of Luther's nursing faculty is to prepare nurses to function autonomously and interdependently with individuals, families, groups, and communities to promote, maintain, and restore optimal health in a variety of health-care settings. The nursing major, therefore, offers an integrated program of liberal arts and professional nursing courses. The program gives students a broad approach to nursing, providing a base for graduate study or immediate entry into the nursing profession.

Following graduation, Luther nursing students may take the National Council Licensure Examination for Registered Nurses (NCLEX-RN). More information is available upon request.

The first year at Luther provides a foundation in the liberal arts and sciences. All nursing majors are assigned a faculty adviser to help each student decide whether to pursue a nursing curriculum plan. All students interested in nursing are invited to participate in the Luther Student Nurses Association (LSNA).

Nursing courses, labs, and clinicals begin in the sophomore year. Nursing courses at this level emphasize health assessment, health promotion, clinical reasoning, and fundamental skills throughout the life span in a variety of settings. These learning experiences develop new communication and interpersonal skills.

Third-year students experience a concentrated study of nursing concepts by caring for children, childbearing families, and adults with physical and emotional problems. The sites for this clinical experience are inpatient and ambulatory care areas at Mayo Clinic; the Federal Medical Center; and a variety of community-based agencies in Rochester, Minnesota. Students also develop leadership, management, and research skills.

The senior year provides final preparation for entry into the practice of professional nursing. Courses focus on promoting health and preventing illness in families and in community groups.

Minimum academic requirements must be met to be considered for enrollment in nursing courses. However, meeting the minimum requirements does not guarantee placement in the courses. Decisions affecting progression in the major are made at the end of each semester.

The study of nursing at Luther incorporates academic classroom learning and clinical experience in several community facilities to provide students with both an urban and rural health-care perspective. These include Winneshiek Medical Center; the Decorah Free Clinic; Mayo Clinic; the Federal Medical

Center; and a variety of community-based health-care agencies in Decorah, Iowa and Rochester, Minnesota.

Nursing scholarships are available to incoming students on a competitive basis upon admission. Selection of recipients is based on academic information submitted on the application and the high school transcript. Scholarship renewal is based on satisfactory academic and clinical performance in the major.

All nursing students benefit from the Bernice Fischer Cross and Bert S. Cross Perpetual Endowment for the Luther College Mayo Nursing Program and Health Sciences Program. This is used for equal-share assistance for the Luther College nursing students enrolled in the curriculum provided at Mayo Clinic in Rochester, Minnesota. The endowment is not a need-based scholarship.

Located in the northeast Iowa town of Decorah (resident population: 8,100), Luther College is an undergraduate liberal arts institution of about 2,400 students that is affiliated with the Lutheran church (ELCA). The Upper Iowa River—the only waterway in the state designated as wild and scenic—flows through the lower portion of Luther's 200-acre central campus and borders Decorah's business district. Decorah is known nationwide for its recreational opportunities, numerous cultural heritage events and festivals, pedestrian-friendly village center, and its conscious efforts to thrive as a small town. Public transportation includes commercial airports in Rochester (Minnesota), Waterloo (Iowa), and La Crosse (Wisconsin); a municipal airport in Decorah; and train and bus depots in La Crosse, Wisconsin.

- *2015–16 UNDERGRADUATE TUITION & FEES:*

  The comprehensive fee was $46,590 ($38,940 tuition, $3,300 room, $4,350 board).

- *APPLICATION DEADLINES:*

  Luther College operates on rolling admission. There is no application deadline.

- *FACULTY INFORMATION:*

  http://www.luther.edu/nursing/faculty

- *MULTIMEDIA:*

  http://www.luther.edu/video

CONTACT INFORMATION

LaDonna McGohan, Head
Department of Nursing
Luther College
700 College Drive
Decorah, Iowa 52101
Phone: 563-387-1057
**   800-458-8437 (toll-free)**
E-mail: mcgola01@luther.edu
Website: http://www.luther.edu/nursing/

Find us on Facebook®: www.facebook.com/luthercollege1861
Follow us on Twitter™: www.twitter.com/luthercollege

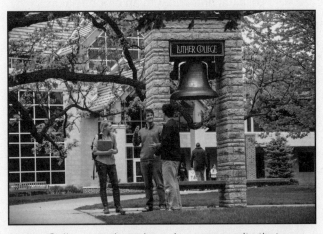

Luther College students learn in a community that emphasizes rigorous academics, a world-class music program, competitive athletics, and opportunities to put their classroom learning to the test through internships, independent research, and study abroad. Typically, 98 percent of Luther graduates are employed, attending graduate school, or engaged in an internship or volunteer work within eight months of graduation.

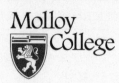

Division of Nursing

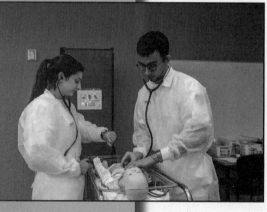

Molloy's new Nursing Center includes seven laboratories with approximately 20 high-tech simulator men/women and children that allow the students to learn and practice clinical procedures.

An Emphasis on Human Compassion, Dignity, and Respect

At Molloy, nursing is both art and science. One of the country's largest and most respected programs, Molloy's Nursing Division curriculum immerses students in clinical practice with an emphasis on human compassion, dignity, and respect for the patient. Molloy's programs proactively respond to the changing needs of today's health-care environment, providing students with individualized attention from an expert faculty that is easily accessible and always committed to students' success.

The opening of the Barbara H. Hagan Center for Nursing in 2016 has only added to the strength of Molloy's Nursing program. The Hagan Center features the latest technology in classrooms and clinical laboratories. Seven laboratories include approximately twenty high-tech simulator men/women and children that allow students to learn and practice clinical procedures, provide nursing care in various clinical situations on these simulated people in preparation for working with real patients in medical facilities. At Molloy, students benefit from a comprehensive array of:

- <u>Undergraduate programs.</u> Offering a wealth of hands-on clinical experiences beginning in a student's sophomore year, Molloy's bachelor's degree program prepares students for a vital role in health care. Already working in health care or in another career? Consider one of Molloy's dual-degree programs, the degree completion program for registered nurses, the LPN to B.S./RN career mobility program, or the accelerated dual-degree program for second degree students holding a non-nursing baccalaureate or higher degree.

- <u>Graduate programs.</u> Focused on advanced theory and its application in a selected area of nursing, Molloy offers seven distinct tracks leading to master's degrees and nine master's certificates concentrating on advanced clinical practice, administrative and informatics expertise, and specialty training in education. Nurse Practitioner tracks are available in Pediatrics, Adult-Gerontology, Family or Psychiatry, Clinical Nurse Specialist (CNS): Adult-Gerontology Health, Nursing Education, or Nursing Administration with Informatics with an option to add an M.B.A. in healthcare management.

- <u>Doctoral programs.</u> Molloy's first two doctoral programs are designed to prepare doctoral students to become leaders, advancing the profession of nursing through research, education, administration, health policy, and clinical practice.

Molloy College launched its first doctoral program, a Ph.D. in Nursing, in 2010. The College began offering its second doctoral program, a Doctor of Nursing Practice (D.N.P.) degree, in 2014. According to Veronica Feeg, Ph.D., RN, FAAN, Associate Dean and Director of the Ph.D. Program, "Doctoral education is important for our profession and the Ph.D. degrees at Molloy will produce the researchers and scholars who will lead the discipline." Joan Ginty, D.N.P., RN, ANP-BC, Associate Dean and Director of the D.N.P. program, adds, "Our new D.N.P. degree has a strong emphasis on inter- and intra-professional collaboration, translating research into practice for populations of patients and the improvement of systems of care delivery."

"We expect that our Ph.D. graduates will leave Molloy prepared to serve our communities, develop the next generation of nursing leaders and have a strong voice in health policy decisions that affect us all," said Jeannine D. Muldoon, Ph.D., RN, Dean of the Division of Nursing. "Armed with the additional knowledge, skills, and acumen to translate research into practice, our D.N.P. students will be leaders in effecting change through evidence-based clinical practice."

A Ph.D. from Molloy prepares nurses for leadership roles in academia, health policy formulation, health-care administration, and clinical practice. The curriculum focuses on theory, research, the humanities, and methodology. Essential elements of the curriculum feature leadership through caring, both in educational and organizational/policy settings, as well as theory and research in the nursing profession. Students are required to complete 45 credits of course work and a dissertation.

Students admitted to the D.N.P. program will complete a total of 37 credits beyond the nurse practitioner specialty track program requirements. The D.N.P. format is composed of nine core courses totaling 27 credits; four residency courses will add 10 credits to the program. In addition to the individual course objectives, the program also addresses policy development, business acumen, translational research, advanced practice, leadership, scholarly writing, informatics, and media relations.

- *2015–16 UNDERGRADUATE TUITION & FEES:*

  Tuition: $26,980

  Fees: $1,050

- *2015–16 GRADUATE TUITION & FEES:*

  Master's program:
  Tuition: $1,025 per credit

  Fees: $740 (if taking 1–4 credits); $900 (if taking 5 or more credits)

  Ph.D. program: $1,150/credit; fees same as for Master's program

- *APPLICATION DEADLINES:*

  Undergraduate: Rolling admissions

  Master's program: Rolling admissions

  Ph.D. program: February 1

CONTACT INFORMATION

Molloy College
1000 Hempstead Avenue
Rockville Centre, New York 11571
Phone: 888-4-MOLLOY (toll-free)
Website: http://www.molloy.edu

Undergraduate Admissions
Phone: 516-323-4000
E-mail: admissions@molloy.edu

Graduate and Ph.D. Admissions
Alina Haitz
Phone: 516-323-4008
E-mail: ahaitz@molloy.edu

Find us on Facebook®: http://www.facebook.com/GoMolloy
Follow us on Twitter™: http://www.twitter.com/MolloyCollege

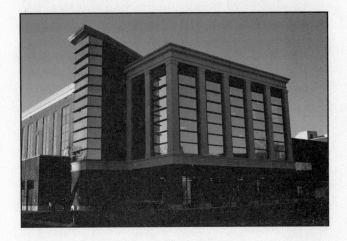

The new Barbara H. Hagan Center for Nursing opened in January 2016.

MOUNT MERCY ✝ UNIVERSITY

Obtain the medical and leadership skills necessary to provide compassionate care.

Nestled in the heart of Cedar Rapids, Iowa's second largest city, Mount Mercy University offers high-quality nursing programs at three levels: Bachelor of Science in Nursing (B.S.N.), RN to B.S.N. (face-to-face or online), and Master of Science in Nursing (M.S.N.). The baccalaureate degree in nursing and master's degree in nursing programs at Mount Mercy University are accredited by the Commission on Collegiate Nursing Education.

The University's Department of Nursing was built upon the compassionate spirit of institution founders, the Sisters of Mercy, and continues a tradition of excellence by caring for and meeting the needs of all people. Through learning the art, science, and culture of nursing, students are prepared to work with patients from various cultures and backgrounds.

Bachelor of Science in Nursing (B.S.N.)

Nursing students are admitted into Mount Mercy's B.S.N. program during their sophomore year, following a year of prerequisite courses. Once in the three-year program, students are offered numerous opportunities for hands-on learning and engagement throughout the surrounding community, gaining exposure to the rapidly changing and diverse healthcare system.

Mount Mercy features a fully equipped Clinical Simulation Laboratory (CSL), which provides students the opportunity to practice newly learned skills through active learning situations in simulated scenarios. By learning in the CSL, students practice their skills before entering the nursing field. Both laboratory time and clinical experiences are critical to a nursing student's success, facilitating the opportunity for professional interaction with faculty, staff, and patients.

RN to B.S.N.

Registered nurses with an associate degree in nursing have the opportunity to earn their B.S.N. through Mount Mercy's accelerated format RN to B.S.N. program—either face-to-face or online.

The University's distinctive face-to-face program is designed with the working professional in mind as it features evening classes over an 18-month completion period. Courses are offered one night a week for either a 5-week or 10-week session. This innovative format allows students to focus on one class at a time. Classroom time allows for high-level discussions, bringing theory and application together while connecting important professional experiences.

Online classes are also offered in 5- and 10-week sessions, with no required log-in days or times. Students are expected to complete weekly deadlines that keep them engaged and on track with their course progress. Typical coursework includes interacting with fellow students and the instructor through discussion forums, submitting written assignments, project-based work (both group and individual), and online quizzes and exams. Mount Mercy's online students have access to all on-campus student resources including Career Services, the Academic Center for Excellence, and the University's expansive Busse Library.

Master of Science in Nursing (M.S.N.)

Mount Mercy offers three tracks within the Master of Science in Nursing program:

- **Health Advocacy:** Prepares graduates to design, implement, manage, continuously

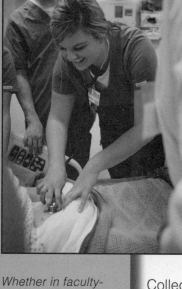

Whether in faculty-supervised clinical groups or independent clinical activities, students are guided, evaluated, and supported in their professional skills development.

improve, and lead innovative healthcare population management programs.

- **Nurse Educator:** Prepares graduates to design, implement, and continuously improve educational initiatives in academic and health care settings.

- **Nurse Administrator:** Prepares graduates to lead and manage complex 21st-century healthcare organizations.

M.S.N. programs focus on the development of nursing skills to prepare graduates for advancement within a healthcare setting or community. Faculty members hold both academic and practical experience, providing students with well-rounded knowledge used in professional and educational environments.

Classes are held at the Mount Mercy University CRST International Graduate Center, allowing graduate students an academic environment to call their own away from main campus.

- **2015–16 TUITION & FEES:**

  Traditional full-time: $28,226 (generous scholarships available)

  Traditional part-time: $768/credit hour

  Online students: $465/credit hour

  Accelerated students: $445/credit hour

  Graduate students: $570/credit hour

- *APPLICATION DEADLINES*

  Traditional students: Rolling deadline

  RN–B.S.N. students: July 1 (fall admission), December 1 (spring admission)

  Graduate students: July 1 (fall admission), December 1 (spring admission)

- *FACULTY INFORMATION: https://www.mtmercy.edu/ nursing-faculty-and-staff*

CONTACT INFORMATION

Admissions, Mount Mercy University

1330 Elmhurst Drive NE

Cedar Rapids, Iowa 52402

Phone: 319-368-6460

800-248-4504

Fax: 319-861-2390

E-mail: admission@mtmercy.edu

Website: www.mtmercy.edu

UNDERGRADUATE NURSING PROGRAM

Mary Tarbox, RN, Ed.D.
Chair, Department of Nursing
Phone: 319-363-1323 x 1527
E-mail: mtarbox@mtmercy.edu

RN–B.S.N. NURSING PROGRAM

Candace Chihak, M.S.N., RN
Director, RN–B.S.N. Program
Phone: 319-363-1323 x 1501
E-mail: cchihak@mtmercy.edu

GRADUATE NURSING PROGRAM

Sharon Guthrie, Ph.D., ARNP, CPNP, NCSN, RN-BC
Director, M.S.N. Graduate Program

Phone: 319-363-1323 x 1538

E-mail: sguthrie@mtmercy.edu

Facebook: www.facebook.com/ mountmercyuniversity

Twittter: twitter.com/mountmercy

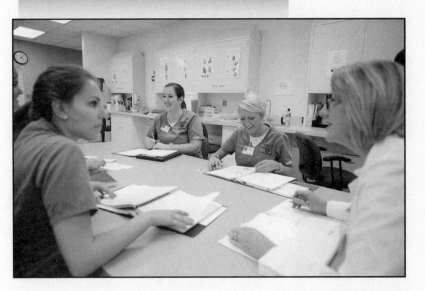

Students learn to read, analyze, and use evidence through ongoing instruction study.

QUINNIPIAC UNIVERSITY

School of Nursing

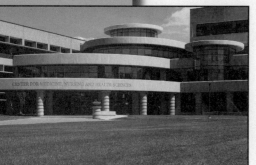

Education with a Personal Touch.

Professional nursing courses take place in the Center for Medicine, Nursing and Health Sciences on Quinnipiac's 104-acre North Haven campus.

Quinnipiac University (QU), located in Hamden and North Haven, Connecticut, just 8 miles from New Haven and midway between New York City and Boston, has 6,982 undergraduate and 2,672 graduate students. QU offers the B.S. in Nursing, an Accelerated B.S.N. for those who hold a non-nursing college degree, an RN to B.S.N Completion Track, a Master's of Science in Nursing (M.S.N. in Nursing), and the Doctorate of Nursing Practice (D.N.P.) for postbaccalaureate and post-master's students. The School of Nursing is located on the North Haven campus along with the Schools of Medicine, Health Sciences, Education, and Law.

Quinnipiac views nursing as a research-based profession that is goal-directed as well as creative and concerned with the health and dignity of the whole person. The art of delivering high-quality nursing care depends on the successful mastery and application of intellectually rigorous nursing knowledge. Quinnipiac goes further by developing a team approach to health care in providing health care to patients of all ages, abilities, and backgrounds.

Accredited by the Commission on Collegiate Nursing Education (CCNE) Quinnipiac's bachelor's degree program in nursing offers the theoretical and clinical education students need to enter professional nursing practice. Graduates of the traditional and accelerated second degree programs are eligible to take the NCLEX-RN exam and are well prepared for graduate study in nursing. The nursing curriculum fosters professional socialization for future roles and responsibilities within the profession. Graduates of the program are prepared as generalists to begin the practice of holistic professional nursing, with sound theoretical foundations and nearly 700 hours of diverse clinical practice and laboratory experiences. In addition to the traditional four-year program, and the accelerated second degree option, an online RN to B.S.N. completion program provides Associate Degree and Diploma trained nurses with an opportunity to develop competencies in research, community and public health, quality, safety, and leadership.

The graduate nursing program, also accredited by CCNE, prepares professional nurses at an advanced theoretical and clinical practice level in order to address present and potential societal health needs. There are six tracks that lead to the Doctor of Nursing Practice degree. Two available post-B.S.N. tracks are Adult-Gerontology Nurse Practitioner and Family Nurse Practitioner. Two post-master's tracks, The Care of Populations and Nursing Leadership, are also available. Two options for post-B.S.N. and post-M.S.N. tracks in nurse anesthesia began in summer of 2014 and are approved by the Commission on Accreditation (COA) as well. A proposed option for an online post-B.S.N. to Master of Science in Nursing (M.S.N.) degree in operational leadership is in the requisite approval process from state authorities. The graduate nursing program broadens the scope of practice and provides for the acquisition of expertise in an area of certified specialization (Adult-Gerontology Nurse Practitioner or Family Nurse Practitioner), as well as leadership roles in advanced specialty practice, population health and health-care systems. The graduate nursing program includes core courses that cover bioethics, Evidence-based practice, organizational systems, epidemiology, and health-care policy.

Quinnipiac's strong affiliates with health-care providers in the area allow students to complete clinical work within institutions such as Yale-New Haven Health system, St. Vincent's Medical Center, Connecticut Children's Medical Center, Mid-State Medical Center, Middlesex Hospital, the Hartford Healthcare system as well as in private practices, clinics, schools, and other community-based settings.

Quinnipiac's Mount Carmel Campus is the primary location for housing, recreation, and course work for undergraduates in their first two years. Starting in the junior year, the professional courses in nursing take place on the nearby 104-acre North Haven campus in the Center for Medicine, Nursing & Health Sciences, a remarkable facility with state-of-the-art technologies to prepare health-care professionals in a variety of fields. The Clinical Simulation Labs house "patients" that are lifelike simulation mannequins. Cameras capture the simulation for student assessment. The variety of labs and technology provide an educational setting for nursing students to learn across the lifespan, across the continuum of care, and across the disciplines. The Physical Diagnosis Lab, Physical Exam Suite, Health Assessment Lab, and the Standardized Patient Center duplicate care in an outpatient primary care setting, such as an emergency room or doctor's office.

For more information on either campus, see www.quinnipiac.edu/about.

Students applying as freshmen into the nursing program should file their application for admission by November 15. Information regarding admission requirements can be found at http://www.quinnipiac.edu/apply. Transfer students must have a minimum 3.0 GPA and are considered on a space-available basis.

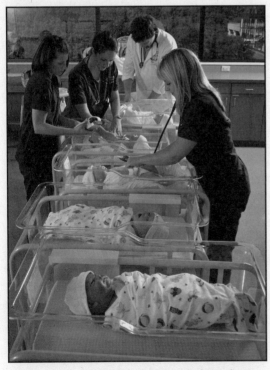

In the pediatrics maternity lab, students learn about fetal development and birthing. Students are taught to bathe and swaddle infants as well as how to educate new mothers about infant care.

The accelerated (second degree) nursing program begins in August. The complete application and all supporting documents must be filed by January 1. See www.quinnipiac.edu/accelerated for details.

Graduate admission information for the M.S., D.N.P., and the various tracks can be found at www.quinnipiac.edu/gradnursing.

- *2016–17 UNDERGRADUATE TUITION & FEES:*

  Full-time: $43,640 (tuition and student fees, covers 12–16 credits per semester); $15,170 (room and board including $2,100 in meals)

  Part-time: $710 per credit; $995 for credits above 16 in a full-time semester

  Technology fee: $300 freshmen, $680 all others

- *2016–17 GRADUATE TUITION: $985 per credit plus $40 per credit student fee.*

- *APPLICATION DEADLINES:*

  Undergraduate applicants should apply by Nov. 15 for fall admission

  Accelerated Nursing applicants (who have a bachelor's degree) applications are due Jan. 1 for fall entrance

  Graduate students should ideally apply by May 1 for summer for the nurse anesthesia program or by June 1 for the fall semester; the program has rolling admissions.

- *FACULTY INFORMATION:*

  http://www.quinnipiac.edu/nursing

- *MULTIMEDIA:*

  http://www.quinnipiac.edu/tour

CONTACT INFORMATION

Joan Isaac Mohr
VP for Admissions & Financial Aid
Admissions Office
Quinnipiac University
275 Mt. Carmel Avenue
Hamden, Connecticut 06518
Phone: 203-582-8600
**   800-462-1944 (toll-free)**
Fax: 203-582-8906
E-mail: admissions@quinnipiac.edu
Website: http://www.quinnipiac.edu

Undergraduate Nursing Program:
Office of Undergraduate Admissions
Phone: 203-582-8600
E-mail: admissions@quinnipiac.edu

Graduate Nursing Program:
Office of Graduate Admissions
Phone: 203-582-8672
E-mail: graduate@quinnipiac.edu

ST. FRANCIS COLLEGE

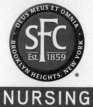

NURSING

Building a foundation of knowledge that will contribute to the development of the nursing profession and society as a whole.

Quality Private Education

St. Francis College (SFC) offers small classes, a technology-rich environment, and professional mentoring that continues well beyond graduation. Graduates of the Nursing Program go on to a wide variety of nursing careers at many of the best hospitals and health-care institutions in the New York area, as well as nationally. St. Francis students are accepted into top graduate programs in nursing that include Columbia University Teacher's College, Long Island University, New York University, Pace University, and SUNY Downstate, among others.

The College's well-rounded nursing program provides access to and affiliations with excellent clinical placements and significantly prepares students for graduate school admission and careers such as nurse practitioners, clinical specialists, administrators, and nurse educators.

Prepare Yourself for the Future of Nursing

The Nursing Program at SFC offers a Bachelor of Science degree with a major in nursing to qualified high school graduates and transfer students interested in preparing for the NCLEX Exam (BSN Pre-Licensure Nursing Program), as well as to qualified students with a valid New York State RN license (RN to BS Program). SFC is registered with the New York State Education Department and accredited by the Commission on Collegiate Nursing Education (CCNE), the accrediting arm of the American Association of Colleges of Nursing (AACN). In addition to a nursing curriculum, students gain valuable knowledge and skills in liberal arts and sciences through courses focused on mathematics, natural sciences, social sciences, advanced writing, and oral communication.

The Pre-Licensure Nursing Program is open to students interested in full-time study only. For those students who are already registered nurses (RN to BS), flexible scheduling allows for full- or part-time study. In fact, the RN to BS program is designed for nurses who wish to keep working while continuing their education. Students in the RN to BS program are required to complete the program within a maximum five-year period.

College Distinctions

St. Francis College consistently makes the grade when it comes to college rankings. *U.S. News & World Report* classifies St. Francis as one of the "Best Regional Colleges in the North" and was selected the fifth-most "Ethnically Diverse Regional College in the North." SFC has also been named by Forbes.com to its "America's Best Colleges" list and was most recently ranked in *Money* magazine's "Best Value for Your Money" category.

Department Mission

The mission of the Department of Nursing is consistent with the overall mission of the College—to promote the development of the whole person by integrating a liberal arts education with pre-professional programs designed to prepare nurses for the rigors of an increasingly technological and globalized marketplace and society. The department's mission encompasses the Franciscan and Catholic traditions that underpin its commitment to academic excellence, spiritual and moral values, physical fitness, social responsibility, and lifelong learning. These traditions include the Franciscan tradition of service, equality, aesthetics, freedom, honor, dignity, justice, and truth that are demonstrated within the context of professional nursing standards at the baccalaureate level (AACN Baccalaureate Essentials; ANA Standards of Clinical Nursing Practice). This nursing program builds a foundation of knowledge that will contribute to the development of the nursing profession as well as society as a whole.

Students who successfully complete the St. Francis Nursing program are able to:

- Integrate knowledge from bio/psycho/social/spiritual dimensions in caring for individuals, families, groups, and communities.

St. Francis is one of the most affordable private colleges in the New York metropolitan area and offers a generous scholarship program.

- Apply the nursing process in the delivery of culturally competent nursing care.

- Apply principles of leadership and management in caring for individuals, families, groups, and communities.

- Demonstrate accountability and responsibility for individual nursing actions.

- Collaborate as a member of a multidisciplinary healthcare team.

- Analyze research findings and technological advances for their applicability to clinical practice.

- Analyze national and international health policy initiatives for their impact on service, equality, aesthetics, freedom, human dignity, justice, and health of populations.

- Critically analyze the rationale for the nursing care provided.

- Incorporate the Franciscan tradition of service, equality, aesthetics, freedom, honor, dignity, justice, and truth into daily nursing practice.

- Recognize the legal and ethical health policy ramifications central to the delivery of health care.

- Demonstrate proficiency in the use of technology in the delivery of nursing care.

- Be prepared to sit for the Registered Nurse Licensing Exam (NCLEX).

- Be prepared for entrance into graduate schools that prepare nurses for advanced nursing roles including nurse practitioner, clinical specialist, and other specialties in the nursing profession that require advanced practice in nursing.

For details on tuition and fees, application deadlines, and additional admission information, please visit the College's website at www.sfc.edu or contact the Office of Admissions. Prospective students are also invited to take the new virtual tour at SFC.EDU.

- *FACULTY:*

The SFC nursing faculty members are highly qualified and are graduates of NYU, Adelphi, Columbia, and Hunter among others.

- *APPLICATION INFORMATION:*

Students are encouraged to apply through the St. Francis College website (free). Students may also apply through the Nursing CAS system affiliated with the American Association of Colleges of Nursing.

CONTACT INFORMATION

Office of Admissions
St. Francis College
180 Remsen Street
Brooklyn Heights, NY 11201
Phone: 718-489-5200
Websites: www.sfc.edu
www.sfc.edu/nursing

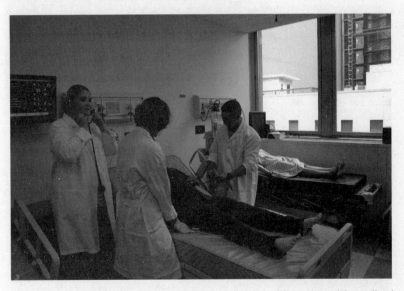

State-of-the-art nursing lab equipped with real-world medical simulators, SimMan, SimMom, and SimBaby.

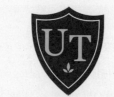

COLLEGE OF NURSING
THE UNIVERSITY OF TOLEDO

Find Your Passion in Nursing and Build Your Career!

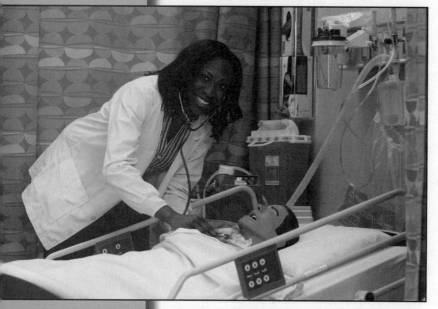

Nursing is among the most versatile, challenging, and rewarding careers across the globe. Firmly on the front-line of health-care delivery, nurses work side-by-side with physicians and health care practitioners. They enact change through evidence-based practice and influence public policy. With convenient classes onsite and online, expert faculty, state-of-the-art learning environments, and affordable tuition, The University of Toledo (UT) is the perfect launching pad for a career in nursing. UT is the perfect environment for registered nurses to pursue an advanced degree and open the door to expand career opportunities.

GRADUATE PROGRAMS

Doctor of Nursing Practice (Post-Master's DNP): In consortium with Wright State University, this program is designed to take master's-prepared advanced practice nurses and nurse leaders to the highest level of clinical practice in order to meet the increasing complexities and challenges of the nation's health-care environment. There are both full- and part-time options in this online degree program.

Doctor of Nursing Practice (BSN–DNP): This program is designed to take BSN-prepared nurses to the highest level of clinical practice. The curriculum includes theoretical and clinical courses to prepare students to lead and develop innovative health-care delivery in a variety of health-care settings. Options include Adult-Gerontology Primary Care Nurse Practitioner, Family Nurse Practitioner, Pediatric Primary Care Nurse Practitioner, and Psychiatric Mental Health Nurse Practitioner. The program is offered in a hybrid model, with both online and campus course work and full- or part-time options. Graduates are eligible to take the National Certification Exam in their specialty area.

Master of Science in Nursing (MSN) Advanced Practice: This program is designed to build on a student's past learning, personal and professional goals, and the insights and experiences gained through practice. It prepares registered nurses with a baccalaureate degree as Adult-Gerontology Primary Care Nurse Practitioners, Family Nurse Practitioners, Pediatric Primary Care Nurse Practitioners or Psychiatric Mental Health Nurse Practitioners. The MSN is a two-year, full-time program with part-time options. Upon completion, students are qualified to take the National Certification Exam in their specialty area.

Nurse Educator: The Nurse Educator major is targeted for baccalaureate graduates with clinical nursing experience who want to become nursing faculty or staff educators. Graduates are envisioned as teachers of undergraduate nursing students in the classroom and clinical setting. This major focuses on: curriculum development, teaching-learning processes, classroom and clinical teaching strategies, and evaluation principles. The nurse educator major offers full-time and part-time options.

Clinical Nurse Leader Program Graduate Entry (Pre-Licensure): This program is designed for the person who holds a bachelor's degree and is not a registered nurse (RN) but desires to become a RN. It is a full-time program with classes offered on campus. The MSN is awarded upon program completion, and graduates are eligible to sit for the NCLEX-RN exam.

GRADUATE CERTIFICATE PROGRAMS

Family Nurse Practitioner (FNP): This program is for those who have completed a master's degree in nursing and who desire to obtain specialized knowledge to seek certification as a FNP. Graduates are qualified to take national FNP certification examinations. The program is offered part-time.

Pediatric Primary Care Nurse Practitioner (PPNP): This program is offered to individuals who have completed a master's degree in nursing and who desire to obtain specialized knowledge to seek certification as a Primary PNP. It is a part-time program and graduates are qualified to take a national certification examination.

Nursing Education Certificate: The program is designed to provide an opportunity for current and potential nurse educators in academic and health-care settings to develop and refine the practice of teaching. Convenient online classes are designed for adult learners with the opportunity for completion within one calendar year. The certificate depicts a commitment to the professional responsibility as an educator in a variety of health-care settings.

UNDERGRADUATE PROGRAMS

Bachelor of Science in Nursing (BSN): This degree program provides the optimal blend for collegiate and academic experience while pursuing a nursing degree. Course work includes the humanities and sciences. Admission is competitive; students may be admitted to the Nursing major in the fall, spring, or summer terms. Clinical experience begins in the first semester of the Nursing major. A variety of settings encompassing the life span are used to promote proficiency in the skills necessary for knowledgeable nursing practice. The program is offered in consortium with Bowling Green State University. Students have the opportunity to be employed as student nurses at the University of Toledo Medical Center during their off semester.

RN–BSN (for individuals who are already registered nurses): This online degree program is available in full- and part-time options with experiential learning opportunities.

- *2015–16 TUITION & FEES:*
  https://www.utoledo.edu/offices/treasurer/index.html

- *APPLICATION DEADLINES:*
  http://www.utoledo.edu/nursing/howtoapply.html

CONTACT INFORMATION:
College of Nursing
The University of Toledo
3000 Arlington Avenue
Toledo, Ohio 43614
Phone: 419-383-5810
E-mail: admitnurse@utoledo.edu
Website: utoledo.edu/nursing

Find us on Facebook: www.facebook.com/UTCON

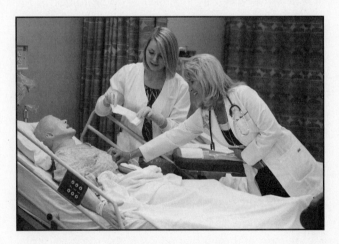

As practitioners, scholars, and educators, the faculty is a knowledgeable—and passionate—resource for students as they strive to become the best in the field.

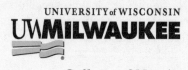

College of Nursing

IDEAS: Innovation, Discovery, Engagement, Access, Solutions.

As Wisconsin's largest nursing program, the University of Wisconsin–Milwaukee College of Nursing has made its home in the commercial, cultural, and economic capital of Wisconsin for over 50 years. The campus is located on 104 acres and offers 188 degree programs. As the seventh-most exciting city in America (Movoto.com), Milwaukee offers students a vibrant city on the shores of beautiful Lake Michigan, just 90 minutes north of Chicago.

UW-Milwaukee's competitive, collaborative nursing program is valued for its ability to prepare science-based, compassionate nurse leaders through innovative, superior educational programs. The College is a vibrant, innovative environment for teaching, research, practice, and service to the community and the profession. The College is one of three universities in the state to offer students the full range of nursing degrees including: Bachelor of Science in Nursing, Master of Nursing, Doctor of Philosophy in Nursing, and Doctor of Nursing Practice. The College of Nursing has an enrollment of over 1,300 undergraduate and 300 graduate students.

The College of Nursing faculty challenges students, creating innovative classroom environments using the latest technology while maintaining over 130 clinical and

Students at UW-Milwaukee engage in experiential learning, clinical training, and high-level critical thinking.

research partnerships throughout Southeast Wisconsin. Faculty members embrace practice by engaging regional and global communities in the development of solutions to improve health care. The College is consistently ranked in the top 10 percent for academic excellence among colleges with graduate nursing programs by *U.S. News & World Report*. Faculty members embrace practice by engaging regional and global communities in the development of solutions to improve health care.

The College of Nursing is one of the most robust scientific research ventures on campus. More than 75 percent of the nursing faculty is funded by public and/or private entities. The global and national perspectives expand the reach of the College's work in key areas, including community-driven research, geriatric health care, self-management, and global health.

The College pioneered and is home to two nurse-managed Community Nursing Centers, serving the uninsured and underinsured communities and providing health-care solutions aligned with their needs. The College provides national leadership in advancing geriatric health care through clinical intervention research and maintains a close relationship with the Jewish Home and Care Center Foundation in Milwaukee. The Self-Management Science Center, funded by the National Institutes of Health (P20NR015339), expands research aimed at enhancing the science of self-management in individuals and families. Faculty members and students have also extended the scope of international research to health care in rural Malawi, Thailand, and Kenya. The College also maintains a 15-year partnership with two sister nursing schools in South Korea.

The undergraduate nursing program maximizes hands-on learning and technological innovation, and requires a dedication to scholarship and a passion for health care. Students master nursing theory and practice through focused clinical cohorts. Teachers are key to student success, providing mentorship, career preparation, and support. The College of Nursing continues to expand and enhance its graduate program opportunities. The College offers a Master in Nursing (M.N.) program with two entry options and a Master of Sustainable Peacebuilding (M.S.P.). The Master of Nursing degree is for nurses and non-nurses who hold a bachelor's degree. The program provides the framework for practice as a clinical nurse leader, public health nurse, clinical research manager, health informatics specialist or nurse manager. The Master of Sustainable Peacebuilding is new to the College of Nursing to prepare practitioners, from any academic background, with skills and concepts required to engage and change issues at a global or local level. In addition to the Master of Nursing, the College offers two doctoral programs: Doctor of Nursing Practice (D.N.P.) and Doctor of Philosophy in Nursing (Ph.D.) in face-to-face and online formats. Students in the doctoral program work closely with faculty mentors to define success early and develop into key clinical and research partners.

To find out more about UW–Milwaukee College of Nursing, visit: www.nursing.uwm.edu.

- *2015–16 UNDERGRADUATE TUITION & FEES:*
  Annual Full-time: $9,428 (residents)
  $19,602 (nonresidents)

  Additional tuition differential fee of $32 per credit is due upon admission to the clinical major.

- *2015–16 GRADUATE TUITION & FEES:*
  Annual Full-time: $11,724 (residents)
  $24,761 (nonresidents)

- *APPLICATION DEADLINES:*
  Undergraduate: December 1 for spring admission; March 1 for fall admission

  Graduate: February 1 for fall admission; October 1 for spring admission

CONTACT INFORMATION

Office of Student Affairs
University of Wisconsin–Milwaukee
College of Nursing
1921 East Hartford Avenue
Milwaukee, Wisconsin 53201
Phone: 414-229-5047
Fax: 414-229-5554
E-mail: uwmnurse@uwm.edu
Web site: www.nursing.uwm.edu

Find us on Facebook®: https://www.facebook.com/UWMNursing
Find us on Twitter: https://twitter.com/UWM_Nursing

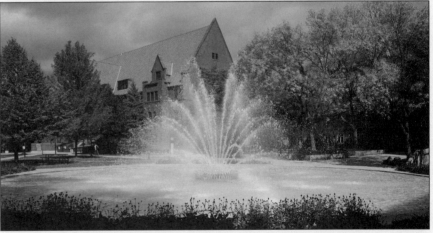

Connect with businesses, corporations and recreational hotspots that make Milwaukee the economic/cultural/entertainment capital of Wisconsin.

INDEXES

BACCALAUREATE PROGRAMS

ACCELERATED BACCALAUREATE

U.S. AND U.S. TERRITORIES

Alabama

University of North Alabama, College of Nursing and Allied Health, *Florence (BSN)*

University of South Alabama, College of Nursing, *Mobile (BSN)*

Arizona

Arizona State University at the Downtown Phoenix campus, College of Nursing, *Phoenix (BSN)*

Chamberlain College of Nursing, *Phoenix (BSN)*

University of Phoenix–Online Campus, Online Campus, *Phoenix (BSN)*

University of Phoenix–Phoenix Campus, College of Health Sciences and Nursing, *Tempe (BSN)*

University of Phoenix–Southern Arizona Campus, College of Social Sciences, *Tucson (BSN)*

California

Azusa Pacific University, School of Nursing, *Azusa (BSN)*

California State University, Northridge, Nursing Program, *Northridge (BSN)*

California State University, San Marcos, School of Nursing, *San Marcos (BSN)*

Mount Saint Mary's University, Department of Nursing, *Los Angeles (BSN, BSc PN)*

Samuel Merritt University, School of Nursing, *Oakland (BSN)*

University of Phoenix–Bay Area Campus, College of Nursing, *San Jose (BSN)*

University of Phoenix–Sacramento Valley Campus, College of Nursing, *Sacramento (BSN)*

University of Phoenix–San Diego Campus, College of Nursing, *San Diego (BSN)*

University of Phoenix–Southern California Campus, College of Health Sciences and Nursing, *Costa Mesa (BSN)*

West Coast University, Nursing Programs, *North Hollywood (BSN)*

Colorado

Denver School of Nursing, *Denver (BSN)*

Platt College, School of Nursing, *Aurora (BSN)*

Regis University, School of Nursing, *Denver (BSN)*

University of Colorado Denver, College of Nursing, *Aurora (BS)*

Connecticut

St. Vincent's College, Nursing Program, *Bridgeport (BSN)*

Southern Connecticut State University, Department of Nursing, *New Haven (BSN)*

Florida

Barry University, Division of Nursing, *Miami Shores (BSN)*

Florida International University, Nursing Program, *Miami (BSN)*

Florida Southern College, School of Nursing & Health Sciences, *Lakeland (BSN)*

Florida State University, College of Nursing, *Tallahassee (BSN)*

Jacksonville University, School of Nursing, *Jacksonville (BSN)*

University of Phoenix–North Florida Campus, College of Nursing, *Jacksonville (BSN)*

University of Phoenix–West Florida Learning Center, College of Nursing, *Temple Terrace (BSN)*

Georgia

Armstrong State University, Program in Nursing, *Savannah (BSN)*

Emory University, Nell Hodgson Woodruff School of Nursing, *Atlanta (BSN)*

Kennesaw State University, School of Nursing, *Kennesaw (BSN)*

Hawaii

University of Phoenix–Hawaii Campus, College of Nursing, *Honolulu (BSN)*

Illinois

Bradley University, Department of Nursing, *Peoria (BSN, BSc PN)*

Olivet Nazarene University, Division of Nursing, *Bourbonnais (BSN)*

Resurrection University, *Chicago (BSN)*

Southern Illinois University Edwardsville, School of Nursing, *Edwardsville (BS)*

Trinity College of Nursing and Health Sciences, *Rock Island (BSN)*

Indiana

Marian University, School of Nursing, *Indianapolis (BSN)*

Purdue University North Central, Department of Nursing, *Westville (BS)*

Valparaiso University, College of Nursing and Health Professions, *Valparaiso (BSN)*

Iowa

Allen College, Graduate Programs, *Waterloo (BSN)*

Kansas

MidAmerica Nazarene University, Division of Nursing, *Olathe (BSN)*

University of Saint Mary, Bachelor of Science in Nursing Program, *Leavenworth (BSN)*

Wichita State University, School of Nursing, *Wichita (BSN)*

Louisiana

University of Phoenix–New Orleans Learning Center, College of Nursing, *Metairie (BSN)*

Maine

University of Maine at Fort Kent, Department of Nursing, *Fort Kent (BSN)*

Maryland

Bowie State University, Department of Nursing, *Bowie (BSN)*

Massachusetts

Elms College, School of Nursing, *Chicopee (BS)*

MCPHS University, School of Nursing, *Boston (BSN)*

MGH Institute of Health Professions, School of Nursing, *Boston (BSN)*

Regis College, School of Nursing, Science and Health Professions, *Weston (BSN)*

Simmons College, School of Nursing and Health Sciences, *Boston (BS)*

Michigan

Baker College, School of Nursing, *Flint (BSN)*

Missouri

Cox College, Department of Nursing, *Springfield (BSN)*

Goldfarb School of Nursing at Barnes-Jewish College, *St. Louis (BSN)*

Graceland University, School of Nursing, *Independence (BSN)*

Maryville University of Saint Louis, The Catherine McAuley School of Nursing, College of Health Professions, *St. Louis (BSN)*

Research College of Nursing, College of Nursing, *Kansas City (BSN)*

Saint Louis University, School of Nursing, *St. Louis (BSN)*

University of Missouri, Sinclair School of Nursing, *Columbia (BSN)*

University of Missouri–St. Louis, College of Nursing, *St. Louis (BSN)*

William Jewell College, Department of Nursing, *Liberty (BS)*

Nebraska

University of Nebraska Medical Center, College of Nursing, *Omaha (BSN)*

Nevada

Roseman University of Health Sciences, College of Nursing, *Henderson (BSN)*

University of Nevada, Las Vegas, School of Nursing, *Las Vegas (BSN)*

University of Nevada, Reno, Orvis School of Nursing, *Reno (BSN)*

New Jersey

Caldwell University, Nursing Programs, *Caldwell (BSN)*

Rutgers, The State University of New Jersey, Camden, Rutgers School of Nursing–Camden, *Camden (BS)*

New Mexico

New Mexico State University, School of Nursing, *Las Cruces (BSN)*

University of Phoenix–New Mexico Campus, College of Nursing, *Albuquerque (BSN)*

New York

Columbia University, School of Nursing, *New York (BS)*

Hartwick College, Department of Nursing, *Oneonta (BS)*

Mount Saint Mary College, School of Nursing, *Newburgh (BSN)*

The Sage Colleges, Department of Nursing, *Troy (BS)*

State University of New York Polytechnic Institute, School of Nursing and Health Systems, *Utica (BS)*

Stony Brook University, State University of New York, School of Nursing, *Stony Brook (BS)*

North Carolina

Queens University of Charlotte, Presbyterian School of Nursing, *Charlotte (BSN)*

The University of North Carolina at Chapel Hill, School of Nursing, *Chapel Hill (BSN)*

Western Carolina University, School of Nursing, *Cullowhee (BSN)*

Ohio

Ashland University, Dwight Schar College of Nursing and Health Sciences, *Ashland (BSN)*

Baldwin Wallace University, Accelerated Bachelor of Science in Nursing, *Berea (BSN)*

Chamberlain College of Nursing, *Columbus (BSN)*

Franklin University, Nursing Program, *Columbus (BSN)*

Kent State University, College of Nursing, *Kent (BSN)*

University of Phoenix–Cleveland Campus, College of Nursing, *Beachwood (BSN)*

Ursuline College, The Breen School of Nursing, *Pepper Pike (BSN)*

Oklahoma

Northwestern Oklahoma State University, Division of Nursing, *Alva (BSN)*

Oklahoma City University, Kramer School of Nursing, *Oklahoma City (BSN)*

Oregon

Oregon Health & Science University, School of Nursing, *Portland (BS)*

Pennsylvania

DeSales University, Department of Nursing and Health, *Center Valley (BSN)*

Drexel University, College of Nursing and Health Professions, *Philadelphia (BSN)*

Edinboro University of Pennsylvania, Department of Nursing, *Edinboro (BSN)*

Holy Family University, School of Nursing and Allied Health Professions, *Philadelphia (BSN)*

Lock Haven University of Pennsylvania, Nursing Program, *Lock Haven (BSN)*

Moravian College, Department of Nursing, *Bethlehem (BSN)*

Thomas Jefferson University, Department of Nursing, *Philadelphia (BSN)*

University of Pennsylvania, School of Nursing, *Philadelphia (BSN)*

Waynesburg University, Department of Nursing, *Waynesburg (BSN)*

Puerto Rico

Inter American University of Puerto Rico, Metropolitan Campus, Carmen Torres de Tiburcio School of Nursing, *San Juan (BSN)*

South Carolina

Anderson University, School of Nursing, *Anderson (BSN)*

Clemson University, School of Nursing, *Clemson (BS)*

Lander University, School of Nursing, *Greenwood (BSN)*

Medical University of South Carolina, College of Nursing, *Charleston (BSN)*

South Dakota

Augustana University, Department of Nursing, *Sioux Falls (BA)*

University of Sioux Falls, School of Nursing, *Sioux Falls (BSN)*

Tennessee

Belmont University, School of Nursing, *Nashville (BSN)*

Carson-Newman University, Department of Nursing, *Jefferson City (BSN)*

Cumberland University, Rudy School of Nursing and Health Professions, *Lebanon (BSN)*

Lincoln Memorial University, Caylor School of Nursing, *Harrogate (BSN)*

University of Memphis, Loewenberg School of Nursing, *Memphis (BSN)*

The University of Tennessee, College of Nursing, *Knoxville (BSN)*

The University of Tennessee Health Science Center, College of Nursing, *Memphis (BSN)*

Texas

Midwestern State University, Wilson School of Nursing, *Wichita Falls (BSN)*

Texas A&M University–Corpus Christi, College of Nursing and Health Sciences, *Corpus Christi (BSN)*

Texas Christian University, Harris College of Nursing, *Fort Worth (BSN)*

Texas Tech University Health Sciences Center El Paso, *El Paso (BSN)*

The University of Texas at Arlington, College of Nursing, *Arlington (BSN)*

The University of Texas at El Paso, School of Nursing, *El Paso (BSN)*

Utah

Western Governors University, Online College of Health Professions, *Salt Lake City (BS)*

Virginia

Eastern Mennonite University, Department of Nursing, *Harrisonburg (BS)*

Hampton University, School of Nursing, *Hampton (BS)*

West Virginia

West Virginia University, School of Nursing, *Morgantown (BSN)*

Wisconsin

Bellin College, Nursing Program, *Green Bay (BSN)*

Milwaukee School of Engineering, School of Nursing, *Milwaukee (BSN)*

CANADA

Alberta

University of Calgary, Faculty of Nursing, *Calgary (BN)*

University of Lethbridge, Faculty of Health Sciences, *Lethbridge (BN)*

British Columbia

The University of British Columbia, Program in Nursing, *Vancouver (BSN)*

New Brunswick

University of New Brunswick Fredericton, Faculty of Nursing, *Fredericton (BN)*

Newfoundland and Labrador

Memorial University of Newfoundland, School of Nursing, *St. John's (BN)*

Nova Scotia

St. Francis Xavier University, Department of Nursing, *Antigonish (BScN)*

Ontario

Lakehead University, School of Nursing, *Thunder Bay (BScN)*

Queen's University at Kingston, School of Nursing, *Kingston (BNSc)*

Trent University, Nursing Program, *Peterborough (BScN)*

University of Toronto, Faculty of Nursing, *Toronto (BScN)*

The University of Western Ontario, School of Nursing, *London (BScN)*

Quebec

Université Laval, Faculty of Nursing, *Québec (BScN)*

Saskatchewan

University of Saskatchewan, College of Nursing, *Saskatoon (BSN)*

ACCELERATED BACCALAUREATE FOR SECOND DEGREE

U.S. AND U.S. TERRITORIES

Alabama

Samford University, Ida V. Moffett School of Nursing, *Birmingham (BSN)*

Arizona

Arizona State University at the Downtown Phoenix campus, College of Nursing, *Phoenix (BSN)*

Brookline College, Baccalaureate Nursing Program, *Phoenix (BSN)*

Chamberlain College of Nursing, *Phoenix (BSN)*

Northern Arizona University, School of Nursing, *Flagstaff (BSN)*

Arkansas

Arkansas State University, Department of Nursing, *State University (BSN)*

California

Concordia University Irvine, Bachelor of Science in Nursing Program, *Irvine (BSN)*

Loma Linda University, School of Nursing, *Loma Linda (BS)*

Colorado

Colorado State University–Pueblo, Department of Nursing, *Pueblo (BSN)*

Denver School of Nursing, *Denver (BSN)*

Metropolitan State University of Denver, Department of Health Professions, *Denver (BSN)*

University of Colorado Colorado Springs, Helen and Arthur E. Johnson Beth-El College of Nursing & Health Sciences, *Colorado Springs (BSN)*

Connecticut

Fairfield University, School of Nursing, *Fairfield (BSN)*

Quinnipiac University, School of Nursing, *Hamden (BSN)*

University of Connecticut, School of Nursing, *Storrs (BS)*

Delaware

University of Delaware, School of Nursing, *Newark (BSN)*

District of Columbia

The Catholic University of America, School of Nursing, *Washington (BSN)*

The George Washington University, School of Nursing, *Washington (BSN)*

Florida

Barry University, Division of Nursing, *Miami Shores (BSN)*

ECPI University, *Lake Mary (BSN)*

Florida Atlantic University, Christine E. Lynn College of Nursing, *Boca Raton (BSN)*

Florida International University, Nursing Program, *Miami (BSN)*

Florida Southern College, School of Nursing & Health Sciences, *Lakeland (BSN)*

Jacksonville University, School of Nursing, *Jacksonville (BSN)*

University of Central Florida, College of Nursing, *Orlando (BSN)*

University of Florida, College of Nursing, *Gainesville (BSN)*

University of Miami, School of Nursing and Health Studies, *Coral Gables (BSN)*

University of North Florida, School of Nursing, *Jacksonville (BSN)*

University of South Florida, College of Nursing, *Tampa (BS)*

Georgia

Albany State University, College of Sciences and Health Professions, *Albany (BSN)*

Armstrong State University, Program in Nursing, *Savannah (BSN)*

Emory University, Nell Hodgson Woodruff School of Nursing, *Atlanta (BSN)*

Kennesaw State University, School of Nursing, *Kennesaw (BSN)*

Idaho

Idaho State University, Department of Nursing, *Pocatello (BS)*

Illinois

Blessing–Rieman College of Nursing and Health Sciences, *Quincy (BSN)*

Bradley University, Department of Nursing, *Peoria (BSN, BSc PN)*

Illinois State University, Mennonite College of Nursing, *Normal (BSN)*

Lewis University, Program in Nursing, *Romeoville (BSN)*

Loyola University Chicago, Marcella Niehoff School of Nursing, *Maywood (BSN)*

Methodist College, *Peoria (BSN)*

Resurrection University, *Chicago (BSN)*

Saint Xavier University, School of Nursing, *Chicago (BSN)*

Trinity College of Nursing and Health Sciences, *Rock Island (BSN)*

Indiana

Indiana State University, Department of Advanced Practice Nursing, *Terre Haute (BS)*

Indiana University Northwest, School of Nursing, *Gary (BSN)*

Indiana University–Purdue University Indianapolis, School of Nursing, *Indianapolis (BSN)*

Indiana University South Bend, Vera Z. Dwyer College of Health Sciences, *South Bend (BSN)*

Indiana Wesleyan University, School of Nursing, *Marion (BSN)*

Marian University, School of Nursing, *Indianapolis (BSN)*

Purdue University, School of Nursing, *West Lafayette (BS)*

Purdue University Calumet, School of Nursing, *Hammond (BSN)*

Purdue University North Central, Department of Nursing, *Westville (BS)*

Saint Joseph's College, St. Elizabeth School of Nursing, *Rensselaer (BSN)*

University of Indianapolis, School of Nursing, *Indianapolis (BSN)*

Iowa

Allen College, Graduate Programs, *Waterloo (BSN)*

Kansas

Wichita State University, School of Nursing, *Wichita (BSN)*

Kentucky

Bellarmine University, Donna and Allan Lansing School of Nursing and Health Sciences, *Louisville (BSN, MSCE)*

Northern Kentucky University, Department of Nursing, *Highland Heights (BSN)*

Spalding University, School of Nursing, *Louisville (BSN)*

Louisiana

Louisiana State University Health Sciences Center, School of Nursing, *New Orleans (BSN)*

Our Lady of the Lake College, Division of Nursing, *Baton Rouge (BSN)*

Southeastern Louisiana University, School of Nursing, *Hammond (BS)*

University of Louisiana at Lafayette, College of Nursing, *Lafayette (BSN)*

Maine

University of Southern Maine, School of Nursing, *Portland (BS)*

Maryland

Salisbury University, Department of Nursing, *Salisbury (BS)*

Massachusetts

American International College, Division of Nursing, *Springfield (BSN)*

Curry College, Division of Nursing, *Milton (BS)*

MCPHS University, School of Nursing, *Boston (BSN)*

Northeastern University, School of Nursing, *Boston (BSN)*

Regis College, School of Nursing, Science and Health Professions, *Weston (BSN)*

Salem State University, Program in Nursing, *Salem (BSN)*

Simmons College, School of Nursing and Health Sciences, *Boston (BS)*

University of Massachusetts Amherst, College of Nursing, *Amherst (BS)*

University of Massachusetts Boston, College of Nursing and Health Sciences, *Boston (BS)*

Michigan

Grand Valley State University, Kirkhof College of Nursing, *Allendale (BSN)*

Michigan State University, College of Nursing, *East Lansing (BSN)*

Oakland University, School of Nursing, *Rochester (BSN)*

University of Detroit Mercy, McAuley School of Nursing, *Detroit (BSN)*

University of Michigan, School of Nursing, *Ann Arbor (BSN)*

University of Michigan–Flint, Department of Nursing, *Flint (BSN)*

Wayne State University, College of Nursing, *Detroit (BSN)*

Minnesota

The College of St. Scholastica, Department of Nursing, *Duluth (BS)*

Concordia College, Department of Nursing, *Moorhead (BA)*

Minnesota State University Mankato, School of Nursing, *Mankato (BS)*

University of Northwestern–St. Paul, School of Nursing, *St. Paul (BSN)*

Mississippi

University of Mississippi Medical Center, School of Nursing, *Jackson (BSN)*

Missouri

Central Methodist University, College of Liberal Arts and Sciences, *Fayette (BSN)*

Cox College, Department of Nursing, *Springfield (BSN)*

Goldfarb School of Nursing at Barnes-Jewish College, *St. Louis (BSN)*

Research College of Nursing, College of Nursing, *Kansas City (BSN)*

Saint Louis University, School of Nursing, *St. Louis (BSN)*

University of Missouri, Sinclair School of Nursing, *Columbia (BSN)*

University of Missouri–Kansas City, School of Nursing and Health Studies, *Kansas City (BSN)*

University of Missouri–St. Louis, College of Nursing, *St. Louis (BSN)*

William Jewell College, Department of Nursing, *Liberty (BS)*

Montana

Montana State University, College of Nursing, *Bozeman (BSN)*

Nebraska

Creighton University, College of Nursing, *Omaha (BSN)*

Nebraska Methodist College, Department of Nursing, *Omaha (BSN)*

Nevada

Nevada State College at Henderson, Nursing Program, *Henderson (BSN)*

Roseman University of Health Sciences, College of Nursing, *Henderson (BSN)*

University of Nevada, Reno, Orvis School of Nursing, *Reno (BSN)*

New Jersey

Fairleigh Dickinson University, Metropolitan Campus, Henry P. Becton School of Nursing and Allied Health, *Teaneck (BSN)*

Felician University, Division of Nursing and Health Management, *Lodi (BSN)*

New Jersey City University, Department of Nursing, *Jersey City (BSN)*

Rutgers, The State University of New Jersey, Newark, Rutgers School of Nursing, *Newark (BSN)*

Seton Hall University, College of Nursing, *South Orange (BSN)*

William Paterson University of New Jersey, Department of Nursing, *Wayne (BSN)*

New York

Adelphi University, College of Nursing and Public Health, *Garden City (BS)*

The College of New Rochelle, School of Nursing, *New Rochelle (BSN)*

Columbia University, School of Nursing, *New York (BS)*

Concordia College–New York, Nursing Program, *Bronxville (BS)*

Dominican College, Department of Nursing, *Orangeburg (BSN)*

Hartwick College, Department of Nursing, *Oneonta (BS)*

Hunter College of the City University of New York, Hunter-Bellevue School of Nursing, *New York (BS)*

Lehman College of the City University of New York, Department of Nursing, *Bronx (BS)*

Le Moyne College, Nursing Programs, *Syracuse (BS)*

Long Island University–LIU Brooklyn, School of Nursing, *Brooklyn (BS)*

Molloy College, Division of Nursing, *Rockville Centre (BS)*

New York University, College of Nursing, *New York (BS)*

Niagara University, Department of Nursing, *Niagara University (BS)*

Pace University, Lienhard School of Nursing, *New York (BS)*

The Sage Colleges, Department of Nursing, *Troy (BS)*

State University of New York Downstate Medical Center, College of Nursing, *Brooklyn (BS)*

University at Buffalo, the State University of New York, School of Nursing, *Buffalo (BS)*

University of Rochester, School of Nursing, *Rochester (BS)*

Utica College, Department of Nursing, *Utica (BS)*

North Carolina

Duke University, School of Nursing, *Durham (BSN)*

East Carolina University, College of Nursing, *Greenville (BSN)*

North Carolina Agricultural and Technical State University, School of Nursing, *Greensboro (BSN)*

Queens University of Charlotte, Presbyterian School of Nursing, *Charlotte (BSN)*

The University of North Carolina at Chapel Hill, School of Nursing, *Chapel Hill (BSN)*

North Dakota

University of North Dakota, College of Nursing, *Grand Forks (BSN)*

Ohio

Ashland University, Dwight Schar College of Nursing and Health Sciences, *Ashland (BSN)*

Capital University, School of Nursing, *Columbus (BSN)*

Chamberlain College of Nursing, *Columbus (BSN)*

Cleveland State University, School of Nursing, *Cleveland (BSN)*

Kent State University, College of Nursing, *Kent (BSN)*

Mount Carmel College of Nursing, Nursing Programs, *Columbus (BSN)*

The University of Akron, School of Nursing, *Akron (BSN)*

University of Cincinnati, College of Nursing, *Cincinnati (BSN)*

Ursuline College, The Breen School of Nursing, *Pepper Pike (BSN)*

Walsh University, Department of Nursing, *North Canton (BSN)*

Oklahoma

Oklahoma City University, Kramer School of Nursing, *Oklahoma City (BSN)*

University of Oklahoma Health Sciences Center, College of Nursing, *Oklahoma City (BSN)*

Oregon

Linfield College, School of Nursing, *McMinnville (BSN)*

Pennsylvania

Bloomsburg University of Pennsylvania, Department of Nursing, *Bloomsburg (BSN)*

Drexel University, College of Nursing and Health Professions, *Philadelphia (BSN)*

Duquesne University, School of Nursing, *Pittsburgh (BSN)*

Edinboro University of Pennsylvania, Department of Nursing, *Edinboro (BSN)*

Holy Family University, School of Nursing and Allied Health Professions, *Philadelphia (BSN)*

Moravian College, Department of Nursing, *Bethlehem (BSN)*

Thomas Jefferson University, Department of Nursing, *Philadelphia (BSN)*

University of Pennsylvania, School of Nursing, *Philadelphia (BSN)*

University of Pittsburgh, School of Nursing, *Pittsburgh (BSN)*

Villanova University, College of Nursing, *Villanova (BSN)*

Waynesburg University, Department of Nursing, *Waynesburg (BSN)*

West Chester University of Pennsylvania, Department of Nursing, *West Chester (BSN)*

Wilkes University, Department of Nursing, *Wilkes-Barre (BS)*

South Carolina

Anderson University, School of Nursing, *Anderson (BSN)*

Lander University, School of Nursing, *Greenwood (BSN)*

Medical University of South Carolina, College of Nursing, *Charleston (BSN)*

Tennessee

Belmont University, School of Nursing, *Nashville (BSN)*

Cumberland University, Rudy School of Nursing and Health Professions, *Lebanon (BSN)*

East Tennessee State University, College of Nursing, *Johnson City (BSN)*

Union University, School of Nursing, *Jackson (BSN)*

University of Memphis, Loewenberg School of Nursing, *Memphis (BSN)*

The University of Tennessee Health Science Center, College of Nursing, *Memphis (BSN)*

Texas

Baylor University, Louise Herrington School of Nursing, *Dallas (BSN)*

Texas A&M Health Science Center, College of Nursing, *College Station (BSN)*

Texas A&M University–Corpus Christi, College of Nursing and Health Sciences, *Corpus Christi (BSN)*

Texas Christian University, Harris College of Nursing, *Fort Worth (BSN)*

Texas Tech University Health Sciences Center, School of Nursing, *Lubbock (BSN)*

University of Houston, School of Nursing, *Houston (BSN)*

The University of Texas at Arlington, College of Nursing, *Arlington (BSN)*

The University of Texas Health Science Center at San Antonio, School of Nursing, *San Antonio (BSN)*

The University of Texas Medical Branch, School of Nursing, *Galveston (BSN)*

Virginia

George Mason University, College of Health and Human Services, *Fairfax (BSN)*

Lynchburg College, School of Health Sciences and Human Performance, *Lynchburg (BS)*

Marymount University, School of Health Professions, *Arlington (BSN)*

Norfolk State University, Department of Nursing, *Norfolk (BSN)*

Shenandoah University, Eleanor Wade Custer School of Nursing, *Winchester (BS)*

Virginia Commonwealth University, School of Nursing, *Richmond (BS)*

Washington

University of Washington, School of Nursing, *Seattle (BSN)*

West Virginia

West Virginia University, School of Nursing, *Morgantown (BSN)*

Wheeling Jesuit University, Department of Nursing, *Wheeling (BSN)*

Wisconsin

Bellin College, Nursing Program, *Green Bay (BSN)*

Edgewood College, Henry Predolin School of Nursing, *Madison (BS)*

Milwaukee School of Engineering, School of Nursing, *Milwaukee (BSN)*

University of Wisconsin–Eau Claire, College of Nursing and Health Sciences, *Eau Claire (BSN)*

University of Wisconsin–Oshkosh, College of Nursing, *Oshkosh (BSN)*

Wyoming

University of Wyoming, Fay W. Whitney School of Nursing, *Laramie (BSN)*

CANADA

Alberta

University of Alberta, Faculty of Nursing, *Edmonton (BScN)*

University of Calgary, Faculty of Nursing, *Calgary (BN)*

British Columbia

Kwantlen Polytechnic University, Faculty of Community and Health Sciences, *Surrey (BSN)*

The University of British Columbia, Program in Nursing, *Vancouver (BSN)*

Nova Scotia

St. Francis Xavier University, Department of Nursing, *Antigonish (BScN)*

Ontario

University of Ottawa, School of Nursing, *Ottawa (BScN)*

University of Toronto, Faculty of Nursing, *Toronto (BScN)*

ACCELERATED LPN TO BACCALAUREATE

U.S. AND U.S. TERRITORIES

California

San Francisco State University, School of Nursing, *San Francisco (BSN)*

West Coast University, Nursing Programs, *North Hollywood (BSN)*

Massachusetts

Fitchburg State University, Department of Nursing, *Fitchburg (BS)*

New York

Dominican College, Department of Nursing, *Orangeburg (BSN)*

Pennsylvania

Wilkes University, Department of Nursing, *Wilkes-Barre (BS)*

South Dakota

Mount Marty College, Nursing Program, *Yankton (BSN)*

Virginia

Norfolk State University, Department of Nursing, *Norfolk (BSN)*

CANADA

Nova Scotia

St. Francis Xavier University, Department of Nursing, *Antigonish (BScN)*

ACCELERATED RN BACCALAUREATE

U.S. AND U.S. TERRITORIES

Arizona

Arizona State University at the Downtown Phoenix campus, College of Nursing, *Phoenix (BSN)*

Arkansas

University of Arkansas for Medical Sciences, College of Nursing, *Little Rock (BSN)*

California

American University of Health Sciences, School of Nursing, *Signal Hill (BSN)*

Azusa Pacific University, School of Nursing, *Azusa (BSN)*

Loma Linda University, School of Nursing, *Loma Linda (BS)*

West Coast University, Nursing Programs, *North Hollywood (BSN)*

Colorado

Colorado State University–Pueblo, Department of Nursing, *Pueblo (BSN)*

Delaware

Wilmington University, College of Health Professions, *New Castle (BSN)*

Georgia

Georgia State University, Byrdine F. Lewis School of Nursing, *Atlanta (BS)*

Thomas University, Division of Nursing, *Thomasville (BSN)*

University of West Georgia, School of Nursing, *Carrollton (BSN)*

Idaho

Boise State University, Department of Nursing, *Boise (BS)*

Illinois

Benedictine University, Department of Nursing, *Lisle (BSN)*

Lakeview College of Nursing, *Danville (BSN)*

Lewis University, Program in Nursing, *Romeoville (BSN)*

Resurrection University, *Chicago (BSN)*

University of St. Francis, Leach College of Nursing, *Joliet (BSN)*

Indiana

Ball State University, School of Nursing, *Muncie (BS)*

Indiana University Kokomo, Indiana University School of Nursing, *Kokomo (BSN)*

Marian University, School of Nursing, *Indianapolis (BSN)*

Saint Joseph's College, St. Elizabeth School of Nursing, *Rensselaer (BSN)*

Iowa

Allen College, Graduate Programs, *Waterloo (BSN)*

Kansas

MidAmerica Nazarene University, Division of Nursing, *Olathe (BSN)*

Tabor College, Department of Nursing, *Hillsboro (BSN)*

Kentucky

Eastern Kentucky University, Department of Baccalaureate and Graduate Nursing, *Richmond (BSN)*

Midway University, Program in Nursing (Baccalaureate), *Midway (BSN)*

Sullivan University, RN to BSN Program, *Louisville (BSN)*

Thomas More College, Program in Nursing, *Crestview Hills (BSN)*

Maine

University of New England, Department of Nursing, *Biddeford (BSN)*

Maryland

Coppin State University, Helene Fuld School of Nursing, *Baltimore (BSN)*

Notre Dame of Maryland University, Department of Nursing, *Baltimore (BS)*

Stevenson University, Nursing Division, *Stevenson (BS)*

Massachusetts

Regis College, School of Nursing, Science and Health Professions, *Weston (BSN)*

Salem State University, Program in Nursing, *Salem (BSN)*

University of Massachusetts Amherst, College of Nursing, *Amherst (BS)*

Minnesota

University of Northwestern–St. Paul, School of Nursing, *St. Paul (BSN)*

Missouri

Chamberlain College of Nursing, *St. Louis (BSN)*

Maryville University of Saint Louis, The Catherine McAuley School of Nursing, College of Health Professions, *St. Louis (BSN)*

Missouri State University, Department of Nursing, *Springfield (BSN)*

Saint Louis University, School of Nursing, *St. Louis (BSN)*

Nebraska

Clarkson College, Master of Science in Nursing Program, *Omaha (BSN)*

Nebraska Methodist College, Department of Nursing, *Omaha (BSN)*

University of Nebraska Medical Center, College of Nursing, *Omaha (BSN)*

New Hampshire

Southern New Hampshire University, Department of Nursing, *Manchester (BS)*

New Jersey

Caldwell University, Nursing Programs, *Caldwell (BSN)*

College of Saint Elizabeth, Department of Nursing, *Morristown (BSN)*

Rutgers, The State University of New Jersey, Camden, Rutgers School of Nursing–Camden, *Camden (BS)*

Seton Hall University, College of Nursing, *South Orange (BSN)*

New York

Binghamton University, State University of New York, Decker School of Nursing, *Vestal (BS)*

The College of New Rochelle, School of Nursing, *New Rochelle (BSN)*

Columbia University, School of Nursing, *New York (BS)*

Daemen College, Department of Nursing, *Amherst (BS)*

Dominican College, Department of Nursing, *Orangeburg (BSN)*

Keuka College, Division of Nursing, *Keuka Park (BS)*

Lehman College of the City University of New York, Department of Nursing, *Bronx (BS)*

Medgar Evers College of the City University of New York, Department of Nursing, *Brooklyn (BSN)*

Mercy College, Programs in Nursing, *Dobbs Ferry (BS)*

Molloy College, Division of Nursing, *Rockville Centre (BS)*

Mount Saint Mary College, School of Nursing, *Newburgh (BSN)*

St. John Fisher College, Wegmans School of Nursing, *Rochester (BS)*

State University of New York Polytechnic Institute, School of Nursing and Health Systems, *Utica (BS)*

University of Rochester, School of Nursing, *Rochester (BS)*

North Carolina

Winston-Salem State University, Department of Nursing, *Winston-Salem (BSN)*

Ohio

Defiance College, Bachelor's Degree in Nursing, *Defiance (BSN)*

Mount St. Joseph University, Department of Nursing, *Cincinnati (BSN)*

Ohio Northern University, Nursing Program, *Ada (BSN)*

Otterbein University, Department of Nursing, *Westerville (BSN)*

The University of Akron, School of Nursing, *Akron (BSN)*

Ursuline College, The Breen School of Nursing, *Pepper Pike (BSN)*

Oklahoma

Bacone College, Department of Nursing, *Muskogee (BSN)*

Northeastern State University, Department of Nursing, *Tahlequah (BSN)*

Oklahoma Wesleyan University, School of Nursing, *Bartlesville (BSN)*

Pennsylvania

Carlow University, College of Health and Wellness, *Pittsburgh (BSN)*

DeSales University, Department of Nursing and Health, *Center Valley (BSN)*

Eastern University, Program in Nursing, *St. Davids (BSN)*

Gwynedd Mercy University, Frances M. Maguire School of Nursing and Health Professions, *Gwynedd Valley (BSN)*

Immaculata University, Division of Nursing, *Immaculata (BSN)*

La Roche College, Department of Nursing and Nursing Management, *Pittsburgh (BSN)*

Misericordia University, Department of Nursing, *Dallas (BSN)*

Mount Aloysius College, Division of Nursing, *Cresson (BSN)*

Neumann University, Program in Nursing and Health Sciences, *Aston (BS)*

Thomas Jefferson University, Department of Nursing, *Philadelphia (BSN)*

Villanova University, College of Nursing, *Villanova (BSN)*

Wilkes University, Department of Nursing, *Wilkes-Barre (BS)*

South Carolina

Lander University, School of Nursing, *Greenwood (BSN)*

University of South Carolina, College of Nursing, *Columbia (BSN)*

South Dakota

South Dakota State University, College of Nursing, *Brookings (BS)*

Tennessee

Cumberland University, Rudy School of Nursing and Health Professions, *Lebanon (BSN)*

East Tennessee State University, College of Nursing, *Johnson City (BSN)*

King University, School of Nursing, *Bristol (BSN)*

University of Memphis, Loewenberg School of Nursing, *Memphis (BSN)*

The University of Tennessee Health Science Center, College of Nursing, *Memphis (BSN)*

Texas

The University of Texas at Arlington, College of Nursing, *Arlington (BSN)*

The University of Texas at Tyler, Program in Nursing, *Tyler (BSN)*

Utah

Western Governors University, Online College of Health Professions, *Salt Lake City (BS)*

West Virginia

Fairmont State University, School of Nursing and Allied Health Administration, *Fairmont (BSN)*

West Liberty University, Department of Health Sciences, *West Liberty (BSN)*

Wisconsin

Cardinal Stritch University, Ruth S. Coleman College of Nursing and Health Sciences, *Milwaukee (BSN)*

Milwaukee School of Engineering, School of Nursing, *Milwaukee (BSN)*

CANADA

Ontario

University of Ottawa, School of Nursing, *Ottawa (BScN)*

University of Toronto, Faculty of Nursing, *Toronto (BScN)*

Quebec

McGill University, School of Nursing, *Montréal (BScN)*

Université du Québec à Chicoutimi, Program in Nursing, *Chicoutimi (BNSc)*

Université Laval, Faculty of Nursing, *Québec (BScN)*

Saskatchewan

University of Saskatchewan, College of Nursing, *Saskatoon (BSN)*

ADN TO BACCALAUREATE

U.S. AND U.S. TERRITORIES

Alabama

Auburn University at Montgomery, School of Nursing, *Montgomery (BSN)*

Tuskegee University, Program in Nursing, *Tuskegee (BSN)*

The University of Alabama at Birmingham, School of Nursing, *Birmingham (BSN)*

University of Mobile, School of Nursing, *Mobile (BSN)*

University of South Alabama, College of Nursing, *Mobile (BSN)*

Arizona

Grand Canyon University, College of Nursing and Health Sciences, *Phoenix (BSN)*

Northern Arizona University, School of Nursing, *Flagstaff (BSN)*

Arkansas

Arkansas Tech University, Program in Nursing, *Russellville (BSN)*

Henderson State University, Department of Nursing, *Arkadelphia (BSN)*

Southern Arkansas University–Magnolia, Department of Nursing, *Magnolia (BSN)*

University of Arkansas, Eleanor Mann School of Nursing, *Fayetteville (BSN)*

University of Arkansas at Monticello, School of Nursing, *Monticello (BSN)*

University of Arkansas for Medical Sciences, College of Nursing, *Little Rock (BSN)*

University of Arkansas–Fort Smith, Carol McKelvey Moore School of Nursing, *Fort Smith (BSN)*

University of Central Arkansas, Department of Nursing, *Conway (BSN)*

California

American University of Health Sciences, School of Nursing, *Signal Hill (BSN)*

Azusa Pacific University, School of Nursing, *Azusa (BSN)*

Biola University, Department of Nursing, *La Mirada (BSN)*

California Baptist University, School of Nursing, *Riverside (BSN)*

California State University, Bakersfield, Program in Nursing, *Bakersfield (BSN)*

California State University, Chico, School of Nursing, *Chico (BSN)*

California State University, East Bay, Department of Nursing and Health Sciences, *Hayward (BS)*

California State University, Fresno, Department of Nursing, *Fresno (BSN)*

California State University, Fullerton, Department of Nursing, *Fullerton (BSN)*

California State University, Long Beach, School of Nursing, *Long Beach (BSN)*

California State University, Northridge, Nursing Program, *Northridge (BSN)*

California State University, Sacramento, Division of Nursing, *Sacramento (BSN)*

California State University, Stanislaus, Department of Nursing, *Turlock (BSN)*

Concordia University Irvine, Bachelor of Science in Nursing Program, *Irvine (BSN)*

Loma Linda University, School of Nursing, *Loma Linda (BS)*

Mount Saint Mary's University, Department of Nursing, *Los Angeles (BSN, BSc PN)*

Pacific Union College, Department of Nursing, *Angwin (BSN)*

Point Loma Nazarene University, School of Nursing, *San Diego (BSN)*

San Diego State University, School of Nursing, *San Diego (BSN)*

San Francisco State University, School of Nursing, *San Francisco (BSN)*

Unitek College, School of Nursing and Allied Health, *Fremont (BSN)*

West Coast University, Nursing Programs, *North Hollywood (BSN)*

Colorado

American Sentinel University, RN to Bachelor of Science Nursing, *Aurora (BSN)*

Colorado Mesa University, Department of Nursing and Radiologic Sciences, *Grand Junction (BSN)*

Colorado State University–Pueblo, Department of Nursing, *Pueblo (BSN)*

Denver School of Nursing, *Denver (BSN)*

Metropolitan State University of Denver, Department of Health Professions, *Denver (BSN)*

Connecticut

Southern Connecticut State University, Department of Nursing, *New Haven (BSN)*

University of Hartford, College of Education, Nursing, and Health Professions, *West Hartford (BSN)*

District of Columbia

The George Washington University, School of Nursing, *Washington (BSN)*

Florida

Barry University, Division of Nursing, *Miami Shores (BSN)*

Jacksonville University, School of Nursing, *Jacksonville (BSN)*

Northwest Florida State College, RN to BSN Degree Program, *Niceville (BSN)*

Palm Beach Atlantic University, School of Nursing, *West Palm Beach (BSN)*

St. Petersburg College, Department of Nursing, *St. Petersburg (BSN)*

State College of Florida Manatee-Sarasota, Nursing Degree Program, *Bradenton (BSN)*

University of Central Florida, College of Nursing, *Orlando (BSN)*

University of South Florida, College of Nursing, *Tampa (BS)*

University of West Florida, Department of Nursing, *Pensacola (BSN)*

Georgia

Albany State University, College of Sciences and Health Professions, *Albany (BSN)*

Armstrong State University, Program in Nursing, *Savannah (BSN)*

Brenau University, College of Health and Science, *Gainesville (BSN)*

Georgia Southern University, School of Nursing, *Statesboro (BSN)*

Georgia State University, Byrdine F. Lewis School of Nursing, *Atlanta (BS)*

Kennesaw State University, School of Nursing, *Kennesaw (BSN)*

Middle Georgia College, School of Nursing and Health Sciences, *Cochran (BSN)*

Thomas University, Division of Nursing, *Thomasville (BSN)*

University of North Georgia, Department of Nursing, *Dahlonega (BSN)*

Guam

University of Guam, School of Nursing and Health Sciences, *Mangilao (BSN)*

Hawaii

University of Hawaii at Hilo, Department in Nursing, *Hilo (BSN)*

University of Hawaii at Manoa, School of Nursing and Dental Hygiene, *Honolulu (BSN)*

Idaho

Idaho State University, Department of Nursing, *Pocatello (BS)*

Lewis-Clark State College, Division of Nursing and Health Sciences, *Lewiston (BSN)*

Illinois

Blessing–Rieman College of Nursing and Health Sciences, *Quincy (BSN)*

Bradley University, Department of Nursing, *Peoria (BSN, BSc PN)*

DePaul University, School of Nursing, *Chicago (BS)*

Eastern Illinois University, Nursing Program, *Charleston (BSN)*

MacMurray College, Department of Nursing, *Jacksonville (BSN)*

McKendree University, Department of Nursing, *Lebanon (BSN)*

Northern Illinois University, School of Nursing and Health Studies, *De Kalb (BS)*

Resurrection University, *Chicago (BSN)*

Rockford University, Department of Nursing, *Rockford (BSN)*

Southern Illinois University Edwardsville, School of Nursing, *Edwardsville (BS)*

Trinity Christian College, Department of Nursing, *Palos Heights (BSN)*

Trinity College of Nursing and Health Sciences, *Rock Island (BSN)*

University of Illinois at Chicago, College of Nursing, *Chicago (BSN)*

Indiana

Bethel College, School of Nursing, *Mishawaka (BSN)*

Indiana University East, School of Nursing, *Richmond (BSN)*

Indiana University–Purdue University Indianapolis, School of Nursing, *Indianapolis (BSN)*

Purdue University, School of Nursing, *West Lafayette (BS)*

Purdue University North Central, Department of Nursing, *Westville (BS)*

University of Saint Francis, Department of Nursing, *Fort Wayne (BSN)*

Iowa

Allen College, Graduate Programs, *Waterloo (BSN)*

Briar Cliff University, Department of Nursing, *Sioux City (BSN)*

Iowa Wesleyan College, Division of Nursing, *Mount Pleasant (BSN)*

Mercy College of Health Sciences, Division of Nursing, *Des Moines (BSN)*

Mount Mercy University, Department of Nursing, *Cedar Rapids (BSN)*

William Penn University, Nursing Division, *Oskaloosa (BSN)*

Kansas

Emporia State University, Newman Division of Nursing, *Emporia (BSN)*

Kansas Wesleyan University, Department of Nursing Education, *Salina (BSN)*

Tabor College, Department of Nursing, *Hillsboro (BSN)*

The University of Kansas, School of Nursing, *Kansas City (BSN)*

Washburn University, School of Nursing, *Topeka (BSN)*

Wichita State University, School of Nursing, *Wichita (BSN)*

Kentucky

Kentucky State University, School of Nursing, *Frankfort (BSN)*

Midway University, Program in Nursing (Baccalaureate), *Midway (BSN)*

Morehead State University, Department of Nursing, *Morehead (BSN)*

Western Kentucky University, School of Nursing, *Bowling Green (BSN)*

Louisiana

McNeese State University, College of Nursing, *Lake Charles (BSN)*

Northwestern State University of Louisiana, College of Nursing and School of Allied Health, *Shreveport (BSN)*

Our Lady of the Lake College, Division of Nursing, *Baton Rouge (BSN)*

University of Louisiana at Lafayette, College of Nursing, *Lafayette (BSN)*

University of Louisiana at Monroe, Nursing, *Monroe (BS)*

Maine

University of Southern Maine, School of Nursing, *Portland (BS)*

Maryland

Salisbury University, Department of Nursing, *Salisbury (BS)*

Stevenson University, Nursing Division, *Stevenson (BS)*

Towson University, Department of Nursing, *Towson (BS)*

University of Maryland, Baltimore, Nursing Programs, *Baltimore (BSN)*

Massachusetts

American International College, Division of Nursing, *Springfield (BSN)*

Anna Maria College, Department of Nursing, *Paxton (BSN)*

Becker College, Nursing Programs, *Worcester (BSN)*

Framingham State University, Department of Nursing, *Framingham (BS)*

Regis College, School of Nursing, Science and Health Professions, *Weston (BSN)*

Salem State University, Program in Nursing, *Salem (BSN)*

Simmons College, School of Nursing and Health Sciences, *Boston (BS)*

Worcester State University, Department of Nursing, *Worcester (BS)*

Michigan

Andrews University, Department of Nursing, *Berrien Springs (BS)*

Baker College, School of Nursing, *Flint (BSN)*

Davenport University, Division of Nursing, *Grand Rapids (BSN)*

Eastern Michigan University, School of Nursing, *Ypsilanti (BSN)*

Grand Valley State University, Kirkhof College of Nursing, *Allendale (BSN)*

Lake Superior State University, Department of Nursing, *Sault Sainte Marie (BSN)*

Madonna University, College of Nursing and Health, *Livonia (BSN)*

Northern Michigan University, College of Nursing and Allied Health Science, *Marquette (BSN)*

Oakland University, School of Nursing, *Rochester (BSN)*

Saginaw Valley State University, College of Health and Human Services, *University Center (BSN)*

Spring Arbor University, Program in Nursing, *Spring Arbor (BSN)*

Western Michigan University, College of Health and Human Services, *Kalamazoo (BSN)*

Minnesota

Augsburg College, Program in Nursing, *Minneapolis (BS)*

The College of St. Scholastica, Department of Nursing, *Duluth (BS)*

Minnesota State University Moorhead, School of Nursing and Healthcare Leadership, *Moorhead (BSN)*

St. Catherine University, Department of Nursing, *St. Paul (BS)*

Southwest Minnesota State University, Nursing Department, *Marshall (BSN)*

Mississippi

Delta State University, School of Nursing, *Cleveland (BSN)*

Mississippi University for Women, College of Nursing and Speech Language Pathology, *Columbus (BSN)*

University of Mississippi Medical Center, School of Nursing, *Jackson (BSN)*

William Carey University, School of Nursing, *Hattiesburg (BSN)*

Missouri

Central Methodist University, College of Liberal Arts and Sciences, *Fayette (BSN)*

Chamberlain College of Nursing, *St. Louis (BSN)*

Cox College, Department of Nursing, *Springfield (BSN)*

Goldfarb School of Nursing at Barnes-Jewish College, *St. Louis (BSN)*

Graceland University, School of Nursing, *Independence (BSN)*

Missouri Southern State University, Department of Nursing, *Joplin (BSN)*

Missouri State University, Department of Nursing, *Springfield (BSN)*

Missouri Western State University, Department of Nursing, *St. Joseph (BSN)*

Saint Louis University, School of Nursing, *St. Louis (BSN)*

University of Central Missouri, Department of Nursing, *Warrensburg (BS)*

University of Missouri, Sinclair School of Nursing, *Columbia (BSN)*

Webster University, Department of Nursing, *St. Louis (BSN)*

Montana

Montana State University–Northern, College of Nursing, *Havre (BSN)*

Nebraska

Clarkson College, Master of Science in Nursing Program, *Omaha (BSN)*

College of Saint Mary, Division of Health Care Professions, *Omaha (BSN)*

Midland University, Department of Nursing, *Fremont (BSN)*

Nebraska Wesleyan University, Department of Nursing, *Lincoln (BSN)*

Union College, Division of Nursing, *Lincoln (BSN)*

Nevada

Great Basin College, BSN Program, *Elko (BSN)*

Touro University, School of Nursing, *Henderson (BSN)*

University of Nevada, Reno, Orvis School of Nursing, *Reno (BSN)*

New Hampshire

Franklin Pierce University, Master of Science in Nursing, *Rindge (BS)*

Rivier University, Division of Nursing, *Nashua (BS)*

New Jersey

Caldwell University, Nursing Programs, *Caldwell (BSN)*

College of Saint Elizabeth, Department of Nursing, *Morristown (BSN)*

Kean University, Department of Nursing, *Union (BSN)*

Monmouth University, Marjorie K. Unterberg School of Nursing, *West Long Branch (BSN)*

Saint Peter's University, Nursing Program, *Jersey City (BSN)*

Seton Hall University, College of Nursing, *South Orange (BSN)*

William Paterson University of New Jersey, Department of Nursing, *Wayne (BSN)*

New Mexico

Eastern New Mexico University, Department of Allied Health–Nursing, *Portales (BSN)*

Western New Mexico University, Nursing Department, *Silver City (BSN)*

New York

The College at Brockport, State University of New York, Department of Nursing, *Brockport (BSN)*

Daemen College, Department of Nursing, *Amherst (BS)*

Lehman College of the City University of New York, Department of Nursing, *Bronx (BS)*

Long Island University–LIU Brooklyn, School of Nursing, *Brooklyn (BS)*

Medgar Evers College of the City University of New York, Department of Nursing, *Brooklyn (BSN)*

Molloy College, Division of Nursing, *Rockville Centre (BS)*

The Sage Colleges, Department of Nursing, *Troy (BS)*

St. John Fisher College, Wegmans School of Nursing, *Rochester (BS)*

State University of New York at Plattsburgh, Department of Nursing, *Plattsburgh (BS)*

State University of New York Polytechnic Institute, School of Nursing and Health Systems, *Utica (BS)*

State University of New York Upstate Medical University, College of Nursing, *Syracuse (BS)*

University of Rochester, School of Nursing, *Rochester (BS)*

York College of the City University of New York, Program in Nursing, *Jamaica (BS)*

North Carolina

Barton College, School of Nursing, *Wilson (BSN)*

East Carolina University, College of Nursing, *Greenville (BSN)*

Gardner-Webb University, School of Nursing, *Boiling Springs (BSN)*

Lees-McRae College, Nursing Program, *Banner Elk (BSN)*

Lenoir-Rhyne University, Program in Nursing, *Hickory (BS)*

Queens University of Charlotte, Presbyterian School of Nursing, *Charlotte (BSN)*

The University of North Carolina at Charlotte, School of Nursing, *Charlotte (BSN)*

The University of North Carolina at Greensboro, School of Nursing, *Greensboro (BSN)*

Winston-Salem State University, Department of Nursing, *Winston-Salem (BSN)*

North Dakota

Dickinson State University, Department of Nursing, *Dickinson (BSN)*

University of Mary, Division of Nursing, *Bismarck (BSN)*

University of North Dakota, College of Nursing, *Grand Forks (BSN)*

Ohio

Ashland University, Dwight Schar College of Nursing and Health Sciences, *Ashland (BSN)*

Capital University, School of Nursing, *Columbus (BSN)*

Defiance College, Bachelor's Degree in Nursing, *Defiance (BSN)*

Kent State University, College of Nursing, *Kent (BSN)*

Lourdes University, School of Nursing, *Sylvania (BSN)*

Malone University, School of Nursing, *Canton (BSN)*

Miami University, Department of Nursing, *Hamilton (BSN)*

Mount Vernon Nazarene University, School of Nursing and Health Sciences, *Mount Vernon (BS)*

Shawnee State University, Department of Nursing, *Portsmouth (BSN)*

The University of Akron, School of Nursing, *Akron (BSN)*

University of Cincinnati, College of Nursing, *Cincinnati (BSN)*

The University of Toledo, College of Nursing, *Toledo (BSN)*

Urbana University, College of Nursing and Allied Health, *Urbana (BSN)*

Ursuline College, The Breen School of Nursing, *Pepper Pike (BSN)*

Youngstown State University, Department of Nursing, *Youngstown (BSN)*

Oklahoma

East Central University, Department of Nursing, *Ada (BS)*

Northwestern Oklahoma State University, Division of Nursing, *Alva (BSN)*

Oklahoma Baptist University, School of Nursing, *Shawnee (BSN)*

Oklahoma City University, Kramer School of Nursing, *Oklahoma City (BSN)*

Oklahoma Panhandle State University, Bachelor of Science in Nursing Program, *Goodwell (BSN)*

Oklahoma Wesleyan University, School of Nursing, *Bartlesville (BSN)*

Oral Roberts University, Anna Vaughn School of Nursing, *Tulsa (BSN)*

Rogers State University, Nursing Program, *Claremore (BSN)*

Southern Nazarene University, School of Nursing, *Bethany (BS)*

Southwestern Oklahoma State University, School of Nursing, *Weatherford (BSN)*

University of Oklahoma Health Sciences Center, College of Nursing, *Oklahoma City (BSN)*

Oregon

Linfield College, School of Nursing, *McMinnville (BSN)*

Pennsylvania

Clarion University of Pennsylvania, School of Nursing, *Oil City (BSN)*

DeSales University, Department of Nursing and Health, *Center Valley (BSN)*

Duquesne University, School of Nursing, *Pittsburgh (BSN)*

Gannon University, Villa Maria School of Nursing, *Erie (BSN)*

Gwynedd Mercy University, Frances M. Maguire School of Nursing and Health Professions, *Gwynedd Valley (BSN)*

Marywood University, Department of Nursing, *Scranton (BSN)*

Mount Aloysius College, Division of Nursing, *Cresson (BSN)*

Neumann University, Program in Nursing and Health Sciences, *Aston (BS)*

Penn State University Park, School of Nursing, *University Park (BS)*

Pennsylvania College of Technology, School of Health Sciences, *Williamsport (BSN)*

Slippery Rock University of Pennsylvania, Department of Nursing, *Slippery Rock (BSN)*

Thomas Jefferson University, Department of Nursing, *Philadelphia (BSN)*

Villanova University, College of Nursing, *Villanova (BSN)*

Widener University, School of Nursing, *Chester (BSN)*

Wilkes University, Department of Nursing, *Wilkes-Barre (BS)*

York College of Pennsylvania, Department of Nursing, *York (BS)*

Puerto Rico

Inter American University of Puerto Rico, Metropolitan Campus, Carmen Torres de Tiburcio School of Nursing, *San Juan (BSN)*

University of Puerto Rico, Medical Sciences Campus, School of Nursing, *San Juan (BSN)*

Rhode Island

University of Rhode Island, College of Nursing, *Kingston (BS)*

South Carolina

Anderson University, School of Nursing, *Anderson (BSN)*

Charleston Southern University, Wingo School of Nursing, *Charleston (BSN)*

Coastal Carolina University, Nursing Completion Program, *Conway (BSN)*

Francis Marion University, Department of Nursing, *Florence (BSN)*

Medical University of South Carolina, College of Nursing, *Charleston (BSN)*

Newberry College, Department of Nursing, *Newberry (BSN)*

University of South Carolina Aiken, School of Nursing, *Aiken (BSN)*

South Dakota

Mount Marty College, Nursing Program, *Yankton (BSN)*

Presentation College, Department of Nursing, *Aberdeen (BSN)*

Tennessee

Aquinas College, School of Nursing, *Nashville (BSN)*

Austin Peay State University, School of Nursing, *Clarksville (BSN)*

Belmont University, School of Nursing, *Nashville (BSN)*

Bethel University, Nursing Program, *McKenzie (BSN)*

Cumberland University, Rudy School of Nursing and Health Professions, *Lebanon (BSN)*

East Tennessee State University, College of Nursing, *Johnson City (BSN)*

Lincoln Memorial University, Caylor School of Nursing, *Harrogate (BSN)*

Milligan College, Department of Nursing, *Milligan College (BSN)*

Southern Adventist University, School of Nursing, *Collegedale (BS)*

Tennessee Technological University, Whitson-Hester School of Nursing, *Cookeville (BSN)*

Tennessee Wesleyan College, Fort Sanders Nursing Department, *Knoxville (BSN)*

University of Memphis, Loewenberg School of Nursing, *Memphis (BSN)*

The University of Tennessee at Chattanooga, School of Nursing, *Chattanooga (BSN)*

The University of Tennessee at Martin, Department of Nursing, *Martin (BSN)*

The University of Tennessee Health Science Center, College of Nursing, *Memphis (BSN)*

Texas

Lamar University, Department of Nursing, *Beaumont (BSN)*

Midwestern State University, Wilson School of Nursing, *Wichita Falls (BSN)*

Sam Houston State University, Nursing Program, *Huntsville (BSN)*

Tarleton State University, Department of Nursing, *Stephenville (BSN)*

Texas A&M Health Science Center, College of Nursing, *College Station (BSN)*

Texas A&M University–Corpus Christi, College of Nursing and Health Sciences, *Corpus Christi (BSN)*

Texas A&M University–Texarkana, Nursing Department, *Texarkana (BSN)*

Texas Tech University Health Sciences Center, School of Nursing, *Lubbock (BSN)*

Texas Tech University Health Sciences Center El Paso, *El Paso (BSN)*

University of Mary Hardin-Baylor, College of Nursing, *Belton (BSN)*

The University of Texas at Arlington, College of Nursing, *Arlington (BSN)*

The University of Texas at Brownsville, Department of Nursing, *Brownsville (BSN)*

The University of Texas at Tyler, Program in Nursing, *Tyler (BSN)*

The University of Texas Health Science Center at Houston, School of Nursing, *Houston (BSN)*

The University of Texas Rio Grande Valley, School of Nursing, *Edinburg (BSN)*

University of the Incarnate Word, Program in Nursing, *San Antonio (BSN)*

West Texas A&M University, Department of Nursing, *Canyon (BSN)*

Utah

University of Utah, College of Nursing, *Salt Lake City (BS)*

Utah Valley University, Department of Nursing, *Orem (BSN)*

Weber State University, Program in Nursing, *Ogden (BSN)*

Vermont

Norwich University, Department of Nursing, *Northfield (BSN)*

Southern Vermont College, Department of Nursing, *Bennington (BSN)*

University of Vermont, Department of Nursing, *Burlington (BS)*

Virgin Islands

University of the Virgin Islands, Division of Nursing, *Saint Thomas (BSN)*

Virginia

Eastern Mennonite University, Department of Nursing, *Harrisonburg (BS)*

Jefferson College of Health Sciences, Nursing Education Program, *Roanoke (BSN)*

Marymount University, School of Health Professions, *Arlington (BSN)*

Shenandoah University, Eleanor Wade Custer School of Nursing, *Winchester (BS)*

University of Virginia, School of Nursing, *Charlottesville (BSN)*

The University of Virginia's College at Wise, Department of Nursing, *Wise (BSN)*

Virginia Commonwealth University, School of Nursing, *Richmond (BS)*

Washington

Saint Martin's University, Nursing Program, *Lacey (BSN)*

University of Washington, School of Nursing, *Seattle (BSN)*

Walla Walla University, School of Nursing, *College Place (BS)*

West Virginia

Bluefield State College, Program in Nursing, *Bluefield (BSN)*

Fairmont State University, School of Nursing and Allied Health Administration, *Fairmont (BSN)*

Shepherd University, Department of Nursing Education, *Shepherdstown (BSN)*

West Virginia University, School of Nursing, *Morgantown (BSN)*

Wisconsin

Alverno College, Division of Nursing, *Milwaukee (BSN)*

Cardinal Stritch University, Ruth S. Coleman College of Nursing and Health Sciences, *Milwaukee (BSN)*

Carroll University, Nursing Program, *Waukesha (BSN)*

Concordia University Wisconsin, Program in Nursing, *Mequon (BSN)*

Marian University, School of Nursing, *Fond du Lac (BSN)*

Silver Lake College of the Holy Family, Nursing Program, *Manitowoc (BSN)*

University of Wisconsin–Eau Claire, College of Nursing and Health Sciences, *Eau Claire (BSN)*

University of Wisconsin–Green Bay, Online Nursing and Health Programs, *Green Bay (BSN)*

University of Wisconsin–Madison, School of Nursing, *Madison (BS)*

University of Wisconsin–Milwaukee, College of Nursing, *Milwaukee (BSN)*

University of Wisconsin–Oshkosh, College of Nursing, *Oshkosh (BSN)*

Wyoming

University of Wyoming, Fay W. Whitney School of Nursing, *Laramie (BSN)*

BACCALAUREATE FOR SECOND DEGREE

U.S. AND U.S. TERRITORIES

Alabama

Auburn University at Montgomery, School of Nursing, *Montgomery (BSN)*

Samford University, Ida V. Moffett School of Nursing, *Birmingham (BSN)*

Spring Hill College, Division of Nursing, *Mobile (BSN)*

The University of Alabama, Capstone College of Nursing, *Tuscaloosa (BSN)*

The University of Alabama at Birmingham, School of Nursing, *Birmingham (BSN)*

The University of Alabama in Huntsville, College of Nursing, *Huntsville (BSN)*

Arizona

Arizona State University at the Downtown Phoenix campus, College of Nursing, *Phoenix (BSN)*

Arkansas

Arkansas Tech University, Program in Nursing, *Russellville (BSN)*

University of Arkansas for Medical Sciences, College of Nursing, *Little Rock (BSN)*

California

California State University, Chico, School of Nursing, *Chico (BSN)*

California State University, Dominguez Hills, Program in Nursing, *Carson (BSN)*

California State University, Fullerton, Department of Nursing, *Fullerton (BSN)*

California State University, Sacramento, Division of Nursing, *Sacramento (BSN)*

Dominican University of California, Program in Nursing, *San Rafael (BSN)*

Loma Linda University, School of Nursing, *Loma Linda (BS)*

National University, Department of Nursing, *La Jolla (BSN)*

University of California, Irvine, Program in Nursing Science, *Irvine (BS)*

Colorado

Colorado State University–Pueblo, Department of Nursing, *Pueblo (BSN)*

University of Northern Colorado, School of Nursing, *Greeley (BS)*

Connecticut

University of Saint Joseph, Department of Nursing, *West Hartford (BS)*

Florida

Barry University, Division of Nursing, *Miami Shores (BSN)*

Florida Southern College, School of Nursing & Health Sciences, *Lakeland (BSN)*

Jacksonville University, School of Nursing, *Jacksonville (BSN)*

Palm Beach Atlantic University, School of Nursing, *West Palm Beach (BSN)*

University of Miami, School of Nursing and Health Studies, *Coral Gables (BSN)*

Georgia

Emory University, Nell Hodgson Woodruff School of Nursing, *Atlanta (BSN)*

Georgia Southwestern State University, School of Nursing, *Americus (BSN)*

Kennesaw State University, School of Nursing, *Kennesaw (BSN)*

Illinois

Bradley University, Department of Nursing, *Peoria (BSN, BSc PN)*

DePaul University, School of Nursing, *Chicago (BS)*

Methodist College, *Peoria (BSN)*

Resurrection University, *Chicago (BSN)*

Saint Anthony College of Nursing, *Rockford (BSN)*

University of Illinois at Chicago, College of Nursing, *Chicago (BSN)*

Western Illinois University, School of Nursing, *Macomb (BSN)*

Indiana

Ball State University, School of Nursing, *Muncie (BS)*

Indiana University Bloomington, Department of Nursing–Bloomington Division, *Bloomington (BSN)*

Marian University, School of Nursing, *Indianapolis (BSN)*

Purdue University, School of Nursing, *West Lafayette (BS)*

Purdue University North Central, Department of Nursing, *Westville (BS)*

Iowa

Allen College, Graduate Programs, *Waterloo (BSN)*

Iowa Wesleyan College, Division of Nursing, *Mount Pleasant (BSN)*

Morningside College, Department of Nursing Education, *Sioux City (BSN)*

Kansas

Washburn University, School of Nursing, *Topeka (BSN)*

Kentucky

Eastern Kentucky University, Department of Baccalaureate and Graduate Nursing, *Richmond (BSN)*

Spalding University, School of Nursing, *Louisville (BSN)*

University of Kentucky, College of Nursing, *Lexington (BSN)*

Western Kentucky University, School of Nursing, *Bowling Green (BSN)*

Maryland

Coppin State University, Helene Fuld School of Nursing, *Baltimore (BSN)*

Stevenson University, Nursing Division, *Stevenson (BS)*

Massachusetts

American International College, Division of Nursing, *Springfield (BSN)*

Regis College, School of Nursing, Science and Health Professions, *Weston (BSN)*

Simmons College, School of Nursing and Health Sciences, *Boston (BS)*

Michigan

Eastern Michigan University, School of Nursing, *Ypsilanti (BSN)*

Saginaw Valley State University, College of Health and Human Services, *University Center (BSN)*

Missouri

Cox College, Department of Nursing, *Springfield (BSN)*

Missouri Southern State University, Department of Nursing, *Joplin (BSN)*

Research College of Nursing, College of Nursing, *Kansas City (BSN)*

Saint Louis University, School of Nursing, *St. Louis (BSN)*

Montana

Montana State University, College of Nursing, *Bozeman (BSN)*

Nebraska

Clarkson College, Master of Science in Nursing Program, *Omaha (BSN)*

University of Nebraska Medical Center, College of Nursing, *Omaha (BSN)*

Nevada

University of Nevada, Reno, Orvis School of Nursing, *Reno (BSN)*

New Jersey

Caldwell University, Nursing Programs, *Caldwell (BSN)*

Seton Hall University, College of Nursing, *South Orange (BSN)*

New York

College of Mount Saint Vincent, Department of Nursing, *Riverdale (BS)*

The College of New Rochelle, School of Nursing, *New Rochelle (BSN)*

Columbia University, School of Nursing, *New York (BS)*

Lehman College of the City University of New York, Department of Nursing, *Bronx (BS)*

Le Moyne College, Nursing Programs, *Syracuse (BS)*

Molloy College, Division of Nursing, *Rockville Centre (BS)*

The Sage Colleges, Department of Nursing, *Troy (BS)*

St. John Fisher College, Wegmans School of Nursing, *Rochester (BS)*

Wagner College, Department of Nursing, *Staten Island (BS)*

North Carolina

Queens University of Charlotte, Presbyterian School of Nursing, *Charlotte (BSN)*

The University of North Carolina at Chapel Hill, School of Nursing, *Chapel Hill (BSN)*

The University of North Carolina at Greensboro, School of Nursing, *Greensboro (BSN)*

Winston-Salem State University, Department of Nursing, *Winston-Salem (BSN)*

North Dakota

University of North Dakota, College of Nursing, *Grand Forks (BSN)*

Ohio

Ashland University, Dwight Schar College of Nursing and Health Sciences, *Ashland (BSN)*

Kent State University, College of Nursing, *Kent (BSN)*

Ursuline College, The Breen School of Nursing, *Pepper Pike (BSN)*

Walsh University, Department of Nursing, *North Canton (BSN)*

Wright State University, College of Nursing and Health, *Dayton (BSN)*

Oklahoma

Northwestern Oklahoma State University, Division of Nursing, *Alva (BSN)*

Oklahoma Baptist University, School of Nursing, *Shawnee (BSN)*

Oklahoma City University, Kramer School of Nursing, *Oklahoma City (BSN)*

Oklahoma Wesleyan University, School of Nursing, *Bartlesville (BSN)*

Southern Nazarene University, School of Nursing, *Bethany (BS)*

Oregon

Linfield College, School of Nursing, *McMinnville (BSN)*

Pennsylvania

Bloomsburg University of Pennsylvania, Department of Nursing, *Bloomsburg (BSN)*

Cedar Crest College, Department of Nursing, *Allentown (BS)*

DeSales University, Department of Nursing and Health, *Center Valley (BSN)*

Eastern University, Program in Nursing, *St. Davids (BSN)*

Gannon University, Villa Maria School of Nursing, *Erie (BSN)*

Holy Family University, School of Nursing and Allied Health Professions, *Philadelphia (BSN)*

Indiana University of Pennsylvania, Department of Nursing and Allied Health, *Indiana (BSN)*

La Salle University, School of Nursing and Health Sciences, *Philadelphia (BSN)*

Misericordia University, Department of Nursing, *Dallas (BSN)*

Moravian College, Department of Nursing, *Bethlehem (BSN)*

Neumann University, Program in Nursing and Health Sciences, *Aston (BS)*

Robert Morris University, School of Nursing and Health Sciences, *Moon Township (BSN)*

Thomas Jefferson University, Department of Nursing, *Philadelphia (BSN)*

University of Pennsylvania, School of Nursing, *Philadelphia (BSN)*

The University of Scranton, Department of Nursing, *Scranton (BSN)*

Villanova University, College of Nursing, *Villanova (BSN)*

York College of Pennsylvania, Department of Nursing, *York (BS)*

Rhode Island

Rhode Island College, Department of Nursing, *Providence (BSN)*

South Carolina

Lander University, School of Nursing, *Greenwood (BSN)*

South Dakota

Presentation College, Department of Nursing, *Aberdeen (BSN)*

South Dakota State University, College of Nursing, *Brookings (BS)*

Tennessee

Austin Peay State University, School of Nursing, *Clarksville (BSN)*

Belmont University, School of Nursing, *Nashville (BSN)*

Cumberland University, Rudy School of Nursing and Health Professions, *Lebanon (BSN)*

East Tennessee State University, College of Nursing, *Johnson City (BSN)*

Milligan College, Department of Nursing, *Milligan College (BSN)*

Tennessee Technological University, Whitson-Hester School of Nursing, *Cookeville (BSN)*

University of Memphis, Loewenberg School of Nursing, *Memphis (BSN)*

The University of Tennessee at Chattanooga, School of Nursing, *Chattanooga (BSN)*

Texas

Sam Houston State University, Nursing Program, *Huntsville (BSN)*

Texas A&M University–Corpus Christi, College of Nursing and Health Sciences, *Corpus Christi (BSN)*

Texas Woman's University, College of Nursing, *Denton (BS)*

The University of Texas at Arlington, College of Nursing, *Arlington (BSN)*

University of the Incarnate Word, Program in Nursing, *San Antonio (BSN)*

Utah

University of Utah, College of Nursing, *Salt Lake City (BS)*

Westminster College, School of Nursing and Health Sciences, *Salt Lake City (BSN)*

Virginia

Eastern Mennonite University, Department of Nursing, *Harrisonburg (BS)*

Radford University, Program in Nursing Practice, *Radford (BSN)*

Shenandoah University, Eleanor Wade Custer School of Nursing, *Winchester (BS)*

Washington

Seattle University, College of Nursing, *Seattle (BSN)*

Wisconsin

Alverno College, Division of Nursing, *Milwaukee (BSN)*

Bellin College, Nursing Program, *Green Bay (BSN)*

Columbia College of Nursing, *Milwaukee (BSN)*

Edgewood College, Henry Predolin School of Nursing, *Madison (BS)*

Milwaukee School of Engineering, School of Nursing, *Milwaukee (BSN)*

CANADA

Alberta

University of Alberta, Faculty of Nursing, *Edmonton (BScN)*

University of Calgary, Faculty of Nursing, *Calgary (BN)*

University of Lethbridge, Faculty of Health Sciences, *Lethbridge (BN)*

Manitoba

Brandon University, School of Health Studies, *Brandon (BN)*

Ontario

McMaster University, School of Nursing, *Hamilton (BScN)*

University of Toronto, Faculty of Nursing, *Toronto (BScN)*

Saskatchewan

University of Saskatchewan, College of Nursing, *Saskatoon (BSN)*

GENERIC BACCALAUREATE

U.S. AND U.S. TERRITORIES

Alabama

Auburn University, School of Nursing, *Auburn University (BSN)*

Auburn University at Montgomery, School of Nursing, *Montgomery (BSN)*

Jacksonville State University, College of Nursing and Health Sciences, *Jacksonville (BSN)*

Oakwood University, Department of Nursing, *Huntsville (BS)*

Samford University, Ida V. Moffett School of Nursing, *Birmingham (BSN)*

Spring Hill College, Division of Nursing, *Mobile (BSN)*

Troy University, School of Nursing, *Troy (BSN)*

Tuskegee University, Program in Nursing, *Tuskegee (BSN)*

The University of Alabama, Capstone College of Nursing, *Tuscaloosa (BSN)*

The University of Alabama at Birmingham, School of Nursing, *Birmingham (BSN)*

The University of Alabama in Huntsville, College of Nursing, *Huntsville (BSN)*

University of Mobile, School of Nursing, *Mobile (BSN)*

University of North Alabama, College of Nursing and Allied Health, *Florence (BSN)*

University of South Alabama, College of Nursing, *Mobile (BSN)*

Alaska

University of Alaska Anchorage, School of Nursing, *Anchorage (BS)*

Arizona

Arizona State University at the Downtown Phoenix campus, College of Nursing, *Phoenix (BSN)*

Brookline College, Baccalaureate Nursing Program, *Phoenix (BSN)*

Northern Arizona University, School of Nursing, *Flagstaff (BSN)*

The University of Arizona, College of Nursing, *Tucson (BSN)*

Arkansas

Arkansas State University, Department of Nursing, *State University (BSN)*

Arkansas Tech University, Program in Nursing, *Russellville (BSN)*

Harding University, College of Nursing, *Searcy (BSN)*

Henderson State University, Department of Nursing, *Arkadelphia (BSN)*

Southern Arkansas University–Magnolia, Department of Nursing, *Magnolia (BSN)*

University of Arkansas, Eleanor Mann School of Nursing, *Fayetteville (BSN)*

University of Arkansas at Monticello, School of Nursing, *Monticello (BSN)*

University of Arkansas for Medical Sciences, College of Nursing, *Little Rock (BSN)*

University of Arkansas–Fort Smith, Carol McKelvey Moore School of Nursing, *Fort Smith (BSN)*

University of Central Arkansas, Department of Nursing, *Conway (BSN)*

California

Azusa Pacific University, School of Nursing, *Azusa (BSN)*

Biola University, Department of Nursing, *La Mirada (BSN)*

California Baptist University, School of Nursing, *Riverside (BSN)*

California State University, Bakersfield, Program in Nursing, *Bakersfield (BSN)*

California State University Channel Islands, Nursing Program, *Camarillo (BSN)*

California State University, Chico, School of Nursing, *Chico (BSN)*

California State University, East Bay, Department of Nursing and Health Sciences, *Hayward (BS)*

California State University, Fresno, Department of Nursing, *Fresno (BSN)*

California State University, Fullerton, Department of Nursing, *Fullerton (BSN)*

California State University, Long Beach, School of Nursing, *Long Beach (BSN)*

California State University, Los Angeles, School of Nursing, *Los Angeles (BSN)*

California State University, Sacramento, Division of Nursing, *Sacramento (BSN)*

California State University, San Bernardino, Department of Nursing, *San Bernardino (BSN)*

California State University, San Marcos, School of Nursing, *San Marcos (BSN)*

California State University, Stanislaus, Department of Nursing, *Turlock (BSN)*

Dominican University of California, Program in Nursing, *San Rafael (BSN)*

Loma Linda University, School of Nursing, *Loma Linda (BS)*

Mount Saint Mary's University, Department of Nursing, *Los Angeles (BSN, BSc PN)*

National University, Department of Nursing, *La Jolla (BSN)*

Point Loma Nazarene University, School of Nursing, *San Diego (BSN)*

Samuel Merritt University, School of Nursing, *Oakland (BSN)*

San Diego State University, School of Nursing, *San Diego (BSN)*

San Francisco State University, School of Nursing, *San Francisco (BSN)*

San Jose State University, The Valley Foundation School of Nursing, *San Jose (BS)*

Sonoma State University, Department of Nursing, *Rohnert Park (BSN)*

University of California, Irvine, Program in Nursing Science, *Irvine (BS)*

University of California, Los Angeles, School of Nursing, *Los Angeles (BS)*

University of San Francisco, School of Nursing and Health Professions, *San Francisco (BSN)*

Colorado

Adams State University, Nursing Program, *Alamosa (BSN)*

Colorado Christian University, Nursing Programs, *Lakewood (BSN)*

Colorado Mesa University, Department of Nursing and Radiologic Sciences, *Grand Junction (BSN)*

Colorado State University–Pueblo, Department of Nursing, *Pueblo (BSN)*

Denver School of Nursing, *Denver (BSN)*

Regis University, School of Nursing, *Denver (BSN)*

University of Colorado Colorado Springs, Helen and Arthur E. Johnson Beth-El College of Nursing & Health Sciences, *Colorado Springs (BSN)*

University of Colorado Denver, College of Nursing, *Aurora (BS)*

University of Northern Colorado, School of Nursing, *Greeley (BS)*

Connecticut

Central Connecticut State University, Department of Nursing, *New Britain (BSN)*

Fairfield University, School of Nursing, *Fairfield (BSN)*

Quinnipiac University, School of Nursing, *Hamden (BSN)*

Sacred Heart University, College of Nursing, *Fairfield (BSN)*

Southern Connecticut State University, Department of Nursing, *New Haven (BSN)*

University of Connecticut, School of Nursing, *Storrs (BS)*

University of Saint Joseph, Department of Nursing, *West Hartford (BS)*

Western Connecticut State University, Department of Nursing, *Danbury (BS)*

Delaware

Delaware State University, Department of Nursing, *Dover (BSN)*

University of Delaware, School of Nursing, *Newark (BSN)*

Wesley College, Nursing Program, *Dover (BSN)*

District of Columbia

The Catholic University of America, School of Nursing, *Washington (BSN)*

Georgetown University, School of Nursing and Health Studies, *Washington (BSN)*

Howard University, Division of Nursing, *Washington (BSN)*

Trinity Washington University, Nursing Program, *Washington (BSN)*

Florida

Adventist University of Health Sciences, Department of Nursing, *Orlando (BSN)*

Barry University, Division of Nursing, *Miami Shores (BSN)*

Bethune-Cookman University, School of Nursing, *Daytona Beach (BSN)*

Florida Agricultural and Mechanical University, School of Nursing, *Tallahassee (BSN)*

Florida Atlantic University, Christine E. Lynn College of Nursing, *Boca Raton (BSN)*

Florida Gulf Coast University, School of Nursing, *Fort Myers (BSN)*

Florida International University, Nursing Program, *Miami (BSN)*

Florida National University, Nursing Division, *Hialeah (BSN)*

Florida Southern College, School of Nursing & Health Sciences, *Lakeland (BSN)*

Florida State University, College of Nursing, *Tallahassee (BSN)*

Jacksonville University, School of Nursing, *Jacksonville (BSN)*

Kaplan University Online, The School of Nursing Online, *Fort Lauderdale (BSN)*

Nova Southeastern University, College of Health Care Sciences, *Fort Lauderdale (BSN)*

University of Central Florida, College of Nursing, *Orlando (BSN)*

University of Florida, College of Nursing, *Gainesville (BSN)*

University of Miami, School of Nursing and Health Studies, *Coral Gables (BSN)*

University of North Florida, School of Nursing, *Jacksonville (BSN)*

University of South Florida, College of Nursing, *Tampa (BS)*

The University of Tampa, Department of Nursing, *Tampa (BSN)*

University of West Florida, Department of Nursing, *Pensacola (BSN)*

Georgia

Albany State University, College of Sciences and Health Professions, *Albany (BSN)*

Armstrong State University, Program in Nursing, *Savannah (BSN)*

Augusta University, School of Nursing, *Augusta (BSN)*

Berry College, Division of Nursing, *Mount Berry (BSN)*

Brenau University, College of Health and Science, *Gainesville (BSN)*

Clayton State University, Department of Nursing, *Morrow (BSN)*

College of Coastal Georgia, Department of Nursing and Health Sciences, *Brunswick (BSN)*

Columbus State University, Nursing Program, *Columbus (BSN)*

Emory University, Nell Hodgson Woodruff School of Nursing, *Atlanta (BSN)*

Georgia College & State University, College of Health Sciences, *Milledgeville (BSN)*

Georgia Southern University, School of Nursing, *Statesboro (BSN)*

Georgia Southwestern State University, School of Nursing, *Americus (BSN)*

Georgia State University, Byrdine F. Lewis School of Nursing, *Atlanta (BS)*

Kennesaw State University, School of Nursing, *Kennesaw (BSN)*

LaGrange College, Department of Nursing, *LaGrange (BSN)*

Mercer University, Georgia Baptist College of Nursing of Mercer University, *Atlanta (BSN)*

Middle Georgia College, School of Nursing and Health Sciences, *Cochran (BSN)*

Piedmont College, School of Nursing, *Demorest (BSN)*

Shorter University, School of Nursing, *Rome (BSN)*

University of North Georgia, Department of Nursing, *Dahlonega (BSN)*

University of West Georgia, School of Nursing, *Carrollton (BSN)*

Valdosta State University, College of Nursing, *Valdosta (BSN)*

Guam

University of Guam, School of Nursing and Health Sciences, *Mangilao (BSN)*

Hawaii

Chaminade University of Honolulu, Nursing Program, *Honolulu (BSN)*

Hawai`i Pacific University, College of Nursing and Health Sciences, *Honolulu (BSN)*

University of Hawaii at Hilo, Department in Nursing, *Hilo (BSN)*

University of Hawaii at Manoa, School of Nursing and Dental Hygiene, *Honolulu (BSN)*

Idaho

Boise State University, Department of Nursing, *Boise (BS)*

Idaho State University, Department of Nursing, *Pocatello (BS)*

Lewis-Clark State College, Division of Nursing and Health Sciences, *Lewiston (BSN)*

Northwest Nazarene University, School of Health and Science, *Nampa (BSN)*

Illinois

Aurora University, School of Nursing, *Aurora (BSN)*

Blessing–Rieman College of Nursing and Health Sciences, *Quincy (BSN)*

Bradley University, Department of Nursing, *Peoria (BSN, BSc PN)*

Chamberlain College of Nursing, Nursing Program, *Addison (BSN)*

Chicago State University, Department of Nursing, *Chicago (BSN)*

Elmhurst College, Deicke Center for Nursing Education, *Elmhurst (BS)*

Illinois State University, Mennonite College of Nursing, *Normal (BSN)*

Illinois Wesleyan University, School of Nursing, *Bloomington (BSN)*

Lakeview College of Nursing, *Danville (BSN)*

Lewis University, Program in Nursing, *Romeoville (BSN)*

Loyola University Chicago, Marcella Niehoff School of Nursing, *Maywood (BSN)*

MacMurray College, Department of Nursing, *Jacksonville (BSN)*

Methodist College, *Peoria (BSN)*

Millikin University, School of Nursing, *Decatur (BSN)*

Northern Illinois University, School of Nursing and Health Studies, *De Kalb (BS)*

North Park University, School of Nursing, *Chicago (BS)*

Olivet Nazarene University, Division of Nursing, *Bourbonnais (BSN)*

Rockford University, Department of Nursing, *Rockford (BSN)*

Saint Anthony College of Nursing, *Rockford (BSN)*

Saint Francis Medical Center College of Nursing, Baccalaureate Nursing Program, *Peoria (BSN)*

St. John's College, Department of Nursing, *Springfield (BSN)*

Saint Xavier University, School of Nursing, *Chicago (BSN)*

Southern Illinois University Edwardsville, School of Nursing, *Edwardsville (BS)*

Trinity Christian College, Department of Nursing, *Palos Heights (BSN)*

Trinity College of Nursing and Health Sciences, *Rock Island (BSN)*

University of Illinois at Chicago, College of Nursing, *Chicago (BSN)*

University of St. Francis, Leach College of Nursing, *Joliet (BSN)*

Western Illinois University, School of Nursing, *Macomb (BSN)*

Indiana

Anderson University, School of Nursing, *Anderson (BSN)*

Ball State University, School of Nursing, *Muncie (BS)*

Bethel College, School of Nursing, *Mishawaka (BSN)*

Goshen College, Department of Nursing, *Goshen (BSN)*

Huntington University, Department of Nursing, *Huntington (BSN)*

Indiana State University, Department of Advanced Practice Nursing, *Terre Haute (BS)*

Indiana University Bloomington, Department of Nursing–Bloomington Division, *Bloomington (BSN)*

Indiana University East, School of Nursing, *Richmond (BSN)*

Indiana University Kokomo, Indiana University School of Nursing, *Kokomo (BSN)*

Indiana University Northwest, School of Nursing, *Gary (BSN)*

Indiana University–Purdue University Fort Wayne, Department of Nursing, *Fort Wayne (BS)*

Indiana University–Purdue University Indianapolis, School of Nursing, *Indianapolis (BSN)*

Indiana University South Bend, Vera Z. Dwyer College of Health Sciences, *South Bend (BSN)*

Indiana University Southeast, School of Nursing, *New Albany (BSN)*

Indiana Wesleyan University, School of Nursing, *Marion (BSN)*

Marian University, School of Nursing, *Indianapolis (BSN)*

Purdue University, School of Nursing, *West Lafayette (BS)*

Purdue University Calumet, School of Nursing, *Hammond (BSN)*

Saint Mary's College, Department of Nursing, *Notre Dame (BS)*

University of Evansville, Department of Nursing, *Evansville (BSN)*

University of Indianapolis, School of Nursing, *Indianapolis (BSN)*

University of Saint Francis, Department of Nursing, *Fort Wayne (BSN)*

University of Southern Indiana, College of Nursing and Health Professions, *Evansville (BSN)*

Valparaiso University, College of Nursing and Health Professions, *Valparaiso (BSN)*

Iowa

Allen College, Graduate Programs, *Waterloo (BSN)*

Briar Cliff University, Department of Nursing, *Sioux City (BSN)*

Clarke University, Department of Nursing and Health, *Dubuque (BSN)*

Coe College, Department of Nursing, *Cedar Rapids (BSN)*

Dordt College, Nursing Program, *Sioux Center (BSN)*

Grand View University, Division of Nursing, *Des Moines (BSN)*

Iowa Wesleyan College, Division of Nursing, *Mount Pleasant (BSN)*

Luther College, Department of Nursing, *Decorah (BA)*

Morningside College, Department of Nursing Education, *Sioux City (BSN)*

Mount Mercy University, Department of Nursing, *Cedar Rapids (BSN)*

Northwestern College, Nursing Program, *Orange City (BSN)*

St. Ambrose University, Program in Nursing (BSN), *Davenport (BSN)*

The University of Iowa, College of Nursing, *Iowa City (BSN)*

Kansas

Baker University, School of Nursing, *Topeka (BSN)*

Benedictine College, Department of Nursing, *Atchison (BSN)*

Bethel College, Department of Nursing, *North Newton (BSN)*

Emporia State University, Newman Division of Nursing, *Emporia (BSN)*

Fort Hays State University, Department of Nursing, *Hays (BSN)*

Kansas Wesleyan University, Department of Nursing Education, *Salina (BSN)*

Newman University, Division of Nursing, *Wichita (BSN)*

Pittsburg State University, Department of Nursing, *Pittsburg (BSN)*

The University of Kansas, School of Nursing, *Kansas City (BSN)*

University of Saint Mary, Bachelor of Science in Nursing Program, *Leavenworth (BSN)*

Washburn University, School of Nursing, *Topeka (BSN)*

Wichita State University, School of Nursing, *Wichita (BSN)*

Kentucky

Bellarmine University, Donna and Allan Lansing School of Nursing and Health Sciences, *Louisville (BSN, MSCE)*

Berea College, Department of Nursing, *Berea (BSN)*

Eastern Kentucky University, Department of Baccalaureate and Graduate Nursing, *Richmond (BSN)*

Kentucky Christian University, School of Nursing, *Grayson (BSN)*

Morehead State University, Department of Nursing, *Morehead (BSN)*

Murray State University, Program in Nursing, *Murray (BSN)*

Northern Kentucky University, Department of Nursing, *Highland Heights (BSN)*

Spalding University, School of Nursing, *Louisville (BSN)*

Thomas More College, Program in Nursing, *Crestview Hills (BSN)*

Union College, School of Nursing & Health Sciences, *Barbourville (BSN)*

University of Kentucky, College of Nursing, *Lexington (BSN)*

University of Louisville, School of Nursing, *Louisville (BSN)*

Western Kentucky University, School of Nursing, *Bowling Green (BSN)*

Louisiana

Dillard University, Division of Nursing, *New Orleans (BSN)*

Grambling State University, School of Nursing, *Grambling (BSN)*

Louisiana College, Department of Nursing, *Pineville (BSN)*

Louisiana State University Health Sciences Center, School of Nursing, *New Orleans (BSN)*

McNeese State University, College of Nursing, *Lake Charles (BSN)*

Nicholls State University, Department of Nursing, *Thibodaux (BSN)*

Northwestern State University of Louisiana, College of Nursing and School of Allied Health, *Shreveport (BSN)*

Our Lady of Holy Cross College, Division of Nursing, *New Orleans (BSN)*

Our Lady of the Lake College, Division of Nursing, *Baton Rouge (BSN)*

Southeastern Louisiana University, School of Nursing, *Hammond (BS)*

Southern University and Agricultural and Mechanical College, School of Nursing, *Baton Rouge (BSN)*

University of Louisiana at Lafayette, College of Nursing, *Lafayette (BSN)*

University of Louisiana at Monroe, Nursing, *Monroe (BS)*

Maine

Husson University, School of Nursing, *Bangor (BSN)*

Saint Joseph's College of Maine, Master of Science in Nursing Program, *Standish (BSN)*

University of Maine, School of Nursing, *Orono (BSN)*

University of Maine at Fort Kent, Department of Nursing, *Fort Kent (BSN)*

University of New England, Department of Nursing, *Biddeford (BSN)*

University of Southern Maine, School of Nursing, *Portland (BS)*

Maryland

Bowie State University, Department of Nursing, *Bowie (BSN)*

Coppin State University, Helene Fuld School of Nursing, *Baltimore (BSN)*

Hood College, BSN Completion Program, *Frederick (BSN)*

Morgan State University, Bachelor of Science in Nursing, *Baltimore (BS)*

Salisbury University, Department of Nursing, *Salisbury (BS)*

Stevenson University, Nursing Division, *Stevenson (BS)*

Towson University, Department of Nursing, *Towson (BS)*

University of Maryland, Baltimore, Nursing Programs, *Baltimore (BSN)*

Massachusetts

American International College, Division of Nursing, *Springfield (BSN)*

Becker College, Nursing Programs, *Worcester (BSN)*

Boston College, William F. Connell School of Nursing, *Chestnut Hill (BS)*

Curry College, Division of Nursing, *Milton (BS)*

Elms College, School of Nursing, *Chicopee (BS)*

Endicott College, Major in Nursing, *Beverly (BS)*

Fitchburg State University, Department of Nursing, *Fitchburg (BS)*

Labouré College, Bachelor of Science in Nursing Program, *Boston (BSN)*

Northeastern University, School of Nursing, *Boston (BSN)*

Regis College, School of Nursing, Science and Health Professions, *Weston (BSN)*

Salem State University, Program in Nursing, *Salem (BSN)*

Simmons College, School of Nursing and Health Sciences, *Boston (BS)*

University of Massachusetts Amherst, College of Nursing, *Amherst (BS)*

University of Massachusetts Boston, College of Nursing and Health Sciences, *Boston (BS)*

University of Massachusetts Dartmouth, College of Nursing, *North Dartmouth (BS)*

University of Massachusetts Lowell, School of Nursing, *Lowell (BS)*

Westfield State University, Nursing Program, *Westfield (BSN)*

Worcester State University, Department of Nursing, *Worcester (BS)*

Michigan

Andrews University, Department of Nursing, *Berrien Springs (BS)*

Baker College, School of Nursing, *Flint (BSN)*

Calvin College, Department of Nursing, *Grand Rapids (BSN)*

Davenport University, Division of Nursing, *Grand Rapids (BSN)*

Davenport University, Bachelor of Science in Nursing Program, *Kalamazoo (BSN)*

Eastern Michigan University, School of Nursing, *Ypsilanti (BSN)*

Ferris State University, School of Nursing, *Big Rapids (BSN)*

Finlandia University, College of Professional Studies, *Hancock (BSN)*

Grand Valley State University, Kirkhof College of Nursing, *Allendale (BSN)*

Hope College, Department of Nursing, *Holland (BSN)*

Lake Superior State University, Department of Nursing, *Sault Sainte Marie (BSN)*

Madonna University, College of Nursing and Health, *Livonia (BSN)*

Michigan State University, College of Nursing, *East Lansing (BSN)*

Northern Michigan University, College of Nursing and Allied Health Science, *Marquette (BSN)*

Oakland University, School of Nursing, *Rochester (BSN)*

Rochester College, School of Nursing, *Rochester Hills (BSN)*

Saginaw Valley State University, College of Health and Human Services, *University Center (BSN)*

Siena Heights University, Nursing Program, *Adrian (BSN)*

University of Detroit Mercy, McAuley School of Nursing, *Detroit (BSN)*

University of Michigan, School of Nursing, *Ann Arbor (BSN)*

Wayne State University, College of Nursing, *Detroit (BSN)*

Western Michigan University, College of Health and Human Services, *Kalamazoo (BSN)*

Minnesota

Bemidji State University, Department of Nursing, *Bemidji (BS)*

Bethel University, Department of Nursing, *St. Paul (BSN)*

College of Saint Benedict, Department of Nursing, *Saint Joseph (BS)*

The College of St. Scholastica, Department of Nursing, *Duluth (BS)*

Concordia College, Department of Nursing, *Moorhead (BA)*

Crown College, Nursing Department, *St. Bonifacius (BSN)*

Globe University–Woodbury, Bachelor of Science in Nursing, *Woodbury (BS)*

Gustavus Adolphus College, Department of Nursing, *St. Peter (BA)*

Herzing University, Nursing Program, *Minneapolis (BSN)*

Metropolitan State University, College of Health, Community and Professional Studies, *St. Paul (BSN)*

Minnesota State University Mankato, School of Nursing, *Mankato (BS)*

St. Catherine University, Department of Nursing, *St. Paul (BS)*

St. Cloud State University, Department of Nursing Science, *St. Cloud (BS)*

St. Olaf College, Nursing Program, *Northfield (BA)*

University of Minnesota, Twin Cities Campus, School of Nursing, *Minneapolis (BSN)*

Winona State University, College of Nursing and Health Sciences, *Winona (BS)*

Mississippi

Alcorn State University, School of Nursing, *Natchez (BSN)*

Delta State University, School of Nursing, *Cleveland (BSN)*

Mississippi College, School of Nursing, *Clinton (BSN)*

Mississippi University for Women, College of Nursing and Speech Language Pathology, *Columbus (BSN)*

University of Mississippi Medical Center, School of Nursing, *Jackson (BSN)*

University of Southern Mississippi, College of Nursing, *Hattiesburg (BSN)*

William Carey University, School of Nursing, *Hattiesburg (BSN)*

Missouri

Avila University, School of Nursing, *Kansas City (BSN)*

Central Methodist University, College of Liberal Arts and Sciences, *Fayette (BSN)*

Chamberlain College of Nursing, *St. Louis (BSN)*

College of the Ozarks, Armstrong McDonald School of Nursing, *Point Lookout (BSN)*

Cox College, Department of Nursing, *Springfield (BSN)*

Goldfarb School of Nursing at Barnes-Jewish College, *St. Louis (BSN)*

Maryville University of Saint Louis, The Catherine McAuley School of Nursing, College of Health Professions, *St. Louis (BSN)*

Missouri Southern State University, Department of Nursing, *Joplin (BSN)*

Missouri State University, Department of Nursing, *Springfield (BSN)*

Missouri Valley College, School of Nursing and Health Sciences, *Marshall (BSN)*

Missouri Western State University, Department of Nursing, *St. Joseph (BSN)*

Research College of Nursing, College of Nursing, *Kansas City (BSN)*

Saint Louis University, School of Nursing, *St. Louis (BSN)*

Saint Luke's College of Health Sciences, Nursing College, *Kansas City (BSN)*

Southeast Missouri State University, Department of Nursing, *Cape Girardeau (BSN)*

Truman State University, Program in Nursing, *Kirksville (BSN)*

University of Central Missouri, Department of Nursing, *Warrensburg (BS)*

University of Missouri, Sinclair School of Nursing, *Columbia (BSN)*

University of Missouri–Kansas City, School of Nursing and Health Studies, *Kansas City (BSN)*

University of Missouri–St. Louis, College of Nursing, *St. Louis (BSN)*

William Jewell College, Department of Nursing, *Liberty (BS)*

Montana

Carroll College, Department of Nursing, *Helena (BS)*

Montana State University, College of Nursing, *Bozeman (BSN)*

Nebraska

Bryan College of Health Sciences, School of Nursing, *Lincoln (BSN)*

Clarkson College, Master of Science in Nursing Program, *Omaha (BSN)*

College of Saint Mary, Division of Health Care Professions, *Omaha (BSN)*

Creighton University, College of Nursing, *Omaha (BSN)*

Midland University, Department of Nursing, *Fremont (BSN)*

Nebraska Methodist College, Department of Nursing, *Omaha (BSN)*

Nebraska Wesleyan University, Department of Nursing, *Lincoln (BSN)*

Union College, Division of Nursing, *Lincoln (BSN)*

University of Nebraska Medical Center, College of Nursing, *Omaha (BSN)*

Nevada

Nevada State College at Henderson, Nursing Program, *Henderson (BSN)*

Roseman University of Health Sciences, College of Nursing, *Henderson (BSN)*

Touro University, School of Nursing, *Henderson (BSN)*

University of Nevada, Reno, Orvis School of Nursing, *Reno (BSN)*

New Hampshire

Colby-Sawyer College, Department of Nursing, *New London (BSN)*

Keene State College, Nursing Program, *Keene (BS)*

Rivier University, Division of Nursing, *Nashua (BS)*

University of New Hampshire, Department of Nursing, *Durham (BS)*

New Jersey

Bloomfield College, Division of Nursing, *Bloomfield (BS)*

Caldwell University, Nursing Programs, *Caldwell (BSN)*

The College of New Jersey, School of Nursing, Health and Exercise Science, *Ewing (BSN)*

Fairleigh Dickinson University, Metropolitan Campus, Henry P. Becton School of Nursing and Allied Health, *Teaneck (BSN)*

Felician University, Division of Nursing and Health Management, *Lodi (BSN)*

Georgian Court University, The Georgian Court-Meridian Health School of Nursing, *Lakewood (BSN)*

Ramapo College of New Jersey, Master of Science in Nursing Program, *Mahwah (BSN)*

Rutgers, The State University of New Jersey, Camden, Rutgers School of Nursing–Camden, *Camden (BS)*

Saint Peter's University, Nursing Program, *Jersey City (BSN)*

Seton Hall University, College of Nursing, *South Orange (BSN)*

Thomas Edison State University, School of Nursing, *Trenton (BSN)*

William Paterson University of New Jersey, Department of Nursing, *Wayne (BSN)*

New Mexico

Brookline College, Department of Nursing, *Albuquerque (BSN)*

New Mexico State University, School of Nursing, *Las Cruces (BSN)*

University of New Mexico, Program in Nursing, *Albuquerque (BSN)*

Western New Mexico University, Nursing Department, *Silver City (BSN)*

New York

Adelphi University, College of Nursing and Public Health, *Garden City (BS)*

Binghamton University, State University of New York, Decker School of Nursing, *Vestal (BS)*

The College at Brockport, State University of New York, Department of Nursing, *Brockport (BSN)*

College of Mount Saint Vincent, Department of Nursing, *Riverdale (BS)*

The College of New Rochelle, School of Nursing, *New Rochelle (BSN)*

Concordia College–New York, Nursing Program, *Bronxville (BS)*

Dominican College, Department of Nursing, *Orangeburg (BSN)*

D'Youville College, School of Nursing, *Buffalo (BSN)*

Elmira College, Program in Nursing Education, *Elmira (BS)*

Farmingdale State College, Nursing Department, *Farmingdale (BS)*

Hartwick College, Department of Nursing, *Oneonta (BS)*

Hunter College of the City University of New York, Hunter-Bellevue School of Nursing, *New York (BS)*

Lehman College of the City University of New York, Department of Nursing, *Bronx (BS)*

Le Moyne College, Nursing Programs, *Syracuse (BS)*

Long Island University–LIU Brooklyn, School of Nursing, *Brooklyn (BS)*

Long Island University–LIU Post, Department of Nursing, *Brookville (BS)*

Molloy College, Division of Nursing, *Rockville Centre (BS)*

Mount Saint Mary College, School of Nursing, *Newburgh (BSN)*

Nazareth College of Rochester, Department of Nursing, *Rochester (BS)*

New York Institute of Technology, Department of Nursing, *Old Westbury (BSN)*

New York University, College of Nursing, *New York (BS)*

Niagara University, Department of Nursing, *Niagara University (BS)*

Nyack College, School of Nursing, *Nyack (BS)*

Pace University, Lienhard School of Nursing, *New York (BS)*

Roberts Wesleyan College, School of Nursing, *Rochester (BScN)*

The Sage Colleges, Department of Nursing, *Troy (BS)*

St. Francis College, Department of Nursing, *Brooklyn Heights (BS)*

St. John Fisher College, Wegmans School of Nursing, *Rochester (BS)*

State University of New York at Plattsburgh, Department of Nursing, *Plattsburgh (BS)*

State University of New York College of Technology at Alfred, Nursing Program, *Alfred (BSN)*

Stony Brook University, State University of New York, School of Nursing, *Stony Brook (BS)*

Touro College, School of Nursing, *New York (BS)*

Trocaire College, Nursing Program, *Buffalo (BS)*

University at Buffalo, the State University of New York, School of Nursing, *Buffalo (BS)*

Utica College, Department of Nursing, *Utica (BS)*

Wagner College, Department of Nursing, *Staten Island (BS)*

North Carolina

Appalachian State University, Department of Nursing, *Boone (BSN)*

Barton College, School of Nursing, *Wilson (BSN)*

East Carolina University, College of Nursing, *Greenville (BSN)*

Fayetteville State University, Program in Nursing, *Fayetteville (BSN)*

Gardner-Webb University, School of Nursing, *Boiling Springs (BSN)*

Lenoir-Rhyne University, Program in Nursing, *Hickory (BS)*

Methodist University, Department of Nursing, *Fayetteville (BSN)*

North Carolina Agricultural and Technical State University, School of Nursing, *Greensboro (BSN)*

North Carolina Central University, Department of Nursing, *Durham (BSN)*

Queens University of Charlotte, Presbyterian School of Nursing, *Charlotte (BSN)*

The University of North Carolina at Chapel Hill, School of Nursing, *Chapel Hill (BSN)*

The University of North Carolina at Charlotte, School of Nursing, *Charlotte (BSN)*

The University of North Carolina at Greensboro, School of Nursing, *Greensboro (BSN)*

The University of North Carolina at Pembroke, Nursing Program, *Pembroke (BSN)*

The University of North Carolina Wilmington, School of Nursing, *Wilmington (BS)*

Western Carolina University, School of Nursing, *Cullowhee (BSN)*

Winston-Salem State University, Department of Nursing, *Winston-Salem (BSN)*

North Dakota

Minot State University, Department of Nursing, *Minot (BSN)*

North Dakota State University, Department of Nursing, *Fargo (BSN)*

University of Mary, Division of Nursing, *Bismarck (BSN)*

University of North Dakota, College of Nursing, *Grand Forks (BSN)*

Ohio

Ashland University, Dwight Schar College of Nursing and Health Sciences, *Ashland (BSN)*

Capital University, School of Nursing, *Columbus (BSN)*

Case Western Reserve University, Frances Payne Bolton School of Nursing, *Cleveland (BSN)*

The Christ College of Nursing and Health Sciences, Department of Nursing, *Cincinnati (BSN)*

Cleveland State University, School of Nursing, *Cleveland (BSN)*

Franciscan University of Steubenville, Department of Nursing, *Steubenville (BSN)*

Franklin University, Nursing Program, *Columbus (BSN)*

Hiram College, Nursing Department, *Hiram (BSN)*

Hondros College, Nursing Programs, *Westerville (BSN)*

Kent State University, College of Nursing, *Kent (BSN)*

Kettering College, Division of Nursing, *Kettering (BSN)*

Lourdes University, School of Nursing, *Sylvania (BSN)*

Malone University, School of Nursing, *Canton (BSN)*

Mercy College of Ohio, Division of Nursing, *Toledo (BSN)*

Miami University, Department of Nursing, *Hamilton (BSN)*

Miami University Hamilton, Bachelor of Science in Nursing Program, *Hamilton (BSN)*

Mount Carmel College of Nursing, Nursing Programs, *Columbus (BSN)*

Mount St. Joseph University, Department of Nursing, *Cincinnati (BSN)*

Mount Vernon Nazarene University, School of Nursing and Health Sciences, *Mount Vernon (BS)*

Muskingum University, Department of Nursing, *New Concord (BSN)*

Notre Dame College, Nursing Department, *South Euclid (BSN)*

Ohio Northern University, Nursing Program, *Ada (BSN)*

The Ohio State University, College of Nursing, *Columbus (BSN)*

Ohio University, School of Nursing, *Athens (BSN)*

Otterbein University, Department of Nursing, *Westerville (BSN)*

The University of Akron, School of Nursing, *Akron (BSN)*

University of Cincinnati, College of Nursing, *Cincinnati (BSN)*

The University of Toledo, College of Nursing, *Toledo (BSN)*

Ursuline College, The Breen School of Nursing, *Pepper Pike (BSN)*

Walsh University, Department of Nursing, *North Canton (BSN)*

Wright State University, College of Nursing and Health, *Dayton (BSN)*

Xavier University, School of Nursing, *Cincinnati (BSN)*

Youngstown State University, Department of Nursing, *Youngstown (BSN)*

Oklahoma

East Central University, Department of Nursing, *Ada (BS)*

Langston University, School of Nursing and Health Professions, *Langston (BSN)*

Northwestern Oklahoma State University, Division of Nursing, *Alva (BSN)*

Oklahoma Baptist University, School of Nursing, *Shawnee (BSN)*

Oklahoma Christian University, Nursing Program, *Oklahoma City (BSN)*

Oklahoma City University, Kramer School of Nursing, *Oklahoma City (BSN)*

Oklahoma Wesleyan University, School of Nursing, *Bartlesville (BSN)*

Oral Roberts University, Anna Vaughn School of Nursing, *Tulsa (BSN)*

Southern Nazarene University, School of Nursing, *Bethany (BS)*

Southwestern Oklahoma State University, School of Nursing, *Weatherford (BSN)*

University of Central Oklahoma, Department of Nursing, *Edmond (BSN)*

University of Oklahoma Health Sciences Center, College of Nursing, *Oklahoma City (BSN)*

The University of Tulsa, School of Nursing, *Tulsa (BSN)*

Oregon

Concordia University, Nursing Program, *Portland (BSN)*

George Fox University, Nursing Department, *Newberg (BSN)*

Linfield College, School of Nursing, *McMinnville (BSN)*

Oregon Health & Science University, School of Nursing, *Portland (BS)*

University of Portland, School of Nursing, *Portland (BSN)*

Pennsylvania

Alvernia University, Nursing, *Reading (BSN)*

Bloomsburg University of Pennsylvania, Department of Nursing, *Bloomsburg (BSN)*

Carlow University, College of Health and Wellness, *Pittsburgh (BSN)*

Cedar Crest College, Department of Nursing, *Allentown (BS)*

DeSales University, Department of Nursing and Health, *Center Valley (BSN)*

Drexel University, College of Nursing and Health Professions, *Philadelphia (BSN)*

Duquesne University, School of Nursing, *Pittsburgh (BSN)*

Eastern University, Program in Nursing, *St. Davids (BSN)*

East Stroudsburg University of Pennsylvania, Department of Nursing, *East Stroudsburg (BS)*

Edinboro University of Pennsylvania, Department of Nursing, *Edinboro (BSN)*

Gannon University, Villa Maria School of Nursing, *Erie (BSN)*

Holy Family University, School of Nursing and Allied Health Professions, *Philadelphia (BSN)*

Immaculata University, Division of Nursing, *Immaculata (BSN)*

Indiana University of Pennsylvania, Department of Nursing and Allied Health, *Indiana (BSN)*

La Salle University, School of Nursing and Health Sciences, *Philadelphia (BSN)*

Mansfield University of Pennsylvania, Department of Health Sciences–Nursing, *Mansfield (BSN)*

Marywood University, Department of Nursing, *Scranton (BSN)*

Messiah College, Department of Nursing, *Mechanicsburg (BSN)*

Misericordia University, Department of Nursing, *Dallas (BSN)*

Moravian College, Department of Nursing, *Bethlehem (BSN)*

Neumann University, Program in Nursing and Health Sciences, *Aston (BS)*

Penn State University Park, School of Nursing, *University Park (BS)*

Robert Morris University, School of Nursing and Health Sciences, *Moon Township (BSN)*

Saint Francis University, Department of Nursing, *Loretto (BSN)*

Temple University, Department of Nursing, *Philadelphia (BSN)*

Thomas Jefferson University, Department of Nursing, *Philadelphia (BSN)*

University of Pennsylvania, School of Nursing, *Philadelphia (BSN)*

University of Pittsburgh, School of Nursing, *Pittsburgh (BSN)*

University of Pittsburgh at Bradford, Department of Nursing, *Bradford (BSN)*

The University of Scranton, Department of Nursing, *Scranton (BSN)*

Villanova University, College of Nursing, *Villanova (BSN)*

Waynesburg University, Department of Nursing, *Waynesburg (BSN)*

West Chester University of Pennsylvania, Department of Nursing, *West Chester (BSN)*

Widener University, School of Nursing, *Chester (BSN)*

Wilkes University, Department of Nursing, *Wilkes-Barre (BS)*

York College of Pennsylvania, Department of Nursing, *York (BS)*

Puerto Rico

Inter American University of Puerto Rico, Arecibo Campus, Nursing Program, *Arecibo (BSN)*

Inter American University of Puerto Rico, Metropolitan Campus, Carmen Torres de Tiburcio School of Nursing, *San Juan (BSN)*

Pontifical Catholic University of Puerto Rico, Department of Nursing, *Ponce (BSN)*

Universidad Adventista de las Antillas, Department of Nursing, *Mayagüez (BSN)*

Universidad del Turabo, Nursing Program, *Gurabo (BS)*

University of Puerto Rico in Arecibo, Department of Nursing, *Arecibo (BSN)*

University of Puerto Rico in Humacao, Department of Nursing, *Humacao (BSN)*

University of Puerto Rico, Mayagüez Campus, Department of Nursing, *Mayagüez (BSN)*

University of Puerto Rico, Medical Sciences Campus, School of Nursing, *San Juan (BSN)*

Rhode Island

Rhode Island College, Department of Nursing, *Providence (BSN)*

Salve Regina University, Department of Nursing, *Newport (BS)*

South Carolina

Anderson University, School of Nursing, *Anderson (BSN)*

Charleston Southern University, Wingo School of Nursing, *Charleston (BSN)*

Clemson University, School of Nursing, *Clemson (BS)*

Francis Marion University, Department of Nursing, *Florence (BSN)*

Lander University, School of Nursing, *Greenwood (BSN)*

Newberry College, Department of Nursing, *Newberry (BSN)*

University of South Carolina, College of Nursing, *Columbia (BSN)*

University of South Carolina Aiken, School of Nursing, *Aiken (BSN)*

University of South Carolina Beaufort, Nursing Program, *Bluffton (BSN)*

University of South Carolina Upstate, Mary Black School of Nursing, *Spartanburg (BSN)*

South Dakota

Augustana University, Department of Nursing, *Sioux Falls (BA)*

Mount Marty College, Nursing Program, *Yankton (BSN)*

National American University, School of Nursing, *Rapid City (BSN)*

Presentation College, Department of Nursing, *Aberdeen (BSN)*

University of Sioux Falls, School of Nursing, *Sioux Falls (BSN)*

The University of South Dakota, Department of Nursing, *Vermillion (BSN)*

Tennessee

Aquinas College, School of Nursing, *Nashville (BSN)*

Austin Peay State University, School of Nursing, *Clarksville (BSN)*

Baptist College of Health Sciences, Nursing Division, *Memphis (BSN)*

Belmont University, School of Nursing, *Nashville (BSN)*

Bethel University, Nursing Program, *McKenzie (BSN)*

Carson-Newman University, Department of Nursing, *Jefferson City (BSN)*

Cumberland University, Rudy School of Nursing and Health Professions, *Lebanon (BSN)*

East Tennessee State University, College of Nursing, *Johnson City (BSN)*

Freed-Hardeman University, Department of Nursing, *Henderson (BSN)*

King University, School of Nursing, *Bristol (BSN)*

Lincoln Memorial University, Caylor School of Nursing, *Harrogate (BSN)*

Lipscomb University, Department of Nursing, *Nashville (BSN)*

Martin Methodist College, Division of Nursing, *Pulaski (BSN)*

Middle Tennessee State University, School of Nursing, *Murfreesboro (BSN)*

Milligan College, Department of Nursing, *Milligan College (BSN)*

South College, Department of Nursing, *Knoxville (BSN)*

Tennessee State University, Division of Nursing, *Nashville (BSN)*

Tennessee Technological University, Whitson-Hester School of Nursing, *Cookeville (BSN)*

Tennessee Wesleyan College, Fort Sanders Nursing Department, *Knoxville (BSN)*

Union University, School of Nursing, *Jackson (BSN)*

University of Memphis, Loewenberg School of Nursing, *Memphis (BSN)*

The University of Tennessee, College of Nursing, *Knoxville (BSN)*

The University of Tennessee at Chattanooga, School of Nursing, *Chattanooga (BSN)*

The University of Tennessee at Martin, Department of Nursing, *Martin (BSN)*

Texas

Abilene Christian University, School of Nursing, *Abilene (BSN)*

Angelo State University, Department of Nursing and Rehabilitation Sciences, *San Angelo (BSN)*

Baylor University, Louise Herrington School of Nursing, *Dallas (BSN)*

Concordia University Texas, School of Nursing, *Austin (BSN)*

East Texas Baptist University, Department of Nursing, *Marshall (BSN)*

Houston Baptist University, School of Nursing and Allied Health, *Houston (BSN)*

Lamar University, Department of Nursing, *Beaumont (BSN)*

Midwestern State University, Wilson School of Nursing, *Wichita Falls (BSN)*

Patty Hanks Shelton School of Nursing, *Abilene (BSN)*

Prairie View A&M University, College of Nursing, *Houston (BSN)*

Sam Houston State University, Nursing Program, *Huntsville (BSN)*

Southwestern Adventist University, Department of Nursing, *Keene (BS)*

Stephen F. Austin State University, Richard and Lucille Dewitt School of Nursing, *Nacogdoches (BSN)*

Tarleton State University, Department of Nursing, *Stephenville (BSN)*

Texas A&M Health Science Center, College of Nursing, *College Station (BSN)*

Texas A&M International University, Canseco School of Nursing, *Laredo (BSN)*

Texas A&M University–Commerce, Nursing Department, *Commerce (BSN)*

Texas A&M University–Corpus Christi, College of Nursing and Health Sciences, *Corpus Christi (BSN)*

Texas Christian University, Harris College of Nursing, *Fort Worth (BSN)*

Texas State University, St. David's School of Nursing, *San Marcos (BSN)*

Texas Tech University Health Sciences Center, School of Nursing, *Lubbock (BSN)*

Texas Woman's University, College of Nursing, *Denton (BS)*

University of Mary Hardin-Baylor, College of Nursing, *Belton (BSN)*

The University of Texas at Arlington, College of Nursing, *Arlington (BSN)*

The University of Texas at Austin, School of Nursing, *Austin (BSN)*

The University of Texas at El Paso, School of Nursing, *El Paso (BSN)*

The University of Texas at Tyler, Program in Nursing, *Tyler (BSN)*

The University of Texas Health Science Center at Houston, School of Nursing, *Houston (BSN)*

The University of Texas Health Science Center at San Antonio, School of Nursing, *San Antonio (BSN)*

The University of Texas Medical Branch, School of Nursing, *Galveston (BSN)*

The University of Texas Rio Grande Valley, School of Nursing, *Edinburg (BSN)*

University of the Incarnate Word, Program in Nursing, *San Antonio (BSN)*

West Texas A&M University, Department of Nursing, *Canyon (BSN)*

Utah

Southern Utah University, Department of Nursing, *Cedar City (BSN)*

University of Utah, College of Nursing, *Salt Lake City (BS)*

Western Governors University, Online College of Health Professions, *Salt Lake City (BS)*

Westminster College, School of Nursing and Health Sciences, *Salt Lake City (BSN)*

Vermont

Castleton State College, Baccalaureate Nursing Program, *Castleton (BS)*

Norwich University, Department of Nursing, *Northfield (BSN)*

Southern Vermont College, Department of Nursing, *Bennington (BSN)*

University of Vermont, Department of Nursing, *Burlington (BS)*

Virgin Islands

University of the Virgin Islands, Division of Nursing, *Saint Thomas (BSN)*

Virginia

Bon Secours Memorial College of Nursing, *Richmond (BSN)*

Eastern Mennonite University, Department of Nursing, *Harrisonburg (BS)*

George Mason University, College of Health and Human Services, *Fairfax (BSN)*

Hampton University, School of Nursing, *Hampton (BS)*

James Madison University, Department of Nursing, *Harrisonburg (BSN)*

Jefferson College of Health Sciences, Nursing Education Program, *Roanoke (BSN)*

Liberty University, Department of Nursing, *Lynchburg (BSN)*

Lynchburg College, School of Health Sciences and Human Performance, *Lynchburg (BS)*

Marymount University, School of Health Professions, *Arlington (BSN)*

Old Dominion University, Department of Nursing, *Norfolk (BSN)*

Radford University, Program in Nursing Practice, *Radford (BSN)*

Sentara College of Health Sciences, Bachelor of Science in Nursing Program, *Chesapeake (BSN)*

Shenandoah University, Eleanor Wade Custer School of Nursing, *Winchester (BS)*

Stratford University, School of Nursing, *Falls Church (BSN)*

University of Virginia, School of Nursing, *Charlottesville (BSN)*

The University of Virginia's College at Wise, Department of Nursing, *Wise (BSN)*

Virginia Commonwealth University, School of Nursing, *Richmond (BS)*

Washington

Gonzaga University, School of Nursing and Human Psychology, *Spokane (BSN)*

Northwest University, The Mark and Huldah Buntain School of Nursing, *Kirkland (BS)*

Pacific Lutheran University, School of Nursing, *Tacoma (BSN)*

Seattle Pacific University, School of Health Sciences, *Seattle (BS)*

Seattle University, College of Nursing, *Seattle (BSN)*

University of Washington, School of Nursing, *Seattle (BSN)*

Walla Walla University, School of Nursing, *College Place (BS)*

WSU College of Nursing, *Spokane (BSN)*

West Virginia

Alderson Broaddus University, Department of Nursing, *Philippi (BSN)*

Marshall University, College of Health Professions, *Huntington (BSN)*

Shepherd University, Department of Nursing Education, *Shepherdstown (BSN)*

University of Charleston, Department of Nursing, *Charleston (BSN)*

West Liberty University, Department of Health Sciences, *West Liberty (BSN)*

West Virginia University, School of Nursing, *Morgantown (BSN)*

West Virginia Wesleyan College, School of Nursing, *Buckhannon (BSN)*

Wheeling Jesuit University, Department of Nursing, *Wheeling (BSN)*

Wisconsin

Alverno College, Division of Nursing, *Milwaukee (BSN)*

Bellin College, Nursing Program, *Green Bay (BSN)*

Cardinal Stritch University, Ruth S. Coleman College of Nursing and Health Sciences, *Milwaukee (BSN)*

Carroll University, Nursing Program, *Waukesha (BSN)*

Columbia College of Nursing, *Milwaukee (BSN)*

Concordia University Wisconsin, Program in Nursing, *Mequon (BSN)*

Edgewood College, Henry Predolin School of Nursing, *Madison (BS)*

Marian University, School of Nursing, *Fond du Lac (BSN)*

Marquette University, College of Nursing, *Milwaukee (BSN)*

Milwaukee School of Engineering, School of Nursing, *Milwaukee (BSN)*

University of Wisconsin–Eau Claire, College of Nursing and Health Sciences, *Eau Claire (BSN)*

University of Wisconsin–Madison, School of Nursing, *Madison (BS)*

University of Wisconsin–Milwaukee, College of Nursing, *Milwaukee (BSN)*

Viterbo University, School of Nursing, *La Crosse (BSN)*

Wisconsin Lutheran College, Nursing Program, *Milwaukee (BSN)*

Wyoming

University of Wyoming, Fay W. Whitney School of Nursing, *Laramie (BSN)*

CANADA

Alberta

Athabasca University, Centre for Nursing and Health Studies, *Athabasca (BN)*

University of Alberta, Faculty of Nursing, *Edmonton (BScN)*

University of Calgary, Faculty of Nursing, *Calgary (BN)*

University of Lethbridge, Faculty of Health Sciences, *Lethbridge (BN)*

British Columbia

Kwantlen Polytechnic University, Faculty of Community and Health Sciences, *Surrey (BSN)*

Trinity Western University, Department of Nursing, *Langley (BScN)*

University of Northern British Columbia, Nursing Programme, *Prince George (BScN)*

Vancouver Island University, Department of Nursing, *Nanaimo (BScN)*

Manitoba

Brandon University, School of Health Studies, *Brandon (BN)*

University of Manitoba, Faculty of Nursing, *Winnipeg (BN)*

New Brunswick

University of New Brunswick Fredericton, Faculty of Nursing, *Fredericton (BN)*

Newfoundland and Labrador

Memorial University of Newfoundland, School of Nursing, *St. John's (BN)*

Nova Scotia

St. Francis Xavier University, Department of Nursing, *Antigonish (BScN)*

Ontario

Brock University, Department of Nursing, *St. Catharines (BScN)*

Lakehead University, School of Nursing, *Thunder Bay (BScN)*

Laurentian University, School of Nursing, *Sudbury (BScN)*

McMaster University, School of Nursing, *Hamilton (BScN)*

Queen's University at Kingston, School of Nursing, *Kingston (BNSc)*

Trent University, Nursing Program, *Peterborough (BScN)*

University of Ottawa, School of Nursing, *Ottawa (BScN)*

The University of Western Ontario, School of Nursing, *London (BScN)*

University of Windsor, Faculty of Nursing, *Windsor (BScN)*

York University, School of Nursing, *Toronto (BScN)*

Prince Edward Island

University of Prince Edward Island, School of Nursing, *Charlottetown (BScN)*

Quebec

McGill University, School of Nursing, *Montréal (BScN)*

Université de Montréal, Faculty of Nursing, *Montréal (BScN)*

Université du Québec à Chicoutimi, Program in Nursing, *Chicoutimi (BNSc)*

Université du Québec à Trois-Rivières, Program in Nursing, *Trois-Rivières (BSN)*

Université du Québec en Outaouais, Département des Sciences Infirmières, *Gatineau (BScN)*

Université Laval, Faculty of Nursing, *Québec (BScN)*

Saskatchewan

University of Saskatchewan, College of Nursing, *Saskatoon (BSN)*

INTERNATIONAL NURSE TO BACCALAUREATE

U.S. AND U.S. TERRITORIES

Colorado

American Sentinel University, RN to Bachelor of Science Nursing, *Aurora (BSN)*

Delaware

Wesley College, Nursing Program, *Dover (BSN)*

Wilmington University, College of Health Professions, *New Castle (BSN)*

District of Columbia

The George Washington University, School of Nursing, *Washington (BSN)*

Georgia

Thomas University, Division of Nursing, *Thomasville (BSN)*

Hawaii

Hawai`i Pacific University, College of Nursing and Health Sciences, *Honolulu (BSN)*

Iowa

Morningside College, Department of Nursing Education, *Sioux City (BSN)*

Massachusetts

Salem State University, Program in Nursing, *Salem (BSN)*

Nebraska

Nebraska Wesleyan University, Department of Nursing, *Lincoln (BSN)*

New Jersey

College of Saint Elizabeth, Department of Nursing, *Morristown (BSN)*

Seton Hall University, College of Nursing, *South Orange (BSN)*

New York

College of Mount Saint Vincent, Department of Nursing, *Riverdale (BS)*

Daemen College, Department of Nursing, *Amherst (BS)*

Lehman College of the City University of New York, Department of Nursing, *Bronx (BS)*

The Sage Colleges, Department of Nursing, *Troy (BS)*

St. Francis College, Department of Nursing, *Brooklyn Heights (BS)*

Oklahoma

Oklahoma City University, Kramer School of Nursing, *Oklahoma City (BSN)*

Oklahoma Wesleyan University, School of Nursing, *Bartlesville (BSN)*

Pennsylvania

Gannon University, Villa Maria School of Nursing, *Erie (BSN)*

Holy Family University, School of Nursing and Allied Health Professions, *Philadelphia (BSN)*

Marywood University, Department of Nursing, *Scranton (BSN)*

Neumann University, Program in Nursing and Health Sciences, *Aston (BS)*

Villanova University, College of Nursing, *Villanova (BSN)*

South Dakota

Mount Marty College, Nursing Program, *Yankton (BSN)*

Texas

Sam Houston State University, Nursing Program, *Huntsville (BSN)*

The University of Texas at Tyler, Program in Nursing, *Tyler (BSN)*

CANADA

Ontario

Ryerson University, Program in Nursing, *Toronto (BScN)*

University of Ottawa, School of Nursing, *Ottawa (BScN)*

LPN TO BACCALAUREATE

U.S. AND U.S. TERRITORIES

Arizona

University of Phoenix–Phoenix Campus, College of Health Sciences and Nursing, *Tempe (BSN)*

University of Phoenix–Southern Arizona Campus, College of Social Sciences, *Tucson (BSN)*

Arkansas

Arkansas State University, Department of Nursing, *State University (BSN)*

Arkansas Tech University, Program in Nursing, *Russellville (BSN)*

Henderson State University, Department of Nursing, *Arkadelphia (BSN)*

University of Arkansas, Eleanor Mann School of Nursing, *Fayetteville (BSN)*

University of Arkansas at Monticello, School of Nursing, *Monticello (BSN)*

University of Arkansas for Medical Sciences, College of Nursing, *Little Rock (BSN)*

University of Central Arkansas, Department of Nursing, *Conway (BSN)*

California

Biola University, Department of Nursing, *La Mirada (BSN)*

California State University, Fullerton, Department of Nursing, *Fullerton (BSN)*

California State University, San Bernardino, Department of Nursing, *San Bernardino (BSN)*

California State University, Stanislaus, Department of Nursing, *Turlock (BSN)*

Loma Linda University, School of Nursing, *Loma Linda (BS)*

National University, Department of Nursing, *La Jolla (BSN)*

University of Phoenix–Sacramento Valley Campus, College of Nursing, *Sacramento (BSN)*

Colorado

Colorado State University–Pueblo, Department of Nursing, *Pueblo (BSN)*

Delaware

Delaware State University, Department of Nursing, *Dover (BSN)*

Wesley College, Nursing Program, *Dover (BSN)*

District of Columbia

Howard University, Division of Nursing, *Washington (BSN)*

Florida

Barry University, Division of Nursing, *Miami Shores (BSN)*

Georgia

Armstrong State University, Program in Nursing, *Savannah (BSN)*

Piedmont College, School of Nursing, *Demorest (BSN)*

Hawaii

Hawai`i Pacific University, College of Nursing and Health Sciences, *Honolulu (BSN)*

University of Phoenix–Hawaii Campus, College of Nursing, *Honolulu (BSN)*

Idaho

Boise State University, Department of Nursing, *Boise (BS)*

Lewis-Clark State College, Division of Nursing and Health Sciences, *Lewiston (BSN)*

Illinois

Bradley University, Department of Nursing, *Peoria (BSN, BSc PN)*

Chicago State University, Department of Nursing, *Chicago (BSN)*

Indiana

Ball State University, School of Nursing, *Muncie (BS)*

Indiana State University, Department of Advanced Practice Nursing, *Terre Haute (BS)*

Purdue University Calumet, School of Nursing, *Hammond (BSN)*

Purdue University North Central, Department of Nursing, *Westville (BS)*

Iowa

Allen College, Graduate Programs, *Waterloo (BSN)*

Briar Cliff University, Department of Nursing, *Sioux City (BSN)*

Iowa Wesleyan College, Division of Nursing, *Mount Pleasant (BSN)*

Morningside College, Department of Nursing Education, *Sioux City (BSN)*

Kansas

Baker University, School of Nursing, *Topeka (BSN)*

Bethel College, Department of Nursing, *North Newton (BSN)*

Emporia State University, Newman Division of Nursing, *Emporia (BSN)*

Newman University, Division of Nursing, *Wichita (BSN)*

Washburn University, School of Nursing, *Topeka (BSN)*

Louisiana

McNeese State University, College of Nursing, *Lake Charles (BSN)*

Nicholls State University, Department of Nursing, *Thibodaux (BSN)*

Northwestern State University of Louisiana, College of Nursing and School of Allied Health, *Shreveport (BSN)*

Our Lady of the Lake College, Division of Nursing, *Baton Rouge (BSN)*

University of Louisiana at Lafayette, College of Nursing, *Lafayette (BSN)*

University of Louisiana at Monroe, Nursing, *Monroe (BS)*

University of Phoenix–New Orleans Learning Center, College of Nursing, *Metairie (BSN)*

Massachusetts

Salem State University, Program in Nursing, *Salem (BSN)*

Simmons College, School of Nursing and Health Sciences, *Boston (BS)*

Worcester State University, Department of Nursing, *Worcester (BS)*

Michigan

Lake Superior State University, Department of Nursing, *Sault Sainte Marie (BSN)*

Madonna University, College of Nursing and Health, *Livonia (BSN)*

Minnesota

Herzing University, Nursing Program, *Minneapolis (BSN)*

Missouri

Cox College, Department of Nursing, *Springfield (BSN)*

Maryville University of Saint Louis, The Catherine McAuley School of Nursing, College of Health Professions, *St. Louis (BSN)*

Missouri Southern State University, Department of Nursing, *Joplin (BSN)*

Montana

Montana State University, College of Nursing, *Bozeman (BSN)*

Nebraska

Clarkson College, Master of Science in Nursing Program, *Omaha (BSN)*

College of Saint Mary, Division of Health Care Professions, *Omaha (BSN)*

Nebraska Methodist College, Department of Nursing, *Omaha (BSN)*

Union College, Division of Nursing, *Lincoln (BSN)*

New Hampshire

Rivier University, Division of Nursing, *Nashua (BS)*

New Jersey

William Paterson University of New Jersey, Department of Nursing, *Wayne (BSN)*

New York

College of Mount Saint Vincent, Department of Nursing, *Riverdale (BS)*

Dominican College, Department of Nursing, *Orangeburg (BSN)*

Molloy College, Division of Nursing, *Rockville Centre (BS)*

Nazareth College of Rochester, Department of Nursing, *Rochester (BS)*

The Sage Colleges, Department of Nursing, *Troy (BS)*

North Carolina

Winston-Salem State University, Department of Nursing, *Winston-Salem (BSN)*

North Dakota

Dickinson State University, Department of Nursing, *Dickinson (BSN)*

North Dakota State University, Department of Nursing, *Fargo (BSN)*

University of Mary, Division of Nursing, *Bismarck (BSN)*

University of North Dakota, College of Nursing, *Grand Forks (BSN)*

Ohio

Kettering College, Division of Nursing, *Kettering (BSN)*

Lourdes University, School of Nursing, *Sylvania (BSN)*

Otterbein University, Department of Nursing, *Westerville (BSN)*

The University of Akron, School of Nursing, *Akron (BSN)*

Oklahoma

Langston University, School of Nursing and Health Professions, *Langston (BSN)*

Northwestern Oklahoma State University, Division of Nursing, *Alva (BSN)*

Oklahoma Baptist University, School of Nursing, *Shawnee (BSN)*

Oklahoma Wesleyan University, School of Nursing, *Bartlesville (BSN)*

Southern Nazarene University, School of Nursing, *Bethany (BS)*

University of Central Oklahoma, Department of Nursing, *Edmond (BSN)*

Pennsylvania

Alvernia University, Nursing, *Reading (BSN)*

Cedar Crest College, Department of Nursing, *Allentown (BS)*

Indiana University of Pennsylvania, Department of Nursing and Allied Health, *Indiana (BSN)*

La Salle University, School of Nursing and Health Sciences, *Philadelphia (BSN)*

Marywood University, Department of Nursing, *Scranton (BSN)*

Neumann University, Program in Nursing and Health Sciences, *Aston (BS)*

Waynesburg University, Department of Nursing, *Waynesburg (BSN)*

South Dakota

Mount Marty College, Nursing Program, *Yankton (BSN)*

Tennessee

Baptist College of Health Sciences, Nursing Division, *Memphis (BSN)*

East Tennessee State University, College of Nursing, *Johnson City (BSN)*

Milligan College, Department of Nursing, *Milligan College (BSN)*

Union University, School of Nursing, *Jackson (BSN)*

Texas

Prairie View A&M University, College of Nursing, *Houston (BSN)*

Sam Houston State University, Nursing Program, *Huntsville (BSN)*

Tarleton State University, Department of Nursing, *Stephenville (BSN)*

The University of Texas at Tyler, Program in Nursing, *Tyler (BSN)*

West Texas A&M University, Department of Nursing, *Canyon (BSN)*

Virgin Islands

University of the Virgin Islands, Division of Nursing, *Saint Thomas (BSN)*

Virginia

Eastern Mennonite University, Department of Nursing, *Harrisonburg (BS)*

Hampton University, School of Nursing, *Hampton (BS)*

Sentara College of Health Sciences, Bachelor of Science in Nursing Program, *Chesapeake (BSN)*

Washington

Pacific Lutheran University, School of Nursing, *Tacoma (BSN)*

Walla Walla University, School of Nursing, *College Place (BS)*

Wisconsin

Alverno College, Division of Nursing, *Milwaukee (BSN)*

CANADA

Manitoba

Brandon University, School of Health Studies, *Brandon (BN)*

Newfoundland and Labrador

Memorial University of Newfoundland, School of Nursing, *St. John's (BN)*

LPN TO RN BACCALAUREATE

U.S. AND U.S. TERRITORIES

Arkansas

University of Arkansas, Eleanor Mann School of Nursing, *Fayetteville (BSN)*

University of Central Arkansas, Department of Nursing, *Conway (BSN)*

California

California State University, Los Angeles, School of Nursing, *Los Angeles (BSN)*

Holy Names University, Department of Nursing, *Oakland (BSN)*

Point Loma Nazarene University, School of Nursing, *San Diego (BSN)*

Colorado

Colorado Mesa University, Department of Nursing and Radiologic Sciences, *Grand Junction (BSN)*

Colorado State University–Pueblo, Department of Nursing, *Pueblo (BSN)*

Denver School of Nursing, *Denver (BSN)*

Florida

Barry University, Division of Nursing, *Miami Shores (BSN)*

Georgia

Georgia Southern University, School of Nursing, *Statesboro (BSN)*

Georgia Southwestern State University, School of Nursing, *Americus (BSN)*

Idaho

Lewis-Clark State College, Division of Nursing and Health Sciences, *Lewiston (BSN)*

Illinois

MacMurray College, Department of Nursing, *Jacksonville (BSN)*

Saint Xavier University, School of Nursing, *Chicago (BSN)*

Indiana

Saint Joseph's College, St. Elizabeth School of Nursing, *Rensselaer (BSN)*

Iowa

Iowa Wesleyan College, Division of Nursing, *Mount Pleasant (BSN)*

Kansas

Wichita State University, School of Nursing, *Wichita (BSN)*

Louisiana

Dillard University, Division of Nursing, *New Orleans (BSN)*

Grambling State University, School of Nursing, *Grambling (BSN)*

McNeese State University, College of Nursing, *Lake Charles (BSN)*

Southeastern Louisiana University, School of Nursing, *Hammond (BS)*

Massachusetts

Salem State University, Program in Nursing, *Salem (BSN)*

Worcester State University, Department of Nursing, *Worcester (BS)*

Michigan

Lake Superior State University, Department of Nursing, *Sault Sainte Marie (BSN)*

Northern Michigan University, College of Nursing and Allied Health Science, *Marquette (BSN)*

Mississippi

Alcorn State University, School of Nursing, *Natchez (BSN)*

Missouri

Chamberlain College of Nursing, *St. Louis (BSN)*

Cox College, Department of Nursing, *Springfield (BSN)*

Nebraska

Clarkson College, Master of Science in Nursing Program, *Omaha (BSN)*

Midland University, Department of Nursing, *Fremont (BSN)*

Nebraska Methodist College, Department of Nursing, *Omaha (BSN)*

New Hampshire

Rivier University, Division of Nursing, *Nashua (BS)*

New York

College of Mount Saint Vincent, Department of Nursing, *Riverdale (BS)*

Molloy College, Division of Nursing, *Rockville Centre (BS)*

Nyack College, School of Nursing, *Nyack (BS)*

North Dakota

Dickinson State University, Department of Nursing, *Dickinson (BSN)*

Ohio

Lourdes University, School of Nursing, *Sylvania (BSN)*

Oklahoma

Northwestern Oklahoma State University, Division of Nursing, *Alva (BSN)*

Oklahoma Baptist University, School of Nursing, *Shawnee (BSN)*

University of Oklahoma Health Sciences Center, College of Nursing, *Oklahoma City (BSN)*

The University of Tulsa, School of Nursing, *Tulsa (BSN)*

Pennsylvania

Alvernia University, Nursing, *Reading (BSN)*

Bloomsburg University of Pennsylvania, Department of Nursing, *Bloomsburg (BSN)*

La Roche College, Department of Nursing and Nursing Management, *Pittsburgh (BSN)*

Mount Aloysius College, Division of Nursing, *Cresson (BSN)*

Neumann University, Program in Nursing and Health Sciences, *Aston (BS)*

The University of Scranton, Department of Nursing, *Scranton (BSN)*

Wilkes University, Department of Nursing, *Wilkes-Barre (BS)*

South Dakota

Mount Marty College, Nursing Program, *Yankton (BSN)*

Presentation College, Department of Nursing, *Aberdeen (BSN)*

Tennessee

Belmont University, School of Nursing, *Nashville (BSN)*

Middle Tennessee State University, School of Nursing, *Murfreesboro (BSN)*

Milligan College, Department of Nursing, *Milligan College (BSN)*

The University of Tennessee at Martin, Department of Nursing, *Martin (BSN)*

Texas

Sam Houston State University, Nursing Program, *Huntsville (BSN)*

Southwestern Adventist University, Department of Nursing, *Keene (BS)*

The University of Texas at Tyler, Program in Nursing, *Tyler (BSN)*

Utah

Western Governors University, Online College of Health Professions, *Salt Lake City (BS)*

Virginia

Hampton University, School of Nursing, *Hampton (BS)*

West Virginia

Alderson Broaddus University, Department of Nursing, *Philippi (BSN)*

Wisconsin

Concordia University Wisconsin, Program in Nursing, *Mequon (BSN)*

CANADA

Alberta

Athabasca University, Centre for Nursing and Health Studies, *Athabasca (BN)*

British Columbia

Vancouver Island University, Department of Nursing, *Nanaimo (BScN)*

RN BACCALAUREATE

U.S. AND U.S. TERRITORIES

Alabama

Auburn University at Montgomery, School of Nursing, *Montgomery (BSN)*

Jacksonville State University, College of Nursing and Health Sciences, *Jacksonville (BSN)*

Oakwood University, Department of Nursing, *Huntsville (BS)*

Troy University, School of Nursing, *Troy (BSN)*

Tuskegee University, Program in Nursing, *Tuskegee (BSN)*

The University of Alabama, Capstone College of Nursing, *Tuscaloosa (BSN)*

The University of Alabama at Birmingham, School of Nursing, *Birmingham (BSN)*

The University of Alabama in Huntsville, College of Nursing, *Huntsville (BSN)*

University of Mobile, School of Nursing, *Mobile (BSN)*

University of North Alabama, College of Nursing and Allied Health, *Florence (BSN)*

University of South Alabama, College of Nursing, *Mobile (BSN)*

Alaska

University of Alaska Anchorage, School of Nursing, *Anchorage (BS)*

Arizona

Arizona State University at the Downtown Phoenix campus, College of Nursing, *Phoenix (BSN)*

Chamberlain College of Nursing, *Phoenix (BSN)*

Grand Canyon University, College of Nursing and Health Sciences, *Phoenix (BSN)*

Northern Arizona University, School of Nursing, *Flagstaff (BSN)*

Arkansas

Arkansas State University, Department of Nursing, *State University (BSN)*

Arkansas Tech University, Program in Nursing, *Russellville (BSN)*

Southern Arkansas University–Magnolia, Department of Nursing, *Magnolia (BSN)*

University of Arkansas, Eleanor Mann School of Nursing, *Fayetteville (BSN)*

University of Arkansas at Little Rock, BSN Programs, *Little Rock (BSN)*

University of Arkansas at Monticello, School of Nursing, *Monticello (BSN)*

University of Arkansas for Medical Sciences, College of Nursing, *Little Rock (BSN)*

University of Central Arkansas, Department of Nursing, *Conway (BSN)*

California

Biola University, Department of Nursing, *La Mirada (BSN)*

Brandman University, School of Nursing and Health Professions, *Irvine (BSN)*

California Baptist University, School of Nursing, *Riverside (BSN)*

California State University Channel Islands, Nursing Program, *Camarillo (BSN)*

California State University, Chico, School of Nursing, *Chico (BSN)*

California State University, Dominguez Hills, Program in Nursing, *Carson (BSN)*

California State University, Fullerton, Department of Nursing, *Fullerton (BSN)*

California State University, Los Angeles, School of Nursing, *Los Angeles (BSN)*

California State University, San Bernardino, Department of Nursing, *San Bernardino (BSN)*

Dominican University of California, Program in Nursing, *San Rafael (BSN)*

Fresno Pacific University, RN to BSN Program, *Fresno (BSN)*

Holy Names University, Department of Nursing, *Oakland (BSN)*

Loma Linda University, School of Nursing, *Loma Linda (BS)*

National University, Department of Nursing, *La Jolla (BSN)*

Pacific College, Bachelor of Science in Nursing, *Costa Mesa (BSN)*

Point Loma Nazarene University, School of Nursing, *San Diego (BSN)*

San Diego State University, School of Nursing, *San Diego (BSN)*

San Francisco State University, School of Nursing, *San Francisco (BSN)*

Stanbridge College, Nursing Program, *Irvine (BSN)*

United States University, School of Nursing, *Chula Vista (BSN)*

University of Phoenix–Central Valley Campus, College of Health and Human Services, *Fresno (BSN)*

Vanguard University of Southern California, Nursing Program, *Costa Mesa (BSN)*

Colorado

Adams State University, Nursing Program, *Alamosa (BSN)*

American Sentinel University, RN to Bachelor of Science Nursing, *Aurora (BSN)*

Colorado Christian University, Nursing Programs, *Lakewood (BSN)*

Colorado Mesa University, Department of Nursing and Radiologic Sciences, *Grand Junction (BSN)*

Colorado State University–Pueblo, Department of Nursing, *Pueblo (BSN)*

Colorado Technical University Online, Nursing Program, *Colorado Springs (BSN)*

Denver School of Nursing, *Denver (BSN)*

Regis University, School of Nursing, *Denver (BSN)*

University of Colorado Colorado Springs, Helen and Arthur E. Johnson Beth-El College of Nursing & Health Sciences, *Colorado Springs (BSN)*

University of Colorado Denver, College of Nursing, *Aurora (BS)*

University of Northern Colorado, School of Nursing, *Greeley (BS)*

Connecticut

Central Connecticut State University, Department of Nursing, *New Britain (BSN)*

Fairfield University, School of Nursing, *Fairfield (BSN)*

Quinnipiac University, School of Nursing, *Hamden (BSN)*

Sacred Heart University, College of Nursing, *Fairfield (BSN)*

Southern Connecticut State University, Department of Nursing, *New Haven (BSN)*

University of Hartford, College of Education, Nursing, and Health Professions, *West Hartford (BSN)*

University of Saint Joseph, Department of Nursing, *West Hartford (BS)*

Western Connecticut State University, Department of Nursing, *Danbury (BS)*

Delaware

Delaware State University, Department of Nursing, *Dover (BSN)*

University of Delaware, School of Nursing, *Newark (BSN)*

Wilmington University, College of Health Professions, *New Castle (BSN)*

District of Columbia

Howard University, Division of Nursing, *Washington (BSN)*

Trinity Washington University, Nursing Program, *Washington (BSN)*

University of the District of Columbia, Nursing Education Program, *Washington (BSN)*

Florida

Adventist University of Health Sciences, Department of Nursing, *Orlando (BSN)*

Barry University, Division of Nursing, *Miami Shores (BSN)*

Bethune-Cookman University, School of Nursing, *Daytona Beach (BSN)*

Broward College, Nursing Program, *Fort Lauderdale (BSN)*

Chipola College, School of Health Sciences, *Marianna (BSN)*

Florida Atlantic University, Christine E. Lynn College of Nursing, *Boca Raton (BSN)*

Florida International University, Nursing Program, *Miami (BSN)*

Florida National University, Nursing Division, *Hialeah (BSN)*

Florida Southern College, School of Nursing & Health Sciences, *Lakeland (BSN)*

Florida SouthWestern State College, Bachelor of Science in Nursing Program, *Fort Myers (BSN)*

Florida State College at Jacksonville, Nursing Department, *Jacksonville (BSN)*

Fortis College, Nursing Department, *Cutler Bay (BSN)*

Gulf Coast State College, Nursing Program, *Panama City (BSN)*

Herzing University, Nursing Program, *Winter Park (BSN)*

Indian River State College, Bachelor of Science in Nursing Program, *Fort Pierce (BSN)*

Keiser University, Nursing Programs, *Fort Lauderdale (BSN)*

Keiser University, Nursing Programs, *Fort Myers (BSN)*

Keiser University, Nursing Programs, *Jacksonville (BSN)*

Keiser University, Nursing Programs, *Lakeland (BSN)*

Keiser University, Nursing Programs, *Melbourne (BSN)*

Keiser University, Nursing Programs, *Miami (BSN)*

Keiser University, Nursing Programs, *Orlando (BSN)*

Keiser University, Nursing Programs, *Port St. Lucie (BSN)*

Keiser University, Nursing Programs, *Sarasota (BSN)*

Keiser University, Nursing Programs, *Tallahassee (BSN)*

Keiser University, Nursing Programs, *Tampa (BSN)*

Miami Dade College, School of Nursing, *Miami (BSN)*

Nova Southeastern University, College of Health Care Sciences, *Fort Lauderdale (BSN)*

Polk State College, RN to BSN Program, *Winter Haven (BSN)*

St. Petersburg College, Department of Nursing, *St. Petersburg (BSN)*

Santa Fe College, Bachelor of Science in Nursing, *Gainesville (BSN)*

State College of Florida Manatee-Sarasota, Nursing Degree Program, *Bradenton (BSN)*

University of Central Florida, College of Nursing, *Orlando (BSN)*

University of Miami, School of Nursing and Health Studies, *Coral Gables (BSN)*

University of North Florida, School of Nursing, *Jacksonville (BSN)*

University of Phoenix–South Florida Campus, College of Nursing, *Miramar (BSN)*

University of West Florida, Department of Nursing, *Pensacola (BSN)*

Georgia

Armstrong State University, Program in Nursing, *Savannah (BSN)*

Brenau University, College of Health and Science, *Gainesville (BSN)*

Clayton State University, Department of Nursing, *Morrow (BSN)*

College of Coastal Georgia, Department of Nursing and Health Sciences, *Brunswick (BSN)*

Columbus State University, Nursing Program, *Columbus (BSN)*

Dalton State College, Department of Nursing, *Dalton (BSN)*

Darton State College, Division of Nursing, *Albany (BSN)*

Georgia College & State University, College of Health Sciences, *Milledgeville (BSN)*

Georgia Highlands College, RN-BSN Online Completion Program, *Rome (BSN)*

Georgia Southwestern State University, School of Nursing, *Americus (BSN)*

Gordon State College, Division of Nursing and Health Sciences, *Barnesville (BSN)*

Herzing University, Nursing Program, *Atlanta (BSN)*

Kennesaw State University, School of Nursing, *Kennesaw (BSN)*

LaGrange College, Department of Nursing, *LaGrange (BSN)*

Mercer University, Georgia Baptist College of Nursing of Mercer University, *Atlanta (BSN)*

Piedmont College, School of Nursing, *Demorest (BSN)*

Thomas University, Division of Nursing, *Thomasville (BSN)*

University of North Georgia, Department of Nursing, *Dahlonega (BSN)*

Valdosta State University, College of Nursing, *Valdosta (BSN)*

Guam

University of Guam, School of Nursing and Health Sciences, *Mangilao (BSN)*

Hawaii

Hawai`i Pacific University, College of Nursing and Health Sciences, *Honolulu (BSN)*

University of Hawaii at Hilo, Department in Nursing, *Hilo (BSN)*

University of Hawaii at Manoa, School of Nursing and Dental Hygiene, *Honolulu (BSN)*

Idaho

Boise State University, Department of Nursing, *Boise (BS)*

Brigham Young University–Idaho, Department of Nursing, *Rexburg (BSN)*

Illinois

Aurora University, School of Nursing, *Aurora (BSN)*

Blessing–Rieman College of Nursing and Health Sciences, *Quincy (BSN)*

Bradley University, Department of Nursing, *Peoria (BSN, BSc PN)*

Chicago State University, Department of Nursing, *Chicago (BSN)*

Elmhurst College, Deicke Center for Nursing Education, *Elmhurst (BS)*

Governors State University, College of Health and Human Services, *University Park (BS)*

Illinois State University, Mennonite College of Nursing, *Normal (BSN)*

Lakeview College of Nursing, *Danville (BSN)*

Loyola University Chicago, Marcella Niehoff School of Nursing, *Maywood (BSN)*

Methodist College, *Peoria (BSN)*

Millikin University, School of Nursing, *Decatur (BSN)*

Northern Illinois University, School of Nursing and Health Studies, *De Kalb (BS)*

North Park University, School of Nursing, *Chicago (BS)*

Olivet Nazarene University, Division of Nursing, *Bourbonnais (BSN)*

Resurrection University, *Chicago (BSN)*

Rockford University, Department of Nursing, *Rockford (BSN)*

Saint Anthony College of Nursing, *Rockford (BSN)*

Saint Francis Medical Center College of Nursing, Baccalaureate Nursing Program, *Peoria (BSN)*

Trinity College of Nursing and Health Sciences, *Rock Island (BSN)*

University of Illinois at Chicago, College of Nursing, *Chicago (BSN)*

Western Illinois University, School of Nursing, *Macomb (BSN)*

Indiana

Bethel College, School of Nursing, *Mishawaka (BSN)*

Goshen College, Department of Nursing, *Goshen (BSN)*

Harrison College, RN to BSN Program, *Indianapolis (BSN)*

Indiana State University, Department of Advanced Practice Nursing, *Terre Haute (BS)*

Indiana University Bloomington, Department of Nursing–Bloomington Division, *Bloomington (BSN)*

Indiana University East, School of Nursing, *Richmond (BSN)*

Indiana University Northwest, School of Nursing, *Gary (BSN)*

Indiana University–Purdue University Fort Wayne, Department of Nursing, *Fort Wayne (BS)*

Indiana University South Bend, Vera Z. Dwyer College of Health Sciences, *South Bend (BSN)*

Indiana University Southeast, School of Nursing, *New Albany (BSN)*

Indiana Wesleyan University, School of Nursing, *Marion (BSN)*

Marian University, School of Nursing, *Indianapolis (BSN)*

Purdue University, School of Nursing, *West Lafayette (BS)*

Purdue University North Central, Department of Nursing, *Westville (BS)*

Saint Joseph's College, St. Elizabeth School of Nursing, *Rensselaer (BSN)*

University of Evansville, Department of Nursing, *Evansville (BSN)*

University of Indianapolis, School of Nursing, *Indianapolis (BSN)*

University of Saint Francis, Department of Nursing, *Fort Wayne (BSN)*

University of Southern Indiana, College of Nursing and Health Professions, *Evansville (BSN)*

Valparaiso University, College of Nursing and Health Professions, *Valparaiso (BSN)*

Vincennes University, Department of Nursing, *Vincennes (BSN)*

Iowa

Allen College, Graduate Programs, *Waterloo (BSN)*

Briar Cliff University, Department of Nursing, *Sioux City (BSN)*

Clarke University, Department of Nursing and Health, *Dubuque (BSN)*

Grand View University, Division of Nursing, *Des Moines (BSN)*

Iowa Wesleyan College, Division of Nursing, *Mount Pleasant (BSN)*

St. Ambrose University, Program in Nursing (BSN), *Davenport (BSN)*

University of Dubuque, School of Professional Programs, *Dubuque (BSN)*

The University of Iowa, College of Nursing, *Iowa City (BSN)*

Upper Iowa University, RN-BSN Nursing Program, *Fayette (BSN)*

Kansas

Bethel College, Department of Nursing, *North Newton (BSN)*

Emporia State University, Newman Division of Nursing, *Emporia (BSN)*

Fort Hays State University, Department of Nursing, *Hays (BSN)*

Kansas Wesleyan University, Department of Nursing Education, *Salina (BSN)*

MidAmerica Nazarene University, Division of Nursing, *Olathe (BSN)*

Newman University, Division of Nursing, *Wichita (BSN)*

Ottawa University–Kansas City, Nursing Program, *Overland Park (BSN)*

Pittsburg State University, Department of Nursing, *Pittsburg (BSN)*

The University of Kansas, School of Nursing, *Kansas City (BSN)*

University of Saint Mary, Bachelor of Science in Nursing Program, *Leavenworth (BSN)*

Washburn University, School of Nursing, *Topeka (BSN)*

Wichita State University, School of Nursing, *Wichita (BSN)*

Kentucky

Bellarmine University, Donna and Allan Lansing School of Nursing and Health Sciences, *Louisville (BSN, MSCE)*

Eastern Kentucky University, Department of Baccalaureate and Graduate Nursing, *Richmond (BSN)*

Lindsey Wilson College, Nursing Division, *Columbia (BSN)*

Midway University, Program in Nursing (Baccalaureate), *Midway (BSN)*

Morehead State University, Department of Nursing, *Morehead (BSN)*

Murray State University, Program in Nursing, *Murray (BSN)*

Northern Kentucky University, Department of Nursing, *Highland Heights (BSN)*

Spalding University, School of Nursing, *Louisville (BSN)*

University of Kentucky, College of Nursing, *Lexington (BSN)*

University of Louisville, School of Nursing, *Louisville (BSN)*

University of Pikeville, RN to BSN Completion Program, *Pikeville (BSN)*

Western Kentucky University, School of Nursing, *Bowling Green (BSN)*

Louisiana

Dillard University, Division of Nursing, *New Orleans (BSN)*

Grambling State University, School of Nursing, *Grambling (BSN)*

Louisiana State University at Alexandria, Nursing Program, *Alexandria (BSN)*

Louisiana State University Health Sciences Center, School of Nursing, *New Orleans (BSN)*

Loyola University New Orleans, School of Nursing, *New Orleans (BSN)*

Nicholls State University, Department of Nursing, *Thibodaux (BSN)*

Northwestern State University of Louisiana, College of Nursing and School of Allied Health, *Shreveport (BSN)*

Our Lady of the Lake College, Division of Nursing, *Baton Rouge (BSN)*

Southeastern Louisiana University, School of Nursing, *Hammond (BS)*

University of Louisiana at Monroe, Nursing, *Monroe (BS)*

Maine

Saint Joseph's College of Maine, Master of Science in Nursing Program, *Standish (BSN)*

University of Maine, School of Nursing, *Orono (BSN)*

University of Maine at Augusta, Nursing Programs, *Augusta (BSN)*

University of Maine at Fort Kent, Department of Nursing, *Fort Kent (BSN)*

University of New England, Department of Nursing, *Biddeford (BSN)*

University of Southern Maine, School of Nursing, *Portland (BS)*

Maryland

Bowie State University, Department of Nursing, *Bowie (BSN)*

Coppin State University, Helene Fuld School of Nursing, *Baltimore (BSN)*

Frostburg State University, Nursing Department, *Frostburg (BSN)*

Hood College, BSN Completion Program, *Frederick (BSN)*

Morgan State University, Bachelor of Science in Nursing, *Baltimore (BS)*

Notre Dame of Maryland University, Department of Nursing, *Baltimore (BS)*

Salisbury University, Department of Nursing, *Salisbury (BS)*

Stevenson University, Nursing Division, *Stevenson (BS)*

Towson University, Department of Nursing, *Towson (BS)*

University of Maryland, Baltimore, Nursing Programs, *Baltimore (BSN)*

Massachusetts

American International College, Division of Nursing, *Springfield (BSN)*

Anna Maria College, Department of Nursing, *Paxton (BSN)*

Becker College, Nursing Programs, *Worcester (BSN)*

Curry College, Division of Nursing, *Milton (BS)*

Elms College, School of Nursing, *Chicopee (BS)*

Emmanuel College, Department of Nursing, *Boston (BS)*

Endicott College, Major in Nursing, *Beverly (BS)*

Fitchburg State University, Department of Nursing, *Fitchburg (BS)*

Northeastern University, School of Nursing, *Boston (BSN)*

Regis College, School of Nursing, Science and Health Professions, *Weston (BSN)*

Simmons College, School of Nursing and Health Sciences, *Boston (BS)*

University of Massachusetts Boston, College of Nursing and Health Sciences, *Boston (BS)*

University of Massachusetts Dartmouth, College of Nursing, *North Dartmouth (BS)*

University of Massachusetts Lowell, School of Nursing, *Lowell (BS)*

Worcester State University, Department of Nursing, *Worcester (BS)*

Michigan

Davenport University, Division of Nursing, *Grand Rapids (BSN)*

Davenport University, Bachelor of Science in Nursing Program, *Kalamazoo (BSN)*

Eastern Michigan University, School of Nursing, *Ypsilanti (BSN)*

Ferris State University, School of Nursing, *Big Rapids (BSN)*

Finlandia University, College of Professional Studies, *Hancock (BSN)*

Grand Valley State University, Kirkhof College of Nursing, *Allendale (BSN)*

Lake Superior State University, Department of Nursing, *Sault Sainte Marie (BSN)*

Madonna University, College of Nursing and Health, *Livonia (BSN)*

Michigan State University, College of Nursing, *East Lansing (BSN)*

Northern Michigan University, College of Nursing and Allied Health Science, *Marquette (BSN)*

Rochester College, School of Nursing, *Rochester Hills (BSN)*

Saginaw Valley State University, College of Health and Human Services, *University Center (BSN)*

Siena Heights University, Nursing Program, *Adrian (BSN)*

University of Detroit Mercy, McAuley School of Nursing, *Detroit (BSN)*

University of Michigan, School of Nursing, *Ann Arbor (BSN)*

University of Michigan–Flint, Department of Nursing, *Flint (BSN)*

Wayne State University, College of Nursing, *Detroit (BSN)*

Minnesota

Bemidji State University, Department of Nursing, *Bemidji (BS)*

Bethel University, Department of Nursing, *St. Paul (BSN)*

Capella University, Nursing Programs, *Minneapolis (BSN)*

Metropolitan State University, College of Health, Community and Professional Studies, *St. Paul (BSN)*

Minnesota State University Mankato, School of Nursing, *Mankato (BS)*

Minnesota State University Moorhead, School of Nursing and Healthcare Leadership, *Moorhead (BSN)*

Rasmussen College Bloomington, School of Nursing, *Bloomington (BSN)*

St. Catherine University, Department of Nursing, *St. Paul (BS)*

Saint Mary's University of Minnesota, B.S. in Nursing, *Winona (BS)*

Walden University, Nursing Programs, *Minneapolis (BSN)*

Winona State University, College of Nursing and Health Sciences, *Winona (BS)*

Mississippi

Alcorn State University, School of Nursing, *Natchez (BSN)*

Mississippi College, School of Nursing, *Clinton (BSN)*

Missouri

Avila University, School of Nursing, *Kansas City (BSN)*

Chamberlain College of Nursing, *St. Louis (BSN)*

Cox College, Department of Nursing, *Springfield (BSN)*

Goldfarb School of Nursing at Barnes-Jewish College, *St. Louis (BSN)*

Graceland University, School of Nursing, *Independence (BSN)*

Hannibal-LaGrange University, Division of Nursing and Allied Health, *Hannibal (BSN)*

Lincoln University, Department of Nursing, *Jefferson City (BSN)*

Maryville University of Saint Louis, The Catherine McAuley School of Nursing, College of Health Professions, *St. Louis (BSN)*

Missouri Southern State University, Department of Nursing, *Joplin (BSN)*

Missouri State University, Department of Nursing, *Springfield (BSN)*

Saint Louis University, School of Nursing, *St. Louis (BSN)*

Southeast Missouri State University, Department of Nursing, *Cape Girardeau (BSN)*

Southwest Baptist University, College of Nursing, *Bolivar (BSN)*

University of Central Missouri, Department of Nursing, *Warrensburg (BS)*

University of Missouri, Sinclair School of Nursing, *Columbia (BSN)*

University of Missouri–Kansas City, School of Nursing and Health Studies, *Kansas City (BSN)*

University of Missouri–St. Louis, College of Nursing, *St. Louis (BSN)*

Webster University, Department of Nursing, *St. Louis (BSN)*

William Jewell College, Department of Nursing, *Liberty (BS)*

Montana

Montana State University–Northern, College of Nursing, *Havre (BSN)*

Montana Tech of The University of Montana, Bachelor of Science in Registered Nursing, *Butte (BS)*

Salish Kootenai College, Nursing Department, *Pablo (BS)*

Nebraska

Bryan College of Health Sciences, School of Nursing, *Lincoln (BSN)*

Clarkson College, Master of Science in Nursing Program, *Omaha (BSN)*

Doane College, Nursing Program, *Crete (BSN)*

Midland University, Department of Nursing, *Fremont (BSN)*

Nebraska Methodist College, Department of Nursing, *Omaha (BSN)*

University of Nebraska Medical Center, College of Nursing, *Omaha (BSN)*

Nevada

Great Basin College, BSN Program, *Elko (BSN)*

Nevada State College at Henderson, Nursing Program, *Henderson (BSN)*

Roseman University of Health Sciences, College of Nursing, *Henderson (BSN)*

Touro University, School of Nursing, *Henderson (BSN)*

University of Nevada, Reno, Orvis School of Nursing, *Reno (BSN)*

New Hampshire

Franklin Pierce University, Master of Science in Nursing, *Rindge (BS)*

Granite State College, Nursing Department, *Concord (BSN)*

Keene State College, Nursing Program, *Keene (BS)*

Plymouth State University, RN-BS Completion Program, *Plymouth (BS)*

Rivier University, Division of Nursing, *Nashua (BS)*

Saint Anselm College, Department of Nursing, *Manchester (BSN)*

New Jersey

Bloomfield College, Division of Nursing, *Bloomfield (BS)*

Caldwell University, Nursing Programs, *Caldwell (BSN)*

The College of New Jersey, School of Nursing, Health and Exercise Science, *Ewing (BSN)*

College of Saint Elizabeth, Department of Nursing, *Morristown (BSN)*

Fairleigh Dickinson University, Metropolitan Campus, Henry P. Becton School of Nursing and Allied Health, *Teaneck (BSN)*

Kean University, Department of Nursing, *Union (BSN)*

Monmouth University, Marjorie K. Unterberg School of Nursing, *West Long Branch (BSN)*

New Jersey City University, Department of Nursing, *Jersey City (BSN)*

Ramapo College of New Jersey, Master of Science in Nursing Program, *Mahwah (BSN)*

Rider University, RN-BSN Program, *Lawrenceville (BSN)*

Rowan University, RN to BSN Program, *Glassboro (BSN)*

Rutgers, The State University of New Jersey, Camden, Rutgers School of Nursing–Camden, *Camden (BS)*

Rutgers, The State University of New Jersey, Newark, Rutgers School of Nursing, *Newark (BSN)*

Saint Peter's University, Nursing Program, *Jersey City (BSN)*

Seton Hall University, College of Nursing, *South Orange (BSN)*

Stockton University, Program in Nursing, *Galloway (BSN)*

William Paterson University of New Jersey, Department of Nursing, *Wayne (BSN)*

New Mexico

New Mexico State University, School of Nursing, *Las Cruces (BSN)*

Northern New Mexico College, College of Nursing and Health Sciences, *Espanola (BSN)*

University of New Mexico, Program in Nursing, *Albuquerque (BSN)*

New York

Adelphi University, College of Nursing and Public Health, *Garden City (BS)*

The College of New Rochelle, School of Nursing, *New Rochelle (BSN)*

College of Staten Island of the City University of New York, Department of Nursing, *Staten Island (BS)*

Daemen College, Department of Nursing, *Amherst (BS)*

Dominican College, Department of Nursing, *Orangeburg (BSN)*

D'Youville College, School of Nursing, *Buffalo (BSN)*

Elmira College, Program in Nursing Education, *Elmira (BS)*

Excelsior College, School of Nursing, *Albany (BS)*

Farmingdale State College, Nursing Department, *Farmingdale (BS)*

Hartwick College, Department of Nursing, *Oneonta (BS)*

Helene Fuld College of Nursing, RN to BSN Program, *New York (BS)*

Hunter College of the City University of New York, Hunter-Bellevue School of Nursing, *New York (BS)*

Lehman College of the City University of New York, Department of Nursing, *Bronx (BS)*

Le Moyne College, Nursing Programs, *Syracuse (BS)*

Long Island University–LIU Post, Department of Nursing, *Brookville (BS)*

Maria College, RN Baccalaureate Completion Program, *Albany (BSN)*

Mercy College, Programs in Nursing, *Dobbs Ferry (BS)*

Molloy College, Division of Nursing, *Rockville Centre (BS)*

Mount Saint Mary College, School of Nursing, *Newburgh (BSN)*

Nazareth College of Rochester, Department of Nursing, *Rochester (BS)*

New York City College of Technology of the City University of New York, Department of Nursing, *Brooklyn (BS)*

New York University, College of Nursing, *New York (BS)*

Niagara University, Department of Nursing, *Niagara University (BS)*

Nyack College, School of Nursing, *Nyack (BS)*

Pace University, Lienhard School of Nursing, *New York (BS)*

Roberts Wesleyan College, School of Nursing, *Rochester (BScN)*

The Sage Colleges, Department of Nursing, *Troy (BS)*

St. Francis College, Department of Nursing, *Brooklyn Heights (BS)*

St. John Fisher College, Wegmans School of Nursing, *Rochester (BS)*

St. Joseph's College, New York, Department of Nursing, *Brooklyn (BSN)*

State University of New York at Plattsburgh, Department of Nursing, *Plattsburgh (BS)*

State University of New York College of Technology at Canton, Nursing Program, *Canton (BS)*

State University of New York College of Technology at Delhi, Bachelor of Science in Nursing Program, *Delhi (BSN)*

State University of New York Downstate Medical Center, College of Nursing, *Brooklyn (BS)*

State University of New York Empire State College, Bachelor of Science in Nursing Program, *Saratoga Springs (BS)*

State University of New York Polytechnic Institute, School of Nursing and Health Systems, *Utica (BS)*

Stony Brook University, State University of New York, School of Nursing, *Stony Brook (BS)*

University at Buffalo, the State University of New York, School of Nursing, *Buffalo (BS)*

University of Rochester, School of Nursing, *Rochester (BS)*

Utica College, Department of Nursing, *Utica (BS)*

York College of the City University of New York, Program in Nursing, *Jamaica (BS)*

North Carolina

Appalachian State University, Department of Nursing, *Boone (BSN)*

Barton College, School of Nursing, *Wilson (BSN)*

Cabarrus College of Health Sciences, Louise Harkey School of Nursing, *Concord (BSN)*

Fayetteville State University, Program in Nursing, *Fayetteville (BSN)*

Methodist University, Department of Nursing, *Fayetteville (BSN)*

North Carolina Agricultural and Technical State University, School of Nursing, *Greensboro (BSN)*

Pfeiffer University, Department of Nursing, *Misenheimer (BS)*

Queens University of Charlotte, Presbyterian School of Nursing, *Charlotte (BSN)*

University of Mount Olive, Department of Nursing, *Mount Olive (BSN)*

The University of North Carolina at Charlotte, School of Nursing, *Charlotte (BSN)*

The University of North Carolina at Greensboro, School of Nursing, *Greensboro (BSN)*

The University of North Carolina at Pembroke, Nursing Program, *Pembroke (BSN)*

The University of North Carolina Wilmington, School of Nursing, *Wilmington (BS)*

Western Carolina University, School of Nursing, *Cullowhee (BSN)*

Wingate University, Department of Nursing, *Wingate (BSN)*

Winston-Salem State University, Department of Nursing, *Winston-Salem (BSN)*

North Dakota

Dickinson State University, Department of Nursing, *Dickinson (BSN)*

Minot State University, Department of Nursing, *Minot (BSN)*

Ohio

Ashland University, Dwight Schar College of Nursing and Health Sciences, *Ashland (BSN)*

Capital University, School of Nursing, *Columbus (BSN)*

Cedarville University, School of Nursing, *Cedarville (BSN)*

Chamberlain College of Nursing, *Columbus (BSN)*

The Christ College of Nursing and Health Sciences, Department of Nursing, *Cincinnati (BSN)*

Cleveland State University, School of Nursing, *Cleveland (BSN)*

Defiance College, Bachelor's Degree in Nursing, *Defiance (BSN)*

Fortis College, School of Nursing, *Centerville (BSN)*

Franciscan University of Steubenville, Department of Nursing, *Steubenville (BSN)*

Good Samaritan College of Nursing and Health Science, Nursing Program, *Cincinnati (BSN)*

Kent State University, College of Nursing, *Kent (BSN)*

Kettering College, Division of Nursing, *Kettering (BSN)*

Lourdes University, School of Nursing, *Sylvania (BSN)*

Malone University, School of Nursing, *Canton (BSN)*

Mercy College of Ohio, Division of Nursing, *Toledo (BSN)*

Miami University, Department of Nursing, *Hamilton (BSN)*

Miami University Hamilton, Bachelor of Science in Nursing Program, *Hamilton (BSN)*

Mount Carmel College of Nursing, Nursing Programs, *Columbus (BSN)*

Notre Dame College, Nursing Department, *South Euclid (BSN)*

Ohio Northern University, Nursing Program, *Ada (BSN)*

The Ohio State University, College of Nursing, *Columbus (BSN)*

Ohio University, School of Nursing, *Athens (BSN)*

Otterbein University, Department of Nursing, *Westerville (BSN)*

Shawnee State University, Department of Nursing, *Portsmouth (BSN)*

University of Cincinnati, College of Nursing, *Cincinnati (BSN)*

University of Rio Grande, Holzer School of Nursing, *Rio Grande (BSN)*

The University of Toledo, College of Nursing, *Toledo (BSN)*

Ursuline College, The Breen School of Nursing, *Pepper Pike (BSN)*

Walsh University, Department of Nursing, *North Canton (BSN)*

Wright State University, College of Nursing and Health, *Dayton (BSN)*

Youngstown State University, Department of Nursing, *Youngstown (BSN)*

Oklahoma

Langston University, School of Nursing and Health Professions, *Langston (BSN)*

Northeastern State University, Department of Nursing, *Tahlequah (BSN)*

Northwestern Oklahoma State University, Division of Nursing, *Alva (BSN)*

Oklahoma Baptist University, School of Nursing, *Shawnee (BSN)*

Oklahoma City University, Kramer School of Nursing, *Oklahoma City (BSN)*

Oklahoma Wesleyan University, School of Nursing, *Bartlesville (BSN)*

Oral Roberts University, Anna Vaughn School of Nursing, *Tulsa (BSN)*

Southwestern Oklahoma State University, School of Nursing, *Weatherford (BSN)*

University of Central Oklahoma, Department of Nursing, *Edmond (BSN)*

The University of Tulsa, School of Nursing, *Tulsa (BSN)*

Oregon

Linfield College, School of Nursing, *McMinnville (BSN)*

Oregon Health & Science University, School of Nursing, *Portland (BS)*

Pennsylvania

Alvernia University, Nursing, *Reading (BSN)*

California University of Pennsylvania, Department of Nursing, *California (BSN)*

Carlow University, College of Health and Wellness, *Pittsburgh (BSN)*

Cedar Crest College, Department of Nursing, *Allentown (BS)*

Chatham University, Nursing Programs, *Pittsburgh (BSN)*

Clarion University of Pennsylvania, School of Nursing, *Oil City (BSN)*

DeSales University, Department of Nursing and Health, *Center Valley (BSN)*

Drexel University, College of Nursing and Health Professions, *Philadelphia (BSN)*

East Stroudsburg University of Pennsylvania, Department of Nursing, *East Stroudsburg (BS)*

Gannon University, Villa Maria School of Nursing, *Erie (BSN)*

Gwynedd Mercy University, Frances M. Maguire School of Nursing and Health Professions, *Gwynedd Valley (BSN)*

Immaculata University, Division of Nursing, *Immaculata (BSN)*

La Roche College, Department of Nursing and Nursing Management, *Pittsburgh (BSN)*

La Salle University, School of Nursing and Health Sciences, *Philadelphia (BSN)*

Lock Haven University of Pennsylvania, Nursing Program, *Lock Haven (BSN)*

Mansfield University of Pennsylvania, Department of Health Sciences–Nursing, *Mansfield (BSN)*

Marywood University, Department of Nursing, *Scranton (BSN)*

Millersville University of Pennsylvania, Department of Nursing, *Millersville (BSN)*

Misericordia University, Department of Nursing, *Dallas (BSN)*

Moravian College, Department of Nursing, *Bethlehem (BSN)*

Mount Aloysius College, Division of Nursing, *Cresson (BSN)*

Penn State University Park, School of Nursing, *University Park (BS)*

Pennsylvania College of Health Sciences, Bachelor of Science in Nursing Program, *Lancaster (BSN)*

Pennsylvania College of Technology, School of Health Sciences, *Williamsport (BSN)*

Robert Morris University, School of Nursing and Health Sciences, *Moon Township (BSN)*

Slippery Rock University of Pennsylvania, Department of Nursing, *Slippery Rock (BSN)*

Temple University, Department of Nursing, *Philadelphia (BSN)*

Thomas Jefferson University, Department of Nursing, *Philadelphia (BSN)*

University of Pittsburgh, School of Nursing, *Pittsburgh (BSN)*

University of Pittsburgh at Bradford, Department of Nursing, *Bradford (BSN)*

The University of Scranton, Department of Nursing, *Scranton (BSN)*

Villanova University, College of Nursing, *Villanova (BSN)*

West Chester University of Pennsylvania, Department of Nursing, *West Chester (BSN)*

Widener University, School of Nursing, *Chester (BSN)*

Wilkes University, Department of Nursing, *Wilkes-Barre (BS)*

York College of Pennsylvania, Department of Nursing, *York (BS)*

Puerto Rico

Inter American University of Puerto Rico, Aguadilla Campus, Nursing Program, *Aguadilla (BSN)*

Universidad Adventista de las Antillas, Department of Nursing, *Mayagüez (BSN)*

Rhode Island

New England Institute of Technology, Nursing Department, *East Greenwich (BSN)*

Rhode Island College, Department of Nursing, *Providence (BSN)*

Salve Regina University, Department of Nursing, *Newport (BS)*

University of Rhode Island, College of Nursing, *Kingston (BS)*

South Carolina

Charleston Southern University, Wingo School of Nursing, *Charleston (BSN)*

Clemson University, School of Nursing, *Clemson (BS)*

Coastal Carolina University, Nursing Completion Program, *Conway (BSN)*

Lander University, School of Nursing, *Greenwood (BSN)*

University of South Carolina Aiken, School of Nursing, *Aiken (BSN)*

University of South Carolina Beaufort, Nursing Program, *Bluffton (BSN)*

University of South Carolina Upstate, Mary Black School of Nursing, *Spartanburg (BSN)*

South Dakota

Dakota Wesleyan University, The Arlene Gates Department of Nursing, *Mitchell (BSN)*

Mount Marty College, Nursing Program, *Yankton (BSN)*

Presentation College, Department of Nursing, *Aberdeen (BSN)*

South Dakota State University, College of Nursing, *Brookings (BS)*

University of Sioux Falls, School of Nursing, *Sioux Falls (BSN)*

The University of South Dakota, Department of Nursing, *Vermillion (BSN)*

Tennessee

Austin Peay State University, School of Nursing, *Clarksville (BSN)*

Baptist College of Health Sciences, Nursing Division, *Memphis (BSN)*

Belmont University, School of Nursing, *Nashville (BSN)*

Carson-Newman University, Department of Nursing, *Jefferson City (BSN)*

Christian Brothers University, RN to BSN Program, *Memphis (BSN)*

Cumberland University, Rudy School of Nursing and Health Professions, *Lebanon (BSN)*

East Tennessee State University, College of Nursing, *Johnson City (BSN)*

Lincoln Memorial University, Caylor School of Nursing, *Harrogate (BSN)*

Middle Tennessee State University, School of Nursing, *Murfreesboro (BSN)*

Milligan College, Department of Nursing, *Milligan College (BSN)*

Tennessee State University, Division of Nursing, *Nashville (BSN)*

Tennessee Technological University, Whitson-Hester School of Nursing, *Cookeville (BSN)*

Tennessee Wesleyan College, Fort Sanders Nursing Department, *Knoxville (BSN)*

Union University, School of Nursing, *Jackson (BSN)*

University of Memphis, Loewenberg School of Nursing, *Memphis (BSN)*

The University of Tennessee, College of Nursing, *Knoxville (BSN)*

The University of Tennessee Health Science Center, College of Nursing, *Memphis (BSN)*

Texas

Angelo State University, Department of Nursing and Rehabilitation Sciences, *San Angelo (BSN)*

Baptist Health System School of Health Professions, RN-BSN Program, *San Antonio (BSN)*

Houston Baptist University, School of Nursing and Allied Health, *Houston (BSN)*

Lamar University, Department of Nursing, *Beaumont (BSN)*

Lubbock Christian University, Department of Nursing, *Lubbock (BSN)*

Midwestern State University, Wilson School of Nursing, *Wichita Falls (BSN)*

Patty Hanks Shelton School of Nursing, *Abilene (BSN)*

Prairie View A&M University, College of Nursing, *Houston (BSN)*

Sam Houston State University, Nursing Program, *Huntsville (BSN)*

Schreiner University, Bachelor of Science in Nursing, *Kerrville (BSN)*

Southwestern Adventist University, Department of Nursing, *Keene (BS)*

Stephen F. Austin State University, Richard and Lucille Dewitt School of Nursing, *Nacogdoches (BSN)*

Texas A&M Health Science Center, College of Nursing, *College Station (BSN)*

Texas A&M International University, Canseco School of Nursing, *Laredo (BSN)*

Texas A&M University–Commerce, Nursing Department, *Commerce (BSN)*

Texas A&M University–Corpus Christi, College of Nursing and Health Sciences, *Corpus Christi (BSN)*

Texas Tech University Health Sciences Center, School of Nursing, *Lubbock (BSN)*

Texas Woman's University, College of Nursing, *Denton (BS)*

University of Houston, School of Nursing, *Houston (BSN)*

University of St. Thomas, Carol and Odis Peavy School of Nursing, *Houston (BSN)*

The University of Texas at Arlington, College of Nursing, *Arlington (BSN)*

The University of Texas at Austin, School of Nursing, *Austin (BSN)*

The University of Texas at El Paso, School of Nursing, *El Paso (BSN)*

The University of Texas at Tyler, Program in Nursing, *Tyler (BSN)*

The University of Texas Medical Branch, School of Nursing, *Galveston (BSN)*

Wayland Baptist University, Bachelor of Science in Nursing Program, *Plainview (BSN)*

Utah

Brigham Young University, College of Nursing, *Provo (BS)*

Dixie State University, Nursing Department, *St. George (BSN)*

Southern Utah University, Department of Nursing, *Cedar City (BSN)*

University of Utah, College of Nursing, *Salt Lake City (BS)*

Western Governors University, Online College of Health Professions, *Salt Lake City (BS)*

Westminster College, School of Nursing and Health Sciences, *Salt Lake City (BSN)*

Vermont

Castleton State College, Baccalaureate Nursing Program, *Castleton (BS)*

Norwich University, Department of Nursing, *Northfield (BSN)*

Southern Vermont College, Department of Nursing, *Bennington (BSN)*

Virgin Islands

University of the Virgin Islands, Division of Nursing, *Saint Thomas (BSN)*

Virginia

Bluefield College, School of Nursing, *Bluefield (BSN)*

Bon Secours Memorial College of Nursing, *Richmond (BSN)*

Eastern Mennonite University, Department of Nursing, *Harrisonburg (BS)*

ECPI University, BSN Program, *Virginia Beach (BSN)*

George Mason University, College of Health and Human Services, *Fairfax (BSN)*

Hampton University, School of Nursing, *Hampton (BS)*

James Madison University, Department of Nursing, *Harrisonburg (BSN)*

Jefferson College of Health Sciences, Nursing Education Program, *Roanoke (BSN)*

Liberty University, Department of Nursing, *Lynchburg (BSN)*

Longwood University, Nursing Program, *Farmville (BSN)*

Marymount University, School of Health Professions, *Arlington (BSN)*

Norfolk State University, Department of Nursing, *Norfolk (BSN)*

Old Dominion University, Department of Nursing, *Norfolk (BSN)*

Radford University, Program in Nursing Practice, *Radford (BSN)*

Sentara College of Health Sciences, Bachelor of Science in Nursing Program, *Chesapeake (BSN)*

Shenandoah University, Eleanor Wade Custer School of Nursing, *Winchester (BS)*

Stratford University, School of Nursing, *Falls Church (BSN)*

University of Virginia, School of Nursing, *Charlottesville (BSN)*

The University of Virginia's College at Wise, Department of Nursing, *Wise (BSN)*

Washington

Bellevue College, Nursing Program, *Bellevue (BSN)*

Northwest University, The Mark and Huldah Buntain School of Nursing, *Kirkland (BS)*

Olympic College, Nursing Programs, *Bremerton (BSN)*

Seattle Pacific University, School of Health Sciences, *Seattle (BS)*

Walla Walla University, School of Nursing, *College Place (BS)*

Western Washington University, RN-to-BSN Program, *Bellingham (BSN)*

WSU College of Nursing, *Spokane (BSN)*

West Virginia

Alderson Broaddus University, Department of Nursing, *Philippi (BSN)*

American Public University System, Bachelor of Science in Nursing, *Charles Town (BSN)*

Bluefield State College, Program in Nursing, *Bluefield (BSN)*

Fairmont State University, School of Nursing and Allied Health Administration, *Fairmont (BSN)*

Marshall University, College of Health Professions, *Huntington (BSN)*

Shepherd University, Department of Nursing Education, *Shepherdstown (BSN)*

West Virginia University, School of Nursing, *Morgantown (BSN)*

Wheeling Jesuit University, Department of Nursing, *Wheeling (BSN)*

Wisconsin

Alverno College, Division of Nursing, *Milwaukee (BSN)*

Columbia College of Nursing, *Milwaukee (BSN)*

Concordia University Wisconsin, Program in Nursing, *Mequon (BSN)*

Herzing University Online, Program in Nursing, *Menomonee Falls (BSN)*

Maranatha Baptist University, Nursing Department, *Watertown (BSN)*

Milwaukee School of Engineering, School of Nursing, *Milwaukee (BSN)*

University of Phoenix–Milwaukee Campus, College of Health and Human Services, *Milwaukee (BSN)*

University of Wisconsin–Eau Claire, College of Nursing and Health Sciences, *Eau Claire (BSN)*

University of Wisconsin–Madison, School of Nursing, *Madison (BS)*

University of Wisconsin–Milwaukee, College of Nursing, *Milwaukee (BSN)*

University of Wisconsin–Oshkosh, College of Nursing, *Oshkosh (BSN)*

Viterbo University, School of Nursing, *La Crosse (BSN)*

CANADA

Alberta

Athabasca University, Centre for Nursing and Health Studies, *Athabasca (BN)*

University of Alberta, Faculty of Nursing, *Edmonton (BScN)*

University of Calgary, Faculty of Nursing, *Calgary (BN)*

British Columbia

British Columbia Institute of Technology, School of Health Sciences, *Burnaby (BSN)*

Kwantlen Polytechnic University, Faculty of Community and Health Sciences, *Surrey (BSN)*

University of Northern British Columbia, Nursing Programme, *Prince George (BScN)*

Manitoba

Brandon University, School of Health Studies, *Brandon (BN)*

University of Manitoba, Faculty of Nursing, *Winnipeg (BN)*

New Brunswick

Université de Moncton, School of Nursing, *Moncton (BScN)*

Nova Scotia

St. Francis Xavier University, Department of Nursing, *Antigonish (BScN)*

Ontario

Lakehead University, School of Nursing, *Thunder Bay (BScN)*

Laurentian University, School of Nursing, *Sudbury (BScN)*

McMaster University, School of Nursing, *Hamilton (BScN)*

Nipissing University, Nursing Department, *North Bay (BScN)*

Ryerson University, Program in Nursing, *Toronto (BScN)*

University of Ottawa, School of Nursing, *Ottawa (BScN)*

The University of Western Ontario, School of Nursing, *London (BScN)*

York University, School of Nursing, *Toronto (BScN)*

Quebec

McGill University, School of Nursing, *Montréal (BScN)*

Université de Montréal, Faculty of Nursing, *Montréal (BScN)*

Université de Sherbrooke, Department of Nursing, *Sherbrooke (BScN)*

Université du Québec à Chicoutimi, Program in Nursing, *Chicoutimi (BNSc)*

Université du Québec à Rimouski, Program in Nursing, *Rimouski (BScN)*

Université du Québec à Trois-Rivières, Program in Nursing, *Trois-Rivières (BSN)*

Université du Québec en Outaouais, Département des Sciences Infirmières, *Gatineau (BScN)*

Université Laval, Faculty of Nursing, *Québec (BScN)*

Saskatchewan

University of Saskatchewan, College of Nursing, *Saskatoon (BSN)*

RPN TO BACCALAUREATE

U.S. AND U.S. TERRITORIES

California

San Jose State University, The Valley Foundation School of Nursing, *San Jose (BS)*

Massachusetts

Curry College, Division of Nursing, *Milton (BS)*

Michigan

Lake Superior State University, Department of Nursing, *Sault Sainte Marie (BSN)*

University of Michigan–Flint, Department of Nursing, *Flint (BSN)*

Missouri

Saint Louis University, School of Nursing, *St. Louis (BSN)*

New York

St. Francis College, Department of Nursing, *Brooklyn Heights (BS)*

Ohio

Franciscan University of Steubenville, Department of Nursing, *Steubenville (BSN)*

Pennsylvania

Chatham University, Nursing Programs, *Pittsburgh (BSN)*

CANADA

Alberta

University of Alberta, Faculty of Nursing, *Edmonton (BScN)*

Ontario

Nipissing University, Nursing Department, *North Bay (BScN)*

Ryerson University, Program in Nursing, *Toronto (BScN)*

University of Ottawa, School of Nursing, *Ottawa (BScN)*

MASTER'S DEGREE PROGRAMS

ACCELERATED AD/RN TO MASTER'S

U.S. AND U.S. TERRITORIES

Alabama

Spring Hill College, Division of Nursing, *Mobile (MSN)*

The University of Alabama at Birmingham, School of Nursing, *Birmingham (MSN, MSN/MPH)*

Arizona

The University of Arizona, College of Nursing, *Tucson (MSN)*

California

University of San Francisco, School of Nursing and Health Professions, *San Francisco (MSN)*

Western University of Health Sciences, College of Graduate Nursing, *Pomona (MSN)*

Delaware

Wesley College, Nursing Program, *Dover (MSN)*

Wilmington University, College of Health Professions, *New Castle (MSN, MSN/MBA, MSN/MS)*

District of Columbia

The George Washington University, School of Nursing, *Washington (MSN)*

Florida

Florida International University, Nursing Program, *Miami (MSN)*

Kentucky

Frontier Nursing University, Nursing Degree Programs, *Hyden (MSN)*

Massachusetts

Regis College, School of Nursing, Science and Health Professions, *Weston (MSN)*

Michigan

Ferris State University, School of Nursing, *Big Rapids (MSN, MSN/MBA)*

Saginaw Valley State University, College of Health and Human Services, *University Center (MSN)*

University of Detroit Mercy, McAuley School of Nursing, *Detroit (MSN)*

Missouri

Missouri State University, Department of Nursing, *Springfield (MSN)*

Nebraska

Nebraska Wesleyan University, Department of Nursing, *Lincoln (MSN, MSN/MBA)*

New York

Daemen College, Department of Nursing, *Amherst (MS)*

State University of New York Polytechnic Institute, School of Nursing and Health Systems, *Utica (MS)*

Ohio

Case Western Reserve University, Frances Payne Bolton School of Nursing, *Cleveland (MSN, MSN/MA, MSN/MPH)*

Walsh University, Department of Nursing, *North Canton (MSN)*

Oklahoma

Oklahoma City University, Kramer School of Nursing, *Oklahoma City (MSN)*

Pennsylvania

DeSales University, Department of Nursing and Health, *Center Valley (MSN, MSN/MBA)*

Gannon University, Villa Maria School of Nursing, *Erie (MSN)*

The University of Scranton, Department of Nursing, *Scranton (MSN)*

Wilkes University, Department of Nursing, *Wilkes-Barre (MS)*

Tennessee

Middle Tennessee State University, School of Nursing, *Murfreesboro (MSN)*

Texas

The University of Texas at Tyler, Program in Nursing, *Tyler (MSN, MSN/MBA)*

University of the Incarnate Word, Program in Nursing, *San Antonio (MSN)*

West Virginia

West Virginia University, School of Nursing, *Morgantown (MSN)*

ACCELERATED MASTER'S

U.S. AND U.S. TERRITORIES

Alabama

University of South Alabama, College of Nursing, *Mobile (MSN)*

Arizona

The University of Arizona, College of Nursing, *Tucson (MSN)*

California

California State University, Fresno, Department of Nursing, *Fresno (MSN)*

University of Phoenix–Sacramento Valley Campus, College of Nursing, *Sacramento (MSN, MSN/MHA)*

West Coast University, Nursing Programs, *North Hollywood (MSN)*

Western University of Health Sciences, College of Graduate Nursing, *Pomona (MSN)*

Georgia

Thomas University, Division of Nursing, *Thomasville (MSN, MSN/MBA)*

Hawaii

University of Hawaii at Manoa, School of Nursing and Dental Hygiene, *Honolulu (MS, MSN/MBA)*

Illinois

Benedictine University, Department of Nursing, *Lisle (MSN)*

Lewis University, Program in Nursing, *Romeoville (MSN, MSN/MBA)*

Rush University, College of Nursing, *Chicago (MSN)*

Maryland

Stevenson University, Nursing Division, *Stevenson (MS)*

Massachusetts

American International College, Division of Nursing, *Springfield (MSN)*

Regis College, School of Nursing, Science and Health Professions, *Weston (MSN)*

Simmons College, School of Nursing and Health Sciences, *Boston (MS)*

Missouri

Saint Louis University, School of Nursing, *St. Louis (MSN)*

Nebraska

Nebraska Wesleyan University, Department of Nursing, *Lincoln (MSN, MSN/MBA)*

New Hampshire

University of New Hampshire, Department of Nursing, *Durham (MS)*

New York

Keuka College, Division of Nursing, *Keuka Park (MS)*

The Sage Colleges, Department of Nursing, *Troy (MS, MS/MBA)*

Oklahoma

Oklahoma City University, Kramer School of Nursing, *Oklahoma City (MSN)*

Southern Nazarene University, School of Nursing, *Bethany (MS)*

Pennsylvania

Holy Family University, School of Nursing and Allied Health Professions, *Philadelphia (MSN)*

Thomas Jefferson University, Department of Nursing, *Philadelphia (MSN)*

Waynesburg University, Department of Nursing, *Waynesburg (MSN, MSN/MBA)*

South Carolina

University of South Carolina, College of Nursing, *Columbia (MSN)*

Tennessee

The University of Tennessee Health Science Center, College of Nursing, *Memphis (MSN)*

Texas

Concordia University Texas, School of Nursing, *Austin (MSN)*

Texas A&M Health Science Center, College of Nursing, *College Station (MSN)*

Utah

Western Governors University, Online College of Health Professions, *Salt Lake City (MS)*

West Virginia

West Virginia University, School of Nursing, *Morgantown (MSN)*

CANADA

Quebec

Université Laval, Faculty of Nursing, *Québec (MSN)*

ACCELERATED MASTER'S FOR NON-NURSING COLLEGE GRADUATES

U.S. AND U.S. TERRITORIES

Alabama

The University of Alabama at Birmingham, School of Nursing, *Birmingham (MSN, MSN/MPH)*

Arizona

The University of Arizona, College of Nursing, *Tucson (MSN)*

California

Azusa Pacific University, School of Nursing, *Azusa (MSN)*

California Baptist University, School of Nursing, *Riverside (MSN)*

San Francisco State University, School of Nursing, *San Francisco (MSN)*

University of San Diego, Hahn School of Nursing and Health Science, *San Diego (MSN)*

University of San Francisco, School of Nursing and Health Professions, *San Francisco (MSN)*

Western University of Health Sciences, College of Graduate Nursing, *Pomona (MSN)*

District of Columbia

Georgetown University, School of Nursing and Health Studies, *Washington (MS)*

Georgia

Augusta University, School of Nursing, *Augusta (MSN)*

Illinois

Millikin University, School of Nursing, *Decatur (MSN)*

Kentucky

University of Louisville, School of Nursing, *Louisville (MSN)*

Massachusetts

Boston College, William F. Connell School of Nursing, *Chestnut Hill (MS, MS/MA, MS/MBA)*

Regis College, School of Nursing, Science and Health Professions, *Weston (MSN)*

Simmons College, School of Nursing and Health Sciences, *Boston (MS)*

University of Massachusetts Medical School, Graduate School of Nursing, *Worcester (MS)*

Missouri

Saint Louis University, School of Nursing, *St. Louis (MSN)*

New Hampshire

University of New Hampshire, Department of Nursing, *Durham (MS)*

New Jersey

Seton Hall University, College of Nursing, *South Orange (MSN, MSN/MBA)*

New York

Columbia University, School of Nursing, *New York (MS, MSN/MBA, MSN/MPH)*

Mercy College, Programs in Nursing, *Dobbs Ferry (MS)*

North Carolina

East Carolina University, College of Nursing, *Greenville (MSN)*

Ohio

Mount St. Joseph University, Department of Nursing, *Cincinnati (MN)*

University of Cincinnati, College of Nursing, *Cincinnati (MSN)*

Xavier University, School of Nursing, *Cincinnati (MSN, MSN/Ed D, MSN/MBA)*

Oregon

Oregon Health & Science University, School of Nursing, *Portland (MN)*

Pennsylvania

University of Pennsylvania, School of Nursing, *Philadelphia (MSN, MSN/MBA, MSN/MPH, MSN/PhD)*

Texas

The University of Texas at Austin, School of Nursing, *Austin (MSN)*

Washington

Pacific Lutheran University, School of Nursing, *Tacoma (MSN, MSN/MBA)*

ACCELERATED MASTER'S FOR NURSES WITH NON-NURSING DEGREES

U.S. AND U.S. TERRITORIES

California

Azusa Pacific University, School of Nursing, *Azusa (MSN)*

California State University, Los Angeles, School of Nursing, *Los Angeles (MSN)*

Charles R. Drew University of Medicine and Science, School of Nursing, *Los Angeles (MSN)*

San Francisco State University, School of Nursing, *San Francisco (MSN)*

West Coast University, Nursing Programs, *North Hollywood (MSN)*

Delaware

Wilmington University, College of Health Professions, *New Castle (MSN, MSN/MBA, MSN/MS)*

Illinois

Lewis University, Program in Nursing, *Romeoville (MSN, MSN/MBA)*

Kentucky

Western Kentucky University, School of Nursing, *Bowling Green (MSN)*

Massachusetts

American International College, Division of Nursing, *Springfield (MSN)*

Regis College, School of Nursing, Science and Health Professions, *Weston (MSN)*

Missouri

Saint Louis University, School of Nursing, *St. Louis (MSN)*

New Jersey

Kean University, Department of Nursing, *Union (MSN, MSN/MPA)*

Seton Hall University, College of Nursing, *South Orange (MSN, MSN/MBA)*

New York

Columbia University, School of Nursing, *New York (MS, MSN/MBA, MSN/MPH)*

Mercy College, Programs in Nursing, *Dobbs Ferry (MS)*

North Carolina

East Carolina University, College of Nursing, *Greenville (MSN)*

Oklahoma

Oklahoma City University, Kramer School of Nursing, *Oklahoma City (MSN)*

Southern Nazarene University, School of Nursing, *Bethany (MS)*

Pennsylvania

University of Pennsylvania, School of Nursing, *Philadelphia (MSN, MSN/MBA, MSN/MPH, MSN/PhD)*

Waynesburg University, Department of Nursing, *Waynesburg (MSN, MSN/MBA)*

Tennessee

University of Memphis, Loewenberg School of Nursing, *Memphis (MSN)*

The University of Tennessee Health Science Center, College of Nursing, *Memphis (MSN)*

Washington

Seattle University, College of Nursing, *Seattle (MSN)*

WSU College of Nursing, *Spokane (MN)*

ACCELERATED RN TO MASTER'S

U.S. AND U.S. TERRITORIES

Arizona

The University of Arizona, College of Nursing, *Tucson (MSN)*

California

California State University, Los Angeles, School of Nursing, *Los Angeles (MSN)*

West Coast University, Nursing Programs, *North Hollywood (MSN)*

Western University of Health Sciences, College of Graduate Nursing, *Pomona (MSN)*

Florida

University of Central Florida, College of Nursing, *Orlando (MSN)*

University of South Florida, College of Nursing, *Tampa (MS, MS/MPH)*

Georgia

Albany State University, College of Sciences and Health Professions, *Albany (MSN)*

Illinois

Lewis University, Program in Nursing, *Romeoville (MSN, MSN/MBA)*

Saint Francis Medical Center College of Nursing, Baccalaureate Nursing Program, *Peoria (MSN)*

Iowa

The University of Iowa, College of Nursing, *Iowa City (MSN, MSN/MBA, MSN/MPH)*

Maryland

Stevenson University, Nursing Division, *Stevenson (MS)*

Massachusetts

American International College, Division of Nursing, *Springfield (MSN)*

Regis College, School of Nursing, Science and Health Professions, *Weston (MSN)*

Michigan

Ferris State University, School of Nursing, *Big Rapids (MSN, MSN/MBA)*

University of Michigan, School of Nursing, *Ann Arbor (MS, MSN/MBA, MSN/MPH)*

University of Michigan–Flint, Department of Nursing, *Flint (MSN)*

Minnesota

Capella University, Nursing Programs, *Minneapolis (MSN)*

Minnesota State University Mankato, School of Nursing, *Mankato (MSN, MSN/MS)*

Nebraska

Nebraska Wesleyan University, Department of Nursing, *Lincoln (MSN, MSN/MBA)*

New Jersey

Fairleigh Dickinson University, Metropolitan Campus, Henry P. Becton School of Nursing and Allied Health, *Teaneck (MSN)*

Felician University, Division of Nursing and Health Management, *Lodi (MA/MSM, MSN)*

Seton Hall University, College of Nursing, *South Orange (MSN, MSN/MBA)*

New York

Daemen College, Department of Nursing, *Amherst (MS)*

Mercy College, Programs in Nursing, *Dobbs Ferry (MS)*

The Sage Colleges, Department of Nursing, *Troy (MS, MS/MBA)*

State University of New York Polytechnic Institute, School of Nursing and Health Systems, *Utica (MS)*

State University of New York Upstate Medical University, College of Nursing, *Syracuse (MS)*

Ohio

Kent State University, College of Nursing, *Kent (MSN, MSN/MBA, MSN/MPA)*

Walsh University, Department of Nursing, *North Canton (MSN)*

Oklahoma

Oklahoma City University, Kramer School of Nursing, *Oklahoma City (MSN)*

Pennsylvania

DeSales University, Department of Nursing and Health, *Center Valley (MSN, MSN/MBA)*

Gannon University, Villa Maria School of Nursing, *Erie (MSN)*

Thomas Jefferson University, Department of Nursing, *Philadelphia (MSN)*

The University of Scranton, Department of Nursing, *Scranton (MSN)*

Waynesburg University, Department of Nursing, *Waynesburg (MSN, MSN/MBA)*

Wilkes University, Department of Nursing, *Wilkes-Barre (MS)*

Tennessee

King University, School of Nursing, *Bristol (MSN, MSN/MBA)*

Southern Adventist University, School of Nursing, *Collegedale (MSN, MSN/MBA)*

Texas

The University of Texas at Tyler, Program in Nursing, *Tyler (MSN, MSN/MBA)*

Utah

Western Governors University, Online College of Health Professions, *Salt Lake City (MS)*

Washington

Gonzaga University, School of Nursing and Human Psychology, *Spokane (MSN)*

WSU College of Nursing, *Spokane (MN)*

West Virginia

West Virginia University, School of Nursing, *Morgantown (MSN)*

Wisconsin

Concordia University Wisconsin, Program in Nursing, *Mequon (MSN)*

CANADA

Quebec

Université de Montréal, Faculty of Nursing, *Montréal (M Sc)*

JOINT DEGREES

U.S. AND U.S. TERRITORIES

Alabama

The University of Alabama at Birmingham, School of Nursing, *Birmingham (MSN, MSN/MPH)*

Arizona

Arizona State University at the Downtown Phoenix campus, College of Nursing, *Phoenix (MS, MS/MPH)*

Grand Canyon University, College of Nursing and Health Sciences, *Phoenix (MS, MSN/MBA)*

University of Phoenix–Online Campus, Online Campus, *Phoenix (MSN, MSN/MBA, MSN/MHA)*

University of Phoenix–Phoenix Campus, College of Health Sciences and Nursing, *Tempe (MSN, MSN/MBA, MSN/MHA)*

California

Holy Names University, Department of Nursing, *Oakland (MSN, MSN/MBA)*

University of California, Los Angeles, School of Nursing, *Los Angeles (MSN, MSN/MBA)*

University of Phoenix–Bay Area Campus, College of Nursing, *San Jose (MSN, MSN/MBA, MSN/MHA)*

University of Phoenix–Sacramento Valley Campus, College of Nursing, *Sacramento (MSN, MSN/MHA)*

University of Phoenix–Southern California Campus, College of Health Sciences and Nursing, *Costa Mesa (MSN, MSN/MBA, MSN/MHA)*

Connecticut

Yale University, School of Nursing, *West Haven (MSN, MSN/MDIV, MSN/MPH)*

Delaware

Wilmington University, College of Health Professions, *New Castle (MSN, MSN/MBA, MSN/MS)*

Florida

Barry University, Division of Nursing, *Miami Shores (MSN, MSN/MBA)*

Florida Southern College, School of Nursing & Health Sciences, *Lakeland (MSN, MSN/MBA)*

Jacksonville University, School of Nursing, *Jacksonville (MSN, MSN/MBA)*

University of Florida, College of Nursing, *Gainesville (MSN, MSN/PhD)*

University of Phoenix–North Florida Campus, College of Nursing, *Jacksonville (MSN, MSN/Ed D, MSN/MHA)*

University of Phoenix–South Florida Campus, College of Nursing, *Miramar (MSN, MSN/MBA, MSN/MHA)*

University of South Florida, College of Nursing, *Tampa (MS, MS/MPH)*

Georgia

Emory University, Nell Hodgson Woodruff School of Nursing, *Atlanta (MSN, MSN/MPH)*

Thomas University, Division of Nursing, *Thomasville (MSN, MSN/MBA)*

Hawaii

Hawai`i Pacific University, College of Nursing and Health Sciences, *Honolulu (MSN, MSN/MBA)*

University of Hawaii at Manoa, School of Nursing and Dental Hygiene, *Honolulu (MS, MSN/MBA)*

Idaho

Boise State University, Department of Nursing, *Boise (MSN, MSN/MS)*

Illinois

Elmhurst College, Deicke Center for Nursing Education, *Elmhurst (MS, MSN/MBA)*

Lewis University, Program in Nursing, *Romeoville (MSN, MSN/MBA)*

Loyola University Chicago, Marcella Niehoff School of Nursing, *Maywood (MSN, MSN/MBA)*

McKendree University, Department of Nursing, *Lebanon (MSN, MSN/MBA)*

Northern Illinois University, School of Nursing and Health Studies, *De Kalb (MS, MSN/MPH)*

North Park University, School of Nursing, *Chicago (MS, MSN/MA, MSN/MBA, MSN/MM)*

Saint Xavier University, School of Nursing, *Chicago (MSN, MSN/MBA)*

Indiana

Anderson University, School of Nursing, *Anderson (MSN, MSN/MBA)*

Valparaiso University, College of Nursing and Health Professions, *Valparaiso (MSN, MSN/MHA)*

Iowa

The University of Iowa, College of Nursing, *Iowa City (MSN, MSN/MBA, MSN/MPH)*

Kansas

The University of Kansas, School of Nursing, *Kansas City (MS, MS/MHSA, MS/MPH)*

Kentucky

Bellarmine University, Donna and Allan Lansing School of Nursing and Health Sciences, *Louisville (Certificate of Completion, MSN, MSN/MBA)*

Maine

Saint Joseph's College of Maine, Master of Science in Nursing Program, *Standish (MSN, MSN/MHA)*

Maryland

Johns Hopkins University, School of Nursing, *Baltimore (MSN, MSN/MBA, MSN/MPH, MSN/PhD)*

University of Maryland, Baltimore, Nursing Programs, *Baltimore (MS, MS/MBA, MS/MPH)*

Massachusetts

Boston College, William F. Connell School of Nursing, *Chestnut Hill (MS, MS/MA, MS/MBA)*

Elms College, School of Nursing, *Chicopee (MSN, MSN/MBA)*

Northeastern University, School of Nursing, *Boston (MS, MS/MBA)*

Salem State University, Program in Nursing, *Salem (MSN, MSN/MBA)*

Michigan

Ferris State University, School of Nursing, *Big Rapids (MSN, MSN/MBA)*

Madonna University, College of Nursing and Health, *Livonia (MSN, MSN/MBA)*

Spring Arbor University, Program in Nursing, *Spring Arbor (MSN, MSN/MBA)*

University of Michigan, School of Nursing, *Ann Arbor (MS, MSN/MBA, MSN/MPH)*

Minnesota

Minnesota State University Mankato, School of Nursing, *Mankato (MSN, MSN/MS)*

Minnesota State University Moorhead, School of Nursing and Healthcare Leadership, *Moorhead (MS, MSN/MHA)*

Missouri

University of Missouri, Sinclair School of Nursing, *Columbia (MSN, MSN/PhD)*

Nebraska

Nebraska Wesleyan University, Department of Nursing, *Lincoln (MSN, MSN/MBA)*

Nevada

University of Nevada, Reno, Orvis School of Nursing, *Reno (MSN, MSN/MPH)*

New Jersey

Felician University, Division of Nursing and Health Management, *Lodi (MA/MSM, MSN)*

Kean University, Department of Nursing, *Union (MSN, MSN/MPA)*

Rutgers, The State University of New Jersey, Newark, Rutgers School of Nursing, *Newark (MSN, MSN/MPH)*

Seton Hall University, College of Nursing, *South Orange (MSN, MSN/MBA)*

New York

Columbia University, School of Nursing, *New York (MS, MSN/MBA, MSN/MPH)*

Hunter College of the City University of New York, Hunter-Bellevue School of Nursing, *New York (MS, MSN/MPA, MSN/MPH)*

Molloy College, Division of Nursing, *Rockville Centre (MS, MS/MBA)*

New York University, College of Nursing, *New York (MS, MS/MPH)*

The Sage Colleges, Department of Nursing, *Troy (MS, MS/MBA)*

State University of New York Downstate Medical Center, College of Nursing, *Brooklyn (MS, MS/MPH)*

North Carolina

Gardner-Webb University, School of Nursing, *Boiling Springs (MSN, MSN/MBA)*

Queens University of Charlotte, Presbyterian School of Nursing, *Charlotte (MSN, MSN/MBA)*

The University of North Carolina at Greensboro, School of Nursing, *Greensboro (MSN, MSN/MBA)*

North Dakota

University of Mary, Division of Nursing, *Bismarck (MSN, MSN/MBA)*

Ohio

Capital University, School of Nursing, *Columbus (MN/MBA, MSN, MSN/JD, MSN/MDIV)*

Case Western Reserve University, Frances Payne Bolton School of Nursing, *Cleveland (MSN, MSN/MA, MSN/MPH)*

Cleveland State University, School of Nursing, *Cleveland (MSN, MSN/MBA)*

Kent State University, College of Nursing, *Kent (MSN, MSN/MBA, MSN/MPA)*

The Ohio State University, College of Nursing, *Columbus (MS, MS/MPH)*

Ursuline College, The Breen School of Nursing, *Pepper Pike (MSN, MSN/MBA)*

Wright State University, College of Nursing and Health, *Dayton (MS, MS/MBA)*

Xavier University, School of Nursing, *Cincinnati (MSN, MSN/Ed D, MSN/MBA)*

Pennsylvania

Bloomsburg University of Pennsylvania, Department of Nursing, *Bloomsburg (MSN, MSN/MBA)*

Carlow University, College of Health and Wellness, *Pittsburgh (MSN, MSN/MBA)*

DeSales University, Department of Nursing and Health, *Center Valley (MSN, MSN/MBA)*

La Salle University, School of Nursing and Health Sciences, *Philadelphia (MSN, MSN/MBA)*

Marywood University, Department of Nursing, *Scranton (MSN, MSN/MPH)*

Penn State University Park, School of Nursing, *University Park (MS, MSN/PhD)*

University of Pennsylvania, School of Nursing, *Philadelphia (MSN, MSN/MBA, MSN/MPH, MSN/PhD)*

Waynesburg University, Department of Nursing, *Waynesburg (MSN, MSN/MBA)*

Widener University, School of Nursing, *Chester (MSN, MSN/PhD)*

Tennessee

King University, School of Nursing, *Bristol (MSN, MSN/MBA)*

Southern Adventist University, School of Nursing, *Collegedale (MSN, MSN/MBA)*

The University of Tennessee, College of Nursing, *Knoxville (MSN, MSN/PhD)*

Vanderbilt University, Vanderbilt University School of Nursing, *Nashville (MSN, MSN/MDIV, MSN/MTS)*

Texas

Lamar University, Department of Nursing, *Beaumont (MSN, MSN/MBA)*

Texas Woman's University, College of Nursing, *Denton (MS, MS/MHA)*

The University of Texas at Arlington, College of Nursing, *Arlington (MSN, MSN/MBA, MSN/MHA, MSN/MPH)*

The University of Texas at Tyler, Program in Nursing, *Tyler (MSN, MSN/MBA)*

The University of Texas Health Science Center at Houston, School of Nursing, *Houston (MSN, MSN/MPH)*

Virginia

University of Virginia, School of Nursing, *Charlottesville (MSN, MSN/PhD)*

Washington

Pacific Lutheran University, School of Nursing, *Tacoma (MSN, MSN/MBA)*

University of Washington, School of Nursing, *Seattle (MN, MN/MPH)*

Wisconsin

Edgewood College, Henry Predolin School of Nursing, *Madison (MS, MSN/MBA)*

Marquette University, College of Nursing, *Milwaukee (MSN, MSN/MBA)*

CANADA

Alberta

Athabasca University, Centre for Nursing and Health Studies, *Athabasca (MN, MN/MHSA)*

British Columbia

The University of British Columbia, Program in Nursing, *Vancouver (MSN, MSN/MPH)*

Ontario

McMaster University, School of Nursing, *Hamilton (M Sc, MSN/PhD)*

MASTER'S

U.S. AND U.S. TERRITORIES

Alabama

Auburn University, School of Nursing, *Auburn University (MSN)*

Auburn University at Montgomery, School of Nursing, *Montgomery (MSN)*

Jacksonville State University, College of Nursing and Health Sciences, *Jacksonville (MSN)*

Samford University, Ida V. Moffett School of Nursing, *Birmingham (MSN)*

Spring Hill College, Division of Nursing, *Mobile (MSN)*

Troy University, School of Nursing, *Troy (MSN)*

The University of Alabama, Capstone College of Nursing, *Tuscaloosa (MSN, MSN/Ed D)*

The University of Alabama at Birmingham, School of Nursing, *Birmingham (MSN, MSN/MPH)*

The University of Alabama in Huntsville, College of Nursing, *Huntsville (MSN)*

University of Mobile, School of Nursing, *Mobile (MSN)*

University of North Alabama, College of Nursing and Allied Health, *Florence (MSN)*

University of South Alabama, College of Nursing, *Mobile (MSN)*

Alaska

University of Alaska Anchorage, School of Nursing, *Anchorage (MS)*

Arizona

Arizona State University at the Downtown Phoenix campus, College of Nursing, *Phoenix (MS, MS/MPH)*

Chamberlain College of Nursing, *Phoenix (MSN)*

Grand Canyon University, College of Nursing and Health Sciences, *Phoenix (MS, MSN/ MBA)*

Northern Arizona University, School of Nursing, *Flagstaff (MS)*

The University of Arizona, College of Nursing, *Tucson (MSN)*

University of Phoenix–Online Campus, Online Campus, *Phoenix (MSN, MSN/MBA, MSN/ MHA)*

University of Phoenix–Phoenix Campus, College of Health Sciences and Nursing, *Tempe (MSN, MSN/MBA, MSN/MHA)*

University of Phoenix–Southern Arizona Campus, College of Social Sciences, *Tucson (MSN)*

Arkansas

Arkansas State University, Department of Nursing, *State University (MSN)*

Arkansas Tech University, Program in Nursing, *Russellville (MSN)*

Harding University, College of Nursing, *Searcy (MSN)*

University of Arkansas, Eleanor Mann School of Nursing, *Fayetteville (MSN)*

University of Arkansas for Medical Sciences, College of Nursing, *Little Rock (MN Sc)*

University of Central Arkansas, Department of Nursing, *Conway (MSN)*

California

Azusa Pacific University, School of Nursing, *Azusa (MSN)*

California Baptist University, School of Nursing, *Riverside (MSN)*

California State University, Chico, School of Nursing, *Chico (MSN)*

California State University, Dominguez Hills, Program in Nursing, *Carson (MSN)*

California State University, Fresno, Department of Nursing, *Fresno (MSN)*

California State University, Fullerton, Department of Nursing, *Fullerton (MSN)*

California State University, Long Beach, School of Nursing, *Long Beach (MSN)*

California State University, Los Angeles, School of Nursing, *Los Angeles (MSN)*

California State University, Sacramento, Division of Nursing, *Sacramento (MS)*

California State University, San Bernardino, Department of Nursing, *San Bernardino (MSN)*

Charles R. Drew University of Medicine and Science, School of Nursing, *Los Angeles (MSN)*

Holy Names University, Department of Nursing, *Oakland (MSN, MSN/MBA)*

Loma Linda University, School of Nursing, *Loma Linda (MS)*

Mount Saint Mary's University, Department of Nursing, *Los Angeles (MSN)*

Point Loma Nazarene University, School of Nursing, *San Diego (MSN)*

Samuel Merritt University, School of Nursing, *Oakland (MSN)*

San Diego State University, School of Nursing, *San Diego (MSN)*

San Francisco State University, School of Nursing, *San Francisco (MSN)*

San Jose State University, The Valley Foundation School of Nursing, *San Jose (MS)*

University of California, Davis, The Betty Irene Moore School of Nursing, *Davis (MS)*

University of California, Irvine, Program in Nursing Science, *Irvine (MS)*

University of California, Los Angeles, School of Nursing, *Los Angeles (MSN, MSN/MBA)*

University of California, San Francisco, School of Nursing, *San Francisco (MS)*

University of Phoenix–Bay Area Campus, College of Nursing, *San Jose (MSN, MSN/ MBA, MSN/MHA)*

University of Phoenix–San Diego Campus, College of Nursing, *San Diego (MSN, MSN/ Ed D)*

University of Phoenix–Southern California Campus, College of Health Sciences and Nursing, *Costa Mesa (MSN, MSN/MBA, MSN/MHA)*

University of San Diego, Hahn School of Nursing and Health Science, *San Diego (MSN)*

Western University of Health Sciences, College of Graduate Nursing, *Pomona (MSN)*

Colorado

American Sentinel University, RN to Bachelor of Science Nursing, *Aurora (MSN)*

Aspen University, Graduate School of Health Professions and Studies, *Denver (MSN)*

Colorado Mesa University, Department of Nursing and Radiologic Sciences, *Grand Junction (MSN)*

Colorado State University–Pueblo, Department of Nursing, *Pueblo (MS)*

Regis University, School of Nursing, *Denver (MS)*

University of Colorado Colorado Springs, Helen and Arthur E. Johnson Beth-El College of Nursing & Health Sciences, *Colorado Springs (MSN)*

University of Colorado Denver, College of Nursing, *Aurora (MS)*

University of Northern Colorado, School of Nursing, *Greeley (MS)*

Connecticut

Fairfield University, School of Nursing, *Fairfield (MSN)*

Quinnipiac University, School of Nursing, *Hamden (MSN)*

Sacred Heart University, College of Nursing, *Fairfield (MSN)*

Southern Connecticut State University, Department of Nursing, *New Haven (MSN)*

University of Connecticut, School of Nursing, *Storrs (MS)*

University of Hartford, College of Education, Nursing, and Health Professions, *West Hartford (MSN)*

University of Saint Joseph, Department of Nursing, *West Hartford (MS)*

Western Connecticut State University, Department of Nursing, *Danbury (MS)*

Yale University, School of Nursing, *West Haven (MSN, MSN/MDIV, MSN/MPH)*

Delaware

Delaware State University, Department of Nursing, *Dover (MS)*

University of Delaware, School of Nursing, *Newark (MSN)*

Wesley College, Nursing Program, *Dover (MSN)*

Wilmington University, College of Health Professions, *New Castle (MSN, MSN/MBA, MSN/MS)*

District of Columbia

The Catholic University of America, School of Nursing, *Washington (MSN)*

Georgetown University, School of Nursing and Health Studies, *Washington (MS)*

The George Washington University, School of Nursing, *Washington (MSN)*

Howard University, Division of Nursing, *Washington (MSN)*

Florida

Barry University, Division of Nursing, *Miami Shores (MSN, MSN/MBA)*

Florida Agricultural and Mechanical University, School of Nursing, *Tallahassee (MSN)*

Florida Atlantic University, Christine E. Lynn College of Nursing, *Boca Raton (MSN)*

Florida Gulf Coast University, School of Nursing, *Fort Myers (MSN)*

Florida International University, Nursing Program, *Miami (MSN)*

Florida Southern College, School of Nursing & Health Sciences, *Lakeland (MSN, MSN/MBA)*

Florida State University, College of Nursing, *Tallahassee (MSN)*

Jacksonville University, School of Nursing, *Jacksonville (MSN, MSN/MBA)*

Kaplan University Online, The School of Nursing Online, *Fort Lauderdale (MSN)*

Keiser University, Nursing Programs, *Fort Lauderdale (MSN)*

Keiser University, Nursing Programs, *Fort Myers (MSN)*

Keiser University, Nursing Programs, *Jacksonville (MSN)*

Keiser University, Nursing Programs, *Lakeland (MSN)*

Keiser University, Nursing Programs, *Melbourne (MSN)*

Keiser University, Nursing Programs, *Miami (MSN)*

Keiser University, Nursing Programs, *Orlando (MSN)*

Keiser University, Nursing Programs, *Port St. Lucie (MSN)*

Keiser University, Nursing Programs, *Sarasota (MSN)*

Keiser University, Nursing Programs, *Tallahassee (MSN)*

Keiser University, Nursing Programs, *Tampa (MSN)*

Nova Southeastern University, College of Health Care Sciences, *Fort Lauderdale (MSN)*

Palm Beach Atlantic University, School of Nursing, *West Palm Beach (MSN)*

University of Central Florida, College of Nursing, *Orlando (MSN)*

University of Florida, College of Nursing, *Gainesville (MSN, MSN/PhD)*

University of Miami, School of Nursing and Health Studies, *Coral Gables (MSN)*

University of North Florida, School of Nursing, *Jacksonville (MSN)*

University of Phoenix–North Florida Campus, College of Nursing, *Jacksonville (MSN, MSN/ Ed D, MSN/MHA)*

University of Phoenix–South Florida Campus, College of Nursing, *Miramar (MSN, MSN/ MBA, MSN/MHA)*

University of South Florida, College of Nursing, *Tampa (MS, MS/MPH)*

The University of Tampa, Department of Nursing, *Tampa (MSN)*

University of West Florida, Department of Nursing, *Pensacola (MSN)*

Georgia

Albany State University, College of Sciences and Health Professions, *Albany (MSN)*

Armstrong State University, Program in Nursing, *Savannah (MSN)*

Augusta University, School of Nursing, *Augusta (MSN)*

Brenau University, College of Health and Science, *Gainesville (MSN)*

Clayton State University, Department of Nursing, *Morrow (MSN)*

Emory University, Nell Hodgson Woodruff School of Nursing, *Atlanta (MSN, MSN/ MPH)*

Georgia College & State University, College of Health Sciences, *Milledgeville (MSN)*

Georgia Southwestern State University, School of Nursing, *Americus (MSN)*

Georgia State University, Byrdine F. Lewis School of Nursing, *Atlanta (MS)*

Kennesaw State University, School of Nursing, *Kennesaw (MSN)*

Mercer University, Georgia Baptist College of Nursing of Mercer University, *Atlanta (MSN)*

Thomas University, Division of Nursing, *Thomasville (MSN, MSN/MBA)*

University of North Georgia, Department of Nursing, *Dahlonega (MS)*

University of West Georgia, School of Nursing, *Carrollton (MSN)*

Valdosta State University, College of Nursing, *Valdosta (MSN)*

Hawaii

Hawai`i Pacific University, College of Nursing and Health Sciences, *Honolulu (MSN, MSN/ MBA)*

University of Hawaii at Manoa, School of Nursing and Dental Hygiene, *Honolulu (MS, MSN/MBA)*

University of Phoenix–Hawaii Campus, College of Nursing, *Honolulu (MSN, MSN/ Ed D)*

Idaho

Boise State University, Department of Nursing, *Boise (MSN, MSN/MS)*

Idaho State University, Department of Nursing, *Pocatello (MS)*

Northwest Nazarene University, School of Health and Science, *Nampa (MSN)*

Illinois

Aurora University, School of Nursing, *Aurora (MSN)*

Benedictine University, Department of Nursing, *Lisle (MSN)*

Blessing–Rieman College of Nursing and Health Sciences, *Quincy (MSN)*

Bradley University, Department of Nursing, *Peoria (MSN)*

Chicago State University, Department of Nursing, *Chicago (MSN)*

Elmhurst College, Deicke Center for Nursing Education, *Elmhurst (MS, MSN/MBA)*

Governors State University, College of Health and Human Services, *University Park (MS)*

Illinois State University, Mennonite College of Nursing, *Normal (MSN)*

Lewis University, Program in Nursing, *Romeoville (MSN, MSN/MBA)*

Loyola University Chicago, Marcella Niehoff School of Nursing, *Maywood (MSN, MSN/ MBA)*

McKendree University, Department of Nursing, *Lebanon (MSN, MSN/MBA)*

Millikin University, School of Nursing, *Decatur (MSN)*

Northern Illinois University, School of Nursing and Health Studies, *De Kalb (MS, MSN/ MPH)*

North Park University, School of Nursing, *Chicago (MS, MSN/MA, MSN/MBA, MSN/ MM)*

Olivet Nazarene University, Division of Nursing, *Bourbonnais (MSN)*

Resurrection University, *Chicago (MSN)*

Saint Anthony College of Nursing, *Rockford (MSN)*

Saint Francis Medical Center College of Nursing, Baccalaureate Nursing Program, *Peoria (MSN)*

Saint Xavier University, School of Nursing, *Chicago (MSN, MSN/MBA)*

Southern Illinois University Edwardsville, School of Nursing, *Edwardsville (MS)*

University of Illinois at Chicago, College of Nursing, *Chicago (MS)*

University of St. Francis, Leach College of Nursing, *Joliet (MSN)*

Indiana

Anderson University, School of Nursing, *Anderson (MSN, MSN/MBA)*

Ball State University, School of Nursing, *Muncie (MS)*

Bethel College, School of Nursing, *Mishawaka (MSN)*

Goshen College, Department of Nursing, *Goshen (MSN)*

Indiana State University, Department of Advanced Practice Nursing, *Terre Haute (MS)*

Indiana University–Purdue University Fort Wayne, Department of Nursing, *Fort Wayne (MS)*

Indiana University–Purdue University Indianapolis, School of Nursing, *Indianapolis (MSN)*

Indiana University South Bend, Vera Z. Dwyer College of Health Sciences, *South Bend (MSN)*

Indiana Wesleyan University, School of Nursing, *Marion (MSN)*

Purdue University, School of Nursing, *West Lafayette (MS)*

Purdue University Calumet, School of Nursing, *Hammond (MS)*

University of Indianapolis, School of Nursing, *Indianapolis (MSN)*

University of Saint Francis, Department of Nursing, *Fort Wayne (MSN)*

University of Southern Indiana, College of Nursing and Health Professions, *Evansville (MSN)*

Valparaiso University, College of Nursing and Health Professions, *Valparaiso (MSN, MSN/ MHA)*

Iowa

Allen College, Graduate Programs, *Waterloo (MSN)*

Briar Cliff University, Department of Nursing, *Sioux City (MSN)*

Grand View University, Division of Nursing, *Des Moines (MS)*

Morningside College, Department of Nursing Education, *Sioux City (MSN)*

Mount Mercy University, Department of Nursing, *Cedar Rapids (MSN)*

St. Ambrose University, Program in Nursing (BSN), *Davenport (MSN)*

The University of Iowa, College of Nursing, *Iowa City (MSN, MSN/MBA, MSN/MPH)*

Kansas

Baker University, School of Nursing, *Topeka (MSN)*

Fort Hays State University, Department of Nursing, *Hays (MSN)*

MidAmerica Nazarene University, Division of Nursing, *Olathe (MSN)*

Newman University, Division of Nursing, *Wichita (MS)*

Pittsburg State University, Department of Nursing, *Pittsburg (MSN)*

Tabor College, Department of Nursing, *Hillsboro (MSN)*

The University of Kansas, School of Nursing, *Kansas City (MS, MS/MHSA, MS/MPH)*

University of Saint Mary, Bachelor of Science in Nursing Program, *Leavenworth (MSN)*

Washburn University, School of Nursing, *Topeka (MSN)*

Kentucky

Bellarmine University, Donna and Allan Lansing School of Nursing and Health Sciences, *Louisville (Certificate of Completion, MSN, MSN/MBA)*

Eastern Kentucky University, Department of Baccalaureate and Graduate Nursing, *Richmond (MSN)*

Murray State University, Program in Nursing, *Murray (MSN)*

Northern Kentucky University, Department of Nursing, *Highland Heights (MSN)*

Spalding University, School of Nursing, *Louisville (MSN)*

University of Kentucky, College of Nursing, *Lexington (MSN)*

Western Kentucky University, School of Nursing, *Bowling Green (MSN)*

Louisiana

Grambling State University, School of Nursing, *Grambling (MSN)*

Loyola University New Orleans, School of Nursing, *New Orleans (MSN)*

McNeese State University, College of Nursing, *Lake Charles (MSN)*

Northwestern State University of Louisiana, College of Nursing and School of Allied Health, *Shreveport (MSN)*

Our Lady of the Lake College, Division of Nursing, *Baton Rouge (MSN)*

Southeastern Louisiana University, School of Nursing, *Hammond (MSN)*

Southern University and Agricultural and Mechanical College, School of Nursing, *Baton Rouge (MSN)*

University of Louisiana at Lafayette, College of Nursing, *Lafayette (MSN)*

Maine

Husson University, School of Nursing, *Bangor (MSN)*

Saint Joseph's College of Maine, Master of Science in Nursing Program, *Standish (MSN, MSN/MHA)*

University of Maine, School of Nursing, *Orono (MSN)*

University of Southern Maine, School of Nursing, *Portland (MS)*

Maryland

Bowie State University, Department of Nursing, *Bowie (MSN)*

Coppin State University, Helene Fuld School of Nursing, *Baltimore (MSN)*

Johns Hopkins University, School of Nursing, *Baltimore (MSN, MSN/MBA, MSN/MPH, MSN/PhD)*

Salisbury University, Department of Nursing, *Salisbury (MS)*

Towson University, Department of Nursing, *Towson (MS)*

University of Maryland, Baltimore, Nursing Programs, *Baltimore (MS, MS/MBA, MS/MPH)*

Massachusetts

American International College, Division of Nursing, *Springfield (MSN)*

Boston College, William F. Connell School of Nursing, *Chestnut Hill (MS, MS/MA, MS/MBA)*

Curry College, Division of Nursing, *Milton (MSN)*

Elms College, School of Nursing, *Chicopee (MSN, MSN/MBA)*

Emmanuel College, Department of Nursing, *Boston (MS)*

Endicott College, Major in Nursing, *Beverly (MSN)*

Fitchburg State University, Department of Nursing, *Fitchburg (MS)*

Framingham State University, Department of Nursing, *Framingham (MSN)*

MGH Institute of Health Professions, School of Nursing, *Boston (MS)*

Northeastern University, School of Nursing, *Boston (MS, MS/MBA)*

Regis College, School of Nursing, Science and Health Professions, *Weston (MSN)*

Salem State University, Program in Nursing, *Salem (MSN, MSN/MBA)*

Simmons College, School of Nursing and Health Sciences, *Boston (MS)*

University of Massachusetts Amherst, College of Nursing, *Amherst (MS)*

University of Massachusetts Boston, College of Nursing and Health Sciences, *Boston (MS)*

University of Massachusetts Dartmouth, College of Nursing, *North Dartmouth (MS)*

University of Massachusetts Lowell, School of Nursing, *Lowell (MS)*

University of Massachusetts Medical School, Graduate School of Nursing, *Worcester (MS)*

Worcester State University, Department of Nursing, *Worcester (MS)*

Michigan

Eastern Michigan University, School of Nursing, *Ypsilanti (MSN)*

Ferris State University, School of Nursing, *Big Rapids (MSN, MSN/MBA)*

Grand Valley State University, Kirkhof College of Nursing, *Allendale (MSN)*

Madonna University, College of Nursing and Health, *Livonia (MSN, MSN/MBA)*

Michigan State University, College of Nursing, *East Lansing (MSN)*

Oakland University, School of Nursing, *Rochester (MSN)*

Saginaw Valley State University, College of Health and Human Services, *University Center (MSN)*

Spring Arbor University, Program in Nursing, *Spring Arbor (MSN, MSN/MBA)*

University of Detroit Mercy, McAuley School of Nursing, *Detroit (MSN)*

University of Michigan, School of Nursing, *Ann Arbor (MS, MSN/MBA, MSN/MPH)*

Wayne State University, College of Nursing, *Detroit (MSN)*

Western Michigan University, College of Health and Human Services, *Kalamazoo (MSN)*

Minnesota

Augsburg College, Program in Nursing, *Minneapolis (MA)*

Bethel University, Department of Nursing, *St. Paul (MA)*

Capella University, Nursing Programs, *Minneapolis (MSN)*

Concordia College, Department of Nursing, *Moorhead (MS)*

Minnesota State University Mankato, School of Nursing, *Mankato (MSN, MSN/MS)*

Minnesota State University Moorhead, School of Nursing and Healthcare Leadership, *Moorhead (MS, MSN/MHA)*

St. Catherine University, Department of Nursing, *St. Paul (MS)*

Saint Mary's University of Minnesota, B.S. in Nursing, *Winona (MS)*

Walden University, Nursing Programs, *Minneapolis (MSN)*

Winona State University, College of Nursing and Health Sciences, *Winona (MS)*

Mississippi

Alcorn State University, School of Nursing, *Natchez (MSN)*

Delta State University, School of Nursing, *Cleveland (MSN)*

Mississippi University for Women, College of Nursing and Speech Language Pathology, *Columbus (MSN)*

University of Mississippi Medical Center, School of Nursing, *Jackson (MSN)*

University of Southern Mississippi, College of Nursing, *Hattiesburg (MSN)*

William Carey University, School of Nursing, *Hattiesburg (MSN)*

Missouri

Central Methodist University, College of Liberal Arts and Sciences, *Fayette (MSN)*

Cox College, Department of Nursing, *Springfield (MSN)*

Goldfarb School of Nursing at Barnes-Jewish College, *St. Louis (MSN)*

Graceland University, School of Nursing, *Independence (MSN)*

Maryville University of Saint Louis, The Catherine McAuley School of Nursing, College of Health Professions, *St. Louis (MSN)*

Missouri Southern State University, Department of Nursing, *Joplin (MSN)*

Missouri State University, Department of Nursing, *Springfield (MSN)*

Missouri Western State University, Department of Nursing, *St. Joseph (MSN)*

Research College of Nursing, College of Nursing, *Kansas City (MSN)*

Saint Louis University, School of Nursing, *St. Louis (MSN)*

Southeast Missouri State University, Department of Nursing, *Cape Girardeau (MSN)*

Southwest Baptist University, College of Nursing, *Bolivar (MSN)*

University of Central Missouri, Department of Nursing, *Warrensburg (MSN)*

University of Missouri, Sinclair School of Nursing, *Columbia (MSN, MSN/PhD)*

University of Missouri–Kansas City, School of Nursing and Health Studies, *Kansas City (MSN)*

University of Missouri–St. Louis, College of Nursing, *St. Louis (MSN)*

Webster University, Department of Nursing, *St. Louis (MSN)*

Montana

Montana State University, College of Nursing, *Bozeman (MN)*

Nebraska

Bryan College of Health Sciences, School of Nursing, *Lincoln (MSN)*

Clarkson College, Master of Science in Nursing Program, *Omaha (MSN)*

College of Saint Mary, Division of Health Care Professions, *Omaha (MSN)*

Creighton University, College of Nursing, *Omaha (MSN)*

Nebraska Methodist College, Department of Nursing, *Omaha (MSN)*

Nebraska Wesleyan University, Department of Nursing, *Lincoln (MSN, MSN/MBA)*

University of Nebraska Medical Center, College of Nursing, *Omaha (MSN)*

Nevada

Touro University, School of Nursing, *Henderson (MSN)*

University of Nevada, Las Vegas, School of Nursing, *Las Vegas (MSN)*

University of Nevada, Reno, Orvis School of Nursing, *Reno (MSN, MSN/MPH)*

New Hampshire

Franklin Pierce University, Master of Science in Nursing, *Rindge (MSN)*

Rivier University, Division of Nursing, *Nashua (MS)*

Southern New Hampshire University, Department of Nursing, *Manchester (MSN)*

University of New Hampshire, Department of Nursing, *Durham (MS)*

New Jersey

The College of New Jersey, School of Nursing, Health and Exercise Science, *Ewing (MSN)*

College of Saint Elizabeth, Department of Nursing, *Morristown (MSN)*

Fairleigh Dickinson University, Metropolitan Campus, Henry P. Becton School of Nursing and Allied Health, *Teaneck (MSN)*

Felician University, Division of Nursing and Health Management, *Lodi (MA/MSM, MSN)*

Kean University, Department of Nursing, *Union (MSN, MSN/MPA)*

Monmouth University, Marjorie K. Unterberg School of Nursing, *West Long Branch (MSN)*

Ramapo College of New Jersey, Master of Science in Nursing Program, *Mahwah (MSN)*

Rowan University, RN to BSN Program, *Glassboro (MSN)*

Rutgers, The State University of New Jersey, Camden, Rutgers School of Nursing–Camden, *Camden (MSN)*

Rutgers, The State University of New Jersey, Newark, Rutgers School of Nursing, *Newark (MSN, MSN/MPH)*

Saint Peter's University, Nursing Program, *Jersey City (MSN)*

Seton Hall University, College of Nursing, *South Orange (MSN, MSN/MBA)*

Thomas Edison State University, School of Nursing, *Trenton (MSN)*

William Paterson University of New Jersey, Department of Nursing, *Wayne (MSN)*

New Mexico

Eastern New Mexico University, Department of Allied Health–Nursing, *Portales (MSN)*

New Mexico State University, School of Nursing, *Las Cruces (MSN)*

University of New Mexico, Program in Nursing, *Albuquerque (MSN)*

University of Phoenix–New Mexico Campus, College of Nursing, *Albuquerque (MSN, MSN/Ed D)*

New York

Adelphi University, College of Nursing and Public Health, *Garden City (MS)*

Binghamton University, State University of New York, Decker School of Nursing, *Vestal (MS)*

College of Mount Saint Vincent, Department of Nursing, *Riverdale (MSN)*

The College of New Rochelle, School of Nursing, *New Rochelle (MS)*

College of Staten Island of the City University of New York, Department of Nursing, *Staten Island (MS)*

Columbia University, School of Nursing, *New York (MS, MSN/MBA, MSN/MPH)*

Daemen College, Department of Nursing, *Amherst (MS)*

Dominican College, Department of Nursing, *Orangeburg (M Sc N)*

D'Youville College, School of Nursing, *Buffalo (MS)*

Excelsior College, School of Nursing, *Albany (MS)*

Hunter College of the City University of New York, Hunter-Bellevue School of Nursing, *New York (MS, MSN/MPA, MSN/MPH)*

Lehman College of the City University of New York, Department of Nursing, *Bronx (MS)*

Le Moyne College, Nursing Programs, *Syracuse (MS)*

Long Island University–LIU Brooklyn, School of Nursing, *Brooklyn (MS)*

Long Island University–LIU Post, Department of Nursing, *Brookville (MS)*

Mercy College, Programs in Nursing, *Dobbs Ferry (MS)*

Molloy College, Division of Nursing, *Rockville Centre (MS, MS/MBA)*

Mount Saint Mary College, School of Nursing, *Newburgh (MS)*

New York University, College of Nursing, *New York (MS, MS/MPH)*

Pace University, Lienhard School of Nursing, *New York (MS)*

Roberts Wesleyan College, School of Nursing, *Rochester (M Sc N)*

The Sage Colleges, Department of Nursing, *Troy (MS, MS/MBA)*

St. John Fisher College, Wegmans School of Nursing, *Rochester (MS)*

St. Joseph's College, New York, Department of Nursing, *Brooklyn (MS)*

State University of New York Downstate Medical Center, College of Nursing, *Brooklyn (MS, MS/MPH)*

State University of New York Empire State College, Bachelor of Science in Nursing Program, *Saratoga Springs (MS)*

State University of New York Polytechnic Institute, School of Nursing and Health Systems, *Utica (MS)*

State University of New York Upstate Medical University, College of Nursing, *Syracuse (MS)*

Stony Brook University, State University of New York, School of Nursing, *Stony Brook (MS)*

University at Buffalo, the State University of New York, School of Nursing, *Buffalo (MS)*

North Carolina

Barton College, School of Nursing, *Wilson (MSN)*

Duke University, School of Nursing, *Durham (MSN)*

East Carolina University, College of Nursing, *Greenville (MSN)*

Gardner-Webb University, School of Nursing, *Boiling Springs (MSN, MSN/MBA)*

Lenoir-Rhyne University, Program in Nursing, *Hickory (MSN)*

Queens University of Charlotte, Presbyterian School of Nursing, *Charlotte (MSN, MSN/MBA)*

The University of North Carolina at Chapel Hill, School of Nursing, *Chapel Hill (MSN)*

The University of North Carolina at Charlotte, School of Nursing, *Charlotte (MSN)*

The University of North Carolina at Greensboro, School of Nursing, *Greensboro (MSN, MSN/MBA)*

The University of North Carolina Wilmington, School of Nursing, *Wilmington (MSN)*

Western Carolina University, School of Nursing, *Cullowhee (MS)*

Winston-Salem State University, Department of Nursing, *Winston-Salem (MSN)*

North Dakota

University of Mary, Division of Nursing, *Bismarck (MSN, MSN/MBA)*

University of North Dakota, College of Nursing, *Grand Forks (MS)*

Ohio

Capital University, School of Nursing, *Columbus (MN/MBA, MSN, MSN/JD, MSN/MDIV)*

Case Western Reserve University, Frances Payne Bolton School of Nursing, *Cleveland (MSN, MSN/MA, MSN/MPH)*

Cedarville University, School of Nursing, *Cedarville (MSN)*

Chamberlain College of Nursing, *Columbus (MSN)*

Cleveland State University, School of Nursing, *Cleveland (MSN, MSN/MBA)*

Franciscan University of Steubenville, Department of Nursing, *Steubenville (MSN)*

Kent State University, College of Nursing, *Kent (MSN, MSN/MBA, MSN/MPA)*

Lourdes University, School of Nursing, *Sylvania (MSN)*

Malone University, School of Nursing, *Canton (MSN)*

Mount Carmel College of Nursing, Nursing Programs, *Columbus (MS)*

Notre Dame College, Nursing Department, *South Euclid (MSN)*

The Ohio State University, College of Nursing, *Columbus (MS, MS/MPH)*

Ohio University, School of Nursing, *Athens (MSN)*

Otterbein University, Department of Nursing, *Westerville (MSN)*

The University of Akron, School of Nursing, *Akron (MSN)*

University of Cincinnati, College of Nursing, *Cincinnati (MSN)*

University of Phoenix–Cleveland Campus, College of Nursing, *Beachwood (MSN)*

The University of Toledo, College of Nursing, *Toledo (MSN)*

Urbana University, College of Nursing and Allied Health, *Urbana (MSN)*

Ursuline College, The Breen School of Nursing, *Pepper Pike (MSN, MSN/MBA)*

Walsh University, Department of Nursing, *North Canton (MSN)*

Wright State University, College of Nursing and Health, *Dayton (MS, MS/MBA)*

Xavier University, School of Nursing, *Cincinnati (MSN, MSN/Ed D, MSN/MBA)*

Youngstown State University, Department of Nursing, *Youngstown (MSN)*

Oklahoma

Northeastern State University, Department of Nursing, *Tahlequah (MSN)*

Oklahoma Baptist University, School of Nursing, *Shawnee (MSN)*

Oklahoma City University, Kramer School of Nursing, *Oklahoma City (MSN)*

University of Central Oklahoma, Department of Nursing, *Edmond (MS)*

University of Oklahoma Health Sciences Center, College of Nursing, *Oklahoma City (MS)*

Oregon

Oregon Health & Science University, School of Nursing, *Portland (MN)*

University of Portland, School of Nursing, *Portland (MS)*

Pennsylvania

Alvernia University, Nursing, *Reading (MSN, MSN/Ed D)*

Bloomsburg University of Pennsylvania, Department of Nursing, *Bloomsburg (MSN, MSN/MBA)*

Carlow University, College of Health and Wellness, *Pittsburgh (MSN, MSN/MBA)*

Cedar Crest College, Department of Nursing, *Allentown (MSN)*

Chatham University, Nursing Programs, *Pittsburgh (MSN)*

Clarion University of Pennsylvania, School of Nursing, *Oil City (MSN)*

DeSales University, Department of Nursing and Health, *Center Valley (MSN, MSN/MBA)*

Drexel University, College of Nursing and Health Professions, *Philadelphia (MSN)*

Duquesne University, School of Nursing, *Pittsburgh (MSN)*

Gannon University, Villa Maria School of Nursing, *Erie (MSN)*

Gwynedd Mercy University, Frances M. Maguire School of Nursing and Health Professions, *Gwynedd Valley (MSN)*

Holy Family University, School of Nursing and Allied Health Professions, *Philadelphia (MSN)*

Immaculata University, Division of Nursing, *Immaculata (MSN)*

Indiana University of Pennsylvania, Department of Nursing and Allied Health, *Indiana (MS)*

La Roche College, Department of Nursing and Nursing Management, *Pittsburgh (MSN)*

La Salle University, School of Nursing and Health Sciences, *Philadelphia (MSN, MSN/MBA)*

Mansfield University of Pennsylvania, Department of Health Sciences–Nursing, *Mansfield (MSN)*

Marywood University, Department of Nursing, *Scranton (MSN, MSN/MPH)*

Messiah College, Department of Nursing, *Mechanicsburg (MSN)*

Millersville University of Pennsylvania, Department of Nursing, *Millersville (MSN)*

Misericordia University, Department of Nursing, *Dallas (MSN)*

Moravian College, Department of Nursing, *Bethlehem (MSN)*

Neumann University, Program in Nursing and Health Sciences, *Aston (MS)*

Penn State University Park, School of Nursing, *University Park (MS, MSN/PhD)*

Robert Morris University, School of Nursing and Health Sciences, *Moon Township (MSN)*

Temple University, Department of Nursing, *Philadelphia (MSN)*

Thomas Jefferson University, Department of Nursing, *Philadelphia (MSN)*

University of Pennsylvania, School of Nursing, *Philadelphia (MSN, MSN/MBA, MSN/MPH, MSN/PhD)*

University of Pittsburgh, School of Nursing, *Pittsburgh (MSN)*

The University of Scranton, Department of Nursing, *Scranton (MSN)*

Villanova University, College of Nursing, *Villanova (MSN)*

West Chester University of Pennsylvania, Department of Nursing, *West Chester (MSN)*

Widener University, School of Nursing, *Chester (MSN, MSN/PhD)*

Wilkes University, Department of Nursing, *Wilkes-Barre (MS)*

York College of Pennsylvania, Department of Nursing, *York (MS)*

Puerto Rico

Inter American University of Puerto Rico, Arecibo Campus, Nursing Program, *Arecibo (MSN)*

University of Puerto Rico, Medical Sciences Campus, School of Nursing, *San Juan (MSN)*

Rhode Island

Rhode Island College, Department of Nursing, *Providence (MSN)*

University of Rhode Island, College of Nursing, *Kingston (MS)*

South Carolina

Charleston Southern University, Wingo School of Nursing, *Charleston (MSN)*

Clemson University, School of Nursing, *Clemson (MS)*

Medical University of South Carolina, College of Nursing, *Charleston (MSN)*

University of South Carolina, College of Nursing, *Columbia (MSN)*

University of South Carolina Upstate, Mary Black School of Nursing, *Spartanburg (MSN)*

South Dakota

Mount Marty College, Nursing Program, *Yankton (MSN)*

South Dakota State University, College of Nursing, *Brookings (MS)*

Tennessee

Aquinas College, School of Nursing, *Nashville (MSN)*

Austin Peay State University, School of Nursing, *Clarksville (MSN)*

Belmont University, School of Nursing, *Nashville (MSN)*

Carson-Newman University, Department of Nursing, *Jefferson City (MSN)*

East Tennessee State University, College of Nursing, *Johnson City (MSN)*

King University, School of Nursing, *Bristol (MSN, MSN/MBA)*

Lincoln Memorial University, Caylor School of Nursing, *Harrogate (MSN)*

Middle Tennessee State University, School of Nursing, *Murfreesboro (MSN)*

Southern Adventist University, School of Nursing, *Collegedale (MSN, MSN/MBA)*

Tennessee Technological University, Whitson-Hester School of Nursing, *Cookeville (M Sc N, MSN)*

Union University, School of Nursing, *Jackson (MSN)*

University of Memphis, Loewenberg School of Nursing, *Memphis (MSN)*

The University of Tennessee, College of Nursing, *Knoxville (MSN, MSN/PhD)*

The University of Tennessee at Chattanooga, School of Nursing, *Chattanooga (MSN)*

The University of Tennessee Health Science Center, College of Nursing, *Memphis (MSN)*

Vanderbilt University, Vanderbilt University School of Nursing, *Nashville (MSN, MSN/MDIV, MSN/MTS)*

Texas

Angelo State University, Department of Nursing and Rehabilitation Sciences, *San Angelo (MSN)*

Baylor University, Louise Herrington School of Nursing, *Dallas (MSN)*

Concordia University Texas, School of Nursing, *Austin (MSN)*

Lamar University, Department of Nursing, *Beaumont (MSN, MSN/MBA)*

Midwestern State University, Wilson School of Nursing, *Wichita Falls (MSN)*

Patty Hanks Shelton School of Nursing, *Abilene (MSN)*

Prairie View A&M University, College of Nursing, *Houston (MSN)*

Tarleton State University, Department of Nursing, *Stephenville (MSN)*

Texas A&M Health Science Center, College of Nursing, *College Station (MSN)*

Texas A&M International University, Canseco School of Nursing, *Laredo (MSN)*

Texas A&M University–Corpus Christi, College of Nursing and Health Sciences, *Corpus Christi (MSN)*

Texas A&M University–Texarkana, Nursing Department, *Texarkana (MSN)*

Texas Christian University, Harris College of Nursing, *Fort Worth (MSN)*

Texas State University, St. David's School of Nursing, *San Marcos (MSN)*

Texas Tech University Health Sciences Center, School of Nursing, *Lubbock (MSN)*

Texas Woman's University, College of Nursing, *Denton (MS, MS/MHA)*

University of Houston, School of Nursing, *Houston (MSN)*

University of Mary Hardin-Baylor, College of Nursing, *Belton (MSN)*

The University of Texas at Arlington, College of Nursing, *Arlington (MSN, MSN/MBA, MSN/MHA, MSN/MPH)*

The University of Texas at Austin, School of Nursing, *Austin (MSN)*

The University of Texas at Brownsville, Department of Nursing, *Brownsville (MSN)*

The University of Texas at El Paso, School of Nursing, *El Paso (MSN)*

The University of Texas at Tyler, Program in Nursing, *Tyler (MSN, MSN/MBA)*

The University of Texas Health Science Center at Houston, School of Nursing, *Houston (MSN, MSN/MPH)*

The University of Texas Health Science Center at San Antonio, School of Nursing, *San Antonio (MSN)*

The University of Texas Medical Branch, School of Nursing, *Galveston (MSN)*

The University of Texas Rio Grande Valley, School of Nursing, *Edinburg (MSN)*

University of the Incarnate Word, Program in Nursing, *San Antonio (MSN)*

West Texas A&M University, Department of Nursing, *Canyon (MSN)*

Utah

Brigham Young University, College of Nursing, *Provo (MS)*

University of Utah, College of Nursing, *Salt Lake City (MS)*

Weber State University, Program in Nursing, *Ogden (MSN)*

Western Governors University, Online College of Health Professions, *Salt Lake City (MS)*

Westminster College, School of Nursing and Health Sciences, *Salt Lake City (MSN)*

Vermont

University of Vermont, Department of Nursing, *Burlington (MS)*

Virginia

Eastern Mennonite University, Department of Nursing, *Harrisonburg (MSN)*

George Mason University, College of Health and Human Services, *Fairfax (MSN)*

Hampton University, School of Nursing, *Hampton (MS)*

James Madison University, Department of Nursing, *Harrisonburg (MSN)*

Jefferson College of Health Sciences, Nursing Education Program, *Roanoke (MSN)*

Liberty University, Department of Nursing, *Lynchburg (MSN)*

Lynchburg College, School of Health Sciences and Human Performance, *Lynchburg (MSN)*

Marymount University, School of Health Professions, *Arlington (MSN)*

Old Dominion University, Department of Nursing, *Norfolk (MSN)*

Radford University, Program in Nursing Practice, *Radford (MSN)*

Shenandoah University, Eleanor Wade Custer School of Nursing, *Winchester (MSN)*

University of Virginia, School of Nursing, *Charlottesville (MSN, MSN/PhD)*

Virginia Commonwealth University, School of Nursing, *Richmond (MS)*

Washington

Gonzaga University, School of Nursing and Human Psychology, *Spokane (MSN)*

Pacific Lutheran University, School of Nursing, *Tacoma (MSN, MSN/MBA)*

Seattle Pacific University, School of Health Sciences, *Seattle (MSN)*

Seattle University, College of Nursing, *Seattle (MSN)*

University of Washington, School of Nursing, *Seattle (MN, MN/MPH)*

WSU College of Nursing, *Spokane (MN)*

West Virginia

Marshall University, College of Health Professions, *Huntington (MSN)*

West Virginia University, School of Nursing, *Morgantown (MSN)*

West Virginia Wesleyan College, School of Nursing, *Buckhannon (MSN)*

Wheeling Jesuit University, Department of Nursing, *Wheeling (MSN)*

Wisconsin

Alverno College, Division of Nursing, *Milwaukee (MSN)*

Bellin College, Nursing Program, *Green Bay (MSN)*

Cardinal Stritch University, Ruth S. Coleman College of Nursing and Health Sciences, *Milwaukee (MSN)*

Columbia College of Nursing, *Milwaukee (MSN)*

Concordia University Wisconsin, Program in Nursing, *Mequon (MSN)*

Edgewood College, Henry Predolin School of Nursing, *Madison (MS, MSN/MBA)*

Herzing University Online, Program in Nursing, *Menomonee Falls (MSN)*

Marian University, School of Nursing, *Fond du Lac (MSN)*

Marquette University, College of Nursing, *Milwaukee (MSN, MSN/MBA)*

Milwaukee School of Engineering, School of Nursing, *Milwaukee (MSN)*

University of Phoenix–Milwaukee Campus, College of Health and Human Services, *Milwaukee (MSN)*

University of Wisconsin–Eau Claire, College of Nursing and Health Sciences, *Eau Claire (MSN)*

University of Wisconsin–Green Bay, Online Nursing and Health Programs, *Green Bay (MSN)*

University of Wisconsin–Milwaukee, College of Nursing, *Milwaukee (MN)*

University of Wisconsin–Oshkosh, College of Nursing, *Oshkosh (MSN)*

Wyoming

University of Wyoming, Fay W. Whitney School of Nursing, *Laramie (MS)*

CANADA

Alberta

Athabasca University, Centre for Nursing and Health Studies, *Athabasca (MN, MN/MHSA)*

University of Alberta, Faculty of Nursing, *Edmonton (MN)*

University of Calgary, Faculty of Nursing, *Calgary (MN)*

University of Lethbridge, Faculty of Health Sciences, *Lethbridge (MN)*

British Columbia

Trinity Western University, Department of Nursing, *Langley (MSN)*

The University of British Columbia, Program in Nursing, *Vancouver (MSN, MSN/MPH)*

University of Northern British Columbia, Nursing Programme, *Prince George (M Sc N)*

University of Victoria, School of Nursing, *Victoria (MN)*

Manitoba

Brandon University, School of Health Studies, *Brandon (MN)*

University of Manitoba, Faculty of Nursing, *Winnipeg (MN)*

New Brunswick

Université de Moncton, School of Nursing, *Moncton (M Sc N)*

University of New Brunswick Fredericton, Faculty of Nursing, *Fredericton (MN)*

Newfoundland and Labrador

Memorial University of Newfoundland, School of Nursing, *St. John's (MN)*

Ontario

Laurentian University, School of Nursing, *Sudbury (M Sc N)*

McMaster University, School of Nursing, *Hamilton (M Sc, MSN/PhD)*

Queen's University at Kingston, School of Nursing, *Kingston (MN Sc)*

Ryerson University, Program in Nursing, *Toronto (MN)*

University of Ottawa, School of Nursing, *Ottawa (M Sc N)*

University of Toronto, Faculty of Nursing, *Toronto (MN)*

The University of Western Ontario, School of Nursing, *London (M Sc N)*

University of Windsor, Faculty of Nursing, *Windsor (M Sc N)*

Quebec

McGill University, School of Nursing, *Montréal (M Sc)*

Université de Montréal, Faculty of Nursing, *Montréal (M Sc)*

Université de Sherbrooke, Department of Nursing, *Sherbrooke (M Sc)*

Université du Québec à Chicoutimi, Program in Nursing, *Chicoutimi (MSN)*

Université du Québec à Rimouski, Program in Nursing, *Rimouski (M Sc N)*

Université du Québec à Trois-Rivières, Program in Nursing, *Trois-Rivières (MSN)*

Université du Québec en Outaouais, Département des Sciences Infirmières, *Gatineau (M Sc N)*

Université Laval, Faculty of Nursing, *Québec (MSN)*

Saskatchewan

University of Saskatchewan, College of Nursing, *Saskatoon (MN)*

MASTER'S FOR NON-NURSING COLLEGE GRADUATES

U.S. AND U.S. TERRITORIES

Alabama

The University of Alabama at Birmingham, School of Nursing, *Birmingham (MSN, MSN/MPH)*

California

California State University, Fullerton, Department of Nursing, *Fullerton (MSN)*

California State University, Los Angeles, School of Nursing, *Los Angeles (MSN)*

Samuel Merritt University, School of Nursing, *Oakland (MSN)*

San Francisco State University, School of Nursing, *San Francisco (MSN)*

University of California, Los Angeles, School of Nursing, *Los Angeles (MSN, MSN/MBA)*

University of California, San Francisco, School of Nursing, *San Francisco (MS)*

Connecticut

Yale University, School of Nursing, *West Haven (MSN, MSN/MDIV, MSN/MPH)*

District of Columbia

Georgetown University, School of Nursing and Health Studies, *Washington (MS)*

Hawaii

University of Hawaii at Manoa, School of Nursing and Dental Hygiene, *Honolulu (MS, MSN/MBA)*

Illinois

DePaul University, School of Nursing, *Chicago (MS)*

Rush University, College of Nursing, *Chicago (MSN)*

University of Illinois at Chicago, College of Nursing, *Chicago (MS)*

Maine

University of Southern Maine, School of Nursing, *Portland (MS)*

Massachusetts

MGH Institute of Health Professions, School of Nursing, *Boston (MS)*

Northeastern University, School of Nursing, *Boston (MS, MS/MBA)*

Regis College, School of Nursing, Science and Health Professions, *Weston (MSN)*

Minnesota

St. Catherine University, Department of Nursing, *St. Paul (MS)*

Missouri

Saint Louis University, School of Nursing, *St. Louis (MSN)*

New Jersey

Seton Hall University, College of Nursing, *South Orange (MSN, MSN/MBA)*

New York

Columbia University, School of Nursing, *New York (MS, MSN/MBA, MSN/MPH)*

Mercy College, Programs in Nursing, *Dobbs Ferry (MS)*

North Carolina

Gardner-Webb University, School of Nursing, *Boiling Springs (MSN, MSN/MBA)*

Ohio

Case Western Reserve University, Frances Payne Bolton School of Nursing, *Cleveland (MSN, MSN/MA, MSN/MPH)*

The Ohio State University, College of Nursing, *Columbus (MS, MS/MPH)*

The University of Toledo, College of Nursing, *Toledo (MSN)*

Oklahoma

University of Oklahoma Health Sciences Center, College of Nursing, *Oklahoma City (MS)*

Pennsylvania

Immaculata University, Division of Nursing, *Immaculata (MSN)*

Thomas Jefferson University, Department of Nursing, *Philadelphia (MSN)*

Wilkes University, Department of Nursing, *Wilkes-Barre (MS)*

South Dakota

Mount Marty College, Nursing Program, *Yankton (MSN)*

Tennessee

University of Memphis, Loewenberg School of Nursing, *Memphis (MSN)*

Vanderbilt University, Vanderbilt University School of Nursing, *Nashville (MSN, MSN/MDIV, MSN/MTS)*

Texas

Angelo State University, Department of Nursing and Rehabilitation Sciences, *San Angelo (MSN)*

Utah

University of Utah, College of Nursing, *Salt Lake City (MS)*

Vermont

University of Vermont, Department of Nursing, *Burlington (MS)*

Virginia

University of Virginia, School of Nursing, *Charlottesville (MSN, MSN/PhD)*

Wisconsin

Marquette University, College of Nursing, *Milwaukee (MSN, MSN/MBA)*

University of Wisconsin–Milwaukee, College of Nursing, *Milwaukee (MN)*

CANADA

Quebec

McGill University, School of Nursing, *Montréal (M Sc)*

MASTER'S FOR NURSES WITH NON-NURSING DEGREES

U.S. AND U.S. TERRITORIES

Alabama

The University of Alabama at Birmingham, School of Nursing, *Birmingham (MSN, MSN/MPH)*

University of South Alabama, College of Nursing, *Mobile (MSN)*

Arizona

University of Phoenix–Online Campus, Online Campus, *Phoenix (MSN, MSN/MBA, MSN/MHA)*

Arkansas

Arkansas Tech University, Program in Nursing, *Russellville (MSN)*

University of Arkansas for Medical Sciences, College of Nursing, *Little Rock (MN Sc)*

California

California State University, Dominguez Hills, Program in Nursing, *Carson (MSN)*

California State University, Sacramento, Division of Nursing, *Sacramento (MS)*

Holy Names University, Department of Nursing, *Oakland (MSN, MSN/MBA)*

Samuel Merritt University, School of Nursing, *Oakland (MSN)*

San Francisco State University, School of Nursing, *San Francisco (MSN)*

University of California, San Francisco, School of Nursing, *San Francisco (MS)*

University of San Francisco, School of Nursing and Health Professions, *San Francisco (MSN)*

Connecticut

University of Hartford, College of Education, Nursing, and Health Professions, *West Hartford (MSN)*

University of Saint Joseph, Department of Nursing, *West Hartford (MS)*

Yale University, School of Nursing, *West Haven (MSN, MSN/MDIV, MSN/MPH)*

Florida

Florida Southern College, School of Nursing & Health Sciences, *Lakeland (MSN, MSN/MBA)*

University of Central Florida, College of Nursing, *Orlando (MSN)*

University of South Florida, College of Nursing, *Tampa (MS, MS/MPH)*

Illinois

Saint Anthony College of Nursing, *Rockford (MSN)*

University of Illinois at Chicago, College of Nursing, *Chicago (MS)*

University of St. Francis, Leach College of Nursing, *Joliet (MSN)*

Indiana

University of Saint Francis, Department of Nursing, *Fort Wayne (MSN)*

Iowa

Allen College, Graduate Programs, *Waterloo (MSN)*

The University of Iowa, College of Nursing, *Iowa City (MSN, MSN/MBA, MSN/MPH)*

Kentucky

Bellarmine University, Donna and Allan Lansing School of Nursing and Health Sciences, *Louisville (Certificate of Completion, MSN, MSN/MBA)*

Frontier Nursing University, Nursing Degree Programs, *Hyden (MSN)*

Louisiana

Loyola University New Orleans, School of Nursing, *New Orleans (MSN)*

Maine

Husson University, School of Nursing, *Bangor (MSN)*

Saint Joseph's College of Maine, Master of Science in Nursing Program, *Standish (MSN, MSN/MHA)*

University of Southern Maine, School of Nursing, *Portland (MS)*

Maryland

Johns Hopkins University, School of Nursing, *Baltimore (MSN, MSN/MBA, MSN/MPH, MSN/PhD)*

Massachusetts

American International College, Division of Nursing, *Springfield (MSN)*

MGH Institute of Health Professions, School of Nursing, *Boston (MS)*

Regis College, School of Nursing, Science and Health Professions, *Weston (MSN)*

Worcester State University, Department of Nursing, *Worcester (MS)*

Michigan

Eastern Michigan University, School of Nursing, *Ypsilanti (MSN)*

University of Detroit Mercy, McAuley School of Nursing, *Detroit (MSN)*

Minnesota

Metropolitan State University, College of Health, Community and Professional Studies, *St. Paul (MSN)*

Minnesota State University Mankato, School of Nursing, *Mankato (MSN, MSN/MS)*

Winona State University, College of Nursing and Health Sciences, *Winona (MS)*

Mississippi

Delta State University, School of Nursing, *Cleveland (MSN)*

Missouri

Saint Louis University, School of Nursing, *St. Louis (MSN)*

Nebraska

Nebraska Methodist College, Department of Nursing, *Omaha (MSN)*

New Hampshire

Franklin Pierce University, Master of Science in Nursing, *Rindge (MSN)*

Rivier University, Division of Nursing, *Nashua (MS)*

University of New Hampshire, Department of Nursing, *Durham (MS)*

New Jersey

College of Saint Elizabeth, Department of Nursing, *Morristown (MSN)*

Kean University, Department of Nursing, *Union (MSN, MSN/MPA)*

Monmouth University, Marjorie K. Unterberg School of Nursing, *West Long Branch (MSN)*

Rutgers, The State University of New Jersey, Newark, Rutgers School of Nursing, *Newark (MSN, MSN/MPH)*

Saint Peter's University, Nursing Program, *Jersey City (MSN)*

Seton Hall University, College of Nursing, *South Orange (MSN, MSN/MBA)*

William Paterson University of New Jersey, Department of Nursing, *Wayne (MSN)*

New Mexico

New Mexico State University, School of Nursing, *Las Cruces (MSN)*

New York

Columbia University, School of Nursing, *New York (MS, MSN/MBA, MSN/MPH)*

Lehman College of the City University of New York, Department of Nursing, *Bronx (MS)*

Mercy College, Programs in Nursing, *Dobbs Ferry (MS)*

Pace University, Lienhard School of Nursing, *New York (MS)*

State University of New York Upstate Medical University, College of Nursing, *Syracuse (MS)*

Ohio

The Ohio State University, College of Nursing, *Columbus (MS, MS/MPH)*

The University of Toledo, College of Nursing, *Toledo (MSN)*

Urbana University, College of Nursing and Allied Health, *Urbana (MSN)*

Xavier University, School of Nursing, *Cincinnati (MSN, MSN/Ed D, MSN/MBA)*

Oklahoma

Oklahoma City University, Kramer School of Nursing, *Oklahoma City (MSN)*

Pennsylvania

Holy Family University, School of Nursing and Allied Health Professions, *Philadelphia (MSN)*

Indiana University of Pennsylvania, Department of Nursing and Allied Health, *Indiana (MS)*

Moravian College, Department of Nursing, *Bethlehem (MSN)*

Thomas Jefferson University, Department of Nursing, *Philadelphia (MSN)*

Widener University, School of Nursing, *Chester (MSN, MSN/PhD)*

South Dakota

Mount Marty College, Nursing Program, *Yankton (MSN)*

Tennessee

University of Memphis, Loewenberg School of Nursing, *Memphis (MSN)*

The University of Tennessee Health Science Center, College of Nursing, *Memphis (MSN)*

Texas

The University of Texas at Austin, School of Nursing, *Austin (MSN)*

The University of Texas at Brownsville, Department of Nursing, *Brownsville (MSN)*

Vermont

University of Vermont, Department of Nursing, *Burlington (MS)*

Virginia

Eastern Mennonite University, Department of Nursing, *Harrisonburg (MSN)*

Jefferson College of Health Sciences, Nursing Education Program, *Roanoke (MSN)*

Old Dominion University, Department of Nursing, *Norfolk (MSN)*

University of Virginia, School of Nursing, *Charlottesville (MSN, MSN/PhD)*

Washington

Gonzaga University, School of Nursing and Human Psychology, *Spokane (MSN)*

Pacific Lutheran University, School of Nursing, *Tacoma (MSN, MSN/MBA)*

Seattle Pacific University, School of Health Sciences, *Seattle (MSN)*

University of Washington, School of Nursing, *Seattle (MN, MN/MPH)*

Wisconsin

Marquette University, College of Nursing, *Milwaukee (MSN, MSN/MBA)*

CANADA

Alberta

Athabasca University, Centre for Nursing and Health Studies, *Athabasca (MN, MN/MHSA)*

Quebec

Université du Québec en Outaouais, Département des Sciences Infirmières, *Gatineau (M Sc N)*

RN TO MASTER'S

U.S. AND U.S. TERRITORIES

Alabama

Samford University, Ida V. Moffett School of Nursing, *Birmingham (MSN)*

Spring Hill College, Division of Nursing, *Mobile (MSN)*

The University of Alabama, Capstone College of Nursing, *Tuscaloosa (MSN, MSN/Ed D)*

The University of Alabama at Birmingham, School of Nursing, *Birmingham (MSN, MSN/MPH)*

The University of Alabama in Huntsville, College of Nursing, *Huntsville (MSN)*

University of North Alabama, College of Nursing and Allied Health, *Florence (MSN)*

Arizona

The University of Arizona, College of Nursing, *Tucson (MSN)*

Arkansas

Arkansas Tech University, Program in Nursing, *Russellville (MSN)*

University of Arkansas for Medical Sciences, College of Nursing, *Little Rock (MN Sc)*

University of Central Arkansas, Department of Nursing, *Conway (MSN)*

California

Holy Names University, Department of Nursing, *Oakland (MSN, MSN/MBA)*

Mount Saint Mary's University, Department of Nursing, *Los Angeles (MSN)*

National University, Department of Nursing, *La Jolla (MSN)*

Point Loma Nazarene University, School of Nursing, *San Diego (MSN)*

University of San Francisco, School of Nursing and Health Professions, *San Francisco (MSN)*

Western University of Health Sciences, College of Graduate Nursing, *Pomona (MSN)*

Colorado

American Sentinel University, RN to Bachelor of Science Nursing, *Aurora (MSN)*

Aspen University, Graduate School of Health Professions and Studies, *Denver (MSN)*

Regis University, School of Nursing, *Denver (MS)*

Connecticut

Sacred Heart University, College of Nursing, *Fairfield (MSN)*

Southern Connecticut State University, Department of Nursing, *New Haven (MSN)*

University of Connecticut, School of Nursing, *Storrs (MS)*

Delaware

University of Delaware, School of Nursing, *Newark (MSN)*

Wesley College, Nursing Program, *Dover (MSN)*

Florida

Jacksonville University, School of Nursing, *Jacksonville (MSN, MSN/MBA)*

Kaplan University Online, The School of Nursing Online, *Fort Lauderdale (MSN)*

Nova Southeastern University, College of Health Care Sciences, *Fort Lauderdale (MSN)*

Palm Beach Atlantic University, School of Nursing, *West Palm Beach (MSN)*

University of North Florida, School of Nursing, *Jacksonville (MSN)*

University of South Florida, College of Nursing, *Tampa (MS, MS/MPH)*

Georgia

Brenau University, College of Health and Science, *Gainesville (MSN)*

Clayton State University, Department of Nursing, *Morrow (MSN)*

Georgia State University, Byrdine F. Lewis School of Nursing, *Atlanta (MS)*

Thomas University, Division of Nursing, *Thomasville (MSN, MSN/MBA)*

Valdosta State University, College of Nursing, *Valdosta (MSN)*

Hawaii

Hawai`i Pacific University, College of Nursing and Health Sciences, *Honolulu (MSN, MSN/MBA)*

University of Hawaii at Manoa, School of Nursing and Dental Hygiene, *Honolulu (MS, MSN/MBA)*

Idaho

Northwest Nazarene University, School of Health and Science, *Nampa (MSN)*

Illinois

Blessing–Rieman College of Nursing and Health Sciences, *Quincy (MSN)*

Bradley University, Department of Nursing, *Peoria (MSN)*

Lewis University, Program in Nursing, *Romeoville (MSN, MSN/MBA)*

Loyola University Chicago, Marcella Niehoff School of Nursing, *Maywood (MSN, MSN/MBA)*

McKendree University, Department of Nursing, *Lebanon (MSN, MSN/MBA)*

North Park University, School of Nursing, *Chicago (MS, MSN/MA, MSN/MBA, MSN/MM)*

Resurrection University, *Chicago (MSN)*

Saint Anthony College of Nursing, *Rockford (MSN)*

Indiana

Ball State University, School of Nursing, *Muncie (MS)*

Indiana University–Purdue University Indianapolis, School of Nursing, *Indianapolis (MSN)*

University of Saint Francis, Department of Nursing, *Fort Wayne (MSN)*

Valparaiso University, College of Nursing and Health Professions, *Valparaiso (MSN, MSN/MHA)*

Kansas

MidAmerica Nazarene University, Division of Nursing, *Olathe (MSN)*

The University of Kansas, School of Nursing, *Kansas City (MS, MS/MHSA, MS/MPH)*

Kentucky

Bellarmine University, Donna and Allan Lansing School of Nursing and Health Sciences, *Louisville (Certificate of Completion, MSN, MSN/MBA)*

Spalding University, School of Nursing, *Louisville (MSN)*

University of Kentucky, College of Nursing, *Lexington (MSN)*

Louisiana

University of Louisiana at Lafayette, College of Nursing, *Lafayette (MSN)*

Maine

Saint Joseph's College of Maine, Master of Science in Nursing Program, *Standish (MSN, MSN/MHA)*

University of Maine, School of Nursing, *Orono (MSN)*

University of Southern Maine, School of Nursing, *Portland (MS)*

Maryland

Salisbury University, Department of Nursing, *Salisbury (MS)*

Stevenson University, Nursing Division, *Stevenson (MS)*

University of Maryland, Baltimore, Nursing Programs, *Baltimore (MS, MS/MBA, MS/MPH)*

Massachusetts

American International College, Division of Nursing, *Springfield (MSN)*

Boston College, William F. Connell School of Nursing, *Chestnut Hill (MS, MS/MA, MS/MBA)*

Curry College, Division of Nursing, *Milton (MSN)*

Elms College, School of Nursing, *Chicopee (MSN, MSN/MBA)*

MGH Institute of Health Professions, School of Nursing, *Boston (MS)*

Regis College, School of Nursing, Science and Health Professions, *Weston (MSN)*

Salem State University, Program in Nursing, *Salem (MSN, MSN/MBA)*

Simmons College, School of Nursing and Health Sciences, *Boston (MS)*

University of Massachusetts Dartmouth, College of Nursing, *North Dartmouth (MS)*

Worcester State University, Department of Nursing, *Worcester (MS)*

Michigan

Ferris State University, School of Nursing, *Big Rapids (MSN, MSN/MBA)*

Saginaw Valley State University, College of Health and Human Services, *University Center (MSN)*

University of Michigan, School of Nursing, *Ann Arbor (MS, MSN/MBA, MSN/MPH)*

University of Michigan–Flint, Department of Nursing, *Flint (MSN)*

Minnesota

Metropolitan State University, College of Health, Community and Professional Studies, *St. Paul (MSN)*

Minnesota State University Mankato, School of Nursing, *Mankato (MSN, MSN/MS)*

Walden University, Nursing Programs, *Minneapolis (MSN)*

Winona State University, College of Nursing and Health Sciences, *Winona (MS)*

Mississippi

University of Mississippi Medical Center, School of Nursing, *Jackson (MSN)*

Missouri

Cox College, Department of Nursing, *Springfield (MSN)*

Graceland University, School of Nursing, *Independence (MSN)*

Missouri State University, Department of Nursing, *Springfield (MSN)*

Research College of Nursing, College of Nursing, *Kansas City (MSN)*

Webster University, Department of Nursing, *St. Louis (MSN)*

Nebraska

Clarkson College, Master of Science in Nursing Program, *Omaha (MSN)*

Nebraska Methodist College, Department of Nursing, *Omaha (MSN)*

Nebraska Wesleyan University, Department of Nursing, *Lincoln (MSN, MSN/MBA)*

New Hampshire

Franklin Pierce University, Master of Science in Nursing, *Rindge (MSN)*

Rivier University, Division of Nursing, *Nashua (MS)*

New Jersey

The College of New Jersey, School of Nursing, Health and Exercise Science, *Ewing (MSN)*

Fairleigh Dickinson University, Metropolitan Campus, Henry P. Becton School of Nursing and Allied Health, *Teaneck (MSN)*

Monmouth University, Marjorie K. Unterberg School of Nursing, *West Long Branch (MSN)*

Rutgers, The State University of New Jersey, Newark, Rutgers School of Nursing, *Newark (MSN, MSN/MPH)*

Seton Hall University, College of Nursing, *South Orange (MSN, MSN/MBA)*

Thomas Edison State University, School of Nursing, *Trenton (MSN)*

New York

The College of New Rochelle, School of Nursing, *New Rochelle (MS)*

Daemen College, Department of Nursing, *Amherst (MS)*

Excelsior College, School of Nursing, *Albany (MS)*

Long Island University–LIU Brooklyn, School of Nursing, *Brooklyn (MS)*

St. John Fisher College, Wegmans School of Nursing, *Rochester (MS)*

State University of New York Polytechnic Institute, School of Nursing and Health Systems, *Utica (MS)*

State University of New York Upstate Medical University, College of Nursing, *Syracuse (MS)*

Stony Brook University, State University of New York, School of Nursing, *Stony Brook (MS)*

North Carolina

Duke University, School of Nursing, *Durham (MSN)*

East Carolina University, College of Nursing, *Greenville (MSN)*

Gardner-Webb University, School of Nursing, *Boiling Springs (MSN, MSN/MBA)*

Lenoir-Rhyne University, Program in Nursing, *Hickory (MSN)*

Queens University of Charlotte, Presbyterian School of Nursing, *Charlotte (MSN, MSN/MBA)*

The University of North Carolina at Chapel Hill, School of Nursing, *Chapel Hill (MSN)*

The University of North Carolina at Charlotte, School of Nursing, *Charlotte (MSN)*

North Dakota

University of Mary, Division of Nursing, *Bismarck (MSN, MSN/MBA)*

Ohio

Capital University, School of Nursing, *Columbus (MN/MBA, MSN, MSN/JD, MSN/MDIV)*

Case Western Reserve University, Frances Payne Bolton School of Nursing, *Cleveland (MSN, MSN/MA, MSN/MPH)*

Franciscan University of Steubenville, Department of Nursing, *Steubenville (MSN)*

Lourdes University, School of Nursing, *Sylvania (MSN)*

The Ohio State University, College of Nursing, *Columbus (MS, MS/MPH)*

The University of Akron, School of Nursing, *Akron (MSN)*

Urbana University, College of Nursing and Allied Health, *Urbana (MSN)*

Xavier University, School of Nursing, *Cincinnati (MSN, MSN/Ed D, MSN/MBA)*

Oklahoma

Oklahoma Baptist University, School of Nursing, *Shawnee (MSN)*

Oklahoma City University, Kramer School of Nursing, *Oklahoma City (MSN)*

Pennsylvania

Alvernia University, Nursing, *Reading (MSN, MSN/Ed D)*

Bloomsburg University of Pennsylvania, Department of Nursing, *Bloomsburg (MSN, MSN/MBA)*

DeSales University, Department of Nursing and Health, *Center Valley (MSN, MSN/MBA)*

Drexel University, College of Nursing and Health Professions, *Philadelphia (MSN)*

Gannon University, Villa Maria School of Nursing, *Erie (MSN)*

Gwynedd Mercy University, Frances M. Maguire School of Nursing and Health Professions, *Gwynedd Valley (MSN)*

La Roche College, Department of Nursing and Nursing Management, *Pittsburgh (MSN)*

La Salle University, School of Nursing and Health Sciences, *Philadelphia (MSN, MSN/MBA)*

Messiah College, Department of Nursing, *Mechanicsburg (MSN)*

Misericordia University, Department of Nursing, *Dallas (MSN)*

Robert Morris University, School of Nursing and Health Sciences, *Moon Township (MSN)*

Thomas Jefferson University, Department of Nursing, *Philadelphia (MSN)*

University of Pittsburgh, School of Nursing, *Pittsburgh (MSN)*

The University of Scranton, Department of Nursing, *Scranton (MSN)*

Wilkes University, Department of Nursing, *Wilkes-Barre (MS)*

Rhode Island

University of Rhode Island, College of Nursing, *Kingston (MS)*

South Carolina

Charleston Southern University, Wingo School of Nursing, *Charleston (MSN)*

South Dakota

Mount Marty College, Nursing Program, *Yankton (MSN)*

South Dakota State University, College of Nursing, *Brookings (MS)*

Tennessee

East Tennessee State University, College of Nursing, *Johnson City (MSN)*

Tennessee State University, Division of Nursing, *Nashville (MSN)*

Vanderbilt University, Vanderbilt University School of Nursing, *Nashville (MSN, MSN/MDIV, MSN/MTS)*

Texas

Angelo State University, Department of Nursing and Rehabilitation Sciences, *San Angelo (MSN)*

Concordia University Texas, School of Nursing, *Austin (MSN)*

Lamar University, Department of Nursing, *Beaumont (MSN, MSN/MBA)*

Midwestern State University, Wilson School of Nursing, *Wichita Falls (MSN)*

Tarleton State University, Department of Nursing, *Stephenville (MSN)*

Texas A&M Health Science Center, College of Nursing, *College Station (MSN)*

Texas A&M University–Corpus Christi, College of Nursing and Health Sciences, *Corpus Christi (MSN)*

Texas Woman's University, College of Nursing, *Denton (MS, MS/MHA)*

University of Houston, School of Nursing, *Houston (MSN)*

The University of Texas at Tyler, Program in Nursing, *Tyler (MSN, MSN/MBA)*

The University of Texas Health Science Center at San Antonio, School of Nursing, *San Antonio (MSN)*

West Texas A&M University, Department of Nursing, *Canyon (MSN)*

Utah

University of Utah, College of Nursing, *Salt Lake City (MS)*

Western Governors University, Online College of Health Professions, *Salt Lake City (MS)*

Vermont

University of Vermont, Department of Nursing, *Burlington (MS)*

Virginia

Hampton University, School of Nursing, *Hampton (MS)*

Shenandoah University, Eleanor Wade Custer School of Nursing, *Winchester (MSN)*

University of Virginia, School of Nursing, *Charlottesville (MSN, MSN/PhD)*

West Virginia

West Virginia University, School of Nursing, *Morgantown (MSN)*

Wheeling Jesuit University, Department of Nursing, *Wheeling (MSN)*

Wisconsin

University of Wisconsin–Eau Claire, College of Nursing and Health Sciences, *Eau Claire (MSN)*

University of Wisconsin–Oshkosh, College of Nursing, *Oshkosh (MSN)*

CANADA

Alberta

University of Calgary, Faculty of Nursing, *Calgary (MN)*

New Brunswick

Université de Moncton, School of Nursing, *Moncton (M Sc N)*

Quebec

Université de Montréal, Faculty of Nursing, *Montréal (M Sc)*

Université du Québec à Chicoutimi, Program in Nursing, *Chicoutimi (MSN)*

CONCENTRATIONS WITHIN MASTER'S DEGREE PROGRAMS

CASE MANAGEMENT

American Sentinel University, CO
Boise State University, ID
Carlow University, PA
Johns Hopkins University, MD
Loyola University New Orleans, LA
Pacific Lutheran University, WA
Regis College, MA
Saint Peter's University, NJ
Samuel Merritt University, CA
San Francisco State University, CA
Seton Hall University, NJ
Université de Moncton, NB
The University of Alabama, AL
University of Kentucky, KY
University of Manitoba, MB
University of New Brunswick Fredericton, NB
University of Utah, UT
Valdosta State University, GA
WSU College of Nursing, WA

CLINICAL NURSE LEADER

Augusta University, GA
Boise State University, ID
California Baptist University, CA
California State University, Sacramento, CA
Central Methodist University, MO
Cleveland State University, OH
The College of New Jersey, NJ
Columbia College of Nursing, WI
Cox College, MO
Creighton University, NE
Curry College, MA
DeSales University, PA
Drexel University, PA
Elmhurst College, IL
Fairfield University, CT
Florida Atlantic University, FL
Georgetown University, DC
Goshen College, IN
Grand Valley State University, MI
Grand View University, IA
Illinois State University, IL
James Madison University, VA
Lynchburg College, VA
Marquette University, WI
MGH Institute of Health Professions, MA
Montana State University, MT
Moravian College, PA
Morningside College, IA
The Ohio State University, OH
Pace University, NY
Pacific Lutheran University, WA
Queens University of Charlotte, NC
Regis College, MA
Research College of Nursing, MO
Resurrection University, IL
Rowan University, NJ
Rush University, IL
Rutgers, The State University of New Jersey, Newark, NJ
Sacred Heart University, CT
Saginaw Valley State University, MI
Saint Anthony College of Nursing, IL
Saint Francis Medical Center College of Nursing, IL
Saint Louis University, MO
Saint Xavier University, IL
Salem State University, MA

Seton Hall University, NJ
South Dakota State University, SD
Southern Connecticut State University, CT
Southern New Hampshire University, NH
Spring Hill College, AL
Texas Christian University, TX
Texas Woman's University, TX
Université de Montréal, QC
Université Laval, QC
The University of Alabama, AL
The University of Alabama at Birmingham, AL
The University of Arizona, AZ
University of California, Los Angeles, CA
University of Connecticut, CT
University of Florida, FL
University of Illinois at Chicago, IL
University of Manitoba, MB
University of Mary Hardin-Baylor, TX
University of Maryland, Baltimore, MD
University of Massachusetts Amherst, MA
University of Nevada, Reno, NV
University of New Hampshire, NH
The University of North Carolina at Chapel Hill, NC
University of Oklahoma Health Sciences Center, OK
University of Pittsburgh, PA
University of Portland, OR
University of San Diego, CA
University of San Francisco, CA
University of South Carolina Upstate, SC
The University of Tennessee Health Science Center, TN
The University of Texas Health Science Center at San Antonio, TX
The University of Texas Medical Branch, TX
University of the Incarnate Word, TX
The University of Toledo, OH
University of Toronto, ON
University of Vermont, VT
University of Virginia, VA
University of West Georgia, GA
University of Windsor, ON
University of Wisconsin–Milwaukee, WI
University of Wisconsin–Oshkosh, WI
Western Governors University, UT
Western University of Health Sciences, CA
Xavier University, OH

CLINICAL NURSE SPECIALIST PROGRAMS

Acute Care

Alvernia University, PA
Arizona State University at the Downtown Phoenix campus, AZ
Inter American University of Puerto Rico, Arecibo Campus, PR
Johns Hopkins University, MD
King University, TN
Liberty University, VA
Loyola University Chicago, IL
McGill University, QC
Rhode Island College, RI
The Sage Colleges, NY
Seattle Pacific University, WA
Thomas Jefferson University, PA
Université de Montréal, QC
Université de Sherbrooke, QC

Université du Québec à Trois-Rivières, QC
Université du Québec en Outaouais, QC
Université Laval, QC
University of Arkansas, AR
University of Arkansas for Medical Sciences, AR
University of Calgary, AB
University of California, Los Angeles, CA
University of Central Florida, FL
University of Kentucky, KY
University of Manitoba, MB
University of Missouri, MO
University of New Brunswick Fredericton, NB
University of Oklahoma Health Sciences Center, OK
University of Ottawa, ON
University of Pennsylvania, PA
University of San Diego, CA
University of South Alabama, AL
University of Toronto, ON
The University of Western Ontario, ON

Adult-Gerontology Acute Care

Alvernia University, PA
California State University, Dominguez Hills, CA
Eastern Michigan University, MI
Indiana University–Purdue University Fort Wayne, IN
Indiana University–Purdue University Indianapolis, IN
Johns Hopkins University, MD
Old Dominion University, VA
Purdue University Calumet, IN
Regis College, MA
St. Joseph's College, New York, NY
Université du Québec en Outaouais, QC
University of Delaware, DE
University of Manitoba, MB
University of Massachusetts Boston, MA
University of Nebraska Medical Center, NE
University of San Diego, CA
University of Virginia, VA
Ursuline College, OH
Widener University, PA
Wright State University, OH
York College of Pennsylvania, PA
Youngstown State University, OH

Adult Health

Alvernia University, PA
Alverno College, WI
Angelo State University, TX
Arizona State University at the Downtown Phoenix campus, AZ
Arkansas State University, AR
Auburn University at Montgomery, AL
Azusa Pacific University, CA
California Baptist University, CA
California State University, Fresno, CA
Capital University, OH
The College of New Jersey, NJ
College of Staten Island of the City University of New York, NY
DeSales University, PA
Florida Southern College, FL
Georgia State University, GA
Governors State University, IL
Grambling State University, LA
Grand Canyon University, AZ

Hunter College of the City University of New York, NY
Johns Hopkins University, MD
Kennesaw State University, GA
Kent State University, OH
King University, TN
La Salle University, PA
Lehman College of the City University of New York, NY
Lewis University, IL
Loma Linda University, CA
Loyola University Chicago, IL
Marquette University, WI
McGill University, QC
Michigan State University, MI
Minnesota State University Mankato, MN
Molloy College, NY
Mount Saint Mary College, NY
Mount Saint Mary's University, CA
Murray State University, KY
Northern Illinois University, IL
The Ohio State University, OH
Otterbein University, OH
Penn State University Park, PA
Rhode Island College, RI
Ryerson University, ON
The Sage Colleges, NY
Saint Anthony College of Nursing, IL
St. John Fisher College, NY
San Diego State University, CA
San Francisco State University, CA
Seattle Pacific University, WA
State University of New York Downstate Medical Center, NY
Stony Brook University, State University of New York, NY
Texas Christian University, TX
Thomas Jefferson University, PA
Troy University, AL
Union University, TN
Université de Montréal, QC
Université du Québec à Trois-Rivières, QC
Université du Québec en Outaouais, QC
Université Laval, QC
The University of Akron, OH
The University of Alabama in Huntsville, AL
University of Arkansas for Medical Sciences, AR
The University of British Columbia, BC
University of Calgary, AB
University of Colorado Denver, CO
The University of Iowa, IA
The University of Kansas, KS
University of Kentucky, KY
University of Louisiana at Lafayette, LA
University of Manitoba, MB
University of Massachusetts Dartmouth, MA
University of Missouri, MO
University of New Brunswick Fredericton, NB
University of North Florida, FL
University of Ottawa, ON
University of Pennsylvania, PA
University of Puerto Rico, Medical Sciences Campus, PR
University of San Diego, CA
The University of Scranton, PA
University of Southern Indiana, IN
The University of Texas at Austin, TX
University of the Incarnate Word, TX
University of Toronto, ON
The University of Western Ontario, ON
University of Wisconsin–Eau Claire, WI

Valdosta State University, GA
Western Connecticut State University, CT
Winona State University, MN
Wright State University, OH

Adult-Psychiatric Mental Health
Georgia State University, GA
Université du Québec à Chicoutimi, QC
Université du Québec en Outaouais, QC
University of Manitoba, MB

Cardiovascular
Alvernia University, PA
McGill University, QC
Université de Montréal, QC
Université du Québec en Outaouais, QC
Université Laval, QC
The University of British Columbia, BC
University of Calgary, AB
University of California, San Francisco, CA
University of Manitoba, MB
University of Missouri, MO
University of New Brunswick Fredericton, NB
University of North Florida, FL
University of Ottawa, ON
University of Toronto, ON

Child/Adolescent Psychiatric-Mental Health
Université du Québec en Outaouais, QC
University of Manitoba, MB

Community Health
Arizona State University at the Downtown Phoenix campus, AZ
Augsburg College, MN
Binghamton University, State University of New York, NY
California State University, San Bernardino, CA
Chicago State University, IL
Cleveland State University, OH
D'Youville College, NY
Hunter College of the City University of New York, NY
Jacksonville State University, AL
Kean University, NJ
McGill University, QC
Mount Mercy University, IA
Mount Saint Mary's University, CA
Northern Illinois University, IL
North Park University, IL
Penn State University Park, PA
Rhode Island College, RI
Ryerson University, ON
Salem State University, MA
San Diego State University, CA
Seattle Pacific University, WA
Seattle University, WA
Stony Brook University, State University of New York, NY
Thomas Jefferson University, PA
Université de Moncton, NB
Université de Montréal, QC
Université de Sherbrooke, QC
Université du Québec à Rimouski, QC
Université du Québec à Trois-Rivières, QC
Université du Québec en Outaouais, QC
Université Laval, QC
University of Alaska Anchorage, AK
The University of British Columbia, BC
University of Calgary, AB
University of California, San Francisco, CA

The University of Iowa, IA
University of Kentucky, KY
University of Manitoba, MB
University of Maryland, Baltimore, MD
University of Massachusetts Dartmouth, MA
University of Michigan, MI
University of Missouri, MO
University of New Brunswick Fredericton, NB
The University of North Carolina at Charlotte, NC
University of North Florida, FL
University of Ottawa, ON
University of Puerto Rico, Medical Sciences Campus, PR
University of South Alabama, AL
University of Toronto, ON
University of Washington, WA
The University of Western Ontario, ON
William Paterson University of New Jersey, NJ
Wright State University, OH
WSU College of Nursing, WA

Critical Care
Alvernia University, PA
Hunter College of the City University of New York, NY
McGill University, QC
Murray State University, KY
San Diego State University, CA
Seattle Pacific University, WA
Stony Brook University, State University of New York, NY
Thomas Jefferson University, PA
Université du Québec à Rimouski, QC
Université du Québec à Trois-Rivières, QC
Université du Québec en Outaouais, QC
Université Laval, QC
University of Calgary, AB
University of California, San Francisco, CA
University of Kentucky, KY
University of Manitoba, MB
University of Missouri, MO
University of New Brunswick Fredericton, NB
University of North Florida, FL
University of Ottawa, ON
University of Puerto Rico, Medical Sciences Campus, PR
University of San Diego, CA
University of Toronto, ON

Family Health
Alvernia University, PA
Auburn University, AL
Binghamton University, State University of New York, NY
Cedarville University, OH
Colorado Mesa University, CO
Cox College, MO
Indiana University–Purdue University Fort Wayne, IN
McGill University, QC
Minnesota State University Mankato, MN
Misericordia University, PA
Missouri Southern State University, MO
Point Loma Nazarene University, CA
Ryerson University, ON
Saginaw Valley State University, MI
Shenandoah University, VA
Southern University and Agricultural and Mechanical College, LA
Stony Brook University, State University of New York, NY
Université de Moncton, NB

Université de Montréal, QC
Université de Sherbrooke, QC
Université du Québec à Trois-Rivières, QC
Université du Québec en Outaouais, QC
Université Laval, QC
The University of British Columbia, BC
University of Calgary, AB
University of Manitoba, MB
University of Massachusetts Boston, MA
University of New Brunswick Fredericton, NB
University of Ottawa, ON
University of South Alabama, AL
University of Toronto, ON
Ursuline College, OH
Valdosta State University, GA
Webster University, MO

Forensic Nursing
Alvernia University, PA
Cleveland State University, OH
Duquesne University, PA
Monmouth University, NJ
National University, CA
Université du Québec en Outaouais, QC
University of Ottawa, ON

Gerontology
Alvernia University, PA
Alverno College, WI
Auburn University at Montgomery, AL
Binghamton University, State University of New York, NY
California State University, Fresno, CA
Capella University, MN
Capital University, OH
College of Staten Island of the City University of New York, NY
DeSales University, PA
Florida Southern College, FL
Gwynedd Mercy University, PA
Lehman College of the City University of New York, NY
Lewis University, IL
McGill University, QC
Michigan State University, MI
Penn State University Park, PA
Point Loma Nazarene University, CA
The Sage Colleges, NY
Saint Francis Medical Center College of Nursing, IL
San Diego State University, CA
Seattle Pacific University, WA
Texas Christian University, TX
Université de Montréal, QC
Université de Sherbrooke, QC
Université du Québec à Rimouski, QC
Université du Québec en Outaouais, QC
Université Laval, QC
The University of Akron, OH
The University of British Columbia, BC
University of Calgary, AB
University of California, San Francisco, CA
The University of Iowa, IA
The University of Kansas, KS
University of Kentucky, KY
University of Manitoba, MB
University of Michigan, MI
University of New Brunswick Fredericton, NB
University of North Dakota, ND
University of North Florida, FL
University of Ottawa, ON

University of Puerto Rico, Medical Sciences Campus, PR
University of Rhode Island, RI
University of San Diego, CA
University of South Alabama, AL
University of Toronto, ON
Wesley College, DE
Wilkes University, PA

Home Health Care
Alvernia University, PA
McGill University, QC
Thomas Jefferson University, PA
Université de Moncton, NB
Université du Québec à Trois-Rivières, QC
Université du Québec en Outaouais, QC
University of Manitoba, MB
University of Michigan, MI
University of Missouri, MO
University of Ottawa, ON

Maternity-Newborn
Grambling State University, LA
Loma Linda University, CA
McGill University, QC
San Diego State University, CA
State University of New York Downstate Medical Center, NY
Troy University, AL
Université de Montréal, QC
Université du Québec à Trois-Rivières, QC
Université du Québec en Outaouais, QC
The University of British Columbia, BC
University of Calgary, AB
University of Manitoba, MB
University of Missouri, MO
University of New Brunswick Fredericton, NB
University of North Florida, FL
University of Ottawa, ON
University of Puerto Rico, Medical Sciences Campus, PR
University of South Alabama, AL
University of Toronto, ON

Medical-Surgical
Alvernia University, PA
Alverno College, WI
Angelo State University, TX
Azusa Pacific University, CA
Inter American University of Puerto Rico, Arecibo Campus, PR
McGill University, QC
Murray State University, KY
Point Loma Nazarene University, CA
The Sage Colleges, NY
Seattle Pacific University, WA
State University of New York Upstate Medical University, NY
Thomas Jefferson University, PA
Université de Montréal, QC
Université du Québec à Trois-Rivières, QC
Université du Québec en Outaouais, QC
University of Arkansas, AR
University of Calgary, AB
University of Central Arkansas, AR
University of Kentucky, KY
University of Manitoba, MB
University of Michigan, MI
University of New Brunswick Fredericton, NB
University of North Florida, FL
University of Ottawa, ON
University of San Diego, CA
University of Toronto, ON

Occupational Health
Université de Moncton, NB
Université de Montréal, QC
Université du Québec en Outaouais, QC
University of California, San Francisco, CA
The University of Iowa, IA
University of Michigan, MI
University of Ottawa, ON
University of Toronto, ON

Oncology
Alvernia University, PA
Case Western Reserve University, OH
Gwynedd Mercy University, PA
King University, TN
McGill University, QC
Seattle Pacific University, WA
Thomas Jefferson University, PA
Université de Montréal, QC
Université du Québec en Outaouais, QC
Université Laval, QC
The University of British Columbia, BC
University of California, San Francisco, CA
University of Kentucky, KY
University of Manitoba, MB
University of Missouri, MO
University of New Brunswick Fredericton, NB
University of Ottawa, ON
University of Toronto, ON

Palliative Care
Case Western Reserve University, OH
D'Youville College, NY
Seattle Pacific University, WA
Université de Montréal, QC
Université du Québec en Outaouais, QC
Université Laval, QC
University of Manitoba, MB
University of Missouri, MO
University of Ottawa, ON
University of San Diego, CA
University of Toronto, ON

Parent-Child
Azusa Pacific University, CA
California State University, Dominguez Hills, CA
Lehman College of the City University of New York, NY
Loma Linda University, CA
McGill University, QC
Seattle Pacific University, WA
Stony Brook University, State University of New York, NY
Université de Montréal, QC
Université du Québec en Outaouais, QC
Université Laval, QC
The University of British Columbia, BC
University of Calgary, AB
University of Kentucky, KY
University of Manitoba, MB
University of New Brunswick Fredericton, NB
University of Ottawa, ON
University of Toronto, ON

Pediatric
Arizona State University at the Downtown Phoenix campus, AZ
Auburn University at Montgomery, AL
Azusa Pacific University, CA
California State University, Fresno, CA
Georgia State University, GA
Grambling State University, LA

Gwynedd Mercy University, PA
Indiana University–Purdue University Indianapolis, IN
Kent State University, OH
Loma Linda University, CA
McGill University, QC
Minnesota State University Mankato, MN
Seattle Pacific University, WA
Stony Brook University, State University of New York, NY
Texas Christian University, TX
Thomas Jefferson University, PA
Union University, TN
Université de Moncton, NB
Université du Québec à Trois-Rivières, QC
Université du Québec en Outaouais, QC
Université Laval, QC
University of Arkansas for Medical Sciences, AR
The University of British Columbia, BC
University of Calgary, AB
University of California, Los Angeles, CA
University of California, San Francisco, CA
University of Delaware, DE
University of Kentucky, KY
University of Manitoba, MB
University of Missouri, MO
University of New Brunswick Fredericton, NB
University of North Florida, FL
University of Ottawa, ON
University of Pennsylvania, PA
University of Puerto Rico, Medical Sciences Campus, PR
University of South Alabama, AL
The University of Tennessee, TN
University of Toronto, ON
Wright State University, OH

Perinatal

Georgia State University, GA
Loma Linda University, CA
McGill University, QC
McMaster University, ON
San Francisco State University, CA
Stony Brook University, State University of New York, NY
Université du Québec à Trois-Rivières, QC
Université du Québec en Outaouais, QC
Université Laval, QC
The University of British Columbia, BC
University of Calgary, AB
University of California, San Francisco, CA
University of Kentucky, KY
University of Manitoba, MB
University of Ottawa, ON
University of Toronto, ON

Psychiatric/Mental Health

Arizona State University at the Downtown Phoenix campus, AZ
Binghamton University, State University of New York, NY
Brandon University, MB
California State University, Los Angeles, CA
Case Western Reserve University, OH
Georgia State University, GA
Gonzaga University, WA
Hunter College of the City University of New York, NY
Husson University, ME
McGill University, QC
Point Loma Nazarene University, CA
The Sage Colleges, NY

Shenandoah University, VA
Stony Brook University, State University of New York, NY
Temple University, PA
Université de Moncton, NB
Université de Montréal, QC
Université du Québec à Chicoutimi, QC
Université du Québec à Rimouski, QC
Université du Québec à Trois-Rivières, QC
Université du Québec en Outaouais, QC
Université Laval, QC
University of Alaska Anchorage, AK
The University of British Columbia, BC
University of Calgary, AB
University of California, San Francisco, CA
University of Florida, FL
University of Hawaii at Manoa, HI
The University of Iowa, IA
University of Kentucky, KY
University of Louisiana at Lafayette, LA
University of Manitoba, MB
University of Michigan, MI
University of New Brunswick Fredericton, NB
University of North Dakota, ND
University of North Florida, FL
University of Ottawa, ON
University of Puerto Rico, Medical Sciences Campus, PR
University of South Alabama, AL
The University of Tennessee, TN
University of Toronto, ON
The University of Western Ontario, ON
Valdosta State University, GA
Wilkes University, PA

Public/Community Health

Cedarville University, OH
Holy Family University, PA
Hunter College of the City University of New York, NY
Université du Québec en Outaouais, QC
University of Manitoba, MB
Worcester State University, MA

Public Health

Adelphi University, NY
Delaware State University, DE
Eastern Kentucky University, KY
Hunter College of the City University of New York, NY
La Salle University, PA
McGill University, QC
Mount Mercy University, IA
Ryerson University, ON
Salem State University, MA
San Francisco State University, CA
Thomas Jefferson University, PA
Université de Moncton, NB
Université de Montréal, QC
Université du Québec à Trois-Rivières, QC
Université du Québec en Outaouais, QC
Université Laval, QC
The University of British Columbia, BC
University of Calgary, AB
University of Florida, FL
University of Kentucky, KY
University of Manitoba, MB
University of Missouri, MO
University of New Brunswick Fredericton, NB
University of North Dakota, ND
University of Ottawa, ON
The University of Texas at Brownsville, TX
University of Toronto, ON

The University of Western Ontario, ON
West Chester University of Pennsylvania, PA
Wright State University, OH

Rehabilitation

McGill University, QC
Salem State University, MA
Université de Montréal, QC
Université du Québec en Outaouais, QC
Université Laval, QC
University of Calgary, AB
University of Manitoba, MB
University of Missouri, MO
University of Ottawa, ON
University of Toronto, ON

School Health

Azusa Pacific University, CA
California State University, Fullerton, CA
Kean University, NJ
Monmouth University, NJ
San Diego State University, CA
Université de Moncton, NB
Université du Québec en Outaouais, QC
University of Manitoba, MB
University of Missouri, MO
University of New Brunswick Fredericton, NB
University of Ottawa, ON
University of Toronto, ON
Wright State University, OH
Youngstown State University, OH

Women's Health

Drexel University, PA
Georgia State University, GA
McGill University, QC
San Diego State University, CA
Seattle Pacific University, WA
Stony Brook University, State University of New York, NY
Université de Montréal, QC
Université du Québec en Outaouais, QC
The University of British Columbia, BC
University of Calgary, AB
University of Kentucky, KY
University of Manitoba, MB
University of Missouri, MO
University of New Brunswick Fredericton, NB
University of North Florida, FL
University of Ottawa, ON
University of South Alabama, AL
University of Toronto, ON
The University of Western Ontario, ON

HEALTH-CARE ADMINISTRATION

Adelphi University, NY
Baker University, KS
Baylor University, TX
Boise State University, ID
California State University, Long Beach, CA
Charleston Southern University, SC
Clarkson College, NE
The College of New Rochelle, NY
Daemen College, NY
DeSales University, PA
Duke University, NC
Emory University, GA
Georgetown University, DC
The George Washington University, DC
Goldfarb School of Nursing at Barnes-Jewish College, MO
Gonzaga University, WA

Hampton University, VA
Johns Hopkins University, MD
Kaplan University Online, FL
Kean University, NJ
Kent State University, OH
Lenoir-Rhyne University, NC
Long Island University–LIU Brooklyn, NY
Loyola University Chicago, IL
Loyola University New Orleans, LA
Mercy College, NY
MGH Institute of Health Professions, MA
MidAmerica Nazarene University, KS
Milwaukee School of Engineering, WI
Minnesota State University Moorhead, MN
Missouri Western State University, MO
The Ohio State University, OH
Oregon Health & Science University, OR
Pacific Lutheran University, WA
Palm Beach Atlantic University, FL
Regis College, MA
Regis University, CO
The Sage Colleges, NY
St. Ambrose University, IA
Salisbury University, MD
San Jose State University, CA
Seton Hall University, NJ
Southern Adventist University, TN
Southern Illinois University Edwardsville, IL
Southern University and Agricultural and
    Mechanical College, LA
Stevenson University, MD
Tabor College, KS
Texas Woman's University, TX
Thomas University, GA
Towson University, MD
Université de Moncton, NB
Université Laval, QC
The University of Alabama in Huntsville, AL
University of Alaska Anchorage, AK
University of Delaware, DE
The University of Kansas, KS
University of Louisiana at Lafayette, LA
University of Maine, ME
University of Manitoba, MB
University of Maryland, Baltimore, MD
University of Michigan, MI
The University of North Carolina at Chapel
    Hill, NC
University of Oklahoma Health Sciences
    Center, OK
University of Pennsylvania, PA
University of Phoenix–Bay Area Campus, CA
University of Phoenix–Hawaii Campus, HI
University of Phoenix–North Florida Campus,
    FL
University of Phoenix–Online Campus, AZ
University of Phoenix–Phoenix Campus, AZ
University of Phoenix–Sacramento Valley
    Campus, CA
University of Phoenix–San Diego Campus, CA
University of Phoenix–Southern Arizona
    Campus, AZ
University of Phoenix–Southern California
    Campus, CA
University of Phoenix–South Florida Campus,
    FL
The University of Texas at Arlington, TX
University of Toronto, ON
The University of Western Ontario, ON
Vanderbilt University, TN
Western Governors University, UT

Wright State University, OH

LEGAL NURSE CONSULTANT
Capital University, OH
Wilmington University, DE

NURSE ANESTHESIA
Arkansas State University, AR
Augusta University, GA
Bloomsburg University of Pennsylvania, PA
Boston College, MA
California State University, Fullerton, CA
Case Western Reserve University, OH
Clarkson College, NE
Columbia University, NY
Drexel University, PA
East Carolina University, NC
Florida Gulf Coast University, FL
Florida International University, FL
Gannon University, PA
Georgetown University, DC
Goldfarb School of Nursing at Barnes-Jewish
    College, MO
La Roche College, PA
La Salle University, PA
Lincoln Memorial University, TN
Loma Linda University, CA
Lourdes University, OH
Michigan State University, MI
Murray State University, KY
National University, CA
Newman University, KS
Northeastern University, MA
Oakland University, MI
Old Dominion University, VA
Oregon Health & Science University, OR
Our Lady of the Lake College, LA
Rutgers, The State University of New Jersey,
    Newark, NJ
Saint Mary's University of Minnesota, MN
Samford University, AL
Samuel Merritt University, CA
Southern Illinois University Edwardsville, IL
State University of New York Downstate
    Medical Center, NY
Thomas Jefferson University, PA
Union University, TN
The University of Akron, OH
The University of Alabama at Birmingham, AL
University of Cincinnati, OH
The University of Iowa, IA
The University of North Carolina at Charlotte,
    NC
University of North Dakota, ND
University of Pennsylvania, PA
University of Pittsburgh, PA
University of Puerto Rico, Medical Sciences
    Campus, PR
The University of Scranton, PA
University of Southern Mississippi, MS
University of South Florida, FL
The University of Tennessee, TN
The University of Tennessee at Chattanooga,
    TN
The University of Texas Health Science Center
    at Houston, TX
University of Toronto, ON
Villanova University, PA
Western Carolina University, NC
York College of Pennsylvania, PA
Youngstown State University, OH

NURSE-MIDWIFERY
California State University, Fullerton, CA
Case Western Reserve University, OH
Columbia University, NY
East Carolina University, NC
Emory University, GA
Frontier Nursing University, KY
Georgetown University, DC
The George Washington University, DC
James Madison University, VA
Marquette University, WI
Marshall University, WV
New York University, NY
The Ohio State University, OH
Old Dominion University, VA
Oregon Health & Science University, OR
Radford University, VA
Rutgers, The State University of New Jersey,
    Newark, NJ
San Diego State University, CA
Shenandoah University, VA
State University of New York Downstate
    Medical Center, NY
Stony Brook University, State University of
    New York, NY
Texas Tech University Health Sciences Center,
    TX
University of California, San Francisco, CA
University of Cincinnati, OH
University of Colorado Denver, CO
University of Florida, FL
The University of Kansas, KS
University of Michigan, MI
University of New Mexico, NM
University of Pennsylvania, PA
Vanderbilt University, TN
Wayne State University, MI
West Virginia Wesleyan College, WV
Yale University, CT

NURSE PRACTITIONER PROGRAMS

Acute Care
Arizona State University at the Downtown
    Phoenix campus, AZ
Armstrong State University, GA
Barry University, FL
California State University, Los Angeles, CA
Case Western Reserve University, OH
The Catholic University of America, DC
Colorado State University–Pueblo, CO
Columbia University, NY
Drexel University, PA
Duke University, NC
Florida Gulf Coast University, FL
Georgetown University, DC
Grand Canyon University, AZ
Hawai'i Pacific University, HI
Johns Hopkins University, MD
Loyola University Chicago, IL
Maryville University of Saint Louis, MO
MGH Institute of Health Professions, MA
The Ohio State University, OH
Rhode Island College, RI
Rutgers, The State University of New Jersey,
    Newark, NJ
The Sage Colleges, NY
Saint Louis University, MO
San Diego State University, CA
Southern Adventist University, TN

Texas Tech University Health Sciences Center, TX
Thomas Jefferson University, PA
Université de Montréal, QC
University of Arkansas for Medical Sciences, AR
University of Calgary, AB
University of California, San Francisco, CA
University of Florida, FL
University of Kentucky, KY
University of Massachusetts Medical School, MA
University of Michigan, MI
University of New Brunswick Fredericton, NB
University of New Mexico, NM
University of Pennsylvania, PA
University of Rhode Island, RI
University of South Alabama, AL
University of Southern Indiana, IN
The University of Tennessee at Chattanooga, TN
The University of Texas at Arlington, TX
The University of Texas Health Science Center at Houston, TX
University of Toronto, ON
Yale University, CT

Adult-Gerontology Acute Care
Allen College, IA
Case Western Reserve University, OH
The Catholic University of America, DC
Daemen College, NY
Duke University, NC
Eastern Michigan University, MI
Emory University, GA
Goldfarb School of Nursing at Barnes-Jewish College, MO
Gonzaga University, WA
Indiana University–Purdue University Indianapolis, IN
Johns Hopkins University, MD
Kent State University, OH
Keuka College, NY
Madonna University, MI
Malone University, OH
Marquette University, WI
MGH Institute of Health Professions, MA
Moravian College, PA
Morningside College, IA
Mount Carmel College of Nursing, OH
New York University, NY
Northeastern University, MA
Northern Kentucky University, KY
Northwestern State University of Louisiana, LA
The Ohio State University, OH
Oregon Health & Science University, OR
Rowan University, NJ
The Sage Colleges, NY
St. John Fisher College, NY
Saint Louis University, MO
Seton Hall University, NJ
Texas Tech University Health Sciences Center, TX
Texas Woman's University, TX
The University of Alabama at Birmingham, AL
The University of Alabama in Huntsville, AL
University of California, Los Angeles, CA
University of Cincinnati, OH
University of Connecticut, CT
University of Massachusetts Boston, MA
University of Miami, FL

University of Mississippi Medical Center, MS
University of Missouri–St. Louis, MO
University of Nebraska Medical Center, NE
University of Nevada, Reno, NV
University of New Mexico, NM
University of Northern Colorado, CO
University of Pennsylvania, PA
University of South Carolina, SC
University of South Florida, FL
The University of Texas at El Paso, TX
University of Virginia, VA
Ursuline College, OH
Vanderbilt University, TN
Virginia Commonwealth University, VA
Walden University, MN
Wright State University, OH
Yale University, CT
York College of Pennsylvania, PA

Adult Health
Adelphi University, NY
Allen College, IA
Arizona State University at the Downtown Phoenix campus, AZ
Armstrong State University, GA
Azusa Pacific University, CA
California State University, Long Beach, CA
California State University, Los Angeles, CA
Case Western Reserve University, OH
The Catholic University of America, DC
Clarkson College, NE
Clemson University, SC
The College of New Jersey, NJ
College of Staten Island of the City University of New York, NY
Columbia University, NY
Concordia University Wisconsin, WI
Drexel University, PA
Duke University, NC
Emory University, GA
Fairleigh Dickinson University, Metropolitan Campus, NJ
Felician University, NJ
Florida Agricultural and Mechanical University, FL
Florida Atlantic University, FL
Florida Gulf Coast University, FL
Florida International University, FL
Florida Southern College, FL
George Mason University, VA
The George Washington University, DC
Georgia State University, GA
Goldfarb School of Nursing at Barnes-Jewish College, MO
Gwynedd Mercy University, PA
Indiana University–Purdue University Fort Wayne, IN
Johns Hopkins University, MD
Kaplan University Online, FL
Kennesaw State University, GA
Kent State University, OH
La Salle University, PA
Lewis University, IL
Long Island University–LIU Brooklyn, NY
Loyola University Chicago, IL
Marian University, WI
Marquette University, WI
Maryville University of Saint Louis, MO
Medical University of South Carolina, SC
Memorial University of Newfoundland, NL
MGH Institute of Health Professions, MA
Michigan State University, MI

Molloy College, NY
Monmouth University, NJ
Moravian College, PA
Mount Saint Mary College, NY
Neumann University, PA
Northern Illinois University, IL
Northern Kentucky University, KY
North Park University, IL
Oakland University, MI
The Ohio State University, OH
Otterbein University, OH
Penn State University Park, PA
Purdue University, IN
Quinnipiac University, CT
Regis College, MA
Research College of Nursing, MO
Resurrection University, IL
Rhode Island College, RI
Rutgers, The State University of New Jersey, Camden, NJ
Rutgers, The State University of New Jersey, Newark, NJ
The Sage Colleges, NY
Saint Anthony College of Nursing, IL
St. Catherine University, MN
St. John Fisher College, NY
Saint Peter's University, NJ
San Diego State University, CA
Seattle Pacific University, WA
Seton Hall University, NJ
Southern Adventist University, TN
Spring Arbor University, MI
State University of New York Polytechnic Institute, NY
State University of New York Upstate Medical University, NY
Stockton University, NJ
Stony Brook University, State University of New York, NY
Temple University, PA
Texas Woman's University, TX
Thomas Jefferson University, PA
Université de Moncton, NB
Université de Montréal, QC
Université Laval, QC
The University of Akron, OH
University of Alberta, AB
University of Calgary, AB
University of California, Irvine, CA
University of California, San Francisco, CA
University of Central Arkansas, AR
University of Central Florida, FL
University of Colorado Colorado Springs, CO
University of Colorado Denver, CO
University of Delaware, DE
University of Florida, FL
University of Hawaii at Manoa, HI
University of Indianapolis, IN
The University of Iowa, IA
The University of Kansas, KS
University of Kentucky, KY
University of Louisiana at Lafayette, LA
University of Michigan, MI
University of New Brunswick Fredericton, NB
The University of North Carolina at Chapel Hill, NC
The University of North Carolina at Charlotte, NC
The University of North Carolina at Greensboro, NC
University of Oklahoma Health Sciences Center, OK

University of Pennsylvania, PA
University of San Diego, CA
The University of Tampa, FL
The University of Texas at Arlington, TX
The University of Texas Health Science Center
   at Houston, TX
University of Toronto, ON
University of Vermont, VT
University of Wisconsin–Eau Claire, WI
Vanderbilt University, TN
Villanova University, PA
Virginia Commonwealth University, VA
Washburn University, KS
Western Connecticut State University, CT
William Paterson University of New Jersey, NJ
Wilmington University, DE
Winona State University, MN
Yale University, CT

Adult-Psychiatric Mental Health

Georgia State University, GA
MGH Institute of Health Professions, MA
Saint Francis Medical Center College of
   Nursing, IL
University of San Diego, CA

Community Health

Allen College, IA
Athabasca University, AB
Binghamton University, State University of
   New York, NY
Hunter College of the City University of New
   York, NY
Johns Hopkins University, MD
The Ohio State University, OH
The Sage Colleges, NY
Université de Moncton, NB
Université de Montréal, QC
The University of British Columbia, BC
University of Hawaii at Manoa, HI
University of New Brunswick Fredericton, NB
The University of Western Ontario, ON

Family Health

Albany State University, GA
Alcorn State University, MS
Allen College, IA
American International College, MA
Angelo State University, TX
Arizona State University at the Downtown
   Phoenix campus, AZ
Armstrong State University, GA
Athabasca University, AB
Auburn University, AL
Augusta University, GA
Austin Peay State University, TN
Azusa Pacific University, CA
Ball State University, IN
Barry University, FL
Belmont University, TN
Binghamton University, State University of
   New York, NY
Bloomsburg University of Pennsylvania, PA
Boston College, MA
Bowie State University, MD
Bradley University, IL
Brenau University, GA
Brigham Young University, UT
California State University, Dominguez Hills,
   CA
California State University, Fresno, CA
California State University, Long Beach, CA
California State University, Los Angeles, CA

Carlow University, PA
Carson-Newman University, TN
Case Western Reserve University, OH
The Catholic University of America, DC
Cedarville University, OH
Clarion University of Pennsylvania, PA
Clarkson College, NE
Clemson University, SC
The College of New Jersey, NJ
The College of New Rochelle, NY
Colorado State University–Pueblo, CO
Columbia University, NY
Concordia University Wisconsin, WI
Coppin State University, MD
Delta State University, MS
DeSales University, PA
Dominican College, NY
Drexel University, PA
Duke University, NC
Duquesne University, PA
D'Youville College, NY
Eastern Kentucky University, KY
East Tennessee State University, TN
Emory University, GA
Fairfield University, CT
Fairleigh Dickinson University, Metropolitan
   Campus, NJ
Felician University, NJ
Florida Atlantic University, FL
Florida Gulf Coast University, FL
Florida International University, FL
Fort Hays State University, KS
Franciscan University of Steubenville, OH
Frontier Nursing University, KY
Gannon University, PA
Gardner-Webb University, NC
George Mason University, VA
Georgetown University, DC
The George Washington University, DC
Georgia College & State University, GA
Georgia Southwestern State University, GA
Georgia State University, GA
Gonzaga University, WA
Goshen College, IN
Graceland University, IA
Grambling State University, LA
Grand Canyon University, AZ
Hampton University, VA
Harding University, AR
Hawai`i Pacific University, HI
Herzing University Online, WI
Holy Names University, CA
Howard University, DC
Husson University, ME
Illinois State University, IL
Indiana State University, IN
Indiana University–Purdue University Fort
   Wayne, IN
Indiana University–Purdue University
   Indianapolis, IN
Indiana University South Bend, IN
Indiana Wesleyan University, IN
Jacksonville University, FL
James Madison University, VA
Johns Hopkins University, MD
Kaplan University Online, FL
Kennesaw State University, GA
Kent State University, OH
La Salle University, PA
Lehman College of the City University of New
   York, NY
Le Moyne College, NY

Lewis University, IL
Lincoln Memorial University, TN
Long Island University–LIU Brooklyn, NY
Long Island University–LIU Post, NY
Loyola University Chicago, IL
Malone University, OH
Marshall University, WV
Marymount University, VA
Maryville University of Saint Louis, MO
McNeese State University, LA
Medical University of South Carolina, SC
Memorial University of Newfoundland, NL
Mercer University, GA
MGH Institute of Health Professions, MA
Michigan State University, MI
Middle Tennessee State University, TN
Midwestern State University, TX
Millersville University of Pennsylvania, PA
Minnesota State University Mankato, MN
Misericordia University, PA
Mississippi University for Women, MS
Molloy College, NY
Monmouth University, NJ
Morningside College, IA
Mount Carmel College of Nursing, OH
Mount Marty College, SD
Murray State University, KY
New York University, NY
Northeastern University, MA
Northern Arizona University, AZ
Northern Illinois University, IL
Northern Kentucky University, KY
North Park University, IL
Northwestern State University of Louisiana,
   LA
Oakland University, MI
The Ohio State University, OH
Ohio University, OH
Old Dominion University, VA
Olivet Nazarene University, IL
Oregon Health & Science University, OR
Otterbein University, OH
Pace University, NY
Pacific Lutheran University, WA
Patty Hanks Shelton School of Nursing, TX
Penn State University Park, PA
Pittsburg State University, KS
Prairie View A&M University, TX
Purdue University Calumet, IN
Quinnipiac University, CT
Radford University, VA
Regis College, MA
Regis University, CO
Research College of Nursing, MO
Resurrection University, IL
Rivier University, NH
Rowan University, NJ
Rutgers, The State University of New Jersey,
   Camden, NJ
Rutgers, The State University of New Jersey,
   Newark, NJ
Sacred Heart University, CT
The Sage Colleges, NY
Saginaw Valley State University, MI
Saint Anthony College of Nursing, IL
Saint Francis Medical Center College of
   Nursing, IL
Saint Louis University, MO
Saint Xavier University, IL
Samford University, AL
Samuel Merritt University, CA
San Francisco State University, CA

Seattle Pacific University, WA
Seattle University, WA
Shenandoah University, VA
Simmons College, MA
South Dakota State University, SD
Southeastern Louisiana University, LA
Southeast Missouri State University, MO
Southern Adventist University, TN
Southern Connecticut State University, CT
Southern Illinois University Edwardsville, IL
Southern University and Agricultural and
    Mechanical College, LA
Spalding University, KY
State University of New York Downstate
    Medical Center, NY
State University of New York Polytechnic
    Institute, NY
State University of New York Upstate Medical
    University, NY
Stony Brook University, State University of
    New York, NY
Temple University, PA
Tennessee State University, TN
Tennessee Technological University, TN
Texas A&M Health Science Center, TX
Texas A&M International University, TX
Texas A&M University–Corpus Christi, TX
Texas State University, TX
Texas Tech University Health Sciences Center,
    TX
Texas Woman's University, TX
Thomas Jefferson University, PA
Troy University, AL
Union University, TN
Université de Moncton, NB
Université de Montréal, QC
The University of Alabama, AL
The University of Alabama at Birmingham, AL
The University of Alabama in Huntsville, AL
University of Alaska Anchorage, AK
University of Arkansas for Medical Sciences,
    AR
The University of British Columbia, BC
University of California, Irvine, CA
University of California, Los Angeles, CA
University of California, San Francisco, CA
University of Central Arkansas, AR
University of Central Florida, FL
University of Central Missouri, MO
University of Cincinnati, OH
University of Colorado Colorado Springs, CO
University of Colorado Denver, CO
University of Connecticut, CT
University of Delaware, DE
University of Detroit Mercy, MI
University of Florida, FL
University of Hawaii at Manoa, HI
University of Indianapolis, IN
The University of Iowa, IA
The University of Kansas, KS
University of Kentucky, KY
University of Maine, ME
University of Mary Hardin-Baylor, TX
University of Massachusetts Boston, MA
University of Massachusetts Lowell, MA
University of Massachusetts Medical School,
    MA
University of Memphis, TN
University of Miami, FL
University of Michigan, MI
University of Mississippi Medical Center, MS
University of Missouri, MO

University of Missouri–St. Louis, MO
University of Nebraska Medical Center, NE
University of Nevada, Las Vegas, NV
University of Nevada, Reno, NV
University of New Brunswick Fredericton, NB
University of New Hampshire, NH
University of New Mexico, NM
The University of North Carolina at Chapel
    Hill, NC
The University of North Carolina at Charlotte,
    NC
The University of North Carolina Wilmington,
    NC
University of North Dakota, ND
University of Northern British Columbia, BC
University of Northern Colorado, CO
University of North Florida, FL
University of North Georgia, GA
University of Oklahoma Health Sciences
    Center, OK
University of Pennsylvania, PA
University of Phoenix–Hawaii Campus, HI
University of Phoenix–Online Campus, AZ
University of Phoenix–Phoenix Campus, AZ
University of Phoenix–Sacramento Valley
    Campus, CA
University of Phoenix–Southern Arizona
    Campus, AZ
University of Phoenix–Southern California
    Campus, CA
University of Rhode Island, RI
University of St. Francis, IL
University of Saint Francis, IN
University of Saint Joseph, CT
University of San Diego, CA
The University of Scranton, PA
University of South Alabama, AL
University of South Carolina, SC
University of Southern Indiana, IN
University of Southern Maine, ME
University of Southern Mississippi, MS
University of South Florida, FL
The University of Tampa, FL
The University of Tennessee, TN
The University of Tennessee at Chattanooga,
    TN
The University of Texas at Arlington, TX
The University of Texas at Austin, TX
The University of Texas at El Paso, TX
The University of Texas at Tyler, TX
The University of Texas Health Science Center
    at Houston, TX
The University of Texas Health Science Center
    at San Antonio, TX
The University of Texas Medical Branch, TX
The University of Texas Rio Grande Valley, TX
The University of Toledo, OH
University of Toronto, ON
University of Vermont, VT
University of Virginia, VA
University of Wisconsin–Eau Claire, WI
Ursuline College, OH
Vanderbilt University, TN
Villanova University, PA
Virginia Commonwealth University, VA
Wagner College, NY
Walden University, MN
Walsh University, OH
Washburn University, KS
Weber State University, UT
West Coast University, CA
Western Carolina University, NC

Western University of Health Sciences, CA
Westminster College, UT
West Texas A&M University, TX
West Virginia University, WV
Wheeling Jesuit University, WV
Widener University, PA
William Paterson University of New Jersey, NJ
Wilmington University, DE
Winona State University, MN
Winston-Salem State University, NC
Wright State University, OH
WSU College of Nursing, WA
Xavier University, OH
Yale University, CT
Youngstown State University, OH

Gerontology
Binghamton University, State University of
    New York, NY
Bloomsburg University of Pennsylvania, PA
California State University, Long Beach, CA
Case Western Reserve University, OH
The Catholic University of America, DC
Clemson University, SC
College of Staten Island of the City University
    of New York, NY
Delta State University, MS
DeSales University, PA
Fairleigh Dickinson University, Metropolitan
    Campus, NJ
Florida Agricultural and Mechanical
    University, FL
Florida Atlantic University, FL
George Mason University, VA
The George Washington University, DC
Hampton University, VA
Hunter College of the City University of New
    York, NY
Johns Hopkins University, MD
Lewis University, IL
Maryville University of Saint Louis, MO
Medical University of South Carolina, SC
MGH Institute of Health Professions, MA
Michigan State University, MI
Moravian College, PA
Oakland University, MI
The Ohio State University, OH
Regis College, MA
Rutgers, The State University of New Jersey,
    Newark, NJ
St. Catherine University, MN
San Diego State University, CA
Seattle University, WA
Spring Arbor University, MI
State University of New York Polytechnic
    Institute, NY
The University of Akron, OH
University of Alberta, AB
University of California, Irvine, CA
University of California, Los Angeles, CA
University of California, San Francisco, CA
University of Hawaii at Manoa, HI
University of Indianapolis, IN
The University of Iowa, IA
The University of Kansas, KS
University of Kentucky, KY
University of Massachusetts Lowell, MA
University of Massachusetts Medical School,
    MA
University of Michigan, MI
University of Mississippi Medical Center, MS
University of Missouri, MO

University of New Brunswick Fredericton, NB
The University of North Carolina at Chapel
  Hill, NC
University of North Dakota, ND
University of Pennsylvania, PA
University of Rhode Island, RI
University of San Diego, CA
University of South Alabama, AL
The University of Texas at Arlington, TX
The University of Texas Health Science Center
  at Houston, TX
The University of Texas Health Science Center
  at San Antonio, TX
The University of Texas Medical Branch, TX
The University of Toledo, OH
University of Toronto, ON
University of Wisconsin–Eau Claire, WI
Walden University, MN
Wayne State University, MI
Wilmington University, DE

Neonatal Health
Arizona State University at the Downtown
  Phoenix campus, AZ
Case Western Reserve University, OH
The College of New Jersey, NJ
Duke University, NC
East Carolina University, NC
Emory University, GA
McGill University, QC
McMaster University, ON
Northeastern University, MA
The Ohio State University, OH
Regis University, CO
Saint Francis Medical Center College of
  Nursing, IL
Stony Brook University, State University of
  New York, NY
Thomas Jefferson University, PA
The University of Alabama at Birmingham, AL
University of Calgary, AB
University of California, San Francisco, CA
University of Cincinnati, OH
University of Connecticut, CT
University of Florida, FL
University of Indianapolis, IN
The University of Iowa, IA
University of Missouri–Kansas City, MO
University of New Brunswick Fredericton, NB
University of Oklahoma Health Sciences
  Center, OK
University of Pennsylvania, PA
University of Pittsburgh, PA
University of South Alabama, AL
The University of Texas at Arlington, TX
The University of Texas Medical Branch, TX
University of Toronto, ON
Vanderbilt University, TN
Wayne State University, MI
West Virginia University, WV
Wright State University, OH

Occupational Health
The University of Alabama at Birmingham, AL
University of California, Los Angeles, CA
University of California, San Francisco, CA
University of Cincinnati, OH
University of South Florida, FL

Oncology
Case Western Reserve University, OH
Duke University, NC
Thomas Jefferson University, PA

Université de Moncton, NB
The University of Alabama at Birmingham, AL
University of Toronto, ON

Pediatric
Arizona State University at the Downtown
  Phoenix campus, AZ
Augusta University, GA
Azusa Pacific University, CA
California State University, Fresno, CA
California State University, Long Beach, CA
California State University, Los Angeles, CA
Case Western Reserve University, OH
The Catholic University of America, DC
Columbia University, NY
Drexel University, PA
Duke University, NC
Emory University, GA
Georgia State University, GA
Grambling State University, LA
Gwynedd Mercy University, PA
Hampton University, VA
Johns Hopkins University, MD
Lehman College of the City University of New
  York, NY
Marquette University, WI
Medical University of South Carolina, SC
MGH Institute of Health Professions, MA
Molloy College, NY
New York University, NY
Northeastern University, MA
The Ohio State University, OH
Old Dominion University, VA
Oregon Health & Science University, OR
Purdue University, IN
Regis College, MA
Seton Hall University, NJ
Spalding University, KY
State University of New York Upstate Medical
  University, NY
Stony Brook University, State University of
  New York, NY
Temple University, PA
Texas Woman's University, TX
Thomas Jefferson University, PA
The University of Akron, OH
University of Arkansas for Medical Sciences,
  AR
University of California, Los Angeles, CA
University of California, San Francisco, CA
University of Cincinnati, OH
University of Colorado Denver, CO
University of Florida, FL
University of Hawaii at Manoa, HI
The University of Iowa, IA
University of Kentucky, KY
University of Michigan, MI
University of Missouri, MO
University of Missouri–St. Louis, MO
University of Nebraska Medical Center, NE
University of New Brunswick Fredericton, NB
University of New Mexico, NM
University of Oklahoma Health Sciences
  Center, OK
University of Pennsylvania, PA
University of South Alabama, AL
The University of Tennessee, TN
The University of Texas at Arlington, TX
The University of Texas at Austin, TX
The University of Texas at Tyler, TX
The University of Texas Health Science Center
  at San Antonio, TX

University of Toronto, ON
University of Virginia, VA
Vanderbilt University, TN
Villanova University, PA
Wayne State University, MI
West Virginia University, WV
Wright State University, OH

Pediatric Primary Care
Boston College, MA
Case Western Reserve University, OH
The Catholic University of America, DC
Duke University, NC
Emory University, GA
Florida International University, FL
Indiana University–Purdue University
  Indianapolis, IN
Johns Hopkins University, MD
Kent State University, OH
Marquette University, WI
Molloy College, NY
Northeastern University, MA
Northern Kentucky University, KY
Northwestern State University of Louisiana,
  LA
The Ohio State University, OH
Oregon Health & Science University, OR
St. Catherine University, MN
Saint Louis University, MO
Seton Hall University, NJ
Texas Tech University Health Sciences Center,
  TX
The University of Akron, OH
The University of Alabama at Birmingham, AL
University of Cincinnati, OH
University of Nevada, Las Vegas, NV
The University of North Carolina at Chapel
  Hill, NC
University of San Diego, CA
University of South Florida, FL
The University of Texas at El Paso, TX
The University of Toledo, OH
Vanderbilt University, TN
Wright State University, OH
Yale University, CT

Primary Care
Arkansas State University, AR
Athabasca University, AB
Auburn University at Montgomery, AL
Azusa Pacific University, CA
California State University, Los Angeles, CA
Case Western Reserve University, OH
The Catholic University of America, DC
Duke University, NC
Eastern Michigan University, MI
Emory University, GA
Florida Atlantic University, FL
Florida Southern College, FL
The George Washington University, DC
Gonzaga University, WA
Hampton University, VA
Indiana University–Purdue University Fort
  Wayne, IN
Johns Hopkins University, MD
Kennesaw State University, GA
Kent State University, OH
Loyola University Chicago, IL
Madonna University, MI
McGill University, QC
Medical University of South Carolina, SC
MGH Institute of Health Professions, MA
Moravian College, PA

New York University, NY
Northeastern University, MA
Northern Kentucky University, KY
The Ohio State University, OH
Regis College, MA
Ryerson University, ON
Saint Louis University, MO
Seton Hall University, NJ
Simmons College, MA
Southern Adventist University, TN
Texas Tech University Health Sciences Center, TX
Université de Moncton, NB
Université de Montréal, QC
Université du Québec à Chicoutimi, QC
Université du Québec à Trois-Rivières, QC
Université du Québec en Outaouais, QC
Université Laval, QC
The University of Akron, OH
The University of British Columbia, BC
University of Colorado Colorado Springs, CO
University of Connecticut, CT
University of Manitoba, MB
University of Massachusetts Medical School, MA
University of Miami, FL
University of Michigan, MI
University of Missouri, MO
University of New Brunswick Fredericton, NB
University of North Dakota, ND
University of North Florida, FL
University of Ottawa, ON
University of Pennsylvania, PA
University of San Diego, CA
University of Saskatchewan, SK
University of Southern Indiana, IN
University of Toronto, ON
University of Vermont, VT
University of Windsor, ON

Psychiatric/Mental Health

Allen College, IA
Arizona State University at the Downtown Phoenix campus, AZ
Binghamton University, State University of New York, NY
Boston College, MA
California State University, Long Beach, CA
California State University, Los Angeles, CA
Case Western Reserve University, OH
Colorado State University–Pueblo, CO
Columbia University, NY
Delta State University, MS
Drexel University, PA
Eastern Kentucky University, KY
Fairfield University, CT
Fairleigh Dickinson University, Metropolitan Campus, NJ
Florida International University, FL
George Mason University, VA
Georgia College & State University, GA
Georgia State University, GA
Gonzaga University, WA
Hunter College of the City University of New York, NY
Indiana University–Purdue University Indianapolis, IN
Jacksonville University, FL
Kent State University, OH
Lincoln Memorial University, TN
Marshall University, WV
McNeese State University, LA

MGH Institute of Health Professions, MA
Midwestern State University, TX
Molloy College, NY
Monmouth University, NJ
New York University, NY
Northeastern University, MA
The Ohio State University, OH
Oregon Health & Science University, OR
Regis College, MA
Rivier University, NH
Rutgers, The State University of New Jersey, Newark, NJ
The Sage Colleges, NY
Saint Francis Medical Center College of Nursing, IL
St. John Fisher College, NY
Saint Louis University, MO
Seattle University, WA
Shenandoah University, VA
Southeastern Louisiana University, LA
Southern Adventist University, TN
State University of New York Upstate Medical University, NY
Stony Brook University, State University of New York, NY
The University of Akron, OH
The University of Alabama, AL
The University of Alabama at Birmingham, AL
University of Alaska Anchorage, AK
University of Arkansas for Medical Sciences, AR
University of California, San Francisco, CA
University of Colorado Denver, CO
University of Florida, FL
The University of Iowa, IA
The University of Kansas, KS
University of Kentucky, KY
University of Louisiana at Lafayette, LA
University of Michigan, MI
University of Mississippi Medical Center, MS
University of Missouri, MO
University of Missouri–Kansas City, MO
University of Missouri–St. Louis, MO
University of Nebraska Medical Center, NE
University of Nevada, Reno, NV
University of New Brunswick Fredericton, NB
The University of North Carolina at Chapel Hill, NC
University of North Dakota, ND
University of Pennsylvania, PA
University of St. Francis, IL
University of Saint Joseph, CT
University of San Diego, CA
University of South Alabama, AL
University of South Carolina, SC
University of Southern Indiana, IN
University of Southern Maine, ME
University of Southern Mississippi, MS
The University of Tennessee, TN
The University of Texas at Arlington, TX
The University of Texas at Austin, TX
The University of Texas Health Science Center at Houston, TX
The University of Texas Health Science Center at San Antonio, TX
The University of Toledo, OH
University of Virginia, VA
Vanderbilt University, TN
Virginia Commonwealth University, VA
Wayne State University, MI
Western Kentucky University, KY
West Virginia Wesleyan College, WV

Winston-Salem State University, NC
Wright State University, OH
WSU College of Nursing, WA
Yale University, CT

School Health

The College of New Jersey, NJ
Seton Hall University, NJ

Women's Health

Arizona State University at the Downtown Phoenix campus, AZ
Boston College, MA
California State University, Fullerton, CA
California State University, Long Beach, CA
Case Western Reserve University, OH
Drexel University, PA
Duke University, NC
Emory University, GA
Florida Agricultural and Mechanical University, FL
Frontier Nursing University, KY
Georgetown University, DC
Georgia State University, GA
Hampton University, VA
Johns Hopkins University, MD
Kent State University, OH
Loyola University Chicago, IL
MGH Institute of Health Professions, MA
Northwestern State University of Louisiana, LA
The Ohio State University, OH
Regis College, MA
Rutgers, The State University of New Jersey, Newark, NJ
Salem State University, MA
San Diego State University, CA
State University of New York Downstate Medical Center, NY
Stony Brook University, State University of New York, NY
Texas Woman's University, TX
The University of Alabama at Birmingham, AL
University of Cincinnati, OH
University of Colorado Denver, CO
University of Indianapolis, IN
University of Missouri–St. Louis, MO
University of Nebraska Medical Center, NE
University of New Brunswick Fredericton, NB
University of Pennsylvania, PA
University of South Alabama, AL
Vanderbilt University, TN
West Virginia University, WV
Yale University, CT

NURSING ADMINISTRATION

Adelphi University, NY
Allen College, IA
American International College, MA
American Sentinel University, CO
Anderson University, IN
Arkansas State University, AR
Arkansas Tech University, AR
Aspen University, CO
Athabasca University, AB
Aurora University, IL
Austin Peay State University, TN
Azusa Pacific University, CA
Ball State University, IN
Barry University, FL
Barton College, NC
Bellarmine University, KY

Bellin College, WI
Bethel College, IN
Bethel University, MN
Binghamton University, State University of New York, NY
Blessing–Rieman College of Nursing and Health Sciences, IL
Bloomsburg University of Pennsylvania, PA
Boise State University, ID
Bradley University, IL
Brenau University, GA
Bryan College of Health Sciences, NE
California State University, Chico, CA
California State University, Dominguez Hills, CA
California State University, Fullerton, CA
California State University, Long Beach, CA
California State University, Los Angeles, CA
California State University, Sacramento, CA
California State University, San Bernardino, CA
Capella University, MN
Capital University, OH
Cardinal Stritch University, WI
Carlow University, PA
Charleston Southern University, SC
Chatham University, PA
Chicago State University, IL
Clarkson College, NE
Clayton State University, GA
Clemson University, SC
The College of New Rochelle, NY
Creighton University, NE
Delta State University, MS
DeSales University, PA
Drexel University, PA
Duke University, NC
East Carolina University, NC
Eastern Mennonite University, VA
East Tennessee State University, TN
Edgewood College, WI
Elms College, MA
Emmanuel College, MA
Endicott College, MA
Excelsior College, NY
Fairleigh Dickinson University, Metropolitan Campus, NJ
Felician University, NJ
Ferris State University, MI
Florida Atlantic University, FL
Florida International University, FL
Florida Southern College, FL
Fort Hays State University, KS
Framingham State University, MA
Franklin Pierce University, NH
Gannon University, PA
Gardner-Webb University, NC
George Mason University, VA
The George Washington University, DC
Georgia Southwestern State University, GA
Georgia State University, GA
Goldfarb School of Nursing at Barnes-Jewish College, MO
Gonzaga University, WA
Grand Canyon University, AZ
Hampton University, VA
Holy Family University, PA
Holy Names University, CA
Hunter College of the City University of New York, NY
Illinois State University, IL
Immaculata University, PA

Indiana University of Pennsylvania, PA
Indiana University–Purdue University Indianapolis, IN
Indiana Wesleyan University, IN
Jacksonville University, FL
James Madison University, VA
Jefferson College of Health Sciences, VA
Kean University, NJ
Lamar University, TX
La Roche College, PA
La Salle University, PA
Lehman College of the City University of New York, NY
Le Moyne College, NY
Lewis University, IL
Loma Linda University, CA
Long Island University–LIU Brooklyn, NY
Lourdes University, OH
Loyola University Chicago, IL
Madonna University, MI
Mansfield University of Pennsylvania, PA
Marquette University, WI
Marshall University, WV
Marywood University, PA
McGill University, QC
McKendree University, IL
McNeese State University, LA
Mercy College, NY
Metropolitan State University, MN
MGH Institute of Health Professions, MA
Middle Tennessee State University, TN
Milwaukee School of Engineering, WI
Minnesota State University Moorhead, MN
Molloy College, NY
Monmouth University, NJ
Moravian College, PA
Mount Carmel College of Nursing, OH
Mount Mercy University, IA
Mount Saint Mary's University, CA
National University, CA
Nebraska Methodist College, NE
Nebraska Wesleyan University, NE
New Mexico State University, NM
New York University, NY
Northeastern University, MA
Northern Kentucky University, KY
North Park University, IL
Northwestern State University of Louisiana, LA
Nova Southeastern University, FL
The Ohio State University, OH
Ohio University, OH
Oklahoma City University, OK
Old Dominion University, VA
Otterbein University, OH
Our Lady of the Lake College, LA
Pacific Lutheran University, WA
Penn State University Park, PA
Pittsburg State University, KS
Prairie View A&M University, TX
Queens University of Charlotte, NC
Regis College, MA
Regis University, CO
Research College of Nursing, MO
Resurrection University, IL
Roberts Wesleyan College, NY
Sacred Heart University, CT
The Sage Colleges, NY
Saginaw Valley State University, MI
St. Ambrose University, IA
Saint Francis Medical Center College of Nursing, IL

Saint Joseph's College of Maine, ME
Saint Peter's University, NJ
Saint Xavier University, IL
Salem State University, MA
Samford University, AL
San Diego State University, CA
San Francisco State University, CA
San Jose State University, CA
Seattle Pacific University, WA
Seton Hall University, NJ
South Dakota State University, SD
Southeastern Louisiana University, LA
Southern Nazarene University, OK
Southwest Baptist University, MO
State University of New York Polytechnic Institute, NY
Stevenson University, MD
Stony Brook University, State University of New York, NY
Tarleton State University, TX
Tennessee State University, TN
Tennessee Technological University, TN
Texas A&M International University, TX
Texas A&M University–Corpus Christi, TX
Texas A&M University–Texarkana, TX
Texas Tech University Health Sciences Center, TX
Texas Woman's University, TX
Thomas University, GA
Troy University, AL
Union University, TN
Université de Moncton, NB
Université de Montréal, QC
Université Laval, QC
University at Buffalo, the State University of New York, NY
The University of Akron, OH
The University of Alabama at Birmingham, AL
University of Arkansas for Medical Sciences, AR
The University of British Columbia, BC
University of California, Los Angeles, CA
University of California, San Francisco, CA
University of Central Florida, FL
University of Cincinnati, OH
University of Colorado Denver, CO
University of Detroit Mercy, MI
University of Hartford, CT
University of Hawaii at Manoa, HI
University of Houston, TX
University of Indianapolis, IN
The University of Iowa, IA
The University of Kansas, KS
University of Kentucky, KY
University of Louisiana at Lafayette, LA
University of Mary, ND
University of Massachusetts Dartmouth, MA
University of Memphis, TN
University of Michigan, MI
University of Mississippi Medical Center, MS
University of Missouri, MO
University of Mobile, AL
University of Nebraska Medical Center, NE
University of New Brunswick Fredericton, NB
University of North Alabama, AL
The University of North Carolina at Charlotte, NC
The University of North Carolina at Greensboro, NC
University of Pennsylvania, PA
University of Phoenix–Bay Area Campus, CA
University of Phoenix–Cleveland Campus, OH

University of Phoenix–Hawaii Campus, HI
University of Phoenix–New Mexico Campus, NM
University of Phoenix–North Florida Campus, FL
University of Phoenix–Online Campus, AZ
University of Phoenix–Phoenix Campus, AZ
University of Phoenix–Sacramento Valley Campus, CA
University of Phoenix–San Diego Campus, CA
University of Phoenix–Southern Arizona Campus, AZ
University of Phoenix–Southern California Campus, CA
University of Phoenix–South Florida Campus, FL
University of Pittsburgh, PA
University of Puerto Rico, Medical Sciences Campus, PR
University of St. Francis, IL
University of Saint Mary, KS
University of San Diego, CA
University of South Alabama, AL
University of South Carolina, SC
University of Southern Indiana, IN
The University of Tennessee, TN
The University of Texas at Arlington, TX
The University of Texas at Austin, TX
The University of Texas at Brownsville, TX
The University of Texas at El Paso, TX
The University of Texas at Tyler, TX
The University of Texas Health Science Center at Houston, TX
The University of Texas Health Science Center at San Antonio, TX
The University of Texas Medical Branch, TX
The University of Texas Rio Grande Valley, TX
University of Toronto, ON
The University of Western Ontario, ON
University of West Florida, FL
University of West Georgia, GA
University of Windsor, ON
University of Wisconsin–Eau Claire, WI
University of Wisconsin–Green Bay, WI
Urbana University, OH
Valdosta State University, GA
Vanderbilt University, TN
Virginia Commonwealth University, VA
Walden University, MN
Washburn University, KS
Waynesburg University, PA
Weber State University, UT
Webster University, MO
West Chester University of Pennsylvania, PA
Western Carolina University, NC
Western Governors University, UT
Western Kentucky University, KY
Western Michigan University, MI
Western University of Health Sciences, CA
West Texas A&M University, TX
West Virginia University, WV
West Virginia Wesleyan College, WV
Wheeling Jesuit University, WV
Wilkes University, PA
William Paterson University of New Jersey, NJ
Wilmington University, DE
Winona State University, MN
Wright State University, OH
WSU College of Nursing, WA
Xavier University, OH

NURSING EDUCATION

Adelphi University, NY
Albany State University, GA
Alcorn State University, MS
Allen College, IA
Alverno College, WI
American International College, MA
American Sentinel University, CO
Anderson University, IN
Angelo State University, TX
Aquinas College, TN
Arkansas State University, AR
Aspen University, CO
Athabasca University, AB
Auburn University, AL
Auburn University at Montgomery, AL
Aurora University, IL
Austin Peay State University, TN
Azusa Pacific University, CA
Baker University, KS
Ball State University, IN
Barry University, FL
Barton College, NC
Bellarmine University, KY
Bellin College, WI
Belmont University, TN
Bethel College, IN
Bethel University, MN
Binghamton University, State University of New York, NY
Blessing–Rieman College of Nursing and Health Sciences, IL
Boise State University, ID
Bowie State University, MD
Bradley University, IL
Brenau University, GA
Briar Cliff University, IA
Bryan College of Health Sciences, NE
California Baptist University, CA
California State University, Chico, CA
California State University, Dominguez Hills, CA
California State University, Fresno, CA
California State University, Fullerton, CA
California State University, Long Beach, CA
California State University, Los Angeles, CA
California State University, Sacramento, CA
California State University, San Bernardino, CA
Capella University, MN
Capital University, OH
Cardinal Stritch University, WI
Carlow University, PA
Carson-Newman University, TN
Case Western Reserve University, OH
Central Methodist University, MO
Charleston Southern University, SC
Chatham University, PA
Chicago State University, IL
Clarkson College, NE
Clayton State University, GA
Clemson University, SC
Cleveland State University, OH
The College of New Rochelle, NY
College of Saint Elizabeth, NJ
College of Saint Mary, NE
Colorado Mesa University, CO
Colorado State University–Pueblo, CO
Concordia College, MN
Concordia University Wisconsin, WI
Cox College, MO
Daemen College, NY

Delaware State University, DE
Delta State University, MS
DeSales University, PA
Drexel University, PA
Duke University, NC
Duquesne University, PA
D'Youville College, NY
East Carolina University, NC
Eastern Kentucky University, KY
Eastern Michigan University, MI
Eastern New Mexico University, NM
East Tennessee State University, TN
Edgewood College, WI
Elmhurst College, IL
Elms College, MA
Emmanuel College, MA
Endicott College, MA
Excelsior College, NY
Fairleigh Dickinson University, Metropolitan Campus, NJ
Felician University, NJ
Ferris State University, MI
Florida Atlantic University, FL
Florida Southern College, FL
Florida State University, FL
Fort Hays State University, KS
Framingham State University, MA
Franciscan University of Steubenville, OH
Franklin Pierce University, NH
Gardner-Webb University, NC
George Mason University, VA
Georgia College & State University, GA
Georgia Southwestern State University, GA
Goldfarb School of Nursing at Barnes-Jewish College, MO
Gonzaga University, WA
Graceland University, IA
Grambling State University, LA
Grand Canyon University, AZ
Hampton University, VA
Herzing University Online, WI
Holy Family University, PA
Holy Names University, CA
Howard University, DC
Husson University, ME
Idaho State University, ID
Immaculata University, PA
Indiana State University, IN
Indiana University of Pennsylvania, PA
Indiana University–Purdue University Indianapolis, IN
Indiana Wesleyan University, IN
Jacksonville University, FL
Jefferson College of Health Sciences, VA
Kaplan University Online, FL
Kent State University, OH
Keuka College, NY
Lamar University, TX
La Roche College, PA
Lehman College of the City University of New York, NY
Le Moyne College, NY
Lenoir-Rhyne University, NC
Lewis University, IL
Liberty University, VA
Loma Linda University, CA
Long Island University–LIU Brooklyn, NY
Long Island University–LIU Post, NY
Lourdes University, OH
Mansfield University of Pennsylvania, PA
Marian University, WI
Marshall University, WV

McKendree University, IL
McNeese State University, LA
Mercy College, NY
Messiah College, PA
Metropolitan State University, MN
MGH Institute of Health Professions, MA
MidAmerica Nazarene University, KS
Middle Tennessee State University, TN
Midwestern State University, TX
Millersville University of Pennsylvania, PA
Millikin University, IL
Minnesota State University Mankato, MN
Minnesota State University Moorhead, MN
Misericordia University, PA
Missouri Southern State University, MO
Missouri State University, MO
Molloy College, NY
Monmouth University, NJ
Moravian College, PA
Mount Carmel College of Nursing, OH
Mount Mercy University, IA
Mount Saint Mary's University, CA
Nebraska Methodist College, NE
Nebraska Wesleyan University, NE
Neumann University, PA
New York University, NY
Northeastern State University, OK
Northern Illinois University, IL
Northern Kentucky University, KY
Northwestern State University of Louisiana, LA
Northwest Nazarene University, ID
Notre Dame College, OH
Nova Southeastern University, FL
Oakland University, MI
Ohio University, OH
Oklahoma Baptist University, OK
Oklahoma City University, OK
Oregon Health & Science University, OR
Otterbein University, OH
Our Lady of the Lake College, LA
Pace University, NY
Pacific Lutheran University, WA
Patty Hanks Shelton School of Nursing, TX
Pittsburg State University, KS
Point Loma Nazarene University, CA
Prairie View A&M University, TX
Queens University of Charlotte, NC
Ramapo College of New Jersey, NJ
Regis College, MA
Regis University, CO
Research College of Nursing, MO
Resurrection University, IL
Rivier University, NH
Robert Morris University, PA
Roberts Wesleyan College, NY
Rutgers, The State University of New Jersey, Newark, NJ
Sacred Heart University, CT
The Sage Colleges, NY
Saginaw Valley State University, MI
Saint Anthony College of Nursing, IL
St. Catherine University, MN
Saint Francis Medical Center College of Nursing, IL
St. Joseph's College, New York, NY
Saint Joseph's College of Maine, ME
Saint Louis University, MO
Salem State University, MA
Salisbury University, MD
Samford University, AL
San Diego State University, CA

San Jose State University, CA
Seattle Pacific University, WA
South Dakota State University, SD
Southeast Missouri State University, MO
Southern Adventist University, TN
Southern Connecticut State University, CT
Southern Illinois University Edwardsville, IL
Southern Nazarene University, OK
Southern New Hampshire University, NH
Southern University and Agricultural and Mechanical College, LA
Southwest Baptist University, MO
Spring Arbor University, MI
State University of New York Empire State College, NY
State University of New York Polytechnic Institute, NY
Stevenson University, MD
Stony Brook University, State University of New York, NY
Tabor College, KS
Tarleton State University, TX
Temple University, PA
Tennessee State University, TN
Tennessee Technological University, TN
Texas A&M Health Science Center, TX
Texas A&M University–Corpus Christi, TX
Texas Christian University, TX
Texas Tech University Health Sciences Center, TX
Texas Woman's University, TX
Thomas Jefferson University, PA
Thomas University, GA
Touro University, NV
Towson University, MD
Troy University, AL
Union University, TN
Université de Moncton, NB
Université de Montréal, QC
The University of Alabama, AL
The University of Alabama at Birmingham, AL
University of Alaska Anchorage, AK
University of Arkansas, AR
University of Arkansas for Medical Sciences, AR
The University of British Columbia, BC
University of Central Arkansas, AR
University of Central Florida, FL
University of Central Missouri, MO
University of Central Oklahoma, OK
University of Detroit Mercy, MI
University of Hartford, CT
University of Hawaii at Manoa, HI
University of Houston, TX
University of Indianapolis, IN
The University of Iowa, IA
University of Louisiana at Lafayette, LA
University of Louisville, KY
University of Maine, ME
University of Manitoba, MB
University of Mary, ND
University of Mary Hardin-Baylor, TX
University of Massachusetts Dartmouth, MA
University of Massachusetts Medical School, MA
University of Memphis, TN
University of Mississippi Medical Center, MS
University of Missouri, MO
University of Missouri–Kansas City, MO
University of Missouri–St. Louis, MO
University of Mobile, AL
University of Nebraska Medical Center, NE

University of Nevada, Las Vegas, NV
University of Nevada, Reno, NV
University of New Brunswick Fredericton, NB
University of New Mexico, NM
University of North Alabama, AL
The University of North Carolina at Chapel Hill, NC
The University of North Carolina at Charlotte, NC
The University of North Carolina at Greensboro, NC
University of North Dakota, ND
University of North Georgia, GA
University of Oklahoma Health Sciences Center, OK
University of Phoenix–Bay Area Campus, CA
University of Phoenix–Hawaii Campus, HI
University of Phoenix–New Mexico Campus, NM
University of Phoenix–North Florida Campus, FL
University of Phoenix–Online Campus, AZ
University of Phoenix–Phoenix Campus, AZ
University of Phoenix–Sacramento Valley Campus, CA
University of Phoenix–San Diego Campus, CA
University of Phoenix–Southern Arizona Campus, AZ
University of Phoenix–Southern California Campus, CA
University of Phoenix–South Florida Campus, FL
University of Portland, OR
University of Puerto Rico, Medical Sciences Campus, PR
University of Rhode Island, RI
University of St. Francis, IL
University of Saint Joseph, CT
University of Saint Mary, KS
University of San Diego, CA
University of Saskatchewan, SK
The University of Scranton, PA
University of South Alabama, AL
University of Southern Indiana, IN
University of Southern Maine, ME
University of South Florida, FL
The University of Texas at Arlington, TX
The University of Texas at Brownsville, TX
The University of Texas at El Paso, TX
The University of Texas at Tyler, TX
The University of Texas Health Science Center at Houston, TX
The University of Texas Health Science Center at San Antonio, TX
The University of Texas Medical Branch, TX
The University of Texas Rio Grande Valley, TX
The University of Toledo, OH
University of Toronto, ON
University of Utah, UT
The University of Western Ontario, ON
University of West Florida, FL
University of West Georgia, GA
University of Wisconsin–Eau Claire, WI
University of Wisconsin–Oshkosh, WI
University of Wyoming, WY
Urbana University, OH
Valdosta State University, GA
Valparaiso University, IN
Villanova University, PA
Wagner College, NY
Walden University, MN
Walsh University, OH

Waynesburg University, PA
Weber State University, UT
Webster University, MO
West Chester University of Pennsylvania, PA
West Coast University, CA
Western Carolina University, NC
Western Governors University, UT
Western Kentucky University, KY
Western Michigan University, MI
Westminster College, UT
West Texas A&M University, TX
West Virginia Wesleyan College, WV
Wheeling Jesuit University, WV
Widener University, PA
Wilkes University, PA
William Carey University, MS
William Paterson University of New Jersey, NJ
Wilmington University, DE
Winona State University, MN
Winston-Salem State University, NC
Worcester State University, MA
Wright State University, OH
WSU College of Nursing, WA
Xavier University, OH
York College of Pennsylvania, PA
Youngstown State University, OH

NURSING INFORMATICS

Adelphi University, NY
American Sentinel University, CO
Anderson University, IN
Austin Peay State University, TN
Chatham University, PA
Duke University, NC
East Tennessee State University, TN
Excelsior College, NY
Fairleigh Dickinson University, Metropolitan
  Campus, NJ
Ferris State University, MI
Georgia Southwestern State University, GA
Georgia State University, GA
Holy Names University, CA
Jacksonville University, FL
Kaplan University Online, FL
Le Moyne College, NY
Loyola University Chicago, IL
Middle Tennessee State University, TN
Molloy College, NY
National University, CA
New York University, NY
Northeastern University, MA
Northern Kentucky University, KY
Nova Southeastern University, FL
Regis College, MA

Rutgers, The State University of New Jersey,
  Newark, NJ
Tabor College, KS
Texas Tech University Health Sciences Center,
  TX
Thomas Jefferson University, PA
Troy University, AL
The University of Alabama at Birmingham, AL
University of Colorado Denver, CO
The University of Iowa, IA
The University of Kansas, KS
University of Manitoba, MB
University of Maryland, Baltimore, MD
University of Miami, FL
University of Michigan, MI
University of New Brunswick Fredericton, NB
The University of North Carolina at Chapel
  Hill, NC
University of Pittsburgh, PA
University of San Diego, CA
University of Toronto, ON
University of Utah, UT
Vanderbilt University, TN
Walden University, MN
Waynesburg University, PA
Xavier University, OH

DOCTORAL PROGRAMS

U.S. AND U.S. TERRITORIES

Alabama

Samford University, Ida V. Moffett School of Nursing, *Birmingham (DNP)*

Troy University, School of Nursing, *Troy (DNP)*

The University of Alabama, Capstone College of Nursing, *Tuscaloosa (DNP)*

The University of Alabama at Birmingham, School of Nursing, *Birmingham (DNP, PhD)*

The University of Alabama in Huntsville, College of Nursing, *Huntsville (DNP)*

Arizona

Arizona State University at the Downtown Phoenix campus, College of Nursing, *Phoenix (DNP)*

Chamberlain College of Nursing, *Phoenix (DNP)*

Northern Arizona University, School of Nursing, *Flagstaff (DNP)*

The University of Arizona, College of Nursing, *Tucson (PhD)*

University of Phoenix–Online Campus, Online Campus, *Phoenix (PhD)*

Arkansas

Arkansas State University, Department of Nursing, *State University (DNP)*

University of Arkansas, Eleanor Mann School of Nursing, *Fayetteville (DNP)*

University of Arkansas for Medical Sciences, College of Nursing, *Little Rock (DNP, PhD)*

California

Azusa Pacific University, School of Nursing, *Azusa (PhD)*

Brandman University, School of Nursing and Health Professions, *Irvine (DNP)*

California State University, Fresno, Department of Nursing, *Fresno (DNP)*

California State University, Fullerton, Department of Nursing, *Fullerton (DNP)*

Loma Linda University, School of Nursing, *Loma Linda (DNP)*

Samuel Merritt University, School of Nursing, *Oakland (DNP)*

University of California, Davis, The Betty Irene Moore School of Nursing, *Davis (PhD)*

University of California, Irvine, Program in Nursing Science, *Irvine (PhD)*

University of California, Los Angeles, School of Nursing, *Los Angeles (PhD)*

University of California, San Francisco, School of Nursing, *San Francisco (PhD)*

University of San Diego, Hahn School of Nursing and Health Science, *San Diego (DNP, PhD)*

University of San Francisco, School of Nursing and Health Professions, *San Francisco (DNP)*

Western University of Health Sciences, College of Graduate Nursing, *Pomona (DNP)*

Colorado

American Sentinel University, RN to Bachelor of Science Nursing, *Aurora (DNP)*

Colorado Mesa University, Department of Nursing and Radiologic Sciences, *Grand Junction (DNP)*

University of Colorado Colorado Springs, Helen and Arthur E. Johnson Beth-El College of Nursing & Health Sciences, *Colorado Springs (DNP)*

University of Colorado Denver, College of Nursing, *Aurora (DNP, PhD)*

University of Northern Colorado, School of Nursing, *Greeley (PhD)*

Connecticut

Fairfield University, School of Nursing, *Fairfield (DNP)*

Quinnipiac University, School of Nursing, *Hamden (DNP)*

Sacred Heart University, College of Nursing, *Fairfield (DNP)*

Southern Connecticut State University, Department of Nursing, *New Haven (EdD)*

University of Connecticut, School of Nursing, *Storrs (DNP, PhD)*

University of Saint Joseph, Department of Nursing, *West Hartford (DNP)*

Yale University, School of Nursing, *West Haven (DNP, PhD)*

Delaware

University of Delaware, School of Nursing, *Newark (PhD)*

District of Columbia

The Catholic University of America, School of Nursing, *Washington (DNP, PhD)*

Georgetown University, School of Nursing and Health Studies, *Washington (DNP)*

The George Washington University, School of Nursing, *Washington (DNP)*

Florida

Barry University, Division of Nursing, *Miami Shores (PhD)*

Florida Agricultural and Mechanical University, School of Nursing, *Tallahassee (PhD)*

Florida Atlantic University, Christine E. Lynn College of Nursing, *Boca Raton (DNP)*

Florida International University, Nursing Program, *Miami (DNP, PhD)*

Florida State University, College of Nursing, *Tallahassee (DNP)*

Jacksonville University, School of Nursing, *Jacksonville (DNP)*

Palm Beach Atlantic University, School of Nursing, *West Palm Beach (DNP)*

University of Central Florida, College of Nursing, *Orlando (DNP, PhD)*

University of Florida, College of Nursing, *Gainesville (PhD)*

University of Miami, School of Nursing and Health Studies, *Coral Gables (DNP)*

University of South Florida, College of Nursing, *Tampa (DNP, PhD)*

Georgia

Augusta University, School of Nursing, *Augusta (DNP, PhD)*

Brenau University, College of Health and Science, *Gainesville (DNP)*

Emory University, Nell Hodgson Woodruff School of Nursing, *Atlanta (PhD)*

Georgia College & State University, College of Health Sciences, *Milledgeville (DNP)*

Georgia Southern University, School of Nursing, *Statesboro (DNP)*

Georgia State University, Byrdine F. Lewis School of Nursing, *Atlanta (PhD)*

Mercer University, Georgia Baptist College of Nursing of Mercer University, *Atlanta (DNP, PhD)*

University of West Georgia, School of Nursing, *Carrollton (EdD)*

Hawaii

University of Hawaii at Manoa, School of Nursing and Dental Hygiene, *Honolulu (PhD)*

Idaho

Idaho State University, Department of Nursing, *Pocatello (DNP, PhD)*

Illinois

Bradley University, Department of Nursing, *Peoria (DNP)*

DePaul University, School of Nursing, *Chicago (DNP)*

Illinois State University, Mennonite College of Nursing, *Normal (DNP, PhD)*

Lewis University, Program in Nursing, *Romeoville (DNP)*

Loyola University Chicago, Marcella Niehoff School of Nursing, *Maywood (DNP, PhD)*

Millikin University, School of Nursing, *Decatur (DNP)*

Rush University, College of Nursing, *Chicago (DNP)*

Saint Anthony College of Nursing, *Rockford (DNP)*

Saint Francis Medical Center College of Nursing, Baccalaureate Nursing Program, *Peoria (DNP)*

Southern Illinois University Edwardsville, School of Nursing, *Edwardsville (DNP)*

University of Illinois at Chicago, College of Nursing, *Chicago (DNP, PhD)*

University of St. Francis, Leach College of Nursing, *Joliet (DNP)*

Indiana

Ball State University, School of Nursing, *Muncie (DNP)*

Indiana State University, Department of Advanced Practice Nursing, *Terre Haute (DNP)*

Indiana University–Purdue University Fort Wayne, Department of Nursing, *Fort Wayne (DNP)*

Indiana University–Purdue University Indianapolis, School of Nursing, *Indianapolis (PhD)*

Purdue University, School of Nursing, *West Lafayette (DNP)*

Saint Mary's College, Department of Nursing, *Notre Dame (DNP)*

University of Indianapolis, School of Nursing, *Indianapolis (DNP)*

University of Southern Indiana, College of Nursing and Health Professions, *Evansville (DNP)*

Valparaiso University, College of Nursing and Health Professions, *Valparaiso (DNP)*

Iowa

Allen College, Graduate Programs, *Waterloo (DNP)*

Briar Cliff University, Department of Nursing, *Sioux City (DNP)*

Clarke University, Department of Nursing and Health, *Dubuque (DNP)*

The University of Iowa, College of Nursing, *Iowa City (PhD)*

Kansas

Pittsburg State University, Department of Nursing, *Pittsburg (DNP)*

The University of Kansas, School of Nursing, *Kansas City (PhD)*

Wichita State University, School of Nursing, *Wichita (DNP)*

Kentucky

Bellarmine University, Donna and Allan Lansing School of Nursing and Health Sciences, *Louisville (DNP)*

Frontier Nursing University, Nursing Degree Programs, *Hyden (DNP)*

Northern Kentucky University, Department of Nursing, *Highland Heights (DNP)*

Spalding University, School of Nursing, *Louisville (DNP)*

University of Kentucky, College of Nursing, *Lexington (PhD)*

University of Louisville, School of Nursing, *Louisville (PhD)*

Western Kentucky University, School of Nursing, *Bowling Green (DNP)*

Louisiana

Louisiana State University Health Sciences Center, School of Nursing, *New Orleans (DNP)*

Loyola University New Orleans, School of Nursing, *New Orleans (DNP)*

Northwestern State University of Louisiana, College of Nursing and School of Allied Health, *Shreveport (DNP)*

Southeastern Louisiana University, School of Nursing, *Hammond (DNP)*

Southern University and Agricultural and Mechanical College, School of Nursing, *Baton Rouge (PhD)*

Maine

University of Southern Maine, School of Nursing, *Portland (DNP)*

Maryland

Johns Hopkins University, School of Nursing, *Baltimore (DNP, PhD)*

Salisbury University, Department of Nursing, *Salisbury (DNP)*

University of Maryland, Baltimore, Nursing Programs, *Baltimore (DNP, PhD)*

Massachusetts

Boston College, William F. Connell School of Nursing, *Chestnut Hill (PhD)*

Elms College, School of Nursing, *Chicopee (DNP)*

MGH Institute of Health Professions, School of Nursing, *Boston (DNP)*

Northeastern University, School of Nursing, *Boston (PhD)*

Regis College, School of Nursing, Science and Health Professions, *Weston (DNP)*

Simmons College, School of Nursing and Health Sciences, *Boston (DNP)*

University of Massachusetts Amherst, College of Nursing, *Amherst (PhD)*

University of Massachusetts Boston, College of Nursing and Health Sciences, *Boston (DNP, PhD)*

University of Massachusetts Dartmouth, College of Nursing, *North Dartmouth (DNP, PhD)*

University of Massachusetts Lowell, School of Nursing, *Lowell (DNP, PhD)*

University of Massachusetts Medical School, Graduate School of Nursing, *Worcester (PhD)*

Michigan

Andrews University, Department of Nursing, *Berrien Springs (DNP)*

Grand Valley State University, Kirkhof College of Nursing, *Allendale (DNP)*

Madonna University, College of Nursing and Health, *Livonia (DNP)*

Michigan State University, College of Nursing, *East Lansing (DNP, PhD)*

Northern Michigan University, College of Nursing and Allied Health Science, *Marquette (DNP)*

Oakland University, School of Nursing, *Rochester (DNP)*

Saginaw Valley State University, College of Health and Human Services, *University Center (DNP)*

University of Michigan, School of Nursing, *Ann Arbor (PhD)*

University of Michigan–Flint, Department of Nursing, *Flint (DNP)*

Wayne State University, College of Nursing, *Detroit (PhD)*

Minnesota

Capella University, Nursing Programs, *Minneapolis (DNP)*

The College of St. Scholastica, Department of Nursing, *Duluth (DNP)*

Metropolitan State University, College of Health, Community and Professional Studies, *St. Paul (DNP)*

Minnesota State University Mankato, School of Nursing, *Mankato (DNP)*

St. Catherine University, Department of Nursing, *St. Paul (DNP)*

University of Minnesota, Twin Cities Campus, School of Nursing, *Minneapolis (DNP, PhD)*

Walden University, Nursing Programs, *Minneapolis (DNP, PhD)*

Winona State University, College of Nursing and Health Sciences, *Winona (DNP)*

Mississippi

Delta State University, School of Nursing, *Cleveland (DNP)*

Mississippi University for Women, College of Nursing and Speech Language Pathology, *Columbus (DNP)*

University of Mississippi Medical Center, School of Nursing, *Jackson (DNP)*

University of Southern Mississippi, College of Nursing, *Hattiesburg (PhD)*

William Carey University, School of Nursing, *Hattiesburg (PhD)*

Missouri

Goldfarb School of Nursing at Barnes-Jewish College, *St. Louis (PhD)*

Graceland University, School of Nursing, *Independence (DNP)*

Maryville University of Saint Louis, The Catherine McAuley School of Nursing, College of Health Professions, *St. Louis (DNP)*

Missouri State University, Department of Nursing, *Springfield (DNP)*

Saint Louis University, School of Nursing, *St. Louis (DNP, PhD)*

University of Missouri, Sinclair School of Nursing, *Columbia (PhD)*

University of Missouri–Kansas City, School of Nursing and Health Studies, *Kansas City (DNP, PhD)*

University of Missouri–St. Louis, College of Nursing, *St. Louis (DNP, PhD)*

Montana

Montana State University, College of Nursing, *Bozeman (DNP)*

Nebraska

Bryan College of Health Sciences, School of Nursing, *Lincoln (EdD)*

Creighton University, College of Nursing, *Omaha (DNP)*

Nebraska Methodist College, Department of Nursing, *Omaha (DNP)*

University of Nebraska Medical Center, College of Nursing, *Omaha (PhD)*

Nevada

Touro University, School of Nursing, *Henderson (DNP)*

University of Nevada, Las Vegas, School of Nursing, *Las Vegas (DNP, PhD)*

University of Nevada, Reno, Orvis School of Nursing, *Reno (DNP)*

New Hampshire

University of New Hampshire, Department of Nursing, *Durham (DNP)*

New Jersey

Fairleigh Dickinson University, Metropolitan Campus, Henry P. Becton School of Nursing and Allied Health, *Teaneck (DNP)*

Rutgers, The State University of New Jersey, Camden, Rutgers School of Nursing–Camden, *Camden (DNP)*

Rutgers, The State University of New Jersey, Newark, Rutgers School of Nursing, *Newark (DNP)*

Seton Hall University, College of Nursing, *South Orange (DNP)*

William Paterson University of New Jersey, Department of Nursing, *Wayne (DNP)*

New Mexico

New Mexico State University, School of Nursing, *Las Cruces (PhD)*

University of New Mexico, Program in Nursing, *Albuquerque (DNP, PhD)*

New York

Adelphi University, College of Nursing and Public Health, *Garden City (PhD)*

Binghamton University, State University of New York, Decker School of Nursing, *Vestal (DNP, PhD)*

Columbia University, School of Nursing, *New York (PhD)*

Daemen College, Department of Nursing, *Amherst (DNP)*

D'Youville College, School of Nursing, *Buffalo (DNP)*

Hunter College of the City University of New York, Hunter-Bellevue School of Nursing, *New York (DNP)*

Lehman College of the City University of New York, Department of Nursing, *Bronx (DNS)*

Molloy College, Division of Nursing, *Rockville Centre (DNP, PhD)*

New York University, College of Nursing, *New York (DNP, PhD)*

Pace University, Lienhard School of Nursing, *New York (DNP)*

The Sage Colleges, Department of Nursing, *Troy (DNS)*

St. John Fisher College, Wegmans School of Nursing, *Rochester (DNP)*

Stony Brook University, State University of New York, School of Nursing, *Stony Brook (DNP)*

University at Buffalo, the State University of New York, School of Nursing, *Buffalo (DNP, PhD)*

North Carolina

Duke University, School of Nursing, *Durham (DNP, PhD)*

East Carolina University, College of Nursing, *Greenville (DNP, PhD)*

Gardner-Webb University, School of Nursing, *Boiling Springs (DNP)*

The University of North Carolina at Chapel Hill, School of Nursing, *Chapel Hill (DNP, PhD)*

The University of North Carolina at Greensboro, School of Nursing, *Greensboro (DNP, PhD)*

North Dakota

North Dakota State University, Department of Nursing, *Fargo (DNP)*

University of Mary, Division of Nursing, *Bismarck (DNP)*

University of North Dakota, College of Nursing, *Grand Forks (PhD)*

Ohio

Ashland University, Dwight Schar College of Nursing and Health Sciences, *Ashland (DNP)*

Case Western Reserve University, Frances Payne Bolton School of Nursing, *Cleveland (PhD)*

Cleveland State University, School of Nursing, *Cleveland (PhD)*

Kent State University, College of Nursing, *Kent (DNP, PhD)*

Mount Carmel College of Nursing, Nursing Programs, *Columbus (DNP)*

The Ohio State University, College of Nursing, *Columbus (DNP, PhD)*

The University of Akron, School of Nursing, *Akron (PhD)*

University of Cincinnati, College of Nursing, *Cincinnati (PhD)*

The University of Toledo, College of Nursing, *Toledo (DNP)*

Ursuline College, The Breen School of Nursing, *Pepper Pike (DNP)*

Walsh University, Department of Nursing, *North Canton (DNP)*

Wright State University, College of Nursing and Health, *Dayton (DNP)*

Xavier University, School of Nursing, *Cincinnati (DNP)*

Oklahoma

Oklahoma City University, Kramer School of Nursing, *Oklahoma City (DNP, PhD)*

University of Oklahoma Health Sciences Center, College of Nursing, *Oklahoma City (PhD)*

Oregon

Oregon Health & Science University, School of Nursing, *Portland (PhD)*

University of Portland, School of Nursing, *Portland (DNP)*

Pennsylvania

Carlow University, College of Health and Wellness, *Pittsburgh (DNP)*

Chatham University, Nursing Programs, *Pittsburgh (DNP)*

Clarion University of Pennsylvania, School of Nursing, *Oil City (DNP)*

DeSales University, Department of Nursing and Health, *Center Valley (DNP)*

Drexel University, College of Nursing and Health Professions, *Philadelphia (Dr NP)*

Duquesne University, School of Nursing, *Pittsburgh (PhD)*

Gannon University, Villa Maria School of Nursing, *Erie (DNP)*

Indiana University of Pennsylvania, Department of Nursing and Allied Health, *Indiana (PhD)*

Penn State University Park, School of Nursing, *University Park (PhD)*

Robert Morris University, School of Nursing and Health Sciences, *Moon Township (DNP)*

Temple University, Department of Nursing, *Philadelphia (DNP)*

Thomas Jefferson University, Department of Nursing, *Philadelphia (DNP)*

University of Pennsylvania, School of Nursing, *Philadelphia (PhD)*

University of Pittsburgh, School of Nursing, *Pittsburgh (PhD)*

Villanova University, College of Nursing, *Villanova (DNP, PhD)*

Waynesburg University, Department of Nursing, *Waynesburg (DNP)*

Widener University, School of Nursing, *Chester (PhD)*

York College of Pennsylvania, Department of Nursing, *York (DNP)*

Rhode Island

University of Rhode Island, College of Nursing, *Kingston (PhD)*

South Carolina

Medical University of South Carolina, College of Nursing, *Charleston (PhD)*

University of South Carolina, College of Nursing, *Columbia (DNP, PhD)*

South Dakota

South Dakota State University, College of Nursing, *Brookings (DNP, PhD)*

Tennessee

Belmont University, School of Nursing, *Nashville (DNP)*

East Tennessee State University, College of Nursing, *Johnson City (DNP, PhD)*

Southern Adventist University, School of Nursing, *Collegedale (DNP)*

The University of Tennessee, College of Nursing, *Knoxville (PhD)*

The University of Tennessee at Chattanooga, School of Nursing, *Chattanooga (DNP)*

The University of Tennessee Health Science Center, College of Nursing, *Memphis (DNP, PhD)*

Vanderbilt University, Vanderbilt University School of Nursing, *Nashville (DNP, PhD)*

Texas

Baylor University, Louise Herrington School of Nursing, *Dallas (DNP)*

Texas Christian University, Harris College of Nursing, *Fort Worth (DNP)*

Texas Tech University Health Sciences Center, School of Nursing, *Lubbock (DNP)*

Texas Woman's University, College of Nursing, *Denton (PhD)*

The University of Texas at Arlington, College of Nursing, *Arlington (PhD)*

The University of Texas at Austin, School of Nursing, *Austin (PhD)*

The University of Texas at El Paso, School of Nursing, *El Paso (DNP)*

The University of Texas at Tyler, Program in Nursing, *Tyler (PhD)*

The University of Texas Health Science Center at Houston, School of Nursing, *Houston (PhD)*

The University of Texas Health Science Center at San Antonio, School of Nursing, *San Antonio (PhD)*

The University of Texas Medical Branch, School of Nursing, *Galveston (DNP)*

University of the Incarnate Word, Program in Nursing, *San Antonio (DNP)*

Utah

University of Utah, College of Nursing, *Salt Lake City (PhD)*

Vermont

University of Vermont, Department of Nursing, *Burlington (DNP)*

Virginia

George Mason University, College of Health and Human Services, *Fairfax (PhD)*

Hampton University, School of Nursing, *Hampton (PhD)*

James Madison University, Department of Nursing, *Harrisonburg (DNP)*

Marymount University, School of Health Professions, *Arlington (DNP)*

Old Dominion University, Department of Nursing, *Norfolk (DNP)*

Radford University, Program in Nursing Practice, *Radford (DNP)*

Shenandoah University, Eleanor Wade Custer School of Nursing, *Winchester (DNP)*

University of Virginia, School of Nursing, *Charlottesville (PhD)*

Virginia Commonwealth University, School of Nursing, *Richmond (DNP, PhD)*

Washington

Gonzaga University, School of Nursing and Human Psychology, *Spokane (DNP)*

Pacific Lutheran University, School of Nursing, *Tacoma (DNP)*

Seattle University, College of Nursing, *Seattle (DNP)*

University of Washington, School of Nursing, *Seattle (DNP, PhD)*

WSU College of Nursing, *Spokane (PhD)*

West Virginia

West Virginia University, School of Nursing, *Morgantown (DNP, PhD)*

Wisconsin

Concordia University Wisconsin, Program in Nursing, *Mequon (DNP)*

Marquette University, College of Nursing, *Milwaukee (DNP, PhD)*

University of Phoenix–Milwaukee Campus, College of Health and Human Services, *Milwaukee (PhD)*

University of Wisconsin–Eau Claire, College of Nursing and Health Sciences, *Eau Claire (DNP)*

University of Wisconsin–Madison, School of Nursing, *Madison (PhD)*

University of Wisconsin–Milwaukee, College of Nursing, *Milwaukee (DNP, PhD)*

University of Wisconsin–Oshkosh, College of Nursing, *Oshkosh (DNP)*

Viterbo University, School of Nursing, *La Crosse (DNP)*

Wyoming

University of Wyoming, Fay W. Whitney School of Nursing, *Laramie (DNP)*

CANADA

Alberta

University of Alberta, Faculty of Nursing, *Edmonton (PhD)*

University of Calgary, Faculty of Nursing, *Calgary (PhD)*

British Columbia

The University of British Columbia, Program in Nursing, *Vancouver (PhD)*

University of Victoria, School of Nursing, *Victoria (PhD)*

Manitoba

University of Manitoba, Faculty of Nursing, *Winnipeg (PhD)*

Newfoundland and Labrador

Memorial University of Newfoundland, School of Nursing, *St. John's (PhD)*

Ontario

McMaster University, School of Nursing, *Hamilton (PhD)*

Queen's University at Kingston, School of Nursing, *Kingston (PhD)*

University of Ottawa, School of Nursing, *Ottawa (PhD)*

University of Toronto, Faculty of Nursing, *Toronto (PhD)*

The University of Western Ontario, School of Nursing, *London (PhD)*

Quebec

McGill University, School of Nursing, *Montréal (PhD)*

Université de Montréal, Faculty of Nursing, *Montréal (PhD)*

Université de Sherbrooke, Department of Nursing, *Sherbrooke (PhD)*

Université Laval, Faculty of Nursing, *Québec (PhD)*

Saskatchewan

University of Saskatchewan, College of Nursing, *Saskatoon (PhD)*

POSTDOCTORAL PROGRAMS

U.S. AND U.S. TERRITORIES

Alabama
The University of Alabama at Birmingham, School of Nursing, *Birmingham*

Arkansas
University of Arkansas for Medical Sciences, College of Nursing, *Little Rock*

California
Brandman University, School of Nursing and Health Professions, *Irvine*

University of California, Davis, The Betty Irene Moore School of Nursing, *Davis*

University of California, Los Angeles, School of Nursing, *Los Angeles*

University of California, San Francisco, School of Nursing, *San Francisco*

Colorado
University of Colorado Denver, College of Nursing, *Aurora*

Connecticut
University of Connecticut, School of Nursing, *Storrs*

Yale University, School of Nursing, *West Haven*

Illinois
Rush University, College of Nursing, *Chicago*

University of Illinois at Chicago, College of Nursing, *Chicago*

Indiana
Indiana University–Purdue University Indianapolis, School of Nursing, *Indianapolis*

Iowa
The University of Iowa, College of Nursing, *Iowa City*

Kansas
The University of Kansas, School of Nursing, *Kansas City*

Maryland
Johns Hopkins University, School of Nursing, *Baltimore*

Salisbury University, Department of Nursing, *Salisbury*

Massachusetts
University of Massachusetts Boston, College of Nursing and Health Sciences, *Boston*

Michigan
Michigan State University, College of Nursing, *East Lansing*

University of Michigan, School of Nursing, *Ann Arbor*

New Jersey
Rutgers, The State University of New Jersey, Camden, Rutgers School of Nursing–Camden, *Camden*

New York
Columbia University, School of Nursing, *New York*

New York University, College of Nursing, *New York*

North Carolina
Duke University, School of Nursing, *Durham*

The University of North Carolina at Chapel Hill, School of Nursing, *Chapel Hill*

Ohio
Case Western Reserve University, Frances Payne Bolton School of Nursing, *Cleveland*

Oregon
Oregon Health & Science University, School of Nursing, *Portland*

Pennsylvania
Penn State University Park, School of Nursing, *University Park*

University of Pennsylvania, School of Nursing, *Philadelphia*

University of Pittsburgh, School of Nursing, *Pittsburgh*

South Carolina
University of South Carolina, College of Nursing, *Columbia*

Tennessee
Vanderbilt University, Vanderbilt University School of Nursing, *Nashville*

Utah
University of Utah, College of Nursing, *Salt Lake City*

Virginia
University of Virginia, School of Nursing, *Charlottesville*

Washington
University of Washington, School of Nursing, *Seattle*

Wisconsin
University of Wisconsin–Madison, School of Nursing, *Madison*

CANADA

British Columbia
The University of British Columbia, Program in Nursing, *Vancouver*

University of Northern British Columbia, Nursing Programme, *Prince George*

Ontario
University of Ottawa, School of Nursing, *Ottawa*

University of Toronto, Faculty of Nursing, *Toronto*

The University of Western Ontario, School of Nursing, *London*

Quebec
McGill University, School of Nursing, *Montréal*

Université de Montréal, Faculty of Nursing, *Montréal*

Université de Sherbrooke, Department of Nursing, *Sherbrooke*

Université du Québec en Outaouais, Département des Sciences Infirmières, *Gatineau*

Université Laval, Faculty of Nursing, *Québec*

ONLINE PROGRAMS

ONLINE BACCALAUREATE PROGRAMS

Adams State University, CO
Adventist University of Health Sciences, FL
Albany State University, GA
Alcorn State University, MS
Allen College, IA
American Public University System, WV
American Sentinel University, CO
Andrews University, MI
Angelo State University, TX
Appalachian State University, NC
Arizona State University at the Downtown
    Phoenix campus, AZ
Arkansas State University, AR
Arkansas Tech University, AR
Ashland University, OH
Aurora University, IL
Bethel College, KS
Bethel University, TN
Blessing–Rieman College of Nursing and
    Health Sciences, IL
Bluefield College, VA
Bluefield State College, WV
Boise State University, ID
Bon Secours Memorial College of Nursing, VA
Brandman University, CA
Brenau University, GA
Caldwell University, NJ
Cardinal Stritch University, WI
Carlow University, PA
Carson-Newman University, TN
Cedar Crest College, PA
Central Methodist University, MO
Chamberlain College of Nursing, AZ
Chamberlain College of Nursing, MO
Charleston Southern University, SC
Clarion University of Pennsylvania, PA
Clarkson College, NE
Clayton State University, GA
Cleveland State University, OH
College of Coastal Georgia, GA
The College of St. Scholastica, MN
Colorado Christian University, CO
Colorado Mesa University, CO
Colorado Technical University Online, CO
Columbus State University, GA
Cox College, MO
Cumberland University, TN
Darton State College, GA
Davenport University, MI
DePaul University, IL
East Carolina University, NC
Eastern Illinois University, IL
Eastern Michigan University, MI
Eastern New Mexico University, NM
East Tennessee State University, TN
ECPI University, VA
Ferris State University, MI
Finlandia University, MI
Fitchburg State University, MA
Florida Atlantic University, FL
Florida International University, FL
Fort Hays State University, KS
Francis Marion University, SC
Frostburg State University, MD
Gannon University, PA
Gardner-Webb University, NC
George Mason University, VA

The George Washington University, DC
Georgia College & State University, GA
Georgia Southern University, GA
Georgia Southwestern State University, GA
Grand Canyon University, AZ
Great Basin College, NV
Hannibal-LaGrange University, MO
Herzing University, GA
Herzing University Online, WI
Hondros College, OH
Howard University, DC
Illinois State University, IL
Immaculata University, PA
Indiana State University, IN
Indiana University Northwest, IN
Indiana University–Purdue University
    Indianapolis, IN
Indiana University Southeast, IN
Jacksonville State University, AL
Jacksonville University, FL
Kettering College, OH
Lakehead University, ON
Lamar University, TX
Lander University, SC
La Roche College, PA
Lees-McRae College, NC
Lehman College of the City University of New
    York, NY
Lewis-Clark State College, ID
Linfield College, OR
Loyola University New Orleans, LA
MacMurray College, IL
Marian University, IN
Marshall University, WV
McKendree University, IL
Mercy College, NY
Mercy College of Ohio, OH
Methodist College, IL
Michigan State University, MI
MidAmerica Nazarene University, KS
Middle Tennessee State University, TN
Midway University, KY
Minnesota State University Moorhead, MN
Minot State University, ND
Mississippi University for Women, MS
Missouri State University, MO
Missouri Valley College, MO
Montana State University–Northern, MT
Morehead State University, KY
Mount Aloysius College, PA
Mount Carmel College of Nursing, OH
Mount Mercy University, IA
Nevada State College at Henderson, NV
Newman University, KS
New Mexico State University, NM
Nipissing University, ON
Northeastern State University, OK
Northern Arizona University, AZ
Northwestern Oklahoma State University, OK
Northwestern State University of Louisiana,
    LA
Notre Dame College, OH
Nova Southeastern University, FL
Nyack College, NY
The Ohio State University, OH
Ohio University, OH
Oklahoma Baptist University, OK
Oklahoma Panhandle State University, OK
Our Lady of the Lake College, LA
Palm Beach Atlantic University, FL

Penn State University Park, PA
Pennsylvania College of Technology, PA
Pittsburg State University, KS
Presentation College, SD
Purdue University Calumet, IN
Queens University of Charlotte, NC
Radford University, VA
Ramapo College of New Jersey, NJ
Rider University, NJ
Rivier University, NH
Robert Morris University, PA
Roberts Wesleyan College, NY
Roseman University of Health Sciences, NV
Ryerson University, ON
Sacred Heart University, CT
Saint Louis University, MO
Saint Mary's University of Minnesota, MN
St. Petersburg College, FL
St. Vincent's College, CT
Sentara College of Health Sciences, VA
Shenandoah University, VA
Siena Heights University, MI
Silver Lake College of the Holy Family, WI
Slippery Rock University of Pennsylvania, PA
South Dakota State University, SD
Southeastern Louisiana University, LA
Southeast Missouri State University, MO
Southern Adventist University, TN
Southern Arkansas University–Magnolia, AR
Southern New Hampshire University, NH
Southwestern Oklahoma State University, OK
Southwest Minnesota State University, MN
State College of Florida Manatee-Sarasota, FL
State University of New York at Plattsburgh,
    NY
State University of New York College of
    Technology at Alfred, NY
State University of New York College of
    Technology at Delhi, NY
State University of New York Empire State
    College, NY
State University of New York Polytechnic
    Institute, NY
Stevenson University, MD
Sullivan University, KY
Tabor College, KS
Texas A&M Health Science Center, TX
Texas A&M University–Corpus Christi, TX
Texas A&M University–Texarkana, TX
Texas Tech University Health Sciences Center,
    TX
Texas Tech University Health Sciences Center
    El Paso, TX
Texas Woman's University, TX
Touro University, NV
Trocaire College, NY
Unitek College, CA
University at Buffalo, the State University of
    New York, NY
The University of Akron, OH
University of Arkansas, AR
University of Arkansas for Medical Sciences,
    AR
University of Arkansas–Fort Smith, AR
University of Central Missouri, MO
University of Colorado Colorado Springs, CO
University of Colorado Denver, CO
University of Delaware, DE
University of Illinois at Chicago, IL
University of Indianapolis, IN

University of Louisiana at Lafayette, LA
University of Louisiana at Monroe, LA
University of Louisville, KY
University of Maine at Fort Kent, ME
University of Mary, ND
University of Maryland, Baltimore, MD
University of Massachusetts Amherst, MA
University of Massachusetts Boston, MA
University of Massachusetts Dartmouth, MA
University of Michigan–Flint, MI
University of Missouri, MO
University of Missouri–Kansas City, MO
University of Missouri–St. Louis, MO
University of Mount Olive, NC
University of North Alabama, AL
The University of North Carolina Wilmington, NC
University of North Georgia, GA
University of Phoenix–Online Campus, AZ
University of Phoenix–Phoenix Campus, AZ
University of Phoenix–Sacramento Valley Campus, CA
University of Phoenix–Southern Arizona Campus, AZ
University of Phoenix–South Florida Campus, FL
University of Phoenix–West Florida Learning Center, FL
University of Rhode Island, RI
University of St. Francis, IL
University of Saint Francis, IN
University of Saint Mary, KS
University of San Francisco, CA
University of Sioux Falls, SD
University of South Carolina, SC
University of South Carolina Aiken, SC
University of South Carolina Upstate, SC
The University of South Dakota, SD
University of Southern Indiana, IN
University of South Florida, FL
The University of Tennessee at Chattanooga, TN
The University of Tennessee Health Science Center, TN
The University of Texas at Arlington, TX
The University of Texas at Brownsville, TX
The University of Texas at Tyler, TX
The University of Texas Rio Grande Valley, TX
University of the Incarnate Word, TX
The University of Toledo, OH
University of Utah, UT
University of Wisconsin–Green Bay, WI
University of Wisconsin–Oshkosh, WI
University of Wyoming, WY
Urbana University, OH
Utica College, NY
Walden University, MN
West Coast University, CA
Western Carolina University, NC
Western Governors University, UT
Western Illinois University, IL
Western New Mexico University, NM
Wheeling Jesuit University, WV
Wichita State University, KS
William Jewell College, MO
Wilmington University, DE

ONLINE ONLY BACCALAUREATE PROGRAMS

Adams State University, CO
Adventist University of Health Sciences, FL

American Public University System, WV
American Sentinel University, CO
Bluefield College, VA
Bluefield State College, WV
Brandman University, CA
Chamberlain College of Nursing, MO
Clarion University of Pennsylvania, PA
Cox College, MO
Darton State College, GA
DePaul University, IL
Eastern Illinois University, IL
Eastern New Mexico University, NM
Florida Atlantic University, FL
Frostburg State University, MD
Great Basin College, NV
Hannibal-LaGrange University, MO
Herzing University Online, WI
Hondros College, OH
Illinois State University, IL
Immaculata University, PA
Kettering College, OH
La Roche College, PA
Loyola University New Orleans, LA
Methodist College, IL
Minnesota State University Moorhead, MN
Missouri Valley College, MO
Montana State University–Northern, MT
Northeastern State University, OK
Oklahoma Baptist University, OK
Oklahoma Panhandle State University, OK
Rider University, NJ
Roseman University of Health Sciences, NV
Saint Mary's University of Minnesota, MN
St. Vincent's College, CT
Slippery Rock University of Pennsylvania, PA
Southern New Hampshire University, NH
Southwest Minnesota State University, MN
State University of New York College of Technology at Delhi, NY
State University of New York Empire State College, NY
Stevenson University, MD
Tabor College, KS
Texas A&M University–Texarkana, TX
Texas Tech University Health Sciences Center, TX
Trocaire College, NY
Unitek College, CA
University of Arkansas–Fort Smith, AR
University of Louisiana at Monroe, LA
University of Mount Olive, NC
University of North Alabama, AL
University of North Georgia, GA
The University of Tennessee at Chattanooga, TN
The University of Texas at Brownsville, TX
The University of Texas at Tyler, TX
Walden University, MN
Western Governors University, UT
William Jewell College, MO

ONLINE MASTER'S DEGREE PROGRAMS

Albany State University, GA
Alcorn State University, MS
Allen College, IA
American International College, MA
American Sentinel University, CO
Angelo State University, TX
Aspen University, CO
Athabasca University, AB

Augusta University, GA
Austin Peay State University, TN
Baker University, KS
Ball State University, IN
Baylor University, TX
Bellin College, WI
Benedictine University, IL
Bradley University, IL
Brandon University, MB
Briar Cliff University, IA
California State University, Dominguez Hills, CA
California State University, Fullerton, CA
The Catholic University of America, DC
Cedar Crest College, PA
Cedarville University, OH
Central Methodist University, MO
Chamberlain College of Nursing, AZ
Charleston Southern University, SC
Chatham University, PA
Clarkson College, NE
Clayton State University, GA
Cleveland State University, OH
Colorado Mesa University, CO
Concordia University Wisconsin, WI
Cox College, MO
Creighton University, NE
Delta State University, MS
Drexel University, PA
Duke University, NC
Duquesne University, PA
East Carolina University, NC
Eastern Mennonite University, VA
Eastern New Mexico University, NM
East Tennessee State University, TN
Excelsior College, NY
Fairleigh Dickinson University, Metropolitan Campus, NJ
Felician University, NJ
Ferris State University, MI
Fitchburg State University, MA
Florida Atlantic University, FL
Florida State University, FL
Frontier Nursing University, KY
Gardner-Webb University, NC
Georgetown University, DC
The George Washington University, DC
Georgia College & State University, GA
Georgia Southwestern State University, GA
Gonzaga University, WA
Grand Canyon University, AZ
Hampton University, VA
Harding University, AR
Herzing University Online, WI
Idaho State University, ID
Illinois State University, IL
Indiana State University, IN
Indiana University–Purdue University Fort Wayne, IN
Indiana University–Purdue University Indianapolis, IN
Indiana Wesleyan University, IN
Jacksonville State University, AL
Jacksonville University, FL
James Madison University, VA
Johns Hopkins University, MD
Kent State University, OH
Lamar University, TX
La Roche College, PA
Lewis University, IL
Liberty University, VA
Loyola University Chicago, IL

Loyola University New Orleans, LA
Lynchburg College, VA
Mansfield University of Pennsylvania, PA
Marshall University, WV
McKendree University, IL
McNeese State University, LA
Medical University of South Carolina, SC
Memorial University of Newfoundland, NL
Mercy College, NY
Messiah College, PA
Metropolitan State University, MN
Michigan State University, MI
MidAmerica Nazarene University, KS
Middle Tennessee State University, TN
Midwestern State University, TX
Minnesota State University Moorhead, MN
Missouri State University, MO
Morningside College, IA
Mount Carmel College of Nursing, OH
Nebraska Methodist College, NE
New Mexico State University, NM
Northeastern State University, OK
Northern Arizona University, AZ
Northern Kentucky University, KY
Northwest Nazarene University, ID
Notre Dame College, OH
Nova Southeastern University, FL
The Ohio State University, OH
Oklahoma Baptist University, OK
Old Dominion University, VA
Olivet Nazarene University, IL
Pace University, NY
Penn State University Park, PA
Purdue University Calumet, IN
Queens University of Charlotte, NC
Ramapo College of New Jersey, NJ
Regis University, CO
Research College of Nursing, MO
Robert Morris University, PA
Roberts Wesleyan College, NY
Rush University, IL
Rutgers, The State University of New Jersey, Newark, NJ
Sacred Heart University, CT
Saint Francis Medical Center College of Nursing, IL
Saint Joseph's College of Maine, ME
Saint Louis University, MO
Saint Xavier University, IL
Samford University, AL
Seton Hall University, NJ
Simmons College, MA
South Dakota State University, SD
Southeastern Louisiana University, LA
Southern Adventist University, TN
Southwest Baptist University, MO
Spring Arbor University, MI
Spring Hill College, AL
State University of New York Empire State College, NY
State University of New York Polytechnic Institute, NY
Stevenson University, MD
Stony Brook University, State University of New York, NY
Tabor College, KS
Tennessee State University, TN
Tennessee Technological University, TN
Texas A&M Health Science Center, TX
Texas A&M University–Corpus Christi, TX
Texas A&M University–Texarkana, TX
Texas Christian University, TX

Texas State University, TX
Texas Tech University Health Sciences Center, TX
Texas Woman's University, TX
Touro University, NV
Troy University, AL
The University of Alabama, AL
The University of Alabama in Huntsville, AL
The University of Arizona, AZ
University of Arkansas, AR
University of Central Arkansas, AR
University of Central Florida, FL
University of Central Missouri, MO
University of Cincinnati, OH
University of Colorado Colorado Springs, CO
University of Colorado Denver, CO
University of Connecticut, CT
University of Delaware, DE
University of Florida, FL
University of Hawaii at Manoa, HI
University of Indianapolis, IN
The University of Kansas, KS
University of Lethbridge, AB
University of Louisiana at Lafayette, LA
University of Mary, ND
University of Maryland, Baltimore, MD
University of Massachusetts Amherst, MA
University of Memphis, TN
University of Michigan–Flint, MI
University of Missouri, MO
University of Nebraska Medical Center, NE
University of Nevada, Las Vegas, NV
University of New Mexico, NM
University of North Alabama, AL
The University of North Carolina at Charlotte, NC
The University of North Carolina at Greensboro, NC
University of North Dakota, ND
University of Northern Colorado, CO
University of Oklahoma Health Sciences Center, OK
University of Phoenix–New Mexico Campus, NM
University of Phoenix–Online Campus, AZ
University of Phoenix–Phoenix Campus, AZ
University of Phoenix–Southern Arizona Campus, AZ
University of Phoenix–South Florida Campus, FL
University of Pittsburgh, PA
University of St. Francis, IL
University of Saint Mary, KS
University of San Francisco, CA
University of South Carolina, SC
University of South Carolina Upstate, SC
University of Southern Indiana, IN
The University of Texas at Arlington, TX
The University of Texas at Brownsville, TX
The University of Texas at El Paso, TX
The University of Texas at Tyler, TX
The University of Texas Medical Branch, TX
The University of Texas Rio Grande Valley, TX
University of Toronto, ON
University of Utah, UT
University of West Florida, FL
University of West Georgia, GA
University of Wisconsin–Green Bay, WI
University of Wisconsin–Oshkosh, WI
University of Wyoming, WY
Urbana University, OH
Vanderbilt University, TN

Walden University, MN
Walsh University, OH
Weber State University, UT
West Coast University, CA
Western Carolina University, NC
Western Governors University, UT
Western Kentucky University, KY
Western University of Health Sciences, CA
West Virginia University, WV
Wheeling Jesuit University, WV
Wilmington University, DE
Wright State University, OH

ONLINE ONLY MASTER'S DEGREE PROGRAMS

Albany State University, GA
American International College, MA
American Sentinel University, CO
Angelo State University, TX
Aspen University, CO
Austin Peay State University, TN
Baker University, KS
Ball State University, IN
Baylor University, TX
Benedictine University, IL
Brandon University, MB
Briar Cliff University, IA
California State University, Dominguez Hills, CA
The Catholic University of America, DC
Central Methodist University, MO
Chamberlain College of Nursing, AZ
Charleston Southern University, SC
Clarkson College, NE
Clayton State University, GA
Cleveland State University, OH
Colorado Mesa University, CO
Concordia University Wisconsin, WI
Cox College, MO
Creighton University, NE
Delta State University, MS
Duquesne University, PA
Eastern Mennonite University, VA
Eastern New Mexico University, NM
East Tennessee State University, TN
Excelsior College, NY
Ferris State University, MI
Fitchburg State University, MA
Florida State University, FL
Frontier Nursing University, KY
Georgetown University, DC
The George Washington University, DC
Georgia College & State University, GA
Georgia Southwestern State University, GA
Gonzaga University, WA
Harding University, AR
Herzing University Online, WI
Idaho State University, ID
Illinois State University, IL
Indiana State University, IN
Indiana University–Purdue University Fort Wayne, IN
Jacksonville State University, AL
Lamar University, TX
La Roche College, PA
Liberty University, VA
Loyola University Chicago, IL
Lynchburg College, VA
Mansfield University of Pennsylvania, PA
McNeese State University, LA
Medical University of South Carolina, SC

Memorial University of Newfoundland, NL
Messiah College, PA
Minnesota State University Moorhead, MN
Missouri State University, MO
Morningside College, IA
Nebraska Methodist College, NE
New Mexico State University, NM
Northeastern State University, OK
Northern Arizona University, AZ
Northern Kentucky University, KY
Northwest Nazarene University, ID
Notre Dame College, OH
Nova Southeastern University, FL
Oklahoma Baptist University, OK
Old Dominion University, VA
Queens University of Charlotte, NC
Ramapo College of New Jersey, NJ
Saint Francis Medical Center College of
  Nursing, IL
Saint Joseph's College of Maine, ME
Saint Louis University, MO
Seton Hall University, NJ
Southern Adventist University, TN
Spring Arbor University, MI
Spring Hill College, AL
State University of New York Empire State
  College, NY
Stevenson University, MD
Tabor College, KS
Tennessee Technological University, TN
Texas A&M Health Science Center, TX
Texas A&M University–Corpus Christi, TX
Texas A&M University–Texarkana, TX
Texas Christian University, TX
Texas State University, TX
Texas Tech University Health Sciences Center,
  TX
Touro University, NV
The University of Alabama, AL
University of Arkansas, AR
University of Central Arkansas, AR
University of Central Missouri, MO
University of Colorado Colorado Springs, CO
University of Lethbridge, AB
University of Louisiana at Lafayette, LA
University of Mary, ND
University of Massachusetts Amherst, MA
University of Missouri, MO
University of Nevada, Las Vegas, NV
University of New Mexico, NM
University of North Alabama, AL
The University of North Carolina at
  Greensboro, NC
University of Northern Colorado, CO
University of Saint Mary, KS
University of South Carolina, SC
University of Southern Indiana, IN
The University of Texas at Brownsville, TX
The University of Texas at El Paso, TX
The University of Texas at Tyler, TX
The University of Texas Medical Branch, TX
University of West Florida, FL
University of West Georgia, GA
University of Wisconsin–Green Bay, WI
University of Wisconsin–Oshkosh, WI
University of Wyoming, WY
Vanderbilt University, TN
Walden University, MN
Walsh University, OH
Western Governors University, UT
Western University of Health Sciences, CA
West Virginia University, WV

Wheeling Jesuit University, WV

ONLINE DOCTORAL DEGREE PROGRAMS

Allen College, IA
Andrews University, MI
Arkansas State University, AR
Ashland University, OH
Ball State University, IN
Binghamton University, State University of
  New York, NY
Bradley University, IL
Brandman University, CA
Briar Cliff University, IA
California State University, Fresno, CA
The Catholic University of America, DC
Chamberlain College of Nursing, AZ
Chatham University, PA
Clarion University of Pennsylvania, PA
Colorado Mesa University, CO
Concordia University Wisconsin, WI
Creighton University, NE
Delta State University, MS
Drexel University, PA
Duke University, NC
Duquesne University, PA
East Carolina University, NC
Frontier Nursing University, KY
Georgia College & State University, GA
Georgia Southern University, GA
Gonzaga University, WA
Graceland University, IA
Hampton University, VA
Idaho State University, ID
Illinois State University, IL
Indiana State University, IN
Indiana University–Purdue University Fort
  Wayne, IN
James Madison University, VA
Lewis University, IL
Loyola University New Orleans, LA
Maryville University of Saint Louis, MO
Medical University of South Carolina, SC
Mercer University, GA
MGH Institute of Health Professions, MA
Missouri State University, MO
Mount Carmel College of Nursing, OH
Nebraska Methodist College, NE
New Mexico State University, NM
North Dakota State University, ND
Northern Arizona University, AZ
Northern Kentucky University, KY
Northwestern State University of Louisiana,
  LA
Old Dominion University, VA
Radford University, VA
Rush University, IL
Saint Francis Medical Center College of
  Nursing, IL
Samford University, AL
Seton Hall University, NJ
Southern Adventist University, TN
Southern Connecticut State University, CT
Texas Christian University, TX
Texas Woman's University, TX
Touro University, NV
Troy University, AL
The University of Alabama, AL
The University of Alabama in Huntsville, AL
University of Alberta, AB
The University of Arizona, AZ

University of Arkansas, AR
University of Colorado Colorado Springs, CO
University of Florida, FL
University of Hawaii at Manoa, HI
University of Indianapolis, IN
The University of Kansas, KS
University of Michigan–Flint, MI
University of Missouri–Kansas City, MO
University of Nebraska Medical Center, NE
University of Nevada, Las Vegas, NV
University of Nevada, Reno, NV
University of New Hampshire, NH
University of New Mexico, NM
University of North Dakota, ND
University of Northern Colorado, CO
University of Phoenix–Online Campus, AZ
University of St. Francis, IL
The University of Tennessee, TN
The University of Tennessee at Chattanooga,
  TN
The University of Tennessee Health Science
  Center, TN
The University of Texas Medical Branch, TX
University of the Incarnate Word, TX
The University of Toledo, OH
University of West Georgia, GA
Virginia Commonwealth University, VA
Walden University, MN
Walsh University, OH
Western University of Health Sciences, CA
Wichita State University, KS
Winona State University, MN
Wright State University, OH

ONLINE ONLY DOCTORAL DEGREE PROGRAMS

Allen College, IA
Andrews University, MI
Arkansas State University, AR
Ashland University, OH
Ball State University, IN
Bradley University, IL
Brandman University, CA
Briar Cliff University, IA
California State University, Fresno, CA
Chamberlain College of Nursing, AZ
Chatham University, PA
Clarion University of Pennsylvania, PA
Colorado Mesa University, CO
Concordia University Wisconsin, WI
Creighton University, NE
Delta State University, MS
Drexel University, PA
Duke University, NC
Duquesne University, PA
Frontier Nursing University, KY
Georgia College & State University, GA
Georgia Southern University, GA
Gonzaga University, WA
Graceland University, IA
Hampton University, VA
Idaho State University, ID
Illinois State University, IL
Indiana State University, IN
Indiana University–Purdue University Fort
  Wayne, IN
James Madison University, VA
Lewis University, IL
Loyola University New Orleans, LA
Maryville University of Saint Louis, MO
Medical University of South Carolina, SC

Mercer University, GA
Mount Carmel College of Nursing, OH
Nebraska Methodist College, NE
New Mexico State University, NM
Northern Arizona University, AZ
Northwestern State University of Louisiana, LA
Old Dominion University, VA
Radford University, VA
Saint Francis Medical Center College of Nursing, IL
Samford University, AL
Southern Adventist University, TN
Southern Connecticut State University, CT
Texas Christian University, TX

Touro University, NV
Troy University, AL
The University of Alabama, AL
The University of Alabama in Huntsville, AL
The University of Arizona, AZ
University of Arkansas, AR
University of Colorado Colorado Springs, CO
University of Hawaii at Manoa, HI
University of Indianapolis, IN
University of Michigan–Flint, MI
University of Missouri–Kansas City, MO
University of Nevada, Las Vegas, NV
University of Nevada, Reno, NV
University of North Dakota, ND
University of Northern Colorado, CO

University of Phoenix–Online Campus, AZ
University of St. Francis, IL
The University of Tennessee, TN
The University of Tennessee at Chattanooga, TN
The University of Tennessee Health Science Center, TN
The University of Texas Medical Branch, TX
University of the Incarnate Word, TX
University of West Georgia, GA
Virginia Commonwealth University, VA
Walden University, MN
Walsh University, OH
Western University of Health Sciences, CA
Winona State University, MN
Wright State University, OH

CONTINUING EDUCATION PROGRAMS

U.S. AND U.S. TERRITORIES

Alabama

Jacksonville State University, College of Nursing and Health Sciences, *Jacksonville*

Samford University, Ida V. Moffett School of Nursing, *Birmingham*

The University of Alabama at Birmingham, School of Nursing, *Birmingham*

The University of Alabama in Huntsville, College of Nursing, *Huntsville*

University of Mobile, School of Nursing, *Mobile*

University of North Alabama, College of Nursing and Allied Health, *Florence*

Arizona

Arizona State University at the Downtown Phoenix campus, College of Nursing, *Phoenix*

Grand Canyon University, College of Nursing and Health Sciences, *Phoenix*

The University of Arizona, College of Nursing, *Tucson*

University of Phoenix–Online Campus, Online Campus, *Phoenix*

University of Phoenix–Phoenix Campus, College of Health Sciences and Nursing, *Tempe*

University of Phoenix–Southern Arizona Campus, College of Social Sciences, *Tucson*

Arkansas

Harding University, College of Nursing, *Searcy*

University of Arkansas for Medical Sciences, College of Nursing, *Little Rock*

California

Azusa Pacific University, School of Nursing, *Azusa*

Brandman University, School of Nursing and Health Professions, *Irvine*

California State University, Bakersfield, Program in Nursing, *Bakersfield*

California State University, Chico, School of Nursing, *Chico*

California State University, Fresno, Department of Nursing, *Fresno*

California State University, Sacramento, Division of Nursing, *Sacramento*

Pacific Union College, Department of Nursing, *Angwin*

Point Loma Nazarene University, School of Nursing, *San Diego*

San Diego State University, School of Nursing, *San Diego*

San Francisco State University, School of Nursing, *San Francisco*

Unitek College, School of Nursing and Allied Health, *Fremont*

University of California, Davis, The Betty Irene Moore School of Nursing, *Davis*

University of California, Irvine, Program in Nursing Science, *Irvine*

University of California, Los Angeles, School of Nursing, *Los Angeles*

University of Phoenix–Sacramento Valley Campus, College of Nursing, *Sacramento*

University of Phoenix–Southern California Campus, College of Health Sciences and Nursing, *Costa Mesa*

West Coast University, Nursing Programs, *North Hollywood*

Colorado

University of Colorado Colorado Springs, Helen and Arthur E. Johnson Beth-El College of Nursing & Health Sciences, *Colorado Springs*

University of Colorado Denver, College of Nursing, *Aurora*

Connecticut

Sacred Heart University, College of Nursing, *Fairfield*

University of Connecticut, School of Nursing, *Storrs*

University of Hartford, College of Education, Nursing, and Health Professions, *West Hartford*

Delaware

University of Delaware, School of Nursing, *Newark*

Wesley College, Nursing Program, *Dover*

Florida

Florida Agricultural and Mechanical University, School of Nursing, *Tallahassee*

Florida Gulf Coast University, School of Nursing, *Fort Myers*

St. Petersburg College, Department of Nursing, *St. Petersburg*

University of Miami, School of Nursing and Health Studies, *Coral Gables*

The University of Tampa, Department of Nursing, *Tampa*

Georgia

Kennesaw State University, School of Nursing, *Kennesaw*

Valdosta State University, College of Nursing, *Valdosta*

Illinois

Lewis University, Program in Nursing, *Romeoville*

Rush University, College of Nursing, *Chicago*

Southern Illinois University Edwardsville, School of Nursing, *Edwardsville*

University of Illinois at Chicago, College of Nursing, *Chicago*

Indiana

Indiana State University, Department of Advanced Practice Nursing, *Terre Haute*

Indiana University Kokomo, Indiana University School of Nursing, *Kokomo*

Indiana University–Purdue University Indianapolis, School of Nursing, *Indianapolis*

Marian University, School of Nursing, *Indianapolis*

Purdue University, School of Nursing, *West Lafayette*

University of Southern Indiana, College of Nursing and Health Professions, *Evansville*

Valparaiso University, College of Nursing and Health Professions, *Valparaiso*

Iowa

Allen College, Graduate Programs, *Waterloo*

Briar Cliff University, Department of Nursing, *Sioux City*

Clarke University, Department of Nursing and Health, *Dubuque*

Grand View University, Division of Nursing, *Des Moines*

Luther College, Department of Nursing, *Decorah*

Mount Mercy University, Department of Nursing, *Cedar Rapids*

St. Ambrose University, Program in Nursing (BSN), *Davenport*

The University of Iowa, College of Nursing, *Iowa City*

Kansas

Pittsburg State University, Department of Nursing, *Pittsburg*

The University of Kansas, School of Nursing, *Kansas City*

Washburn University, School of Nursing, *Topeka*

Kentucky

Bellarmine University, Donna and Allan Lansing School of Nursing and Health Sciences, *Louisville*

Kentucky Christian University, School of Nursing, *Grayson*

Midway University, Program in Nursing (Baccalaureate), *Midway*

Murray State University, Program in Nursing, *Murray*

Northern Kentucky University, Department of Nursing, *Highland Heights*

Spalding University, School of Nursing, *Louisville*

University of Kentucky, College of Nursing, *Lexington*

University of Louisville, School of Nursing, *Louisville*

Western Kentucky University, School of Nursing, *Bowling Green*

Louisiana

Dillard University, Division of Nursing, *New Orleans*

Louisiana State University Health Sciences Center, School of Nursing, *New Orleans*

McNeese State University, College of Nursing, *Lake Charles*

Nicholls State University, Department of Nursing, *Thibodaux*

Northwestern State University of Louisiana, College of Nursing and School of Allied Health, *Shreveport*

Our Lady of the Lake College, Division of Nursing, *Baton Rouge*

University of Louisiana at Lafayette, College of Nursing, *Lafayette*

University of Louisiana at Monroe, Nursing, *Monroe*

Maine

Saint Joseph's College of Maine, Master of Science in Nursing Program, *Standish*

University of New England, Department of Nursing, *Biddeford*

University of Southern Maine, School of Nursing, *Portland*

Maryland

Johns Hopkins University, School of Nursing, *Baltimore*

University of Maryland, Baltimore, Nursing Programs, *Baltimore*

Massachusetts

Anna Maria College, Department of Nursing, *Paxton*

Becker College, Nursing Programs, *Worcester*

Boston College, William F. Connell School of Nursing, *Chestnut Hill*

Endicott College, Major in Nursing, *Beverly*

Framingham State University, Department of Nursing, *Framingham*

MCPHS University, School of Nursing, *Boston*

Northeastern University, School of Nursing, *Boston*

Regis College, School of Nursing, Science and Health Professions, *Weston*

Salem State University, Program in Nursing, *Salem*

University of Massachusetts Amherst, College of Nursing, *Amherst*

University of Massachusetts Boston, College of Nursing and Health Sciences, *Boston*

University of Massachusetts Dartmouth, College of Nursing, *North Dartmouth*

University of Massachusetts Medical School, Graduate School of Nursing, *Worcester*

Worcester State University, Department of Nursing, *Worcester*

Michigan

Grand Valley State University, Kirkhof College of Nursing, *Allendale*

Michigan State University, College of Nursing, *East Lansing*

Northern Michigan University, College of Nursing and Allied Health Science, *Marquette*

Oakland University, School of Nursing, *Rochester*

Saginaw Valley State University, College of Health and Human Services, *University Center*

Western Michigan University, College of Health and Human Services, *Kalamazoo*

Minnesota

Bemidji State University, Department of Nursing, *Bemidji*

Minnesota State University Mankato, School of Nursing, *Mankato*

University of Minnesota, Twin Cities Campus, School of Nursing, *Minneapolis*

Mississippi

University of Mississippi Medical Center, School of Nursing, *Jackson*

Missouri

Cox College, Department of Nursing, *Springfield*

Missouri State University, Department of Nursing, *Springfield*

Missouri Western State University, Department of Nursing, *St. Joseph*

Saint Louis University, School of Nursing, *St. Louis*

University of Missouri, Sinclair School of Nursing, *Columbia*

University of Missouri–Kansas City, School of Nursing and Health Studies, *Kansas City*

Nebraska

Clarkson College, Master of Science in Nursing Program, *Omaha*

Creighton University, College of Nursing, *Omaha*

Nebraska Methodist College, Department of Nursing, *Omaha*

University of Nebraska Medical Center, College of Nursing, *Omaha*

Nevada

University of Nevada, Las Vegas, School of Nursing, *Las Vegas*

New Hampshire

Saint Anselm College, Department of Nursing, *Manchester*

New Jersey

The College of New Jersey, School of Nursing, Health and Exercise Science, *Ewing*

College of Saint Elizabeth, Department of Nursing, *Morristown*

Monmouth University, Marjorie K. Unterberg School of Nursing, *West Long Branch*

Ramapo College of New Jersey, Master of Science in Nursing Program, *Mahwah*

Rutgers, The State University of New Jersey, Newark, Rutgers School of Nursing, *Newark*

New York

Binghamton University, State University of New York, Decker School of Nursing, *Vestal*

Columbia University, School of Nursing, *New York*

Elmira College, Program in Nursing Education, *Elmira*

Hunter College of the City University of New York, Hunter-Bellevue School of Nursing, *New York*

Lehman College of the City University of New York, Department of Nursing, *Bronx*

Le Moyne College, Nursing Programs, *Syracuse*

Molloy College, Division of Nursing, *Rockville Centre*

New York University, College of Nursing, *New York*

The Sage Colleges, Department of Nursing, *Troy*

State University of New York Downstate Medical Center, College of Nursing, *Brooklyn*

State University of New York Polytechnic Institute, School of Nursing and Health Systems, *Utica*

State University of New York Upstate Medical University, College of Nursing, *Syracuse*

Stony Brook University, State University of New York, School of Nursing, *Stony Brook*

North Carolina

Queens University of Charlotte, Presbyterian School of Nursing, *Charlotte*

The University of North Carolina at Chapel Hill, School of Nursing, *Chapel Hill*

Winston-Salem State University, Department of Nursing, *Winston-Salem*

Ohio

Case Western Reserve University, Frances Payne Bolton School of Nursing, *Cleveland*

Cleveland State University, School of Nursing, *Cleveland*

Kent State University, College of Nursing, *Kent*

The Ohio State University, College of Nursing, *Columbus*

Otterbein University, Department of Nursing, *Westerville*

Shawnee State University, Department of Nursing, *Portsmouth*

The University of Akron, School of Nursing, *Akron*

University of Cincinnati, College of Nursing, *Cincinnati*

The University of Toledo, College of Nursing, *Toledo*

Urbana University, College of Nursing and Allied Health, *Urbana*

Wright State University, College of Nursing and Health, *Dayton*

Oklahoma

Oklahoma City University, Kramer School of Nursing, *Oklahoma City*

University of Oklahoma Health Sciences Center, College of Nursing, *Oklahoma City*

Oregon

Linfield College, School of Nursing, *McMinnville*

Oregon Health & Science University, School of Nursing, *Portland*

Pennsylvania

Alvernia University, Nursing, *Reading*

DeSales University, Department of Nursing and Health, *Center Valley*

Drexel University, College of Nursing and Health Professions, *Philadelphia*

Duquesne University, School of Nursing, *Pittsburgh*

Holy Family University, School of Nursing and Allied Health Professions, *Philadelphia*

La Roche College, Department of Nursing and Nursing Management, *Pittsburgh*

La Salle University, School of Nursing and Health Sciences, *Philadelphia*

Marywood University, Department of Nursing, *Scranton*

Mount Aloysius College, Division of Nursing, *Cresson*

Penn State University Park, School of Nursing, *University Park*

Temple University, Department of Nursing, *Philadelphia*

Thomas Jefferson University, Department of Nursing, *Philadelphia*

University of Pittsburgh, School of Nursing, *Pittsburgh*

Villanova University, College of Nursing, *Villanova*

Widener University, School of Nursing, *Chester*

Wilkes University, Department of Nursing, *Wilkes-Barre*

Puerto Rico

Universidad Adventista de las Antillas, Department of Nursing, *Mayagüez*

University of Puerto Rico, Mayagüez Campus, Department of Nursing, *Mayagüez*

University of Puerto Rico, Medical Sciences Campus, School of Nursing, *San Juan*

Rhode Island

Salve Regina University, Department of Nursing, *Newport*

South Carolina

University of South Carolina, College of Nursing, *Columbia*

South Dakota

South Dakota State University, College of Nursing, *Brookings*

Tennessee

East Tennessee State University, College of Nursing, *Johnson City*

Southern Adventist University, School of Nursing, *Collegedale*

Union University, School of Nursing, *Jackson*

The University of Tennessee, College of Nursing, *Knoxville*

The University of Tennessee Health Science Center, College of Nursing, *Memphis*

Texas

Lamar University, Department of Nursing, *Beaumont*

Midwestern State University, Wilson School of Nursing, *Wichita Falls*

Patty Hanks Shelton School of Nursing, *Abilene*

Tarleton State University, Department of Nursing, *Stephenville*

Texas A&M Health Science Center, College of Nursing, *College Station*

Texas A&M University–Corpus Christi, College of Nursing and Health Sciences, *Corpus Christi*

Texas Christian University, Harris College of Nursing, *Fort Worth*

The University of Texas at Brownsville, Department of Nursing, *Brownsville*

The University of Texas Health Science Center at Houston, School of Nursing, *Houston*

The University of Texas Health Science Center at San Antonio, School of Nursing, *San Antonio*

Virginia

George Mason University, College of Health and Human Services, *Fairfax*

Jefferson College of Health Sciences, Nursing Education Program, *Roanoke*

Shenandoah University, Eleanor Wade Custer School of Nursing, *Winchester*

Washington

Pacific Lutheran University, School of Nursing, *Tacoma*

University of Washington, School of Nursing, *Seattle*

WSU College of Nursing, *Spokane*

West Virginia

Fairmont State University, School of Nursing and Allied Health Administration, *Fairmont*

Shepherd University, Department of Nursing Education, *Shepherdstown*

West Virginia University, School of Nursing, *Morgantown*

Wisconsin

Alverno College, Division of Nursing, *Milwaukee*

Milwaukee School of Engineering, School of Nursing, *Milwaukee*

University of Wisconsin–Eau Claire, College of Nursing and Health Sciences, *Eau Claire*

University of Wisconsin–Madison, School of Nursing, *Madison*

University of Wisconsin–Oshkosh, College of Nursing, *Oshkosh*

Wisconsin Lutheran College, Nursing Program, *Milwaukee*

CANADA

British Columbia

British Columbia Institute of Technology, School of Health Sciences, *Burnaby*

Thompson Rivers University, School of Nursing, *Kamloops*

Vancouver Island University, Department of Nursing, *Nanaimo*

New Brunswick

Université de Moncton, School of Nursing, *Moncton*

University of New Brunswick Fredericton, Faculty of Nursing, *Fredericton*

Nova Scotia

St. Francis Xavier University, Department of Nursing, *Antigonish*

Ontario

Laurentian University, School of Nursing, *Sudbury*

Ryerson University, Program in Nursing, *Toronto*

University of Toronto, Faculty of Nursing, *Toronto*

University of Windsor, Faculty of Nursing, *Windsor*

York University, School of Nursing, *Toronto*

Quebec

Université de Montréal, Faculty of Nursing, *Montréal*

Université du Québec à Chicoutimi, Program in Nursing, *Chicoutimi*

Université du Québec à Rimouski, Program in Nursing, *Rimouski*

Université du Québec en Outaouais, Département des Sciences Infirmières, *Gatineau*

Université Laval, Faculty of Nursing, *Québec*

Saskatchewan

University of Saskatchewan, College of Nursing, *Saskatoon*

ALPHABETICAL LISTING OF INSTITUTIONS